James F. Crow

WA Dove.

Perspectives on Genetics

○ **Perspectives on Genetics** ○

Anecdotal, Historical, and Critical Commentaries, 1987–1998

Edited by

James F. Crow and William F. Dove

THE UNIVERSITY OF WISCONSIN PRESS

The University of Wisconsin Press
2537 Daniels Street
Madison, Wisconsin 53718

3 Henrietta Street
London WC2E 8LU, England

All essays in this volume were originally published in the journal *Genetics*
and are reprinted here by permission of the Genetics Society of America.

The publication of this volume was made possible by generous grants from the
Brittingham Fund, Inc. of the University of Wisconsin and from the Genetics Society of America.

Cataloging-in-Publication Data
Perspectives on genetics: anecdotal, historical, and critical commentaries, 1987–1998
edited by James F. Crow and William F. Dove
pp.   cm.
Includes bibliographical references and index.
ISBN 0–299–16604–X (paper: alk. paper)
1. Genetics. 2. Genetics—Anecdotes. 3. Genetics—History.
I. Crow, James F. (James Franklin), 1916– II. Dove, W. F. (William Franklin), 1936–
QH438 P47   2000
576.5—dc21   99–049567

Contents

Introduction

IN 1986 John (Jan) Drake, the editor of *Genetics,* had the idea of including in each issue an introductory essay under the general heading, "Perspectives: Anecdotal, Historical, and Critical Commentaries on Genetics." We were asked to be the editors and cheerfully accepted. In this volume, the first 12 years of "Perspectives" are reprinted.

The great majority of articles were commissioned by us. We wrote some ourselves, sometimes because a commissioned essay failed to appear, and a few essays were volunteered. Over the years the concept was broadened to include mini-reviews and essays by contemporary investigators on the issues in which they were involved. Thus the collection is quite heterogeneous. Some essays are short and anecdotal. Some are historical. Some set the record straight by righting an injustice. A few are scholarly reviews. Some have been obituaries, and one is the GSA Medal Essay. Several are follow-ups by the original authors of important papers, usually from *Genetics.*

In short, the collection as a whole is diverse in content, style, and depth of treatment. Yet, we believe that by reprinting this 12-year series, we have made available a "birds' eye" view of the subject of genetics during a time of spectacular advances. The series has also played a unifying role by presenting a view of the broad range of subjects at a time when the field is becoming an increasingly fragmented collection of specialty groups; the broader view is lost in the primary research articles or papers at specialized meetings.

Several authors have taken advantage of the opportunity to provide brief updates; these are included as Addenda et Corrigenda at the end of the collection. The updates should be especially useful to those readers who would like to know what has happened in the interval since the original essay was published, especially when the original was some years ago. Also, it should be noted that the authors' institutional affiliations and addresses, including e-mail, are those at the time of the original publication of the particular essays and may no longer be current.

We are indebted to Jan Drake, not only for instigating the idea, but for his continued support. His eye for good writing, as well as that of Pamela Drake, show up in the quality of the final product. Since Jan's retirement, the editing function has been taken over by Elizabeth Jones and Leah Kauffman. In Madison, Ilse Riegel has been responsible for the copyediting process. Her ability to spot stylistic infelicities and inconsistencies has enhanced the readability and greatly reduced the number of errors in both text and references.

We happily acknowledge the financial support of the Genetics Society of America and the Brittingham Fund of the University of Wisconsin for the publication of this volume. This has helped make it available at a reasonable price, and we hope that many (including students) will avail themselves of the opportunity.

Our greatest debt is to the numerous authors who have responded, almost always with enthusiasm, to our invitations to write essays. Some have responded more than once. We look forward to the continuation of the series and in due course to additional collections.

James F. Crow
jfcrow@facstaff.wisc.edu

William F. Dove
dove@oncology.wisc.edu

Madison, Wisconsin
November 1999

∘   **Perspectives on Genetics**   ∘

Sewall Wright and Physiological Genetics

James F. Crow

Genetics Department, University of Wisconsin–Madison, Madison, Wisconsin 53706

SEWALL WRIGHT celebrated his 97th birthday anniversary on December 21, 1986. He is the last survivor of the pioneers who founded twentieth-century genetics. His first genetical paper was published in 1914, his first in this journal in 1918, and his most recent in 1984. These 70 years saw the production of 210 articles and four books. Within the past few months a full-length biography (PROVINE 1986) has appeared, along with a reprint of some of WRIGHT's best and hardest-to-obtain papers (WRIGHT 1986). Furthermore, his four-volume treatise on population and evolutionary genetics is now available in paperback form (WRIGHT 1968, 1969, 1977, 1978). It seems timely and fitting to make him the subject of this first "Perspectives."

WRIGHT's writings in mathematical population genetics, inbreeding, and evolutionary theory are known to all geneticists and his inbreeding coefficient is a standard part of elementary courses. Yet he devoted the major share of his time to physiological and developmental genetics, and this work is much less known. He worked on pigment genetics of guinea pigs from his graduate student days until his retirement from the University of Chicago in 1955, and produced a stream of papers from 1916 to 1960. He also studied a number of developmental problems. He sometimes thought of switching to the mouse or Drosophila, but there were always more guinea pig experiments to do.

I recently asked WRIGHT how he happened to choose the guinea pig. He replied that he did not choose it; it was assigned to him by WILLIAM E. CASTLE, his mentor at Harvard. C. C. LITTLE had started graduate work earlier in the same laboratory and was already working on mice. CASTLE himself worked with rats and rabbits. I have often wondered how different the history of genetics in the United States might have been had WRIGHT and LITTLE arrived at Harvard in reverse order. Surely the early work on mouse genetics would have been more chemical and physiological, and there would have been much greater emphasis on gene interaction. LITTLE emphasized the development of inbred lines and the

study of transplantable tumors. Their most striking contrast, however, was personal. WRIGHT was, and is, shy and retiring. LITTLE was a politician and organizer. After being fired as President of the University of Michigan, he was able, through persistence and personal charm, to raise enough money to found the Jackson Laboratory in Bar Harbor, Maine, now a world center for mouse genetics. Guinea pigs would have been much less suitable. In any case, the genetics world owes a vote of thanks to the trustees of the University of Michigan for unintentionally starting a great research laboratory.

WRIGHT published an extensive review of physiological genetics in 1941 (WRIGHT 1941a). He planned to expand it into a book, but this was also the year that biochemical genetics of Neurospora began (BEADLE and TATUM 1941). WRIGHT foresaw that this would forever alter the nature of genetical research and abandoned his project as *passé*. Perhaps it is time to resurrect WRIGHT's kind of quantitative studies of gene action and interaction, utilizing the enormous advances in molecular genetics and changed viewpoints since that time.

At the 1932 International Congress of Genetics, H. J. MULLER (1932) showed how, by judicious use of deletions and duplications to vary gene dosage, he could classify mutant gene action relative to that of the normal allele. He introduced the words that are now part of the standard vocabulary of genetics: *amorph* (producing a phenotypic effect equivalent to that of a deletion), *hypomorph* (producing an effect like that of the normal allele, but weaker), *hypermorph* (stronger than the normal allele), *antimorph* (producing an effect antagonistic to that of the normal allele), and *neomorph* (producing a new effect). It is to MULLER's credit that he did not speculate about intermediate mechanisms, knowing that the only available information came from external phenotypes. In the MULLER tradition, but using newer techniques, is an article in this issue (BARTON, SCHEDL and KIMBLE 1987).

By 1939, having quantitative chemical and colorimetric information on guinea pig coat pigments, WRIGHT was able to carry MULLER's analysis further. Using then-current theory of enzyme kinetics, he derived a series of differential equations from which various interactions caused by dominance and epistasis could be inferred (WRIGHT 1941b). For example, he pointed out an addition to MULLER's classes—a *mixomorph*, an allele that acts as a hypomorph with respect to less active alleles, but as an antimorph with respect to more active ones. This, WRIGHT suggested, would happen if the mutant gene product were effective in combining with the substrate but ineffective in producing the product of the reaction. Such a mutant, *pearl* eye color (w^p), was in fact found in Drosophila by A. STEINBERG and studied by a puzzled GOLDWEBER (1939). In combination with an amorph, *white* (w), and a hypomorph, *eosin* (w^e), the genotypes in order of eye pigmentation are

$$ww < w^p w < w^p w^p < w^e w^p < w^e w < w^e w^e.$$

Thus, w^p increases the pigment in combination with the amorph w, but decreases it in combination with the hypomorph w^e, as a mixomorph should.

WRIGHT earlier had observed that alleles at the C locus, which affects coat and eye color in the guinea pig, could not be arrayed in a single order when both yellow and black pigments were considered. But, by using a complex model involving two substrates and interacting genes, WRIGHT was able to assign numbers to individual reaction-rate constants and predict *quantitatively* the pigment measures of genotypes involving alleles at six loci. It represented a major *tour de force* in quantitative physiological genetics, and represents a high point for this kind of model building. Yet it has received little attention. I might note that both MULLER's and WRIGHT's articles are now hard to find, although part of MULLER's has been reprinted (1962).

WRIGHT's later work (1960 and references therein) was more quantitative in the measurements and more sophisticated in the statistical analysis, but the story got to be too complicated for a single overall quantitative interpretation. As the biochemical information becomes more precise, we can expect to add mechanistic details to WRIGHT's kind of analysis. He could only measure phenotypes; now intermediate products can be taken into account. For example, KACSER and BURNS (1981) have continued in the WRIGHT tradition to explain the ubiquity of dominance, using a "sensitivity coefficient" defined as the ratio of the proportional changes of flux and enzyme activity.

One more example, this time showing the continuing relevance of WRIGHT's experimental work: KINGHORN (1987) has developed an analysis that combines molecular models of polymer formation with traditional analysis of epistatic variance components. And where did he go for the best data on life history and production traits? To WRIGHT's guinea pig measurements published in 1922 (WRIGHT 1922a,b).

LITERATURE CITED

BARTON, M. K., T. B. SCHEDL and J. KIMBLE, 1987 Gain-of-function mutations of *fem-3*, a sex determination gene in *Caenorhabditis elegans*. Genetics 115: 107–119.

BEADLE, G. W. and E. L. TATUM, 1941 Genetic control of biochemical reactions in *Neurospora*. Proc. Natl. Acad. Sci. USA 27: 499–506.

GOLDWEBER, S., 1939 A new allele in the white series of Drosophila and its relationship to some other white alleles. Am. Nat. 73: 568–572.

KACSER, H. and J. A. BURNS. 1981 The molecular basis of dominance. Genetics 97: 639–666.

KINGHORN, B., 1987 The nature of epistatic interactions in animals: evidence from Sewall Wright's guinea pig data. Theor. Appl. Gen. In press.

MULLER, H. J., 1932 Further studies on the nature and causes of gene mutations. Proc. 6th Int. Congr. Genet. 1: 213–255.

MULLER, H. J., 1962 *Studies in Genetics.* Indiana University Press, Bloomington.

PROVINE, W. B., 1986 *Sewall Wright and Evolutionary Biology.* University of Chicago Press, Chicago.

WRIGHT, S., 1914 Duplicate genes. Am. Nat. 49: 140–148.

WRIGHT, S., 1918 On the nature of size factors. Genetics 3: 367–374.

WRIGHT, S., 1922a The effects of inbreeding and crossbreeding on guinea pigs. I. Decline in vigor. II. Differentiation among inbred families. U.S. Dep. Agric. Bull. 1090.

WRIGHT, S., 1922b The effects of inbreeding and crossbreeding on guinea pigs. III. Crosses between highly inbred families. U.S. Dep. Agric. Bull. 1121.

WRIGHT, S., 1941a The physiology of the gene. Physiol. Rev. 21: 487–527.

WRIGHT, S., 1941b A quantitative study of the interactions of the major colour factors of the guinea-pig. Proc. 7th Int. Genet. Congr. 1939, pp. 319–329.

WRIGHT, S., 1960 Postnatal changes in the intensity of coat color in diverse genotypes of the guinea pig. Genetics 45: 1503–1529.

WRGHT, S., 1968, 1969, 1977, 1978 *Evolution and the Genetics of Populations,* Vols. 1–4. University of Chicago Press, Chicago.

WRIGHT, S., 1984 The first Meckel oration: On the causes of morphological differences in a population of guinea pigs. Am. J. Med. Genet. 18: 591–616.

WRIGHT, S., 1986 *Evolution, Selected Papers,* Edited by W. B. PROVINE. University of Chicago Press, Chicago.

Paradox Found

○ ○

William F. Dove

McArdle Laboratory for Cancer Research, University of Wisconsin–Madison, Madison, Wisconsin 53706

False facts are highly injurious to the progress of science, for they often endure long; but false views, if supported by some evidence, do little harm, for everyone takes a salutary pleasure in proving their falseness.

C. Darwin, *The Descent of Man*

IT seems only yesterday that I took my deproteinized bacterial DNAs, worked up in the Caltech Chemistry Building, down to the Delbrück phage laboratory where HARRIETT EPHRUSSI-TAYLOR helped me to assay individual markers by pneumococcal DNA transformation. There I encountered BOB EDGAR and CHARLEY STEINBERG, deep in debate after tabulating data from a gigantic phage cross. Over the summer they were joined by DICK FEYNMAN who, I had learned on my first day at Caltech, was the fun-loving intellectual hero of the student body.

Today, to my surprise, I observe that it was 25 years ago that GENETICS published a pair of papers by EDGAR and STEINBERG, the first also involving FEYNMAN. Each of these three investigators has remained active, EDGAR now working on *Caenorhabditis elegans*, STEINBERG serving as a resident energizer and critic at the Basel Institute of Immunology and FEYNMAN, as followers of the inquiry into the *Challenger* disaster will know, still wearing a Joseph's coat (see FEYNMAN 1985). Meanwhile, the two GENETICS papers that were so novel in 1962 have since been fully woven into the tapestry of molecular genetics.

It is interesting to reexamine these 1962 papers in a 1987 perspective. To some readers of GENETICS a 1962 phage paper no doubt merely signals a part of the transition from Mendelian genetics to DNA sequencing. To others it may seem a relic of a distant past, a time when formal, rigorous model building, free of specific molecular content, was used to divine whether the gene was linear in fine structure and whether recombination involved heteroduplex DNA. These papers, however, played key roles in the rapid advance of modern genetics.

"Mapping experiments with *r* mutants of bacteriophage T4D" (EDGAR *et al.* 1962) supplemented BENZER's (1961) just-published analysis of the *rII* locus,

both showing that the locus was internally linear; while BENZER used the method of deletion mapping, EDGAR *et al.* used quantitative two-factor crosses and also neatly demonstrated high negative interference in two-factor crosses. However, the superb complexity and richness of *rII* genetics was to be in part eclipsed by experimental systems having an important additional feature, one required to reveal the relationship between gene structure and polypeptide structure. These systems, *Escherichia coli* tryptophan synthetase, T4 head protein and T4 lysozyme, provided direct access to gene products, a deficiency of *rII* genetics that persists to this day.

"A critical test of a current theory of genetic recombination in bacteriophage" (STEINBERG and EDGAR 1962) reports a paradoxically negative result. The "current theory" under test was based on EDGAR's strong experimental evidence that phage recombinants which have experienced clustered recombination events were the offspring of heterozygotes. If these heterozygous intermediates involved overlap structures (DNA heteroduplexes), then outside markers should have recombined. Instead, clustered recombinants showed classical segregation patterns: double crossovers were parental for outside markers. This paradox, inexorably argued in their paper, shortly succumbed to the discovery that T4 sports two classes of heterozygotes, heteroduplex "hets" and terminal-redundancy "hets" (SÉCHAUD *et al.* 1965; STAHL *et al.* 1965; STREISINGER 1966). Thus the paradox rapidly provoked its resolution.

It is rare to find a classic paper reporting a simple negative result. However, this era of active ferment in molecular genetics offers repeated examples of inoculation by negative result, by footnote and by unpublished observation. The formal possibility of two classes of heterozygotes had been put forward in an appendix to a paper by NOMURA and BENZER (1961), but was brought into focus only by concrete molecular modeling at the hands of STREISINGER and his colleagues. In the "mapping experiments" paper of EDGAR *et al.*, a set of *rII* mutations, *s1*, *s2* and *s3*, was isolated by FEYNMAN as intragenic suppressors of other *rII* mutations, "to be reported elsewhere." This suppression pattern, analyzed by FEYNMAN using the notion of side-chain interactions at the protein level and never published (see FEYNMAN 1985), was independently discovered and then magnified by the Cambridge group in its germinal analysis of frameshift mutations and the nonoverlapping triplet code (CRICK *et al.* 1961). The Cambridge group also began erroneously, starting with the notion that intragenic suppression reflected base pairing interactions in mRNA (S. BRENNER, personal communication), but soon found their way. The circle was eventually closed by the Cambridge work on tRNA stems (SMITH *et al.* 1970).

At the time these two phage papers appeared, genetics could proceed in a world of its own and with a precision far exceeding that of the molecular analysis of gene and chromosome structure. On the molecular side, however, doubt persisted as to whether T4 contained but a single, uninterrupted duplex DNA molecule, and even as to whether the subunit for semiconservative DNA replication was a single polynucleotide chain rather than a duplex (CAVALIERI and ROSENBERG 1961). The STEINBERG-EDGAR paradox focused attention on these lacunae, which were then filled by hard-won technical progress in the controlled shearing of long DNA molecules (RUBENSTEIN, THOMAS and HERSHEY 1961) and in measuring the mass per unit length of prokaryotic chromosomes (DAVISON *et al.* 1961; CAIRNS 1961, 1962), both of which created a solid molecular springboard for gymnastics such as terminal redundancy [see STREISINGER (1966) for other aspects of these gymnastics].

My musings over old papers and old science bring me, finally, to something for today. At the end of my walk to the phage laboratory, JEAN WEIGLE shared an enthusiasm from a letter from AL HERSHEY on the latter's continual efforts to determine the structure of phage DNA molecules: "There's nothing like technical progress! Ideas come and go, but technical progress cannot be taken away."

LITERATURE CITED

BENZER, S., 1961   On the topography of the genetic fine structure. Proc. Natl. Acad. Sci. USA **47:** 403–415.

CAIRNS, J., 1961   An estimate of the length of the DNA molecular of T2 bacteriophage by autoradiography. J. Mol. Biol. **3:** 756–761.

CAIRNS, J., 1962   A proof that the replication of DNA involves separation of the strands. Nature **194:** 1274.

CAVALIERI, L. F. and B. H. ROSENBERG, 1961   The replication of DNA. I. Two molecular classes of DNA. II. The number of polynucleotide strands in the conserved unit of DNA. III. Changes in the number of strands in *E. coli* DNA during its replication cycle. Biophys. J. **1:** 317–351.

CRICK, F. H. C., L. BARNETT, S. BRENNER and R. J. WATTS-TOBIN, 1961   General nature of the genetic code for proteins. Nature **192:** 1227–1232.

DAVISON, P. F., D. FREIFELDER, R. HEDE and C. LEVINTHAL, 1961   The structural unity of the DNA of T2 bacteriophage. Proc. Natl. Acad. Sci. USA **47:** 1123–1129.

EDGAR, R. S., R. P. FEYNMAN, S. KLEIN, I. LIELAUSIS and C. M. STEINBERG, 1962   Mapping experiments with *r* mutants of bacteriophage T4D. Genetics **47:** 179–186.

FEYNMAN, R. P., 1985   pp. 72–76. In *Surely You're Joking, Mr. Feynman.* Norton, New York.

NOMURA, M. and S. BENZER, 1961   The nature of the "deletion" mutants in the *r*II region of phage T4. J. Mol. Biol. **3:** 684–692.

RUBENSTEIN, I. C. A., THOMAS and A. D. HERSHEY, 1961   The molecular weights of T2 bacteriophage DNA and its first and second breakage products. Proc. Natl. Acad. Sci. USA **47:** 1113–1122.

SÉCHAUD, J., G. STREISINGER, J. EMRICH, J. NEWTON, H. LANFORD, H. REINHOLD and M. M. STAHL, 1965   Chromosome structure in phage T4. I. Terminal redundancy and heterozygosis. Proc. Natl. Acad. Sci. USA **54:** 1333–1339.

SMITH, J. D., L. BARNETT, S. BRENNER and R. L. RUSSELL, 1970   More mutant tyrosine transfer ribonucleic acids. J. Mol. Biol. **54:** 1–14.

STAHL, F. W., H. MODERSOHN, B. E. TERZAGHI and J. M. CRASEMANN, 1965   The genetic structure of complementation heterozygotes. Proc. Natl. Acad. Sci. USA **54:** 1342–1345.

STEINBERG, C. M. and R. S. EDGAR, 1962   A critical test of a current theory of genetic recombination. Genetics **47:** 187–208.

STREISINGER, G., 1966   Terminal redundancy, or all's well that ends well. pp. 335–340. In: *Phage and the Origins of Molecular Biology,* Edited by J. CAIRNS, G. S. STENT and J. D. WATSON. Cold Spring Harbor Laboratory, Cold Spring Harbor, New York.

March 1987

Seventy Years Ago in *Genetics*
H. S. Jennings and Inbreeding Theory

James F. Crow

Genetics Department, University of Wisconsin–Madison, Madison, Wisconsin 53706

IN 1917 GENETICS was in its second year. The March issue contained a 58-page article by H. S. JENNINGS, analyzing mathematically the consequences of inbreeding and selection. He had a 37-page article on the same subject in the very first issue of the journal, January 1916, and the entire September issue that year (127 pages) was devoted to his article on the genetics of Difflugia, a shelled rhizopod. In those days GENETICS was not so crowded.

JENNINGS was the first to use microorganisms to study behavior and genetics. He foresaw the value of using simple species to attack basic biological problems, and in the process founded Paramecium genetics. In Difflugia he demonstrated templated replication of some shell structures. Only after the discovery of DNA replication was the significance of such a supramolecular copying process appreciated. His contributions to population genetics are less well known, but had a significant place in its history.

HERBERT SPENCER JENNINGS (1868–1947), named by a father who was caught up in the new wave of Darwinism (another son was named Darwin), spent most of his childhood in Tonica, Illinois. He taught himself to read at age 3, soon read biology texts and Shakespeare, and continued to devour books the rest of his life. Too poor to go to college, he spent 4 years in various jobs, including three rural teaching posts. His first class had half a dozen students, "one totally ineducable and the others little better." The pay was $25 per month, and he walked 7 miles each morning and evening. Characteristically, he used the noon recesses to study *The Decline and Fall*. Then a bizarre thing happened. His former high school teacher, by then a Professor at Texas A & M, remembered his brilliance and got him a position there as assistant professor of botany. JENNINGS, who had never been to college, was teaching college students! He started many lectures, he said, with knowledge an hour ahead of those in the class "and came out even." In 1888 Texas A & M had 227 students, fewer than its 1987 Cotton Bowl marching band. The experience was not entirely happy. The serious, shy scholar found a student body more interested in horseplay than learning and a faculty split into two warring factions. His last article (1946) was a wryly humorous account of life at Texas A & M 58 years earlier. At the end of the year he was fired.

He had, however, earned enough to enroll at the University of Michigan, and with the later help of an assistantship he graduated in 1893 at age 25. After one postgraduate year there he went to Harvard, getting his Ph.D. in 2 years. After a year in Germany, he taught successively at Montana, Dartmouth and Michigan. Among his writings during this period was a 486-page book on the anatomy of the cat (REIGHARD and JENNINGS 1901). (I write this with nostalgia: this book and formaldehyde fumes are among my vivid memories of an anatomy course in the hot Kansas summer of 1935.) Later, JENNINGS was appointed to the faculty of the University of Pennsylvania, and finally to Johns Hopkins. He was promised that he would eventually succeed W. K. BROOKS as director of the Johns Hopkins Zoological Laboratory. Conveniently, BROOKS died 2 years later. The search committee recommended T. H. MORGAN for the position, but JENNINGS documented the earlier commitment and got the job in 1910. He retired in 1938 and stayed on as professor emeritus. He continued to write until shortly before his death in 1947.

JENNINGS' academic career can be divided into three phases. The first decade was devoted to the study of behavior. He was convinced that behavior, including human, was determined by the physical structure and its responses to previous experience. He held the monistic view, then still controversial, that mind and matter were inseparable. He thought that the route to understanding behavior in higher forms was through lower ones. His book *Behavior of the Lower Organisms*, published in 1906, became a classic and was reprinted as recently as 1976.

In 1907 he shifted his interest to genetics, the initial object being to test the generality of Mendelism. Again he decided that the optimum strategy would be to concentrate on the simplest organisms and chose his favorite, Paramecium. His judgment was good but his luck was bad, for Paramecium turned out to be more reluctant than Drosophila to reveal its genetic mechanisms. JENNINGS' breeding experiments were frustrated by his being unable to obtain conjugation except within a type. This greatly restricted the range of genetic experiments, yet he was able to obtain a remarkable amount of information by clever indirect methods. The complications of mating type were not fully understood until 30 years later when his student, T. M. SONNEBORN, made the key discoveries. JENNINGS was now retired, but the two of them wrote back-to-back papers on two species of Paramecium (JENNINGS 1939; SONNEBORN 1939). The analytical power of genetics was now at hand, but JENNINGS did not live to see its fruition at the hands of SONNEBORN and his students.

The third phase of JENNINGS' life, from World War I until his retirement in 1938, was spent mainly in teaching, administration, and public activities. He wrote a prize-winning book, *The Biological Basis of Human Nature* (1930), that was both authoritative and popular. His *The Universe and Life* (1933) represented his mature general and philosophical thought. SONNEBORN (1975), in a detailed and admiring biography, called it his "greatest and perhaps the most enduring" book. JENNINGS accepted the social aim of trying to improve, or at least not worsen, the quality of human genes in future generations. He was one of the first to express concern about the accumulation of deleterious mutations with relaxed selection. In those years there was a large group, including many influential geneticists, who had idealistic hopes for a better human society through eugenics. There were also those, mostly nongeneticists, who naively mistook the consequences of poor environment and unfamiliarity with English for innate stupidity. JENNINGS took the lead in emphasizing the complexities of the problem. He urged caution and pointed out the slowness of genetic changes compared to those brought about by environmental improvement. In the early 1920s he appeared before a Congressional committee to argue against geographically restrictive immigration laws. Although the great majority of geneticists probably shared his views, he was the most outspoken early critic of the simplicity and crudity of the old eugenics movement.

This essay was stimulated by JENNINGS' paper of 70 years ago. At that time the genetic consequences of inbreeding were of great interest, and not well understood. While the reduction of heterozygosity with repeated self-fertilization had been known since MENDEL, the well known RAYMOND PEARL (1913) tried to extend this to sib-mating. Starting with an *AA* × *aa* mating, he noted that the progeny were 100% heterozygous, and the two following sib-mated generations were both 50% homozygous. He saw no need to

calculate further and concluded that the 50% homozygosity remained indefinitely. HAROLD FISH, a modest, intelligent graduate student of WILLIAM CASTLE at Harvard, realized that this was wrong and laboriously worked out the correct results, showing that the homozygosity in the fourth generation was 62.5%, the fifth was 68.75%, and so on, reaching 99.5% after 25 generations. PEARL was so annoyed at the possibility of being publicly corrected by a graduate student that he asked that FISH be fired. Nevertheless, not only FISH and PEARL, but WHITING, DETLEFSEN and JENNINGS all published the correct results in the same year, 1914. It seems that almost everyone took "salutary pleasure" in correcting PEARL's error, in accordance with the Darwinian dictum quoted in this space last month. Yet none of the acrimony comes through in the published papers, which are exceedingly polite and generous.

How does JENNINGS fit in? He was the first to publish a general formula and to show that FISH's proportion of homozygotes in successive generations of sib-mating could be expressed in terms of the famous and well understood Fibonacci sequence. The relation is most transparent when written as the proportion of heterozygotes. In successive generations this is 1/1, 1/2, 2/4, 3/8, 5/16, 8/32, etc., in which each numerator is the sum of the two preceding. JENNINGS then studied more complicated systems, giving correct results for parent-offspring mating and for some kinds of selection and assortative mating.

The 1917 paper extends the analysis to two loci, where linkage enormously complicates the picture. This paper, 58 pages long, tries the patience of a contemporary geneticist, who knows how to obtain the results much more easily. Yet JENNINGS got there first. His work represents the high point of the method of the time, which was to calculate a few generations by strong-arm methods and hope to find a pattern. Soon afterward, HALDANE, FISHER and WRIGHT introduced more powerful and fruitful ways of looking at inbreeding and selection problems, and population genetics was under way.

SEWALL WRIGHT was FISH's office-mate at Harvard. FISH filled many pages with calculations, covering not only his desk but the floor. After helping FISH, WRIGHT decided that there had to be a better way and in 1922 published his simple algorithm for computing the inbreeding coefficient for any pedigree, however complex. What took FISH and JENNINGS pages of calculations can now be done on the back of an envelope by elementary genetics students.

Although PEARL, JENNINGS and WRIGHT became leading scientists, FISH all but disappeared. As a graduate student he was already married and had two children. Financial problems, and perhaps an unwillingness to stay with one problem, led him to drop out of graduate school and take a position at Denison University, where he soon had a reputation as an excellent teacher. To complete the circle, one of his masters-degree students, LOUISE WILLIAMS, taught genetics at Smith College and later became MRS. SEWALL WRIGHT.

Although he had no training in mathematics, JENNINGS enjoyed doing calculations. Very late in his life he had his first encounter with the calculus, a joyous love affair. But JENNINGS recognized his mathematical limitations and soon realized that his elementary methods would no longer suffice. The concluding words of his 1917 paper are: "The present writer would find it a relief if someone else would deal thoroughly with the laborious problem of the effects of inbreeding on two pairs of linked factors." I ruefully empathize. The influx of skilled mathematicians into population genetics has greatly advanced the field, but it has made it tough for amateurs.

LITERATURE CITED

DETLEFSEN, J. A., 1914   Genetic studies on a cavy species cross. Carnegie Inst. Wash. Pub. **205**: 1–134.

FISH, H. D., 1914   On the progressive increase of homozygosis in brother-sister matings. Am. Nat. **48**: 759–761.

JENNINGS, H. S., 1906   *Behavior of the Lower Organisms.* Macmillan, New York. Reprinted 1923, Columbia University Press, New York. Reprinted 1962, 1976, Indiana University Press, Bloomington, Indiana.

JENNINGS, H. S., 1914   Formulae for the results of inbreeding. Am. Nat. **48**: 693–696.

JENNINGS, H. S., 1916   Numerical results of diverse systems of breeding. Genetics **1**: 53–89.

JENNINGS, H. S., 1916   Heredity, variation and the results of selection on the uniparental reproduction of *Difflugia corona.* Genetics **1**: 407–534.

JENNINGS, H. S., 1917   The numerical results of diverse systems of breeding, with respect to two pairs of factors, linked or independent, with special relation to the effects of linkage. Genetics **2**: 97–154.

JENNINGS, H. S., 1930   *The Biological Basis of Human Nature.* W. W. Norton, New York.

JENNINGS, H. S., 1933   *The Universe and Life.* Yale University Press, New Haven, Connecticut.

JENNINGS, H. S., 1939   *Paramecium bursaria*: mating types and groups, mating behavior, self sterility; their development and inheritance. Am. Nat. **73**: 414–431.

JENNINGS, H. S., 1946   Stirring days at A. and M. Southwest Rev. **31**: 341–344.

PEARL, R., 1913   A contribution towards an analysis of the problem of inbreeding. Am. Nat. **47**: 557–614.

PEARL, R., 1914   On the results of inbreeding a Mendelian population; a correction and extension of previous conclusions. Am. Nat. **48**: 57–62.

REIGHARD, J., and H. S. JENNINGS, 1901   *The Anatomy of the Cat.* Henry Holt, New York.

SONNEBORN, T. M., 1939   *Paramecium aurelia*: mating types and groups; lethal interactions; determination and inheritance. Am. Nat. **73**: 390–413.

SONNEBORN, T. M., 1975   Herbert Spencer Jennings, 1868–1947. Bibliographical Memoirs, Natl. Acad. Sci. USA **47**: 142–223.

WHITING, P. W., 1914   Heredity of the bristles in the common greenbottle fly, *Lucilia sericata*: a study of factors governing distribution. Am. Nat. **48**: 339–355.

WRIGHT, S., 1922   Coefficients of inbreeding and relationship. Am. Nat. **56**: 330–338.

April 1987

Twenty Years of Illegitimate Recombination

Philip Anderson

Department of Genetics, University of Wisconsin–Madison, Madison, Wisconsin 53706

NAOMI FRANKLIN (1967) described "normal" recombination events as "those which occur with regularity and relatively high frequency between homologous DNA segments." Such recombination, familiar to us all, occurs with high fidelity and results in crossing over and gene conversion. Molecular mechanisms of homologous recombination are understood in at least outline form (DRESSLER and POTTER 1982).

FRANKLIN (1971) described "extraordinary" or "illegitimate" recombination, on the other hand, as being "rare, haphazard, and not obviously dependent upon genetic homology." Such recombination is typically termed "nonhomologous," indicating that *extended* regions of base sequence homology are not present at the crossover point. Examples of illegitimate recombination include the DNA rearrangements leading to deletions and duplications, and specialized transducing phages. This issue of GENETICS marks the 20th anniversary of a paper by FRANKLIN (1967) in which she investigated the relationship of illegitimate to homologous recombination. This *Perspectives* will consider how our understanding of illegitimate recombination—especially that which relates to formation of spontaneous deletions—has matured during these two decades.

The goal of FRANKLIN's 1967 experiments was to determine whether spontaneous deletions are generated using the enzymatic machinery of homologous recombination. Her experiments were made possible by the isolation of mutants in which homologous recombination is abolished (CLARK and MARGULIES 1965; HOWARD-FLANDERS and THERIOT 1966). FRANKLIN's experiments were simple and direct: the frequency of spontaneous deletions was measured in recombination-proficient and recombination-deficient backgrounds. Her results were equally direct: a recombination deficiency had no effect on the frequency of spontaneous deletions. Similar results have been obtained subsequently by numerous investigators (see, for example, INSELBURG 1967; SPUDICH, HORN and YANOFSKY 1970; MÜLLER-HILL and KANIA 1974; GHOSAL and SAEDLER 1979; FOSTER *et al.* 1981).

FRANKLIN proposed two general models to explain deletion formation. First, "slipped mispairing" during DNA replication might cause regions of the DNA to be bypassed. FRANKLIN's formulation of this model, like all others since, derives from the work of STREISINGER *et al.* (1966). His appealing and persuasive models account for the formation of frameshift mutations in bacteriophage T4 but are applicable to a wide variety of DNA arrangements. Second, FRANKLIN proposed that errors of DNA breakage and reunion might lead to deletions. In this model, enzymes that break and join DNA as part of their normal functions would do so on sequences that share little or no homology.

How have our thoughts concerning illegitimate recombination changed in these years? Surprisingly little. Contemporary models are more explicit, and specific enzymatic activities have been implicated in the deletion process. Yet, FRANKLIN's 1967 models remain the more general formations of today's specific ideas. The difference between "legitimate" and "illegitimate" recombination, however, has become vague. Illegitimate recombination is less frequent than normal recombination, but it is certainly not haphazard. Illegitimate recombination, furthermore, *does* depend upon base sequence homology, but this was not apparent using the genetic techniques available to FRANKLIN.

The importance of base sequence homology to deletion formation was recognized only when techniques of DNA sequencing became available. FARABAUGH *et al.* (1978) were the first to demonstrate that the break points of spontaneous deletions are not random. Rather, deletion termini are usually located within pairs of fortuitous, short, direct repeats (5–10 base pairs). The material between the repeats is deleted, and the resulting chromosome contains a single copy of what originally was the repeat. Similar results have been obtained by many investigators. The association of direct repeats with deletion termini in prokaryotes is very striking and contemporary models always involve base pairing at some level to account for this.

If homologous sequences participate in forming a deletion, why then is $recA^+$ function, which is essential for all homologous recombination, not required for spontaneous deletion? Obviously, $recA$-independent mechanisms exist for these sequences to interact. GLICKMAN and RIPLEY (1984) argue that base pairing between inverted repeats, or involving both direct and inverted repeats simultaneously, can generate structural intermediates for deletions, leading either to enzymatic removal of a single-strand loop or to replication across a cruciform structure formed transiently in single-stranded DNA. Inverted repeats of the transposon Tn*10* have dramatic effects on the frequency of Tn*10* excision (FOSTER et al. 1981); Tn*10* excision is a deletion process that is unrelated to transposition. Certain deletions could be generated by site-specific recombination. Sequence repeats in this case might reflect protein-DNA recognition, rather than direct base pairing alone. However, the immense variety of deletion termini argues that, except in special circumstances, site-specific recombination is not responsible for most spontaneous deletions.

In fact, some deletions *do* depend upon $recA^+$ for their formation. In an elegant series of experiments, ALBERTINI et al. (1982) investigated the involvement of short homologies and general recombination in the formation of *lacI* deletions. Deletion termini in this system are often located within typical direct repeats. Mutational disruption of these repeats reduces the frequency of the corresponding deletion. Deletions in this system depend upon $recA^+$ function; such events occur at much lower frequencies in $recA^-$ than in $recA^+$ strains. Surprisingly, deletions obtained in a $recA^-$ background have their termini located at direct repeats that are identical to those utilized in $recA^+$ cells. The $recA^+$ function, therefore, must facilitate (but not required for) some step in the deletion process.

What other enzymatic activities might be involved in deletion formation? DNA polymerases, copying an *Escherichia coli lacZ* template *in vitro* and unassisted by any other proteins, frequently generate deletions, often between short direct repeats (KUNKEL 1985a,b). DNA topoisomerases can also covalently join DNA molecules *in vitro*. DNA topoisomerases modify the topological states of DNA by catalyzing specific types of coupled breakage/rejoining reactions (reviewed by WANG 1985). Type I topoisomerases catalyze transient single-strand breaks, whereas type II topoisomerases catalyze transient double-strand breaks. *E. coli* DNA gyrase (a type II topoisomerase) catalyzes illegitimate recombination of DNAs *in vitro* (IKDEA, MORIYA and MATSUMOTO 1981; IKEDA, AOKI and NAITO 1982). IKEDA et al. propose that such recombination occurs when two covalent DNA-gyrase complexes exchange subunits before the rejoining step. T4 DNA topoisomerase (another type II enzyme) also catalyzes illegitimate recombination *in vitro* (IKEDA 1986). In neither case do these *in vitro* recombinations require $recA^+$ function.

Are these *in vitro* reactions relevant in *in vivo* deletions? The answer is probably yes. MARVO, KING and JASKUNAS (1983) describe a series of deletions arising *in vivo* that are very similar to the recombinants isolated *in vitro* by IKEDA et al. and present a "gyrase cascade model" to account for their structures. They suggest that sequence repeats at deletion termini arise because the protruding single strand of a DNA-gyrase complex is more likely to be rejoined to a second DNA-gyrase complex with which it shares base-sequence homology. An unresolved problem with this idea is that deletion termini should correspond to DNA gyrase cleavage sites (MORRISON and COZZARELLI 1979). The sequences around deletion crossover points occasionally but inconsistently confirm this (MARVO, KING and JASKUNAS 1983).

Deletions affecting bacteriophage M13 directly suggest the involvement of a type I DNA topoisomerase. The M13 gene *II* protein has enzymatic activities that are similar to those of a type I DNA topoisomerase (MEYER and GEIDER 1982). Gene *II* enzyme initiates DNA replication by introducing a site-specific nick at the M13 origin of replication and terminates replication by cleaving a newly synthesized strand and sealing it to form the circular viral molecule. Spontaneous deletions near the M13 origin of replication depend upon gene *II* for their formation. The termini of these deletions are located within typical direct-repeat sequences, but one endpoint is always located precisely at the site of gene *II* nicking (MICHEL and EHRLICH 1986). Such structures demonstrate convincingly that site-specific enzymatic activities can be involved in certain types of deletions.

It emerges from this discussion that at least two and perhaps several pathways exist for spontaneous deletion in prokaryotes. The short homologous sequences found at deletion termini can interact in either a $recA$-dependent or $recA$-independent manner. Features that distinguish these two pathways are unknown. Inverted repeat structures can facilitate the deletion of nearby sequences, but the details of this process are unclear. Which of the *in vivo* pathways involve DNA topoisomerases is unknown. Some of these uncertainties might be clarified if a wider variety of mutations affecting the deletion process were available. Mutants selected because they exhibit either altered frequencies or altered termini of spontaneous deletions would be valuable. Such mutants would identify components of the deletion process and possibly indicate the relationship of DNA deletion to replication, recombination and repair. Mutants affecting excision of the transposon Tn*10*, for example, have implicated genes involved in methylation-directed mismatch repair as being important for certain types of deletion (LUND-BLAD and KLECKNER 1985).

Are deletions in eukaryotes formed by mechanisms similar to those in prokaryotes? DNA topoisomerase I has been implicated in the eukaryotic deletion process. The crossover points leading to excision of SV40 from the mammalian chromosome correspond to topoisomerase I cleavage sites (BULLOCK, CHAMPOUX and BOTCHAN 1985). The sequence features of deletion termini in eukaryotes, however, are much less striking than those in prokaryotes. Sequence repeats, if present, are generally quite small. NALBANTOGLU *et al.* (1986) observe repeats that are 2–5 base pairs long at the termini of five spontaneous deletions affecting the *aprt* locus of CHO cells. R. PULAK and P. ANDERSON (unpublished results) observed repeats that are at most 4 base pairs long at the termini of 16 spontaneous deletions affecting a nematode myosin heavy chain gene. ROTH, PORTER and WILSON (1985) have summarized the repeat sizes associated with a large number of published eukaryotic illegitimate recombinations. Their summary indicates that crossover points contain on average slightly more homology than that predicted by completely random breakage and rejoining. ROTH and WILSON (1986) demonstrate that the slight bias toward sequence repeats at points of illegitimate recombination can be explained by a minor role for short sequence homologies in the DNA joining reaction. Thus, deletions in eukaryotes are similar to those in prokaryotes, but the DNA repeats are much less striking. This could indicate either a fundamental or superficial difference in their mechanisms of formation.

LITERATURE CITED

ALBERTINI, A. M., M. HOFER, M. P. CALOS and J. H. MILLER, 1982 On the formation of spontaneous deletions: the importance of short sequence homologies in the generation of large deletions. Cell **29:** 319–328.

BULLOCK, P., J. J. CHAMPOUX and M. BOTCHAN, 1985 Association of crossover points with topoisomerase I cleavage sites: a model for nonhomologous recombination. Science **230:** 954–958.

CLARK, A. J. and A. D. MARGULIES, 1965 Isolation and characterization of recombination deficient mutants of *E. coli* K12. Proc. Natl. Acad. Sci. USA **53:** 451–459

DRESSLER, D. and H. POTTER, 1982 Molecular mechanisms in genetic recombination. Annu. Rev. Biochem. **51:** 727–761.

FARABAUGH, P. J., U. SCHMEISSNER, M. HOFER and J. H. MILLER, 1978 Genetic studies of the *lac* repressor. VII. On the molecular nature of spontaneous hotspots in the *lacI* gene of *Escherichia coli.* J. Mol. Biol. **126:** 847–857.

FOSTER, T. J., V. LUNDBLAD, S. HANLEY-WAY, S. M. HALLING and N. KLECKNER, 1981 Three Tn10-associated excision events: relationship to transposition and role of direct and inverted repeats. Cell **23:** 215–227.

FRANKLIN, N. C., 1967 Extraordinary recombinational events in

Escherichia coli. Their independence of the *rec*+ function. Genetics **55:** 699–707.

FRANKLIN, N. C., 1971 Illegitimate recombination. pp. 175–194. In: *The Bacteriophage Lambda*, Edited by A. D. HERSHEY. Cold Spring Harbor Laboratory, Cold Spring Harbor, New York.

GHOSAL, D. and H. SAEDLER, 1979 IS2-61 and IS2-611 arise by illegitimate recombination from IS2-6. Mol. Gen. Genet. **176:** 233–238.

GLICKMAN, B. W. and L. S. RIPLEY, 1984 Structural intermediates of deletion mutagenesis: a role for palindromic DNA. Proc. Natl. Acad. Sci. USA **81:** 512–516.

HOWARD-FLANDERS, P. and L. THERIOT, 1966 Mutants of *Escherichia coli* K-12 defective in DNA repair and in genetic recombination. Genetics **53:** 1137–1150.

IKEDA, H., 1986 Bacteriophage T4 DNA topoisomerase mediates illegitimate recombination *in vitro*. Proc. Natl. Acad. Sci. USA **83:** 922–926.

IKEDA, H., K. AOKI and A. NAITO, 1982 Illegitimate recombination mediated *in vitro* by DNA gyrase of *Escherichia coli*: structure of recombinant DNA molecules. Proc. Natl. Acad. Sci. USA **79:** 3724–3728.

IKEDA, H., K. MORIYA and T. MATSUMOTO, 1981 In vitro study of illegitimate recombination: involvement of DNA gyrase. Cold Spring Harbor Symp. Quant. Biol. **45:** 399–408.

INSELBERG, J., 1967 Formation of deletion mutations in recombination-deficient mutants of *Escherichia coli*. J. Bacteriol. **94:** 1266–1267.

KUNKEL, T. A., 1985a The mutational specificity of DNA polymerase-β during *in vitro* DNA synthesis. Production of frameshift, base substitution, and deletion mutations. J. Biol. Chem. **260:** 5787–5796.

KUNKEL, T. A., 1985b The mutational specificity of DNA polymerases-α and -γ during *in vitro* DNA synthesis. J. Biol. Chem. **260:** 12866–12874.

LUNDBLAD, V. and N. KLECKNER, 1985 Mismatch repair mutations of *Escherichia coli* K12 enhance transposon excision. Genetics **109:** 3–19.

MARVO, S. L., S. R. KING and S. R. JASKUNAS, 1983 Role of short regions of homology in intermolecular illegitimate recombination events. Proc. Natl. Acad. Sci. USA **80:** 2452–2456.

MEYER, T. F. and K. GEIDER, 1982 Enzymatic synthesis of bacteriophage fd viral DNA. Nature **296:** 828–832.

MICHEL, B. and S. D. EHRLICH, 1986 Illegitimate recombination at the replication origin of bacteriophage M13. Proc. Natl. Acad. Sci. USA **83:** 3386–3390.

MORRISON, A. and N. R. COZZARELLI, 1979 Site-specific cleavage of DNA by *E. coli* DNA gyrase. Cell **17:** 175–184.

MÜLLER-HILL, B. and J. KANIA, 1974 *Lac* repressor can be fused to beta-galactosidase. Nature **249:** 561–563.

NALBANTOGLU, J., D. HARTLEY, G. PHEAR, G. TEAR and M. MEUTH, 1986 Spontaneous deletion formation at the *aprt* locus of hamster cells: the presence of short sequence homologies and dyad symmetries at deletion termini. EMBO J. **5:** 1199–1204.

ROTH, D. B., T. N. PORTER and J. H. WILSON, 1985 Mechanisms of nonhomologous recombination in mammalian cells. Mol. Cell. Biol. **5:** 2599–2607.

ROTH, D. B. and J. H. WILSON, 1986 Nonhomologous recombination in mammalian cells: role for short sequence homologies in the joining reaction. Mol. Cell. Biol. **6:** 4295–4304.

SPUDICH, J., V. HORN and C. YANOFSKY, 1970 On the production of deletions in the chromosome of *E. coli*. J. Mol. Biol. **53:** 49–67.

STREISINGER, G., Y. OKADA, J. EMRICH, J. NEWTON, A. TSUGITA, E. TERZAGHI and M. INOUYE, 1966 Frameshift mutations and the genetic code. Cold Spring Harbor Symp. Quant. Biol. **31:** 77–84.

WANG, J. C., 1985 DNA topoisomerases. Annu. Rev. Biochem. **54:** 665–697.

May 1987

Molecular Genetics of *Mus musculus*
Point Mutagenesis and Millimorgans

William F. Dove

McArdle Laboratory for Cancer Research, University of Wisconsin–Madison, Madison, Wisconsin 53706

THE world of genetics resembles an intellectual food chain. Approaches and attitudes developed in phage genetics are used in turn to study yeasts, slime molds, nematodes, plants, Drosophila or mammals. Only rarely does this chain circularize, since investigators nowadays most commonly move from the simpler to the more complex organisms. I vividly recall one exception, a talk at a Cold Spring Harbor phage meeting in which the presenter spoke of "sacrificing" phage-infected bacterial cultures for an enzyme analysis. From rat liver to phage, I thought.

This month's column traces the movement of molecular genetics into mouse genetics along a chain in which phage, yeast and Drosophila genetics provide successive nourishment.

Natural variants with heterozygous phenotypes: Much of classical mouse genetics rests on natural variants, often mutations expressing heterozygous phenotypes that beget more severe homozygous phenotypes. The well known alleles *Agouti-yellow* (*A'*), *Steel* (*Sl*) and dominant *White-spotting* (*W*) illustrate this proclivity. HALDANE (1956) suggested the term "patent lethal" for alleles with dominant visible and recessive lethal phenotypes, usefully avoiding the ambiguous terms "dominant lethal" and "semidominant." The series of recessive *t* haplotypes is an intricate version of patent lethals: each displays a heterozygous visible phenotype, tailless, in repulsion to the *brachyury* mutation (*T*) and, commonly, a homozygous lethal phenotype. Starting with the discovery of *T* 60 years ago (DOBROVOLSKAÏA-ZAVADSKAÏA 1927), L. C. DUNN and his colleagues collected much of the natural variant *t* material defining the *t* complex, culminating in a paper in GENETICS 25 years ago this spring in which the complementary interactions and rare recombinations with wild type were summarized (DUNN, BENNETT and BEASLEY 1962). It is now becoming plain that the *t* haplotypes share a set of inversions with one another. The *t* inversions account for the suppression of recombination between *t* haplotypes and wild-type chromatin. The genetic isolation of *t* haplotypes from wild type (and even from one another) has permitted each to accumulate polymorphisms of both the deletion/addition and the base pair substitution variety. Sequencing particular regions of *t* chromatin indicates that substitutions have accumulated to a level of 0.007 per base pair (FIGUEROA *et al.* 1985; UEHARA *et al.* 1987). Thus, a single transcribed 10-kb region may carry about 70 base-pair changes with respect to wild type. Two recent papers in GENETICS (MAINS 1986; SKOW *et al.* 1987) deal with this highly polymorphic aspect of *t* haplotypes.

In summary, the natural variants of the mouse *t* complex accumulated under conditions of blocked recombination and segregation distortion (LYON 1986) are a rich lode of developmental defects but an embarrasing plethora of changes at molecular resolution. For a geneticist working with a microorganism, or even with Drosophila, the reflex response might well be to induce new mutations on a standard background. In this issue of GENETICS (LEE *et al.* 1987), the laboratories of CHOVNICK and BENDER take just this approach to the controlling region of the *rosy* locus in Drosophila.

One powerful strategy employs insertional mutagenesis. For mouse genetics, this approach is being successfully used over the whole genome by JAENISCH, LEDER, JENKINS, and COPELAND, and their collaborators. Mutations induced by cloned DNA elements give direct access to the affected region of the genome. However, detailed studies of retroviral insertions indicate that such elements exert position effects over at least kilobasepair distances (BREINDL, HARBERS and JAENISCH 1984; RINCHIK *et al.* 1986). These position effects increase the target size for affecting a locus of interest but they confound the search for the DNA sequence that is responsible for the normal function of a gene. More crucial to the logistics of a mouse mutagenesis program, however, is the currently estimated efficiency of insertional mutagenesis, 10^{-4} to 10^{-5} per locus (DOVE 1984; JENKINS and COPELAND 1985). For a specific locus, it is vastly more difficult to screen

10,000 or more mouse pedigrees than the 1000–2000 required to find a new allele of the locus after chemical mutagenesis by ethylnitrosourea (ENU).

The second experimental paradigm comes directly from Drosophila genetics: to induce recessive mutations at a locus by using recessive visible markers and balancers to follow the pedigree of a mutated chromosome. The historical time scale is informative: MULLER and ALTENBURG published the first Drosophila experiments using recessive visible markers in 1919, SNELL carried out the first search for recessive lethals in the mouse in 1935, HALDANE (1956) worked out breeding systems for optimal scanning of the whole genome and CARTER (1957, 1959) used such systems in pilot experiments, detecting one X-ray-induced recessive lethal mutation. The efficiency of mutagenesis was clearly the limiting parameter, particularly for a mouse genetics facility of ordinary size that might screen only 300 mutagenized gametes per year.

ENU and 2000 mutagenized gametes: The nitrosamides have been championed by the Chester Beatty carcinogenesis workers LOVELESS, BROOKES and LAWLEY as penetrating alkylating agents needing no metabolic activation and more predisposed than is EMS to O-alkylation of guanine and thymine, generating base pair substitutions (LOVELESS 1969). In microorganisms, nitrosamides produce a favorable mutant frequency per unit of cell killing. Though these compounds are highly carcinogenic and mutagenic, they are so rapidly inactivated under mild conditions that safe handling requires only short-term chemical hazard containment.

Consistent with chemical expectations, mutations induced by ENU in the controlling region of the Drosophila *rosy* locus are predominantly $G \cdot C \rightarrow A \cdot T$ transitions (see LEE *et al.* in this issue). In contrast to the clustered mutations often found after nitrosoguanidine mutagenesis, only one of these *rosy* mutations was complex, an $A \cdot T \rightarrow C \cdot G$ transversion plus a nearby $A \cdot T$ deletion. RUSSELL and his colleagues (1979), working in the large-scale mutagen testing program at the Oak Ridge National Laboratory, established conditions in which ENU is a highly efficient germline mutagen for the mouse, particularly to spermatogonia. At visible loci, forward mutant frequencies average 0.0007 per locus. These frequencies make a crucial difference for a mouse laboratory that can handle only a few hundred parallel pedigrees emerging from mutagenized gametes.

BODE (1984) and JUSTICE and BODE (1986) have initiated a mutagenic attack on the *t* region by recovering induced alleles of its known visible loci, *tct*, *qk* and *tf*. As in the specific locus test, this involves only single-generation screens that detect recessive mutant phenotypes after mating a mutagenized wild-type male to a homozygous mutant female. Our Wisconsin laboratory and that of JEAN-LOUIS GUÉNET at the Institut Pasteur have collaborated on the efficient use of MULLER/HALDANE breeding protocols to recover numerous recessive lethal mutations in the *t* complex (SHEDLOVSKY *et al.* 1986). (One crucial component of this scheme is the fecundity of L. C. DUNN's mouse strain BTBR). This constitutes the first attempt to saturate a particular region of the mouse genome with induced mutant alleles and reflects a spirit spreading in mouse genetics: it is now feasible to induce mutations in a system of interest rather than merely to depend on natural variants.

The number of lethal complementation groups identified by ENU-induced mutations in the *t* region seems to be large, perhaps 50–100 (SHEDLOVSKY *et al.* 1986). These mutations must first be characterized by mapping rather than by complementation, because the number of mapping experiments increases linearly with the number of isolates rather than quadratically as do complementation tests. An increasing number of DNA markers (HERRMANN *et al.* 1986) and cDNA clones (WILLISON, DUDLEY and POTTER 1986) are becoming available for such mapping, with no limit in sight (POUSTKA and LEHRACH 1986). The question then becomes, what level of map resolution is necessary to assign point mutations to cloned segments?

Gene density in the mouse genome *vs.* the cosmid: Extrapolating the frequency of *t*-region recessive lethals induced by ENU suggests that there are 5,000–10,000 single-copy vital genes in the mouse genome (SHEDLOVSKY *et al.* 1986). [Previous measurements of lethals, with less efficient mutagenesis, had given estimates ranging from 1,000 (LYON, PHILLIPS and SEARLE 1964; RODERICK 1983; SHERIDAN 1983) to 10,000 (LYON 1956).] One imponderable in the ENU estimates is whether the average target size for generating a lethal allele is the same as that for producing a visible allele. A factor complicating interpretation of the X-ray induction of recessive lethals is the generally unknown size of deletions induced by X-rays. If the average deletion is large compared with the spacing between vital genes, then each induced recessive lethal mutation hits more than one vital locus and the number of vital loci will be underestimated (CHAKRABARTI *et al.* 1983).

The direct estimate of only 50–100 single-copy vital genes in the *t* region would correspond to a spacing no closer than 250 kb between such genes. The unique assignment of point mutations to loci would then require mapping to a resolution of 0.1–0.2 cM. There is reason to believe, however, that the frequency of transcribed regions in the mammalian genome is threefold to tenfold higher than this estimate of single-copy vital genes. Indeed, the number of known genes in the *t* region already approaches 100. OHNO (1986) has estimated the average spacing of transcribed regions to be 35 kb. BIRD (1986) and BROWN and BIRD (1986) have found that unmethylated CpG clusters (*Hpa*II tiny fragments of "HTF islands") occur on average every 90 kb; however, HTF islands may only mark genes that are expressed constitutively, thus underestimating the total frequency of transcribed regions. Detailed analysis of the *H-2K* region of the *t* complex shows nine class I and class II genes in 600 kb of DNA (STEINMETZ, STEPHAN and LINDAHL 1986). If we take 50 kb as the spacing of active genes—that is, the size of a DNA cosmid clone—then mapping of point mutations to segments of cosmid size would require resolution to about 0.02 cM. The analysis of the *agouti* locus reported in the April issue (LOVETT *et al.* 1987) well illustrates this gap in mapping resolution: markers generated from a linked retroviral insertion may lie at least 1 cM (50 cosmid lengths) from the DNA segment of interest.

In summary, molecular genetic analysis in the mouse currently straddles a challenging chasm. On one side, the direct advantage of insertional mutagenesis is compromised by the unknown distances over which position effects are exerted and by low insertion frequencies per locus compared with the number of gametes that can realistically be screened in pedigrees. On the other side, the high efficiency and point character of nitrosamide mutagenesis must be coupled with heroic mapping efforts to achieve molecular assignments for any of the biologically interesting mutations that now regularly turn up in ENU mutagenesis programs. The intrinsic biological interest of the newly induced mutations must drive our efforts to bridge this chasm.

Number of vital genes *vs.* the number of active genes: I close by wondering why the estimated frequency of vital loci in the mammalian genome is lower, by up to an order of magnitude, than the frequency of transcribed regions or HTF islands. A prime possibility is the one recently presented for the streamlined genome of *Saccharomyces cerevisiae* by GOEBL and PETES (1986). Gene disruption of putative single-copy sequences leads to a detectable phenotype only 30% of the time, though at least 50% of the yeast genome is transcribed and introns are rare (KABACK, ANGERER and DAVIDSON 1979). The putative single-copy sequences may actually belong to functionally redundant sets of genes (multigene families in which sufficient neutral drift has occurred to eliminate hybridization under the stringencies used) or to genes unrelated in DNA sequence but convergent in function. Analogous possibilities for Drosophila and for the mouse are discussed by GOEBL and PETES. It seems possible that, for each of these genetically tamed organisms, only a minority of the active loci are identified by recessive mutations. The rest of the iceberg is

invisible to us. Perhaps some useful variations can be played on the theme of the patent lethal from which mouse genetics began [see SUZUKI and PROCUNIER (1969) and KENNISON and RUSSELL in this issue].

I thank VERN BODE for cheerful company on the long walk from lambda to mouse genetics and MARY LYON for constructive suggestions.

LITERATURE CITED

BIRD, A. P., 1986 CpG-rich islands and the function of DNA methylation. Nature **321:** 209–213.

BODE, V. C., 1984 Ethylnitrosourea mutagenesis and the isolation of mutant alleles for specific genes located in the *t* region of mouse chromosome *17*. Genetics **108:** 457–470.

BREINDL, M., K. HARBERS and R. JAENISCH, 1984 Retrovirus-induced lethal mutation in collagen 1 gene of mice is associated with an altered chromatin structure. Cell **38:** 9–16.

BROWN, W. R. A. and A. P. BIRD, 1986 Long-range restriction site mapping of mammalian genomic DNA. Nature **322:** 477–481.

CARTER, T. C., 1957 Recessive lethal mutation induced in the mouse by chronic γ-irradiation. Proc. R. Soc. B **147:** 402–411.

CARTER, T. C., 1959 A pilot experiment with mice, using Haldane's method for detecting induced autosomal recessive lethal genes. J. Genet. **56:** 353–362.

CHAKRABARTI, S., G. STREISINGER, F. SINGER and C. WALKER, 1983 Frequency of γ-ray induced specific locus and recessive lethal mutations in mature germ cells of the zebrafish, *Brachydanio rerio*. Genetics **103:** 109–123.

DOBROVOLSKAÏA-ZAVADSKAÏA, N., 1927 Sur la mortification spontanée de la queue chez la souris nouveau-née et sur l'existence d'un caractère (facteur) héréditaire "non viable." C. R. Soc. Biol. **97:** 114–116.

DOVE, W. F., 1984 Developmental molecular genetics of the mouse and its embryonal carcinoma. Cell Differ. **15:** 205–213.

DUNN, L. C., D. BENNETT and A. B. BEASLEY, 1962 Mutation and recombination in the vicinity of a complex gene. Genetics **47:** 285–303.

FIGUEROA, F., M. GOLUBIĆ, D. NIŽETIĆ and J. KLEIN, 1985 Evolution of mouse major histocompatibility complex genes borne by *t* chromosomes. Proc. Natl. Acad. Sci. USA **82:** 2819–2823.

GOEBL, M. G. and T. D. PETES, 1986 Most of the yeast genomic sequences are not essential for cell growth and division. Cell **46:** 983–992.

HALDANE, J. B. S., 1956 The detection of autosomal lethals in mice induced by mutagenic agents. J. Genet. **54:** 327–342.

HERRMANN, B., M. BUĆAN, P. E. MAINS, A.-M. FRISCHAUF, L. M. SILVER and H. LEHRACH, 1986 Genetic analysis of the proximal portion of the mouse *t* complex: evidence for a second inversion within *t* haplotypes. Cell **44:** 469–476.

JENKINS, N. A. and N. G. COPELAND, 1985 High frequency germline acquisition of ecotropic MuLV proviruses in SWR/J-RF/J hybrid mice. Cell **43:** 811–819.

JUSTICE, M. J., and V. C. BODE, 1986 Induction of new mutations in a mouse *t*-haplotype using ethylnitrosourea mutagenesis. Genet. Res. **47:** 187–192.

KABACK, D. B., L. M. ANGERER and N. DAVIDSON, 1979 Improved

methods for the formation and stabilization of R-loops. Nucleic Acids Res. **6:** 2499–2517.

KENNISON, J. A. and M. A. RUSSELL, 1987 Dosage-dependent modifiers of homoeotic mutations in *Drosophila melanogaster*. Genetics **116:** 75–86.

LEE, C. S., D. CURTIS, M. MCCARRON, C. LOVE, M. GRAY, W. BENDER and A. CHOVNICK, 1987 Mutations affecting expression of the *rosy* locus in *Drosophila melanogaster*. Genetics **116:** 55–66.

LOVELESS, A., 1969 Possible relevance of *O*-6 alkylation of deoxyguanosine to the mutagenicity and carcinogenicity of nitrosamines and nitrosamides. Nature **223:** 206–207.

LOVETT, M., Z.-Y. CHENG, E. M. LAMELA, T. YOKOI and C. J. EPSTEIN, 1987 Molecular markers for the *agouti* coat color locus of the mouse. Genetics **115:** 747–754.

LYON, M. F., 1956 Some evidence concerning the "mutational load" in inbred strains of mice. Heredity **13:** 341–352.

LYON, M. F., 1986 Male sterility of the mouse *t*-complex is due to homozygosity of the distorter genes. Cell **44:** 357–363.

LYON, M. F., R. J. S. PHILLIPS and A. G. SEARLE, 1964 The overall rates of dominant and recessive lethal and visible mutation induced by spermatogonial x-irradiation of mice. Genet. Res. **5:** 448–467.

MAINS, P. E., 1986 The *cis-trans* test shows no evidence for a functional relationship between two mouse *t* complex lethal mutations: implications for the evolution of *t* haplotypes. Genetics **114:** 1225–1237.

MULLER, H. J. and E. ALTENBURG, 1919 The rate of change of hereditary factors in Drosophila. Proc. Soc. Exp. Biol. Med. **17:** 10–14.

OHNO, S., 1986 The total number of genes in the mammalian genome. Trends Genet. **2:** 8.

POUSTKA, A. and H. LEHRACH, 1986 Jumping libraries and linking libraries: the next generation of molecular tools in mammalian genetics. Trends Genet. **2:** 174–179.

RINCHIK, E. M., L. B. RUSSELL, N. G. COPELAND and N. A. JENKINS, 1986 Molecular genetic analysis of the *dilute-short ear* (*d-se*) region of the mouse. Genetics **112:** 321–342.

RODERICK, T. H., 1983 Using inversions to detect and study recessive lethals and detrimentals in mice. pp. 135–137. In: *Utilization of Mammalian Specific Locus Studies in Hazard Evaluation and Estimation of Genetic Risk*, Edited by F. J. DE SERRES and W. SHERIDAN. Plenum, New York.

RUSSELL, W. L., E. M. KELLY, P. R. HUNSICKER, J. W. BANGHAM, S. C. MADDUX and E. L. PHIPPS, 1979 Specific-locus test shows ethylnitrosourea to be the most potent mutagen in the mouse. Proc. Natl. Acad. Sci. USA **76:** 5818–5819.

SHEDLOVSKY, A., J.-L. GUÉNET, L. L. JOHNSON and W. F. DOVE, 1986 Induction of recessive lethal mutations in the *T/t-H-2* region of the mouse genome by a point mutagen. Genet. Res. **47:** 135–142.

SHERIDAN, W., 1983 The detection of induced recessive lethal mutations in mice. pp. 125–134. In: *Utilization of Mammalian Specific Locus Studies in Hazard Evaluation and Estimation of Genetic Risk*, Edited by F. J. DE SERRES and W. SHERIDAN. Plenum, New York.

SKOW, L. C., J. N. NADEAU, J. C. AHN, H.-S. SHIN, K. ARTZT and D. BENNETT, 1987 Polymorphism and linkage of the αA-crystallin gene in *t*-haplotypes of the mouse. Genetics **116:** 107–111.

SNELL, G. D., 1935 The induction by X-rays of hereditary changes in mice. Genetics **20:** 545–567.

STEINMETZ, M., D. STEPHAN and K. F. LINDAHL, 1986 Gene organization and recombinational hotspots in the murine major histocompatibility complex. Cell **44:** 895–904.

SUZUKI, D. T. and D. PROCUNIER, 1969 Temperature-sensitive mutations in *Drosophila melanogaster*. III. Dominant lethals and semilethals on chromosome 2. Proc. Natl. Acad. Sci. USA **62:** 369–376.

UEHARA, H., K. ABE, C.-H. T. PARK, H.-S. SHIN, D. BENNETT and K. ARTZT, 1987 The molecular organization of the *H-2K* region of two *t*-haplotypes: implications for the evolution of genetic diversity. EMBO J. **6:** 83–90.

WILLISON, K. R., K. DUDLEY and J. POTTER, 1986 Molecular cloning and sequence analysis of a haploid expressed gene encoding *t* complex polypeptide 1. Cell **44:** 727–738.

June 1987

Twenty-five Years Ago in *Genetics*
Motoo Kimura and Molecular Evolution

James F. Crow

Genetics Department, University of Wisconsin–Madison, Madison, Wisconsin 53706

THE June 1962 issue of GENETICS contained an article by MOTOO KIMURA entitled "On the probability of fixation of mutant genes in a population." In this paper he gave a very general treatment of the probability that a mutant allele with a specified frequency will eventually replace the existing allele(s). Although the problem had long attracted mathematical interest, it was not at the time regarded as of central evolutionary importance. FISHER (1930) had called attention to the considerable chance of stochastic loss of any new mutant, even a favorable one. Yet, in any large population, mutations at the same locus occur repeatedly, so he assumed that the chances of fixation of one or another of them is near certainty. WRIGHT (1931, 1942, 1945) was mainly interested in the steady-state distribution of allele frequencies, these being relevant to his shifting-balance theory. The only serious use for the fixation probability was in animal breeding theory, where it arises in connection with determining selection limits (ROBERTSON 1960). Remarkably, KIMURA's work turned out to be pre-adapted for the later study of molecular evolution.

As early as 1927, HALDANE used a method of FISHER (1922) to show that the probability of ultimate fixation of a mutant allele with a selective advantage s is approximately $2s$. FISHER (1930), WRIGHT (1931, 1942), and MALÉCOT (1952) all provided refinements. (MALÉCOT shared MENDEL's fate of being for a long time ignored by most geneticists; his pioneering work was published in an out of the way place, and in French.) KIMURA (1957, 1962, 1964) solved the problem, using a diffusion model, for arbitrary dominance and fluctuating selection coefficients. A simple version of KIMURA's formula for the probability of fixation of a new mutation, sufficient for consideration of molecular evolution, is

$$P = (1 - e^{-2s})/(1 - e^{-4Ns})$$

in which N is the size of the breeding population. When $s \to 0$ while $Ns > 1$, $P \approx 2s$, HALDANE's result. For a neutral mutant ($s \to 0$), $P = 1/2N$, as might be expected. (Recall that, for small x, $e^{-x} \approx 1 - x$.)

In the late 1960s it became increasingly clear that nucleotide and amino acid substitutions are marching to a different drummer than that of traditional morphological evolution. The latter is characterized by widely different rates, within and between lineages, by strong environmental influences, by dependence on availability of ecological niches, and possibly by association with speciation events. Molecular evolution, on the contrary, is roughly constant for the same protein within and between lineages, and is essentially independent of the environment. KIMURA had the happy insight that the average rate of nucleotide substitutions in a long evolutionary period does not depend on the time required for an individual mutation to be fixed, the problem addressed by classical population genetics. Rather it depends on the frequency of occurrence of ultimately fixed mutations. This requires that the mutation rate be small and that we view the process over a time period that is long relative to the number of generations required for a successful mutation to go to fixation, later shown by KIMURA and OHTA (1969) to be about four times the population number. Nucleotide and amino acid substitutions occurring over periods of several hundred million years meet these criteria.

The simplest and oldest hypothesis for molecular evolution is that it is a succession of substitutions of selectively favored mutations. We can use KIMURA's equation to examine this hypothesis. In a diploid population there will be $2N\mu$ new mutations each generation, where μ is the mutation rate per site per generation and again N is the population number. Each mutation has a probability P of ultimately being fixed in the population, so that the long-time average rate of substitution is $2N\mu P$ per generation. Substituting $2s$ for P gives a rate $4\mu s N$. That the rate should be proportional to μ and s is reasonable, but the proportionality to N is dubious. Furthermore, it is contrary to fact; carnivores with small populations evolve molecularly just as rapidly as do herbivores with large ones, and those invertebrates with enormous population numbers change no more rapidly than do mammals. This argues strongly against molecular evolution being the result of successive incorporation of favorable mutations.

KIMURA's well known alternative is that molecular substitutions are mainly neutral. If $s = 0$, $P = 1/2N$ and the rate is simply μ. Although there are uncertainties and exceptions, the data fit this hypothesis much better than that invoking favorable mutations. KIMURA argues that molecular evolution is mainly the random fixation of neutral, or possibly slightly deleterious mutations (OHTA 1973; KIMURA 1983).

This is only one argument. KIMURA (1983) has given many other reasons for believing that the overwhelming majority of nucleotide changes and a large fraction of amino acid changes are the result of chance fixation of lucky mutations, whose fitness effects are so slight that chance predominates. The process becomes mutation-driven rather than selection-driven. That a great deal of nucleotide and amino acid evolution is of this sort seems to me to be well established. The exact fraction remains to be determined.

I first heard of KIMURA's mathematical work in the early 1950s through a student, NEWTON MORTON, who was temporarily working in Hiroshima. I first met KIMURA at a Genetics Society meeting in Madison in 1953, at which time he brought a manuscript on the difficult problem of gene frequency drift due to fluctuating selection intensities. He had found a transformation that converted this into a partial differential equation like that for heat conduction, which could readily be solved. The paper was soon published in GENETICS (KIMURA 1954). To my surprise, I discovered that KIMURA had a master's degree in cytogenetics but that his mathematics and population genetics were self-taught. After a year of graduate work at Iowa State University he joined my group and received his Ph.D. two years later. This was the beginning of a happy professional and personal association that still continues.

More than any other person, KIMURA carried the theoretical work of FISHER and WRIGHT into the second half of the century. He is largely responsible for popularizing diffusion equations in population genetics and has used them to solve a host of problems. But this is only part of his work. He has contributed to the theory of inbreeding, selection of multifactorial

traits, population structure, linkage and epistasis, multigene families, truncation selection, selection for altruism, and more. His neutral theory and ramifications therefrom have generated a flood of theoretical and observational studies. His work has been a major catalyst for the high level of mathematical analysis that now characterizes the field. Equations such as he introduced in that 1962 GENETICS paper are now part of standard population genetics theory.

Whether MOTOO KIMURA will best be remembered for the neutral theory or for his work in extending the general theory of population genetics remains to be seen. But that he will be remembered is not in doubt.

LITERATURE CITED

FISHER, R. A., 1922 On the dominance ratio. Proc. R. Soc. Edinb. **42:** 321–341.

FISHER, R. A., 1930 *The Genetical Theory of Natural Selection.* Clarendon Press, Oxford, Rev. ed. 1958, Dover Publ., New York.

HALDANE, J. B. S., 1927 A mathematical theory of natural and artificial selection. Part V. Selection and mutation. Proc. Camb. Phil. Soc. **23:** 838–844.

KIMURA, M., 1954 Process leading to quasi-fixation of genes in natural populations due to random fluctuations of selection intensities. Genetics **39:** 280–295.

KIMURA, M., 1957 Some problems of stochastic processes in genetics. Ann. Math. Stat. **28:** 882–901.

KIMURA, M., 1962 On the probability of fixation of mutant genes in a population. Genetics **47:** 713–719.

KIMURA, M., 1964 Diffusion models in populations genetics. J. Appl. Prob. **1:** 177–232.

KIMURA, M., 1983 *The Neutral Theory of Molecular Evolution.* Cambridge University Press, Cambridge.

KIMURA, M. and T. OHTA, 1969 The average number of generations until fixation of a mutant gene in a finite population. Genetics **61:** 763–771.

MALÉCOT, G., 1952 Les processus stochastiques et al méthode des fonctions génératices ou caractéristiques. Pub. Inst. Stat. Univ. de Paris **1** (3): 1–16.

OHTA, T., 1973 Slightly deleterious mutant substitutions in evolution. Nature **246:** 96–98.

ROBERTSON, A., 1960 A theory of limits in artificial selection. Proc. R. Soc. B **153:** 234–249.

WRIGHT, S., 1931 Evolution in Mendelian populations. Genetics **16:** 97–159.

WRIGHT, S., 1942 Statistical genetics and evolution. Bull. Am. Math. Soc. **48:** 223–246.

WRIGHT, S., 1945. The differential equation of the distribution of gene frequencies. Proc. Natl. Acad. Sci. USA **31:** 382–389.

July 1987

The *waxy* Locus in Maize Twenty-five Years Later

Oliver E. Nelson

Laboratory of Genetics, University of Wisconsin–Madison, Madison, Wisconsin 53706

TWENTY-FIVE years ago it was reported in GE-NETICS that the frequency of nonmutant *Wx* gametes estimated by scoring pollen produced by maize plants heteroallelic for two *wx* alleles (*wx-C* and *wx-90*) of independent mutational origin could be validated by using the pollen from such plants to fertilize a *wx/wx* tester stock and showing that a similar frequency of seeds with a Wx phenotype resulted (NELSON 1962). Since this was the first demonstration that a fine structure study was feasible in a higher plant, the corroboration of intragenic recombination inferred from pollen assays in a conventional genetic backcross stimulated a more extensive study of intragenic recombination within the locus and an investigation of the enzymatic lesion produced by the mutations. In the intervening years, the *wx* locus has been a fruitful source of material for investigations into the molecular genetics of maize.

The *waxy* locus in maize came first to the attention of geneticists in seeds of an unusual phenotype in a maize variety that COLLINS (1909) collected and brought back from China. The designation as *waxy* derived from the soft wax-like sheen of kernels homozygous for a *waxy* allele, although it became apparent later that the mutation affected the type of starch produced in the endosperm tissue.

The reference *wx* allele (*wx-C*) has been a most useful genetic marker because it conditions an unmistakable seed phenotype and is linked on the short arm of chromosome *9* to other loci, *aleurone color-1* (*c1*), *shrunken-1* (*sh1*) and *bronze-1* (*bz1*), which affect seed phenotype (NEUFFER, JONES and ZUBER 1968).

WEATHERWAX (1922) reported that the starch in *waxy* endosperms gave an anomalous reaction with an I_2,KI stain, producing a reddish-brown color instead of the intense blue-black color observed with ordinary starch. He reported also that the dissimilarity in starches produced in *waxy* and nonwaxy endosperms did not extend to the embryos of seeds of these genotypes, because the starch grains in embryo tissue of both genotypes reacted with the iodine stain to produce a blue-black color. WEATHERWAX referred to the polysaccharide product in *waxy* endosperms as "erythrodextrin" but it was not until 1943 that the nature of the change in *waxy* starch was understood when SPRAGUE, BRIMHALL and HIXON reported that *waxy* lacked the straight-chain component of starch, amylose, and was composed entirely of the branched-chain component, amylopectin.

BRINK and MACGILLIVRAY (1924) and DEMEREC (1924) reported, independently but in the same number of the *American Journal of Botany*, that *Wx/wx* plants produced equal numbers of *Wx* and *wx* pollen grains as shown by their reaction with the I_2,KI stain. It was thus apparent that not only was the *Wx* allele necessary for the production in pollen of starch staining blue-black with an iodine stain but that the phenotype after staining of a pollen grain was conditioned by its own haploid genotype and not that of the plant by which it was produced.

These observations of BRINK and MACGILLIVRAY and of DEMEREC suggested that the *wx* locus might be a useful system in which to ascertain whether the intragenic recombination that had been shown to occur in prokaryotic organisms and in the filamentous fungi Aspergillus and Neurospora was also a feature of a plant species that was a traditional favorite for genetic investigations (NELSON 1957). A maize plant produces about 2.5×10^7 pollen grains, some five orders of magnitude more than the number of seeds produced by that plant. If different mutant sites were affected in *wx* mutants of independent origin and if recombination occurred between these sites, then a heteroallelic F$_1$ plant should produce a characteristic frequency of *Wx* pollen grains easily distinguished among the *wx* pollen grains. To eliminate the possibility of *Wx* pollen in the air settling on the anthers being sampled, a protocol was devised to release about 5×10^4 pollen grains from anthers in unopened florets into a mixture of I_2,KI stain and a gelatin solution that can be spread over the surface of a large slide. Upon gelling, this mixture fixes the pollen grains in position prior to estimating the population size and counting the *Wx* pollen.

The initial test of this hypothesis revealed that each F_1 cross between two *wx* alleles of independent origin produced a characteristic frequency of *Wx* pollen ranging from 0 to 80×10^{-5} (NELSON 1958). Also, the numbers of *Wx* pollen grains packaged within each anther of an F_1 plant were in close agreement with a Poisson distribution, as would be expected if the events giving rise to *Wx* pollen grains were independent and occurred after DNA replication. Furthermore, backcrosses of an F_1 with a high frequency of *Wx* pollen to either homoallelic parent produced about equal numbers of progeny plants with 0 *Wx* pollen grains and with a *Wx* frequency approximating that of the F_1 cross, as expected if a heteroallelic constitution at the *wx* locus were required to generate a *Wx* frequency above those of the *wx* parents. However, a further test was desirable. If the pollen grains whose phenotype indicated that they were *Wx* were indeed the product of a recombinational event reconstituting a functional *Wx* allele, then the pollen from an F_1 cross fertilizing a *wx/wx* tester stock should produce a frequency of seeds with a *Wx* phenotype close to the frequency of *Wx* pollen grains found in the pollen produced by plants of that F_1 cross. Such validation for the *wx-C/wx-90* heteroallelic F_1 was reported 25 years ago (NELSON 1962). Since flanking markers were present (*bronze-1* distal to *wx* and *virescent-1* proximal), it could also be shown that the most frequent class of *Wx* recombinants had the distal marker that entered the cross with *wx-90* and the proximal marker that entered with *wx-C*. Thus, the mutational sites in these two alleles could be ordered relative to the outside markers. The second most frequent class of *Wx* recombinants had the flanking markers that entered with the *wx-C* allele, suggesting that these might have arisen by gene conversion. The results of a later study using heterozygosity for several chromosomal aberrations to reduce recombination frequencies on the short arm of chromosome *9* were consistent with the hypothesis that those *Wx* recombinants with the flanking markers that entered the cross with *wx-C* (the second most numerous class of *Wx* recombinants) resulted from gene conversion events and not from double exchanges, one within the *wx* locus and one outside (NELSON 1975).

In subsequent years, numerous crosses were conducted with 31 *wx* mutants in order to ascertain whether mutations resulting from the insertions of transposable elements in the *wx* locus could be mapped. To this end, a number of *wx* alleles isolated by BARBARA MCCLINTOCK and resulting from the insertion of a defective transposable element in a *Wx* allele were included. These were nonautonomous mutable alleles that require the presence in the genome of a transacting element of the same family in order to transpose. In the absence of such an element, they are completely stable and can be used in recombination experiments in the same fashion as any other allele. The results of these intercrosses showed clearly that the mutations induced by the transposable elements recombined with each other and with many other spontaneous mutations. Their positions within the locus could be specified and they occupied different sites (NELSON 1968). Because recombination frequencies were not additive in this series of crosses (probably owing to the occurrence of the mutations in different genetic backgrounds), the map of the locus was constructed via the method of overlapping deletions as used by BENZER (1959) for the *rII* region of bacteriophage T4. This was possible since several of the mutations behaved as though they occupied a segment of the locus.

Studies of the enzymatic deficiency in *wx* mutants were conducted concomitantly with the genetic investigations. NELSON and RINES reported in 1962 that the developing endosperms of *waxy* seeds lacked a nucleoside diphosphate glucose:starch glucosyl transferase that is tightly bound to the starch granules and that adds glucose to the nonreducing ends of starch molecules. The starch granules of nonmutant endosperms have high glucosyl transferase activity. Later studies showed that the functional alleles at the *wx* locus are expressed only in the pollen and endosperm tissue and that the starch granules in the embryos of *waxy* seeds have as high activity as those from the embryos of nonwaxy seeds (NELSON and TSAI 1964). The glucosyl transferase bound to embryo starch granules can be distinguished on biochemical grounds from that bound to the endosperm starch granules. This demonstrated that the *Wx* alleles at the *wx* locus are not regulatory alleles that allow expression of the glucosyl transferase in embryo, pollen, megaspore and endosperm while the *wx* alleles permit expression only in the embryo (AKATSUKA and NELSON 1966).

After solubilizing the proteins bound to starch granules, ECHT and SCHWARTZ (1981) demonstrated that the extract from *wx-C* starch lacked a 60-kd protein that was present in the extracts from *Wx* starch. The demonstration that the *wx* locus is the structural gene for the 60-kd protein came from the observation that four of the *wx* alleles mapped by NELSON (1968) produced altered forms of this protein. The connection between the 60-kd protein and the glucosyl transferase was affirmed by showing that the amount of protein increased in triploid endosperms through the dosage series *wx/wx/wx*, *wx/wx/Wx*, *Wx/Wx/wx* and *Wx/Wx/Wx* in the same manner in which the enzymatic activity had been shown to increase (TSAI 1974). Fortuitously, two mutations mapping at opposite extremes of the locus (*90* and *R*) condition the production of altered proteins. Thus, it was apparent that these alleles are located within the structural gene and so are all the alleles located between them. The gate to using the *waxy* locus alleles in molecular genetics was then opened when SHURE, WESSLER and FEDOROFF (1983) employed the methods of ECHT and SCHWARTZ to solubilize and purify *Wx* protein against which antiserum could be raised. The antiserum was used to identify the RNA that supported the synthesis of a polypeptide which was immunoprecipitable and to identify the cDNA clones which would hybridize to *Wx* mRNA. Genomic clones of *Wx* were then isolated. The cDNA clones of *Wx* enabled FEDOROFF, WESSLER and SHURE (1983) to identify a restriction fragment from *Ac wx-m9*, an autonomous mutable allele resulting from the insertion of the transposable element *Ac* into a *Wx* allele. This was the initial isolation of *Ac* which was shown to be a 4.3-kb element. The same report showed that, while there were numerous sequences in the maize genome with homology to the termini of *Ac*, there were relatively few with homology to the center of *Ac*. This observation has been crucial in using *Ac* as a tag to identify the clones of other loci (FEDOROFF, FURTEK and NELSON 1984).

The *wx* locus has also been the key to isolating the autonomous member *En* (a.k.a. *Spm*) of the second well studied family of maize transposable elements, *Suppressor-mutator* (*I,En*). PEREIRA *et al.* (1985) used the *wx* locus to isolate an insertion of *En* in a *Wx* allele that had produced a mutable *wx* allele, thus enabling the demonstration that *En* is 8.4 kb long, has 13-bp perfect inverted repeats at the termini and produces a 3-bp duplication of host sequences upon insertion. The same laboratory has shown that the *wx* coding region contains 3718 bp and 14 exons (KLOESGEN *et al.* 1986).

WESSLER and VARAGONA (1985) have analyzed further by Southern blots 22 of the *wx* mutations mapped by NELSON (1968) and found excellent correlation between the genetic and molecular maps. Twelve of the 17 spontaneous mutations resulted from deletions or insertions of size sufficient to be detected by this type of analysis. It is notable that insertion mutants (7) were more numerous than deletion mutants (5) in this small sample.

FREELING (1976) demonstrated that the *adh1* locus of maize could also be used in fine structure studies because the phenotype of a pollen grain following ethanol-dependent reduction of *para*-nitrobluetetrazolium chloride depends on the genotype of the pollen grain at that locus.

There are *wx* mutants in barley, rice, and sorghum (ERIKSSON 1969) but in none of these species has the locus been subjected to the searching scrutiny accorded the *wx* locus in maize where it has enabled a study of intragenic recombination in a higher plant and has facilitated access to the fascinating transposable element systems *Ac, Ds* and *Spm* (*I,En*).

LITERATURE CITED

AKATSUKA, T. and O. E. NELSON, 1966 Starch granule-bound adenosine diphosphate glucose-starch glucosyl transferases of maize seeds. J. Biol. Chem. **241:** 2280–2286.

BENZER, S., 1959 On the topology of the genetic fine structure. Proc. Natl. Acad. Sci. USA **45:** 1607–1620.

BRINK, R. and J. M. MacGILLIVRAY, 1924 Segregation for the waxy character in maize pollen and differential development of the male gametophyte. Am. J. Bot. **11:** 465–469.

COLLINS, G. N., 1909 A new type of Indian corn from China. U.S. Dept. Agric. Bur. Plant Indust. Bull. **161:** 7–30.

DEMEREC, M., 1924 A case of pollen dimorphism in maize. Am. J. Bot. **11:** 461–464.

ECHT, C. and D. SCHWARTZ, 1981 Evidence for the inclusion of controlling elements within the structural gene at the waxy locus in maize. Genetics **99:** 275–284.

ERICKSSON, G., 1969 The waxy character. Hereditas **63:** 180–204.

FEDOROFF, N., D. B. FURTEK and O. E. NELSON, 1984 Cloning of the *bronze* locus in maize by a simple and generalizable procedure using the transposable controlling element *Ac*. Proc. Natl. Acad. Sci. USA **81:** 3825–3829.

FEDOROFF, N., S. WESSLER and M. SHURE, 1983 Isolation of the transposable maize controlling elements *Ac* and *Ds*. Cell **35:** 235–242.

FREELING, M., 1976 Intragenic recombination in maize: pollen analysis method and the effect of parental *Adh1+* isoalleles. Genetics **83:** 701–717.

KLOESGEN, R. B., A. GIERL, Z. SCHWARZ-SOMMER and H. SAEDLER, 1986 Molecular analysis of the waxy locus of *Zea mays*. Mol. Gen. Genet. **203:** 237–244.

NELSON, O. E., 1957 The feasibility of investigating "genetic fine structure" in higher plants. Am. Nat. **91:** 331–332.

NELSON, O. E., 1958 Intracistron recombination in the Wx/wx region of maize. Science **130:** 794–795.

NELSON, O. E., 1962 The *waxy* locus in maize. I. Intralocus recombination frequency estimates by pollen and conventional analyses. Genetics **47:** 737–742.

NELSON, O. E., 1968 The *waxy* locus in maize. II. The location of the controlling element alleles. Genetics **60:** 507–524.

NELSON, O. E., 1975 The *waxy* locus in maize. III. Effect of structural heterozygosity on intragenic recombination and flanking marker assortment. Genetics **79:** 31–44.

NELSON, O. E. AND H. W. RINES, 1962 The enzymatic deficiency in the waxy mutant of maize. Biochem. Biophys. Res. Commun. **9:** 297–300.

NELSON, O. E. and C. Y. TSAI, 1964 Glucose transfer from adenosine diphosphate glucose to starch in preparations of waxy seeds. Science **145:** 1194–1195.

NEUFFER, M. G., L. JONES and M. S. ZUBER, 1968 *The Mutants of Maize.* Crop Science Society, Madison, Wisc.

PEREIRA, A., Z. SCHWARZ-SOMMER, A. GIERL, I. BERTRAM, P. A. PETERSON and H. SAEDLER, 1985 Genetic and molecular analysis of the Enhancer (*En*) transposable element system of *Zea mays*. EMBO J. **5:** 835–841.

SHURE, M., S. WESSLER and N. FEDOROFF, 1983 Molecular identification and isolation of the *waxy* locus in maize. Cell **35:** 225–233.

SPRAGUE, G. F., B. BRIMHALL and R. M. HIXON, 1943 Some effects of the waxy gene in corn on properties of the endosperm starch. J. Am. Soc. Agron. **35:** 817–822.

TSAI, C. Y., 1974 The function of the Waxy locus in starch synthesis in maize endosperm. Biochem. Genet. **11:** 83–96.

WEATHERWAX, P., 1922 A rare carbohydrate in waxy maize. Genetics **7:** 568–572.

WESSLER, S. and M. J. VARAGONA, 1985 Molecular basis of mutations at the *waxy* locus of maize: correlation with the fine structure map. Proc. Natl. Acad. Sci. USA **82:** 4177–4181.

August 1987

Doing Behavioral Genetics with Bacteria

John S. Parkinson

Biology Department, University of Utah, Salt Lake City, Utah 84112

MOTILE microorganisms exhibit surprisingly sophisticated sensory behaviors. They migrate toward food sources, flee from noxious chemicals, and generally seek out optimum environments for their metabolic activities. These behaviors came to light in the pioneering work of ENGELMANN, PFEFFER and others in the 1880s [see BERG (1975) for a review of this early work] but were largely overlooked until JULIUS ADLER (1965, 1966) initiated work on the chemotaxis system of *Escherichia coli* in the mid-1960s. ADLER chose *E. coli* primarily for the genetic methods that could be brought to bear on the problem, reasoning that the flow of sensory information through stimulus transduction components should be amenable to genetic dissection much like a conventional biochemical pathway. The first report from the ADLER group on motility mutants of *E. coli* appeared just 20 years ago in GENETICS (ARMSTRONG and ADLER 1967). Subsequent work by the chemotaxis community, much of it inspired by ADLER's lead, has elucidated many of the molecular events underlying stimulus detection and signal processing in bacteria. Because genetic methods have played a central role in this endeavor, it seems appropriate to reflect on the early days of behavioral genetics in bacteria, when obtaining chemotaxis mutants was the only game in town and one that proved to be no simple task.

I first learned about the psychic life of *E. coli* in a seminar that ADLER presented at Caltech shortly after that first GENETICS paper appeared. I was a graduate student in BOB EDGAR's phage group at the time, and had probably come to regard bacteria as little more than a means for making plaques. Nevertheless, I was immediately captivated by the animated behavior of these little creatures and by the prospect of using genetic techniques to understand their antics at the molecular level. Consequently, I enlisted for a postdoctoral stint in ADLER's laboratory and arrived in Madison in 1970 along with two other postdocs, BOB READER from LOU SIMONIVITCH's lab and GEORGE ORDAL from DALE KAISER's lab. What follows is the story of three expatriate phage workers who tried to match wits with *E. coli*.

E. coli swims by rotating flagellar filaments. In the absence of chemotactic stimuli, the flagellar motors reverse directions about once per second, causing the cell to move in a three-dimensional random flight. In the presence of chemical gradients, net chemotactic movements are produced by modulating the pattern of flagellar reversals in response to changing attractant or repellent concentrations. This behavior can be assayed by directly observing the responses of individual cells to temporal chemoeffector gradients in the light microscope, or by measuring the rate or extent of migration of an entire bacterial population in spatial chemoeffector gradients. The simplest assay involves the use of semisolid agar "swarm" plates, in which the cells themselves set up and follow attractant gradients by consuming nutrient compounds as they grow.

Since neither motility nor chemotaxis is essential for viability, at least in laboratory-reared *E. coli*, it seemed at the outset that doing behavioral genetics would be a straightforward undertaking. In order to reconstruct the "wiring diagram" of *E. coli*, we simply needed to isolate and characterize large numbers of mutants defective in the receptors responsible for detecting chemical stimuli and in the transduction components needed to relay chemoreceptor signals to the flagellar motors. A handful of chemotaxis mutants had already been isolated by repeatedly cycling cells that remained in the center of swarming colonies (ARMSTRONG, ADLER and DAHL 1967), so we knew that it was possible. However, that original procedure was poorly suited for large-scale mutant hunts. First, the yield of desired mutants was very low; most of the selected cells simply had motility or growth defects. Second, the chemotaxis mutants could (and sometimes did) arise in several steps owing to the many generations of growth during the course of the enrichment process. Clearly, more efficient mutant isolation methods were needed.

A variety of clever schemes were devised, employing preformed gradients to eliminate metabolism mutants, but none proved very successful. Although reconstruction tests with the chemotaxis mutants on hand indicated that these selection methods did work, the enrichment factor was very low. Why did so many wild-type chemotactic cells come through? The problem stems from the fact that wild-type cultures invariably contain a relatively high proportion of phenocopies, individuals that have suffered temporary loss of flagella or some other physiological misfortune. These "perverts" refused to perform, even though they possessed a wild-type genome, and their descendants wreaked havoc with our selection schemes.

Another inventive approach involved exposing *E. coli* to mind-altering drugs. It seemed likely that if the sensory apparatus of bacteria was similar to that of higher organisms, bacterial behavior might be perturbed by anesthetics, stimulants, tranquilizers or hallucinogens. If such compounds interfered with chemotaxis, it should then be possible to identify their molecular targets by isolating mutants whose behavior was no longer sensitive to inhibition. To pursue this possibility, ADLER acquired (through proper channels) an extensive collection of pyschoactive compounds, which he kept locked in the Biochemistry Department safe "to prevent undergraduates from experimenting with them." Unfortunately, none of them had any useful effect on *E. coli* behavior, although I do recall that 1 M LSD inhibited motility a bit.

Having exhausted our bag of tricks, we finally resorted to the inelegant strategy of brute-force screening. An assembly line was set up for pouring swarm plates and picking individual colonies to test chemotactic responses. Now the mutants began to trickle in, often several useful ones per day. After several months we realized that, rather than transferring colonies to swarm plates one at a time with toothpicks, the swarms could be initiated from single cells by embedding them in the agar as the plate was poured. Such "miniswarm" methods permitted us to screen several hundred colonies per plate, and the trickle became a torrent.

The mutants isolated during those early days of *E. coli* chemotaxis were widely disseminated to workers in the chemotaxis field and have served to define most of the known components of the sensory transduction machinery: receptors, transducers, signaling elements and flagellar switching components (*cf.* PARKINSON 1981). They have been used to identify, purify and characterize the various chemotaxis proteins and to detect interactions among them. They have also been used to clone and sequence the structural genes for those proteins and to explore their regulation and functional activity. Today, the goal of understanding a simple behavior at the molecular level is well within sight (*cf.* MACNAB 1987). Although many groups participated in these discoveries, we owe special thanks to JULIUS ADLER for having the foresight to pick an organism with good genetics.

LITERATURE CITED

ADLER, J., 1965 Chemotaxis in *Escherichia coli*. Cold Spring Harbor Symp. Quant. Biol. **30:** 289–292.

ADLER, J., 1966 Chemotaxis in bacteria. Science **153:** 708–716.

ARMSTRONG, J. B. and J. ADLER, 1967 Genetics of motility in *Escherichia coli*: complementation of paralyzed mutants. Genetics **56:** 363–373.

ARMSTRONG, J. B., J. ADLER and M. M. DAHL, 1967 Nonchemotactic mutants of *Escherichia coli*. J. Bacteriol. **93:** 390–398.

BERG, H. B., 1975 Chemotaxis in bacteria. Annu. Rev. Biophys. Bioeng. **4:** 119–136.

MACNAB, R. M., 1987 Motility and chemotaxis. In: *Escherichia coli and Salmonella typhimurium: Cellular and Molecular Biology*, Edited by J. INGRAHAM, K. B. LOW, B. MAGASANIK, H. E. UMBARGER and F. C. NEIDHARDT. American Society for Microbiology, Washington, D.C.

PARKINSON, J. S., 1981 Genetics of bacterial chemotaxis. Symp. Soc. Gen. Microbiol. **31:** 265–290.

Gene Recombination and Linked Segregations in *Escherichia coli*

Joshua Lederberg

The Rockefeller University, New York, New York 10021–6399

A N article with this title was published in GENETICS just 40 years ago[1] (LEDERBERG 1947), following soon after the first discovery of recombination in *Escherichia coli* strain K-12 (LEDERBERG and TATUM 1946). Its appearance coincided with my arrival at the University of Wisconsin to become an assistant professor of genetics. The work had been completed in E. L. TATUM's laboratory at Yale University between March 1946 and June 1947. I then spent the summer at the Marine Biological Laboratory at Woods Hole writing my Ph.D. dissertation and the 1947 article[2] (which was its most important chapter). These studies had begun at Columbia University (in the Zoology Department!) in FRANCIS J. RYAN's laboratory in July of 1945. Although his name does not appear in the authorship, I had benefited enormously from his tutelage, encouragement and discipline. Homage to Francis has been expressed more fully in my own reminiscences (LEDERBERG 1986, 1987) and by others as well (MOORE 1964; RAVIN 1976). I was equally fortunate to have had TATUM take me in his laboratory and share the then hard-won auxotrophic mutants of *E. coli* K-12 that greatly facilitated the experiments (LEDERBERG 1977, 1988).

Our first presentation about crossing in K-12 had been to the Symposium on Heredity and Variation in Microorganisms at Cold Spring Harbor in July, 1946. Although it elicited many critical questions, I was most fortunate to have had such an extraordinary forum in which to respond to them. With the notable intransigence of MAX DELBRÜCK aside, I encountered little further entrenched skepticism about the result, except from some few who had not participated in that debate. What could be reported that July included:

1. The production of prototrophic recombinants from the admixture of various auxotrophs. Stringent selection allowed the detection of as few as one per million recombinants and these occurred even from parents doubly marked to forfend occasional spontaneous one-locus reversions.

2. The segregation among selected recombinants of unselected markers, including auxotrophy (*e.g.*, proline-less in proline-supplemented medium) and resistance to phage T1.

The fact that T1 resistance segregated among prototrophs was an important datum, for it seemed to rule out additive cell-mixture or nuclear-mixture (heterokaryosis) as an artefact. If the prototrophic isolate was pure and stably sensitive, it could hardly contain resistant cells. If it were a heterokaryon, it might be either sensitive or resistant (in fact sensitivity is dominant), but one would not expect a sharp segregation into two stable categories of prototrophs, pure sensitive and pure resistant. However, not everyone at Cold Spring Harbor was so persuaded by these genetic arguments, and I was compelled to promise to do explicit single-cell isolations. MAX ZELLE helped me to learn that technique, and it was to do good service in later studies (ZELLE and LEDERBERG 1951; LEDERBERG 1956, 1957; NOSSAL and LEDERBERG 1958).

So many new questions were now opened up by these thrilling observations! How to react? For one thing, I had to seek another year's leave from medical school; who in his right mind would leave the problem at that stage? The entire project had been motivated by AVERY, MACLEOD and McCARTY's discovery (1944) of DNA as the transforming principle in the pneumococcus. This could not be assimilated as the chemistry of the gene without a broader base of genetics in bacteria. We were disappointed, however, not to find a way to use DNA directly in *E. coli* genetics. (It took some years before a witch's brew was concocted to condition the cells.) Deoxyribonuclease did not influence the K-12 crosses, arguing for some direct cell-to-cell interaction—perhaps like conjugation in ciliates, so brilliantly investigated by T. M. SONNEBORN (1947; *cf.* WENRICH 1954). But it was hard to design direct approaches to the physical mech-

---

[1] It will be awkward to cite original sources at every point of historical attribution: see especially LEDERBERG (1987), BACHMANN (1983), IPPEN-IHLER and MINKLEY (1986), and JACOB and WOLLMAN (1961) for comprehensive reviews. An important overview of *E. coli* and *Salmonella* genetics has just been announced (NEIDHARDT 1987).

[2] It is time to correct a typographical error in my 1947 paper: N. T. J. BAILEY has pointed out to me that "203" on the first line of Table 5 should be "303."

anism of crossing when it remained such a rare, sporadic phenomenon. Even with hyperfertile strains, this remains something of a difficulty today, compared to the massive synchronization that facilitates kinetic studies of viral infection.

The main issues that could be addressed at that point, and which would contribute to the "Mendelization" of bacteria, were:

1. What is the range of markers that participate in crossing? and

2. Are they organized in linkage groups or chromosomes?

The work of 1946–1947 was then devoted to accumulating a wider panoply of markers and to improving the methods for handling them. Besides the auxotrophs and virus resistance, sugar fermentation mutants were particularly attractive: they could be acquired by visual inspection of the colonies on indicator media (such as eosin-methylene blue agar), and similar methods could be used to score the segregants in numbers. The relevant enzymes, especially the disaccharases, would also be most readily amenable to further studies. [The β-D-galactosidase of E. coli K-12 (LEDERBERG 1950) has certainly made its contributions to our understanding of gene action!]

Table 1 of the 1947 paper lists eight markers, in addition to another eight auxotrophies used for recombinant selection. The former all segregated, and recombined in every imaginable fashion, but not at random. The statistics of co-segregation implied a single linkage group, and permitted the figuring of the first map, substantially consistent with today's very nearly complete mappings of over a thousand markers (BACHMANN 1983) and the expectation that E. coli K-12 will have its DNA completely sequenced (about 5 megabase pairs) within this decade. Reverse crosses were used to show that the segregation ratios were intrinsic to the locus rather than to the physiology of the allele. Four-strand crossing-over was also looked for as prototroph colonies containing two clones of different crossover classes. These were rare, partly because of the stringencies of selection. A later study on microscopically isolated zygotic pairs corroborated the loss of chromosome segments and gave evidence of recurrent cycles of recombination in the exconjugant clone (LEDERBERG 1957; ANDERSON and MAZÉ 1957). Needless to say, these efforts to graft the classical concepts of chromosomal behavior in meiosis onto recombination in bacteria have been overtaken by molecular genetic perspectives.

A great and continuing puzzle was the failure to find chromosomal aberrations even in heavily irradiated stocks, in contrast to the results typical of Drosophila and other eukaryotes. Yes, deletions (COOK and LEDERBERG 1962) and, of course, insertions are now well known, but inversions are rare indeed, apart from those involved in adaptive gene regulations (BORST and GREAVES 1987). I am not aware of any systematic study of the production of inversions in bacteria by physical or chemical mutagens. I had thought at the time that bacteria might lack explicit enzymatic machinery for heterologous translocational repairs of broken DNA. One also had to think of differences in chromosomal organization: there was no evidence of histones in bacteria. Later, the discovery of species-specific repeated-sequence DNA in eukaryotes opened the possibility that this might furnish homologous stretches for reunion modelled on crossing-over. (Repetitious DNA is far less abundant in bacteria.) I have looked in vain for published reports on the distribution of chromosome rearrangements in interspecific somatic cell hybrids that might test that hypothesis; it is, however, supported by the correlation of chromosome breakpoints in Drosophila rearrangements with repetitious DNA (LEE 1975; cf. DAVIS, SHEN and JUDD 1987). The matter was of some consequence in our efforts, starting in the late 1960s, to design ways of splicing foreign DNA into the bacterial genome (LEDERBERG 1969; CIFERRI, BARLATI and LEDERBERG 1970; SGARAMELLA 1972; EHRLICH, SGARAMELLA and LEDERBERG 1977; HARRIS-WARRICK and LEDERBERG 1978). To this day we rely mainly upon interaction of homologous sequences in designing for DNA integration. The relative paucity of inversions may also be a perspective of scale: there is little intergenic spacing in E. coli. Most pairs of breaks would do potentially lethal intragenic damage in two places (not to mention the problems of reversing the direction of transcription). SCHMIDT and ROTH (1983) have discussed these and other contingencies in connection with the rarity of inversions in Salmonella.

The overall maps of distantly related species, like Salmonella and E. coli, are remarkably well conserved despite their large divergence in DNA homology. It has then been proposed (RILEY and ANILIONIS 1978) that the large-scale organization of the map in bacteria may be functionally constrained, as it surely is in viruses.

Our original linear map started to fall apart when additional markers were recruited, especially xylose and maltose fermentation and streptomycin resistance. They just did not fit: in 1951, I published a map needing three branches (LEDERBERG et al. 1951). Despite my admonition at the symposium, and in the caption, that "This diagram is purely formal and does not imply a true branched chromosome," the model was taken as a concrete proposal rather than as a portent of problems. J. D. WATSON and W. HAYES (1953) thought that three chromosomes would suit better than a branched monstrosity. Fortunately, WOLLMAN and JACOB (1958; reviewed by JACOB and

WOLLMAN 1961) soon resolved these and other confusions with their kinetic studies of progressive chromosome transfer, sometimes interrupted in midpassage, and the now accepted circular map. In my 1947 paper, the selective markers had provided operational termini for the map, as noted in the discussion.

There are some points of tenderness here. Other data (on persistent heterozygotes with hemizygous reaches, NELSON and LEDERBERG 1954) implied that chromosome segments might be deleted from either parent. For some time (LEDERBERG 1955), I believed that this post-zygotic elimination (shades of SCIARA or the MARY LYON effect!) was an alternative to progressive transfer. That was plainly wrong-headed; but the data still pertain, although interruptable progressive transfer is clearly the first-order mechanism. Very probably, both processes operate: the issue has been virtually forgotten and has not been cogently addressed for almost 30 years. (I left K-12 behind when I moved from Wisconsin to Stanford in 1959, and there concentrated on DNA-amenable systems like *Bacillus subtilis*.)

It is many years since WOLLMAN and JACOB illuminated the kinetic mechanism of DNA transfer. We are approaching the completion of the *E. coli* map in a way that portends the sequencing of the human genome. *E. coli* today is perhaps exploited almost as much as its technological potential as for fundamental studies. Nevertheless, some elementary aspects remain unsettled, in particular the precise physical conduit of the DNA strand as it is progressively passed from one cell to the other, and what happens to it on its way to the formation of recombinants.

LITERATURE CITED

ANDERSON, T. F., and R. MAZÉ, 1957 Analyse de la descendance de zygotes formés par conjugaison chez *Escherichia coli* K 12. Ann. Inst. Pasteur **93**: 194–198.

AVERY, O. T., C. M. MacLEOD and M. McCARTY, 1944 Studies on the chemical nature of the substance inducing transformation of pneumococcal types. J. Exptl. Med. **79**: 137–158.

BACHMANN, B. J., 1983 Linkage map of *Escherichia coli* K-12, Edition 7. Microbiol. Rev. **47**: 180–230.

BORST, P., and D. R. GREAVES, 1987 Programmed gene rearrangements altering gene expression. Science **235**: 658–667.

CIFERRI, O., S. BARLATI and J. LEDERBERG, 1970 Uptake of synthetic polynucleotides by competent cells of *Bacillus subtilis*. J. Bacteriol. **104**: 684–688.

COOK, A., and J. LEDERBERG, 1962 Recombination studies of lactose nonfermenting mutants in *Escherichia coli* K-12. Genetics **47**: 1335–1353.

DAVIS, P. S., M. W. SHEN and B. H. JUDD, 1987 Asymmetrical pairings of transposons in and proximal to the white locus of *Drosophila* account for four classes of regularly occurring exchange products. Proc. Natl. Acad. Sci. USA **84**: 174–178.

EHRLICH, S. D., V. SGARAMELLA and J. LEDERBERG, 1977 T4

ligase joins flush-ended DNA duplexes generated by restriction endonucleases. pp. 261–268. In: *Nucleic Acid-Protein Recognition*, Edited by H. J. VOGEL. Academic Press, New York.

HARRIS-WARRICK, R. M., and J. LEDERBERG, 1978 Interspecies transformation in *Bacillus*: sequence heterology as the major barrier. J. Bacteriol. **133**: 1237–1245.

IPPEN-IHLER, K. A., and E. G. MINKLEY, 1986 The conjugation system of F, the fertility factor of *Escherichia coli*. Annu. Rev. Genet. **20**: 593–624.

JACOB, F., and E. L. WOLLMAN, 1961 *Sexuality and the Genetics of Bacteria*. Academic Press, New York.

LEDERBERG, J., 1947 Gene recombination and linked segregations in *Escherichia coli*. Genetics **32**: 505–525.

LEDERBERG, J., 1950 The *beta*-D-galactosidase of *Escherichia coli*, strain K-12. J. Bacteriol. **60**: 381–392.

LEDERBERG, J., 1955 Genetic recombination in bacteria. Science **122**: 920.

LEDERBERG, J., 1956 Linear inheritance in transductional clones. Genetics **41**: 845–871.

LEDERBERG, J., 1957 Sibling recombinants in zygote pedigrees of *Escherichia coli*. Proc. Natl. Acad. Sci. USA **43**: 1060–1065.

LEDERBERG, J., 1969 *Health in the World of Tomorrow*. PAHO/WHO Lectures on the Biomedical Sciences, 1968. Pan American Health Organization, Scientific Publication No. 175. Washington, D.C.

LEDERBERG, J., 1977 Edward Lawrie Tatum (1909–1975). Annu. Rev. Genet. **13**: 1–5.

LEDERBERG, J., 1986 Forty years of genetic recombination in bacteria. A fortieth anniversary reminiscence. Nature **324**: 627–628.

LEDERBERG, J., 1987 Genetic recombination in bacteria: a discovery account. Annu. Rev. Genet. **21**: 23–46.

LEDERBERG, J., 1988 Edward Lawrie Tatum. Biogr. Mem. Natl. Acad. Sci. USA. In press.

LEDERBERG, J., and E. L. TATUM, 1946 Novel genotypes in mixed cultures of biochemical mutants of bacteria. Cold Spring Harbor Symp. Quant. Biol. **11**: 113–114.

LEDERBERG, J., E. M. LEDERBERG, N. D. ZINDER and E. R. LIVELY, 1951 Recombination analysis of bacterial heredity. Cold Spring Harbor Symp. Quant. Biol. **16**: 413–443.

LEE, C. S., 1975 A possible role of repetitious DNA in recombinatory joining during chromosome rearrangement in *Drosophila melanogaster*. Genetics **79**: 467–470.

MOORE, J. A., 1964 Francis Joseph Ryan, 1916–1963. Genetics **50**: s15–s17.

NEIDHARDT, F. C. (Editor), 1987 *Escherichia coli and Salmonella typhimurium: Cellular and Molecular Biology*, Vols. 1–2. American Society for Microbiology, Washington, D.C.

NELSON, T. C., and J. LEDERBERG, 1954 Postzygotic elimination of genetic factors in *Escherichia coli*. Proc. Natl. Acad. Sci. USA **40**: 415–419.

NOSSAL, G. J. V., and J. LEDERBERG, 1958 Antibody production by single cells. Nature **181**: 1419–1420.

RAVIN, A. W., 1976 Francis Joseph Ryan (1916–1963). Genetics **84**: 1–25.

RILEY, M., and A. ANILIONIS, 1978 Evolution of the bacterial genome. Annu. Rev. Microbiol. **32**: 519–560.

SCHMIDT, M. B., and J. R. ROTH, 1983 Genetic methods for analysis and manipulation of inversion mutations in bacteria. Genetics **105**: 517–537.

SGARAMELLA, V., 1972 Enzymatic oligomerization of bacteriophage P22 DNA and of linear simian virus 40 DNA. Proc. Natl. Acad. Sci. USA **69**: 3389–3393.

SONNEBORN, T. M., 1947 Recent advances in the genetics of Paramecium and Euplotes. Adv. Genet. **1**: 263–358.

WATSON, J. D., and W. HAYES, 1953 Genetic exchange in *Escherichia coli* K12: evidence for three linkage groups. Proc. Natl. Acad. Sci. USA **39**: 416–426.

WENRICH, D. H. (Editor), 1954   *Sex in Microorganisms*. American Association for the Advancement of Science, Washington, D.C.

WOLLMAN, E. L., and F. JACOB, 1958   Sur les processus de conjugaison et de recombinaison chez E. coli. V. Le méchanisme du

transfert de matériel génétique. Ann. Inst. Pasteur **95**: 641–666.

ZELLE, M. R., and J. LEDERBERG, 1951   Single-cell isolations of diploid heterozygous *Escherichia coli*. J. Bacteriol. **61**: 351–355.

See also page 704 in Addenda et Corrigenda.

A Mouse Phoenix Rose from the Ashes

Elizabeth S. Russell

The Jackson Laboratory, Bar Harbor, Maine 04609

FORTY years ago, in October of 1947, the State of Maine experienced a short-term disaster which developed, at least for biomedical research and mammalian genetics, into a long-term benefit. To appreciate this situation, one must be aware of oddities of Maine weather, the status of biological research shortly after World War II, and the very special qualities of CLARENCE COOK LITTLE, mentioned in this column in January, 1987.

Down-easterners are fond of saying, "If you don't like Maine weather, wait a minute." Usually it does change frequently and usually there is plenty of rain and fog, but all of 1947 was dry, and in the fall the weather continued to be entirely too beautiful—nothing but glorious sunny days from late August until late October. Trees and bushes became dry tinder, and tiny brush smudges grew into raging forest fires. Most of the state was declared a disaster area, including Mt. Desert Island where both Acadia National Park and The Jackson Laboratory are located.

A brush fire started October 12 or 13 in a swamp about eight miles from the main Jackson Laboratory near Bar Harbor. I can remember seeing its small plume of smoke of October 14 while sitting in a staff meeting at nearby Hamilton Station, the newly acquired dog and rabbit branch of the Laboratory. We were told then that the fire was under control, but I also remember seeing this same fire, three days later, spreading to capture the crowns of successive pine trees, despite concerted fire-fighting efforts of local and imported fire engines. The tiny fire we had seen from the Hamilton Station continued to grow, fanned by strong winds, burning much of Acadia National Park and the middle of Mt. Desert Island. The fire extended to mountains east of the main laboratory, mercifully heading toward the sea.

On the afternoon of October 23, however, a sudden wind shift turned the flames directly back toward Bar Harbor and the Jackson Laboratory. The population of Bar Harbor was evacuated that evening in a car-convoy, driving 15 miles westward, often with burning trees on both sides of the road, to the only bridge connecting to the mainland. Next day we learned that most of the Jackson Laboratory was gutted, with roof, inner partitions, floors, and mouse boxes completely gone.

Would there ever again be a Jackson Laboratory? C. C. LITTLE never doubted. He called us together in Ellsworth, on the mainland not far from the Island, assured mouse box-changers that they still had jobs, and assigned responsibilities to staff and research assistants. When he viewed the ashes around the wreck of the old Lab, he said, "Now we can see the sea." He saw to it that money appeared to continue building the new animal wing. Our needs were dramatic, and inspired both publicity and very welcome assistance.

In 1947, the young, small but growing Jackson Laboratory was emerging from serious financial struggles. It had been founded in 1929 by LITTLE with a group of seven researchers who had worked in the mouse genetics laboratory which he had maintained in Ann Arbor while President of the University of Michigan (1925–1929). The beginning of the great depression was not an ideal time to establish what the concerned group of Detroit industrialists had intended to be a research institute supported entirely by private funds. When anticipated support failed to materialize, LITTLE persuaded his coworkers to "live sparsely" while pushing forward with research on genetics and cancer.

Despite its precarious situation, the early Laboratory was a happy place. Prexy, as LITTLE was called, appreciated and supported everyone's research efforts. Every month, staff, box-changers and their families loved to go to the All-Lab Party. The Laboratory managed to survive, and in 1933 the entire staff jointly published an important scientific contribution ("The existence of non-chromosomal influences on the incidence of mammary tumors in mice," Science **78**: 465–466). LITTLE devoted great efforts to seeking money for the Laboratory and to persuading the federal government and the public that support of research was a national responsibility. Providing genetically controlled mice, gleaned from each researcher's own colony to supply other institutions, became one of the Lab's means of support.

In 1947, the Jackson Laboratory was still a small place with 18 doctoral-level investigators plus a few research assistants and animal caretakers. College and pre-college students and visiting investigators came in the summer months. But the Laboratory showed potential for growth in the post-war expanding world of science. In the summer of 1947 foundations had been laid for a big new animal wing, with much of the construction supported by the new National Cancer Institute which LITTLE had helped found.

Living through the winter of 1947–1948 was quite an experience. Until the end of December we were all piled on top of one another in a hallway at the Hamilton Station. Most of the records, as well as the animals, were lost. I was very lucky because a fine assistant, KAY HAMILTON, had rescued an invaluable file of data on pigment granules. However, most of the others' research at that time involved waiting for cancers to appear. With treated and control mice destroyed, all experiments in progress had to be repeated from the very beginning. We also needed to build up animal resources to supply critical needs of researchers in other institutions. Where would the necessary mice come from?

Almost immediately after the fire, a very welcome pile of letters began to pour in. Investigators who had recently received pedigreed mice from the Jackson Laboratory, and geneticists who maintained inbred mouse colonies stemming from our stocks, wrote to offer "starts" of almost all the strains we had lost, plus some valuable new types. LITTLE assigned to me the exciting responsibility of accepting the most pertinent offers, and as quickly as possible we built up a common foundation colony from which both in-house individ-

ual research colonies and a separate animal resources colony were supplied on an equal basis. By spring of 1948, mice were moved into the new animal wing. Ground was also broken for a new research wing, with funding from the National Cancer Institute and the American Cancer Society. The Ladies Auxiliary of the Veterans of Foreign Wars provided us with a Summer Laboratory and living quarters for summer students. From that time on, the size and productivity of The Jackson Laboratory increased rapidly. During the next five years the research staff increased from 19 to 33, resulting in broader research programs and increased scientific publication. More and more mice were provided to outside investigators.

The 1947 fire came at a propitious time for the scientific community. Just as large numbers of researchers were coming to depend on animals from outside suppliers, disruption by the fire focused attention on the importance of selecting the right animals for a particular project. The Laboratory's losses in the fire, and rescue by gifts from other mouse geneticists, gave the staff a heightened sense of genetic responsibility. In addition to contributing through their own research, they now wanted to apply genetic know-how to guarantee ready availability and continuity of pertinent, genetically uniform, well-characterized mice for the growing biomedical research community. The Laboratory had added a new phase to its scientific mission.

Biomedical and genetic research are deeply indebted to the foresight of C. C. LITTLE in establishing inbred lines of mice. The Jackson Laboratory was both founded and rescued by his confidence, his personality, and his unfailing optimism.

November 1987

"In the Air"—Theodosius Dobzhansky's
Genetics and the Origin of Species

Jeffrey R. Powell

Department of Biology, Yale University, New Haven, Connecticut 06511

Theodosius Dobzhansky's *Genetics and the Origin of Species* was first published 50 years ago. Many, myself included, would argue that it is the most important and influential book on evolution of the twentieth century. Certainly, taken together with later editions as well as with *Genetics of the Evolutionary Process* (1970) (which was meant to be a fourth edition), the book has been the cornerstone of genetic studies of evolutionary change for much of the last 50 years. It is perhaps difficult for us today to understand why a book integrating Mendelian genetics and Darwinian evolution was so important—or, indeed, even necessary—some 37 years after the rediscovery of Mendel and 25 years after Morgan and his associates confirmed and so elegantly extended Mendelian principles. Perhaps equally difficult to appreciate is how this book continues to influence not only genetical studies of evolution but also such fields as systematics and paleontology.

To understand the book's initial impact, it is necessary to realize that in the 1930s it was far from established that Mendelian genetics could account for evolutionary changes observed in nature [see Mayr (1980) for thought-provoking documentation]. In particular, two factors delayed the synthesis (as it was to be called) between the Darwinian tradition and Mendelism. The first was misunderstanding, lack of communication and, at times, mistrust between geneticists and evolutionists (the latter group consisting primarily of systematists, natural historians and paleontologists). As Bateson stated in a famous lecture in 1922:

I am convinced that biology would greatly gain by some cooperation among workers in several branches. I had expected that genetics would provide at once common ground for the systematist and laboratory worker. This hope has been disappointed. Each still keeps apart. Systematic literature grows precisely as if the genetical discoveries had never been made and the geneticists more and more withdraw each into his special "claim"—a most lamentable result. Both are to blame.

A main issue of contention was the genetic basis for the origin of species, the phrase from both Dobzhansky's and Darwin's major contributions. It was clear enough that Mendelian rules of inheritance could predict patterns of inheritance of many traits within populations, but could Mendelian factors account for the origin of new species, genera, and all higher taxa? One problem before 1937 was that some geneticists who often wrote about evolution (deVries, Bateson and Goldschmidt) believed that new species (and all higher taxa) arose by some form of special "mutation" (macromutations, hopeful monsters, systemic mutations, etc.) which immediately established a recognizably discontinuous form of a new species. Yet the evolutionist studying nature saw a quite different pattern: there were subtle geographic differences blending into subspecific recognition followed by the gradual accumulation of sufficient distinctness to warrant the designation of a new species. This continuous, gradual formation of species was a far cry from the genetic explanation offered by deVries, Bateson and Goldschmidt. No wonder evolutionists doubted that the new Mendelian genetics was their key to the mechanism of evolution. This led evolutionists to consider other forms of inheritance, in particular what Mayr (1980) has termed "soft inheritance" theories including various forms of Lamarckism, Geoffroyism, and other environmentally induced adaptive changes. That this was still an issue is illustrated by the serious consideration given to the infamous case of Kammerer (1924).

A second cause of the schism between geneticists and evolutionists is illustrated by T. H. Morgan, the most influential geneticist of his time. Contrary to some population notions, Morgan had a keen interest in evolution and, in fact, wrote three books on the subject (1903, 1925, 1932). Why did Morgan fail to bridge the gap and set in motion the synthesis? His books reveal at least three reasons. First, he did not believe in species. He felt that species designations were arbitrary, the result of "a scholastic distinction that arose when species were regarded as specially created" (MORGAN 1932, p. 105). Second, MORGAN had an unorthodox view of natural selection [see WEINSTEIN (1980) for detailed discussion] and felt that it was not the primary force of change. He emphasized the role of mutation as the driving force of evolution—indeed, the creative force. After discussing his view of the importance of mutation, he states:

> This consideration shows that even without natural selection evolution might have taken place. What the theory does account for is the absence of many kinds of living things that could not survive . . . Natural selection may then be invoked to explain the absence of a vast array of forms that appeared, but this is saying no more than that most of them have not had a survival value. The argument shows that natural selection does not play the role of a creative principle in evolution (MORGAN 1932, p. 131).

Finally, MORGAN was one of the original staunch reductionists in approaching all biological problems. He believed that the key to understanding evolution was a more thorough knowledge of the physicochemical basis of heredity. Two examples will suffice. In discussing the origin of sterility of the mule, he points out that great strides have been made in discovering that the sterility is due to failure of proper synapsis of chromosomes. Then he states, "Until we learn more concerning the conditions that bring about the union of chromosomes, it may be unsafe to offer any explanation of the process" (MORGAN 1925, p. 50). In his 1932 book he devotes a whole chapter to "The Theory of Sexual Selection and Hormones." He makes a plea that the key to understanding sexual dimorphism is to learn more about ways in which hormones differentially affect development in the sexes. Nowhere in his writings on evolution is there a serious concern for populational phenomena. Evolutionists would be concerned with trying to understand what population histories might have caused the horse and donkey to possess different chromosomes. What interaction with the environment might have caused selection, drift, or whatever, to fix these differences? Such issues did not concern MORGAN. In this context it is interesting to see how MORGAN treated the emerging field of population genetics as exemplified by WRIGHT, FISHER and HALDANE. By 1932 he must certainly have been aware of their writings, yet none of their theoretical papers is referenced or discussed. (Curiously, none of MORGAN's books on evolution and genetics is cited by DOBZHANSKY despite the fact that MORGAN was the chairman of DOBZHANSKY's department!)

MORGAN was not alone among geneticists in not appreciating populational phenomena. MAYR (1980, p. 29) states: "GOLDSCHMIDT thought of the origin of new types in terms of proximate causation. In 1952 I asked GOLDSCHMIDT how the population in which a new hopeful monster occurred would react to it. He answered, after considerable pause, 'I have never thought of it that way.'"

Why, then, did DOBZHANSKY succeed in 1937 when his predecessors had failed to bridge the gap? The usual (e.g., GOULD 1982) and probably largely valid explanation is that he was trained in and understood genetics, systematics and natural history. This was due to his initial education in natural history and systematics in Russia followed by training in MORGAN's laboratory. Thus, he could appreciate as could few others the different approaches, concerns, and vocabularies of the two groups of biologists. (A. H. STURTEVANT was perhaps another who had the required breadth and background; however, he was not one to indulge in the necessarily speculative arguments which were needed. In England, J. HUXLEY had gone very far toward realizing the beginning of a synthesis, although his definitive treatise, *Evolution, The Modern Synthesis*, did not appear until 1943. However, in his Preface, HUXLEY states that "DOBZHANSKY's valuable and distinctive book did not appear until much of the present volume was in proof.") The highlights of DOBZHANSKY's 1937 book are, briefly:

- The various theories of "soft inheritance" were untenable, whereas the geneticists' insistence on the importance of spontaneous mutations as the source of variation was valid.
- While mutation was the source of variation, natural selection was the prime agent of adaptation. Thus, DOBZHANSKY reinstated the Darwinian tradition (as practiced by natural historians) as the central tenet in understanding the "creative" aspect of evolution.
- The integration of genetics with systematics and natural history could best be achieved by adopting a populational approach. The theoretical basis for this approach was being developed by WRIGHT, FISHER and HALDANE. WRIGHT's models in particular appealed to DOBZHANSKY because they emphasized population structure (size, fluctuations, geographic isolation, etc.) which students of natural populations saw as vital in understanding evolution.
- Species, as a stage in the evolutionary process, are real and are one of the crucial steps in all evolutionary change. The biological species concept was introduced and defended. The importance of isolating mechanisms was emphasized: with the establishment of genetic isolation (speciation), lineages are free to independently explore new adaptive peaks, *sensu* WRIGHT.
- For the first time it was emphasized that, in addition to being an adaptive process, evolutionary change leads to diversity (thus DOBZHANSKY's emphasis on the speciation process as a multiplication of life forms).
- The genetic basis for species differences and, by extension, the speciation process, is not qualitatively

different from intraspecific genetic variation.

Thus, in a sense, there was something for everyone. Concepts like soft inheritance and macromutations or hopeful monsters were discounted. The familiar Mendelian genes and chromosomes geneticists studied in the laboratory were more than trivial curiosities; they could account for larger biological phenomena. For the natural historian, the gradual changes observed in nature were shown to be perfectly compatible with Mendelian genetics, natural selection regained its central role as the agent of adaptive change, and populational concepts were brought to the forefront. For the systematist, the reality of species as natural units was defended and their importance as a crucial stage of evolutionary change was emphasized. Thus, systematics took on greater importance than the merely "pigeon-holing" role detractors had assigned to the field. To be sure, each group had to relinquish some cherished beliefs, but many were willing to, given the logic, internal consistency and supportive data that weave through the book.

It is often said that timing is important in presenting new ideas and 1937 seemed to be the right time for this first attempt to present the synthesis. "It was, so to speak, in the air" (DOBZHANSKY 1962). This is not to imply that the 1937 book was the final word, far from it. DOBZHANSKY himself stated in 1962: "As I look it (the First Edition) over now, I see quite a lot of things which are simply naive, and a lot of other things which are plain wrong." What it did supply was a common ground, a starting point for the next several decades of attempting to fully integrate genetics with evolution. Several seminal books were directly inspired by DOBZHANSKY's book: E. MAYR's *Systematics and the Origin of Species* (1942), G. G. SIMPSON's *Tempo and Mode in Evolution* (1944) and G. L. STEBBINS' *Variation and Evolution in Plants* (1950). These books and their successors greatly broadened the synthesis to include paleontology, systematics and botanical studies. Thus, the authors and work stimulated by *Genetics and the Origin of Species* have been at least as important as the book itself.

A second major impact of this book, especially in its later editions, was to establish the field of experimental population and evolutionary genetics. Largely through his own experimental work, DOBZHANSKY was able to show that many problems of evolution were amenable to experimental study. His earlier exposure to the Russian school of CHETVERIKOV, TIMOFEEF-RESSOVSKY, SEREBROVSKY, etc., who had begun programs in experimental evolutionary genetics, no doubt predisposed him to pursue such studies. (The rise of LYSENKO snuffed out this pioneering Russian research program; had it not, the history of evolutionary genetics would have been very different.) Probably the best illustration in the 1937 edition is

the study of the genetic basis of the sterility of F_1 males from crosses of *Drosophila pseudoobscura* and *D. persimilis* (then called Races A and B). Using mutant markers, he was able to demonstrate that the factors causing sterility resided on the chromosomes and that many factors spread over the genome were involved. This was clearly at odds with many theories of species differences. Perhaps more importantly, he showed that the degree of sterility varied with the geographic origin of the strains used in the crosses. A similar study by HOLLINGSHEAD (1930) demonstrated that geographic variation in the production of viable hybrids in the plant *Crepis* was due to a single Mendelian factor. These were crucial demonstrations that intraspecific variation existed for the very traits which define interspecific distinctions. This was the key in demonstrating the microevolution (intraspecific) and macroevolution (interspecific or higher taxonomic level) were qualitatively the same in the sense that they relied on the same genetic basis: Mendelian genes and chromosomal rearrangements.

A final observation worth considering, especially in light of contemporary ideas, is the role of random genetic drift in evolution. An insistence on the primacy of natural selection in adaptive evolution does not exclude a role for drift. Indeed, DOBZHANSKY was very much enamored of WRIGHT's views on the importance of random changes, especially for characters under weak or no selection. DOBZHANSKY began his study of the third-chromosome inversion polymorphism of *D. pseudoobscura* precisely because he wanted to test WRIGHT's theories. He thought the inversion polymorphism to be the ideal candidate for a neutral trait; no gene mutations were thought to be involved, only a rearrangement of existing genetic information. As the evidence became overwhelming that this polymorphism is under remarkably strong selection, DOBZHANSKY began to de-emphasize a role for drift in later editions. After all, if precisely the character one chooses to study as the ideal neutral trait turns out to be under strong selection, it is quite understandable that one would begin to doubt the importance of genetic drift. GOULD (1982) has called this the "hardening of the synthesis," by which he means the panselectionist attitudes so prevalent in the 1950s and 1960s.

With the introduction of molecular techniques to the study of natural genetic variation in the 1960s and 1970s, the attitude toward the importance of drift changed radically. With so much genetic variation at the nucleotide level, it seems virtually impossible that all such variation is subject to selection at all times. The theories of neutral molecular evolution, especially as developed by KIMURA and his associates, have been most influential. While DOBZHANSKY initially resisted, he eventually recognized the importance of these new developments. He told me in 1974, "I began as a drifter and then became a selectionist. Now, in my old age, I find myself becoming a drifter again."

Most evolutionary geneticists today have a healthy respect for the interaction of the various forces which can drive evolutionary change. The days of panselectionism, or pan anything, are over. The first edition of DOBZHANSKY's *Genetics and the Origin of Species* has, in this context, a curiously modern ring to it. It is still worth reading. It was crucial in helping to set into motion one of the great advances in biology as well as an agenda for research which continues today.

I thank H. CARSON, J. CROW, D. FUTUYMA, E. MAYR and W. PROVINE for comments on an earlier draft of this essay. Needless to state, not all of their advice was heeded.

LITERATURE CITED

BATESON, W., 1922 Evolutionary faith and modern doubts. Science **55:** 55–61.

DOBZHANSKY, TH., 1937 *Genetics and the Origin of Species.* Columbia University Press, New York. Second edition, 1941; third edition, 1951; first edition republished, 1982.

DOBZHANSKY, TH., 1962 The reminiscences of Theodosius Dobzhansky. Transcript of interview conducted by B. LAND for the Oral History Research Office of Columbia University, New York.

DOBZHANSKY, TH., 1970 *Genetics of the Evolutionary Process.* Columbia University Press, New York.

GOULD, S. J., 1982 Introduction. pp. xvii–xli. In: *Genetics and the Origin of Species* by TH. DOBZHANSKY. Columbia University Press, New York.

HOLLINGSHEAD, L., 1930 A lethal factor in Crepis effective only in interspecific hybrids. Genetics **15:** 114–140.

HUXLEY, J., 1943 *Evolution, The Modern Synthesis.* Harper & Brothers, New York.

KAMMERER, P., 1924 *The Inheritance of Acquired Characteristics.* Boni & Liveright, New York.

MAYR, E., 1942 *Systematics and the Origin of Species.* Columbia University Press, New York.

MAYR, E., 1980 Prologue: Some thoughts on the history of the evolutionary synthesis. pp. 1–48. In: *The Evolutionary Synthesis,* Edited by E. MAYR and W. PROVINE. Harvard University Press, Cambridge, Mass.

MORGAN, T. H., 1903 *Evolution and Adaptation.* Macmillan, New York.

MORGAN, T. H., 1925 *Evolution and Genetics.* Princeton University Press, Princeton, N. J.

MORGAN, T. H., 1932 *The Scientific Basis of Evolution.* W. W. Norton, New York.

SIMPSON, G. G., 1944 *Tempo and Mode in Evolution.* Columbia University Press, New York.

STEBBINS, G. L., 1950 *Variation and Evolution in Plants.* Columbia University Press, New York.

WEINSTEIN, A., 1980 Morgan and the theory of natural selection. pp. 432–445. In: *The Evolutionary Synthesis,* Edited by E. MAYR and W. PROVINE. Harvard University Press, Cambridge, Mass.

Quantitative Genetics in 1987

B. S. Weir

Department of Statistics, North Carolina State University, Raleigh, North Carolina 27695–8203

IN 1976, an International Conference on Quantitative Genetics was held at Iowa State University (POLLAK, KEMPTHORNE and BAILEY 1977). Although that Conference was regarded as being successful, it did have the nature of a review of the field and there was a feeling that quantitative genetics was not about to make great progress in the future. Of course, the whole field of genetics has changed greatly since 1976, and several developments in quantitative genetics suggested the need for the Second International Conference, held at North Carolina State University in 1987 (WEIR *et al.* 1987). The present vitality of the field was demonstrated by the attendance of over 500 quantitative geneticists from around the world.

Three major new directions were evident at the 1987 conference: quantitative geneticists are aware of the potential benefits and problems of introducing foreign genes into domestic species; the techniques of quantitative genetics are being applied to natural populations in order to address evolutionary questions; and human geneticists are tackling quantitative genetic problems of increasing complexity.

With much attention currently being focused on "biotechnology" (generally meaning the application of advances in molecular biology), it was interesting to hear the ways in which new technology may impact on quantitative genetics. Prior to these technologies, plant and animal breeding had achieved great gains in food and fiber production by identifying individuals with superior breeding values and using them as parents for the next generation, although M. BICHARD pointed out that even this basic procedure is still not used on much of the world's livestock.

Technological changes available to plant and animal breeders include those in statistics, such as mixed fixed and random effects models; in reproductive physiology, such as multiple ovulation and embryo transplants; and in molecular biology, such as the use of transgenes. In reviewing likely progress in animals, C. SMITH contrasted transgenes with large effects (on disease resistance, for example, or which restrict metabolic pathways or produce novel products) *vs.* those

which affect economic merit in conventional production systems. With present uncertainty over the locations or copy numbers of inserted elements, using the latter type of transgenes will require traditional quantitative genetic methods to identify and exploit unique superior transgenic genotypes. For crop plants, R. D. SHILLITO believes that initial gains will come from those inserted genes that reduce losses from weed competition or from predation rather than from increases in yield *per se*, and he is optimistic that genetic engineering will provide means to permanently alter the genetic makeup of these plants.

L. B. CRITTENDEN has been able to introduce mobile genetic elements into the chicken germ line with retroviruses, a process which may be as valuable for providing insertional mutagens for gene tagging at the molecular level as for providing vectors to insert specific genes. A similar idea has been pursued by T. F. C. MACKAY in suggesting that transposable element-induced mutations (from hybrid dysgenesis) in *Drosophila melanogaster* generate quantitative genetic variation. This renewed interest in the role of mutation in maintaining variation, which may play a role in the continued response found in long-term selection programs, suggested a cyclical trend to F. D. ENFIELD who was reminded of the focus on mutational breeding among plant breeders in the 1960s.

While molecular biology is causing changes in quantitative genetics, ecological biology is adding most notably to the ranks of quantitative geneticists. The number of contributed papers at the conference that concerned natural populations was only slightly fewer than the number concerned with each of the more conventional quantitative genetic areas of plant and animal breeding. R. LANDE remarked that most of the characters studied by evolutionary biologists are continuously varying or meristic traits that can be analyzed by quantitative genetic methods. He reviewed the growth in empirical studies on correlated characters in natural populations, particularly for life-history traits, and made the interesting claim that attempts to model the maintenance of genetic variation by mutation in natural populations has reawakened interest by more traditional quantitative geneticists in the role of mutation in artificial selection programs. Such interest was displayed in the theory presented by W. G. HILL.

M. TURELLI relaxed the assumption, of LANDE and others, of normality for the distribution of quantitative characters and S. KARLIN also discussed theory to accommodate non-Gaussian distributions. TURELLI's conclusion that quantitative variation in natural populations cannot all be explained by mutation-selection balance theories indicates that the debates among population geneticists a decade ago on the forces responsible for observed levels of protein polymorphisms have now shifted to the more complex polygenic situation.

Complexity is also a feature of quantitative genetic work on human traits. In a review of progress, R. C. ELSTON stated that most advances over the past decade have been in the development of increasingly sophisticated models to distinguish between genetic and familial or environmental effects. D. W. FULKER presented a path analysis of genetic and cultural contributions to personality development and L. ISELIUS evaluated the genetic epidemiology of several common diseases, including coronary heart disease. In discussing alcoholism, C. R. CLONINGER referred to the need for a developmental perspective, a theme elaborated in the theory described by L. J. EAVES.

With so much attention being paid recently to plans to sequence the human genome, it is obvious that human quantitative genetic studies stand to gain greatly from the increased availability of marker and sequence data. C. F. SING reported on work using restriction markers in a strategy that incorporates measures of allelic variability to determine the genetic architecture underlying phenotypic variability for complex diseases.

The above selection of speakers highlights activities in quantitative genetics that represent a departure from those discussed in the 1976 conference, but only hint at the whole spectrum of activities. New work was reported on selection strategies and accounting for inbreeding in domestic species. Theories were presented to accommodate genotype-environment in-

teraction, heterosis and epistasis. Applications of quantitative genetic techniques to species as diverse as Monterey pine and Atlantic salmon were described, as was work in countries as separated as Brazil and the People's Republic of China. Quantitative genetics as a field embraces a great diversity of disciplines and organisms but has as its unifying feature the study of traits controlled by many genes.

International conferences are as valuable for the personal contacts they foster as for the knowledge communicated, and participants at the 1987 conference were sorry that illness prevented O. KEMPTHORNE, the host of the 1976 conference, from attending. They were greatly saddened that J. L. JINKS, one of the leaders in the field and who had planned to present a paper, succumbed to cancer just a day after the conference concluded.

For us at North Carolina State University, as well as for many of his colleagues around the world, a highlight of the conference was the opportunity it allowed us to honor C. CLARK COCKERHAM for his many contributions to quantitative genetics. His work has been at the forefront since his classic partitioning of genetic variances in 1954 and his description of methods of estimating variance components, using the covariances among relatives, in 1963. As readers of this journal are aware, his contributions continue. It was my particular pleasure to chair a session of papers, by A. J. WRIGHT, T. MUKAI and P. E. SMOUSE, that described theory for selfing species of crop plants, experiments on *D. melanogaster*, and surveys of tribal human populations, respectively—all work that used methodology developed by COCKERHAM.

See also page 706 in Addenda et Corrigenda.

LITERATURE CITED

POLLAK, E., O. KEMPTHORNE and T. B. BAILEY, JR. (Editors), 1977 *Proceedings of the International Conference on Quantitative Genetics.* Iowa State University Press, Ames, Iowa.

WEIR, B. S., E. J. EISEN, M. M. GOODMAN and G. NAMKOONG (Editors), 1987 *Proceedings of the Second International Conference on Quantitative Genetics.* Sinauer Associates, Sunderland, Mass.

A Diamond Anniversary
The First Chromosome Map

James F. Crow

Genetics Department, University of Wisconsin–Madison, Madison, Wisconsin 53706

SEVENTY-FIVE years ago this month A. H. STUR-TEVANT (1913) published the first linkage map. It involved five X-chromosomal loci in *Drosophila ampelophila*, now called *Drosophila melanogaster*. This was early genetics at its most exquisite. From seemingly irrelevant counts of the number of different kinds of offspring from various matings, and with no idea of the nature of the genes, STURTEVANT could nevertheless infer their sequence and relative distances apart on the chromosome.

These quiet beginnings stand in abrupt contrast to the current hubbub over the human linkage map and the proper definition of a map (ROBERTS 1987). With its rival factions and the glare of publicity, the mapping race is almost a genetic Olympics. One other contrast: the 1913 Drosophila paper had one author, the 1987 paper on the human map has 33 (DONIS-KELLER *et al.* 1987).

STURTEVANT was still an undergraduate student at Columbia University when he had the key idea. In his words (1965):

In the latter part of 1911, in conversation with MORGAN . . ., I suddenly realized that the variations in strength of linkage, already attributed by MORGAN to differences in the spatial separation of the genes, offered the possibility of determining sequences in the linear dimension of a chromosome. I went home and spent most of the night (to the neglect of my undergraduate homework) in producing the first chromosome map.

The first publication in 1913 was a masterpiece of clarity. Here is a sample:

By determining the distances . . . between A and B and between B and C, one should be able to predict AC. For, if proportion of cross-overs really represents distance, AC must be, approximately, either AB plus BC or AB minus BC.

Figure 1 shows STURTEVANT's original map, together with the current distances as given by LINDSLEY and GRELL (1968). Considering the primitive laboratory conditions and large distances between markers, the agreement is remarkable. This pathbreaking paper and 32 more of STURTEVANT's most important contributions have been reprinted (STURTEVANT 1961).

STURTEVANT and C. B. BRIDGES were both students in MORGAN's course in elementary zoology at Columbia in 1909. They were both given places to work in the "fly room" and immediately became members of the research team. This room was only 16 by 23 feet and, somehow, eight desks were crowded into it. The room also included fly food preparation, with an always-present stalk of bananas. It soon became filled with additional geneticists, notably H. J. MULLER who joined the group in 1912. Included in this close-packed area was PHOEBE REED, who washed glassware, prepared media, and later became MRS. STURTEVANT.

Each of the researchers made important contributions, of both data and ideas, to the rapid mapping of the Drosophila genome. MULLER introduced the ideas of coincidence and interference. BRIDGES concerned himself with the technology, working out standardized culture conditions and mating systems designed to minimize viability complications. Curiously, the MORGAN school made no use of mathematical mapping functions, which would have been very useful in the early days when distances between known genes were large. Such functions were developed in England (HALDANE 1919) but did not make it across the Atlantic for many years.

The free exchange of data, the continuous discussion of each other's results and the scientific excellence of the group created a situation in which new results came at an enormous rate. Within a few years the rules of transmission genetics and the mechanical basis of sex-linked inheritance, crossing over, nondis-

b c		p r		m
0.0 1.0		30.7 33.7		57.6
0.0 1.5		33.0 36.1		54.5
y w		v m		r

FIGURE 1.—STURTEVANT's original linkage map of the Drosophila X chromosome, with his placements and the symbols used at the time (*upper*) compared to the current locations and symbols (*lower*). The loci are *yellow* body, *white* eyes, *vermilion* eyes, *miniature* wings and *rudimentary* wings.

junction and chromosome aberrations were worked out.

There was always complete openness, with no ideas or data held back. MULLER suggested measuring distance as percent recombinants; MORGAN first suggested that "crossover reducers" might be inversions, a point that was confirmed by STURTEVANT when he found that the gene order in *Drosophila simulans* differed from that in *D. melanogaster*. STURTEVANT suggested to MULLER that lethals might be an objective way to measure mutation rates. However, it is very difficult to trace the origins of many of the ideas, since all were discussed freely from the beginning.

STURTEVANT's work did not stop with chromosome mapping. He did a key early experiment in multigeneration selection. His finding that the *vermilion* eyecolor gene was nonautonomous in gynandromorphs paved the way for the studies by BEADLE and EPHRUSSI on Drosophila eye pigments. These in turn led to the Neurospora studies of BEADLE and TATUM and the beginnings of modern biochemical genetics. STURTEVANT's analysis of cell lineage by using mosaic flies was the direct antecedent of fate mapping as developed by GARCIA-BELLIDO and MERRIAM (1969); in fact, their analysis was based on 379 drawings that STURTEVANT had prepared from a high-nondisjunction strain of *D. simulans*. BENZER later used fatemapping to study neurological mutants. Recognizing the origins of the idea, he coined the term "sturt" to measure abstract embryological distances. STURTEVANT's discovery of the sex-transforming mutant *tra* is a forerunner of recent work by BAKER, CLINE and others on sex differentiation. He inspired a school of chromosome mechanics carried on by COOPER, NOVITSKI, LINDSLEY and SANDLER. In a totally different area, STURTEVANT was the first to measure the frequency of concealed lethals in natural populations and to note that their frequency was less than expected; he suggested what has turned out to be the correct mechanism, that "recessive" lethals are not completely recessive.

Although Drosophila was his major interest, STURTEVANT also studied the genetics of other organisms. He started out with an interest in horses and his first paper was on color inheritance in the American harness horse. He showed that the puzzling inheritance of the Himalayan coat color in rabbits could easily be explained by multiple alleles. He demonstrated that the strange inheritance of direction of coiling in snails fell into place when one assumed that the direction was determined by the genotype of the mother rather than of the individual itself. He had a long-time hobby of iris breeding and some of his products still adorn the Caltech campus.

STURTEVANT was also deeply interested in insect taxonomy and biogeography and he knew the native plants. He was an excellent taxonomist and wrote monographs and original descriptions of a number of insects. Of all the MORGAN group, he was the one with the greatest interest in *D. melanogaster* as an organism and in its relationship to other species. He was also interested in the history of genetics and his book on the subject has become a classic (STURTEVANT 1965).

No discussion of STURTEVANT is complete without a discussion of his contributions to others. He was most generous with his time and usually had useful, often key suggestions about experiments and their interpretation. He read widely, spending a regular part of each day in the library, and it showed. Until shortly before his death, he kept up with the evergrowing literature of genetics. This knowledge was of enormous value to his colleagues.

The relationship between STURTEVANT and DOBZHANSKY is a matter of endless fascination for historians of genetics. According to DOBZHANSKY, STURTEVANT was an early hero and saved his lifed by making it possible for DOBZHANSKY to stay in the United States rather than having to return to Russia where he was in dangerous disrepute. The two enjoyed an active collaboration and were pioneers in the genetic study of natural populations; their joint paper on inferrring phylogenetic relationships from overlapping inversions is a classic. Together they started *Drosophila pseudoobscura* on its way to fame. Then something went wrong. One possibility is that STURTEVANT, whose careful work was always absolutely reliable, became disillusioned with the work of DOBZHANSKY, who in his enthusiasm to get things done quickly was less careful. In any case, there was a schism and STURTEVANT, who had outlined a whole program of research in evolutionary genetics of *D. pseudoobscura* (PROVINE 1981), ceased to work on this species, leaving the field to be developed by DOBZHANSKY.

STURTEVANT was an interesting conversationalist and enjoyed telling stories from the early days of Drosophila genetics. He especially liked to relate the "omelet incident" in the fly lab at Columbia. He and his associates were playing bridge on a Saturday afternoon when a package arrived addressed to E. B. WILSON. They found that it contained an ostrich egg and, thinking that WILSON wanted the embryo, removed this and fixed it. Then, what to do with the rest of the egg? The obvious answer was to make an omelet, which they did; it provided an enjoyable meal. Soon after, WILSON appeared asking if he had received a package. It turned out that WILSON wanted not just the embryo, but the whole egg to use as an illustration of the largest single cell. He was not pleased. A possible rift between the MORGAN and WILSON groups at Columbia was averted by the timely intervention of an ostrich at the Bronx Zoo, which produced an egg at the opportune moment.

STURTEVANT enjoyed talking about his scientific friends. Knowing this, I once asked him if he could provide me with some anecdotes about my crusty and earthy major professor, J. T. PATTERSON, that could be used in dedicating the new Patterson Building at the University of Texas. He replied that he knew dozens of anecdotes by and about PATTERSON, none of which was suitable for such an occasion.

STURTEVANT did more than his share for GENETICS. In addition to serving on its Editorial Board, he reviewed many manuscripts and was especially valuable when decisions were difficult. On one occasion he was sent two manuscripts to review, one by a young cytogeneticist and one by DOBZHANSKY. His reply went somewhat as follows (I am quoting from memory): "The first paper is not quite up to GENETICS standards but is a good effort by a young investigator who should be encouraged. I say, reject with regrets. The DOBZHANSKY paper is not his best but I suppose has to be published. I say, accept with regrets."

I am indebted to E. B. LEWIS and DAN LINDSLEY for a number of useful suggestions.

LITERATURE CITED

DONIS-KELLER, H., P. GREEN, C. HELMS, *et al.*, 1987 A genetic linkage map of the human genome. Cell **51**: 319–337.

GARCIA-BELLIDO, A., and J. R. MERRIAM, 1969 Cell lineage of the imaginal disks in Drosophila gynandromorphs. J. Exptl. Zool. **170**: 61–75.

HALDANE, J. B. S., 1919 The combination of linkage values, and the calculation of distance between loci of linked factors. J. Genet. **8**: 299–309.

LINDSLEY, D. L., and E. H. GRELL, 1968 *Genetic Variations of Drosophila melanogaster.* Carnegie Inst. Wash. Publ. 527.

PROVINE, W. B., 1981 Origins of the Genetics of Natural Populations series. pp. 1–76. In: *Dobzhansky's Genetics of Natural Populations*, Edited by R. C. LEWONTIN, J. A. MOORE, W. B. PROVINE and B. WALLACE. Columbia University Press, New York.

ROBERTS, L., 1987 Flap arises over genetic map. Science **238**: 750–752.

STURTEVANT, A. H., 1913 The linear arrangement of six sex-linked factors in *Drosophila*, as shownl by their mode of association. J. Exptl. Zool. **14**: 43–59.

STURTEVANT, A. H., 1961 *Genetics and Evolution: Selected Papers of A. H. Sturtevant*, Edited by E. B. LEWIS. W. H. Freeman, New York.

STURTEVANT, A. H., 1965 *A History of Genetics.* Harper & Row, New York.

February 1988

∘ The Year of the Fly ∘

William F. Dove

McArdle Laboratory for Cancer Research, University of Wisconsin–Madison, Madison, Wisconsin 53706

BARELY three years have passed since the discovery of the near-perfect homeodomain identities between Drosophila developmental regulators and vertebrate proteins. These observations scattered clues that still guide searches for the developmental regulators of vertebrates (see HART *et al.*, this issue). We are accustomed to the nearly universal alphabet in molecular biology—the genetic code. Could it be that the sentences of metazoan development include some universal syllables (domains), or even complete words (genes) (see GOULD 1986)? On the Chinese New Year, February 17, we shall look back upon a year in which extended functional domains in developmental genes of Drosophila have been compared with regions within vetebrates genes that can mutate to participate in neoplastic transformation. Some of these relationships extend over entire genes, warranting a literal use of the Greek word *homolog*.

The identities between these Drosophila and vertebrate amino acid sequences range from 47 to 75%, less complete than those of the homeodomains which range from 90 to 95%. In the 469-residue amino-subterminal segment of the Abelson proto-oncogene protein and its Drosophila cognate, the 75% identity and 85% similarity in amino acid sequence clearly reflect common descent of the regions. Furthermore, these genes are functionally related, as judged by autophosphorylation of tyrosine in both products (HENKEMEYER *et al.* 1988). The Drosophila locus is now known to have multiple developmental functions (HENKEMEYER *et al.* 1987). But its strict relationship to the c-*Abl* vertebrate proto-oncogene does not cover the entire gene sequence: the carboxy-terminal segments of the mammalian and the Drosophila proteins differ by 244 residues in size and resemble one another only in being proline-rich.

A relationship spanning an entire gene has been found between the *wingless* homeotic gene of Drosophila and the integration region *int-1* that is activated by the murine mammary tumor virus in mammary carcinomas (RIJSEWIJK *et al.* 1987). The relationship includes nucleic acid cross-hybridization, extended amino acid sequence similarity (54%), and conservation of 23 out of 25 cysteine sites. The biochemical function is not yet known, so that this final proof of homology is not yet available. However, the *int-1* products are glycoproteins that may be secreted (PAPKOFF, BROWN and VARMUS 1987) and the *wingless* gene has nonautonomous action in Drosophila development (see BENDER and PEIFER 1987).

Numerous segmental sequence relationships between expressed developmental genes of Drosophila and transforming oncogenes of vertebrates join the 1987 list. The amino-terminal third of the inferred protein product of the *Dorsal* maternal-effect locus is 47% identical and 80% similar to a segment lying at a similar position in the v-*rel* oncogene carried by the avian reticuloendotheliosis virus (STEWARD 1987). Again, the functions of these proteins are not yet known. The carboxy-terminal quarter of the 220-kD product of the *sevenless* gene of Drosophila is similar (and identical in 56 out of the 65 residues) to the tyrosine kinase domain of the 43-kD cellular proto-oncogene product related to the *Ros* oncogene of the avian UR2 retrovirus (HAFEN *et al.* 1987).

Comparisons of genes involved in neoplasia between Drosophila and vertebrates are becoming two-way. The Drosophila genome includes perhaps 25 loci that can mutate to recessive alleles generating embryonic hyperplasias (GATEFF 1982). In at least some of these cases, when affected homozygous mutant tissue is transplanted to the abdomen of adults, it proliferates autonomously, is invasive, and is lethal to the host. Interestingly, the aberrant growth of such Drosophila neoplasms is corrected if the host is carried through metamorphosis. The Drosophila cDNA sequence for one such locus, *lethal(2)-giant-larvae*, has been determined by both SCHMIDT and his collaborators in Freiburg and MECHLER and his collaborators in Mainz (LÜTZELSCHWAB *et al.* 1987; JACOB *et al.* 1987). The former group has found scattered amino acid sequence resemblances among three entities: the inferred *l(2)gl* product, cell adhesion proteins of the chick, and contact site A protein of *Dictyostelium*. However, the latter group has shown that, when the gene *l(2)gl* product lacks most of the cognate "cell-adhesion" amino acid residues, it apparently retains full functionality in Drosophila development. Beware computers bearing gifts!

Can the fly talk with the mouse about neoplasia? Here we combine two earlier but still unanswered questions: are there syllables, or even complete words, used universally in the sentences of invertebrate and vertebrate developmental biology? And can an understanding of the normal functions of the cellular proto-oncogenes help to understand the functions of their aberrant derivatives, the transforming oncogenes, in the chaos of neoplasia?

Prima facie evidence that neoplasia in vertebrates involves a different set of genes than its analog in Drosophila comes from the observation that all known Drosophila mutations leading to transplantable proliferative states are recessive and none map to loci that hybridize to vertebrate oncogene sequences (GATEFF 1982). However, one might expect not to find germline mutations in the elements that can mutate to the dominant neoplasm-inducing alleles, because of dominant lethality (but see SINN *et al.* 1987). The question of relatedness between vertebrate and Drosophila neoplasia then becomes: are the recessive Drosophila alleles counterparts to the vertebrate "recessive oncogenes" such as retinoblastoma and Wilms' tumor (CAVENEE, KOPUFOS and HANSEN 1986)? Although these human conditions are transmitted as highly penetrant dominant characters, their cellular action is recessive, through somatic loss of heterozygosity. The high penetrance implies that the somatic processes whereby heterozygosity is lost occur with high probability in each carrier of the recessive allele. For Drosophila, the probability of spontaneous hemizygosity or homozygosity for a recessive marker distalmost to the centromere on chromosome *1* is only 0.35 (GARCIA-BELLIDO 1972). Thus, it is possible that the set of recessive mutations predisposing Drosophila neoplasia includes lesions in genes homologous to the vertebrate retinoblastoma/Wilms' family. Surely this will become known soon.

Inspection of the pathways to neoplasia in the fly and the mouse generates a reciprocal issue: is one underestimating the number of vertebrate developmental genes that act in the manner of the retinoblastoma/Wilms' family? In this case, recessive mutations in such vertebrate genes would be uncovered too efficiently or too early in development. Consequently, they would be removed from the population by the dominant-lethal filter. In transgenic mouse lines carrying normal or activated proto-oncogenes, tumor formation remains focal rather than systematic, even when two elements predisposing to neoplasia are brought into the same zygote (SINN *et al.* 1987). If the dominant somatic penetrance of a "recessive oncogene" is similarly incomplete, the mutant allele would be spared from the dominant-lethal filter.

This pair of considerations of the possible relationships between recessive neoplasm-inducing alleles and the dominant-lethal filter creates an experimental challenge shared by fly and mouse geneticists: to find conditions of background genotype or environment that increase or decrease the dominant somatic penetrance of recessive neoplasm-inducing alleles. These conditions might involve factors that affect the fidelity of mitotic segregation.

The prospects of a fuller biological conversation about neoplasia between the fly and the mouse are compromised by two experimental limitations: the genetics of vertebrates and their cultured somatic cells does not permit facile isolation of recessive loss-of-function alleles, and limitations in the ability to culture cells from Drosophila restrict assays for neoplastic transformation in this material. If there is to be an extended hybrid conversation, we wonder which Isadora Duncan—G. B. Shaw hybrid it will resemble.

On the side of Drosophila genetics, there may be the opportunity to identify by selectional genetics those loci whose products lie in the regulatory pathways in which activated proto-oncogenes work. On the side of the genetics of mammals and their somatic cells, improvements in chemical mutagenesis of the germline (BODE *et al.* this issue; SHEDLOVSKY, KING and DOVE 1988) and in the efficiency of gene-targeting through homologous integration of transforming DNA (THOMAS and CAPECCHI 1987; DOETSCHMAN *et al.* 1987) may create the opportunity to generate null alleles of the mouse counterparts to the control loci that are discovered in Drosophila by its selectional genetics. Thus, an extended genetical dialog can be envisaged in which concrete molecular entities identified in Drosophila can be investigated in vertebrate biology by gene-targeting in the mouse or its somatic cell lines.

Dramatic technical advances have combined with the long-term scientific capital of Drosophila and mouse biology to create a great deal of momentum for this exchange on neoplasia. We can expect at least metaphorical substance, even if not literal content from these investigations. To paraphrase Adlai Stevenson, "Metaphor is all right, if you don't inhale." The next year on the Chinese calendar is The Year of the Dragon.

LITERATURE CITED

BENDER, W., and M. PEIFER, 1987 Oncogenes take wing. Cell **50:** 519–520.

BODE, V. C., J. D. McDONALD, J.-L. GUENET and D. SIMON, 1988 *hph-1:* A mouse mutant with hereditary hyperphenyl-alaninemia induced by ethylnitrosourea mutagenesis. Genetics **118:** 299–305.

CAVENEE, W. K., A. KOUFOS and M. F. HANSEN, 1986 Recessive mutant genes predisposing to human cancer. Mutat. Res. **168:** 3–14.

DOETSCHMAN, T., R. G. GREGG, N. MAEDA, M. L. HOOPER, D. W. MELTON, S. THOMPSON and O. SMITHIES, 1987 Targeted correction of a mutant HPRT gene in mouse embryonic stem cells. Nature **330:** 576–578.

GARCIA-BELLIDO, A., 1972 Some parameters of mitotic recombination in *Drosophila melanogaster.* Mol. Gen. Genet. **115:** 54–72.

GATEFF, E., 1982 Cancer, genes, and development: the Drosophila case. Adv. Cancer Res. **37:** 33–74.

GOULD, S. J., 1986 Geoffroy and the homeobox. pp. 205–218. In: *Progress in Developmental Biology, Part A,* Edited by H. C. SLAVKIN. Alan R. Liss, New York.

HAFEN, E., K. BASLER, J.-E. EDSTROEM and G. M. RUBIN, 1987 *Sevenless,* a cell-specific homeotic gene of Drosophila, encodes a putative transmembrane receptor with a tyrosine kinase domain. Science **236:** 55–63.

HART, C. P., D. K. DALTON, L. NICHOLS, L. HUNIHAN, T. H. RODERICK, S. H. LANGLEY, B. A. TAYLOR and F. H. RUDDLE, 1988 The *Hox-2* homeo box gene complex on mouse chromosome *11* is closely linked to *Re.* Genetics **118:** 319–327.

HENKEMEYER, M. J., F. B. GERTLER, W. GOODMAN and F. M. HOFFMANN, 1987 The Drosophila Abelson proto-oncogene homolog: identification of mutant alleles that have pleiotropic effects late in development. Cell **51:** 821–828.

HENKEMEYER, M. J., R. L. BENNETT, F. B. GERTLER and F. M. HOFFMANN, 1988 DNA sequence, structure, and tyrosine kinase activity of the Drosophila Abelson proto-oncogene homolog. Mol. Cell. Biol. **8:** In press.

JACOB, L., M. OPPER, B. METZROTH, B. PHANNAVONG and B. M. MECHLER, 1987 Structure of the *l(2)gl* gene of Drosophila and delimitation of its tumor suppressor domain. Cell **50:** 215–225.

LÜTZELSCHWAB, R., C. KLÄMBT, R. ROSSA and O. SCHMIDT, 1987 A protein product of the Drosophila recessive tumor gene, *l(2)gl,* potentially has cell adhesion properties. EMBO J. **6:** 1791–1797.

PAPKOFF J., A. M. C. BROWN and H. E. VARMUS, 1987 The *int*-1 proto-oncogene products are glycoproteins that appear to enter the secretory pathway. Mol. Cell. Biol. **7:** 3978–3984.

RIJSEWIJK, F., M. SCHUERMANN, E. WAGENAAR, P. PARREN, D. WEIGEL and R. NUSSE, 1987 The Drosophila homolog of the mouse mammary oncogene *int*-1 is identical to the segment polarity gene *wingless.* Cell **50:** 649–657.

SHEDLOVSKY, A., T. R. KING and W. F. DOVE, 1988 Saturation germline mutagenesis of the murine *t*-region, including a lethal allele at the quaking locus. Proc. Natl. Acad. Sci. USA **85:** 180–184.

SINN, E., W. MULLER, P. PATTENGALE, I. TEPLER, R. WALLACE and P. LEDER, 1987 Coexpression of MMTV/v-Ha-*ras* and MMTV/c-*myc* genes in transgenic mice: synergistic action of oncogenes in vivo. Cell **49:** 465–475.

STEWARD, R., 1987 *Dorsal,* an embryonic polarity gene in Drosophila, is homologous to the vertebrate proto-oncogene, c-*rel.* Science **238:** 692–694.

THOMAS, K. R., and M. R. CAPECCHI, 1987 Site-directed mutagenesis by gene targeting in mouse embryo-derived stem cells. Cell **51:** 503–512.

The Ultraselfish Gene

James F. Crow

Genetics Department, University of Wisconsin–Madison, Madison, Wisconsin 53706

I N 1957 L. SANDLER and E. NOVITSKI published an article entitled "Meiotic drive as an evolutionary force" in which they wrote:

As the study of the genetics of higher organisms becomes more precise and extensive, an increasing number of cases is found in which heterozygotes of certain constitutions fail to produce the two kinds of gametes with equal frequency. Such a pattern of behavior will drastically alter frequencies of alleles in a population; where such a force, potentially capable of altering gene frequencies, is a consequence of the mechanics of the meiotic divisions, we suggest that the name *meiotic drive* be applied.

They called attention to the excess of daughters produced by "sex ratio" males of *Drosophila pseudoobscura,* preferential segregation of knobbed chromosomes in maize (caused by neocentromeres, which are selectively included in the egg nucleus), nonrandom disjunction in heteromorphic chromosomes in female *Drosophila melanogaster,* and the excess of progeny carrying *t* alleles from male mice.

The meiotic drive paper appeared in the spring of 1957 at about the time SANDLER had obtained a fellowship to work at the University of Wisconsin. Coincidentally, and unknown to him, Y. HIRAIZUMI had just discovered a case of extreme meiotic drive in a natural population of *D. melanogaster.* The two of them made a superb team and in the next few years they worked out the basic phenomenology of *Segregation distortion* (*SD*), as they named it.

In the intervening three decades a great deal more has been learned about meiotic-drive systems and, on January 6–8 of this year, a conference on this subject was held at the University of Hawaii. The organizers were T. LYTTLE, D. PERKINS and T. PROUT. The success of the conference can be attributed to its narrow focus on transmission-ratio distortion and to the knowledge and active interest of the roughly 50 attendees. To the regret of the participants, neither NOVITSKI nor SANDLER was able to attend. Both were sorely missed. Especially distressing to his many friends and admirers was the death of LARRY SANDLER only a few months earlier. He had been one of the original organizers of the Conference. Several of the

participants spoke of his scientific ingenuity, his depth and breadth of knowledge and his friendly guidance.

The subject matter was broader than originally encompassed by the term *meiotic drive.* The discussions included a plethora of mechanisms by which a genetic entity is able to increase in the population without regard to, or in spite of, its effect on the fitness of the host organism. Some of the examples were: B chromosomes in a large number of plants, gametocidal genes in cereals, Spore-killer in Neurospora, sex-ratio genes in mosquitos, sex-ratio factors in parasitic hymenoptera, preferential transmission of structurally abnormal chromosomes in *D. melanogaster,* and chromosome drive in *Lucilia cuprina.* The mechanisms are diverse but the common element is that, in each case, the driven entity is preferentially transmitted to the next generation. For example, some B chromosomes accomplish this by regular nondisjunction followed by nonrandom inclusion in the sperm nucleus destined to fuse with the egg nucleus. The systems range from preferential segregation in maize, which is meiotic drive by the strictest definition, to parasitic microorganisms. Ideas and data flowed freely during the conference. The origins of some are identified in parentheses below.

The past year has been one of great progress in the *SD* complex in *D. melanogaster* (B. GANETZKY). As shown in Figure 1, the system includes (besides numerous modifiers) *Segregation distorter* (*Sd*), Responder (*Rsp*) and *Enhancer* (*E*(*SD*), here designated

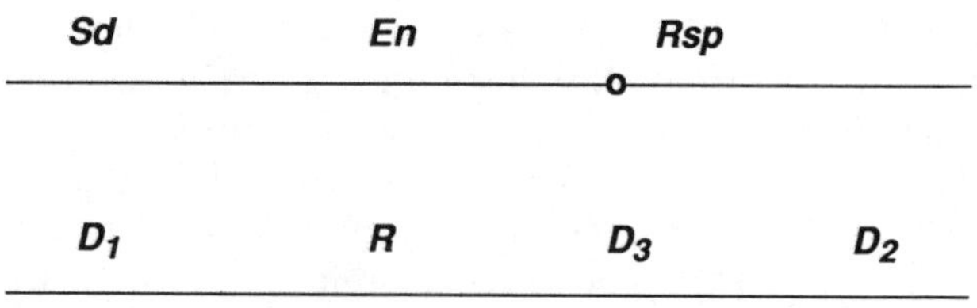

FIGURE 1.—Rough maps of the gene orders for the *SD* region in Drosophila (upper) and the *t* region in the mouse (lower). The symbols are: *Sd, Segregation distorter; En, Enhancer; o, centromere; Rsp, Responder; D₁, D₂, D₃, distorters; R, Responder.*

En). *Responder* may be sensitive (*Rsp^s*) or insensitive (*Rsp^i*). In the presence of *Sd*, sperms carrying *Rsp^s* fail to develop normally, leading to distorted transmission ratios. *En* is similar to *Sd*; each is independently capable of causing dysfunction of *Rsp^s* sperms but their effect is greater when they are combined (R. TEMIN). The driven chromosome found in natural populations is *Sd En Rsp^i*. Being insensitive, it has no dysfunctional effect on its own sperm, but in heterozygous males it is highly destructive to sperms carrying *Rsp^s*.

The *t* system in mice is quite similar, as can be seen in Figure 1 (M. LYON, D. BENNETT). The three distorter alleles, *D₁, D₂*, and *D₃*, are comparable to *Sd* and *En* in their cumulative effect. In the presence of one or more distorter alleles, sperms containing *R⁺* are dysfunctional while sperms carrying *R* are resistant. Thus, *R⁺* is comparable to *Rsp^s* and *R* to *Rsp^i*. In both systems the responder locus exists in various degrees of responsiveness. And, in both systems there are crossover-suppressing inversions. This hints that the special property of distorter genes in both mouse and Drosophila is not the specific nature of their product, but rather their tight linkage to a responder locus.

Both *Sd* and *Rsp* have been cloned. *Sd⁺* and *Sd* chromosomes have 7-kb and 12-kb *Eco*RI fragments, respectively, and detailed restriction mapping reveals that *Sd* carries a duplicated segment. There is a 4.2-kb *Sd*-specific transcript (P. POWERS). The structure of *Responder* turns out to be particularly suggestive. It was first shown to be divisible (T. LYTTLE), then multiple (S. PIMPINELLI), and finally to comprise repeated 120-bp units (C.-I. WU). The sensitivity increases with the number of repeats up to several hundred for "supersensitive" chromosomes. Although it does not reveal a specific mechanism of *Sd*-*Rsp* interaction, this molecular insight encourages the hope that such knowledge will be forthcoming. The underlying cause of sperm dysfunction remains obscure in both Drosophila and mouse.

The sex-determining systems of hymenoptera, where diploids are female and haploids male, are a particularly inviting target for entities that distort the sex ratio. A rather small sample from a wild population of the parasitic wasp, *Nasonia vitripennis* (familiar to genetic oldsters as *Mormoniella*), yielded no fewer than three different systems. In each case the intruding entity shifts the sex ratio in the direction that furthers its own perpetuation. "Son-killer" is a maternally transmitted bacterium that causes the unfertilized eggs not to hatch, thus producing all-female progeny. The maternally transmitted "Maternal sex ratio" (MSR) induces the inseminated female, which has control over whether or not eggs are fertilized, to fertilize all her eggs, producing only female offspring. MSR differs from Son-killer in that

there is no egg lethality. "Paternal sex ratio" (PSR) causes degeneration of the paternal chromosomes so that all the progeny are male. It had previously been thought that the causative agent was extrachromosomal. It turns out, however, that it is a supernumerary chromosome that destroys all paternally derived chromosomes except itself (J. WERREN). In this way the fratricidal chromosome perpetuates itself by causing the production of male offspring, which carry it to the next generation.

Meiotic drive leads to all sorts of interesting evolutionary questions. It is easily shown that PSR can increase only if the proportion of eggs fertilized is greater than ½; this happens when MSR is present. The *t* region in the mouse regularly carries a number of lethals, in contrast to a small number or none in *SD* chromosomes of Drosophila. There is an obvious advantage to the population in converting useless sterile males into embryonic lethals. But how can one explain this without committing the sin of invoking group selection? The clue may lie in mice being litter-bearing with possible reproductive compensation and having a demic population structure; these might favor some form of kin selection (B. CHARLESWORTH). Mice also seem to have behavioral modifications that weaken the *t*-locus drive system; females appear to prefer +/+ males (S. LENNINGTON). Could such kinds of behavior be found with other systems? Meiotic-drive systems are a fertile field for population genetics theory; many results are counter-intuitive to one used to thinking in Mendelian terms, especially in linked multilocus systems (M. FELDMAN). One particularly interesting result is that drive-reducing modifiers are more readily incorporated into the population when they are independent of the drive system. Thus, organisms having a large number of chromosomes with individually long linkage maps would be those most capable of tolerating drive systems. An autosomal drive system that is otherwise harmless, or nearly so, can be carried to fixation with little permanent harm. This is not true for a driven *Y* chromosome, which can only lead to extinction through an excess of males. Is hedging against such a disaster a reason for the genetic inertness of *Y* chromosomes (W. HAMILTON)?

A deletion of *Sd* behaves like *Sd⁺* and a deletion of *Rsp* is insensitive. Neither locus is required for normal development. Yet it seems likely that *Sd⁺* has some function; this notion is strengthened by finding the 7-kb restriction pattern in *D. simulans*. But such a function may have nothing to do with segregation distortion. Population studies of the *SD* system have been inhibited by the absence of an overt phenotype. The necessity for progeny testing has made experiments very labor-intensive. Recent molecular knowledge makes it possible to determine the genotypes of individual flies. It seems obvious that *Rsp^s* must have a selective advantage compared to Rsp^i; otherwise it would not be as common as it is in natural populations. Only with molecular methods has it been feasible to test this, and early studies with population cages seem to bear out the conjecture. In theory, the SD system produces the kind of cyclical trajectories of chromosome frequency change that have long fascinated population ecologists. But experimental tests of this depend on the kinds of precise measures of fitnesses of the different components that have only recently become feasible.

What is the conclusion from such a Conference? I think it is this: Mendelism is a magnificent invention for fairly testing genes in many combinations, like an elegant factorial experimental design. Yet it is vulnerable at many points and is in constant danger of subversion by cheaters that seem particularly adept at finding such points.

LITERATURE CITED

SANDLER, L., and E. NOVITSKI, 1957 Meiotic drive as an evolutionary force. Am. Nat. **41:** 105–110.

April 1988

Notes of a Bigamous Biologist

Gerald R. Fink

Whitehead Institute, Massachusetts Institute of Technology, Cambridge, Massachusetts 02139

GENETICISTS, like other biologists, have a passionate attraction to organisms but, unlike their colleagues, they are usually monogamous, wedded to one organism for much of their careers. This fidelity is not a manifestation of dreamy romanticism, but rather a consequence of the dedication required to create a standard organism suitable for genetic studies. The emphasis is on "create" because, contrary to the common perception, good genetic organisms are not found in nature; they are shaped by geneticists. There are, however, intrinsically bad genetic organisms, those that have long life cycles and are difficult to study in the laboratory (whales) or those with no sexual stage (Penicillium). Clearly, one must begin with an organism that is easily cultured in the laboratory and has a tractable sexual cycle. But all the rest is hard work. Mutant strains must be designed so that the biochemistry, physiology, and even the genotype can be manipulated at will. Once the organism has been redesigned so that crosses, complementation, recombination and transformation can be carried out with facility, the modified organism can be used by all biologists. Witness the use of bacteriophage lambda, *Escherichia coli*, yeast and Drosophila in genetic engineering experiments by evolutionists, biophysicists, crystallographers and embryologists. None of these standard organisms exists in nature; all have been painstakingly altered to perform the scientist's bidding.

The goal of this single-minded devotion is the creation of a standard organism that can be used to reveal themes fundamental to all organisms or groups of organisms. A great deal is known about all bacteria because of the millions of laboratory hours that have been invested in a single bacterium, *E. coli*. The encyclopedic knowledge about *E. coli*, its genetics and biochemistry make it an invaluable standard, akin to the meter stick, against which other procaryotes and even eucaryotes can be compared. A system of knowledge based on the *E. coli* standard in no way diminishes our interest in other microorganisms. In fact, it intensifies interest and increases the quality of questions that can be posed. The answer to the question, "Is this like *E. coli*?" has profound meaning because the quality and quantity of work on this model organism elevate the criteria for comparison. If the answer is "Yes," then the question has been answered to a first approximation. If the answer is "No," then a new phenomenon has been uncovered. So fruitful has been this approach that geneticists are reluctant to stray from their model systems no matter how alluring another organism seems.

In view of this commitment to sophisticated genetic systems, it is impressive that many *E. coli*, yeast and Drosophila geneticists are initiating studies on the cruciform plant *Arabidopsis thaliana*. The attraction of Arabidopsis is the pioneering of a new paradigm for plants. As has been pointed out in several excellent reviews (REDEI 1975; MEYEROWITZ and PRUITT 1985; ESTELLE and SOMERVILLE 1986), this flowering plant has many attributes that bode well for its use as an object of molecular-genetic research. It is easily cultivated, even in laboratories located in urban centers with erratic climatic conditions. Because of its small size and minimal nutritional requirements, it is possible to grow large numbers of plants in petri dishes or pots without recourse to greenhouse or field. When grown at room temperature and under constant illumination, a generation (seed → plant → seed) takes 5–6 weeks. The plants are self-fertilizing and extremely hardy, needing little tending to produce abundant seed (as many as 10^4/ plant). Mutations can be identified among the progeny of plants derived from seed mutagenized with EMS.

In the laboratory, Arabidopsis is compatible with any of the other standard genetic organisms. Its ease of cultivation and modest demands on space relieve the domestic tensions usually engendered by such bigamous relationships. Although the duration of the Arabidopsis life cycle seems at first interminable to the microbial geneticist, it becomes less of a psychological shock as one learns to initiate experiments in parallel rather than in series. Once this new rhythm has been acquired, the results arrive in the rapid succession to which microbial geneticists are accustomed.

Arabidopsis also has many biochemical features that facilitate the application of the powerful techniques of molecular genetics. It has a remarkably small genome (70,000 kb), only 15 times that of *E. coli*. The small genome coupled with the absence of substantial repeated DNA facilitates the cloning and mapping of genes. Several laboratories are mapping restriction polymorphisms and a high resolution RFLP map should be available soon. Of the handful of genes that have been cloned and sequenced, most are present in only one or two copies and either have but a few short introns or lack them completely. A seemingly trivial coincidence between the base composition of Arabidopsis DNA (41% G+C) and that of *Saccharomyces cerevisiae* provides a crucial route to the cloning of Arabidopsis genes. The identity in base composition between Saccharomyces and Arabidopsis means that the third-position codon biases (As and Ts) in Arabidopsis will be similar to those of Saccharomyces. Therefore, if there is extensive amino acid conservation between a Saccharomyces protein and an Arabidopsis protein, the Arabidopsis gene should have stretches of DNA sequences in common with the Saccharomyces gene. Indeed, several Arabidopsis genes have already been cloned by hybridization to a Saccharomyces gene. Vital information about the function of the newly cloned Arabidopsis gene can be inferred because the function of the cognate Saccharomyces gene is usually known.

Despite these attributes, many problems must be overcome before Arabidopsis can be considered a good genetic system. For one thing, there is a paucity of good genetic markers. Although many mutations have been isolated, few permit selection at the level of resolution required for reversion, recombination, and transformation experiments. This problem could be alleviated if auxotrophic mutations and the corresponding genes could be isolated. Second, there is no rapid method for constructing and maintaining the large numbers of heterozygotes required for the key genetic manipulations of complementation, recombination, and mutagenesis. Because Arabidopsis is naturally self-fertilizing, every outcross requires manual pollination, removing the anthers from one parent and subsequently dusting the stigma of that flower with mature anthers from the other parent. Moreover, the hybrid plant resulting from cross-fertilization will self, producing a genetically mixed population in the next generation. These difficulties could be resolved by constructing a set of strains containing balanced lethal chromosomes. Finally, the transformation system needs to be improved. A procedure for leaf-disc transformation with *Agrobacterium tumefaciens* has been worked out (LLOYD *et al.* 1986). However, transformation with Agrobacterium not only requires the regeneration of plants from transformed cells (a process that takes considerable time) but also occurs by nonhomologous integration events that preclude gene replacements. A more rapid transformation system that did not depend on Agrobacterium might uncover a route to homologous recombination. In the search for a strain that transforms well, many lines from different geographical locations have been introduced into the laboratory. It will be important to converge on one strain so that isogenicity can be maintained.

Progress in overcoming these problems should be rapid because Arabidopsis workers are enthusiastic and cooperative, freely exchanging strains, clones and information. The congenial atmosphere may be attributed to the character of the individual scientists as well as to the fact that, thus far, Arabidopsis has no known practical agricultural or medical value.

The day is not far off when scientists will say, "Is it like Arabidopsis?"

LITERATURE CITED

ESTELLE M. A., and C. R. SOMERVILLE, 1986 The mutants of *Arabidopsis*. Trends Genet. **2:** 89–93.

LLOYD, A. M., A. R. BARNASON, S. G. ROGERS, M. C. BYRNE, R. T. FRALEY and R. B. HORSCH, 1986 Transformation of *Arabidopsis thaliana* with *Agrobacterium tumifaciens*. Science **234:** 464–466.

MEYEROWITZ, E. M., and R. E. PRUITT, 1985 *Arabidopsis thaliana* and plant molecular genetics. Science **229:** 1214–1218.

REDEI, G. P., 1975 *Arabidopsis* as a genetic tool. Annu. Rev. Genet. **9:** 111–127.

May 1988

Cytogenetics and Karl Sax

Carl P. Swanson

Department of Botany, University of Massachusetts, Amherst, Massachusetts 01002

CYTOGENETICS is a science of correlations, of the presence and transmission of a predictable trait with the presence of a physical entity. It is but a matter of degree whether the physical unit is a cloned oncogene related to a particular malignancy, a single extra chromosome responsible for Down's syndrome or altered fruit morphology in the Jimsonweed, or elimination of male chromosomes determining maternal inheritance in the fungus gnat Sciara. All are comfortably embraced under the aegis of cytogenetics. However, the breadth of cytogenetics, the diversity of its test organisms and the vigor of its cutting edge sometimes promote easy fragmentation, sequestering one or another portion as a new discipline.

As a science, cytogenetics followed a typical path as it gained identity. The early papers were descriptive, their correlations couched in tentative terms and their conclusions cautious. Only later would cytogenetic presentations become more quantitative and more critically analytical. Scientists have been urged to be audacious in speculations but only when meticulous in observation and experiment. Meticulous, to be sure, but audacious hardly seems characteristic of cytogeneticists of my own and earlier generations. (There are, of course, exceptions: C. D. DARLINGTON leaps to mind.) But let me illustrate my points by discussing two papers by KARL SAX, a leading cytogeneticist of a past generation. They appeared 70 and 50 years ago in GENETICS.

SAX's 1918 paper was entitled "The behavior of the chromosomes in fertilization." SAX was a graduate student under E. M. EAST at the Bussey Institute at Harvard University. Obviously, the problems then addressed differed from those currently unresolved and may, from this distance in time, seem naive. But from a historical point of view, the paper is interesting because of the questions raised, the doubts expressed and the convictions enbraced. Cytogenetics can be assumed to have had its origins around 1902–1903, when the SUTTON-BOVERI chromosome theory of inheritance was enunciated. SUTTON had concluded that the meiotic segregation of chromosomes of the male insect Brachystola followed the segregation rules of the abstract factors of Mendelian inheritance, while BOVERI, through cleavage studies in Ascaris, had earlier demonstrated the influence of each chromosome on developmental processes. McCLUNG had also established that the X chromosome, previously of unknown significance, was concerned with sex determination (although sex had yet to be defined as a genetic trait). In the years immediately preceding SAX's paper, the linkage of genetic factors was established; STURTEVANT defined map distances by means of the three-point cross; BRIDGES, through his nondisjunction studies, provided proof of the chromosome theory of inheritance; ELEANOR CAROTHERS, examining the meiotic distribution of heteromorphic homologs in grasshoppers, provided a chromosomal basis for the independent assortment of factors; and the MORGAN school demonstrated that chromosomal rearrangements, gains and losses could be deduced by genetic means.

All these pieces of information were derived by examining animal species; however, a degree of confusion still reigned among plant cytogeneticists. There was a clear need to reliably describe events from meiosis through the first few zygotic divisions, to which end SAX chose the flowering plant Fritillaria with its large liliaceous chromosomes. Additional data were added from his studies of Triticum, but these would be more fully explored in his later classical papers on wheat hybrids.

Some of the confusion stemmed from the known process of double fertilization and its consequences, but more perplexing were the meaning and origin of the doubleness of chromosomes in meiotic and mitotic prophase, plus a report by HUTCHINSON claiming transverse segmentation of the chromosomes of *Abies balsamea*. These were related to the alternation of n and $2n$ chromosome numbers during gametogenesis and fertilization, and to the inheritance of genetic traits. After demonstrating by illustration and argument that doubleness in meiosis results from the pairing of homologs, and that separating homologs halves the number of chromosomes, SAX pointed out that doubleness in mitosis, followed by the longitudinal segregation of the halves, does not alter the number of chromosomes. He then disposed of the question of transverse segregation in the following manner: "If we assume that not only are the hereditary factors located in the chromosomes, but also in a definite linear arrangement in the chromosomes, it is evident that the chromosomes cannot divide longitudinally at one time and transversely at another time . . . without causing chaos in the distribution of hereditary factors." He then cautioned, "To be sure the latter theory"—the linear arrangement of a factors in the chromosomes—"is only a working hypothesis."

SAX also addressed the problem, stemming from a report by ATKINSON, of whether the segregation of factors in the first zygotic division was responsible for the appearance of unusual F_1 hybrid types. ATKINSON had proposed that "a shock (resulting) from the meeting of egg and sperm, particularly when there is genotypic difference between the two germ plasms" would lead to more than one hybrid type "due to interchange, crossing over, dominance, as well as blending, of factors in the zygote." SAX was apparently skeptical of such hypothetical explanations and offered pollen contamination as the most likely source of the aberrant hybrids.

A purely cytological problem surfaced in this paper: the nature of the spireme (a continuous thread comprising all the chromosomes of the genome), and when and how the individual chromosomes lost and regained their identity. SAX attempted to trace the course of a spireme through the prophase nucleus but could not do so, thus raising in his mind the question of its reality. But he was reluctant to discard the term and assumed that the many ends of chromosomes in early prophase were introduced by the microtome as he prepared his material. The smear technique had not yet been devised, so that doubts remained in his mind during his graduate student days.

In the 20 years between 1918 and 1938, SAX published extensively, with 13 papers in GENETICS alone. The projects he undertook were varied and included his studies of hybrid wheat, inheritance of agronomic factors in a number of crop plants, cytotaxonomic examination of plants in the Arnold Arboretum (of which he would eventually become director), translocations in *Rheo discolor*, and inversions in the mouton peony. But most important for this story was his collaboration with EDGAR ANDERSON, during which he was introduced to the cytological advantages of the microspore division of the genus *Tradescantia* as revealed by the acetocarmine smear

technique. *Tradescantia* would join *Drosophila* and *Zea* as a superb genus for experimental studies, and SAX's 1938 paper, "Chromosome aberrations induced by X-rays," represented a significant shift from the generally descriptive nature of his earlier studies to that of a quantitative and analytical character.

It is worthy of mention that Volume 23 of GENETICS (1938) was of more than passing interest. In the issue preceding that of SAX's paper were BARBARA MCCLINTOCK's study of the behavior of ring chromosomes in maize and their relation to phenotypic deficiencies, and MARCUS RHOADES' paper on the *Dt* gene and its effect on mutability of the *a* locus in another chromosome.

SAX, of course, was not a pioneer in opening up the field of radiation biology; he was preceded by a number of well known figures (To mention but a few whom he cited in his bibiliography: MULLER and STADLER, BAUER, KAUFMANN and DEMEREC, HUSKINS, CATCHESIDE, MATHER and MARSHAK.) What was significant, however, was his entry into an emerging field of experimental endeavor with an organism ideally suited for quantitative studies at a time when a host of questions were in need of answers. The data he provided dealt with the effect of dosage on the frequency of various kinds of aberrations, leading to the concept of "one-hit" and "two-hit" phenomena; the lack of a temperature effect on chromosome breakage, a position that he would later qualify as wider temperature ranges were explored; the differential sensitivity of chromosomes to breakage in meiotic and mitotic divisions, as well as during the stages of division; the lack of a differential effect of X-ray quality, another position that had to be modified as very soft and very hard X-rays (and γ-rays) were tested; the mechanism involved in generating translocations, rings and inversions, leading him to develop the "breakage-first" concept rather than support the idea of fusion followed by breakage; and the timing of chromosome doubling, also making clear the distinction between chromosome and chromatid aberrations. The problem of chromosome doubling was one SAX had explored in the 1918 paper, but with less success. The use of X-rays narrowed the timing of doubling a bit, but this was a problem that would not yield until radioactive tracers became available. Finally, relating his studies to the mutation data of MULLER and STADLER, he supported the idea, proposed by others, that most mutations induced by radiation were chromatin losses or rearrangements on a submicroscopic scale.

KARL SAX had an active group of graduate students around him at Harvard just before the start of World War II, most of us trained in some aspect of radiation biology at a time when atomic bombs and nuclear power were not household words. However, for reasons I do not know, none of us was associated with the Manhattan Project, although from 1947 onward, as the center of radiation biology shifted to the national laboratories of the Atomic Energy Commission, most of us spent varying lengths of time at Oak Ridge with ALEXANDER HOLLAENDER. As one who came under SAX's wing during the years 1937–1940, I can only say that it was an exciting and fruitful period to be doing research.

In the first paragraph I mentioned the fragmentation of a science and its acquisition of new names. This need not always be the case. Several years ago at a dinner, I sat next to another biologist much younger than I. By way of conversation he asked me what I was doing in the Department of Botany. When I indicated my continuing interest in cytogenetics, he remarked in a pleasant sort of way that he thought it was a dead subject that had outlived its intellectual usefulness. When I demurred that, on the contary, cytogenetics was still very active, that the new techniques of chromosome and gene manipulation had, in essence, created a species-wide gene pool whose potential for industrial, agricultural, and human use was only beginning to be explored, he replied, "But that's molecular biology." I prefer to regard it as a part of cytogenetics, an old science gaining a set of new and powerful tools. Whatever it is called, it builds on foundations laid by people like KARL SAX.

LITERATURE CITED

SAX, K., 1918   The behavior of the chromosomes in fertilization. Genetics 3: 309–327.

SAX, K., 1938   Chromosome aberrations induced by X-rays. Genetics 23: 494–516.

H. J. Muller, Communism, and the Cold War

Diane Paul

Department of Political Science, University of Massachusetts, Boston, Massachusetts 02125

THE OFFICE OF CENSORSHIP
THE CABLE AND RADIO CENSOR

IN REPLY REFER TO: MV/011/17516

67 BROAD STREET
NEW YORK 4 N.Y.

June 23, 1943

Mr. Henry Muller
Amherst College
Amherst, Massachusetts

Dear Mr. Muller:

It has come to our attention that you have recently received the following message from LANCELOT HOGBEN, BIRMINGHAM:

"ARISTALESS DEAD WANTS ARISTALESS AND ARISTAPEDIA BADLY LUV"

Will you please be so kind as to furnish this office with the complete explanation of the text, including the location, the full name and identity of the parties mentioned therein.

Please also briefly identify yourself and the sender.

Kindly direct your reply to the attention of the Service Division.

Very truly yours,

S. W. HUBBEL
By direction

THE wartime censor was not alone in suspecting the political sympathies of H. J. MULLER. MULLER's communist past worried many people, and as a result caused him no small amount of difficulty. But already by the time of the war, MULLER had discarded his communist views, a change of heart that was either not generally recognized or not appreciated.

Among the least forgiving was a host of university deans and trustees, an important factor in MULLER's long inability to find a permanent academic job. Notwithstanding a powerful patron in the Rockefeller Foundation, which offered to contribute to both his salary and research costs, few institutions were willing to take the risk. At the age of 53, MULLER had not held a regular position since leaving the University of Texas in 1932 at the age of 42; he thus had neither savings nor pension.

MULLER's difficulties trace back to various unhappy experiences at the University of Texas. In early 1932 he suffered a nervous breakdown, culminating in a nearly successful suicide attempt. Shortly thereafter he received a Guggenheim fellowship to work with N. W. TIMOFÉEFF-RESSOVSKY in Berlin. Just before he left Texas, the F.B.I. sent the university's president and all the members of its board of regents evidence purporting to prove that MULLER not only was "mixed up in Russian propaganda and was receiving money for this from Russian sources," but also that he was involved in the publication of a student communist newspaper (W. WEAVER, Diary excerpts, October 30, 1933 and March 2, 1936, Rockefeller Foundation Archives. R.G. 1.2. Series 249. Box 1. Folder 6; see also CARLSON 1981). At the time, Texas was not a very comfortable place for academics with liberal, much less communist, sympathies. WARREN WEAVER, director of the Rockefeller Foundation's Natural Sciences Division, described the atmosphere of the campus in 1933: "The still present Dean of the Engineering College called, a few years ago, a student meeting to give himself the opportunity to make a patriotic speech. He referred ... to the fact that a foreign government had tried to present a medal to his son ... and said that he would rather see his son 'dead and white and in his coffin than accept decorations from any other country.' He concluded his speech by opening wide his coat, revealing an American flag wrapped about his body" (Diary excerpt, October 30, 1933).

The following year, MULLER accepted an offer from NIKOLAI VAVILOV to work at the Institute of Genetics in Leningrad, in the process publicly confirming his communist sympathies. MULLER would ultimately clash with Soviet authorities—over both Lysenkoism and eugenics—and leave disillusioned in 1937 (CARLSON 1981). But the incidents at Texas, combined with his subsequent acceptance of a position in the USSR, damaged his chances of finding employment at home. MULLER would not find a permanent job (at Indiana University) until 1945, the year before he won the Nobel Prize.

Indiana's offer was also prompted by the Rockefeller Foundation, which followed up with an appropriation of $95,000 to the genetics group (which also included TRACY SONNEBORN and RALPH CLELAND) in the hope that "it would stabilize MULLER once and for all" (F. B. HANSON, Diary excerpt, January 28, 1946, Rockefeller Foundation Archives, 1. 200. 143. 1760). By the time MULLER left for Indiana, the Foundation's officers had been actively engaged for eight years in the effort to find him a permanent appointment. His positions at Edinburgh (following his departure from the USSR) and, following that, Amherst College were both supported by Rockefeller grants. But most places did not even want MULLER for free.

In 1939, MILISLAV DEMEREC told FRANK BLAIR HANSON (of the Rockefeller Foundation) that "it would be impossible to place M. in a State institution in this country and that most privately endowed institutions would also reject him. His long residence in Russia and his widely known book on Communism would militate against his acceptance here" (HANSON, Diary excerpt, September 25, 1939, 1.1. 405. 4. 45). The "widely known book on communism" was presumably *Out of the Night*, a eugenics manifesto with a distinctly socialist twist: MULLER envisioned a social revolution equalizing environments, after which differences among people could be presumed to be heritable and hence selectable. DEMEREC suggested placing MULLER at Cold Spring Harbor. This was attractive for another reason: MULLER could be his own boss and thus avoid conflict with others, as was assumed would occur in a university department. But, after a long period of negotiation, the deal fell through, in large part as a result of the Carnegie trustees' "fear of MULLER's past political background" (HANSON, Diary excerpt, January 8, 1942, 1.1. 200. 128. 1571). An attractive opportunity at Cornell was lost for similar reasons.

During the war, while at Amherst, MULLER did manage to get enough clearance to receive "consultant" status on CURT STERN's Manhattan District project on genetic effects of radiation at very low doses. As supplier of the stocks that STERN was using, MULLER had information crucial to the project. He coauthored none of the manuscripts that resulted from the work and were subsequently published. But he was rather proud of his involvement in such "secret and confidential" work. He feared that roles of an advisory nature might not often come his way as a result of his "having been abroad so long." His association with the Manhattan District provided legitimization in this regard (see, for example, the letter from MULLER to U. FANO, October 1, 1946, MULLER Papers).

Although MULLER could have advanced his cause by disavowing his communist past, he refused to do so. He considered it degrading. He also feared that, in light of the rise of LYSENKO, to do so might draw unnecessarily dangerous attention to his former Russian associates, especially VAVILOV (CARLSON 1981).

However, MULLER's problems were not simply political. While greatly admired as a scientist, he was not generally well liked. He was widely considered to be obsessed with questions of priority (see also CARLSON 1981), neurotic, and touchy in his personal relationships. His appointments at Edinburgh and Amherst began with high hopes and ended with fault-finding on both sides. Even those most concerned to help considered him "difficult." He also had a reputation as an overdemanding, uninspiring undergraduate teacher. The Rockefeller officers' diaries and reports include numerous references to the tangle of "personal and political deficiencies" that made it so difficult to find him a place, notwithstanding about a dozen possibilities over the years and the concerted efforts of many geneticists such as DEMEREC, L. C. DUNN, THEODOSIUS DOBZHANSKY, CURT STERN, RICHARD GOLDSCHMIDT, LEWIS STADLER, JULIAN HUXLEY and SEWALL WRIGHT.

In August of 1948, TROFIM D. LYSENKO finally succeeded in wresting control of Soviet biology. MULLER no longer had reason to keep political silence. He organized tirelessly to expose Lysenkoism. During the 1940s, MULLER's attitude toward the USSR (and not just LYSENKO) had hardened considerably. In the wake of LYSENKO's victory, he emerged as a fervent cold warrior; for example, testifying before the House Un-American Activities Committee, where he opposed having communists teach in most fields, including science (*Chicago Sunday Tribune*, March 15, 1953, Part 1, p. 18).

MULLER's anti-communism shows up most prominently in his assessment of the genetic risks associated with military uses of nuclear energy. It is certainly true that MULLER placed great emphasis on the long-term consequences of an increase in mutations resulting from exposure to fallout. But his concern about fallout, in and of itself, did not lead him to oppose nuclear weapons testing (see also CARLSON 1981). For some years after the war, MULLER's fear of the Soviets was stronger than his fear of the genetic consequences of weapons testing, even the consequences, genetic or otherwise, of nuclear war. By the mid-fifties, his position had become more moderate: he favored a bilateral ban on testing. Failing that, however, he considered the genetic consequences of continued nuclear weapons testing to be an affordable way of checking Soviet aggression [see, for example, MULLER (1955); see also his testimony before the Joint Committee on Atomic Energy (1957)]. The following passage from an address to the National Academy of Sciences typifies his views. He complained, "It is natural that those in opposition to us should be making every effort to have nuclear arms prohibited *selectively*. For that would change the military balance greatly in their (the Soviets') favor, in view of the fact that at present we are ahead in nuclear arms and they in conventional arms and armies . . . But for many of us who abhor totalitarianism, that form of slavery appears to be a condition as miserable and as hopeless, if grown worldwide, as the barbarism which total war might bring" (MULLER 1955, p. 212).

But not even such strong anticommunist pronouncements could dissuade some of those who had branded MULLER a communist. AEC Commissioner WILLARD LIBBY, who is reported to have played a major role in excluding MULLER from the International Conference on Peaceful Uses of Atomic Energy in Geneva in 1955, never trusted him (CARLSON 1981).

By the mid-fifties, MULLER was making himself heard in an advisory capacity at the most important forums on radiation and social policy: on committees of the National Academy of Sciences, the United Nations and the World Health Organization, and on the National Committee on Radiation Protection. By 1957 MULLER was politically legitimate enough to represent the community of geneticists (along with JAMES CROW, BENTLEY GLASS, WILLIAM L. RUSSELL and A. H. STURTEVANT) before a special session of the Congressional Joint Committee on Atomic Energy dedicated to "The Nature of Radioactive Fallout and Its Effects on Man" (Joint Committee on Atomic Energy, 1957). MULLER had an opportunity there to reiterate his cost-benefit analysis of nuclear weapons testing. When it came to his own experiences in the Soviet Union, members of Congress expressed an interest only in what MULLER knew about the state of Soviet genetics, wanting to know in particular what the Soviets thought about the genetic effects of fallout. MULLER was no longer a goat for "having been abroad so long"—rather, he was a resource. The hearing closed with a request that MULLER make available for the record the paper that was excluded by the AEC from the Geneva conference. That paper follows MULLER's testimony.

JOHN BEATTY has stubbornly refused to be listed as coauthor despite his extensive substantive and stylistic contributions. This work was supported in part by a grant from the Division of Research Programs of the National Endowment for the Humanities.

LITERATURE CITED

The letter from the Office of Censorship and the letter from MULLER to U. FANO are from MULLER's papers located in the Manuscripts Department of the Lilly Library, Indiana University, Bloomington. All other unpublished materials are from the Rockefeller Foundation Archives at the Rockefeller Archive Center, North Tarrytown, New York

CARLSON, E. A., 1981 *Genes, Radiation, and Society: The Life and Work of H. J. Muller.* Cornell University Press, Ithaca, N.Y.

Joint Committee on Atomic Energy, 1957 *The Nature of Radioactive Fallout and Its Effects on Man.* U.S. Government Printing Office, Washington, D.C.

MULLER, H. J., 1955 The genetic damage produced by radiation. Bull. At. Sci. **11:** 210–230.

See also page 706 in Addenda et Corrigenda.

Eighty Years Ago
The Beginnings of Population Genetics

James F. Crow

Genetics Department, University of Wisconsin–Madison, Madison, Wisconsin 53706

I suppose that every teacher of elementary genetics has at one time or another encountered the belief that in the absence of counteracting factors there should be three times as many dominant as recessive phenotypes in the population. It was this statement that induced G. H. HARDY in 1908 to write his famous paper. He started out somewhat apologetically, saying: "I am reluctant to intrude in a discussion concerning matters of which I have no expert knowledge, and I should have expected the very simple point which I wish to make to have been familiar to biologists."

The principle was independently published a few months earlier by WEINBERG (1908), but this paper remained unknown to most English-speaking geneticists, so for many years the principle was called HARDY's law. Since the 1940s, thanks to CURT STERN's (1943) setting the record straight, it is referred to as the HARDY-WEINBERG law. It is so self-evident that it hardly needed to be "discovered"; SEWALL WRIGHT, among others, used it before he had heard of either HARDY or WEINBERG. Yet, trivial as it appears, the H-W principle is the foundation for diploid population genetics.

The law can be stated in two ways. First, it says that if mating is at random in a large population and mutation, migration, and selection are absent, the genotype proportions do not change from generation to generation. This is almost a tautology: if nothing changes the frequencies, they won't change. But the principle does make clear that, with inbreeding or assortative mating, the genotype frequencies can change while the allele frequencies do not. Second, and much more usefully, the law permits the prediction of genotype frequencies from knowledge of gene frequencies. If alleles A and a are in the proportions p and q, the three zygotic types AA, Aa, and aa are in the proportions p^2, $2pq$, and q^2. Thus, equations can be written in terms of the more basic units of allele frequencies, and hypotheses about how phenotypes are inherited can be tested from population data.

Most natural populations show approximate agreement with HARDY-WEINBERG expectations. The main reason for this is that, unlike most equilibria, this one is attained within a single generation rather than asymptotically. Thus, there is no cumulative departure from H-W proportions; although allele frequencies may change cumulatively by random drift, each generation is close to H-W expectations for *its* allele frequencies. Furthermore, a single generation of random mating undoes all the effects of nonrandom mating that may have gone before. All this was clearly pointed out by HARDY in his two-page paper.

In his 1908 paper WEINBERG generalized the law to multiple alleles and in his 1909 paper he extended it to multiple loci. He realized that with more than one locus the equilibrium is not attained in a single generation as it is with one locus but is approached asymptotically at a rate determined by the amount of recombination. By this date the basic foundations of diploid, randomly mating populations had been established. The only problem was that WEINBERG's work was hardly noticed, mainly I suspect because most British and American geneticists were not fluent in German. WEINBERG suffered from a neglect similar to that of MENDEL.

The H-W principle has been most useful for studying inheritance in nonexperimental populations. It has been especially helpful in working out the mode of inheritance of common Mendelian traits, which do not lend themselves to pedigree studies. As far as I know, the earliest application of this law to elucidate the inheritance of a trait was WRIGHT's (1917) demonstration, from herdbook records, of the single-locus inheritance of red, roan, and white colors in Shorthorn cattle, now a standard textbook example. Another example is the human ABO blood groups. Although it was known from the turn of the century that these are inherited, the mode of inheritance was not known until BERNSTEIN (1924, 1925) applied gene frequency methods. Still another is FISHER's analysis of the Rh factors, summarized by him in 1947. Now, of course, these techniques are part of the standard equipment of human geneticists.

HARDY was a British mathematician, one of the greatest, and WEINBERG was a German physician. As far as I know, they never met, although WEINBERG did review HARDY's paper; he didn't think much of the derivation.

HARDY spent most of his life at Cambridge and, along with his friend J. E. LITTLEWOOD, formed the most productive mathematical partnership of all time. Some of their greatest work was in number theory and complex analysis, very deep and very creative work. HARDY was also the first to recognize the greatness of the self-taught Indian genius RAMANU-JAN; other mathematicians had failed to understand and appreciate him. RAMANUJAN's hundredth birth-day anniversary was recently celebrated. HARDY, a confirmed bachelor who lived for mathematics, cricket, and conversation, said that the discovery of RAMANUJAN was the one romantic event in his life. When he first saw the letter from RAMANUJAN con-taining several hand-scrawled theorems, he was as-tounded. "I had never seen anything in the least like them before. A single look at them is enough to show that they could only be written down by a mathe-matician of the highest class. They must be true because, if they were not true, no one would have had the imagination to invent them." RAMANUJAN's rapidly converging expression for π, which included a five-digit numerical constant, was recently used to compute the value to 17 million decimal places; only after this was a rigorous proof worked out. What concatenation of genes can produce such special genius?

RAMANUJAN lived only a short time after being brought to England by HARDY, who tells a story about visiting him while he was hospitalized. In an effort to make conversation, HARDY told RAMANUJAN that the taxi on which he had ridden had the license number 1729, a rather dull number. RAMANUJAN replied that, on the contrary, it was a very interesting number, the smallest that can be expressed as the sum of two cubes in two different ways. In summa-rizing his life, HARDY said: "I still say to myself when I am depressed, and find myself forced to listen to pompous and tiresome people, 'Well, I have done one thing you could never have done, and that is to have collaborated with both LITTLEWOOD and RA-MANUJAN on something like equal terms.'"

HARDY was a pure mathematician's pure math-ematician. He abhored any "practical" mathematics. For him, pure mathematics was beautiful and useless, while useful mathematics was dull and ugly. In his acerbic, opinionated, idiosyncratic, yet charming *A Mathematician's Apology* (1940) he writes: "I have never done anything 'useful.' No discovery of mine has made, or is likely to make, directly or indirectly, for

good or ill, the least difference to the amenity of the world." He took the same view of physics; practical physics was ugly. Curiously, the branches of physics that he regarded as most beautiful, and hence most useless, were relativity and quantum mechanics.

It must have embarrassed him that his mathe-matically most trivial paper is not only far and away his most widely known, but has been of such distaste-fully practical value. He published this paper not in the obvious place, *Nature*, but across the Atlantic in *Science*. Why? It has been said that he didn't want to get embroiled in the bitter argument between the Mendelists and biometricians. I would like to think that he didn't want it to be seen by his mathematician colleagues.

WEINBERG was a physician, general practitioner and obstetrician, in Stuttgart. He attended at more than 3500 births. Despite this busy life, he somehow found the time and energy to make fundamental discoveries. He published a method for calculating the proportion of monozygotic and dizygotic twins from the proportion of like-sexed twins as early as 1901, at a time when the biological origin of the two types of twins was still only an assumption. He also concluded, correctly, that a propensity to dizygotic twinning, but not to monozygotic, is inherited.

WEINBERG was the first to recognize and correct ascertainment bias. In his 1901 paper on the inherit-ance of twinning he astutely used the sibs of twins to determine the proportion of twinning in families that had been identified through a twin pair. Later (1912), on reading BATESON's comment that there are more than ¼ albinos among children of heterozygous parents, he realized that this was also an ascertain-ment problem. Families with no affected children were not discovered, and thus the proportion of albinos is inflated in those families that are included. He invented the sib and proband methods to correct for it; both utilize the ratio in the sibs of affected, with the probands removed. WEINBERG was the foun-der of segregation analysis. It was developed further by HALDANE and FISHER, and greatly extended by MORTON (1982), who worked out methods, now in wide use, for separating out sporadic and polygenic components.

In 1910 WEINBERG published an article[1] on the correlations between relatives in a randomly mating population. At this time, PEARSON and other biome-tricians thought that the observed correlations be-tween relatives were inconsistent with Mendelian inheritance. WEINBERG showed this to be wrong. He also took environmental effects into account and

[1] Part of this remarkable paper has been translated by KARIN MEYER (see pp. 42–57 of HILL 1984). HILL (*ibid.*, pg. 13) has also provided a useful table of correspondences between WEINBERG's sometimes confusing notation and that now in common use.

utilized the additivity of squared standard deviations, anticipating the analysis of variance.

While WEINBERG was writing in Germany, R. A. FISHER was beginning his studies in England. FISHER was later to become the greatest statistician of his generation if not the greatest ever. While still an undergraduate he had written a paper (1912) that foreshadowed the use of maximum likelihood as an estimating procedure. Yet, for all his promise, he was not able to find a job that suited his talents. He was turned down for military service in World War I because of poor eyesight, and finally found employment teaching physics and mathematics. He taught at Rugby and Haileybury Schools, on a naval training ship, and at Bradfield College. He hated it, and undoubtedly was no good at bringing the subject down to the level of his students.

In these years there was a raging argument in Britain between the "Mendelists" and the "Biometricians." In retrospect the disagreement seems a bit silly, for it now seems obvious that quantitative traits can be explained by postulating a large number of Mendelian factors. In fact the argument never took place in the United States, where this assumption was made from the beginning. The continuing vituperation probably had more to do with the personal differences and sensitive egos of PEARSON and WELDON, representing the biometricians, and BATESON and PUNNETT, representing the Mendelists, than on the scientific evidence.

While still a student at Cambridge, FISHER became convinced that the large number of Mendelian factors was a sufficient explanation of metrical traits. He decided to see if the observed correlations between relatives were consistent with Mendelism. His blockbuster, "The correlation between relatives on the supposition of Mendelian inheritance," was published in 1918. FISHER wrote the paper while teaching school students and completed it in 1916, but it was not accepted for publication by the Royal Society of London. For creativity and depth by someone out of the academic mainstream, this is reminiscent of EINSTEIN's great papers written while he worked in a patent office. FISHER's reviewers were PEARSON and PUNNETT, bitter opponents in the Mendelism-biometrics debate, and neither recommended publication. It has been said that this was the only time that the two ever agreed. The paper was finally published in the *Transactions of the Royal Society of Edinburgh*, and only through the financial help of LEONARD DARWIN, CHARLES DARWIN's son. Ironically, by the time the paper was published, the point had been settled and the paper's main argument was moot.

Yet this paper is remarkable, and more important, in other ways. Not only did FISHER show that biometry and Mendelism were compatible, but he worked out in full detail the theory of correlations between relatives and the apportionment of variance— a term he invented in this paper—between genetic and environmental factors. He further showed that dominance contributed to sib correlations but not to those of parent-offspring, thus accounting for the greater observed value of sib correlations. Nowadays, we would give more emphasis to the greater environmental correlations of sibs, but FISHER's analysis was a remarkable theoretical breakthrough. He also showed how to include epistatic interactions as a component of variance. Finally, he considered in great detail the consequences of assortative mating, in some ways more thoroughly than anyone since.

Although this paper is in many ways the foundation of quantitative genetics, FISHER did little more on this subject. Perhaps he thought he had answered most of the major questions. He did write one more paper, with IMMER and TEDIN (1932), in which he carried the analysis to third moments. It has not been used widely.

In 1919 FISHER finally got a job. This was at the Rothamsted Experiment Station, and it was in connection with this work that he worked out the procedures—analysis of variance and covariance, factorial design, field plot arrangements, design of experiments—that are now everyday practice. He also laid the mathematical foundations for the statistics of small samples. His biological interests turned to evolution, and his book *The Genetical Theory of Natural Selection* (1930) is in many ways the natural successor to *The Origin of Species*. A book-length biography of FISHER is available, written by his daughter (BOX 1978).

1918 is significant for another paper, this time in GENETICS. In this year WRIGHT published a paper with the innocent title, "The nature of size factors." This is the forerunner of path analysis, WRIGHT's technique for using partial regression coefficients to assign relative importance to different paths in a complex causal pattern. This method became his greatest contribution to statistical methodology.

Finally, 1988 is the bicentennial of the completion of GIBBON's *Decline and Fall*. Other than as a numerical coincidence, why mention *this* book in *this* context? The reason is that FISHER was greatly influenced by it, and the last chapters of his 1930 book are devoted to the conditions for stability of civilizations. To FISHER's regret his genetically based theory was ignored by both biologists and historians. The last chapters of his otherwise highly influential book are largely unread.

The years 1908 and 1918 are important ones in the history of genetics. FISHER's 1918 paper is still discussed and WRIGHT's method of path analysis is widely applied in the social sciences. And we are still learning things about the HARDY-WEINBERG relationship. In this issue of GENETICS, C. C. LI shows that random mating is a sufficient, not a necessary condition for H-W ratios.

LITERATURE CITED

BERNSTEIN, F., 1924 Ergebnisse einer biostatischen zusammenfassenden Betrachtung über die Erblichen Blustrukturen des Menshen. Wien. Klin. Wochenschr. **3:** 1495–1497.

BERNSTEIN, F., 1925 Zusammenfassende Betrachtungen über die erblichen Blutstructuren des Menschen. Z. Indukt. Abstammungs Vererbungsl. **37:** 237–270.

BOX, J. F., 1978 *R. A. Fisher: The Life of a Scientist.* John Wiley & Sons. New York.

FISHER, R. A., 1912 On an absolute criterion for fitting frequency curves. Messenger Math. **41:** 155–160.

FISHER, R. A., 1918 The correlation between relatives on the supposition of Mendelian inheritance. Trans. R. Soc. Edinb. **42:** 399–433.

FISHER, R. A., 1930 *The Genetical Theory of Natural Selection.* Oxford University Press, Oxford.

FISHER, R. A., 1947 The Rhesus factor. Am. Sci. **35:** 95–102, 113.

FISHER, R. A., F. R. IMMER and O. TEDIN, 1932 The genetical interpretation of statistics of the third degree in the study of quantitative inheritance. Genetics **17:** 107–124.

HARDY, G. H., 1908 Mendelian proportions in a mixed population. Science **28:** 49–50.

HARDY, G. H., 1940 *A Mathematician's Apology.* Cambridge University Press, Cambridge.

HILL, W. G. (Editor), 1984 *Quantitative Genetics.* Benchmark Papers in Genetics. Van Nostrand Reinhold, New York.

MORTON, N. E., 1982 *Outline of Genetic Epidemiology.* S. Karger, Basel.

STERN, C., 1943 The Hardy-Weinberg law. Science **97:** 137–138.

WEINBERG, W., 1901 Beiträgae zur Physiologie und Pathologie der Mehrlingsgeburten beim Menschen. Arch. Ges. Physiol. **88:** 346–430.

WEINBERG, W., 1908 Über den Nachweis der Vererbung beim Menshen. Jahresh. Ver. Vaterl. Naturkd. Wuerttemb. **64:** 368–382.

WEINBERG, W., 1909 Über Vererbungsgesetze beim Menschen. Z. Indukt. Abstammungs Vererbungsl. **1:** 277–330.

WEINBERG, W., 1910 Weitere Beiträge zur Theorie der Vererbung. Arch. Rass. Ges. Biol. **7:** 35–49.

WEINBERG, W., 1912 Über Methode und Fehlerquellen der Untersuchung auf Mendelsche Zahlen beim Menschen. Arch. Rass. Ges. Biol. **9:** 165–174.

WRIGHT, S., 1917 Color inheritance in mammals. VI. Cattle. J. Hered. **8:** 521–527.

WRIGHT, S., 1918 On the nature of size factors. Genetics **3:** 367–374.

A Diamond in a Desert

Herschel Roman

Department of Genetics, University of Washington, Seattle, Washington 98195

I first met LEWIS J. STADLER in 1936, in the spring of my senior year as an undergraduate at the University of Missouri in Columbia. I was told by a faculty member in the Department of Chemistry that he had recommended me to STADLER to fill a vacancy as a technical assistant. After a brief interview, I was offered and accepted the job. I later became his graduate student.

STADLER was in mid-career when I joined his group. His principal goal in research was to identify the material basis of the gene. To this end he devoted himself to the study of mutations, those induced by X-rays and ultraviolet light and those which arose spontaneously. I was hired to help develop filters that would screen out successive bands of ultraviolet light for the ultimate purpose of seeing which bands induced gene mutations, so that a profile of frequency of mutations as a function of wavelength could be obtained. Many substances of biological significance had known absorption spectra and it was his hope that the genic material could be identified by finding the relationship between mutations and the wavelengths that were effective in producing them.

STADLER's investigation of gene mutation induced by X-rays, published in 1928, was a historical landmark in plant genetics. H. J. MULLER earlier (1927) had published a more complete account of similar results with Drosophila. The two men arrived at their results independently but MULLER was favored in the choice of material, Drosophila having a generation time of about 12 days whereas, at that time, only one crop of corn (or barley, used by STADLER for his early experiments) could be grown each year. Many of his contemporaries thought that STADLER should have shared the Nobel Prize that was awarded to MULLER in 1946. STADLER himself extolled the achievements of MULLER in his posthumous article in *Science* (1954).

Drosophila was excellent experimental material for X-ray studies but was inadequate for studies with ultraviolet light because the tissues overlying the testes were relatively opaque to the wavelengths that proved to be effective in causing genetic effects. Corn pollen did not have this shortcoming but there were technical difficulties to which I will refer in more detail later.

Although I was unaware of it at the time, the spring of 1936 saw the beginnings of the flowering of genetics at the University of Missouri. ERNEST R. SEARS and JOSEPH G. O'MARA came to the University to join STADLER, GEORGE F. SPRAGUE and LUTHER SMITH. BARBARA MCCLINTOCK came in the fall of 1936 to a position in the Department of Botany. FRED M. UBER arrived at about the same time to a position in the Department of Physics. His research, in collaboration with STADLER, was concerned with the genetic effects of ultraviolet light. I was aware that LEWIS STADLER must have had an important hand in these appointments. The effect of his influence was obvious and it was also obvious that he was the acknowledged leader of the group. His leadership was subtle since he held no official position that entitled him to assume such a role. The group was not departmentalized; there was no formal organization. I think he was recognized for his intellectual force and that this was the basis for his preeminence. He was easy-going, imperturbable and, above all, brilliant.

STADLER was becoming more and more involved in the use of ultraviolet light for the induction of chromosomal effects. The sunlamp that he was using was soon replaced by a quartz monochromator, which permitted him to treat pollen grains with individual wavelengths of ultraviolet light, thereby disposing of the need for filters. The lines of the ultraviolet spectrum could also be measured for the energy of emission. The two sperm nuclei of each pollen grain are eccentrically disposed, with a layer of starch and the outer layer of the pollen grain between the nuclei and the radiation. The loss of energy due to absorption or scattering by the overlying materials varied with the wavelength and was a significant factor in evaluating the radiation's effects. Since the spherical pollen grains assumed all possible orientations with respect to the sperm nuclei, correction had to be made for the amount of overlying material as a function of the position of the sperm nuclei. In fact, it could be reasonably assumed that when the nuclei were farthest from the radiation source, that is, when the overlying material was maximal, most of the ultraviolet radiation failed to reach the nuclei, the greatest loss occurring at the shorter wavelengths.

When these corrections were applied—the distribution of sperm nuclei by a formula devised by SEWALL WRIGHT and the loss of energy due to the pollen grain contents above the nuclei, measured experimentally by UBER—an experimental curve was obtained relating the effectiveness of the various wavelengths in inducing chromosomal effects (STADLER and UBER 1942). The curve could be construed as denoting that the absorbing material responsible for the genetic effects was DNA. This remarkable achievement takes on a new significance when one understands that the results were published decades in advance of the discovery of the structure of DNA (WATSON and CRICK 1953) and the interpretation that DNA was the genetic material. Small wonder that STADLER did not jump to this conclusion and in fact turned his attention to other ways of getting clues to the structure of the gene. DNA was then regarded not as an informational polymer but as a molecule too simple in structure to account for gene replication or the effects of the gene.

In a series of persuasive papers, STADLER pointed out that radiation-induced mutations could not be assumed to be true gene mutations, that is, those of consequence in the evolutionary process. True mutations could not be easily distinguished from other genetic effects induced by radiation, such as chromosomal aberrations, including small deletions and position effects. Thus their frequency could not be determined precisely, but a very low upper limit could be set.

STADLER next turned to spontaneous mutation, that is, mutation whose origin was unknown but which, in his estimation, offered a greater possibility of establishing criteria for the true gene mutation. He chose the R locus for this purpose because this locus was sufficiently variable in the different strains of corn that were under cultivation, because it had a mutation rate that was not so rare as to be unmanageable, and because it had well defined phenotypes. The R locus affected anthocyanin pigmentation in various parts of the plant and in the seed.

After an extensive series of experiments with different strains of maize, collected from presumably independent sources, STADLER concluded that the R locus consisted of two sets of elements, those that affected pigmentation in the plant (P) and those that affected pigmentation of the seed (S). The number of such elements could not be ascertained but each had enough homology to the other so that the two could be separated by unequal crossing over. If P was absent, under the appropriate genetic background, the plant lacked anthocyanin; if the S element was lacking, the seed was devoid of anthocyanin. Both P and S could mutate independently, but there was an interaction between them revealed by their rates of mutation, each of which fluctuated under the influence of changes in the other element. Thus the P and S elements were not only related, but the composition of one element or array of elements affected the rate of mutation of the other. By one criterion—the fact that the one could mutate independently of the other—the two elements appeared to be separable as two genes; by the other criterion—the interdependence of the two elements—the R locus appeared to house a single gene (STADLER 1954; STADLER and EMMERLING 1956). The slight but constant variation in phenotype of the many alleles tested indicated further that these might be the elusive true gene mutations of evolutionary significance. This was the state of his investigations at the time of his death as a consequence of Hodgkin's disease on May 12, 1954, at the age of 58.

The quality of the group that he had assembled, or was influential in assembling, is indicated by the honors that were awarded to members of the group, either before or after his death. STADLER himself was elected to the National Academy of Sciences, the American Academy of Arts and Sciences and the Philosophical Society. McCLINTOCK, SPRAGUE, and SEARS were also elected to the National Academy of Sciences. SPRAGUE (1978), McCLINTOCK (1981) and SEARS (1986) each shared the Wolf Prize. In addition, McCLINTOCK was awarded the Nobel Prize in 1983 in recognition of her discovery of what are now known as transposable elements.

I am reminded at this juncture of a conversation I had with MAX DELBRÜCK on the occasion of his first visit to the United States, in 1937. I asked him why he had chosen to come to the University of Missouri, which was out of the way in his extensive itinerary. He replied that one had to come to Columbia if one was interested in the nature of the gene, no matter if it were out of the way. "It's a diamond in a desert."

What more can be added to describe this remarkable man? He was a master of experimental design. His lectures and writings were noted for their clarity and lucidity. He was always approachable. He was a gentle man, quiet but sure of himself. I never knew him to be angry with his colleagues or to speak ill of anyone. He and his wife CORNELIA were cordial hosts and it was a great pleasure to be a guest in their home. A memoir published for the National Academy of Sciences provides information about STADLER's background and family life, and brings together aspects of the scientist and the private man in a way that gives a more complete portrait of an extraordinary person (RHOADES 1957).

I am indebted to my wife CARYL for her help in recalling events of some 50 years ago and her expert editing of the manuscript. Thanks are also due to E. R. SEARS, who made valuable comments in its preparation.

LITERATURE CITED

MULLER, H. J., 1927   Artificial transmutation of the gene. Science 46: 84–87.

RHOADES, M. M., 1957   Lewis John Stadler 1896–1954. Biogr. Mem. Natl. Acad. Sci. 30: 329–347.

STADLER, L. J., 1928   Mutations in barley induced by X-rays and radium. Science 68: 186–187.

STADLER, L. J., 1954   The gene. Science 120: 811–819.

STADLER, L. J., and M. M. EMMERLING, 1956   Relation of unequal crossing over to the interdependence of R^r elements (P) and (S). Genetics 41: 124–137.

STADLER, L. J., and F. M. UBER, 1942   Genetic effects of ultraviolet radiation in maize. IV. Comparison of monochromatic radiations. Genetics 27: 84–118.

WATSON, J. D., and F. H. C. CRICK, 1953   Genetic implications of the structure of deoxyribonucleic acid. Nature 171: 737–738.

Unequal Crossing Over Then and Now

Kenneth D. Tartof

Institute for Cancer Research, Fox Chase Cancer Center, 7701 Burholme Avenue, Philadelphia, Pennsylvania 19111

THE *Bar* eye mutation of Drosophila occupies a rather special place in the history of genetics. As the experiments of STURTEVANT and MORGAN (1923) and STURTEVANT (1925) showed, it was the first example of unequal crossing over and also the first demonstration of position effect. Over the past 65 years our understanding of position effects has remained largely unresolved, but our knowledge and appreciation of the importance of unequal crossing over has grown substantially. While much remains to be learned, I think it is now clear that the phenomenon of unequal recombination is a matter of considerable significance for genetic biology. It is, therefore, the subject of this *Perspectives* on the occasion of the 65th anniversary of its discovery.

I am going to focus on two basic modes by which unequal crossing over occurs. One involves direct tandem redundancy, whereas the other is mediated by transposons. My purpose is to illustrate these two situations with examples from diverse organisms in order to provide a sense of the context in which they occur and to understand the questions they raise. Because our concept of unequal crossing over derives directly from studies of the *Bar* mutation, it is useful to consider these in some detail.

Bar is a dominant, homozygous viable, sex-linked mutation that reduces, in heterozygotes, the number of facets in the compound eye to about half their usual value. By 1921 ZELENY had shown that *Bar* was unstable and could mutate at considerable frequency (6×10^{-4}) to either wild type or to a more severe phenotype he referred to as *ultra Bar*. However, no mechanism to explain this anomalous behavior seemed obvious until STURTEVANT and MORGAN (1923) reported the results of a disarmingly simple experiment. They marked chromosomes carrying *Bar* (*B*, 57.0 cM) with the flanking mutations *forked* (*f*, 56.5 cM) and *fused* (*fu*, 59.5 cM) to produce $f^+ B\ fu/f\ B\ fu^+$ heterozygotes and found that the *Bar$^+$* revertant progeny were also recombinant for the adjacent markers, being either $f^+ fu^+$ or $f fu$. Their conclusion was unequivocal: "... reversion of *Bar* to normal is associated with crossing over at or near the *Bar* locus."

But the matter was not to rest there. Two years later, in 1925, STURTEVANT solved the riddle of the unusual properties of *Bar* in a publication entitled "The effects of unequal crossing over at the Bar locus in Drosophila." It is a remarkable paper. At the outset, STURTEVANT advances the hypothesis that both the *ultra Bar* mutants and the wild-type revertants arise from $f^+ B\ fu^+/f\ B\ fu$ individuals by unequal crossing over at *Bar*. He proposed that if the site of recombination lies to the left of *Bar* in one chromosome, but to the right of it on the other, then the *ultra Bar* mutants should be more properly referred to as *double Bar* because they would be genotypically $f\ BB\ fu^+$ or $f^+ BB\ fu$ and, hence, duplicated for *Bar*. The wild-type revertants, on the other hand, would be $f^+ fu$ or $f\ fu^+$ and deficient for *Bar*. Accordingly, *double Bar* and wild-type revertants are necessarily reciprocal products of the same exchange event and should be recovered in equal numbers. In fact, they are not. This is probably due to the reduced viability of *double Bar* and the difficulty of distinguishing it from *Bar* alone. However, what made the unequal crossing over hypothesis so compelling was STURTEVANT's discovery and use of a new allele of *Bar* known as *Bar-infrabar* (B^i). This mutation arose spontanteously in a *Bar* stock and reduces the number of eye facets to a value intermediate between *B* and wild type and thereby made it possible to devise a crucial test of the unequal crossing over mechanism. STURTEVANT was able to derive, for example, the tandem arrangement of BB^i from B/B^i heterozygotes and then to recover separately the *B* and B^i alleles in their proper order with respect to flanking markers.

It would be 11 years, until the discovery of polytene chromosomes, before STURTEVANT's unequal crossing over hypothesis could be confirmed. MULLER, PROKOFIEVA-BELGOVSKAYA and KOSSIKOV (1936) and BRIDGES (1936) found that the *Bar* mutation itself is a direct tandem duplication of seven bands that compose section 16A1-7 of the polytene map. Unequal crossing over results when the distal repeat of one chromosome recombines with the proximal repeat in the opposite homolog to yield *Bar$^+$* revertants and

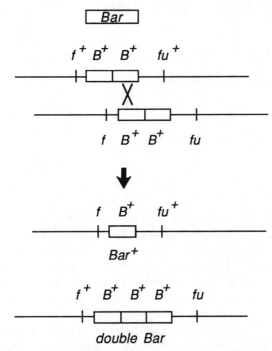

FIGURE 1.—Unequal crossing over at *Bar*. The large open rectangle at the top represents the *Bar* tandem duplication whereas each smaller rectangle below denotes one copy of the *Bar*[+] (*B*[+]) locus which spans section 16A1-7 on the polytene map. One of two possible misalignments of the *Bar* duplication is illustrated. In this case, unequal exchange in *f*[+] *B fu*[+]/*f B fu* heterozygotes produces *f B*[+] *fu*[+] (*Bar*[+]) and *f*[+] *BB fu* (*double Bar*) progeny that possess one and three copies of the *Bar*[+] locus, respectively. Recently, STUART TSUBOTA (personal communication) has observed the presence of a 7.5-kb transposon inserted at the 16A7-16A1 breakpoint in the middle of the *Bar* duplication. This suggests that the duplication itself may have been formed in the process of transposon mobilization.

double Bar progeny (Figure 1). Thus, the reversion of *Bar* does not involve a loss of the *Bar* locus as initially thought, but rather a loss of the duplicate copy of section 16A; conversely, *double Bar* actually contains three doses of the *Bar*[+] region.

Since recombination was known to take place at the four-strand stage, STURTEVANT considered the possibility that unequal sister chromatid exchange might be responsible for some of the changes in *Bar*. However, after examining more than 36,000 offspring from homozygous *B* or *B*[i] females, every instance of either reversion or augmentation of *Bar* was also accompanied by crossing over between *f* and *fu*. If unequal sister chromatid exchange ever occurs here, it is a rather rare event. Nevertheless, PETERSON and LAUGHNAN (1963) pursued the issue further in an elegant series of experiments. They searched for exceptional nonrecombinant *B*[+] male offspring produced from females that were either: (1) hemizygotes, carrying *f B fu* on one *X* chromosome and a deficiency for *Bar* on the other; (2) heterozygotes, bearing *f B os* on one *X* (*os*, outstretched small eye, 59.2 cM), and the other an inversion containing *f*[+] *B os*[+]; or finally (3), heterozygotes of the genotype *f B os/f*[+] *B os*[+]. In

total, they obtained 9 nonrecombinant *B* to *B*[+] revertant males among 215,376 progeny for a frequency of about 4×10^{-5}. This value is 15 times lower than the comparable interchromatid event which they found to be 6×10^{-4} (46 recombinant revertants among 78,433 progeny).

Similarly, JACKSON and FINK (1985) have shown that in Saccharomyces the occurrence of unequal sister chromatid exchange between two copies of a direct tandem duplication of the *HIS4* gene is also 10–20-fold less frequent than the comparable rate of interchromosomal recombination. Although the cause of this striking suppression of intrachromatid unequal exchange in both flies and yeast is unknown, it does suggest the presence of a well regulated pathway controlling these events. JACKSON and FINK have proposed that suppressing sister chromatid crossing over might be selectively advantageous by reducing the production of deficiencies and inversions that would otherwise result from intrastrand exchange between direct or inverted repeats on the same chromosome. This speculation may be particularly relevant to micro-repeats, sequences 2–10 bp in length and separated from each other by less than 1 kb, that participate in the generation of spontaneous deletions through illegitimate exchange as previously discussed in these *Perspectives* by ANDERSON (1987).

In contrast to the situation for unique genes like *Bar* and *HIS4*, highly redundant sequences such as the ribosomal RNA genes (rDNA) have a propensity for unequal sister chromatid exchange. RITOSSA et al. (1966) showed that in Drosophila there is a 100–200 copy array of these genes imbedded within the centric heterochromatin of the *X* chromosome and another on the short arm of the *Y* and that partial deficiencies of rDNA result in a short-bristle phenotype known as *bobbed* (*bb*). He subsequently made the remarkable discovery that when *X* chromosome *bb* mutants are maintained for several generations with a *Y* chromosome deficient for most of its rDNA (*Ybb*[−]), as in *bb/Ybb*[−] males, phenotypically *bb*[+] flies containing a wild-type amount of rDNA appear (RITOSSA 1968). This phenomenon has been referred to as "magnification."

In order to explain the very existence of *bobbed* mutants, RITOSSA et al. (1966) speculated that they might arise by unequal crossing over. However, the possibility that unequal exchange was responsible for magnification was rejected by both RITOSSA (1968, 1972, 1973) and ATWOOD (1969). Part of the difficulty in understanding this phenomenon was that it occurred only in males, a gender in which meiotic recombination is virtually absent. However, as a result of examining the frequency of magnification in single males rather than in populations of flies, I proposed that the mechanism by which magnification occurs is unequal mitotic sister chromatid exchange (TARTOF 1974). I demonstrated that rDNA magnification arises primarily in mitotically active germ cells and at a frequency such that 80% of the offspring of some *bb/Ybb⁻* individuals are *bb^{m+}* (magnified wild type *bb⁺*). This frequency of magnification is several orders of magnitude higher than expected for interchromosomal meiotic recombination events. Moreover, the *Ybb⁻* chromosome not only induces rDNA magnification of *bb* mutants but is also able to decrease the rDNA content of the wild-type *bb⁺* locus, a phenomenon referred to as "reduction." It was further shown that magnification and reduction are reciprocal events in *bb/Ybb⁻* germ cells, although *bb^{m+}* progeny are recovered more frequently than their reduction-produced lethal counterparts (*bb^{rlethal}*). This might be expected owing to selection against *bb^{rlethal}* germ cells in a manner reminiscent of the under-representation of *double Bar* recombinants observed by STURTEVANT. Finally, magnification of a *bb* mutation when present in a ring *X* chromosome is diminished as might be expected because single (or odd-number) crossovers are lost as double-size dicentric chromosomes. More recently, we have shown that under nonselective conditions, recovery of *bb^{m+}* and *bb^{rlethal}* products is equal and that, although the vast majority of the magnified *bb⁺* progeny from *bb/Ybb⁻* males arise premeiotically, some of these magnifying events also occur at meiosis (HAWLEY and TARTOF 1985).

There are two genetic factors crucial to the process of ribosomal gene magnification and reduction. First, the presence of the *Ybb⁻* chromosome is required. What makes this chromosome so mutagenic is not clear. It is deficient for most of its own rDNA, but this alone does not explain its behavior because *Ybb⁻* chromosomes have been constructed with a wild-type rDNA content and they are still effective at inducing magnification (HAWLEY and TARTOF 1983). However, it may be that *Ybb⁻* is deficient for a critical pairing site and this leads to misalignment between the rDNA clusters when homologous regions of the *X* and *Y* synapse. Second, some of the genes (*mei-41, mus-101, mus-108*) that control meiotic recombination and DNA repair are also required for magnification-reduction, whereas others (*mei-9, mus-102, mus-109*) are not (HAWLEY and TARTOF 1983; HAWLEY *et al.* 1985). It is interesting to note that those genes affecting rDNA magnification and reduction are also involved in post-replication repair.

Just as the rDNA of Drosophila may undergo unequal sister chromatid exchange in both mitotic and meiotic cells, similar events occur in Saccharomyces. By virtue of site-specific transformation, it has been possible to insert a single *LEU2* gene into the tandemly arrayed rDNA cluster located on chromosome *XII* of yeast. Measurement of the frequency of increase and decrease in *LEU2* copy number has provided an unequivocal genetic and molecular demonstration of the regular occurrence of unequal sister strand exchange

within the rDNA cluster of mitotic cells (SZOSTAK and WU 1980) as well as meiotic cells (PETES 1980). In mitotic cells, about 10^{-2} unequal sister chromatid exchange event is observed per generation. In meiotic cells, the frequency of unequal sister strand exchange is at least 10^{-1} per meiosis, while recombination between nonsister chromatids is suppressed.

A somewhat similar situation has also been observed in the mouse. The distal ends of mammalian *X* and *Y* chromosomes frequently pair and undergo reciprocal exchange in gametogenesis. As a consequence, the pattern of inheritance of markers located in this region is not strictly sex-linked and is called pseudoautosomal. HARBERS *et al.* (1986) have isolated a mouse containing a single Moloney murine leukemia virus (M-MuLV) genome inserted in the pseudoautosomal region of the *Y*. The M-MuLV proviral sequence is readily transferred from the *Y* to the *X* and back again at a frequency of about 10^{-1}. Moreover, approximately 7% of the offspring from males homozygous for M-MuLV (*X^{Mov}/Y^{Mov}*) contain either no provirus or two copies of it. Since the proviral insert is flanked by a tandemly redundant sequence (repeat length ~1.3 kb), a plausible explanation for the gain and loss of proviral DNA is unequal crossing over between the repeated elements. It is not known if some of these events are premeiotic or involve sister chromatids. Such issues may be resolved, both in this case and in mammalian systems in general, by using restriction fragment length polymorphisms (RFLPs) as chromosome markers flanking the site of unequal exchange to determine precisely the source of alteration in gene copy number.

In humans, too, there is evidence for unequal crossing over. JEFFREYS, WILSON and THEIN (1985) have described a probe that detects hypervariable, dispersed, tandemly redundant "minisatellite" regions whose repeat lengths vary from 16 to 64 bp and are highly polymorphic in the human genome. In fact, these repeat lengths are so polymorphic from one person to the next that they provide a means for detecting individual-specific DNA. The likely source of such polymorphism is unequal crossing over. In an incisively direct experiment, JEFFREYS *et al.* (1988) examined human pedigrees with five different minisatellite probes to determine the rate at which new alleles (DNA restriction fragments) appear. For each individual probe, the mutation rate per gamete varied from undetectable to as high as 5×10^{-2} for the most unstable locus.

The examples of unequal crossing over at *Bar*, in rDNA, in the pseudoautosomal region of the mouse and in the minisatellites of humans all share a common structural feature: direct tandem repetition of genetic sequence. It is conceptually straightforward to understand how unequal crossing over among repeated sequences arises when there are two or more identical sites, and hence, substantial opportunity for misalignment between the iterated copies. But what causes unequal crossing over in genetically unique portions of the genome where tandem duplication is not apparent? What sort of homology is required, and how extensive must it be, to effect asymmetric exchange?

Considerable progress toward answering these questions has been provided by GOLDBERG et al. (1983) and DAVIS, SHEN and JUDD (1987). They examined the molecular structure of reciprocal duplications and deficiencies produced by interchromosomal unequal exchange in Drosophila females heterozygous for various white (w) alleles. In the experiments of GOLDBERG et al. it was found that a 7.2-kb transposable element (BEL) was present in both w^a and w^{a4} mutants but inserted at slightly different locations in each mutant, about 60 kb apart and in the same orientation. Further analysis demonstrated that asymmetric pairing and exchange between the staggered BEL sequences are responsible for the observed duplications and deficiencies. The frequency of unequal exchange between these two white alleles is about 2×10^{-4}. DAVIS, SHEN and JUDD examined unequal crossing over in w^{ric}/w^{bf} heterozygotes. w^{ric} possesses an 8.7-kb roo transposon located at 0 kb on the molecular map of white whereas w^{bf} contains two roo elements, one at −1.1 kb and the other at +31.9 kb. All three roo inserts are oriented in the same direction. Here, too, unequal crossing over is transposon-mediated. In w^{ric}/w^{bf} heterozygotes the frequency of unequal exchange between the roo elements at 0 and −1.1 is four times higher (2×10^{-4}) than between the roo transposons located at 0 and +31.9 (5×10^{-5}). This indicates that the interaction between transposons may be inversely related to the distance that separates them.

What is perhaps most astonishing about these results is that small (8-kb) displaced regions of homology, in the form of transposons, are able to pair with each other at considerable frequency despite separation by 60 kb and despite being surrounded by extensive regions of standard homology. At present, we do not understand how transposons participate in this process. Anecdotal observations (BURKE JUDD, personal communication) indicate that the heterozygosity of transposon locations may be important because w^{bf} homozygotes, with their two roo elements only 33 kb apart, seem to show no evidence of asymmetric exchange. This would suggest a mechanism of transposon-mediated unequal crossing over whereby homolog pairing in heterozygotes results in looped-out unpaired transposons that recombine with each other in a distance-dependent manner. Still, the extent to which heterozygosity affects this process needs to be clearly defined. It is also possible that a transposase is involved. The genes that control transposon-mediated unequal exchange are yet to be identified. In this regard it would be useful to examine the effect of overexpression of the appropriate transposase as well as the impact that various recombination and DNA repair mutations might have on transposon-mediated unequal crossing over.

Because small, slightly displaced transposons appear to be such a significant feature of unequal crossing over, the question arises of how many times per genome one might expect members of the same transposon family to be sufficiently close (for instance, within 60 kb) to pair with each other and undergo unequal exchange. In Drosophila melanogaster there are about 70 different mobile element families, each represented on average about 33 times in the euchromatic portion of the genome (YOUNG 1979). Given these parameters, SAM LITWIN and I have calculated, by both analytical means (LITWIN 1974) and by computer simulation, the frequency distribution of two identical transposons located on the same chromosome arm and displaced by ≤60 kb. Assuming all transposons to be randomly distributed, our results predict about 13 instances per Drosophila genome, similar to the w^a/w^{a4} situation where two members of the same transposon family reside within 60 kb or less of each other and in the same orientation. It follows, then, that the average genomic frequency of transposon-mediated unequal crossing over per meiosis in Drosophila might be (2×10^{-4}) $\times$ 13 or about 3×10^{-3}. This is a very high rate for a mutagenic process.

Since the frequency of unequal exchange is so high and so ubiquitous, it is not surprising to observe its impact on human disease. Either tandem duplications (as in Bar) or transposons (as in w^a/w^{a4}) may be involved.

Color blindness, an X-linked disease that affects about 8% of Caucasian males, in an example of unequal crossing over mediated by gene duplication. This locus codes for the red and green visual pigment apoproteins and is organized as a head-to-tail tandem array composed of a single red-pigment gene at the 5′ end followed by a variable number (one, two or three) of green-pigment genes (NATHANS, THOMAS and HOGNESS 1986; VOLLRATH, NATHANS and DAVIS 1988). The polymorphism for the number of green-pigment genes is probably explained by unequal crossing over. Examination of genomic DNA from males with two different forms of color blindness revealed the presence of an interesting pattern of rearrangements (NATHANS et al. 1986). One class of color blindness, anomalous trichromacy, has been thought to result from the presence of photopigment with an altered absorption spectrum. In fact, analysis of the DNA from such individuals demonstrates the presence of either a 5′ red—3′ green or a 5′ green—3′ red hybrid photopigment gene. These data are most easily explained by unequal crossing over between red-pigment and green-pigment loci. This seems likely given the fact that their DNA sequences are 98% identical and that the number of green-pigment genes is so variable. In a second type of color blindness, referred to as dichromacy, the red or green photopigment is missing as a consequence of either gene deletion or red-green gene fusion. Here, too, the mutations can be most easily explained by unequal crossing over, although gene conversion may sometimes occur. Similarly, hemoglobinopathies, such as certain α-thalassemias, hemoglobin Lepore and hemoglobin Kenya, illustrate the concept of unequal exchange between tandemly related loci (for a review see COLLINS and WEISSMAN 1984).

Perhaps the clearest human example of unequal crossing over involving displaced transposons comes from studies of familial hypercholesterolemia. This malady is a consequence of a defect in the gene coding for the LDL (low density lipoprotein) receptor, a transmembrane glycoprotein responsible for the binding of LDL and its eventual endocytosis in coated pits. LEHRMAN et al. (1987a,b) have described a duplication and a deletion mutation that appear to result from unequal crossing over between Alu sequences located in different introns of the locus.

From the foregoing discussion is is apparent that the eukaryotic genome is constantly expanding and contracting in size. Results from Drosophila indicate that, for the genetically unique portion of the genome, transposon-mediated unequal exchange may result in duplications or deficiencies of at least 60 kb or so once in every 300 meioses. This will have special consequences for wild-type genes whose phenotypes are sensitive to dosage. In Drosophila, dosage-sensitive loci include *Bar*, the *bithorax* complex, *runt*, *Notch*, *Enhancer-Suppressor of Hairless*, modifiers of *Polycomb*, *Minutes*, and *Enhancer-Suppressors of variegation*. For the repetitous component of the genome, evidence from Drosophila, yeast, mice and humans indicates that the frequency of unequal crossing over per meiosis is on the order of 10^{-1} for some sequences. While it has been suggested that continual unequal exchange provides a means for maintaining the homogeneity of tandemly repeated sequences (SMITH 1973), other processes such as gene conversion may be as important, if not more so, in this regard (JACKSON and FINK 1981; KLEIN and PETES 1981).

In the context of evolution, new proteins are derived from older ones by gene duplication. Proteins, particularly those with extracellular function such as the LDL receptor, the serum albumin family and the epidermal growth factor family, are often built up from a smaller unit of amino acid sequence that is then reiterated as a tandem array. The duplication of an entire gene, or portions of its internal structure, may be considered simply a consequence of unequal crossing over where the exchange event requires regions of homology either in the form of multiple gene copies or interspersed transposons. Thus, the pathologic manifestations of duplication and deletion mutations as they occur in the human LDL receptor are but a reflection of the mechanism by which the gene itself was created. It might be reasonably argued that as the number of gene copies or transposons increases, so should the rate of unequal exchange. But unequal crossing over is a mutagenic event that would be expected to have negative, often lethal consequences as a result of altering gene dosage or producing novel gene fusions. Thus, the tendency to constantly accumulate gene duplications may be limited by the adverse impact these extra DNA sequences usually have. Likewise, increases in transposon copy number may also be constrained by their potential for deleterious effects through unequal exchange (LANGLEY et al. 1988).

We know embarrassingly little about the role unequal crossing over plays in the genetic life of somatic cells. Even in Drosophila, where it should be possible to obtain some information on the frequency of this process, there are few compelling facts. However, malignant cells by their very nature clonally amplify rare genetic events and therefore provide a useful source of biological material with which to investigate this problem. An interesting example in this regard concerns the homogeneously staining regions (HSRs) of mammalian chromosomes that are found only in tumor and drug-resistant cells. They represent a form of gene amplification which evidence suggests is a product of unequal sister chromatid exchange (HOLDEN et al. 1987). Although direct evidence is lacking, unequal crossing over may also be one of the several means by which potentially malignant cells establish homozygosity or hemizygosity for somatically recessive cancer genes (KNUDSON 1971).

In his book *A History of Genetics*, STURTEVANT (1965) modestly regarded the *Bar* eye case as ". . . too special to serve as a basis for any general picture of mutation. . . ." Indeed, it is a special paradigm, but not in the restrictive sense. I suspect STURTEVANT would be pleased with the broad and general importance of his contribution, and how things are turning out.

LITERATURE CITED

ANDERSON, P., 1987 Twenty years of illegitimate recombination. Genetics **115**: 581–584.

ATWOOD, K. C., 1969 Some aspects of the *bobbed* problem in Drosophila. Genetics **61** (Suppl.): 319–327.

BRIDGES, C. B., 1936 The bar "gene" a duplication. Science **83**: 210–211.

COLLINS, F. S., AND S. M. WEISSMAN, 1984 The molecular genetics of human hemoglobin. Prog. Nucleic Acid Res. Mol. Biol. **31:** 317–462.

DAVIS, P. S., M. W. SHEN AND B. H. JUDD, 1987 Asymmetrical pairings of transposons in and proximal to the white locus of *Drosophila* account for four classes of regularly occurring exchange products. Proc. Natl. Acad. Sci. USA **84:** 174–178.

GOLDBERG, M. L., J-Y. SHEEN, W. J. GEHRING AND M. M. GREEN, 1983 Unequal crossing-over associated with asymmetrical synapsis between nomadic elements in the *Drosophila melanogaster* genome. Proc. Natl. Acad. Sci. USA **80:** 5017–5021.

HARBERS, K., P. SORIANO, U. MÜLLER AND R. JAENISCH, 1986 High frequency of unequal recombination in pseudoautosomal region shown by proviral insertion into transgenic mouse. Nature **324:** 682–685.

HAWLEY, R. S., AND K. D. TARTOF, 1983 The effect of *mei-41* on rDNA redundancy in *Drosophila melanogaster*. Genetics **104:** 63–80.

HAWLEY, R. S., AND K. D. TARTOF, 1985 A two-stage model for the control of rDNA magnification. Genetics **109:** 691–700.

HAWLEY, R. S., C. H. MARCUS, M. L. CAMERON, R. L. SCHWARTZ AND A. E. ZITRON, 1985 Repair-defect mutations inhibit rDNA magnification in *Drosophila* and discriminate between meiotic and premeiotic magnification. Proc. Natl. Acad. Sci. USA **82:** 8095–8099.

HOLDEN, J. J. A., M. R. HOUGH, D. L. REIMER AND B. N. WHITE, 1987 Evidence for unequal crossing-over as the mechanism for amplification of some homogeneously staining regions. Cancer Genet. Cytogenet. **29:** 139–149.

JACKSON, J. A., AND G. R. FINK, 1981 Gene conversion between duplicated genetic elements in yeast. Nature **292:** 306–311.

JACKSON, J. A., AND G. R. FINK, 1985 Meiotic recombination between duplicated genetic elements in *Saccharomyces cerevisiae*. Genetics **109:** 303–332.

JEFFREYS, A. J., V. WILSON AND S. L. THEIN, 1985 Hypervariable "minisatellite" regions in human DNA. Nature **314:** 67–73.

JEFFREYS, A. J., N. J. ROYLE, V. WILSON AND Z. WONG, 1988 Spontaneous mutation rates to new length alleles at tandem-repetitive hypervariable loci in human DNA. Nature **332:** 278–281.

KLEIN, H. L., AND T. D. PETES, 1981 Intrachromosomal gene conversion in yeast. Nature **289:** 144–148.

KNUDSON, A. J. JR., 1971 Mutation and cancer: statistical study of retinoblastoma. Proc. Natl. Acad. Sci. USA **68:** 820–823.

LANGLEY, C. H., E. MONTGOMERY, R. HUDSON AND N. KAPLAN, 1988 On the role of unequal exchange in the containment of transposable element copy number. Genet. Res. (in press).

LEHRMAN M. A., J. L. GOLDSTEIN, D. W. RUSSELL AND M. S. BROWN, 1987a Duplication of seven exons in LDL receptor gene caused by Alu-Alu recombination in a subject with familial hypercholesterolemia. Cell **48:** 827–835.

LEHRMAN, M. A., D. W. RUSSELL, J. L. GOLDSTEIN AND M. S. BROWN, 1979b Alu-Alu recombination deletes splice acceptor sites and produces secreted low density lipoprotein receptor in a subject with familial hypercholesterolemia. J. Biol. Chem. **262:** 3354–3361.

LITWIN, S., 1974 The distribution on the shortest distance between random cuts on opposite strands of DNA. J. Appl. Prob. **11:** 363–368.

MULLER, H. J., A. A. PROKOFIEVA-BELGOVSKAYA AND K. V. KOSSIKOV, 1936 Unequal crossing over in the bar mutant as a result of duplication of a minute chromosome section. C. R. (Dokl.) Acad. Sci. USSR **1:** 87–88.

NATHANS, J., D. THOMAS AND D. S. HOGNESS, 1986 Molecular genetics of human color vision: the genes encoding blue, green and red pigments. Science **232:** 193–202.

NATHANS, J., T. P. PIANTANIDA, R. L. EDDY, T. B. SHOWS AND D. S. HOGNESS, 1986 Molecular genetics of inherited variation in human color vision. Science **232:** 203–210.

PETERSON, H. M., AND J. R. LAUGHNAN, 1963 Intrachromosomal exchange at the bar locus in Drosophila. Proc. Natl. Acad. Sci. USA **50:** 126–133.

PETES, T. D., 1980 Unequal meiotic recombination within tandem arrays of yeast ribosomal DNA genes. Cell **19:** 765–774.

RITOSSA, F. M., 1968 Unstable redundancy of genes for ribosomal RNA. Proc. Natl. Acad. Sci. USA **60:** 509–516.

RITOSSA, F., 1972 Procedure for magnification of lethal deletions of genes for ribosomal RNA. Nature New Biol. **240:** 109–111.

RITOSSA, F., 1973 Crossing-over between X and Y chromosomes during ribosomal DNA magnification in *Drosophila melanogaster*. Proc. Natl. Acad. Sci. USA **70:** 1950–1954.

RITOSSA, F. M., K. C. ATWOOD, D. L. LINDSLEY AND S. SPIEGELMAN, 1966 On the chromosomal distribution of DNA complementary to ribosomal and soluble RNA. Natl. Cancer Inst. Monogr. **23:** 449–472.

SMITH, G. P., 1973 Unequal crossover and the evolution of multigene families. Cold Spring Harbor Symp. Quant. Biol. **38:** 507–513.

STURTEVANT, A. H., 1925 The effects of unequal crossing over at the bar locus in Drosophila. Genetics **10:** 117–147.

STURTEVANT, A. H., 1965 A *History of Genetics*. Harper & Row, New York.

STURTEVANT, A. H., AND T. H. MORGAN, 1923 Reverse mutation of the bar gene correlated with crossing over. Science **57:** 746–747.

SZOSTAK, J. W., AND R. WU, 1980 Unequal crossing over in the ribosomal DNA of *Saccharomyces cerevisiae*. Nature **284:** 426–430.

TARTOF, K. D., 1974 Unequal mitotic sister chromatid exchange as the mechanism of ribosomal RNA gene magnification. Proc. Natl. Acad. Sci. USA **71:** 1272–1276.

VOLLRATH, D., J. NATHANS AND R. W. DAVIS, 1988 Tandem array of human visual pigment genes at Xq28. Science **240:** 1669–1672.

YOUNG, M. W., 1979 Middle repetitive DNA: a fluid component of the *Drosophila* genome. Proc. Natl. Acad. Sci. USA **76:** 6274–6278.

ZELENY, C., 1921 The direction and frequency of mutation in the bar-eye series of multiple allelomorphs of Drosophila. J. Exptl. Zool. **34:** 203–233.

The Genesis of Dysgenesis

James F. Crow

Genetics Department, University of Wisconsin–Madison, Madison, Wisconsin 53706

IN 1972 MARGARET KIDWELL from Providence and JOHN SVED from Sydney chanced to attend an informal summer conference on population biology at the University of Massachusetts in Amherst. To their surprise they found themselves reporting almost identical results. Each had found striking increases in mutability and male crossing over in certain Drosophila matings. This brief encounter was the beginning of a trans-Pacific collaboration that produced the name *hybrid dysgenesis*, defined as "a syndrome of correlated genetic traits that is spontaneously induced in hybrids between certain mutually interacting strains, usually in one direction only" (KIDWELL and KIDWELL 1976; KIDWELL, KIDWELL and SVED 1977). The name caught on and the syndrome was soon expanded to include chromosome breakage and temperature-dependent sterility. The sharp difference in reciprocal crosses facilitated genetic analysis, and at the same time molecular methods were rapidly being adapted to Drosophila. It soon became apparent that the syndrome was the result of transposable elements, which in the experiments of SVED and the KIDWELLs turned out to be the *P* element. Hybrid dysgenesis ushered in a new generation of genetic tools for Drosophila.

Mutable genes have been known from the early days of Mendelian genetics. EMERSON studied variegated pericarp in maize as long ago as 1914. The first detailed report of a highly mutable gene in Drosophila was published 60 years ago in this journal (DEMEREC 1928). The species was *Drosophila virilis* and the mutable allele was *reddish-alpha* at the *yellow* locus. DEMEREC also found two other mutable genes in this species. All three were *X*-linked, probably because of ease of detection, and all had the characteristic mutator property of reverting from mutant to normal and from recessive to dominant. Furthermore, among the *miniature* wing alleles, all of which arose from a single mutant gene, one was unstable in somatic tissues only, another was unstable in both germ and somatic cells, and a third was stable in both. In a summary of this and other work, DEMEREC (1935) said that he knew of at least 63 examples of mutable genes in plants. DEMEREC, the subject of next month's *Perspectives*, hoped that mutable loci would provide insights as to the nature of the gene. He did as good a genetic analysis as could be done at the time. He also tried various environmental agents, and in particular found that the system was insensitive to radiation. He, and others, also found that a strain of *Drosophila melanogaster* from Florida had a very high mutation rate (DEMEREC 1937). The stock rather quickly lost its high mutability and flies collected a year later from the same locality had normal mutation rates. DEMEREC was ahead of his time; the techniques of the day weren't adequate.

Although many geneticists regarded mutation as a possible avenue into the mysteries of the gene, most of the emphasis was on genes with normal mutation rates. I don't recall ever hearing any discussion of DEMEREC's work during my student days in the late 1930s. More in tune with the times was the work of STADLER, discussed in a recent *Perspectives* (ROMAN 1988). STADLER preferred to work with ultraviolet radiation, rather than the more drastic ionizing radiation, and with spontaneous mutations. A paper by STURTEVANT (1939) attracted much attention. He reported a high mutation rate in backcrosses from hybrids between races A and B of *Drosophila pseudoobscura* (now called *pseudoobscura* and *persimilis*). The rationale for this experiment made sense. STURTEVANT believed that natural selection would tend to minimize the mutation rate. Different populations would be expected to accomplish this reduction by different means and gene interactions producing such an effect would be broken up by recombination in the hybrids.

The next three decades saw a number of reports of high mutability in Drosophila. Typically the cause was obscure. Efforts to map the genes were usually inconclusive, and the mutability property was often lost after a few generations. NEEL (1942) reported a strain of *D. melanogaster* with a high mutation rate. IVES (1950) found a strain (hi), derived from a wild population in Florida, that greatly increased the lethal mutation rate and also produced chromosome rearrangements. A striking example is the chromosome-breaking system in *Drosophila robusta*, first reported in 1962 (summarized by LEVITAN and VERDONCK 1986). The inheritance is maternal and only the paternal chromosomes are broken. The mechanistic basis of this curious phenomenon remains obscure. These and other early examples of high mutation and chromosome breakage in Drosophila were reviewed by GREEN (1976).

An awakened interest in mutability and chromosome breakage came in the 1960s following the widely heralded work of MCCLINTOCK (1956) on transposable elements in maize and the discovery of insertion sequences and transposons in bacteria. More and more, attention turned to transposable elements as a basis for high rates of mutation and chromosome breakage (GREEN 1969, 1977; ISING and RAMEL 1976). This soon came to be the preferred explanation for the various manifestations of hybrid dysgenesis.

Who first observed hybrid dysgenesis? Undoubtedly several workers found one or another of the associated phenomena, but the properties were so variable both in appearance and persistence as to preclude making sense out of the observations. It is quite likely that RAISSA BERG in the Soviet Union was first. She had studied with H. J. MULLER while he was in Russia in the 1930s, and on his advice had examined the frequency of mutant alleles in natural populations of *D. melanogaster*. She is notable for her persistence through several difficult decades. The life of a Mendelian geneticist in the LYSENKO period was not easy, and hers was no exception. She not only found high frequencies of mutant alleles later found to be associated with *P* elements, notably at the *singed* bristle locus, but also showed that the cause was indeed high mutability and not selection. Very probably she was observing hybrid dysgenesis (for a summary, see BERG 1982).

The first unequivocal observation of hybrid dysgenesis due to *P* elements was made by HIRAIZUMI (1971) whose earlier adherence to the BRIDGES principle of treasuring exceptions led to the discovery of segregation distortion (SANDLER, HIRAIZUMI and SANDLER 1959; HIRAIZUMI and CROW 1960). He found a high rate of male recombination (MR) following crosses between laboratory females and males from a natural population in Texas. Soon after, he discovered high mutability in this stock (SLATKO and HIRAIZUMI 1973). Later on it was shown that the MR strain carries *P* elements. Also 1971 was the year in which a similar system of hybrid dysgenesis, the I-R system, was first reported (PICARD 1971, 1976; PICARD and L'HERITIER 1971).

The time was ripe for a unifying concept and it came with the catchy words "hybrid dysgenesis" and the influential paper by KIDWELL, KIDWELL and SVED (1977). It seemed reasonable that all the associated traits—high mutability, male crossing over, temperature-dependent sterility, and chromosome breakage—had their basis in chromosome damage, likely to be the consequence of insertion and excision of a transposable element. It was soon evident that there were two quite independent systems with somewhat similar properties. In the P-M system the dysgenic conditions arose from crosses between P (paternal contributing) males and M (maternal contributing) females; in the I-R system the dysgenic cross was I (inducer) male by R (responder) female.

The property that made these two systems particularly amenable to research was the occurrence of dysgenesis in only one type of mating; the reciprocal mating was normal. The temperature dependence of the sterility was also useful. Thus the instability was conditional; it could be suppressed at will, greatly facilitating genetic analysis. It was soon shown that the dysgenic effects in the P-M system depended on chromosomal elements interacting with a maternally transmitted "cytotype" (ENGELS 1979). Strong early evidence that the P strain carried a family of transposable elements came from localization of breakage hot spots to specific points on the chromosome. Additional evidence came from the strikingly high mutability of the *singed* allele *sn^w* which was under cytotype control and which in dysgenic condition mutated at an extraordinarily high rate to two stable forms. Furthermore, this locus was a chromosome-breakage site (reviewed by ENGELS 1983).

A molecular breakthrough was not long in coming. The transposon hypothesis could be confirmed by finding an insertion in a dysgenesis-induced allele of a gene that had been cloned. The first such instance was reported by RUBIN, KIDWELL and BINGHAM (1982). This immediately made possible the molecular identification of *P* elements. The various confirming tests were soon to come, for example, the demonstration that the hot spots for chromosome breakage did indeed contain *P* elements. P strains were found to have numerous such elements and M strains to lack them. It was also found that the elements were of two classes, a homogeneous class of complete 2907-bp elements and a heterogeneous group of smaller incomplete ones. Only the complete elements produced the transposase required for dysgenic activity.

The P-M system quickly lent itself to molecular trickery. Mutations can readily be induced. Any transposon-induced mutation can be identified and recovered, thus making feasible the molecular analysis of otherwise inaccessible loci. After a gene has been cloned it can be reinserted into the genome by the use of *P* elements. This was first exploited by SPRAD-

LING and RUBIN (1982) who injected a bacterial plasmid containing a complete *P* element into the blastoderm of *sn^w* embryos. The induced mutability of *sn^w*, which contains only incomplete elements, proved that a complete element had been incorporated somewhere in the system. At the same time, RUBIN and SPRADLING (1982) inserted a wild-type *rosy* gene into a *P* element. By introducing such an element into a mutant *rosy* embryo, the *rosy* genetic defect could be permanently cured.

At the next Drosophila meeting RUBIN and SPRADLING explained their transformation techniques and agreed to make the necessary materials available to any who wished them. The result was an instantaneous spread of *P* element methodology throughout the Drosophila world. It quickly became a standard method for molecular manipulation of genes, and is in no small part responsible for recent rapid progress in Drosophila genetics. The technical advantages of *P* factors and similar elements for the study of developmental genetics means that there is now more emphasis on their use than on the elements themselves. Yet those interested in the elements for their own sakes are also making rapid progress in understanding detailed mechanisms. For a recent review of the P-M system, see ENGELS (1988).

I regret giving short shrift to other transposable elements, due to both personal and space limitations. The I-R system has recently been reviewed by FINNEGAN (1988). For a general review of mobile elements, see BERG and HOWE (1988).

The free exchange of information, techniques, and stocks in Drosophila has a long tradition dating back to the MORGAN school. The continuation of this custom as molecular methods have become more sophisticated has been an important reason for current rapid advances and the popularity of Drosophila. I hope that increased numbers, competition, pressure to publish, desire to protect priority, and unaccustomed publicity will not lead to an erosion of this grand tradition.

This article is much better for my having received helpful suggestions from MARGARET KIDWELL, RAYLA TEMIN, BILL ENGELS and BILL EGGLESTON.

LITERATURE CITED

BERG, R. L., 1982 Mutability changes in *Drosophila melanogaster* populations of Europe, Asia, and North America and probable mutability changes in human populations of the U.S.S.R. Jpn. J. Genet. **57:** 171–183.

BERG, D. E., and M. M. HOWE, 1988 *Mobile DNA.* American Society for Microbiology, Washington, D.C.

DEMEREC, M., 1928 Mutable characters of *Drosophila virilis.* I. Reddish-alpha body character. Genetics **13:** 359–388.

DEMEREC, M., 1935 Unstable genes. Bot. Rev. **1:** 233–248.

DEMEREC, M., 1937 Frequency of spontaneous mutations in certain stocks of *Drosophila melanogaster.* Genetics **22:** 469–478.

EMERSON, R. A., 1914 The inheritance of a recurring variation in variegated ears of maize. Am. Nat. **48:** 87–115.

ENGELS, W. R., 1979 Hybrid dysgenesis in *Drosophila melanogaster*: rules of inheritance of female sterility. Genet. Res. **33:** 219–236.

ENGELS, W. R., 1983 The P family of transposable elements in Drosophila. Annu. Rev. Genet. **17:** 315–344.

ENGELS, W. R., 1988 P elements in Drosophila. In: *Mobile DNA,* Edited by D. E. BERG and M. M. HOWE. American Society for Microbiology, Washington, D.C. (in press).

FINNEGAN, D. J., 1988 The I factor and I-R hybrid dysgenesis in *Drosophila melanogaster.* In: *Mobile DNA,* Edited by D. E. BERG and M. M. HOWE. American Society for Microbiology, Washington D.C. (in press).

GREEN, M. M., 1969 Controlling element mediated transpositions of the *white* gene in *Drosophila melanogaster.* Genetics **61:** 429–441.

GREEN, M. M., 1976 Mutable and mutator loci. pp. 929–946. In: *The Genetics and Biology of Drosophila.* Edited by M. ASHBURNER and E. NOVITSKI. Academic Press, New York.

GREEN, M. M., 1977 Genetic instability in *Drosophila melanogaster: de novo* induction of putative insertion mutations. Proc. Natl. Acad. Sci. USA **74:** 3490–3493.

HIRAIZUMI, Y., 1971 Spontaneous recombination in *Drosophila melanogaster* males. Proc. Natl. Acad. Sci. USA **68:** 268–270.

HIRAIZUMI, Y., and J. F. CROW, 1960 Heterozygous effects on viability, fertility, rate of development, and longevity of Drosophila chromosomes that are lethal when homozygous. Genetics **45:** 1071–1083.

ISING, G., and C. RAMEL, 1976 The behavior of a transposing element in *Drosophila melanogaster.* pp. 947–954. In: *The Genetics and Biology of Drosophila,* Edited by M. ASHBURNER and E. NOVITSKI. Academic Press, New York.

IVES, P. T., 1950 The importance of mutation rate genes in evolution. Evolution **4:** 236–252.

KIDWELL, M. G., and J. F. KIDWELL, 1976 Selection for male recombination in *Drosophila melanogaster.* Genetics **84:** 333–351.

KIDWELL, M. G., J. F. KIDWELL and J. A. SVED, 1977 Hybrid dysgenesis in *Drosophila malanogaster*: a syndrome of aberrant traits including mutation, sterility and male recombination. Genetics **86:** 813–833.

LEVITAN, M., and M. VERDONCK, 1986 25 years of a unique chromosome-breaking system. I. Principal features and comparison to other systems. Mutat. Res. **161:** 135–142.

McCLINTOCK, B., 1956 Controlling elements and the gene. Cold Spring Harbor Symp. Quant. Biol. **21:** 197–216.

NEEL, J. V., 1942 A study of a case of high mutation rate in *Drosophila melanogaster.* Genetics **27:** 519–536.

PICARD, G., 1971 Un cas de stérlité femelle, chez *Drosophila melanogaster*, lié à un agent transmis maternellement. C. R. Acad. Sci. Paris D **272:** 2482–2487.

PICARD, G., 1976 Non-Mendelian female sterility in *Drosophila melanogaster*: hereditary transmission of *I* factor. Genetics **83:** 107–123.

PICARD, G., and P. L'HERITIER, 1971 A maternally inherited factor inducing sterility in *Drosophila melanogaster.* Drosophila Inform. Serv. **46:** 54.

ROMAN, H., 1988 A diamond in a desert. Genetics **119:** 739–741.

RUBIN, G. M., and A. C. SPRADLING, 1982 Genetic transmission of Drosophila with transposable element vectors. Science **218:** 348–353.

RUBIN, B. M., M. G. KIDWELL and P. M. BINGHAM, 1982 The molecular basis of P-M hybrid dysgenesis: the nature of induced mutations. Cell **29**: 987–994.

SANDLER, L., Y. HIRAIZUMI and I. SANDLER, 1959 Meiotic drive in natural populations of *Drosophila melanogaster*. I. The cytogenetic basis of segregation-distortion. Genetics **44**: 233–250.

SLATKO, B. E., and Y. HIRAIZUMI, 1973 Mutation induction in the male recombination strains of *Drosophila melanogaster*. Genetics **75**: 643–649.

SPRADLING, A. C., and G. M. RUBIN, 1982 Transposition of cloned P elements into *Drosophila* germ line chromosomes. Science **218**: 341–347.

STURTEVANT, A. H., 1939 High mutation frequency induced by hybridization. Proc. Natl. Acad. Sci. USA **25**: 308–310.

Between Novembers
Demerec, Cold Spring Harbor, and the Gene

Philip E. Hartman

Department of Biology, The Johns Hopkins University, Baltimore, Maryland 21218

EXACTLY fifty years ago my father-in-law, MILISLAV DEMEREC, coauthored a GENETICS paper on X-ray-induced chromosomal breaks in Drosophila (BAUER, DEMEREC and KAUFMANN 1938). Then, exactly 25 years ago, he authored a paper on bacterial genetics DEMEREC (1963), again in the November issue of GENETICS. Why this migration from eukaryote to prokaryote, the opposite of present-day trends? What happened during those intervening 25 years? This is mainly the story of a man deeply involved in a search for the structure of the gene and who, at the same time, quietly developed two institutions at Cold Spring Harbor that emerged under his leadership as a hub of what is now known as molecular genetics. It is also the story of a man whose name is misspelled in at least two histories of genetics and whose last name is more often than not mispronounced ("Demer-etts" comes close to the Croatian).

Profiles of DEMEREC have appeared elsewhere [GLASS (1971); five profiles are reprinted in CASPARI (1971)] and GLASS (1971) has compiled a list of his publications. That list is an underestimate because DEMEREC encouraged younger collaborators to publish as sole authors, thus encouraging their independence (*e.g.*, seven of nine papers in DEMEREC *et al.* 1956). Some 5000 items of DEMEREC correspondence and 56 volumes of research notes are housed at the American Philosophical Society Library in Philadelphia, along with the files of other prominent geneticists (GLASS 1988). It is amazing to me to find such a paper trail because most of DEMEREC's communications were either in person or over the phone. As ALEXANDER HOLLAENDER said to me, "It's faster, and they can't say no."

Shortly after immigrating to the United States from Yugoslavia, DEMEREC studied for his Ph.D. at Cornell and completed his work in 1923. He was one of a number of young geneticists, destined to become well known, who were associated with the maize genetics group of R. A. EMERSON (STURTEVANT 1965). He then joined C. W. METZ, A. F. BLAKESLEE, E. G. ANDERSON (another Cornell graduate) and others at Cold Spring Harbor in 1923. There he continued with the genetics of maize, at the same time initiating pioneering studies of unstable genes in Drosophila (DEMEREC 1935). At that time a gene was defined by three operational criteria: it affected a particular phenotype, it was recombinationally indivisible but could recombine with other genes, and it could suddenly and permanently change, *i.e.*, mutate. DEMEREC focused on the last, believing that studies of the mutational process would ultimately lead to an understanding of gene structure. In fact, his work on mutable loci led him to infer that a gene was a linear array containing "different structural components of a molecule" (DEMEREC 1938). Earlier he had used DNA as an example of such a molecule (DEMEREC 1933) but the then general belief was that DNA was a monotonous series of tetranucleotides.

Besides studying mutable genes in Drosophila and in the plant Delphinium, DEMEREC added an additional approach, one that was almost universally popular at the time (DELBRÜCK 1970). He took up the observations of HERMAN J. MULLER (1927) and used X-rays to induce mutations in Drosophila. One outgrowth of the Drosophila work predominating in DEMEREC's laboratory was the founding, with CALVIN B. BRIDGES in 1934, of *Drosophila Information Service.* This was an innovation in its day and still is a valuable mode of communication. DEMEREC continued as editor of the increasingly popular *DIS* through the 33rd issue in 1960, a full decade after his own laboratory had abandoned Drosophila. By then, the *DIS* directory listed 989 workers and the issue contained short communications from 191 laboratories in 29 countries (DEMEREC 1942–1960).

While involved with this and numerous other outside endeavors, DEMEREC became increasingly concerned with the operations of the laboratory itself. He took active roles in an attempt in 1932 and again in 1936 to attract to Cold Spring Harbor the young plant and Drosophila geneticist GEORGE W. BEADLE (MILLER 1978). BEADLE declined the offers and went on to share the Nobel Prize in 1958; one can only conjecture whether the same result would have en-sued had BEADLE accepted one of DEMEREC's invitations and proceeded through approaches different from those used in his actual career.

DEMEREC became formally involved with the administration of the Department of Genetics of the Carnegie Institution of Washington (located, despite its name, in Cold Spring Harbor) when, in 1935, A. F. BLAKESLEE was appointed Director (previously Acting Director) and DEMEREC's appointment was changed from Investigator to Assistant Director. During this transition period, DEMEREC also served as secretary-treasurer (1935–1938), vice president (1938) and president (1939) of the Genetics Society of America.

B. P. KAUFMANN joined the Carnegie staff in 1937, rounding out the collaboration on that November 1938 paper (BAUER, DEMEREC and KAUFMANN 1938). Some 1038 induced breaks were located in euchromatic regions of Drosophila chromosomes. BAUER, one of numerous guest investigators to migrate through Cold Spring Harbor, did most or all of the described work on-site. An illustrious array of visiting researchers was to continue passing through Cold Spring Harbor (recorded in DEMEREC 1941–1960).

The introduction to the 1938 paper tells exactly what each of the coauthors contributed and goes on to mention that some of the slides of 1765 pairs of salivary glands were prepared by Mr. HERSCHEL RO-MAN who had been sent there by L. J. STADLER (ROMAN 1988) to learn a little about Drosophila. One very important aspect of the Cold Spring Harbor laboratories that was established in the DEMEREC years was a tradition of catering to bright and eager young minds.

Research on effects of X-rays and important studies on spreading of gene inactivation along the chromosome in variegated position effects (STURTEVANT 1965) kept DEMEREC occupied in the laboratory in the late 1930s. He also was active in many other areas. The first edition of DEMEREC and KAUFMANN's widely used *Drosophila Guide* appeared in 1940 and this collaboration continued through the sixth edition published in 1957. A selected set of Drosophila stocks useful in teaching was assembled and made available to high school and college biology and genetics teachers. As many as 1876 stocks were sent out per year in the late 1950s. Also, from about 1935 the laboratory maintained specialized Drosophila stocks for research workers, sending out about 300 cultures per year in the late 1940s and early 1950s (DEMEREC 1942–1960) and preserving a valuable resource used today in molecular studies. From 1939 to 1942 DEMEREC provided impetus in an attempt to secure an appointment for H. J. MULLER at the Carnegie, a move blocked by the trustees (PAUL 1988) just 4 years before MULLER was awarded a Nobel Prize.

The year 1941 saw DEMEREC, already Assistant Director at the Carnegie, become Director of the adjacent Biological Laboratory. This year also witnessed the arrival of BARBARA MCCLINTOCK to the Carnegie staff. (She was to serve as President of the Genetics Society of America in 1945. It was about this latter time when she commenced her crucial studies, initially appreciated by few, that won her a Nobel Prize in 1983.) In 1941 and extending to his retirement in 1960, DEMEREC also played a major role in organizing and supervising the Cold Spring Harbor Symposium on Quantitative Biology. For the 1941 (ninth) meeting, DEMEREC squeezed what previously had been 5-week marathons into a streamlined 2-week period so that "biologists, biophysicists and biochemists interested in the gene problem" would remain together and interact (DEMEREC 1941). Wide conjecture not only was allowed but was invited; it included physicist M. DELBRÜCK's thoughts on autocatalytic synthesis and chromosome reproduction. This and later symposia had broad visions and crossed disciplines, stimulating novel interactions and thoughts. The "CSHSQB" volumes of this era are notable for the way in which discussions were captured so that distant students might mull over the outstanding controversies. DELBRÜCK was not only invited to be a symposium speaker but also to spend the summer at Cold Spring Harbor (LURIA 1966). His driving interests, his conviction that bacteriophages were organisms of major importance in genetics (ELLIS and DELBRÜCK 1939) and his contacts with key phage workers were to have a major impact at Cold Spring Harbor.

In the latter part of 1941 DEMEREC became Acting Director and in 1943 Director of the Department of Genetics of the Carnegie, replacing A. F. BLAKESLEE who retired. This move consolidated activities of the two institutions at Cold Spring Harbor, much to the benefit of each. These two laboratories had not shared a common Director since 1923. The consolidation added to DEMEREC's duties because he quietly supervised everything from budgets to mowing the grass to maintaining aging laboratory buildings to arranging purchase of laboratory land along Bungtown Road. In those days the Director could not hire a new staff person to cover each new responsibility; he had to do much of it himself. There were also formal annual reports to be written and compiled, both for the Carnegie (DEMEREC 1942–1960) and for the Biological Laboratory (DEMEREC 1941–1960). Both reports required an introduction and synopsis as well as a résumé of ongoing research. DEMEREC's Carnegie research section includes the names of 62 people in the 19 years he was Carnegie Director; few people are listed more than 2 years in a row. This is an indication of the flow and vitality of the laboratory and the man.

He also engineered similar visits from both younger and more senior scientists through positions at the Biological Laboratory, being indirectly responsible for a high percentage of the research accomplishments of the temporary staff at Cold Spring Harbor (DEMEREC 1941–1960).

DEMEREC managed these jobs, participated in various international scientific activities (MILLER 1978) and ran a tightly supervised laboratory by carefully and systematically partitioning his day. Into the lab early, he completed a lot of scientific concentration before laboratory rounds began around 9 am, by which time everyone else was supposed to be in. As a postdoc I was asked by DEMEREC one morning why I wasn't in at 9 am. I explained that the previous day's experiments hadn't been completed until about 2 am, only to receive the reply, "*That's* no excuse!" While my story was true, I'm sure that DEMEREC had heard it before and was skeptical. And, besides, he was always excited by each new research result and was anxious to have a full and free discussion on the spot, a fine training exercise for younger scientists like me.

DEMEREC and his wife MARY constantly entertained the flow of visitors through the laboratories. But, if parties lasted too late, DEMEREC excused himself and went to bed in order to rise early the next morning. MARY and her sister VERA ZIEGLER always cordially carried on the gatherings with friends who took such a happening expectedly, or at least with good grace. MARY and VERA were teachers at a local grade school. MARY was a teacher of science who gained national recognition for her innovative, hands-on laboratory experiments in physics and in biology. I remember her excitement at obtaining beautifully colored mutant silkworm eggs. These were kindly supplied by Japanese scientists. The eggs had been pasted to white cardboard and formed letters in a striking poster at the Tenth International Congress of Genetics in Montreal. Silkworms love mulberry leaves. Thus, mulberry trees were always included among the fruit trees that were one of DEMEREC's hobbies. DEMEREC was a member of both the Organizing Committee and the Program Committee for that Tenth Congress in 1958. Much of the Congress paperwork was done at home at his card table, often set up in the middle of the living room where he could follow the day's comings and goings and visit with the family. He never seemed to be in a hurry.

The early 1940s witnessed a decided shift in DEMEREC's interests toward microorganisms as tools for genetic study. Partly this stemmed from contributions during World War II when his laboratory made a very important practical discovery: they obtained a derivative of Penicillium that would grow when submerged instead of only on the surface of liquid medium. This allowed greatly increased penicillin pro-

duction in large vats (MILLER 1978). There were also ongoing collaborations with A. HOLLAENDER, then at the National Institutes of Health, on the induction of mutations in Neurospora with X-rays and ultraviolet light. DEMEREC studied mechanisms and patterns of bacterial mutations to antibiotic resistance. Also, following the classic LURIA and DELBRÜCK (1943) paper in a November issue of GENETICS, he took up studies of mutations to bacteriophage resistance. In 1945 DELBRÜCK was a temporary member of the Biological Laboratory and initiated the phage course, an instant success that was superbly taught for a number of years by MARK H. ADAMS. This course greatly enhanced interest among young people in the new genetic system and helped to move Cold Spring Harbor to the center of microbial genetics by the mid-1950s.

The year 1946 was crucial for the two laboratories. A long-range plan for future activities was prepared at the request of V. BUSH (DEMEREC 1942–1960). This plan paved the way for further consolidation of research focus, interlaboratory collaboration, and construction of new laboratories and a lecture hall beginning in 1951. The laboratory building was later to be named after DEMEREC following his retirement. The auditorium housed the annual Symposium and other meetings in the summers and was a center for seminars and badminton in winters. The old laboratory building was converted to a library which, by the time of DEMEREC's retirement in 1960, was to hold close to 20,000 bound books focusing on genetics (DEMEREC 1942–1960). The library has served as a quiet and useful workshop for staff and numerous summer visitors.

In 1947 the first issue of *Advances in Genetics* appeared with DEMEREC as editor. His editorship continued through volume 9 (1958), after which E. W. CASPARI and J. M. THODAY took over. The first volume of *Annual Review of Genetics* was not published until 1967. Thus, for 20 years *Advances* remained the lone, key American outlet for timely reviews in genetics.

The latter 1940s saw DEMEREC's interests shift from radiations to chemical mutagens. While some of the first work was done with Drosophila (DEMEREC 1948), there was a gradual shift toward emphasis on *Escherichia coli* so that, by 1950, the DEMEREC lab was almost exclusively working with this organism. *E. coli* genetics also was the center of interest in the laboratories of E. M. WITKIN, who received a full staff appointment at the Carnegie in 1949 after several years as a Fellow, and of V. BRYSON and W. SZYBALSKI of the Biological Laboratory. The next year saw the arrival of A. D. HERSHEY at the Carnegie where he initiated the studies on phages that were to lead to a share of the Nobel Prize with M. DELBRÜCK and S. E. LURIA in 1969. In the summer of 1950, the first informal and highly successful summer course in bacterial genetics was established by DEMEREC, BRYSON and WITKIN. A short conference on bacteriophages was organized by DELBRÜCK. Also in 1950, *The Biology of Drosophila*, edited by DEMEREC, was published in its one and only edition. Supplemented more recently by various treatises, that classic still remains a valuable resource.

By 1951 DEMEREC's journey from maize and delphiniums to Drosophila to prokaryotes was complete; his scientific section of the annual reports (DEMEREC 1942–1960), which had always been entitled "The Gene," was changed in 1951 to "Bacterial Genetics." This is not to say that DEMEREC had suddenly become technique-oriented rather than problem-oriented. In fact, a final transition was to come, engendered once again by the search for the gene. Stimulated by ZINDER and LEDERBERG's (1952) description of transduction in Salmonella, DEMEREC suddenly converted his entire laboratory operation to this close cousin of *E. coli* with almost immediate success (CARLSON 1966). These studies satisfied DEMEREC's long-term goal of highly definitive analyses of gene structure. They critically complemented other work of that mini-era, studies performed with phages and fungi. Furthermore, they revealed the presence in bacteria of linkages among genes with related functions (DEMEREC *et al.* 1956). This finding was one important precursor of modern descriptions of gene function (JACOB and MONOD 1961). DEMEREC's jackpot spilled over so fast that he decided to produce a book (DEMEREC *et al.* 1956) where his work could be viewed collectively. However, a peak year of this work, 1955, saw V. BUSH, a firm backer during the DEMEREC years at Cold Spring Harbor, retire as President of the Carnegie Institution.

The mid-1950s work included contributions by several young Japanese guests, beginning with T. YURA and H. OZEKI, who were to found new schools of microbial genetics in Japan. Both F. J. RYAN at Columbia University and DEMEREC were interested in such a development. However, it is my understanding that RYAN trained bright individuals who had written to him directly and who, with the prominent exception of T. WATANABE, mostly stayed in the United States. In contrast, DEMEREC had firm contacts among more established Japanese geneticists and asked for their best students who were expected to return to their native land. DEMEREC used the same approach through the years with Yugoslavs, including D. KANAZIR, now President of the Serbian Academy of Science and Arts; unfortunately that country has not been able to mobilize and afford substantial molecular biology, although the nucleus and talent is in place.

In 1956 DEMEREC was a member of an important National Academy of Sciences Committee on the Biological Effects of Atomic Radiation. The committee, chaired by W. WEAVER, included such luminaries as G. W. BEADLE, J. F. CROW, H. B. GLASS, H. J. MULLER, A. H. STURTEVANT and S. WRIGHT. This group prepared the first major risk assessment for ionizing radiation, a prototype of more recent assessments for exposure to other agents such as chemical mutagens.

Over the next few years the DEMEREC laboratory continued to describe new bacterial genes and operons as well as to examine genetic homologies between Salmonella and *E. coli*. But at age 65, DEMEREC was facing obligatory retirement as Director in 1960, and there was no smooth transition in sight analogous to the DAVENPORT→BLAKESLEE→DEMEREC eras. Perhaps the absence of a younger leader, combined with financial constraints, led the post-BUSH Carnegie to the 1962 decision to phase out its presence at Cold Spring Harbor, supporting only those on-deck until their impending retirements. In any event, DEMEREC sought to carry on with grant support using space in the Biological Laboratory at Cold Spring Harbor. However, he was turned down at the last moment and moved to the Brookhaven National Laboratories where H. J. CURTIS was Chairman of the Department of Biology. For Cold Spring Harbor it was the end of the *zlatno doba*—the golden age—of DEMEREC.

An active laboratory immediately sprang up at Brookhaven where the Salmonella studies were continued. The second November GENETICS paper, published out of Brookhaven (DEMEREC 1963), summarizes and analyzes a wealth of data on "selfing." Selfing is the unexpected ability of transducing phage grown on particular mutants to convert the respective mutants to the wild type. Because some deletion mutants were found to be selfers, this is a phenomenon that should now be analyzed with the tools of molecular biology. Just as he had earlier helped to establish a Drosophila stock center at Cold Spring Harbor, DEMEREC now set up a similar Salmonella center at Brookhaven and initiated comprehensive reviews of Salmonella genetics (DEMEREC and SANDERSON 1965). Both ventures have been competently carried on to the present by K. E. SANDERSON. DEMEREC also set standards for nomenclature that now are almost universally used by bacterial geneticists (DEMEREC *et al.* 1956, 1966). This nomenclature is easy to understand and eliminates an almost infinite number of subscripts, superscripts, and Greek symbols.

When he reached 70 in 1965, DEMEREC again retired, only to open a new laboratory at C. W. Post College near his home in Laurel Hollow. Again an active laboratory was generated in a short amount of time, before DEMEREC quietly passed away. He died of a sudden heart attack while in his sleep in April 1966 after a full and productive day at work. At Post he had taken in three novice technicians and trained them, without help, in the ways of science and the intricacies of the bacterial genome. All three went on to Ph.D. degrees and to successful careers in biology. HERSHEY (1966) has said, "When it came to decisions of importance to research, to the laboratory, or to science at large, he seemed to call on an infallible instinct." Perhaps that's because he had an infillable instinct about honest people, upon whom all the rest depends.

LITERATURE CITED

BAUER, H., M. DEMEREC and B. P. KAUFMANN, 1938 X-ray induced chromosomal alteration in *Drosophila melanogaster*. Genetics **23**: 610–630.

CARLSON, E. A., 1966 *The Gene: A Critical History*. W. B. Saunders, Philadelphia.

CASPARI, E. W. (Editor) (1971) Milislav Demerec (1895–1966). Adv. Gen. **16**: xv–xl.

DELBRÜCK, M., 1970 A physicist's renewed look at biology: twenty years later. Science **168**: 1312–1315.

DEMEREC, M., 1933 What is a gene? J. Hered. **24**: 368–378.

DEMEREC, M., 1935 Unstable genes. Bot. Rev. **1**: 233–248.

DEMEREC, M., 1938 Eighteen years of research on the gene. Carnegie Inst. Wash. Publ. **501**: 295–314.

DEMEREC, M., 1941 Forward. Cold Spring Harbor Symp. Quant. Biol. **9**: v–vii.

DEMEREC, M., 1941–1960 Annual Report of the Biological Laboratory, Long Island Biological Laboratory, Cold Spring Harbor, N.Y.

DEMEREC, M., 1942–1960 Annual Report of the Director of the Department of Genetics. Carnegie Inst. Wash. Year Book, vols. 41–59.

DEMEREC, M., 1948 Mutations induced by carcinogens. Br. J. Cancer **2**: 114–117.

DEMEREC, M. (Editor), 1950 *The Biology of Drosophila*. John Wiley & Sons, New York.

DEMEREC, M., 1957 The Biological Laboratory, Cold Spring Harbor. Am. Inst. Biol. Sci. Bull. **7**: 20–21.

DEMEREC, M., 1963 Selfer mutants of *Salmonella typhimurium*. Genetics **48**: 1519–1531.

DEMEREC, M., and K. E. SANDERSON, 1965 The linkage map of *Salmonella typhimurium*. Genetics **51**: 897–913.

DEMEREC, M., *et al.*, 1956 *Genetic Studies With Bacteria*. Carnegie Inst. Wash. Publ. 612.

DEMEREC, M., E. A. ADELBERG, A. J. CLARK and P. E. HARTMAN, 1966 A proposal for a uniform nomenclature in bacterial genetics. Genetics **54**: 61–76.

ELLIS, E. L., and M. DELBRÜCK, 1939 The growth of bacteriophage. J. Gen. Physiol. **22**: 365–384.

GLASS, B., 1971 Milislav Demerec, January 11, 1895–April 12, 1966. Biogr. Mem. Natl. Acad. Sci. **42**: 1–27.

GLASS, H. B., 1988 M. Demerec. pp. 39–44. In: *Guide to the Genetics Collections of the American Philosophical Society*, Library Publ. #13. American Philosophical Society, Philadelphia.

HERSHEY, A. D., 1966 Milislav Demerec. Carnegie Inst. Wash. Year Book **65**: 558.

JACOB, F., AND J. MONOD, 1961 Genetic regulatory mechanisms in the synthesis of proteins. J. Mol. Biol. **3**: 381–356.

LURIA, S., 1966 Mutations of bacteria and of bacteriophage. pp. 173–179. In: *Phage and the Origins of Molecular Biology*, Edited by J. CAIRNS, G. S. STENT and J. D. WATSON. Cold Spring Harbor Laboratory of Quantitative Biology, Cold Spring Harbor, N.Y.

LURIA, S. E., and M. DELBRÜCK, 1943 Mutations of bacteria from virus sensitivity to virus resistance. Genetics **28**: 491–511.

MILLER, M., 1978 The Milislav Demerec papers at the American Philosophical Society Library. American Philosophical Society, Philadelphia.

MULLER, H. J., 1927 Artificial transmutation of the gene. Science **66**: 84–87.

PAUL, D., 1988 H. J. Muller, communism, and the cold war. Genetics **119**: 223–225.

ROMAN, H. 1988 A diamond in a desert. Genetics **119**: 739–741.

STURTEVANT, A. H., 1965 pp. 92, 142. In: *A History of Genetics*. Harper & Row, New York.

ZINDER, N. D., AND J. LEDERBERG, 1952 Genetic exchange in *Salmonella*. J. Bacteriol. **64**: 679–699.

The Hawthorne Deletion
Twenty-five Years Later

Ira Herskowitz

Department of Biochemistry and Biophysics, University of California, San Francisco, California 94143

IN a three-page paper published in GENETICS in December 1963, DON HAWTHORNE (1963a) described a simple observation concerning yeast mating types that confronted geneticists with both a paradox and a puzzle. He described a mutation, the "HAWTHORNE deletion," that affects the mating type locus of an α cell and causes the cell to exhibit the **a** mating type.

The paradox concerns the relationship between **a** and α alleles of the mating type locus. First, let us look at what was known about the mating type locus at the time. There are two alleles: $MAT\mathbf{a}$ confers the **a** cell phenotype and $MAT\alpha$ confers the α cell phenotype (LINDEGREN and LINDEGREN 1943). $MAT\mathbf{a}$ and $MAT\alpha$ are truly alleles: sporulation of a $MAT\mathbf{a}/MAT\alpha$ diploid yields two **a** and two α segregants in essentially all tetrads. ROMAN, PHILLIPS and SANDS (1955) provided the other concrete piece of information about the alleles of the mating type locus: they are codominant. They constructed diploid strains of three genotypes, $MAT\mathbf{a}/MAT\mathbf{a}$, $MAT\alpha/MAT\alpha$ and $MAT\mathbf{a}/MAT\alpha$. All three exhibited distinctive phenotypes. The $MAT\mathbf{a}/MAT\mathbf{a}$ and $MAT\alpha/MAT\alpha$ strains behaved like their haploid counterparts with respect to mating and could not sporulate. In contrast, the $MAT\mathbf{a}/MAT\alpha$ strains did not mate but could sporulate. These observations indicate that $MAT\mathbf{a}$ is not simply the absence of $MAT\alpha$ and that $MAT\alpha$ is not simply the absence of $MAT\mathbf{a}$.

Given the codominance of $MAT\alpha$ and $MAT\mathbf{a}$, HAWTHORNE's finding—that it is possible to change $MAT\alpha$ to $MAT\mathbf{a}$ by a deletion of the mating type locus—is paradoxical. We expect that deletions should remove genes and thus create recessive mutations. The paradox is how to convert an α cell to an **a** cell by a deletion when the alleles of MAT are codominant.

The puzzle concerns the ability of cells to change from one mating type to the other. α cells, by and large, give rise to progeny α cells. However, at low frequency (something like 10^{-6}), α cells can give rise to progeny that are **a**. The first report of such a change in mating type was by ROMAN and SANDS (1953). Subsequently, a "rare mating" protocol, described below, was used to identify changes in mating type. This was the approach used by HAWTHORNE to identify the deletion. In actuality, two types of changes from α to **a** are found. The first is a "simple" switch to **a** and the second (the HAWTHORNE deletion) is a switch to **a** that is accompanied by a recessive lethal mutation.

In the rare mating experiment, α cells with two auxotrophic mutations are mixed with other α cells that have complementary auxotrophic mutations. The mixed culture is allowed to incubate awhile and is then assayed for the presence of prototrophs (growth on minimal medium). One class of prototrophs is unable to mate but is able to sporulate efficiently and yields two **a** and two α segregants. These prototrophs are apparently formed by the following sequence of events: first, one of the original α cells changes its mating type to **a**; next, this **a** mates with an α cell carrying complementary mutations and forms a $MAT\mathbf{a}/MAT\alpha$ diploid able to grow on minimal medium.

The ability of strains to switch mating types is a fundamental genetic puzzle: how can cells be stably α but then switch to become stably **a**? As noted above, the frequency of the switching event is rather low. Hence, it can be suggested that the change may be due simply to a standard mutational event, for example, a base substitution. This explanation is difficult to reconcile with another remarkable aspect of the switching process: in closely related yeast strains, the switching frequency is vastly higher and cells can switch from **a** to α or from α to **a** almost every cell division (STRATHERN and HERSKOWITZ 1979). These strains carry a gene, originally termed D (for *diploidization*) and later termed HO (for *homothallism*), that catalyzes switching of mating types, and it is merely the presence or absence of HO that determines the stability of the mating type (WINGE and ROBERTS 1949; reviewed by HERSKOWITZ and OSHIMA 1981). As HAWTHORNE describes in another of his 1963 publications (HAWTHORNE 1963b), a paper even shorter than the HAWTHORNE deletion paper, strains carrying *HO* actually change the allele of the mating type locus. "Slow-motion" demonstrations of this (including segregation data) are presented by TAKANO and OSHIMA (1970), OSHIMA and TAKANO (1971), HICKS and HERSKOWITZ (1976, 1977) and STRATHERN and HERSKOWITZ (1979). The puzzle, if mutation is ruled out, is how cells switch from one *MAT* allele to the other.

In the deletion paper, HAWTHORNE (1963a) described a sporulation-proficient, nonmating prototroph that gives a striking result upon sporulation: only two of the four spores grow into colonies, the viable segregants invariably being *α*. Even though two spores could not grow into colonies, their mating types could be examined by cell-to-cell mating tests which show that both are **a**. It is these segregants that contain the HAWTHORNE deletion, a deletion on the right arm of chromosome *III*, extending from the mating type locus rightward, that removes the *THR4* locus and comes close to the *MAL2* locus. Although HAWTHORNE described only one such deletion, it is straightforward to repeat the rare mating procedure and obtain other mutants in which cells have switched from *α* to **a** by an event that creates a recessive lethal mutation (RABIN 1970; STRATHERN 1977). The lethality was presumed to result from deletion of essential genes, which has turned out to be the case.

The original explanation: Faced with the enigmas posed by the switching process and by what he termed the "**a**-lethal" mutation, HAWTHORNE explained his deletion by proposing that the mating type locus is bipartite: *MAT* contains information that is capable of conferring the *α* phenotype and information that is capable of conferring the **a** phenotype. In his words, "the mating type locus is a complex with an operator and structural cistrons for both the *α* and **a** products." The difference between **a** and *α* strains was thus a matter of which information was expressed. He imagined that the deletion removed "enough of the *α* cistron to render it inoperative while leaving the **a** portion functional."

The other end of the deletion: HAWTHORNE's explanation involved the left end of the deletion: it removed part of the mating type locus and led to activation of the **a** regulatory determinant. The ultimate explanation for HAWTHORNE's deletion required understanding the other end of the deletion. Work from laboratories in Japan, Spain and the U.S.S.R. had identified two loci, in addition to *HO*, that play important roles in the ability of yeast cells to switch mating types at high frequency (TAKANO and OSHIMA 1967; SANTA MARIA and VIDAL 1970; NAUMOV and TOLSTORUKOV 1973; HARASHIMA, NOGI and OSHIMA 1974). One of these loci is necessary for cells to switch from **a** to *α*; the other is necessary for cells to switch

from *α* to **a**. When JEFF STRATHERN, then a graduate student in my laboratory, learned about the map positions of these loci (HARASHIMA and OSHIMA 1976), several things immediately clicked into place. The new fact was that the gene necessary for switching from *α* to **a** was located on the right arm of chromosome *III*; JEFF's insight was that this gene might simply be an ordinarily silent form of the **a** mating type locus itself. HAWTHORNE's deletion caused a switch from *MATα* to *MAT***a** by deleting the information at *MATα* and activating the information at this ordinarily silent locus, which is now known as *HMR***a**.

Some immediate predictions of the cassette model: STRATHERN's explanation for the HAWTHORNE deletion was crucial in the development of the cassette model for mating type interconversion (HICKS, STRATHERN and HERSKOWITZ 1977; HICKS and HERSKOWITZ 1977). The key feature of this hypothesis is that *HMR* and *HML* contain silent versions of *MAT* information which become activated by transposition to the "playback locus," the mating type locus. This hypothesis led to many predictions, elaborations, and tests, which included the following: (1) The proposal of silent copies of mating types locus information beautifully explained a truly puzzling observation that JIM HICKS and DON HAWTHORNE had made: cells with a defective *α* mating type locus could switch from *α*⁻ to **a** and then to a perfectly functional *α* (HICKS and HERSKOWITZ 1977; D. HAWTHORNE, personal communication). (2) The proposal that *HML* and *HMR* contain silent *MAT* information led us to search for a rearrangement that could activate the ordinarily silent information at *HMLα*. R. MORTIMER and D. HAWTHORNE (personal communication) had found at least one example of a switch from **a** to *α* that was associated with a recessive lethal event. We were readily able to identify more strains of this type (STRATHERN *et al.* 1979). We imagined that one way to produce such rearrangements would be by forming a large circular derivative of chromosome *III* and were able to enlist the talents of CAROL NEWLON to look for such a circle, which she found (STRATHERN *et al.* 1979).

What we now know: Of course, the mating type locus alleles and the silent versions have now been cloned and sequenced (STRATHERN *et al.* 1980; NASMYTH and TATCHELL 1980; ASTELL *et al.* 1981). We know much about the mating type locus itself—it codes for regulatory proteins that govern transcription of other genes (STRATHERN, HICKS and HERSKOWITZ 1981; JOHNSON and HERSKOWITZ 1985; BENDER and SPRAGUE 1987). We know what *HO* does—it codes for a site-specific double-strand endonuclease that initiates mating type interconversion by cleaving the mating type locus (KOSTRIKEN *et al.* 1983; KOSTRIKEN and HEFFRON 1984). And we know the outlines of mating type interconversion—*HO* protein

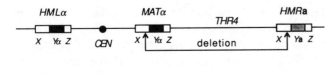

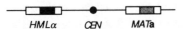

FIGURE 1.—Formation of the HAWTHORNE deletion. The diagram on the top line shows the structure, arrangement and orientation of the *HML*, *MAT* and *HMR* loci on chromosome *III* for a *MATα* cell (STRATHERN *et al.* 1980; NASMYTH and TATCHELL 1980; ASTELL *et al.* 1981). The central regions of the cassette loci—*Ya* (stippled rectangle) or *Yα* (filled rectangle)—are 642 and 747 bp, respectively. The *X* region is 707 bp and the *Z* region is 239 bp. Not drawn are additional regions of identity to the left of *HML* and *MAT* (*W*, 723 bp) and to the right of *HML* and *MAT* (*Z2*, 89 bp). The distance between *MAT* and *HML* is approximately 200 kbp (STRATHERN *et al.* 1979; NEWLON *et al.* 1986) and the distance between *MAT* and *HMR* is approximately 150 kbp (NEWLON *et al.* 1986). The HAWTHORNE deletion appears to have been formed by recombination between the *X* regions at *MATα* and *HMRa*, which results in a fusion of *MAT* and *HMR* and a deletion of the region between these loci, as shown in the lower line.

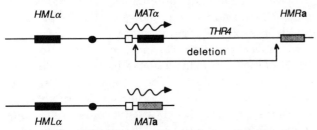

FIGURE 2.—Original proposal for activation of silent **a** cassette by the HAWTHORNE deletion. According to the original proposal (HICKS, STRATHERN and HERSKOWITZ 1977), the HAWTHORNE deletion activates the cassette at *HMRa* by hooking up the **a** cassette to an essential site (such as a promoter or ribosome binding site, drawn as an open box) present at *MAT*. This picture has been modified in two respects—the reason why cassettes at *HML* and *HMR* are silent and the orientation of transcription from mating type locus cassettes (Figure 3).

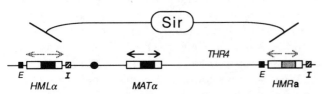

FIGURE 3.—The current view of transcription from mating type locus cassettes and how the silent cassettes are repressed. As described in the text, *MATa* and *MATα* each produce two transcripts which are initiated from the *Y* region and transcribed as indicated. Dotted lines above *HML* and *HMR* indicate the transcripts whose synthesis is blocked by action of Sir. Sir acts at sites to the left of *HML* and *HMR* (*E*, "essential" sites) and to the right of *HML* and *HMR* (*I*, "important" sites) to repress transcription from these loci.

cleaves *MAT* and this break is then healed by a repair process that copies in the information from *HML* or *HMR* (STRATHERN *et al.* 1982). The molecular details of these processes are discussed in the papers just cited and need not be reviewed here. But what I would like

to do in closing is to make a few comments about some of the original questions that were raised by HAWTHORNE's deletion and how we understand them now.

Codominance. The key observation indicating that *MATa* and *MATα* are codominant is the novel behavior of *MATa/MATα* strains, which had been interpreted to indicate that both *MAT* alleles code for distinctive products that function in these cells (see KASSIR and SIMCHEN 1976). This interpretation is fully correct: the novel properties of **a**/α cells result from the production of a novel molecular regulatory species, termed "**a**1-α2," that requires the α2 polypeptide coded by *MATα* and the **a**1 polypeptide coded by *MATa* (STRATHERN, HICKS and HERSKOWITZ 1981; KASSIR and SIMCHEN 1976). The most recent biochemical studies on **a**1-α2 are described by GOUTTE and JOHNSON (1988).

Formation of the HAWTHORNE deletion. We proposed that the HAWTHORNE deletion removes DNA to the right of *MATα* and extends to *HMRa*. Based on the structure of *MATα* and *HMRa*, it appears that the deletion resulted from recombination between tandemly repeated sequences located at *MAT* and *HMR* (STRATHERN *et al.* 1980). As shown in Figure 1, *MATα* and *HMLα* have a segment of DNA "*Yα*" that is distinct from the "*Ya*" segment present at *MATa* and *HMRa*. Flanking the *Y* regions at all three loci is an identical sequence of 707 bp, the *X* region; flanking the *Y* regions on the other side is an identical sequence of 239 bp, the *Z1* region (ASTELL *et al.* 1981). The orientations of *X*, *Y* and *Z* for all three loci (*HML*, *MAT* and *HMR*) are the same (STRATHERN *et al.* 1980). Hence, the likely explanation for formation of the HAWTHORNE deletion is simply that it resulted from recombination between directly repeated *X* sequences at *MAT* and *HMR* (Figure 1). Formation of the circular derivative of chromosome *III* can be similarly explained as recombination between directly repeated sequences to the left of *HMLα* and *MATa*.

Activation of the silent cassettes. We originally proposed that the mating type locus contains a promoter (or other essential site) that governs rightward expression of the mating type locus and that the **a** cassette at *HMRa* lacks this essential site and is thereby silent. According to this view, the HAWTHORNE deletion activates *HMRa* by hooking up its **a** cassette to the mating type locus (Figure 2). Subsequent work (KLAR *et al.* 1981; NASMYTH *et al.* 1981) showed that expression of the cassettes at *HML* and *HMR* is blocked at the transcriptional level. It turns out that the cassettes at *HML* and *HMR* are silent not because they lack an essential site but rather because they contain sites that cause them to be repressed. This repression is brought about by the Sir products of the *silent-information regulator* (*SIR*) genes (RINE and HERSKOWITZ 1987):

mutations that inactivate a *SIR* gene allow expression of the ordinarily silent cassettes. Hence, the information at *HML* and *HMR* is intact and potentially functional. Much work has been done on identifying the sites next to *HML* and *HMR* that are necessary for repression of the cassettes located at these positions (ABRAHAM *et al.* 1984; FELDMAN, HICKS and BROACH 1984; BRAND, MICKLEM and NASMYTH 1987). The most important site (the "*E*," essential, site) is located to the left of the *HML* and *HMR* loci (Figure 3): the HAWTHORNE deletion activates the information at *HMR*a by removing the *E* site.

Molecular analysis of the mating type locus has revealed a surprise about Sir and repression of the silent cassettes. Both *MAT*a and *MAT*α contain two genes (STRATHERN, HICKS and HERSKOWITZ 1981; TATCHELL *et al.* 1981). The surprise is that transcription of these genes is divergent, originating from the *Y* region and extending outward (Figure 3) (ASTELL *et al.* 1981; NASMYTH *et al.* 1981). Thus Sir exerts repression by acting downstream of the transcription initiation site in the *Y* region, more than 1400 bp from this site. One intriguing possibility is that Sir turns off the silent cassettes by condensing their DNA (BRAND *et al.* 1985; SCHNELL and RINE 1986). A biochemical attack on this problem is underway (SHORE *et al.* 1987; BUCHMAN *et al.* 1988).

We see that the HAWTHORNE deletion activates cryptic **a** information by an alteration downstream of its transcription initiation site. Insertions of retroviruses upstream or downstream of chicken c-*myc* and mouse *int*-1 proto-oncogenes can likewise activate these genes (PAYNE, BISHOP and VARMUS 1982; NUSSE *et al.* 1984). A further understanding of the HAWTHORNE deletion may shed light on such activation events. HAWTHORNE's deletion lives on.

It is a pleasure to acknowledge several stimulating conversations over the years with DON HAWTHORNE. I thank JASPER RINE and FLORA BANUETT, as well as others from my laboratory, for comments on the manuscript, and I thank TOM KING for help with the illustrations.

LITERATURE CITED

ABRAHAM, J., K. A. NASMYTH, J. N. STRATHERN, A. J. S. KLAR and J. B. HICKS, 1984 Regulation of mating-type information in yeast. Negative control requiring sequences both 5' and 3' to the regulated region. J. Mol. Biol. **176:** 307–331.

ASTELL, C. R., L. AHLSTROM-JONASSON, M. SMITH, K. TATCHELL, K. A. NASMYTH and B. D. HALL, 1981 The sequence of the DNAs coding for the mating type loci of *Saccharomyces cerevisiae.* Cell **27:** 15–23.

BENDER, A., and G. F. SPRAGUE, JR., 1987 MATα1 protein, a

yeast transcription activator, binds synergistically with a second protein to a set of cell-type-specific genes. Cell **50:** 681–691.

BRAND, A. H., G. MICKLEM and K. NASMYTH, 1987 A yeast silencer contains sequences that can promote autonomous plasmid replication and transcriptional activation. Cell **51:** 709–719.

BRAND, A. H., L. BREEDEN, J. ABRAHAM, R. STERNGLANZ and K. NASMYTH, 1985 Characterization of a "silencer" in yeast: a DNA sequence with properties opposite to those of a transcriptional enhancer. Cell **41:** 41–48.

BUCHMAN, A. R., W. J. KIMMERLEY, J. RINE and R. D. KORNBERG, 1988 Two DNA-binding factors recognize specific sequences at silencers, upstream activating sequences, autonomously replicating sequences, and telomeres in *Saccharomyces cerevisiae.* Mol. Cell. Biol. **8:** 210–225.

FELDMAN, J. B., J. B. HICKS and J. R. BROACH, 1984 Identification of sites required for repression of a silent mating type locus in yeast. J. Mol. Biol. **178:** 815–834.

GOUTTE, C., and A. D. JOHNSON, 1988 **a**1 protein alters the DNA binding specificity of α2 repressor. Cell **52:** 875–882.

HARASHIMA, S., and Y. OSHIMA, 1976 Mapping of the homothallic genes, *HM*α and *HM***a** in Saccharomyces yeasts. Genetics **84:** 437–451.

HARASHIMA, S., Y. NOGI and Y. OSHIMA, 1974 The genetic system controlling homothallism in Saccharomyces yeasts. Genetics **77:** 639–650.

HAWTHORNE, D. C., 1963a A deletion in yeast and its bearing on the structure of the mating type locus. Genetics **48:** 1727–1729.

HAWTHORNE, D. C., 1963b Directed mutation of the mating type alleles as an explanation of homothallism in yeast. Proc. 11th Intern. Congr. Genet. **1:** 34–35.

HERSKOWITZ, I., AND Y. OSHIMA, 1981 Control of cell type in *Saccharomyces cerevisiae:* mating type and mating type interconversion. pp. 181–209. In: *The Molecular Biology of the Yeast Saccharomyces: Life Cycle and Inheritance,* Edited by J. N. STRATHERN, E. W. JONES and J. R. BROACH. Cold Spring Harbor Laboratory Press, Cold Spring Harbor, N.Y.

HICKS, J. B., and I. HERSKOWITZ, 1976 Interconversion of yeast mating types. I. Direct observations of the action of the homothallism (*HO*) gene. Genetics **83:** 245–258.

HICKS, J. B., and I. HERSKOWITZ, 1977 Interconversion of yeast mating types. II. Restoration of mating ability to sterile mutants in homothallic and heterothallic strains. Genetics **85:** 373–393.

HICKS, J. B., J. N. STRATHERN and I. HERSKOWITZ, 1977 The cassette model of mating type interconversion. pp. 457–462. In: *DNA Insertion Elements, Plasmids and Episomes,* Edited by A. BUKHARI, J. SHAPIRO and S. ADHYA. Cold Spring Harbor Laboratory Press, Cold Spring Harbor, N.Y.

JOHNSON, A. D., and I. HERSKOWITZ, 1985 A repressor (*MAT*α2 product) and its operator control expression of a set of cell type specific genes in yeast. Cell **42:** 237–247.

KASSIR, Y., and G. SIMCHEN, 1976 Regulation of mating and meiosis in yeast by the mating-type region. Genetics **82:** 187–206.

KLAR, A. J. S., J. N. STRATHERN, J. R. BROACH and J. B. HICKS, 1981 Regulation of transcription in expressed and unexpressed mating type cassettes of yeast. Nature **289:** 239–244.

KOSTRIKEN, R., and F. HEFFRON, 1984 The product of the *HO* gene is a nuclease: purification and characterization of the enzyme. Cold Spring Harbor Symp. Quant. Biol. **49:** 89–96.

KOSTRIKEN, R., J. N. STRATHERN, A. J. S. KLAR, J. HICKS and F. HEFFRON, 1983 A site-specific endonuclease essential for mating-type switching in *Saccharomyces cerevisiae.* Cell **35:** 167–174.

LINDEGREN, C. C., and G. LINDEGREN, 1943 A new method for hybridizing yeast. Proc. Natl. Acad. Sci. USA **29:** 306–308.

NASMYTH, K. A., and K. TATCHELL, 1980 The structure of transposable yeast mating type loci. Cell **19:** 753–764.

NASMYTH, K. A., K. TATCHELL, B. D. HALL, C. ASTELL and M. SMITH, 1981 A position effect in the control of transcription at yeast mating type loci. Nature **289:** 244–250.

NAUMOV, G. I., and I. I. TOLSTORUKOV, 1973 Comparative genetics of yeast. X. Reidentification of mutators of mating types in Saccharomyces. Genetika **9:** 82–91.

NEWLON, C. S., R. P. GREEN, K. J. HARDEMAN, K. E. KIM, L. R. LIPSCHITZ, T. G. PALZKILL, S. SYNN and S. T. WOODY, 1986 Structure and organization of yeast chromosome III. pp. 211–223. In: *Yeast Cell Biology*, Edited by J. B. HICKS. Alan R. Liss, New York.

NUSSE, R., A. VAN OOYEN, D. COX, Y. K. T. FUNG and H. VARMUS, 1984 Mode of proviral activation of a putative mammary oncogene (*int-*1) on mouse chromosome 15. Nature **307:** 131–136.

OSHIMA, Y., and I. TAKANO, 1971 Mating types in Saccharomyces: their convertibility and homothallism. Genetics **67:** 327–335.

PAYNE, G. S., J. M. BISHOP and H. E. VARMUS, 1982 Multiple arrangements of viral DNA and an activated host oncogene (*c-myc*) in bursal lymphomas. Nature **295:** 209–213.

RABIN, M., 1970 Mating type mutations obtained from "rare matings" of cells of like mating type. M.S. thesis, University of Washington, Seattle.

RINE, J., and I. HERSKOWITZ, 1987 Four genes responsible for a position effect on expression from *HML* and *HMR* in *Saccharomyces cerevisiae*. Genetics **116:** 9–22.

ROMAN, H., and S. SANDS, 1953 Heterogeneity of clones of Saccharomyces derived from haploid ascospores. Proc. Natl. Acad. Sci. USA **39:** 171–179.

ROMAN, H., M. M. PHILLIPS and S. M. SANDS, 1955 Studies of polyploid Saccharomyces. I. Tetraploid segregation. Genetics **40:** 546–561.

SANTA MARIA, J., and D. VIDAL, 1970 Segregación anormal del "mating type" en Saccharomyces. Inst. Nac. Invest. Agron. Conf. **30:** 1–21.

SCHNELL, R., and J. RINE, 1986 A position effect on the expression of a tRNA gene mediated by the *SIR* genes in *Saccharomyces cerevisiae*. Mol. Cell Biol. **6:** 494–501.

SHORE, D., D. J. STILLMAN, A. H. BRAND and K. A. NASMYTH, 1987 Identification of silencer binding proteins from yeast: possible roles in SIR control and DNA replication. EMBO J. **6:** 461–467.

STRATHERN, J. N., 1977 Regulation of cell type in *Saccharomyces cerevisiae*. Ph.D. thesis, University of Oregon, Eugene.

STRATHERN, J. N., and I. HERSKOWITZ, 1979 Asymmetry and directionality in production of new cell types during clonal growth: the switching pattern of homothallic yeast. Cell **17:** 371–381.

STRATHERN, J., J. HICKS, and I. HERSKOWITZ, 1981 Control of cell type in yeast by the mating type locus: the α1-α2 hypothesis. J. Mol. Biol., **147:** 357–372.

STRATHERN, J. N., C. S. NEWLON, I. HERSKOWITZ and J. B. HICKS, 1979 Isolation of a circular derivative of yeast chromosome III: implications for the mechanism of mating type interconversion. Cell **18:** 309–319.

STRATHERN, J. N., E. SPATOLA, C. MCGILL and J. B. HICKS, 1980 The structure and organization of transposable mating type cassettes in *Saccharomyces cerevisiae*. Proc. Natl. Acad. Sci. USA **77:** 2839–2843.

STRATHERN, J. N., A. J. S. KLAR, J. B. HICKS, J. A. ABRAHAM, J. M. IVY, K. A. NASMYTH and C. MCGILL, 1982 Homothallic switching of yeast mating type cassettes is initiated by a double-stranded cut in the *MAT* locus. Cell **31:** 183–192.

TAKANO, I., and Y. OSHIMA, 1967 An allele specific and a complementary determinant controlling homothallism in *Saccharomyces oviformis*. Genetics **57:** 875–885.

TAKANO, I., and Y. OSHIMA, 1970 Mutational nature of an allele-specific conversion of the mating type by the homothallic gene *HOα* in Saccharomyces yeasts. Genetics **65:** 421–427.

TATCHELL, K., K. A. NASMYTH, C. ASTELL and M. SMITH, 1981 *In vitro* mutation analysis of the mating-type locus in yeast. Cell **27:** 25–35.

WINGE, Ö., and C. ROBERTS, 1949 A gene for diploidization in yeasts. C. R. Lab. Carlsberg Ser. Physiol. **24:** 341–346.

See also page 703 in Addenda et Corrigenda.

Early Worms

Jonathan Hodgkin

MRC Laboratory of Molecular Biology, Hills Road, Cambridge CB2 2QH, England

JUST over 21 years ago, in October of 1967, SYD-NEY BRENNER soaked a culture of hermaphroditic nematodes of the species *Caenorhabditis elegans* in a solution of ethyl methane sulfonate. A week later, examining their F_2 descendants, he noticed a short, "dumpy" animal among the long, thin wild-type worms. The dumpy animal was picked to a separate culture plate and allowed to produce self-progeny, which were also dumpy: it was a true-breeding mutant. The new strain was given the name E1. Crosses with the parental wild-type strain showed that the mutant phenotype was due to a single autosomal recessive mutation—in modern nomenclature, allele *e1* of the gene *dpy-1*.

BRENNER went on to analyze many other mutants, finding that they were easy to generate, assign to complementation groups and map genetically. The results of hundreds of mutagenesis experiments and crosses were meticulously recorded in rows of green files that came to occupy almost 20 feet of shelf space. This work culminated in the definitive paper he published in GENETICS 15 years ago. Thus, in a very real sense, the isolation of *e1* marks the birth of nematode genetics. Over the past two decades, research in *C. elegans* has expanded inexorably and with an increasing sense of excitement. Today, strain E1 is only the first of at least 10,000 genetic variants of *C. elegans* stored in some 70 different laboratories and studied in ever increasing detail by over 300 investigators. There seems to be no limit to the variety of problems that can be studied using *C. elegans*, and "the worm" now stands second only to Drosophila as a favorite invertebrate for geneticists.

Why should this have happened? As with so many other experimental systems, the success of *C. elegans* has been the result of both luck and design. The initial choice was dictated by certain useful properties of this species, but subsequent work revealed unforeseen advantages which have played a major role in its popularization.

The original reasons for choosing *C. elegans* were that it is small, anatomically simple and suitable for electron microscopy. It is also easy to grow and to manipulate genetically, being able to reproduce either by self-fertilization or by cross-fertilization. Despite its simplicity, it has the full range of differentiated cell types found in more complicated animals. In addition, *C. elegans* had been the subject of research by several nematologists (E. DOUGHERTY and V. NIGON in particular), so that some background knowledge was available.

Among the additional advantages was the extremely small size of the genome, about 80,000 kb (SULSTON AND BRENNER 1974). No other metazoon is known to have so little DNA. At the time the measurement was made, it was not appreciated just how useful this would prove to be. The consequences of a small genome are that the genes are correspondingly smaller, introns are fewer and shorter, gene families are smaller and repeated sequences are less numerous than in other animals. All of this makes molecular genetics—cloning, sequencing, hybridization, walking and so on—much easier and simpler than in organisms with large genomes. The small genome has also permitted a project that would be daunting in any other animal: constructing a complete physical map of the genome (COULSON *et al.* 1988). As of late 1988, this project has reached a point where 90% of the genome has been assembled into "contigs" (regions of overlapping DNA clones ranging from 50 to 4000 kb). The ultimate aim is to reduce the number of contigs (now about 250) to six, the haploid number of chromosomes.

A second fortuitous advantage has been the ability to store worms frozen in liquid nitrogen. Some nematode species do not survive freezing, or else require inconvenient freezing protocols. *C. elegans*, however, is easy to freeze (by slow cooling in dilute glycerol) and stocks that have been frozen for over 18 years can still be thawed to yield viable worms. In terms of human generations, this is the equivalent of resurrecting people from 40,000 BC. Freezing means that stocks can be maintained essentially forever without genetic alteration and at little cost. Parental lines for any given mutant should always be available and stocks that might otherwise be abandoned can be preserved on the off chance that they may later become useful (for example, the transgenic lines now being generated in great numbers).

An advantage related to the ability to freeze worms, but more to the fact that *C. elegans* genetics was founded by one man, is the single defined and universally agreed wild type, which is homozygous, permanently preserved and stable. Almost all mutant lines have a defined pedigree that traces back to this single stock. Consequently, genetic background effects can be controlled, phenotypes can always be compared to the same wild type and alterations in the DNA sequence of mutants can be referred back to the original wild-type sequence. In contrast, most other standard genetic organisms (*Escherichia coli, Saccharomyces cerevisiae*, Arabidopsis, Drosophila) do not have a single, agreed wild-type strain.

A third benefit that only gradually became clear is the superior optical qualities of *C. elegans*, which permit the transparent living worms to be examined at high resolution using Nomarski microscopy. Some nematode species of comparable size contain excess refractile material which severely limits light microscopy. Without the good optical qualities of *C. elegans*, the complete description of the somatic cell lineages (by J. E. SULSTON, H. R. HORVITZ, J. E. KIMBLE and collaborators) would have been harder or impossible to obtain. Also, laser microsurgery (developed by J. G. WHITE) would be a less powerful technique.

A final advantage that has emerged over the years has been the establishment of a group of enthusiastic and dedicated workers. All of the early genetic work was due to BRENNER, but the appeal of the system was such that more and more disciples began to accumulate. As with the mutant strains, so with the scientists: almost every worker in the field has an intellectual pedigree that traces back to a single source. Moreover, most of the early workers had a common background in either bacterial or phage genetics—especially T4, like BRENNER himself. He remarked that switching from phage to nematodes was a comfortable transition because both T4 and *C. elegans* live by eating *E. coli*, the one from the inside and the other from the outside. Scientists who had worked only on prokaryotes usually were briefly disconcerted at having to deal with a diploid organism but thereafter took to worm genetics like ducks to water.

The "phage" influence colored a lot of the early work, for example, the emphasis on powerful selections and rare events, the usefulness of conditional mutants (both temperature sensitive and suppressible nonsense) and the need for long-term storage. Not all of these influences lasted, one instance being the use of wooden toothpicks for transfers and crosses. The average toothpick, fine for picking plaques, is too blunt for manipulating individual worms less than 1 mm long, Thus, early workers spent excessive amounts of time sharpening wooden picks to a fine point with a razor blade and autoclaving them to prevent the spread of fungal and bacterial contamination. Only after some years did R. K. HERMAN introduce the now universal platinum worm pick: a wire with a flattened scoop or loop at the end, ideal for picking up worms and instantly sterilized by flaming.

There also were unsuccessful attempts to turn the worm into an honorary microbe by making it a colonial organism. Some paralyzed mutants of *C. elegans* move so little on a lawn of bacterial food that each worm plus its descendants forms a small separate mound. In principle these could be treated as colonies and replica-plated to a different medium, but in practice the idea never really worked. Perhaps if there had been more interest in developing biochemical genetics (still a neglected area of *C. elegans* research), schemes like this might have been pursued further.

It is interesting to compare the original aims of research on *C. elegans* with the present state of the field. Initially there was a strong emphasis on behavioral genetics with the hope of using mutants as a means of decoding both how the neuroanatomy is specified genetically and in turn how this neuroanatomy dictates the behavior of the animal. Several investigators were particularly interested in sensory behavior such as chemotaxis (*e.g.*, WARD 1973). Here again the prokaryotic influence was felt, in this case as a result of the beautiful work of J. ADLER on bacterial chemotaxis. Both sensory and locomotory mutants were found and studied, but it became apparent that it was going to be hard to understand them without more information on the normal development of the animal and its complete structure.

Gradually it became clear that it was both feasible and desirable to study the biology and development of the whole animal. Many research groups have tried to concentrate on one single aspect of *C. elegans* biology, but it has been striking how frequently findings in one area have affected research in another and the field as a whole has adopted a rather holistic attitude. Information and techniques have continued to accumulate steadily, so that it now seems possible that some parts of the development of this animal will be completely understood in terms of genes and proteins, the ultimate goal of molecular developmental biology.

Another early goal was to use *C. elegans* to analyze the nature of eukaryotic genes, which appeared to be disproportionately larger than prokaryotic genes. Even in this animal, there was far more DNA than seemed to be necessary. This, of course, is a problem that has been solved with the advent of molecular cloning. Introns, transposable elements, repeated sequences and large regulatory regions all contribute to the greater size of eukaryotic genomes, and the "C value paradox" has essentially vanished. However, there remain many questions about the large-scale organization and evolution of animal genomes, and the study of *C. elegans* is likely to contribute useful information on these questions. For example, it should soon be possible to use the physical map of the genome in order to ask if there is any significant long-range ordering of repeated sequences.

In some ways, the wheel has come full circle: attention is once more being focused on the construction and function of the nervous system because the tools for detailed molecular analysis of these problems are now available. At the same time, *C. elegans* will continue to be used for studying a host of other problems in genetics and in cellular, developmental and molecular biology (for a general review, see WOOD 1988). Given the appeal of the system and the fact that it is

still largely virgin territory with respect to research areas such as evolutionary genetics, population biology and physiological and biochemical genetics, we can expect to see expansion and diversification in the years to come.

See also page 703 in Addenda et Corrigenda.

LITERATURE CITED

BRENNER, S., 1974 The genetics of *Caenorhabditis elegans*. Genetics **77:** 71–94.

COULSON, A., R. WATERSTON, J. KIFF, J. SULSTON, AND Y. KOHARA, 1988 Genomic linking with yeast artificial chromosomes. Nature **235:** 184–186.

SULSTON, J. E., and S. BRENNER, 1974 The DNA of *Caenorhabditis elegans*. Genetics **77:** 95–104.

WARD, S., 1973 Chemotaxis by the nematode *Caenorhabditis elegans:* identification of attractants and the analysis of the response by use of mutants. Proc. Natl. Acad. Sci. USA **70:** 817–821.

WOOD, W. B. (Editor), 1988 *The Nematode Caenorhabditis elegans.* Cold Spring Harbor Laboratory, Cold Spring Harbor, N.Y.

February 1989

There's a Whole Lot of Shaking Going On

Barry Ganetzky

Laboratory of Genetics, University of Wisconsin–Madison, Madison, Wisconsin 53706

MOLECULAR neurobiology is a field whose time has come. Thanks to advances in recombinant DNA techniques, investigators are for the first time getting a glimpse at the molecular hardware responsible for electrical signaling in the nervous system. Considerable interest has focused on ion channels—transmembrane proteins that permit the selective permeation of particular species of ions (*e.g.*, Na^+, Ca^{2+} or K^+, depending on the channel type), thereby mediating action potentials and synaptic transmission in neurons. Until recently, the molecular details of the structure and function of these proteins were largely inaccessible. Now, by using toxins and other ligands that bind to certain types of ion channels with very high affinity and specificity, it has been possible to purify some of these proteins, obtain a partial amino acid sequence and subsequently isolate cDNAs from which the entire primary sequence has been deduced. This method has worked well for the study of several different channels, including sodium and calcium channels (see review by CATTERALL 1988). But what about those channels that cannot be readily purified? For example, potassium channels comprise a diverse group responsible for the repolarization phase of an action potential and they play major roles in determining the characteristic electrical properties of nerve and muscle. However, little is known about these channels at the protein level for lack of suitable affinity ligands for purification.

A biochemical method that can overcome some of these difficulties takes advantage of the expression of functional channels in Xenopus oocytes injected with the appropriate mRNA. Using this system it is possible, though laborious, to identify a cDNA whose transcript when injected into oocytes directs the production of the channel of interest (LÜBBERT *et al.* 1987; JULIUS *et al.* 1988).

Fortunately, genetics offers still another option. In an organism such as *Drosophila melanogaster*, mutations can be identified that disrupt the structure or function of ion channels and the corresponding genes can be cloned without any *a priori* information about

the encoded product. Another important feature that distinguishes the genetic approach from all biochemical strategies is that the analysis of mutant phenotypes can provide insight into the biological role of a particular channel type in the nervous system. For example, what are the *in vivo* consequences for the function and development of the nervous system when the activity of a particular ion channel is eliminated or altered?

The recent cloning and characterization of the Drosophila *Shaker* (*Sh*) locus represents the first successful application of this genetic strategy to the study of ion channels. The success of this approach, the demonstration that *Sh* represents a potassium channel structural gene and the surprises that fell out of these studies have therefore generated considerable excitement among neurobiologists (including many who harbored initial doubts about the potential contribution of Drosophila genetics to neurobiology).

In February of 1969, when KAPLAN and TROUT published a description in GENETICS of four behavioral mutants of *D. melanogaster* whose most distinctive phenotype was a rapid leg shaking under ether anesthesia, they could hardly have anticipated all the fanfare that would surround one of these genes 20 years later. The mutations, which were discovered fortuitously in a screen for X-linked lethals, identified three different loci: *Shaker* (*Sh*), *Hyperkinetic* (*Hk*) and *ether à go-go* (*eag*). *Hk* and *eag* represented previously undescribed genes. The first *Sh* mutation in *D. melanogaster* had been isolated earlier by CATSCH (1944) and resembled one first described by LUERS in *Drosophila funebris* (1936). However, there was little work on these mutants and the stocks appear to have been lost in the years before KAPLAN and TROUT reported their studies.

By 1969 a fledgling field fusing genetics with neurobiology was beginning to emerge in which *Sh* and related mutants would soon find a happy niche. In 1967, BENZER was charting the way by isolating behavioral mutants in Drosophila using a countercurrent apparatus. Also in Drosophila, PAK was embarking on a genetic dissection of visual transduction (PAK,

GROSSFIELD and WHITE 1969). At about the same time, ADLER (1966, 1969) was the first to employ a mutational analysis to dissect chemotaxis in bacteria. Within the next few years KUNG (1971a, b) had isolated mutations disrupting membrane excitability in Paramecium and, as discussed last month by HODGKIN (1988), BRENNER (1974) had amassed a collection of behavioral mutants in *Caenorhabditis elegans*.

Following up the isolation of the shaking mutants, IKEDA and KAPLAN (1970) pioneered the application of electrophysiological techniques to Drosophila to characterize abnormal electrical activity in the motor neurons in *Hk* mutants. Although these experiments helped to demonstrate that Drosophila was not hopelessly small for such studies, the methods were technically demanding; few if any investigators could match IKEDA's skill in penetrating the small neurons of the adult thoracic ganglion with an intracellular electrode. In another breakthrough, JAN and JAN (1976) introduced the use of the Drosophila larva for electrophysiological studies. The body wall muscles in mature third-instar larvae are large single cells that can readily be impaled with glass microelectrodes and the nerves innervating these muscles can be stimulated by an extracellular electrode. This experimental paradigm permitted more straightforward assays of electrical signaling in the Drosophila nervous system in mutant and wild-type larvae (JAN, JAN and DENNIS 1977; WU *et al.* 1978).

The first mutant analyzed was an allele of the *Sh* locus isolated in BENZER's laboratory. JAN, JAN and DENNIS (1977) demonstrated abnormally prolonged release of neurotransmitter at the larval neuromuscular junction in this mutant, owing to the failure of the nerve terminal to repolarize normally following an electrical stimulus. A variety of electrophysiological and pharmacological evidence suggested a defect in potassium channels (JAN, JAN and DENNIS 1977; TANOUYE, FERRUS and FUJITA 1981). Further experiments using more sophisticated electrophysiological methods provided direct evidence that a particular class of potassium channels (referred to as I_A channels) was altered in *Sh* mutants (SALKOFF and WYMAN 1981; WU and HAUGLAND 1985).

Phenotypic analysis of a collection of mutant alleles suggested that *Sh* was probably a structural gene for I_A potassium channels. Several alleles cause the total elimination of the A current, others a partial loss. Sh^5, isolated by KAPLAN and TROUT, is a unique allele that alters the kinetic and voltage-dependent properties of the current (SALKOFF and WYMAN 1981; WU and HAUGLAND 1985). The genetic and electrophysiological studies of *Sh* mutants thus provided a strong impetus to pursue molecular analysis of this gene.

Chromosome rearrangements that are now known to disrupt the *Sh* coding region (including an inversion and several translocations) and a *Sh* deletion provide additional information about the *Sh* phenotype (TANOUYE, FERRUS and FUJITA 1981; TIMPE and JAN 1987). Although these mutations completely eliminate the A current in muscle cells, the flies are viable when homozygous. Thus, *Sh* is not an essential gene. When heterozygous, these null mutations partially reduce I_A and produce a dominant leg-shaking phenotype. That known loss-of-function *Sh* alleles have a dominant effect on leg shaking permits the inference that the dominance or semidominance of all other *Sh* alleles with respect to this phenotype also results from complete or partial loss of function. Nonetheless, how a reduction or loss of the A current produces the leg-shaking behavior remains unexplained.

Most importantly, the chromosome rearrangements with breaks in the *Sh* region enabled precise cytological mapping of the *Sh* locus to polytene bands 16F1-4 on the *X* chromosome (TANOUYE, FERRUS and FUJITA 1981). This information proved essential for cloning *Sh*. Three groups independently cloned the genomic region containing this locus by chromosome walking using an unrelated cDNA that mapped to region 16F (KAMB, IVERSON and TANOUYE 1987; PAPAZIAN *et al.* 1987; BAUMANN *et al.* 1987). *Sh* alleles associated with chromosome rearrangements or transposon insertions were localized on the molecular map and found to span a region of about 60 kb, indicating that the *Sh* transcription unit was potentially quite large. Isolation of cDNAs from the *Sh* region confirmed this conclusion. When genomic DNA from the chromosome walk was probed with the *Sh* cDNAs, the cDNAs hybridized to portions that spanned more than 65 kb and encompassed the sites of all the *Sh* mutations that had been localized on the molecular map.

The deduced amino acid sequence left little doubt that *Sh* encoded a structural component of potassium channels (KAMB, IVERSON and TANOUYE 1987; TEMPEL *et al.* 1987; BAUMANN *et al.* 1987). The predicted protein contains six potential membrane-spanning domains, a characteristic feature of other channel proteins. Remarkably, the *Sh* protein also contains one region of high sequence similarity to the vertebrate sodium and calcium channels. This region (the "S4 domain") consists of a stretch of 22 amino acids in which positively charged arginine residues are spaced at every third position and are separated by hydrophobic residues. It has previously been suggested that the S4 domains represent the voltage sensors by which the sodium and calcium channels respond to voltage changes across the membrane (see review by CATTERALL 1988). The discovery that potassium channels share this motif with sodium and calcium channels supports the notion that all voltage-dependent ion channels share a common mechanism of activation as well as a common evolutionary origin, as originally proposed by HILLE (1984). One important distinction between the *Sh* protein *vs.* sodium and calcium channels is that the latter comprise four internally homologous domains each containing six apparent membrane spanning regions (see review by CATTERALL 1988). In contrast, the *Sh* product does not contain these internally duplicated regions and appears to correspond to just a single homology unit of the sodium or calcium channel polypeptides. Proof that *Sh* cDNAs encode a potassium channel was provided by the demonstration that expression of these cDNAs in Xenopus oocytes results in the production of a voltage-dependent potassium current with appropriate kinetic and voltage-dependent properties (TIMPE *et al.* 1988; IVERSON *et al.* 1988).

Perhaps the most surprising result is the discovery that differential splicing of the primary *Sh* transcript apparently generates at least ten, and perhaps more, distinct products (SCHWARZ *et al.* 1988; KAMB, TSENG-CRANK and TANOUYE 1988; PONGS *et al.* 1988). The general pattern consists of variable 3′ and 5′ ends spliced onto a constant central portion (which contains all the membrane-spanning regions) to yield distinct cDNAs encoding different but functionally related proteins. Several of these cDNAs have been individually expressed in Xenopus oocytes and each gives rise to an I_A-type potassium current but with somewhat different physiological properties (TIMPE *et al.* 1988; IVERSON *et al.* 1988). It thus appears that alternative splicing is one mechanism generating the diversity of potassium channels in the nervous system.

It remains unknown when and where these potentially different forms of *Sh* protein are expressed *in vivo* and whether they each subserve distinct biological roles. Also unknown is the subunit composition of I_A channels *in vivo*. Because the *Sh* products, in contrast to sodium and calcium channels, do not contain four repeat segments within the same polypeptide, it is likely that a multimeric (perhaps tetrameric) assembly of polypeptide subunits is required to produce functional I_A channels. Whether such a multi-subunit assembly is homomultimeric or heteromultimeric in composition remains to be determined.

The *Sh* cDNAs have also provided the first molecular probes for potassium channel genes in vertebrate organisms. By screening with a probe derived from a *Sh* cDNA, TEMPLE, JAN and JAN (1988) isolated a cDNA from mouse brain that specified an amino acid sequence very similar to that of the *Sh* protein. Similarly, five cDNAs, which have distinct but closely related nucleotide sequences and apparently represent different genes, were isolated from rat brain on the basis of their homology to *Sh* probes (A. BAUMANN and O. PONGS, personal communication). The amino acid sequences specified by these cDNAs show remarkably high conservation to each other and to the

Sh protein. So far there is no evidence that the transcripts from any of these mammalian genes undergo alternative processing to generate a number of distinct products, as occurs with *Sh*. One possibility is that the diversity of I_A channels in mammalian systems is generated by a large multigene family rather than by multiple products from one or a few genes.

Although they have yet to achieve the superstar status of *Sh*, the other loci identified by KAPLAN and TROUT are also proving to be interesting. Electrophysiological studies of *eag* (WU *et al.* 1983; GANETZKY and WU 1983) and *Hk* (STERN and GANETZKY 1989) indicate that they, too, disrupt potassium currents, leading to neuronal hyperexcitability. Molecular analysis of these loci is now in progress (R. DRYSDALE, K. SCHLIMGEN and B. GANETZKY, unpublished data) and should further advance our understanding of potassium channels in Drosophila and other organisms.

In the opening paragraph of their paper, KAPLAN and TROUT remark that the leg-shaking mutants were recovered serendipitously. Serendipity in this case was probably essential because it is doubtful that anyone back in 1969 would have thought to screen deliberately for so peculiar a mutant phenotype. Yet, it is to their credit that KAPLAN and TROUT were sufficiently observant to notice these mutants while looking for something else and sufficiently prescient to recognize their potential importance. Were it not for the attention they drew to their funny flies, we might still have no idea what a potassium channel looks like or how to get our hands on one.

LITERATURE CITED

ADLER, J., 1966   Chemotaxis in bacteria. Science **153**: 708–716.

ADLER, J., 1969   Chemoreceptors in bacteria. Science **166**: 1588–1597.

BAUMANN, A., I, KRAH-JENTGENS, R. MULLER, F. MULLER-HOLT-KAMP, R. SEIDEL, N. KECSKEMETHY, J. CASAL, A. FERRUS and O. PONGS, 1987   Molecular organization of the maternal effect region of the *Shaker* complex of Drosophila: characterization of an I_A channel transcript with homology to vertebrate Na^+ channel. EMBO J. **6**: 3419–3429.

BENZER, S., 1967   Behavioral mutants of Drosophila isolated by countercurrent distribution. Proc. Natl. Acad. Sci. USA **58**: 1112–1119.

BRENNER, S., 1974   The genetics of *Caenorhabditis elegans*. Genetics **77**: 71–94.

CATSCH, A., 1944   Eine erbliche Störung des Bewegungsmechanismus bei *Drosophila melanogaster*. Z. Indukt. Abstammungs Verebungsl. **82**: 64–66.

CATTERALL, W. A., 1988   Structure and function of voltage-sensitive ion channels. Science **242**: 50–61.

GANETZKY, B., and C.-F. WU, 1983 Neurogenetic analysis of potassium currents in Drosophila: synergistic effects on neuromuscular transmission in double mutants. J. Neurogenet. **1:** 17–28.

HILLE, B., 1984 *Ionic Channels of Excitable Membranes.* Sinauer, Sunderland, Mass.

HODGKIN, J., 1988 Early worms. Genetics **121:** 1–3.

IKEDA, K., and W. D. KAPLAN, 1970 Patterned neural activity of a mutant *Drosophila melanogaster.* Proc. Natl. Acad. Sci. USA **66:** 765–772.

IVERSON, L. E., M. A. TANOUYE, H. A. LESTER, N. DAVIDSON and B. RUDY, 1988 A-type potassium channels expressed from *Shaker* locus cDNAs. Proc. Natl. Acad. Sci. USA **85:** 5723–5728.

JAN, L. Y., and Y. N. JAN, 1976 Properties of the larval neuromuscular junction in *Drosophila melanogaster.* J. Physiol. **262:** 189–214.

JAN, Y. N., L. Y. JAN and M. J. DENNIS, 1977 Two mutations of synaptic transmission in Drosophila. Proc. R. Soc. London Ser. B **198:** 87–108.

JULIUS, D., A. B. MacDERMOTT, R. AXEL and T. M. JESSELL, 1988 Molecular characterization of a functional cDNA encoding the serotonin 1c receptor. Science **241:** 558–564.

KAMB, A., L. E. IVERSON and M. A. TANOUYE, 1987 Molecular characterization of *Shaker,* a Drosophila gene that encodes a potassium channel. Cell **50:** 405–413.

KAMB, A., J. TSENG-CRANK and M. A. TANOUYE, 1988 Multiple products of the Drosophila Sh gene may contribute to potassium channel diversity. Neuron **1:** 421–430.

KAPLAN, W. D., and W. E. TROUT III, 1969 The behavior of four neurological mutants of Drosophila. Genetics **61:** 399–409.

KUNG, C., 1971a Genic mutations with altered system of excitation in *Paramecium aurelia.* I. Phenotypes of the behavioral mutants. Z. Vergl. Physiol. **71:** 142–164.

KUNG, C., 1971b Genic mutations with altered system of excitation in *Paramecium aurelia.* II. Mutagenesis, screening and genetic analysis of the mutants. Genetics **69:** 29–45.

LÜBBERT, H., B. J. HOFFMAN, T. P. SNUTCH, T. VAN DYKE, A. J. LEVINE, P. R. HARTIG, H. A. LESTER and N. DAVIDSON, 1987 cDNA cloning of a serotonin 5-HT$_{1c}$ receptor by electrophysiological assays of mRNA-injected *Xenopus* oocytes. Proc. Natl. Acad. Sci. USA **84:** 4332–4336.

LUERS, H., 1936 *Shaker,* eine erbliche Bewegungsstorung bei *Drosophila funebris.* Z. Indukt. Abstammungs Verebungsl. **72:** 119–126.

PAK, W. L., J. GROSSFIELD, and N. V. WHITE, 1969 Non-

phototactic mutants in a study of vision in Drosophila. Nature **222:** 351–354.

PAPAZIAN, D. M., T. L. SCHWARZ, B. L. TEMPEL, Y. N. JAN and L. Y. JAN, 1987 Cloning of genomic and complementary DNA from *Shaker,* a putative potassium channel gene from Drosophila. Science **237:** 749–753.

PONGS, O., N. KECSKEMETHY, R. MULLER, I. KRAH-JENTJENS, A. BAUMANN, H. H. KILTZ, I. CANAL, S. LLAMAZARES and A. FERRUS, 1988 *Shaker* encodes a family of putative potassium channel proteins in the nervous system of Drosophila. EMBO J. **7:** 1087–1096.

SALKOFF, L., and R. WYMAN, 1981 Genetic modification of potassium channels in Drosophila *Shaker* mutants. Nature **293:** 228–230.

SCHWARZ, T. L., B. L. TEMPEL, D. M. PAPAZIAN, Y. N. JAN and L. Y. JAN, 1988 Multiple potassium-channel components are produced by alternative splicing at the *Shaker* locus in Drosophila. Nature **331:** 137–142.

STERN, M. J., and B. GANETZKY, 1989 Altered synaptic transmission in Drosophila hyperkinetic mutants. J. Neurogenet. In press.

TANOUYE, M. A., A. FERRUS and S. FUJITA, 1981 Abnormal action potentials associated with the *Shaker* complex locus of Drosophila. Proc. Natl. Acad. Sci. USA **78:** 6548–6552.

TEMPEL, B. L., Y. N. JAN and L. Y. JAN, 1988 Cloning of a probable potassium channel from mouse brain. Nature **332:** 837–839.

TEMPEL, B. L., D. M. PAPAZIAN, T. L. SCHWARZ, Y. N. JAN, and L. Y. JAN, 1987 Sequence of a probable potassium channel component encoded at the *Shaker* locus of Drosophila. Science **237:** 770–774.

TIMPE, L. C., and L. Y. JAN, 1987 Gene dosage and complementation analysis of the *Shaker* locus in Drosophila. J. Neurosci. **7:** 1307–1317.

TIMPE, L. C., T. L. SCHWARZ, B. L. TEMPEL, D. M. PAPAZIAN, Y., N. JAN and L. Y. JAN, 1988 Expression of functional potassium channels from *Shaker* cDNA in Xenopus oocytes. Nature **331:** 143–145.

WU, C.-F., and F. HAUGLAND, 1985 Voltage-clamp analysis of membrane currents in larval muscle fibers of Drosophila: alteration of potassium currents in *Shaker* mutants. J. Neurosci. **5:** 2626–2640.

WU, C.-F., B. GANETZKY, Y. N. JAN, L. Y. JAN and S. BENZER, 1978 A Drosophila mutant with a temperature-sensitive block in nerve conduction. Proc. Natl. Acad. Sci. USA **75:** 4047–4051.

WU, C.-F., B. GANETZKY, F. HAUGLAND and N. LIU, 1983 Potassium currents in Drosophila: different components affected by mutations in two genes. Science **220:** 1076–1078.

See also page 703 in Addenda et Corrigenda.

March 1989

Replica Plating and Indirect Selection of Bacterial Mutants
Isolation of Preadaptive Mutants in Bacteria by Sib Selection

Joshua Lederberg

The Rockefeller University, New York, New York 10021

HISTORICALLY and conceptually, the two themes in these titles (LEDERBERG and LEDERBERG 1952; CAVALLI-SFORZA and LEDERBERG 1956) are complexly intertwined. *Replica plating* is a homely methodology to ease the technical burdens of screening large numbers of bacterial colonies for mutants to use in genetic analysis. This was sometimes easy. For example, phage or drug resistance could be readily obtained with positive selection using phage or a drug, respectively. But many other kinds of mutants were desired, and replica plating facilitated their discovery. Furthermore, the broader philosophical question remained open, whether the resistance was a preadaptive or a postadaptive change: did it emerge by natural selection of rare preexisting mutants or did the agent somehow induce the heritable change? I elaborate first on this second broader question and its resolution by *indirect (sib) selection*.

LURIA and DELBRÜCK (1943) introduced a carefully thought out quantitative kinetics into the study of bacterial mutation. The jackpot theory (LURIA 1984) was a consequence of clonal expansion. Spontaneous mutations, in a culture started from a small inoculum, would occur rarely among the few cells present at early stages of exponential growth. But when this happened they would have a disproportionate number of mutant offspring. Hence, while the distribution of mutational *events* should follow a Poisson distribution over a series of similar cultures, the distribution of mutant *cells* would show occasional jackpots. Uncited by and perhaps unknown to LURIA and DELBRÜCK, YANG and BRUCE WHITE (1934) had previously noted such fluctuations and remarked that they signified the spontaneous occurrence of "rough" mutants in Shigella.

Nevertheless, the theoretical rigor of LURIA and DELBRÜCK's analysis and its concurrence with the quantitative data were for many the decisive stimulus to look seriously at mutation in bacteria, to think about a bacterial genetics. In my own development, this paper was one of the key impulses to inquire about genetic recombination in bacteria (LEDERBERG 1987).

By 1950 it was no longer controversial among geneticists. *Pace* periodic selection, the monotonic increase of mutant number with time in long-term chemostat cultures observed by NOVICK and SZILARD (1950) sealed lacunae in the 1943 experiments. (Otherwise, one could have entertained some labored hypothetical alternatives like uncontrolled environmental variation from tube to tube, or a subset of that: temporal fluctuations within a culture in its overall propensity to turn resistant on exposure to a selective agent.) Nevertheless, many, perhaps most, readers of the 1943 article did not understand its abstruse mathematical argument and would respond either with uncritical acceptance or uncritical rejection. Notable for the latter, the last holdout, was the prestigious Sir CYRIL HINSHELWOOD, President of the Royal Society of London, who denounced every assertion of genes in bacteria in favor of an extended reaction network model of biological continuity and adaptivity (HINSHELWOOD 1946; DEAN and HINSHELWOOD 1957). As inappropriate as these network models have proven to be for the fundamental elements of genetic structure, they have been revived for the explanation of developmental switches, where one gene product reinforces its own synthesis and represses an alternative gene's and *vice versa* (DELBRÜCK 1949; PTASHNE 1986).

Meanwhile, bacterial genetics had grown to the point of needing ever larger libraries of mutants, most of which bore biochemical defects and were not readily amenable to positive selection. Today we apply many ingenious tricks to this game (VINOPAL 1987). In 1948, the penicillin method (LEDERBERG and ZINDER 1948; DAVIS 1948) partly answered this need by selectively killing cells actively growing in minimal medium. Penicillin could exert positive selection in favor of auxotrophic mutants. But many bacterial strains were relatively recalcitrant to the feeble mutagens than available, and even after penicillin selection there was still the tedious task of screening thousands of colonies for the 1% or so that might be growth-factor dependent. In addition, the escalation of recombination studies imposed the equally tedious task of classifying vast numbers of individual recombinant colonies to score them on a series of growth factors, sugars, drugs and bacteriophages. For the first several years of my work at the University of Wisconsin, starting in the fall of 1947, I was deeply preoccupied with these technical and doctrinal issues and eager to follow other leads.

L. SZILARD and A. NOVICK, at the University of Chicago, faced similar problems in scoring the phenotypes of an abundance of colonies. In February 1951, at one of the monthly phage seminars that SZILARD had organized, they remarked that they had been using multipronged inoculators, even a wire brush, for a primitive kind of what I later called replica plating (NOVICK 1972). This was not very satisfactory owing to the poor resolution available with that material.

For a couple of years prior to that point, possibly as the result of a serendipitous accident, it had been common practice in our laboratory to make impressions of the dark and light colonies on eosin-methylene blue agar plates simply by pressing a piece of paper onto the agar surface and then mounting this under cellulose tape in our laboratory notebooks. This was far more convenient and cheaper than photography for retaining a permanent record of the actual colony distribution when this was manifest in a pigment difference. We had the idea of trying to use such prints as inocula for fresh plates, but there was far too much smearing on the paper to allow this to be useful (as was also found by N. VISCONTI at the Cold Spring Harbor Laboratory). (Have no fear about the biological hazard in these notebooks: we have never been able, alas, to recover viable organisms from these impressions, and we do not advocate such a procedure for spore formers or pathogens. Even so, this practice is probably disallowed under present-day regulations.)

Meanwhile, HOWARD NEWCOMBE (1949) evoked a still more graphic image of the clonal expansion of spontaneous mutants. Allowing a lawn of bacterial growth on an agar surface, he would count the number of mutational events by directly spraying the mature plate with phage. Each individual resistant cell, or the clone clustered around it, would be scored as a single colony. However, if the plate were respread prior to selection, there was always a substantial increase in the number of mutant colonies: this was a direct translation of the clonal expansion of the individual mutational stem cells. Sometime thereafter, I elaborated on his experiment by making a single streak of growth rather than a two-dimensional lawn. I would then move a spreader perpendicular to the stroke, and each clone would then be represented by a line of resistant colonies along the direction of the second stroke. These findings engendered still more intense preoccupation with the imagery of what was happening to mutant clones buried within the bacterial population. If only there were some constructive method to sample those clones prior to exposing them to the selective agent!

Perhaps the multipoint sampling technology of NOVICK and SZILARD could be applied to this broader problem as well as to the tedium of colony scoring! But: how to improve upon the poor resolution and handling properties of the wire brush? ED TATUM had taught me to use a beakerful of sterilized tooth picks, one by one, for colony picking; that saved the time needed to flame a platinum loop between picks. The brush was conceptually an ordered array of tooth-picks. What might be a functional equivalent?

Paper was unsatisfactory: its lateral capillarity and its compression of the colonies distorted and broke up the original growth pattern. It occurred to me that some fabric with a vertical pile would be an analog of the paper on one hand and the wire brush on the other, and I soon collected a wide variety of remnants from the local dry goods shops to put them to empirical tests. (The predictable myth that I invaded my wife's wardrobe for this purpose is pure fantasy.) Also helpful were books on fabric structure (like STRONG 1947) which helped me to focus on cotton velveteen as the most desirable material. (Nylon velvets were then far more expensive and their stiffer fibers caused some problems.) The cotton velveteen has become quite standardized and the material can, if necessary, be conveniently laundered and resterilized for repeated use. The experimental trials soon confirmed that one could rapidly enrich the proportion of resistant mutants by fishing the growth at the point on the original plate where a replica demonstrated the presence of a resistant clone. Without difficulty, one can exclude about 99% of the irrelevant growth on a bacterial lawn, which offers the prospect of a 100-fold enrichment at every cycle. This means that one can achieve a pure culture of resistant organisms in three or four cycles based on selection applied to the sibling clones that have been exposed to the selective agent. This procedure thus accomplished a constructive proof that had been so long elusive, namely, the preadaptive initiation of these rare resistant mutant clones. One can argue that this need never have been in doubt, but here for the first time was a general procedure that could be applied to any such problematical situation.

JAMES CROW, my colleague in the Wisconsin Genetics Department, enjoyed being able to analogize bacterial indirect selection with sibling selection as practiced in dairy and poultry husbandry. Bulls and roosters are selected by indices of milk and egg production by their sisters and daughters (LUSH 1945). At a time when the genetic basis of altruism is in question (MICHOD 1982), we can reflex on a system whereby replica-platefuls of clones, sensitive and resistant alike, were relegated to the autoclave once they had given the locational cues for their indirectly selected cousins.

As satisfying as this demonstration was, I lamented that it depended on a new technology (that of replica plating). An Euclidean bent has always led me to seek for proofs that came closer to the use of nothing more than a straight edge and a compass. Furthermore, it was difficult to quantitate the progress of indirect selection on agar plates. It was difficult to maintain rigorous control over the proportion of cells that were transferred during replica plating or the proportion that could be plucked by going back to the source plate. There was no reason, I thought, that the same methodology could not be used with an array of test tubes taking the place of the agar plate, with pipettes transferring well defined volumes from tube to tube in place of the velvet transfer. This was the burden of CAVALLI-SFORZA and LEDERBERG (1956): during one of several visits to our laboratory, CAVALLI took an interest in following the quantitative aspects of selection using that methodology. If one starts, say, with 100 tubes so adjusted that a mutational event will have occurred in only one of them, one can find out which tube that was by testing a sample of each for drug resistance. Discarding the other 99 tubes would in principle then give a 100-fold enrichment of the proportion of mutant cells within that tube compared to the overall population. Then one knows what dilution to make of the culture in that tube for a second cycle of inocula and can recycle from there with progressive enrichment. CAVALLI found that this procedure worked very well, although this progress of selection was often not as rapid as predicted by the first-order theory. This could be explained by the observed growth lags of the resistant mutants and thus offers no great problem.

Replica plating has grown into a major industry, its progeny including the various blots around the compass—Northern, Southern, etc.—as well as its direct application to a number of microbiological problems. Sib selection by serial dilution has been used in several genetic engineering enterprises where a special producing clone is a needle in the haystack but its products can be sensitively detected (KEDES et al. 1975; NAGATA et al. 1980).

A 1989 perspective on postadaptive mutation: The concept of the gene as immutable in the course of hereditary transmission (MORGAN 1926) was an idealization that played a constructive role in the emergence of Mendelian genetics. As HALDANE (1949)

pointed out, this view taken to an extreme contradicts the understanding of the gene as a material substance (we would now say as DNA). We must have an open mind about evolutionary specializations where metabolic alterations can target the DNA itself. This might sometimes lead to postadaptations, that is, adaptive genetic changes specifically induced by an environmental stress. As specialized evolutionary developments, one does not expect them to be a routine occurrence. They have been hard to find and authenticate, with one generic exception: lysogenizing viruses typically confer immunity to the lytic function of the virus, a subset of lysogenic inductions (HERSHEY 1971; PTASHNE 1986). The frequency of "processed pseudogenes" in eukaryotic genomes is particular testimony to a history of RNA insertions (see pp. 448ff. in DARNELL, LODISH and BALTIMORE 1986). With site-directed mutagenesis we know today how to expose, or even directly use, DNA sequences so as to achieve mutation by intelligent design.

To turn to less specific responses, mutational storms hypothetically related to insertional transposons may also be mediated by RNA in train of environmental stress (MCDONALD 1983). In addition, contemporary with the development of replica plating, my own laboratory had concluded that UV mutagenesis was probably a secondary physiological response during recovery and DNA repair (LEDERBERG et al. 1951). We know now how environmental DNA damage can evoke the "SOS" response (WALKER 1987) leading to several categories of genetic instability. One could argue that UV resistance was a postadaptive mutation, but this is to ignore the broad-ranging nonspecificity of the mutations that occur during the SOS response.

It is too early to answer many questions that have been raised during the past few months about postadaptive mutational responses claimed to occur in glycosidase-deficient *Escherichia coli* mutants incubated in the presence of lactose or salicin (CAIRNS, OVERBAUGH and MILLER 1988; CAIRNS et al. 1988; HALL 1988). There are many pitfalls in the exclusion of artefacts in mutagenesis experiments (LEDERBERG 1948) and each has entrapped unwary investigators in the course of microbial genetics. Such artefacts aside, cells starved for carbon but receiving a trickle of nutrient through spontaneous or allospecific enzymatic hydrolysis of the substrate are in a metabolic state that requires critical examination. As a reducing sugar, unmetabolized lactose might well be expected to react with the DNA of such mutants (LEE 1987). Even if it should be verified that lactose is a mutagen for *lac⁻* mutants, its specificity, *i.e.*, lactose at the *lac* locus *vs.* salicin at the *bgl* locus in a common genetic background, should be corroborated before further evolutionary speculation.

Specific DNA alterations are achieving higher credibility in a role in epigenesis, in reaction against long-held dogmas of the uniformity of the genome of somatic cells (LEDERBERG 1958). Segmental DNA excisions responding to an environmentally induced, site-specific DNA recombinase are associated with terminal heterocyst differentiation in Anabaena (HASELKORN et al. 1987). A similar story has just been reported for the terminal differentiation of the mother cell during sporulation in *Bacillus subtilis* (STRAGIER et al. 1989).

In microbial genetics, two other phenomena also fit the paradigm of directed mutation. Bacteria can be cured of many plasmids under the influence of acridine dyes (HIROTA 1960) or other chemical and physical agents (TREVORS 1986). Acridine dyes alter mitochondria in yeast and also remove kinetoplasts from trypanosomes, and streptomycin ablates chloroplasts from Euglena and other green plants (reviewed in LEDERBERG 1952). Acridine sensitivity of bacterial plasmids depends on the presence of specific DNA sequences (WECHSLER and KLINE 1980). LEDERBERG and ST. CLAIR (1958) showed that *E. coli* cells could be converted *en masse* into spheroplasts with penicillin in hypertonic media, and that these spheroplasts could be propagated as wall-deficient clones in agar but promptly reverted in the absence of penicillin. LANDMAN (1968) has reported, however, that wall-deficient "L forms" of *B. subtilis* induced by lysozyme were clonally propagated as L-forms in the absence of lysozyme, although they would revert in solid media. This is evidently an extranucleic event and deserves further study as a unique instance in bacteria of morphogenetic continuity of a cytoplasmic organelle, so long the focus of study in the genetics of Paramecium (SAPP 1987).

These exceptions notwithstanding, reinforcing the Darwinian model of adaptive resistance mutation in bacteria bolstered the eventual discard of instructional theories of induced enzyme formation (MONOD 1956, 1966) and antibody formation (LEDERBERG 1989). Any heuristic can be treacherous, but a Darwinian explanation is the first I would seek in explaining a biological enigma. I do not insist that it will always be the last, but it has had enormous power in bringing us to our present understanding.

LITERATURE CITED

CAIRNS, J., J. OVERBAUGH and S. MILLER, 1988 The origin of mutants. Nature **335:** 142–145.

CAIRNS, J., et al., 1988 Origin of mutants disputed. (Correspondence of several authors pertaining to CAIRNS, OVERBAUGH and MILLER 1988). Nature **336:** 525–528.

CAVALLI-SFORZA, L. L., and J. LEDERBERG, 1956 Isolation of preadaptive mutants in bacteria by sib selection. Genetics **41:** 367–381.

DARNELL, J., H. LODISH and D. BALTIMORE, 1986 *Molecular Cell Biology*. Scientific American Books, New York.

DAVIS, B. D, 1948 Isolation of biochemically deficient mutants of bacteria by penicillin. J. Am. Chem. Soc. **70:** 4267.

DEAN, A. C. R., and C. HINSHELWOOD, 1957 Aspects of the problem of drug resistance in bacteria, pp. 4–24 in *Drug Resistance in Micro-Organisms* (Ciba Foundation Symposium), edited by G. E. W. WOLSTENHOLME and C. M. O'CONNOR. J. & A Churchill, London.

DELBRÜCK, M., 1949 Enzyme systems with alternative steady states, pp. 33-4 in *Unités Biologiques Douées de Continuité Génétique* (International Symposium CNRS No. 8). Editions du CNRS, Paris.

HALDANE, J. B. S., 1949 In defence of genetics. Mod. Q. **4:** 194–202.

HALL, B. G., 1988 Adaptive evolution that requires multiple spontaneous mutations. I. Mutations involving an insertion sequence. Genetics **120:** 887–897.

HASELKORN, R., J. W. GOLDEN, P. J. LAMMERS and M. E. MULLIGAN, 1987 Rearrangement of *nif* genes during cyanobacterial heterocyst differentiation. Phil. Trans. R. Soc. **B 317:** 173–181.

HERSHEY, A. D. (Editor), 1971 *The Bacteriophage Lambda*. Cold Spring Harbor Laboratory, Cold Spring Harbor, N.Y.

HINSHELWOOD, C. N., 1946 *The Chemical Kinetics of the Bacterial Cell*. Clarendon Press, Oxford.

HIROTA, Y., 1960 The effect of acridine dyes on mating type factors in *Escherichia coli*. Proc. Natl. Acad. Sci. USA **46:** 57–64.

KEDES, L. H., A. C. Y. CHANG, D. HOUSEMAN and S. N. COHEN, 1975. Isolation of histone genes from unfractionated sea urchin DNA by subculture cloning in *E. coli*. Nature **255:** 533–538.

LANDMAN, O. E., 1968 Protoplasts, spheroplasts and L-forms viewed as a genetic system, pp. 319–332 in *Microbial Protoplasts, Spheroplasts and L-Forms*, edited by L. B. GUZE. Williams & Wilkins, Baltimore.

LEDERBERG, J., 1948 Problems in microbial genetics. Heredity **2:** 145–198.

LEDERBERG, J., 1952 Cell genetics and hereditary symbiosis. Physiol. Rev. **32:** 403–430.

LEDERBERG, J., 1958 Genetic approaches to somatic cell variation: summary comment. J. Cell. Comp. Physiol. **1:** 383–402.

LEDERBERG, J., 1987 Perspectives: gene recombination and linked segregations in *Escherichia coli*. Genetics **117:** 1–4.

LEDERBERG, J., 1989 Reflections on Darwin and Ehrlich: the ontogeny of the clonal selection theory of antibody formation. Ann. NY Acad Sci. (in press).

LEDERBERG, J., and E. M. LEDERBERG, 1952 Replication plating and indirect selection of bacterial mutants. J. Bacteriol. **63:** 399–406.

LEDERBERG, J., and J. ST. CLAIR, 1958 Protoplasts and L-type growth of *Escherichia coli*. J. Bacteriol. **75:** 143–160.

LEDERBERG, J., and N. D. ZINDER, 1948 Concentration of biochemical mutants of bacteria with penicillin. J. Am. Chem. Soc. **70:** 4267–4268.

LEDERBERG, J., E. M. LEDERBERG, N. D. ZINDER and E. R. LIVELY, 1951 Recombination analysis of bacterial heredity. Cold Spring Harbor Symp. Quant. Biol. **16:** 413–443.

LEE, A. T., 1987 The nonenzymatic glycosylation of DNA by reducing sugars in vivo may contribute to the DNA damage associated with aging. Age **10:** 150–155.

LURIA, S. E., 1984 *A Slot Machine, a Broken Test Tube: an Autobiography*. Harper & Row, New York.

LURIA, S. E., and M. DELBRÜCK, 1943 Mutations of bacteria from virus sensitivity to virus resistance. Genetics **28:** 491–511.

LUSH, J. L., 1945   *Animal Breeding Plans*, Ed. 3. Iowa State College Press, Ames.

McDONALD, J. F., 1983   The molecular basis of adaptation. A critical review of relevant ideas and observations. Annu. Rev. Ecol. Syst. **14:** 77–102.

MICHOD, R. E., 1982   The theory of kin selection. Annu. Rev. Ecol. Syst. **13:** 23–55.

MONOD, J., 1956   Remarks on the mechanism of enzyme induction, pp. 7–28 in *Enzymes: Units of Biological Structure and Function*, edited by O. H. GAEBLER. Academic Press, New York.

MONOD, J., 1966   From enzymatic adaptation to allosteric transitions. Science **154:** 465–483.

MORGAN, T. H., 1926   *The Theory of the Gene.* Yale University Press, New Haven, Conn.

NAGATA, S., H. TAIRA, A. HALL, L. JOHNSRUD, M. STREULI, J. ECSODI, W. BOLL, K. CANTELL and C. WEISSMANN, 1980   Synthesis in *E. coli* of a polypeptide with human leukocyte interferon activity. Nature **284:** 316–320.

NEWCOMBE, H. B., 1949   Origin of bacterial variants. Nature **164:** 50.

NOVICK, A., 1972   Introduction, pp. 389–392 in *The Collected Works of Leo Szilard. Part IV. Scientific Papers*, edited by B. T. FELD and G. W. SZILARD. MIT Press, Cambridge, Mass.

NOVICK, A., and L. SZILARD, 1950   Experiments with the chemostat on spontaneous mutations of bacteria. Proc. Natl. Acad. Sci. USA **36:** 708–719.

PTASHNE, M., 1986   *A Genetic Switch: Gene Control and Phage* λ. Cell Press and Blackwell Scientific Publ., Palo Alto, Calif.

SAPP, J., 1987   *Beyond the Gene. Cytoplasmic Inheritance and the Struggle for Authority in Genetics.* Oxford University Press.

STRAGIER, P., B. KUNKEL, L. KROOS and R. LOSICK, 1989   Chromosomal rearrangement generating a composite gene for a developmental regulatory protein. Science (in press).

STRONG, J. H., 1947   *Fabric Structure.* Chemical Publishing Co., New York.

TREVORS, J. T., 1986   Plasmid curing in bacteria. FEMS Microbiol. Rev. **32:** 149–157.

VINOPAL, R. T., 1987   Selectable phenotypes, pp. 990–1015 in *Escherichia coli and Salmonella typhimurium: Cellular and Molecular Biology*, Vol. 2, edited by F. C. NEIDHARDT. American Society for Microbiology, Washington, D.C.

WALKER, G. C., 1987   The SOS response of *Escherichia coli*, pp. 1346–1357 in *Escherichia coli and Salmonella typhimurium: Cellular and Molecular Biology*, Vol. 2, edited by F. C. NEIDHARDT. American Society for Microbiology, Washington, D.C.

WECHSLER, J., and B. C. KLINE, 1980   Mutation and identification of the F plasmid locus determining resistance to acridine orange curing. Plasmid **4:** 276–280.

YANG, Y. N., and P. BRUCE WHITE, 1934   Rough variation in *V. cholerae* and its relation to resistance to cholera-phage (type A). J. Pathol. Bacteriol. **38:** 187–200.

See also page 704 in Addenda et Corrigenda.

Twenty-five Years Ago in *Genetics*
The Infinite Allele Model

James F. Crow

Genetics Department, University of Wisconsin–Madison, Madison, Wisconsin 53706

THE model of a mutational repertoire of infinitely many alleles, nicknamed the "infinite allele model," was published in the April 1964 issue of GENETICS. Six years earlier, on April 4, 1958, I had written a letter to MOTOO KIMURA, then in Japan, asking this question:

Have you ever considered this problem? Suppose every mutant is to an entirely different allele (or at least is counted this way, so that the only homozygosity is homozygosity by descent). Under such a system with a finite population of size *n* what is the proportion of homozygous loci at equilibrium? Perhaps you have already solved this, but I am not sure. Some of Josh's work suggests that every mutant is distinguishable from every other one if a careful enough test is made; at least this is true for a large number.

"Josh," of course, was my colleague JOSHUA LEDERBERG. I don't remember what experiments I had in mind, but this was a time of high resolution recombination studies in microorganisms. He was finding that most "point" mutations at the *Gal* and *Lac* loci showed some recombination, and at the same time BENZER was doing his fine structure mapping of phage T4. The number of potential alleles promised to be very large.

I knew of KIMURA's uncanny ability to solve such problems, and was not disappointed. On July 24, 1959, he wrote a letter giving the answer. For neutral alleles he found the equilibrium expression

$$\varphi(x) = 4N\mu x^{-1}(1 - x)^{4N\mu-1} \tag{1}$$

in which $\varphi(x)dx$ is the expected number of alleles whose frequency lies between x and $x + dx$, N is the effective population number, and μ is the mutation rate per gene per generation. The probability F that an individual is homozygous at the locus under consideration is readily obtained from this and is

$$F = \int_0^1 x^2\varphi(x)dx = \frac{1}{4N\mu + 1}. \tag{2}$$

The heterozygosity, then, is

$$H = 1 - F = \frac{4N\mu}{4N\mu + 1}. \tag{3}$$

KIMURA rejoined me at the University of Wisconsin from 1961 to 1963. The results were eventually published (KIMURA and CROW 1964) in a paper that began:

It has sometimes been suggested that the wild-type allele is not a single entity, but rather a population of different isoalleles that are indistinguishable by any ordinary procedure. With hundreds of nucleotides, each presumably capable of base substitutions and with additional permutations possible through sequence rearrangements, gains, and losses, the number of possible gene states becomes astronomical. It is known that a single nucleotide substitution can have the most drastic consequences, but there are also mutations with very minute effects and there is the possibility that many are so small as to be undetectable. It is not the purpose of this article to discuss the plausibility of such a system of isoalleles, or the evidence for or against. Instead, we propose to examine some of the population consequences of such a system if it does exist. The probability seems great enough to warrant such an inquiry.

In this context, "neutral" means that the selective differences are sufficiently small that allele frequencies are determined mainly by mutation and random processes; operationally, the selection difference $s \ll 1/N$. It is easy to modify Equations 2 and 3 when there is a fixed number of allelic states, but the formulas then lose some of their appeal.

Of course the "infinite allele" sobriquet does not mean that the mutational repertoire is really infinite; only that it is sufficiently large that a new allele does not duplicate one already in the population. An immediate advantage of this assumption is that, at equilibrium, identity by descent and identity in state become the same thing. *H* becomes an absolute measure of heterozygosity, not simply relative as in WRIGHT's classical theory. One can then employ MALÉCOT's (1948) identity-by-descent methods. Shortly thereafter, with the development of techniques to measure isozyme polymorphisms (LEWONTIN and HUBBY 1966; HARRIS 1966), the launching of the neutral theory (KIMURA 1968, 1983), and the treatment of polymorphism as a phase of molecular evolution (KIMURA and OHTA 1971), Equations 2 and 3 came into wide use. The neutral, infinite allele model provided a convenient null hypothesis for testing alternative selective models. It was preadapted to molecular data. As molecular technology provides finer resolution of allelic differences, down to the nucleotide level, the assumption that each new mutation represents a state not already existing in the population becomes increasingly realistic.

KIMURA and I defined the *effective* number of alleles, n_e, as the reciprocal of the homozygosity. If all alleles are equally frequent this is the actual number; otherwise it is less. It may be much less. In May 1964, WARREN EWENS visited the Wisconsin laboratory. He was especially interested in the *actual* number of alleles and had worked out a formula, which involves integrating (1). Thus the mean of the actual number, ignoring any distinction between actual and effective number, is

$$n = \int_{1/2N}^{1} \varphi(x)dx. \qquad (4)$$

He published this the same year in GENETICS (EWENS 1964). The difference between the actual and the effective number can be enormous because of the large number of alleles maintained at very low frequency. For example, with an effective population number 250,000 and mutation rate 10^{-6}, the actual number of alleles is about 13.1 (a slight correction of EWENS' value) while the effective number is only 2. The reason for the difference is the large number of very rare alleles which make negligible contributions to homozygosity. Which allele number is most useful depends, of course, on one's purpose. KIMURA and I were interested in homozygosity and genetic loads, hence the emphasis on n_e.

After receiving KIMURA's letter I was impressed that, despite the complexity of its derivation, the homozygosity formula was remarkably simple. I have always cherished the perhaps dubious principle that if there is a simple result there ought to be a simple way of getting it. We quickly found this to be true in this case and derived $F = 1/(4N\mu + 1)$ by an elementary, MALÉCOT-like method (see MALÉCOT 1948) which is included in the 1964 paper. MALÉCOT, a sadly underrecognized French population geneticist, is the subject of June's *Perspectives*.

The infinite allele model, with its useful properties, might well have been thought of earlier. Indeed it was. In 1951 MALÉCOT published the same idea: "Nous raisonnerons comme si chaque mutation faisant apparaître un gène différent de tous ceux qui existent déjà dans la population." It is perhaps excusable to have overlooked a statement in a French publication not ordinarily read by English-speaking geneticists. But the idea goes back still further. WRIGHT (1949) had proposed the same idea in an article in, of all places, the *Encyclopedia Britannica*. He had discovered

Equation 1 and if we substitute $1/2N$ for dx and replace integration by summation, (4) reduces to WRIGHT's formula for the number of alleles at equilibrium. Why would WRIGHT present a totally new idea in such a place? It never occurred to me to read an encyclopedia to find a new thought in population genetics theory! Typically, WRIGHT never mentioned it, although we saw each other almost every day and must have discussed the model many times. Asserting priority was not his bent. In 1949 and 1951 the idea was ahead of its time; in 1964 the time was ripe.

The mathematics becomes much more difficult when selection is introduced. I suspect that most readers of our 1964 paper stopped after the easy neutral part rather than going on to see KIMURA's more recondite analysis. He solved the problem approximately for two cases: an overdominance model in which all heterozygotes have relative fitness 1 and all homozygotes $1 - s$, and a mixture of overdominant and deleterious mutations. (I prefer FISHER's word "superdominant" but it hasn't caught on.) We were especially interested in the average homozygosity (and its reciprocal, the effective allele number) and in the reduced fitness brought about by inferior homozygotes (segregation load). KIMURA was able to get an approximate numerical solution that was quite accurate for large $N\mu$, although less so for small values. The results show a striking effect of random drift. When $\mu = 10^{-6}$ and $s = 0.01$, the segregation load increases by a factor >10 as the effective population number decreases from 10^7 to 10^5.

The 1960s were a time when overdominance was a popular idea and there was much discussion of the large segregation load introduced by numerous heterotic loci. We noted that in a population with $N = 10^4$, $s = 0.01$ and 5000 segregating loci, the mean fitness would be 0.002 times that of a multiple heterozygote. Several writers, quite appropriately, criticized the assumption of independent gene action and suggested that truncation selection, *i.e.*, selection based on rank order with a sharp cutoff between selected and rejected, could greatly reduce the load. The discussion has lost relevance in recent years as evidence for the postulated widespread overdominance has failed to appear.

As more and more molecular data accumulated in the 1960s, it became important to develop a theory for observations of individual nucleotides. KIMURA (1969) developed such a theory, sometimes called the "infinite site model." This also appeared in an April issue of GENETICS, exactly 20 years ago. The number of nucleotide sites is, of course, enormous while the mutation rate per site is very small. The model assumes that, whenever a mutation appears, it occurs at a new, previously homoallelic site. Since the observed heterozygosity per site in higher organisms ranges from 0.002 to 0.02 (NEI 1987), the model is a reasonable approximation to the real world.

Succeeding years have brought refinements. For example, WATTERSON (1977) found improved formulas for the frequency spectrum and therefore could make more accurate calculations. For a general theoretical review, see EWENS (1979). One of the principal uses of this theory has been to test the predictions of KIMURA's neutral model. Using Equation 3 as a null hypothesis, estimating μ from evolution rates and N from census data, the neutral theory predicts considerably more heterozygosity than is observed. One reason is that the effective population number may be much smaller than the census number, especially if there have been fluctuations in population sizes in the past. Also there is a contribution from deleterious mutations held in the population by mutation-selection balance. More explicit tests based on Equation 1 have shown a distribution much closer to the neutral model than to an overdominance model (KIMURA 1983; NEI 1988). I think the best current interpretation is that most of the observed protein polymorphism is a mixture of nearly neutral alleles, whose frequency is determined by mutation and random drift, and rare deleterious alleles maintained by mutation-selection balance. Despite some conspicuous examples, such as histocompatibility and self-sterility loci, there seems to be very little molecular polymorphism maintained by balancing selection, such as overdominance for fitness or rarity advantage. Overdominance as a major factor seems to be largely ruled out by the finding that haploids have a level of polymorphism comparable to that of diploids (YAMAZAKI 1981). The amount of variability and the neutral fraction increase greatly when synonymous changes and introns are included (for example, KREITMAN 1983).

KIMURA's (1983) neutral equations have been used widely. Perhaps the most far-out example comes from DYSON (1982, 1985), who found the equations useful in developing his hypothesis about the origin of life and argues that neutrality was widely prevalent when life was just beginning. (In DYSON's numerical example a basic quantity, Δ, related to the probability of a shift from disorder to order, turns out to be $\log 3 - (19/12) \log 2$, which he notes is the proportional difference between a perfect and a tempered fifth. Musicians and Pythagorean numerologists, take note.)

The infinite allele model has been extended in several directions, of which I shall mention three. For several years OHTA has been applying a similar theory to the evolution of multigene families. For her recent work, see OHTA (1986) and references therein; for more mathematical analysis, see NAGYLAKI (1988). MARUYAMA (1970, 1971) extended the theory to a geographically structured population using several models of population structure. He found that, at equilibrium for mutation, migration and random drift, for several population models, the effective number of alleles in the total population, n_e, is

$$n_e = \frac{4N\mu}{1 - f_0} \tag{5}$$

in which N is the effective total population size, μ is the mutation rate and f_0 is the local homozygosity. These analyses were quite loose, and many of the results have been put on a much sounder mathematical basis by NAGYLAKI (1982). A third extension of the infinite allele model is an application to mitochondrial and chloroplast genes in last month's GENETICS (BIRKY, FUERST and MARUYAMA 1989).

The model of infinitely many alleles has turned out to be a serviceable starting point for many investigations, far more than could have been anticipated at the time of my casual letter to KIMURA back in 1958.

TAKEO MARUYAMA (1936–1987) was a leading figure in mathematical population genetics. On December 11, 1987, he died, suddenly and unexpectedly, at the height of his career. This article is dedicated to his memory.

I am indebted to MOTOO KIMURA, WARREN EWENS and THOMAS NAGYLAKI for a number of valuable suggestions.

LITERATURE CITED

BIRKY, C. W., P. FUERST and T. MARUYAMA, 1989 Organelle gene diversity under migration, mutation, and drift: equilibrium expectations, approach to equilibrium, effects of heteroplasmic cells, and comparison to nuclear genes. Genetics **121:** 613–627.

DYSON, F. J., 1982 A model for the origin of life. J. Mol. Evol. **18:** 344–350.

DYSON, F., 1985 *Origins of Life.* Cambridge University Press, Cambridge.

EWENS, W. J., 1964 The maintenance of alleles by mutation. Genetics **50:** 891–898.

EWENS, W. J., 1979 *Mathematical Population Genetics.* Springer-Verlag, Berlin.

HARRIS, H., 1966 Enzyme polymorphism in man. Proc. R. Soc. Lond. Ser. B **164:** 298–310.

KIMURA, M., 1968 Evolutionary rate at the molecular level. Nature **217:** 624–626.

KIMURA, M., 1969 The number of heterozygous nucleotide sites maintained in a finite population due to steady flux of mutations. Genetics **61:** 893–903.

KIMURA, M., 1983 *The Neutral Theory of Molecular Evolution.* Cambridge University Press, Cambridge.

KIMURA, M., and J. CROW, 1964 The number of alleles that can be maintained in a finite population. Genetics **49:** 725–738.

KIMURA, M., and T. OHTA, 1971 Protein polymorphism as a phase of molecular evolution. Nature **229:** 467–469.

KREITMAN, M., 1983 Nucleotide polymorphism at the alcohol

dehydrogenase locus of *Drosophila melanogaster*. Nature **304:** 412–417.

LEWONTIN, R. C., and J. L. HUBBY, 1966   A molecular approach to the study of genic heterozygosity in natural populations. II. Amount of variation and degree of heterozygosity in natural populations of *Drosophila psuedoobscura*. Genetics **54:** 595–609.

MALÉCOT, G., 1948   *Les Mathématiques de l'Hérédité*. Masson & Cie, Paris. English translation by D. M. YERMANOS, 1969, W. H. Freeman, San Francisco.

MALÉCOT, G., 1951   Un traitement stochastique des problèmes linéaires (mutation, linkage, migration) en génétique de population. Ann. Univ. Lyon Sci. A **14:** 79–117.

MARUYAMA, T., 1970   Effective number of alleles in a subdivided population. Theor. Popul. Biol. **1:** 173–306.

MARUYAMA, T., 1971   Analysis of population structure. II. Two-dimensional stepping stone models of finite length and other geographically structured populations. Ann. Hum. Genet. **35:** 179–196.

NAGYLAKI, T., 1982   Geographical invariance in population genetics. J. Theor. Biol. **99:** 159–172.

NAGYLAKI, T., 1988   Gene conversion, linkage, and the evolution of multigene families. Genetics **120:** 291–301.

NEI, M., 1987   *Molecular Evolutionary Genetics*. Columbia University Press, New York.

NEI, M., 1988   Relative roles of mutation and selection in the maintenance of genetic variability. Phil. Trans. R. Soc. Lond. B **319:** 615–629.

OHTA, T., 1986   Actual number of alleles contained in a multigene family. Genet. Res. **48:** 119–123.

WATTERSON, G. A., 1977   Heterosis or neutrality? Genetics **85:** 789–814.

WRIGHT, S., 1949   Genetics of populations, in *Encyclopedia Britannica*, Ed. 14, Vol. 10, pp. 111–115. Reprinted in S. WRIGHT, 1986, *Evolution: Selected Papers*, edited by W. B. PROVINE. University of Chicago Press, Chicago.

YAMAZAKI, T., 1981   Genetic variabilities in natural populations of a haploid plant, *Conocephalum conicum*. I. The amount of heterozygosity. Jpn. J. Genet. **56:** 373–383.

May 1989

Evolving Theories of Enzyme Evolution

Daniel L. Hartl

Department of Genetics, Washington University School of Medicine, St. Louis, Missouri 63110–1095

FIFTEEN years ago in GENETICS, BARRY HALL and I published a paper on the evolved β-galactosidase in *Escherichia coli* (HALL and HARTL 1974). Thanks to previous work by JOHN H. CAMPBELL and his collaborators at the University of California in Los Angeles, this system for experimental enzyme evolution seemed especially promising for exploring the evolution of a novel catalytic activity using an organism with a well developed system for genetic manipulation. It seemed a way out of the dilemma that many of the deepest processes in evolutionary biology appeared almost inaccessible to direct experimental investigation. These included the origin of life itself and the evolution of new enzyme functions. Although experiments were possible, they were often indirect and their relevance speculative. Against this background, the prospect of the experimental evolution of β-galactosidase seemed to provide a great opportunity both to determine the evolutionary potential of a specific enzyme in a well adapted and well studied organism and to define the nature of these potentials at the molecular level. We assumed that understanding the molecular basis of enzyme adaptation to utilize novel substrates would also provide some insight into the fundamental processes by which new enzyme activities can arise in the course of evolution.

The evolution of novel catalytic activities was well recognized as paradoxical. As expressed by EDEN (1967) in the Wistar Symposium on *Mathematical Challenges to the Neo-Darwinian Interpretation of Evolution*, the problem was in the infinitesimal probability that catalytically useful proteins containing hundreds of amino acids could result from the random assembly of their amino acid subunits. For example, the probability that a particular sequence of 100 amino acids in a functional polypeptide would occur by chance combination is only 20^{-100} or 10^{-130} which, even allowing for some freedom in the amino acids that can occupy individual positions, is pretty small. While the probability paradox was not emphasized in evolutionary thinking, it remained unresolved in the major theories of enzyme evolution, including the classical theory of duplication and divergence in which new catalytic activities were supposed to evolve by random amino acid changes resulting from nucleotide substitutions in duplicate copies of preexisting genes. If the acquisition of a new enzyme function requires more than a few substitutions, then it is extremely improbable to occur by chance. The dilemma was that "either functionally useful proteins are very common . . . so that almost any polypeptide [of random amino acid sequence] . . . has a useful function to perform, or else . . . there exist certain strong regularities for finding useful paths [of protein evolution]" (EDEN 1967, p. 7). Of course, polypeptides are not assembled at random but are selected step by step from preexisting ones, and in the same book WRIGHT (1967) likened natural selection to the game of Twenty Questions, in which it is possible to arrive at the correct sequence of 100 amino acids in a polypeptide by a series of 500 questions answered yes or no. Nevertheless, there is a paradox in that acquisition of new enzyme functions may require multiple amino acid substitutions and therefore may not be selectable step by step.

The evolved β-galactosidase was first discovered by the microbial evolutionary biologist JOHN H. CAMPBELL, who had noticed that colonies of *E. coli* with a *lacZ* deletion mutation often gave rise to lactose-fermenting papillae when the plates were incubated for two weeks or so. By contrast, typical *lacZ* missense mutations usually yielded *Lac*+ revertant papillae within a few days. Overcoming considerable skepticism in the orthodox microbial genetics community, CAMPBELL and collaborators showed that the papillae in the aged plates grew from mutants containing a novel β-galactosidase activity coded by a gene designated *ebg* (evolved *b*eta *g*alactosidase), currently positioned at 67.5 min on the genetic map, not quite directly across the chromosome from *lacZ* at 8.0 min (CAMPBELL, LENGYEL and LANGRIDGE 1973).

BARRY HALL and I were both quite taken with these observations and were all the more impressed after an all-night brainstorming session in CAMPBELL's room at a Lake Arrowhead Meeting in February of 1972 when CAMPBELL laid out the details and our eyes were opened to the experimental possibilities. We resolved to exploit the system to study experimental enzyme evolution. In October 1972, CAMPBELL visited my laboratory at Minnesota to help get things started and in June 1973, BARRY transferred his NIH Postdoctoral Fellowship there and the work began in earnest.

The first discovery was that *ebg* mutants were very easy to get. Although the β-galactosidase enzyme in the evolved strains was indistinguishable from that discovered by CAMPBELL, our mutants fell into two types according to whether their β-galactosidase activity was constitutive or inducible by lactose. The lactose inducibility suggested that the normal product of the *ebg* structural gene is a lactose-inducible β-galactosidase, but one that does not hydrolyze lactose well enough to allow growth on lactose as the sole carbon source. The problem was to prove it, because Lac⁻ cells failed to grow on lactose and Lac⁺ cells growing on lactose produced so much *lacZ* β-galactosidase that any *ebg* enzyme produced could not be detected. The experimental trick was to grow *lacZ*⁻ cells on a very poor carbon source in the presence of excess lactose, plus isopropyl thiogalactoside (IPTG) to induce the *lacY* permease; out of context the experiment makes no sense, but under these conditions the *ebg* enzyme was induced sufficiently that its presence could be detected by its ability to hydrolyze the chromogenic β-galactoside ONPG (HARTL and HALL 1974). The ability of the *ebg* β-galactosidase to hydrolyze lactose, or a number of other β-galactosides that BARRY studied later (HALL 1977, 1981), evidently resulted from just one or a small number of amino acid replacements, and this was something of a disappointment at the time.

After a year of happy collaboration, BARRY moved to Newfoundland to pursue *ebg* and I moved to Purdue and soon became interested in naturally occurring enzyme polymorphisms in *E. coli*. BARRY showed that the *ebg* strains we had selected for growth on lactose also contained regulatory mutations in the closely linked gene *ebgR* encoding a repressor that regulates transcription of the *ebg* structural gene (HALL and CLARKE 1977). Comparisons of the amount of enzyme synthesized in the wild-type and mutant strains showed that all mutant strains synthesized more molecules of enzyme per cell than did the wild type. Some strains had become constitutive for *ebg* but most were still regulated by a mutant repressor more sensitive to lactose as inducer. Mutations in the repressor were necessary for growth on lactose because none of the mutant enzymes had sufficient lactase activity to permit growth unless the level of expression was increased above the normal level of induction. A fully induced wild-type *ebg* operon produces only about 5% as much enzyme as an *ebgR*-constitutive strain (HALL 1983).

BARRY also showed that the *ebg* β-galactosidase had a remarkable potential for acquiring new substrate specificities according to rather specific rules. For example, strains that constitutively synthesized the wild-type *ebg* enzyme gave rise to two distinct types of mutants capable of growth on lactose. The mutant enzymes were designated class I and class II. The class I enzyme enabled good growth on lactose but not on lactulose (galactosyl-fructose), whereas the class II enzyme enabled good growth on lactulose but moderate growth on lactose. The kinetic properties and substrate specificities of the class I and class II enzymes were different and correlated well with the growth characteristics of the strains (HALL 1981). Genetic studies demonstrated that the class I and class II enzymes differed from the wild type by mutations at opposite ends of the structural gene (HALL and ZUZEL 1980), which has since been confirmed directly by DNA sequencing.

Remarkably, when both the class I and class II mutations in the structural *ebg* gene were brought together in the same gene, the doubly mutant enzyme, designated class IV, exhibited two new substrate specificities (HALL and ZUZEL 1980). The first was the ability to allow growth on galactosyl-arabinose. Although the wild-type *ebg* enzyme exhibits some activity toward galactosyl-arabinose (as well as toward lactose and lactulose), these wild-type activities were too feeble to allow growth on any of these substrates. The class IV enzyme also exhibited a novel activity that could not be demonstrated in the wild type or in class I or class II mutants. This was the ability to hydrolyze lactobionic acid. While the lactobionic acid activity was too weak to allow growth, it could be increased by a third mutation so that growth on this substrate became possible.

The class IV enzyme could also do something else that neither of the others could—it could produce allolactose as a side product of lactose hydrolysis (HALL 1982a). Allolactose is the *in vivo* inducer of the *lac* operon and it is normally produced as a side reaction by the *lacZ* enzyme. Growth of most *ebg* mutants on lactose requires the presence of IPTG or some other gratuitous (nonmetabolized) inducer to enable synthesis of the *lacY* permease. However, strains with the class IV enzyme produce enough allolactose to induce the *lac* operon on their own. The finale was the production of a strain with the two structural mutations in class IV plus a mutation in the *ebg* repressor increasing the level of enzyme induced by lactose (HALL 1982b). This strain was able to grow on lactose alone without added gratuitous inducer— the lactose induced the class IV enzyme, which in turn produced enough allolactose to induce the *lacY* permease.

One of the important findings of the *ebg* work was

that identical enzymes occurred repeatedly in replicate experiments, suggesting that selection for growth on novel substrates favored only a very few of the large number of possible amino acid replacements. In addition, the different amino acid replacements had different evolutionary potentials as defined by their abilities to sustain growth on different substrates, and some mutations that enhanced activity toward one substrate had no detectable effect toward another substrate. Although the *ebg* mutations occurred in the laboratory, different potentials for selection also occur among naturally occurring amino acid polymorphisms in a variety of enzymes. ROGER MILKMAN (1973) had shown that electrophoretic variation in enzymes among *E. coli* isolates was widespread—more so, in fact, than in eukaryotes. If single amino acid replacements could have such profound effects on *ebg* function, then it seemed possible that natural variants of enzymes might also have important functional effects.

The experimental system to study natural enzyme variants made use of the power of *E. coli* genetics to create isogenic pairs of strains differing only in the enzyme gene of interest. These pairs were placed in chemostats in strong competition for substrates that require the target enzyme in their metabolism. DANIEL DYKHUIZEN was the chemostat expert who made this system work. The main finding was that naturally occurring enzyme variants usually produced no detectable effects on growth rate under growth conditions usually considered optimal for *E. coli* but that many did produce significant effects on growth rate when the conditions were altered, for example under competition for an unusual substrate (DYKHUIZEN and HARTL 1980; HARTL and DYKHUIZEN 1981). This situation was in many ways analogous to the various forms of *ebg*. The interpretation was that naturally occurring genetic variants, many of which may be selectively neutral or nearly neutral under the prevailing mosaic of environments, may nevertheless have a latent potential for selection that can be expressed under alternative environmental conditions (HARTL and DYKHUIZEN 1984, 1985). The implications of this principle for general evolution have been discussed by STEBBINS and HARTL (1988) and by KIMURA (1989).

Even though the selective effects of many naturally occurring enzyme polymorphisms are often too small to detect in chemostats, their effects under natural conditions can nevertheless be estimated from DNA sequences. This approach was made possible through an important theoretical analysis by STANLEY SAWYER, who analyzed the sample configurations (number of occurrences of each possible nucleotide) at 768 homologous nucleotide positions within the DNA coding for 6-phosphogluconate dehydrogenase in seven natural isolates (SAWYER, DYKHUIZEN and HARTL 1987).

The sequenced regions included 12 amino acid polymorphisms and 78 silent nucleotide polymorphisms. On the hypothesis that amino acid polymorphisms are as weakly selected as are the silent-site polymorphisms in the same genes, their sampling configurations among the genes should be the same as at the silent sites. This hypothesis could be rejected, and indeed it could be asserted with 95% confidence that no more than half of the amino acid polymorphisms in this enzyme are selectively neutral. The data are also consistent with a model in which all of the observed amino acid polymorphisms are mildly deleterious with an estimated average selection coefficient of 1.6×10^{-7}. This is smaller by several orders of magnitude than the minimum amount of selection detectable in chemostats. (I know of no experimental system in which selection of such small magnitude could be detected directly.)

The finding that many naturally occurring enzyme variants have very small effects on fitness makes considerable sense in light of metabolic control theory, an approach to understanding integrated metabolic systems that was pioneered by KACSER and BURNS (1973). Metabolic control theory also helps to explain why all of the *ebg* variants so far isolated exhibit only a small fraction of the lactase activity found in strains that contain the β-galactosidase coded by *lacZ*.

In their mathematical analysis of the flux across a metabolic pathway at steady state, KACSER and BURNS (1973, 1979) developed several important principles with wide applicability to complex metabolic systems, and their metabolic control theory has been widely cited because of its straightforwardness and intuitive appeal (KACSER and PORTEOUS 1987; HARTL, DYKHUIZEN and DEAN 1985; DEAN, DYKHUIZEN and HARTL 1988a; HARTL 1989). Some of the evolutionary implications of metabolic control theory have been discussed by HARTL, DYKHUIZEN and DEAN (1985) and STEBBINS and HARTL (1988). The KACSER-BURNS analysis demonstrated that the control of metabolic flux through a pathway is not usually through a single rate-limiting enzyme, but instead is shared among all enzymes in the pathway through control coefficients that are functions of the kinetic parameters. As the activity of any enzyme in the pathway increases, the flux becomes less sensitive to small perturbations in the activity and the control coefficient of the enzyme decreases. This is the familiar diminishing-returns or saturation phenomenon encountered in many complex systems with interacting components. Under rather general conditions the summation of all control coefficients in a pathway must equal unity, which implies that large control coefficients of some enzymes must be accompanied by small control coefficients of others. In the example of *E. coli* growing on lactose, the control coefficient of the β-galactosidase permease with respect to growth rate is greater than that of the β-galactosidase by a factor of approximately 30 (DYKHUIZEN, DEAN and HARTL 1987). This implies that cells with as little as 5% of wild-type *lacZ* activity can grow on lactose almost as well as does the wild type (DEAN, DYKHUIZEN and HARTL 1986), so that the relatively low β-galactosidase activities that occur in *ebg* strains are nevertheless compatible with virtually normal growth.

The relatively large control coefficient of the β-galactoside permease also helps to explain an unexpected result obtained by ANTHONY DEAN in his studies of the effects of spontaneous amino acid replacements in the *lacZ* β-galactosidase (DEAN, DYKHUIZEN and HARTL 1988b). These essentially random replacements were obtained in the laboratory as revertants of nonsense codons that restored enzyme synthesis but altered its electrophoretic mobility or thermostability as compared with wild type. The unexpected result was that most of the amino acid replacements produced effects too small to be detected in chemostats. Among 25 amino acid replacements occurring in 17 codons distributed approximately uniformly along the gene, only three produced selective effects large enough to be statistically significant. The remaining 22 produced effects that could not be detected under conditions in which the limit of resolution was a selection coefficient of approximately 0.4% per generation. It seemed reasonable to assume that many of the amino acid replacements actually resulted in small differences in enzyme activity but that these gave undetectable effects in chemostats owing to the relatively small control coefficient of β-galactosidase with respect to fitness (DEAN, DYKHUIZEN and HARTL 1986).

The experiments with *ebg* helped to define the alterations in substrate specificity resulting from simple amino acid replacements. As noted at the outset, we had assumed that these studies would also provide some insight into the mechanisms by which novel enzyme activities are created during the course of evolution. However, as things turned out, the *ebg* system proved to be a better model for the refinement of enzyme activity than for the evolution of catalytic novelty. Indeed, it now appears that novel catalytic activities are often acquired by a process quite beyond anything that we, or anyone else, had imagined at the time.

It now appears that enzymes with truly novel functions, rather than being derived from single amino acid replacements, are often assembled piecemeal from smaller functional units. One indication that protein evolution may involve a combinatorial process came from the finding of similar folding domains with similar functions in otherwise unrelated proteins (PHILLIPS, STERNBERG and SUTTON 1983). Another

indication came from the discovery that many genes in eukaryotes are split into exons and introns, often with a correlation between exons and protein-folding domains suggestive of piecemeal assembly from smaller units capable of somewhat autonomous folding and function (GILBERT 1978). The powerful combinatorial possibilities help to overcome the odds against protein evolution by random amino acid replacement. Strong support for this model of protein evolution came from the finding that the low-density lipoprotein receptor gene contains exons that are clearly paralogous (homologous because of gene duplication) with exons in genes for components of complement, blood-clotting factors and epidermal growth factor (SÜDHOF *et al.* 1985). A combinatorial mechanism of protein evolution provides a resolution of EDEN's probability paradox mentioned earlier, because piecemeal combination gives "strong regularities for finding useful paths" of protein evolution.

The genes-in-pieces mechanism of protein evolution has been further elaborated by BRENNER (1988) in a principle of local functionality, according to which the folding of small segments of a polypeptide is determined mainly by local interactions within each segment. Brenner has argued that the principle of local functionality allowed discrete functions of individual peptides to continue undisturbed in composite molecules and eventually resulted in the formation of present-day exons.

One implication of local functionality is that certain polypeptide segments of proteins may be interchangeable with segments of comparable local structure from totally unrelated proteins. This prediction is subject to direct experimental test using oligonucleotide site-directed mutagenesis to interchange comparable local segments of proteins whose three-dimensional structure is well determined. ROBERT DUBOSE has succeeded in doing this with α-helical segments in the alkaline phosphatase of *E. coli*, each seven amino acids in length. The helical segments were obtained either from different domains within the alkaline phosphatase or from a helical segment within the bacteriophage T4 lysozyme. Three such replacements were carried out, and in all three cases the activity of the alkaline phosphatase was retained, although it was different from the wild-type enzyme (R. DUBOSE and D. L. HARTL, unpublished results). This result provides strong support for the principle of local functionality, at least with regard to helical segments. If the principle can be demonstrated more generally, then it supports the hypothesis that combinations of units with novel functions can be assembled piecemeal and their activity and specificity can later be improved and refined by individual amino acid replacements.

In addition to the evolutionary implications of *ebg*, the locus also presents some interesting molecular biology. At the protein level, HALL and collaborators have demonstrated that the *ebg* β-galactosidase contains multiple subunits of two polypeptides coded by the partially overlapping cistrons *ebgA* and *ebgC*. The major polypeptide is the *ebgA* gene product of 1032 amino acids (STOKES, BETTS and HALL 1985) and the minor polypeptide is the *ebgC* gene product of 173 amino acids. Expression of the *ebgA* and *ebgC* cistrons is negatively regulated by the *ebg* repressor produced from the tightly linked *ebgR* gene which codes for a polypeptide of 328 amino acids.

The mutations responsible for the class I and class II *ebg* enzymes have also been identified at the nucleotide level. Class I mutations in *ebg* include the *ebgA2* and *ebgA4* alleles described in the 1974 paper. As noted earlier, they significantly increase the activity of the enzyme toward lactose but not toward lactulose. The dramatic change in substrate specificity of the class I alleles results from a single amino acid replacement of asparagine for aspartic acid at position 92. In the class II enzymes, which significantly increase activity toward lactulose as well as lactose, one mutation always results in the replacement of a cysteine for a tryptophan at position 977, and in some alleles there is also a serine-to-glycine replacement at position 978. The positions of these replacements have no apparent proximity to the region implicated in the active site of the enzyme, which should perhaps not be too surprising because refinement of enzyme function may often involve long-range interactions between residues in different domains. Selection may result in a molecular coadaptation that promotes the particular domains to function well in combination. This principle supervenes that of local functionality for the fine tuning of enzyme function.

As RILEY, SOLOMON and ZIPKAS (1978) predicted from the relative map positions of the genes in the *E. coli* chromosome, *ebgA* is paralogous with *lacZ* and *ebgR* is paralogous with *lacI*. At the amino acid level, the sequences of the *ebgA* and *lacZ* polypeptides are about 34% identical and those of the *ebgR* and *lacI* polypeptides are about 25% identical. The relatively large divergence suggests that the duplication of the common ancestors of these genes was ancient. The *ebgA* gene has, however, retained its β-galactosidase activity and sufficient potential for lactose hydrolysis that direct selection for growth on lactose is successful. Interestingly, *E. coli* strains containing deletions of both *ebgA* and *lacZ* do not give rise to a third β-galactosidase, even after heavy mutagen treatment and prolonged selection on lactose (unpublished results of D. L. HARTL and of B. G. HALL). Comparisons of gene sequences and functions around the *E. coli* chromosome suggest that genes paralogous to *lacZ* and *ebg* should exist midway between them on both sides of the chromosome (RILEY, SOLOMON and ZIPKAS

1978) and perhaps even at 7-min intervals (KUNISAWA and OTSUKA 1988). Evidently, these other paralogous genes are so divergent that no single or small number of amino acid replacements are sufficient to generate a β-galactosidase with enough lactose hydrolysis to survive direct selection for growth on lactose.

The results of experiments with *ebg* vindicate JOHN CAMPBELL's perspicacity in pursuing the unexpected papillae that emerged from decrepit Lac⁻ colonies after prolonged incubation on lactose indicator plates. Anyone who has studied old bacterial plates knows that a lot of strange things can appear, most of them grungy, many of them uninteresting, some unanalyzable and a few downright hazardous to one's research career if not to one's health. While CALVIN BRIDGE's admonition to treasure your exceptions is often quoted to encourage students not to ignore unexpected observations that might conceivably be significant, the image of an old bacterial plate may signify the important corollary that it takes a specific kind of genius to foresee which exceptions should be treasured among the many that are dross.

I thank BARRY G. HALL for his important contributions to this *Perspective* and ROBERT DuBOSE for his many helpful comments. I am also grateful to the collaborators mentioned in the text who have made the scientific odyssey from *ebg* not only possible but also very agreeable. BARRY G. HALL was typically generous in permitting the use of unpublished data on *ebg* sequences. This work is presently supported by National Institutes of Health grants GM30201 and M40322.

LITERATURE CITED

BRENNER, S., 1988 A tale of two serines. Nature **334:** 528–530.

CAMPBELL, J. H., J. A. LENGYEL and J. LANGRIDGE, 1973 Evolution of a second gene for β-galactosidase in *Escherichia coli*. Proc. Natl. Acad. Sci. USA **70:** 1841–1845.

DEAN, A. M., D. E. DYKHUIZEN and D. L. HARTL, 1986 Fitness as a function of β-galactosidase activity in *Escherichia coli*. Genet. Res. **48:** 1–8.

DEAN, A. M., D. E. DYKHUIZEN and D. L. HARTL, 1988a Theories of metabolic control in quantitative genetics, pp. 536–548 in *Proceedings of the Second International Conference on Quantitative Genetics*, edited by B. S. WEIR, E. J. EISEN, M. M. GOODMAN and G. NAMKOONG. Sinauer Associates, Sunderland, Mass.

DEAN, A. M., D. E. DYKHUIZEN and D. L. HARTL, 1988b. Fitness effects of amino-acid replacements in the β-galactosidase of *Escherichia coli*. Mol. Biol. Evol. **5:** 469–485.

DYKHUIZEN, D. E., A. M. DEAN and D. L. HARTL, 1987 Metabolic flux and fitness. Genetics **115:** 25–31.

DYKHUIZEN, D., and D. L. HARTL, 1980 Selective neutrality of 6PGD allozymes in *E. coli* and the effects of genetic background. Genetics **96:** 801–817.

EDEN, M., 1967 Inadequacies of neo-darwinian evolution as a scientific theory, pp. 5–19 in *Mathematical Challenges to the Neo-Darwinian Interpretation of Evolution*, edited by P. S. MOORHEAD and M. M. KAPLAN. Wistar Institute Press, Philadelphia. Reprinted (1985) by Alan R. Liss, New York.

GILBERT, W., 1978 Why genes in pieces? Nature **271:** 501.

HALL, B. G., 1977 Number of mutations required to evolve a new lactase function in *Escherichia coli.* J. Bacteriol. **129:** 540–543.

HALL, B. G., 1981 Changes in the substrate specificities of an enzyme during directed evolution of new functions. Biochemistry **20:** 4042–4049.

HALL, B. G., 1982a Transgalatosylation activity of the *ebg* β-galactosidase synthesizes allolactose from lactose. J. Bacteriol. **150:** 132–140.

HALL, B. G., 1982b Evolution of a regulated operon in the laboratory. Genetics **101:** 335–344.

HALL, B. G., 1983 Evolution of new metabolic functions in laboratory organisms, pp. 234–257 in *Evolution of Genes and Proteins,* edited by M. NEI and R. KOEHN. Sinauer Associates, Sunderland, Mass.

HALL, B. G., and N. D. CLARKE, 1977 Regulation of newly evolved enzymes. III. Evolution of the *ebg* repressor during selection for enhanced lactase activity. Genetics **85:** 193–201.

HALL, B. G., and D. L. HARTl, 1974 Regulation of newly evolved enzymes. I. Selection of a novel lactase regulated by lactose in *Escherichia coli.* Genetics **76:** 391–400.

HALL, B. G., and T. ZUZEL, 1980 Evolution of a new enzymatic function by recombination within a gene. Proc. Natl. Acad. Sci. USA **77:** 3529–3533.

HARTL, D. L., 1989 The physiology of weak selection. Genome (in press).

HARTL, D. L., and D. E. DYKHUIZEN, 1981 Potential for selection among nearly neutral allozymes of 6-phosphogluconate dehydrogenase in *Escherichia coli.* Proc. Natl. Acad. Sci. USA **78:** 6344–6348.

HARTL, D. L., and D. E. DYKHUIZEN, 1984 The population genetics of *Escherichia coli.* Annu. Rev. Genet. **18:** 31–68.

HARTL, D. L., and D. E. DYKHUIZEN, 1985 The neutral theory and the molecular basis of preadaptation, pp. 107–124 in *Population Genetics and Molecular Evolution,* edited by T. OHTA and K. AOKI. Japan Scientific Societies Press, Tokyo.

HARTL, D. L., D. E. DYKHUIZEN and A. M. DEAN, 1985 Limits of adaptation: the evolution of selective neutrality. Genetics **111:** 655–674.

HARTL, D. L., and B. G. HALL, 1974 Second naturally occurring β-galactosidase in *E. coli.* Nature **248:** 152–153.

KACSER, H., and J. A. BURNS, 1973 The control of flux. Symp. Soc. Expt. Biol. **32:** 65–104.

KACSER, H., and J. A. BURNS, 1979 Molecular democracy: who shares the controls? Biochem. Rev. **7:** 1150–1160.

KACSER, H., and J. W. PORTEOUS, 1987 Control of metabolism: what do we have to measure? Trends Biochem. Sci. **12:** 5–14.

KIMURA, M., 1989 The present status of the neutral theory, in press in *Population Biology of Genes and Molecules,* edited by N. TAKAHATA and J. F. CROW. Cambridge University Press, Cambridge, England.

KUNISAWA, T., and J. OTSUKA, 1988 Periodic distribution of homologous genes or gene segments on the *Escherichia coli* K12 genome. Protein Seq. Data Anal. **1:** 263–267.

MILKMAN, R., 1973 Electrophoretic variation in *Escherichia coli* from natural sources. *Science* **182:** 1024–1026.

PHILLIPS, D. C., M. J. E. STERNBERG and B. J. SUTTON, 1983 Intimations of evolution from the three-dimensional structures of proteins, pp. 145–173 in *Evolution from Molecules to Men,* edited by D. S. BENDALL. Cambridge University Press, Cambridge, England.

RILEY, M., L. SOLOMON and D. ZIPKAS, 1978 Relationship between gene function and gene location in *Escherichia coli.* J. Mol. Evol. **11:** 47–56.

SAWYER, S. A., D. E. DYKHUIZEN and D. L. HARTL, 1987 A confidence interval for the number of selectively neutral amino acid polymorphisms. Proc. Natl. Acad. Sci. USA **84:** 6225–6228.

STEBBINS, G. L., and D. L. HARTL, 1988 Comparative evolution: latent potentials for anagenic advance. Proc. Natl. Acad. Sci. USA **85:** 5141–5145.

STOKES, H. W., P. W. BETTS and B. G. HALL, 1985 Sequence of the *ebgA* gene of *Escherichia coli*: comparison with the *lacZ* gene. Mol. Biol. Evol. **2:** 469–477.

SÜDHOF, T. C., J. L. GOLDSTEIN, M. S. BROWN and D. W. RUSSELL, 1985 The LDL receptor gene: a mosaic of exons shared with different proteins. Science **228:** 815–822.

WRIGHT, S., 1967 Comments on the preliminary working papers of EDEN and WADDINGTON, pp. 117–120 in *Mathematical Challenges to the Neo-Darwinian Interpretation of Evolution,* edited by P. S. MOORHEAD and M. M. KAPLAN. Wistar Institute Press, Philadelphia. Reprinted (1985) by Alan R. Liss, New York.

Gustave Malécot and the Transition from Classical to Modern Population Genetics

Thomas Nagylaki

Department of Molecular Genetics and Cell Biology, The University of Chicago, Chicago, Illinois 60637

ABSTRACT

The contributions of Gustave Malécot to theoretical population genetics are described, discussed, and put into perspective relative to earlier and later work. In this context, certain aspects of the theory of inbreeding, the correlation between relatives, the evolution of finite panmictic populations, and (in more depth) spatial variation are reviewed. A brief biographical sketch of Malécot is also presented.

SELDOM does a doctoral dissertation substantially advance its field. Nevertheless, just such a rare dissertation, *Théorie mathématique de l'hérédité mendélienne generalisée*, was submitted fifty years ago, to the Faculty of Sciences of the University of Paris, by GUSTAVE MALÉCOT (1939a). Despite the breadth, depth, originality, power, and elegance of the contributions of this great French theoretical population geneticist, much of his work is known even now only to a small minority of researchers in his area. Therefore, it seems appropriate on this semicentennial to delineate and discuss MALÉCOT's contributions and to place them into perspective relative to earlier and later work, especially that of FISHER, WRIGHT, and KIMURA. It is also of interest to inquire why his contributions have not diffused more rapidly and widely.

MALÉCOT has written articles on the philosophy of science, on statistics, and on the theory of stochastic processes and its application to economics and physics. These will not be discussed here. About 45 of his papers fully or partly concern population genetics. They include brief research announcements; some items, such as lecture notes, whose aim is primarily didactic, but which often contain important new results and approaches; and long, detailed, powerful original papers. It is interesting to note, and an indication of MALÉCOT's intellectual independence and of the relative isolation in which he worked, that he is

the sole author of every one of his papers in genetics.

MALÉCOT's work focuses on stochastic processes in population genetics. His doctoral research on the correlation between relatives (MALÉCOT 1939a) led him to the gradual discovery of one of the most basic and fruitful concepts in population genetics: *identity by descent* (MALÉCOT 1941, 1942, 1946, 1948). He used this idea to prove and interpret probabilistically WRIGHT's formulas for the genotypic frequencies under inbreeding (which he generalized to multiple alleles) and for the inbreeding coefficient of an individual with an arbitrary pedigree (MALÉCOT 1941, 1942, 1948), to derive the correlation between relatives for traits without epistasis (MALÉCOT 1948), to examine the evolution of finite panmictic populations (MALÉCOT 1946, 1948, 1951), and to investigate his original models for the genetic structure of populations distributed discretely or continuously in space (MALÉCOT 1948, 1949, 1950, 1951, 1965, 1967, 1975). Before molecular genetics might have motivated him, MALÉCOT (1946, 1948, 1951) introduced mutation by proposing that every allele mutates at the same rate and no mutant is identical by descent to any preexisting allele, and he employed this beautifully simple hypothesis in many of his studies. He deduced the asymptotic distribution of the gene frequency for pure random genetic drift (MALÉCOT 1944), the complete time-dependent diffusion approximation for the gene-frequency distribution with reversible mutation (MALÉCOT 1948), and the probability of ultimate fixation for selection without dominance (MALÉCOT 1952).

MALÉCOT's 1948 classic, *Les mathématiques de l'hérédité*, is one of the most original, elegant, concise, and

---

This paper is dedicated to the memory of CHARLES W. COTTERMAN (1914–1989), one of the most lucid, rigorous, and original thinkers in mathematical genetics, who was always exceeding generous with his deep understanding and extensive unpublished research.

stimulating books every written on population genetics. His achievement is even more remarkable than
it seems: MALÉCOT wrote a section of the book each
week for a mathematical genetics course he was teaching at the Institute of Statistics of the University of
Paris. For many readers, a slightly revised and extended English translation (MALÉCOT 1969) may provide the easiest entrée to MALÉCOT's oeuvre. The
translation, however, contains some errors that do not
appear in the original, both in the text and in the
displays.

MALÉCOT's dissertation, his book, and some of his
more didactic papers have been reprinted (with new
typesetting) in *Probabilités et hérédité* (MALÉCOT 1966),
which includes also a list of his publications complete
to May 1, 1966. Unfortunately, financial exigencies
have prevented the publication of a planned companion volume of his most important research papers. In
particular, none of the papers cited above is reprinted
in MALÉCOT (1966). FELSENSTEIN's (1981) superb bibliography is also useful.

After a brief biographical sketch, MALÉCOT's contributions will be described in more detail. This entails
reviewing certain aspects of the theory of inbreeding,
the correlation between relatives, the evolution of
finite panmictic populations, and (in more depth) spatial variation. The final section comprises a broader
discussion of the style and significance of his work and
its relation to earlier and later research.

BIOGRAPHICAL SKETCH

GUSTAVE MALÉCOT was born in la Grand-Croix
(Loire), near Saint-Étienne, on December 28, 1911.
In 1932, after his secondary education at the Lycée
de Saint-Étienne, he entered the École Normale Su-
périeure to study mathematics, with the intention of
teaching it at the secondary level. At this "grande
école," his professors included ÉMILE BOREL, ÉLIE
CARTAN, GEORGES DARMOIS, and MAURICE FRÉCHET.
He graduated in 1935 (Agrégé des sciences mathématiques), second in his class.

MALÉCOT then proceeded to the Institut Henri
Poincaré of the University of Paris, where he had a
research fellowship. His research was guided by DAR-
MOIS, and in 1939 MALÉCOT received his Doctorat
d'État for a thesis that elucidated, rigorized, systematized, and generalized FISHER's (1918) seminal but
notoriously difficult reconciliation of biometry and
Mendelian inheritance ("obscur et génial, comme tout
ce qu'a écrit Sir Ronald" is MALÉCOT's description in
a personal communication).

MALÉCOT taught mathematics first at the Lycée de
Saint-Étienne (1940–1942) and then at the University
of Montpellier (1942–1944), where he was maître de
conférences. The work of WRIGHT (1921a, b, 1922a,
1931, 1933a, b) stimulated him to develop the concept
of identity by descent (MALÉCOT 1941, 1942, 1946,

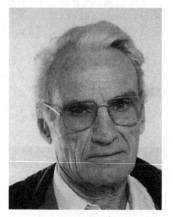

GUSTAVE MALÉCOT

1948) and to apply it to inbreeding (MALÉCOT 1941,
1942, 1948), the correlation between relatives (MA-
LÉCOT 1948), and random mating in a finite population (MALÉCOT 1946, 1948, 1951). In graduate
school, he had already studied the research of KOL-
MOGOROV, FRÉCHET, and DOEBLIN on Markov processes. Their probabilistic methods, together with the
pertinent work of FISHER (1922, 1930a, b) and
WRIGHT (1931, 1937, 1938a, 1939), inspired his powerful investigations of gene-frequency fluctuations in
a finite population (MALÉCOT 1937, 1944, 1945,
1948, 1952).

In 1944, MALÉCOT became maître de conférences
at the University of Lyon (Université Claude Bernard); from 1945 until his retirement in 1981, he was
professor of applied mathematics there. At Lyon, he
taught probability, mechanics, and mathematical economics. For many years, he lectured on population
genetics at the Institute of Statistics of the University
of Paris. Among those who have studied with MALÉ-
COT are GILLOIS, JACQUARD, LALOUEL, MARCHAND,
PICARD, and SERANT. WRIGHT's island model
(WRIGHT 1931) and treatment of isolation by distance
(WRIGHT 1943a, b, 1946) and discussions with MAX-
IME LAMOTTE concerning geographical variation in
the snail *Cepaea nemoralis* motivated MALÉCOT's extensive and important research on the genetic structure of populations with discrete or continuous spatial
distributions (MALÉCOT 1948, 1949, 1950, 1951,
1965, 1967, 1975). He is still working on these problems.

MALÉCOT has received a number of honors for his
work: Prix Montyon de l'Académie des Sciences, Officier des Palmes Académiques, Chevalier de la Légion
d'Honneur (1962), and Officier de la Légion d'Honneur (1982).

CONTRIBUTIONS TO POPULATION GENETICS

This section comprises the description of MALÉ-
COT's research on identity by descent, inbreeding, the
correlation between relatives, panmixia in finite populations, the balance between mutation and random

drift, the random drift of gene frequencies, and spatial variation. These subjects are discussed in the above order, rather than chronologically.

Identity by descent: Two homologous genes are identical by descent if and only if they are derived from the same gene or one is derived from the other (in both cases without mutation). This fundamental idea was discovered independently by COTTERMAN (1940) and MALÉCOT (1941, 1942, 1946, 1948); it had been foreshadowed by HALDANE and MOSHINSKY (1939). It is an essential ingredient of all of MALÉCOT's major contributions except those that deal directly with the random fluctuation of gene frequencies. COTTERMAN (1940, 1983) employed identity by descent to specify precisely the genetic relation between arbitrary relatives and to solve many interesting problems of particular importance in human genetics; KARLIN (1969), JACQUARD (1974), and CANNINGS and THOMPSON (1981) present extensions and other applications. Identity by descent lies at the heart of the powerful genealogical approach to population genetics (see DONNELLY and TAVARÉ 1987; HOPPE 1987; HUDSON and KAPLAN 1988; KAPLAN, DARDEN and HUDSON 1988; EWENS 1989; and references therein). Finally, extensions and variants of identity arguments have served vitally in many analyses of genome evolution (see OHTA 1985; NAGYLAKI 1988a; and references therein).

Inbreeding: This subsection covers MALÉCOT's definitions of the inbreeding coefficient and of the coefficient of consanguinity, his derivation of the genotypic frequencies under inbreeding, and his proof of WRIGHT's formula for the inbreeding coefficient of an individual with an arbitrary pedigree.

The inbreeding coefficient: The introduction of the inbreeding coefficient is only one of WRIGHT's (1921b, 1922a) many extremely important and highly creative contributions to population genetics. WRIGHT's definition, as the correlation between uniting gametes, however, involves irrelevant numerical values and (implicitly) gene frequencies, thereby disguising the basic facts that the inbreeding coefficient is a function only of ancestry, and is therefore the same for all (autosomal) loci and independent of gene frequencies. The definition of COTTERMAN (1940) and MALÉCOT (1941, 1942, 1946, 1948) exhibits these facts immediately and leads to a more concise, lucid, and rigorous theory of inbreeding. Therefore, it is the preferred approach for modern exposition and research. An individual is *autozygous* at a locus if and only if his two genes at that locus are identical by descent. The inbreeding coefficient, F, of an individual is the probability that he is autozygous.

A measure of the relatedness of two individuals is MALÉCOT's (1941, 1942, 1946, 1948) *coefficient of consanguinity.* The coefficient of consanguinity of individuals I and J, F_{IJ}, is the probability that a randomly chosen gene from I and a homologous randomly chosen gene from J are identical by descent. Hence, if O is the offspring of I and J, then $F_{IJ} = F_O$, the inbreeding coefficient of O.

Genotypic frequencies: Consider an infinite population with discrete, nonoverlapping generations. Assume this population is initially in Hardy-Weinberg proportions and it practices pure inbreeding thereafter (*i.e.*, all other evolutionary forces are absent). If p_i and P_{ij} denote denote the respective frequencies of A_i alleles and ordered A_iA_j genotypes, then

$$P_{ii} = p_i^2 + Fp_i(1 - p_i), \tag{1a}$$

$$P_{ij} = (1 - F)p_ip_j, \quad i \neq j. \tag{1b}$$

This equation holds also for a finite population if the initial generation is sampled at random from an infinite population in Hardy-Weinberg proportions and the gene and genotypic frequencies are interpreted as expectations. The fundamental result (1), which encapsulates the biological significance of the inbreeding coefficient, was derived by WRIGHT (1921b, 1922b) for two alleles. COTTERMAN (1940) and MALÉCOT (1946) deduced (1) for two alleles by probabilistic arguments, which MALÉCOT (1948) soon extended to multiple alleles.

Pedigrees: WRIGHT (1922a) obtained his beautiful formula for the inbreeding coefficient of an individual with an arbitrary pedigree by examining special cases with his method of path coefficients (WRIGHT 1921a, b, 1934, 1968). Special cases, of course, cannot prove a general result. Furthermore, although WRIGHT recognized that the method of path coefficients requires linear determination of the dependent variables by the independent variables (*cf.* TUKEY 1954; MORAN 1961), he did not demonstrate this linearity in any of his genetic applications. COTTERMAN (1940) supported WRIGHT's formula by probabilistic reasoning. MALÉCOT (1941) noted the inadequacy of WRIGHT's analysis and established the formula by a subtle inductive argument. Consult BOUCHER (1988) for a more detailed and explicit proof.

The correlation between relatives: As noted above, MALÉCOT's (1939a) dissertation on the analysis of the phenotypic variance and the correlation between relatives was inspired by FISHER's (1918) classic treatment of these problems. MALÉCOT's concise, suggestive conditional-expectation arguments greatly simplified the calculation of the correlations, for which FISHER had used association tables. MALÉCOT (1938a, b, 1939b, c) reported his results in a series of short notes. In his elegant and seminal second investigation of this subject (MALÉCOT 1948), he used identity by descent. In both studies, he posited equilibrium, an arbitrary number of diallelic loci with independent assortment, and an additive, stochastically independent environmental contribution.

Random mating, inbreeding, and assortative mating will be discussed separately.

Random mating: Suppose first that the trait is determined without dominance or epistasis. WRIGHT (1922a) assumed further that the trait is not influenced by the environment and employed path coefficients to derive the formula $r_{IJ} = 2F_{IJ}$ for the correlation r_{IJ} between arbitrary relatives I and J whose coefficient of consanguinity is F_{IJ}. In his thesis, MALÉCOT (1939a) demonstrated how to calculate the correlation for any specified relationship. Later, he proved that $r_{IJ} = 2F_{IJ}h^2$, where h^2 is the heritability (MALÉCOT 1948).

FISHER (1918) included dominance and derived the correlation for the three closest ancestral relatives (*i.e.*, parent and offspring, grandparent and grandchild, and great grandparent and great grandchild), full siblings, uncle-niece, and single and double first cousins. (He showed as well that his results for the analysis of variance and the parental and sibling correlations hold for multiple alleles.) MALÉCOT (1939a) first evaluated the correlation for two classes of relatives: (i) those related only through one parent of one of them (*e.g.*, parent-offspring and uncle-niece) and (ii) those for which no parent of either individual is related to both parents of the other (*e.g.*, full siblings and double first cousins). A false assumption (MALÉCOT 1948, p. 21) unfortunately restricts the validity of his subsequent treatment to category (ii), which excludes, *inter alia*, the above examples of category (i). In any case, neither category includes relatives such as quadruple half-first cousins (TRUSTRUM 1961; VAN AARDE 1975). KEMPTHORNE (1955a, b, 1957, pp. 330–332) used identity by descent to derive the formula for arbitrary relatives.

The results described above do not, in fact, depend on the linkage map. If there is epistasis, this independence still holds for the decomposition of the variance (COCKERHAM 1954; KEMPTHORNE 1954, 1955a, b, 1957, pp. 413–419), but not for the correlation between relatives. FISHER (1918) generalized his formulae to two-factor epistasis, and MALÉCOT (1939a) indicated how to include three-factor epistasis. COCKERHAM (1954) extended FISHER's work to arbitrary relatives and arbitrary epistasis, but identity by descent was the crucial tool in KEMPTHORNE's (1954, 1955a, b, 1957, pp. 419–420) derivation of a concise and informative general formula. Identity by descent was equally vital in the incorporation of linkage (COCKERHAM 1956; SCHNELL 1963; VAN AARDE 1975).

Inbreeding: In the case of purely additive gene action, both WRIGHT (1922a) and MALÉCOT (1948) included inbreeding. MALÉCOT obtained the formula

$$r_{IJ} = 2F_{IJ}h^2/[(1 + F_I h^2)(1 + F_J h^2)]^{1/2}, \qquad (2)$$

where h^2 denotes the heritability with random mating and F_I and F_J designate the respective inbreeding

coefficients of individuals I and J. WRIGHT had derived (2) in the absence of an environmental effect ($h = 1$).

For a single locus, (2) is certainly correct. For two or more loci, however, all derivations of (2) tacitly assume that *allelic effects* at different loci are uncorrelated. But this is not obvious: as a rule, *genotypes* at different loci are mutually dependent under inbreeding. Although the equilibria of examples such as partial selfing (KIMURA 1963; NARAIN 1966; WEIR and COCKERHAM 1973) support the implicit conjecture, the general validity of (2) remains to be proved (or disproved).

Assortative mating: FISHER (1918) was the first to treat assortative mating for a quantitative character. He posited stochastic independence of the environment, control of the character by many unlinked loci with contributions of the same order of magnitude, and the absence of epistasis. Using ingenious intuitive arguments, he evaluated approximately the genotypic variance at the equilibrium determined by assortative mating in terms of the initial, panmictic genotypic variance, and calculated the equilibrium correlation between sundry close relatives in terms of the marital correlation and the broad and narrow heritabilities.

MALÉCOT (1939a) proved for diallelic loci that FISHER's formulas for the variance and the parental and sibling correlations hold in the limit as the number of loci tends to infinity. FISHER's work had suggested that assortative mating increases the additive genetic variance, leaving the dominance variance approximately unaltered, and FISHER (1918) implicitly made this assumption in his study of the correlation between relatives. This result was also established by MALÉCOT (1939a).

This subject is difficult, and many challenging problems remain open (NAGYLAKI 1982a).

Random mating in a finite population: WRIGHT used path coefficients to deduce many basic properties of the evolution of a population under pure random genetic drift. Employing probabilities of identity instead of correlations as his dynamical variables, MALÉCOT derived equations equivalent to WRIGHT's and established some important new results. Although MALÉCOT's one-locus probabilities refer to identity by descent, he did not assume that they all vanish initially, as is conventional, but rather treated arbitrary initial conditions. Thus, his analyses differ only in interpretation from the later approach of KIMURA (1963), whose probabilities refer to identity in state. It is identity in state that is (at least in principle) measurable and, as far as probabilities of identity are concerned, more general, If the initial population is a random sample from an infinite population in Hardy-Weinberg proportions, then (1) and similar equations yield probabilities of identity in state in terms of probabilities of identity by descent.

MALÉCOT investigated evolution at a single locus in a monoecious population as well as at single autosomal and sex-linked loci and at a pair of autosomal loci in a dioecious population. In the important case of a single autosomal locus in a dioecious population, he studied also the effects of rapid population growth and arbitrary distribution of the number of progeny per individual.

Ideal population: Each of N monoecious individuals produces the same extremely large number of gametes, which fuse wholly at random (including self-fertilization); N randomly chosen zygotes survive to reproductive age. Thus, the rate of selfing is $1/N$. If at least one generation of panmixia precedes the initial generation, in which the heterozygosity is h_0, then the expected heterozygosity in generation t $(=0,1,2,\cdots)$ reads (WRIGHT 1931; MALÉCOT 1946, 1948; KIMURA 1963)

$$h_t = h_0\left(1 - \frac{1}{2N}\right)^t. \tag{3}$$

Therefore, the characteristic time for the loss of genetic variability is $2N$ generations. This is the first fundamental result of the theory of random genetic drift, and it motivated (in different directions!) the development of the evolutionary theories of both FISHER (1930b) and WRIGHT (1931, 1977, Ch. 13).

The distribution of the allelic numbers in any generation, conditioned on those in the previous generation, is multinomial. This is usually called the WRIGHT-FISHER model. On account of its simplicity, it is the reference model for random drift.

An autosomal locus in a dioecious population: MALÉCOT (1946, 1948) demonstrated that (3) approximates the expected heterozygosity in a panmictic population of N_1 males and N_2 females if the following five conditions hold: h_0 is replaced by k_0, the probability that two genes chosen at random from distinct individuals in the initial generation are different alleles, N is replaced by the effective population number

$$N_e = \frac{4N_1 N_2}{N_1 + N_2}, \tag{4}$$

$k_0 > 0$, $N_e \gg 1$, and $t \geq 1$. WRIGHT (1931) had shown only that replacing N by N_e approximates the asymptotic decay rate of the expected heterozygosity.

MALÉCOT (1946, 1948) proved also that if the population numbers N_1 and N_2 are deterministic functions of time, then some genetic variability is preserved (*i.e.*, $h_t \nrightarrow 0$ as $t \to \infty$) if and only if

$$\sum_{t=0}^{\infty} \frac{1}{N_e(t)} < \infty. \tag{5}$$

Thus, sufficiently rapid population growth preserves some genetic diversity. It is easy to show that the criterion (5) applies as well to ideal populations. This beautiful result has stimulated much work on the

more difficult problem of stochastically varying population number (see DONNELLY 1986; KLEBANER 1988; and references therein). Furthermore, if $N_e(t)$ is reinterpreted as the number of ancestors t generations in the past of a specified individual, then (5) is necessary but not sufficient for the preservation of some genetic heterogeneity in certain classes of regular inbreeding systems (ARZBERGER 1988).

In an ideal population, the number of successful gametes produced by a specified individual is binomially distributed. To take deviations from the binomial distribution into account, WRIGHT (1938b, 1939) devised the inbreeding effective population number. MALÉCOT (1951) derived an inbreeding effective population number for a dioecious population; his formula, a generalization of (4), closely approximates the exact one if the total population number is much greater than one (KIMURA and CROW 1963; CROW and KIMURA 1970, pp. 349–352; POLLAK 1977; CROW and DENNISTON 1988).

Sex-linked loci: Instead of (4), the effective population number is now (WRIGHT 1933a, MALÉCOT 1951, KIMURA 1963)

$$N_e = \frac{9N_1 N_2}{2(2N_1 + N_2)}. \tag{6}$$

Two loci: MALÉCOT (1951) derived the recursion relations for the two-locus probabilities of specified alleles (in the same gamete, in uniting gametes, or in randomly chosen gametes) in a dioecious population. Obvious averages of his variables and recursion relations yield those of KIMURA (1963); simple transformations establish agreement with WRIGHT's (1933b) recursions for correlations. Whereas WRIGHT and KIMURA investigated the equilibrium, MALÉCOT calculated the rate of convergence.

The balance between mutation and random drift: MALÉCOT (1946, 1948, 1951) introduced mutation by proposing that every allele mutates at rate u and no mutant is identical by descent to any preexisting allele. He proved for an ideal population (MALÉCOT 1946) and for autosomal (MALÉCOT 1946, 1948) and sex-linked (MALÉCOT 1951) loci in a dioecious population that the autozygosity converges as $t \to \infty$ to

$$\hat{F} \approx 1/(1 + 4N_e u), \tag{7}$$

where the approximation holds if the mutation rate $u \ll 1$, and the effective population number N_e is given in the three cases by the actual population number N, (4), and (6), respectively.

MALÉCOT's (1951) lucid discussion demonstrates that he considered the same elegant postulate for identity in state but, lacking empirical motivation, did not pursue it. Similarly, WRIGHT (1948) mentioned this possibility only fleetingly. It was KIMURA and CROW (1964) who, with molecular genetics to support them, posited that each mutant is of a novel allelic type—the model of infinitely many alleles—and began the investigation of the consequences of this hypothesis. Since the probabilities of the two kinds of identity differ only in their initial conditions, the first major result of this model is precisely (7), in which $\hat{F}$ is now interpreted as the expected homozygosity. Thus, MALÉCOT's idea led to one of the most important and thoroughly analyzed models of molecular population genetics (EWENS 1979, 1989; KINGMAN 1980; KIMURA 1983; HOPPE 1987).

The random drift of gene frequencies: The probabilities of identity discussed in the last two subsections are functionals of the Markov chain that describes the evolution of the population. These probabilities yield some basic results quite easily, but the more difficult direct analysis of the Markov chain is more informative. This subsection concerns MALÉCOT's studies of the random fluctuation of the gene frequency at a diallelic autosomal locus in a finite population. Although he first formulated a general Poisson model for these fluctuations (MALÉCOT 1937), his subsequent papers treat various aspects of the Wright-Fisher model: the asymptotic probability distribution for pure random drift, the general stationary distribution, the (time-dependent) probability distribution for reversible mutation, and the fixation probability for genic selection (*i.e.*, selection without dominance).

Mathematical research in diffusion theory influenced population genetics only gradually. As described in more detail below, WRIGHT was unaware of KOLMOGOROV's (1931) pioneering paper, and WRIGHT, MALÉCOT, and KIMURA were all apparently unacquainted with KHINTCHINE's (1933) book. The work of these two great Russian mathematicians would have led these population geneticists to easier, more rigorous, and sometimes more general analyses. Thus, the mutually beneficial cross-fertilization between diffusion theory and population genetics did not start until FELLER published his seminal 1951 paper. But this probably still represents relatively rapid communication between fields.

A general Poisson model: FISHER (1922, 1930a, b) suggested that if an organism produces an exceedingly large number of progeny, of which only a small fraction survives, then (at least approximately) the number of surviving progeny should have a Poisson distribution, and he used this idea to examine the behavior of rare alleles. In his first publication, MALÉCOT (1937) extended FISHER's hypothesis to incorporate (random or nonrandom) mating, fertility differences among mating types, and viability differences among genotypes. Had he fixed the total number of offspring, his trivariate probability-generating function would have been of the same type as those of FELDMAN (1966), WATTERSON (1970), and ETHIER and NAGYLAKI (1980), who were all apparently unaware of MALÉCOT's model.

The asymptotic probability distribution for pure random drift: FISHER (1922, 1930a, b) and WRIGHT (1931) employed rough, intuitive methods to seek the distribution of the gene frequency (excluding absorption) in a large ideal population after a long time has elapsed.

In the first application of the diffusion approximation in population genetics, FISHER (1922) derived a partial differential equation for the gene-frequency distribution and deduced that as $t \to \infty$ this distribution becomes uniform and decays at the rate $1/(4N)$ per generation. However, comparison with a preliminary version of WRIGHT (1931) led FISHER (1930a, b) to discover an error in his 1922 derivation; the corrected asymptotic distribution is still uniform, but decays twice as fast, in agreement with (3). It must be noted that FISHER's analysis of the diffusion equation was still incomplete.

WRIGHT (1931) examined directly the Chapman-Kolmogorov equations (whose general validity for Markov chains was unknown to him) for steady decay at the rate (3) and observed that a uniform distribution satisfies them approximately. This does not suffice, however, to demonstrate that (3) gives the maximal eigenvalue of the Markov chain of gene frequencies.

Neither FISHER nor WRIGHT obtained the normalization of the uniform distribution and, as MALÉCOT (1944) pointed out, neither of them fully established convergence to this distribution. MALÉCOT (1944) appealed to the theory of Markov chains—the first time this was done explicitly in population genetics (SENETA 1974)—to show that for $t \gg N \gg 1$ and initial gene frequency p, the distribution of the gene frequency x $(0 < x < 1)$ can be approximated by the probability density

$$\phi(p,x,t) \approx 6p(1 - p)e^{-t/(2N)}. \tag{8}$$

This is precisely the leading term as $t \to \infty$ in KIMURA's (1955) complete solution of the Kolmogorov forward equation. Equation 8 approximates also the probability that the locus is still segregating in generation t.

The general stationary distribution: WRIGHT (1929) first presented without derivation a formula for the stationary distribution of the gene frequency under reversible mutation and genic selection. He showed later (WRIGHT 1931) that in the absence of selection his formula approximately satisfies the stationary CHAPMAN-KOLMOGOROV equations. Comparison with results of FISHER (1930b) for extremely low mutation rates revealed, however, that his selection factor was wrong. WRIGHT (1931) corrected his formula by enforcing constancy of the mean gene frequency. Subsequently, he obtained the stationary distribution for arbitrary selection by enforcing constancy of both the mean and the variance (WRIGHT 1937). Then he used the same method to derive the general formula

(WRIGHT 1938a)

$$\hat{\phi}(x) = \frac{C}{V(x)} \exp\left[2 \int^x \frac{M(y)}{V(y)} dy \right] \qquad (9)$$

for the stationary distribution (in modern terminology) of a diffusion with drift and diffusion coefficients $M(x)$ and $V(x)$. (C is a normalization constant.)

In his classic 1931 paper, KOLMOGOROV showed that his forward equation yields the stationary result

$$\frac{1}{\hat{\phi}} \frac{d\hat{\phi}}{dx} = \frac{2M}{V} - \frac{1}{V} \frac{dV}{dx}, \qquad (10)$$

from which (9) follows immediately. In 1935, he applied (10) to reversible mutation without selection, and about ten years later sent this biological paper (KOLMOGOROV 1935) to WRIGHT (1945). However, KOLMOGOROV did not cite his earlier paper, and therefore WRIGHT did not realize that KOLMOGOROV had proved both the forward equation and (9) in complete generality. The distributions in WRIGHT (1931, 1937, 1938a, 1945) follow easily and rigorously from the forward equation and (9).

MALÉCOT (1945) noted that invariance of the first two moments does not establish invariance of the probability distribution. By an original method (described below), he rederived the stationary case of the forward equation and from this easily deduced both the general formula (9) and its application to reversible mutation and arbitrary selection.

The probability distribution for reversible mutation: Reversible mutation without selection is the only process for which the time-dependent solution of the KOLMOGOROV forward equation was obtained before the extensive and systematic investigations of KIMURA (reviewed in KIMURA 1964; CROW and KIMURA 1970). This was accomplished independently by MALÉCOT (1948) and (slightly more explicitly) by GOLDBERG (1950). KIMURA calculated all the moments of the gene frequency, and from these he reconstructed GOLDBERG's solution (CROW and KIMURA 1956).

MALÉCOT's (1945, 1948) derivation of the KOLMOGOROV forward equation is of independent interest. Instead of following KOLMOGOROV (1931), he assumed that the drift and diffusion coefficients are polynomials and established a partial differential equation for the moment-generating function, from which he deduced the forward equation. Partial differential equations for the moment-generating function are often useful in the analysis of stochastic processes. MALÉCOT did not know that PALM (1943, pp. 56–66) had used them earlier in special cases. Independently of PALM and MALÉCOT, BARTLETT (1947, 1949) developed the method quite generally.

The fixation probability for genic selection: Fixation probabilities directly affect the rate of evolution and illuminate the fluctuation of gene frequencies. FISHER

(1922, 1930a, b) was the first to examine the fixation probability of a favorable mutation. HALDANE (1927) used FISHER's branching-process method to show that for a Poisson offspring distribution in an infinite population, if s designates the selective advantage of the heterozygote Aa over the homozygote aa and selection is weak (*i.e.*, $0 \leq s \ll 1$), then the probability that the descendants of a single new mutant A are ultimately fixed (rather than lost) is $u \approx 2s$. For genic selection, by a rather complicated and indirect argument, FISHER (1930a, b) extended this result to a finite population of size N:

$$u \approx 2s/(1 - e^{-4Ns}), \qquad (11)$$

provided $|s| \ll 1$ and $N \gg 1$. WRIGHT (1931) simplified FISHER's argument and confirmed (11).

Discussions with HALDANE prompted MALÉCOT (1952) to generalize (11) to an arbitrary initial frequency, p, of A. Invoking his derivation of the forward equation (MALÉCOT 1948), he showed easily that the moment-generating function

$$g(p,\xi,t) = E[e^{\xi X(t)} | X(0) = p] \qquad (12)$$

of the gene frequency $X(t)$ satisfies the partial differential equation

$$\frac{\partial g}{\partial t} = \xi\left(s + \frac{\xi}{4N_e} \right)\left(\frac{\partial g}{\partial \xi} - \frac{\partial^2 g}{\partial \xi^2} \right), \qquad (13)$$

in which N_e denotes the variance effective population number (CROW and DENNISTON 1988). Clearly, (13) implies that $g(p, -\sigma, t)$, where $\sigma = 4N_e s$, is constant. Appealing to (12) to evaluate $g(p, -\sigma, t)$ at $t = 0$ and as $t \to \infty$ demonstrates immediately that the fixation probability $u(p)$ satisfies

$$u(p)e^{-\sigma} + 1 - u(p) = e^{-\sigma p},$$

whence (MALÉCOT 1952)

$$u(p) = \frac{1 - e^{-\sigma p}}{1 - e^{-\sigma}}. \qquad (14)$$

This approach does not extend readily to arbitrary dominance, and KIMURA (1957, 1962) used a more powerful method to deduce the general formula: he demonstrated that $u(p)$ satisfies the ordinary differential equation $Lu = 0$, where L represents the generator of the diffusion (the operator in the KOLMOGOROV backward equation), and solved for $u(p)$ with the appropriate boundary conditions. This method (for diffusions in one and two dimensions) goes back to KHINTCHINE (1933, pp. 32, 41); it was also treated by DARLING and SIEGERT (1953) and FELLER (1954).

Spatial variation: Since many, perhaps most, natural populations are distributed in space and mate at random only locally, it is important to study under what conditions the effects of population subdivision are negligible (NAGYLAKI 1980, 1983) and to seek quantities that, under suitable restrictions, are invariant under population subdivision (NAGYLAKI 1982b and references therein). In the model of infinitely many neutral alleles, population subdivision produces interdeme differentiation and increases the mean homozygosity and the effective number of alleles (NAGYLAKI 1985, 1986). Only the investigation of particular migration patterns, however, can yield a detailed understanding of the stationary and transient patterns of genetic variability in spatially distributed populations.

MALÉCOT has devoted far more effort to this problem than to any other. His research has stimulated an extensive theoretical literature, much of which is discussed in this subsection. The rest of the literature on neutral models of spatial variation can be traced from the references. His results have been widely compared with data from natural populations (LAMOTTE 1951, 1959; CAVALLI-SFORZA and BODMER 1971; MORTON 1982; WIJSMAN and CAVALLI-SFORZA 1984; SLATKIN 1985).

After some general remarks about the sundry models for spatial variation, infinite and finite populations will be treated successively.

Models: The first idea was again WRIGHT's (1931): in his island model, infinitely many finite, panmictic colonies exchange migrants wholly at random, *i.e.*, with no spatial effect on dispersal. Much later, this model was formulated and analyzed for finitely many islands (MARUYAMA 1970a; MAYNARD SMITH 1970; NAGYLAKI 1983, 1986).

A more elaborate model is required to study the decrease of relationship with distance. WRIGHT's (1943a, b, 1946, 1951, 1969, pp. 295–324) model of isolation by distance in a spatially continuous population is a rough, intuitive scheme without detailed, explicit derivation of the fundamental equations from clearly specified assumptions. These equations depend only on the variance of the migration distribution (through the neighborhood size), whereas an exact discrete-time model must depend on the entire distribution (*cf.* MALÉCOT 1948, p. 61). This reduction occurs because WRIGHT treats a continuously distributed population as if it were a hierarchy of panmictic neighborhoods from which ancestors are drawn at random. It is also difficult to see why the demographic fluctuations discussed below would not occur in WRIGHT's scheme.

Like WRIGHT's, MALÉCOT's models are selectively neutral. Although his most recent papers concern continuous-time, birth-and-death migration models (MALÉCOT 1977, 1980, 1981), in the work described below he almost invariably posits discrete, nonoverlapping generations. To maximize biological interest and simplify the exposition, mutation to new alleles at rate u will be assumed. The theory is similar for the covariance of gene frequencies in a diallelic model with reversible mutation (MALÉCOT 1949, 1971; KIMURA

and WEISS 1964; WEISS and KIMURA 1965; FLEMING and SU 1974; NAGYLAKI 1978a); in this case, small fluctuations around a space-independent overdominant equilibrium can also be included (MALÉCOT 1948).

In most of his research on spatial variation, MALÉCOT postulates discrete distribution of the population into (finitely or infinitely many) panmictic colonies, often called demes. MALÉCOT (1949) first deduced the recursion relations for the covariances in the diallelic model under the reasonable approximation that all evolutionary forces (*i.e.*, mutation, migration, and random drift) are weak. Soon thereafter, he wrote the recursion relations satisfied by the probabilities of identity for the migration of nonselfing diploids (MALÉCOT 1950). If all the evolutionary forces are weak, these equations are close to the exact ones (SAWYER 1976; NAGYLAKI 1983). It was in his 1951 paper that MALÉCOT obtained the system to which he and others subsequently devoted so much attention. This system turns out to be exact for the following life cycle.

First, every one of the N_i monoecious, diploid adults in deme i produces the same very large number of gametes, which then disperse. Complete random union of gametes within each deme follows. Therefore, a proportion $1/N_i$ of the zygotes whose gametes both originated in deme i are produced by self-fertilization. Mutation is next, and finally population regulation returns the number of individuals in deme i to N_i. Let $f_{ij}(t)$ denote the probability that two distinct genes chosen at random from adults just before gametogenesis in generation t, one from colony i and one from colony j, are the same allele. Define m_{ij} as the probability that a gamete in deme i after dispersion was produced in deme j. After one generation, the probabilities of identity satisfy (MALÉCOT 1951, 1975; NAGYLAKI 1976a, 1980, 1983; SAWYER 1976)

$$f'_{ij} = v\left[\sum_{k,l} m_{ik}m_{jl}f_{kl} + \sum_k m_{ik}m_{jk}(2N_k)^{-1}(1 - f_{kk})\right], \quad (15)$$

where $v = (1 - u)^2$ and the prime signifies the next generation. Actually, (15) holds if mutation occurs at any time between gametogenesis and regulation. Population regulation during this period would have no effect if it were sufficiently weak to leave very large numbers of gametes and zygotes. As SAWYER (1976) has noted, (15) also applies to a model with $2N_i$ haploid individuals in deme i.

If $0 \le f_{ij}(0) \le 1$ for every i and j, then $0 \le f_{ij}(t) \le 1$ for every i, j, and t. In addition, if $f_{ij}(0) = f_{ji}(0)$ for every i and j, then $f_{ij}(t) = f_{ji}(t)$ for every i, j, and t. Thus, biologically sensible initial conditions are preserved. If mutation is present ($u > 0$), then as $t \to \infty$, $f_{ij}(t) \to \hat{f}_{ij}$, the unique equilibrium of (15), at least as fast as v^t (NAGYLAKI 1980). Furthermore, some genetic variability is preserved: from (15) it follows that $\hat{f}_{ij} < 1$ for some i and j.

For the unbounded and circular stepping-stone models and for the island model with a finite number of islands, if mutation or random drift is weak, then the unique equilibrium of the gametic-dispersion model (15) is close to that of the exact diploid-migration model (SAWYER 1976; NAGYLAKI 1983). Consult NAGYLAKI (1983) for other results on this type of robustness.

Subdivision of a population into discrete colonies was proposed independently by KIMURA (1953). Although he presented no explicit formulation of his "stepping-stone" model for spatially homogeneous migration between nearest neighbors, it is clear that he focused directly on gene-frequency fluctuations, as he did in his subsequent collaborative analyses of the general homogeneous model (KIMURA and WEISS 1964; WEISS and KIMURA 1965).

In his more expository writings, MALÉCOT (1948, 1955, 1959, 1967) postulated continuous spatial distribution of the population. Independent reproduction and migration yield random fluctuations in the population density. Whereas in the above discrete model this difficulty can be obviated by population regulation, this has not been accomplished for any biologically reasonable continuous model (FELSENSTEIN 1975; KINGMAN 1977; SUDBURY 1977; SAWYER and FELSENSTEIN 1981). Furthermore, the lack of rigor in the formulation of the continuous model is reflected in the devastating fact that biologically sensible initial conditions in the continuous analog of (15) can lead (at least for low population densities) to probabilities of identity that are negative or greater than one (NAGYLAKI 1976a).

Despite these serious difficulties, it can be shown that the equilibrium probabilities of identity in the continuous analogs of the unbounded and circular stepping-stone models are between zero and one. Furthermore, approximating these equilibrium probabilities of identity for weak mutation in an infinite population (MALÉCOT 1948, 1955, 1959, 1967; NAGYLAKI 1974a, 1976b, 1978b) yields correct results (NAGYLAKI 1976a, SAWYER 1977a). Approximate formulas for the rate and pattern of convergence (as $t \to \infty$) in the special case of identity by descent without mutation (NAGYLAKI 1978b) are also correct (NAGYLAKI 1976a, SAWYER 1976).

Although the spatial distribution of a population obviously cannot be exactly continuous, in many cases the stepping-stone model surely overestimates the degree of clustering. Therefore, it would be highly desirable to formulate a biologically reasonable model for a population distributed with a finite, continuous density.

Diffusion approximation of the basic system (15) provides another route toward the derivation of a continuous model. This approach applies if all evolutionary forces are weak, and it leads to a partial differential equation, which is more tractable than (15). Early work in this direction, initiated by MALÉCOT (1959, 1967, 1969) and continued by MARUYAMA (1971a), FLEMING and SU (1974), and NAGYLAKI (1974a, b) was heuristic, but in one spatial dimension more rigorous derivations have been presented (NAGYLAKI 1978a, 1986, 1988b). Unfortunately, the diffusion approximation fails in more than one dimension (FLEMING and SU 1974; NAGYLAKI 1974a, 1978a), essentially because the required scalings yield $N_i \to \infty$ only in one dimension (NAGYLAKI 1978a).

Organisms confined to a river, riverbank, seashore, mountain range, etc., do occupy essentially one-dimensional habitats, but most natural populations are distributed over two dimensions. Therefore, it would be important to develop a continuous-time, continuous-space model in two dimensions.

Infinite populations: Suppose there are demes of N individuals each at the points of the infinite integer lattice in d dimensions. Migration is homogeneous, *i.e.*, the migration rates depend only on displacement, rather than on the initial and final positions separately (MALÉCOT 1949, 1950, 1951; KIMURA 1953). Probabilistic formulation and investigations of this stepping-stone model are extremely illuminating (SAWYER 1976, 1977b, 1979; RUSINEK 1982; SHIGA 1985; SHIGA and UCHIYAMA 1986), but, as in MALÉCOT's work, the emphasis here is on the probabilities of identity.

Consider first the *equilibrium* of (15). To express the results in simple form, first rotate coordinates so as to diagonalize the covariance matrix of the migration distribution m. Write the eigenvalues of this matrix as $\frac{1}{2} \sigma_i^2$ ($i = 1, \cdots, d$), let $\mathbf{w}$ denote the separation (in the rotated coordinates) between the demes from which genes are sampled, and introduce the scaled coordinates $x_i = w_i / \sigma_i$ ($i = 1, \cdots, d$). Finally, define

$$c = \prod_{i=1}^{d} \sigma_i, \tag{16a}$$

$$x = \left(\sum_{i=1}^{d} x_i^2 \right)^{1/2}, \quad \xi = 2\sqrt{u}x. \tag{16b}$$

The product Nc is essentially WRIGHT's (1946) neighborhood size. In natural populations, Nc always seems to exceed 30 and is usually at least about 300 (WRIGHT 1978, Ch. 2). The equilibrium probability of identity $\hat{f}$ is spatially homogeneous, *i.e.*, it depends on the coordinates of the two demes sampled only through their scaled separation $\mathbf{x}$. Under some biologically trivial technical restrictions, $\hat{f}(\mathbf{x})$ can be approximated for weak mutation; consult NAGYLAKI (1976a) and, especially, SAWYER (1977a) for the most detailed and precise results. Although the exact value of $\hat{f}(\mathbf{x})$ depends on the entire migration distribution m, the approximations below depend on m only through the variances σ_i^2.

In one dimension, the mean heterozygosity is given by

$$1 - \hat{f}(\mathbf{0}) \sim 4Nc\sqrt{u} \qquad (17a)$$

as $u \to 0$. (The notation means that the ratio of the two sides tends to one as $u \to 0$.) The probability of identity decays exponentially in space:

$$\hat{f}(\mathbf{x}) \sim e^{-\xi} \qquad (17b)$$

as $u \to 0$ and $x \to \infty$ with ξ fixed. If $u \ll 1$ and $Nc \gg 1$ (and ξ is bounded above), the approximation

$$\hat{f}(\mathbf{x}) \approx \frac{e^{-\xi}}{1 + 4Nc\sqrt{u}} \qquad (17c)$$

is adequate.

In two dimensions, the mean heterozygosity reads

$$1 - \hat{f}(\mathbf{0}) \sim -4\pi Nc/\ln(2u) \qquad (18a)$$

as $u \to 0$. As $u \to 0$ and $x \to \infty$ with ξ fixed,

$$\hat{f}(\mathbf{x}) \sim -\frac{2}{\ln(2u)} K_0(\xi), \qquad (18b)$$

where K_0 designates the modified Bessel function of the second kind of order zero. If $\xi \gg 1$, (18b) becomes

$$\hat{f}(\mathbf{x}) \approx -\frac{1}{\ln(2u)} \sqrt{\frac{2\pi}{\xi}} e^{-\xi}, \qquad (18c)$$

which decays more rapidly than the unidimensional result (17b). If $u \ll 1$ and $Nc \gg 1$ (and ξ is bounded below and above), the approximation

$$\hat{f}(\mathbf{x}) \approx \frac{2K_0(\xi)}{4\pi Nc - \ln(2u)} \qquad (18d)$$

suffices.

The three-dimensional case may apply to some aquatic or subterranean organisms. There is no simple formula for the expected heterozygosity. If $u \ll 1$, $Nc \gg 1$, and ξ is bounded away from 0 and ∞, then

$$\hat{f}(\mathbf{x}) \approx \frac{e^{-\xi}}{4\pi Ncx}. \qquad (19)$$

This decreases faster than (18c) by a factor of $\sqrt{x}$.

In his very first paper on subdivided populations, MALÉCOT (1949) already presented an intuitive preliminary analysis of the unbounded, linear stepping-stone model; for symmetric nearest-neighbor migration, he obtained the rate of decay in (17c), but his approximation misses the 1 in the denominator. Next, he derived (17c) for symmetric nearest-neighbor migration and showed that the rate of decay is the same for arbitrary symmetric migration (MALÉCOT 1950). In his 1951 paper, MALÉCOT deduced (17c) in full generality. WEISS and KIMURA (1965) also obtained the numerator in (17c); as discussed in NAGYLAKI (1974a), their asymptotic analysis contains some er-

rors. See NAGYLAKI (1976a) and SAWYER (1977a) for proofs of (17) with error estimates.

The more difficult two-dimensional problem has a more complicated history. First, MALÉCOT (1948) established (18a) in the continuous model with isotropic Gaussian migration. Unfortunately, an error in the asymptotics of the stepping-stone model with symmetric nearest-neighbor migration led MALÉCOT (1950) to the pure exponential decay $e^{-\xi}$. Subsequently, he found the more rapid rate $e^{-\xi}/\sqrt{\xi}$ for isotropic Gaussian migration (MALÉCOT 1959). He misinterpreted this discrepancy, however, as an actual difference between the asymptotics of the discrete and continuous models. For symmetric nearest-neighbor migration, the mean heterozygosity (18a) can be extracted from the results of WEISS and KIMURA (1965). These authors also obtained the behavior $K_0(\xi)$ in (18b) for arbitrary symmetric migration, though not entirely correctly (cf. NAGYLAKI 1974a). It is fairly easy to prove (18a) in the most general case (NAGYLAKI 1976a; SAWYER 1977a), but a rigorous demonstration of the full result (18), with error estimates, is more delicate (SAWYER 1977a).

MALÉCOT did not examine the three-dimensional problem. WEISS and KIMURA (1965) and NAGYLAKI (1976b) investigated special cases; the general formula (19) is due to SAWYER (1977a).

The results are more accurate in one dimension than in two or more. For the same values of u and Nc, the mean heterozygosity increases with the number of dimensions. Note that the characteristic length of the decay of $\hat{f}(\mathbf{x})$ is greater than that of migration by the large factor $1/(2\sqrt{u}) \gtrsim 200$.

The work of WRIGHT (1943a, 1951, 1969) suggests that in the absence of mutation one- and two-dimensional populations tend to genetic homogeneity. Indeed, perhaps the most interesting qualitative property of the stepping-stone model is that as $u \to 0$, $\hat{f}(\mathbf{x}) \to 1$ for $d = 1,2$, but $\hat{f}(\mathbf{x}) \nrightarrow 1$ for $d \geq 3$ (WEISS and KIMURA 1965; NAGYLAKI 1976a; SAWYER 1976). Since the population is infinite, the ultimate loss of genetic variability in one or two dimensions is a consequence of spatial structure. The underlying distinction between $d = 1,2$ and $d \geq 3$ is recurrence of the associated migration random walk (SAWYER 1976).

If $u = 0$, in a finite population ultimately the descendants of one of the genes initially present are *fixed* with probability one. In the stepping-stone model, the interpretation of $\hat{f}(\mathbf{x}) \equiv 1$ is more subtle (SAWYER 1976): the descendants of any particular initial gene ultimately become *extinct* with probability one. Apparently, every bounded region is eventually occupied by single dynasties (i.e., the descendants of a single initial gene) for increasingly long periods of time, and the periods of transition between dynasties become too rare to produce $\hat{f}(\mathbf{x}) < 1$.

The equilibrium results are biologically important

only if *convergence* occurs on an evolutionarily reasonable time scale. Convergence will be treated here only in one or two dimensions; SAWYER's (1976) theorems are very general and could be applied in three or more dimensions. For long times, the asymptotic behavior depends on the recurrent potential $\psi(\mathbf{x})$ of the associated random walk (NAGYLAKI 1976a; SAWYER 1976; SPITZER 1976, Chs. 2, 7). This complicated functional of the migration distribution satisfies $\psi(\mathbf{0}) = 0$ and

$$\psi(\mathbf{x}) \sim x, \qquad d = 1, \tag{20a}$$

$$\psi(\mathbf{x}) \sim \frac{\ln x}{\pi}, \qquad d = 2, \tag{20b}$$

as $x \to \infty$ (NAGYLAKI 1976a; SAWYER 1976; SPITZER 1976, pp. 124, 345).

Let $f_t(\mathbf{y},\mathbf{z})$ represent the probability of identity for genes sampled from demes at $\mathbf{y}$ and $\mathbf{z}$ (in the rotated and scaled coordinates) in generation t. The probability of nonidentity

$$h_t(\mathbf{y},\mathbf{z}) = 1 - f_t(\mathbf{y},\mathbf{z}) \tag{21}$$

yields the mean heterozygosity at $\mathbf{y}$ if $\mathbf{y} = \mathbf{z}$. The separation between the demes is $\mathbf{x} = \mathbf{y} - \mathbf{z}$. The results are much simpler for $u = 0$ than for $u > 0$.

If there is no mutation ($u = 0$), it suffices to impose the exceedingly mild decay condition

$$\lim_{r \to \infty} \sup_{x=r} f_0(\mathbf{y},\mathbf{z}) = 0 \tag{22}$$

on the initial probability of identity. Notice that for identity by descent, $f_0(\mathbf{y},\mathbf{z}) = 0$, so (22) holds trivially. Then

$$h_t(\mathbf{y},\mathbf{z}) \sim [1 + (2Nc)^{-1}\psi(\mathbf{x})]h_t(\mathbf{0},\mathbf{0}) \tag{23a}$$

as $t \to \infty$ with $\mathbf{y}$ and $\mathbf{z}$ fixed, and the expected heterozygosity

$$h_t(\mathbf{0},\mathbf{0}) \sim 2Nc\sqrt{\frac{2}{\pi t}}, \qquad d = 1, \tag{23b}$$

$$h_t(\mathbf{0},\mathbf{0}) \sim \frac{4\pi Nc}{\ln t}, \qquad d = 2, \tag{23c}$$

as $t \to \infty$.

If mutation is present ($u > 0$), assume initial spatial homogeneity:

$$f_0(\mathbf{y},\mathbf{z}) = f_0(\mathbf{x},\mathbf{0}) \tag{24}$$

for every $\mathbf{y}$ and $\mathbf{z}$. Then $f_t(\mathbf{y},\mathbf{z}) = f_t(\mathbf{x},\mathbf{0})$ for every $\mathbf{y},\mathbf{z}$, and t, and one can set

$$\hat{f}(\mathbf{x}) - f_t(\mathbf{y},\mathbf{z}) = v^t\phi_t(\mathbf{x}). \tag{25}$$

Instead of (22), now impose the stronger but still weak decay condition, $f_0(\mathbf{x},\mathbf{0}) = O(x^{-2-\eta})$ as $x \to \infty$, for some $\eta > 0$. Both hypotheses hold trivially for identity by descent. Finally, suppose that $t\phi_t(\mathbf{x})$ is monotone de-

creasing in t for sufficiently large t, for every $\mathbf{x}$. Then

$$\phi_t(\mathbf{x}) \sim [1 + (2Nc)^{-1}\psi(\mathbf{x})]\phi_t(\mathbf{0}) \tag{26a}$$

as $t \to \infty$ with $\mathbf{x}$ fixed, and

$$\phi_t(\mathbf{0}) \sim ANc\sqrt{\frac{2}{\pi t^3}}, \qquad d = 1, \tag{26b}$$

$$\phi_t(\mathbf{0}) \sim \frac{4\pi ANc}{t(\ln t)^2}, \qquad d = 2, \tag{26c}$$

as $t \to \infty$, where the constant A is given by

$$A = -\phi_0(\mathbf{0}) + \frac{1}{c}\sum_{\mathbf{x}}\phi_0(\mathbf{x})[2Nc + \psi(\mathbf{x})]. \tag{26d}$$

For identity by descent,

$$A = \frac{v}{1-v} \sim \frac{1}{2u} \tag{26e}$$

as $u \to 0$.

In one dimension, the diffusion limit exists, and under the simplifying assumption (24), it leads to an explicit solution for $\phi_t(\mathbf{x})$ for every $\mathbf{x}$ and t (NAGYLAKI 1974a, 1978b, 1986). Approximating this solution as $t \to \infty$ yields (23a, b) and, without the monotonicity assumption on $t\phi_t(\mathbf{x})$, (26a, b); in the diffusion limit, $\psi(\mathbf{x}) = x$ exactly and (26d) is replaced by an integral (NAGYLAKI 1974a, 1978b, 1986).

MALÉCOT confined himself to identity by descent in one dimension. He used generating functions and a Tauberian theorem to deduce (20a) and (23a, b) (MALÉCOT 1975); in later, unpublished research, he obtained (26a, b) with his methods (G. MALÉCOT, personal communication).

Equations 20 to 26 were derived in NAGYLAKI (1976a). For $u = 0$, however, the assumptions in NAGYLAKI (1976a) are stronger than the very weak ones—due to SAWYER (1976)—presented here. For $u > 0$ and identity by descent, (26) follows from SAWYER (1976). His outstanding paper contains powerful methods, interesting ideas, and other important results.

The most important biological conclusion from these results is that in the absence of mutation, the rate of loss of genetic variability in two dimensions is negligibly slow: (23c) shows that even if Nc were only 10, after 10^{500} generations the mean heterozygosity would still be about 0.11! If there is mutation, the rate of convergence to equilibrium is much faster; convergence is faster in one dimension than in two.

If $u = 0$, subject to (22), the results are spatially homogeneous and independent of the initial condition f_0; if $u > 0$, they depend on f_0 only through the constant A.

Under the assumptions made here, the spatial dependence is the same for $u = 0$ and $u > 0$. In the usual biological situation $Nc \gg 1$, so $\psi(x) \ll 2Nc$ unless $d = 1$ and x is at least of the same order as Nc. Therefore,

(23a) and (26a) reveal that the spatial dependence is sometimes negligible if $d = 1$ and often negligible if $d = 2$.

If part of the habitat is bounded, spatial homogeneity is lost and the analysis becomes much more difficult. The boundary may be either a barrier impenetrable to migration, or a point or line of contact with a region of extremely high population density or dispersal rate (a density-mobility boundary). For a semi-infinite linear habitat with either type of boundary, a complete analysis of the equilibrium has been obtained in the diffusion approximation (NAGYLAKI and BARCILON 1988).

SAWYER (1978) has studied migration models in a (topological) tree, which may describe some populations in river systems. SAWYER and FELSENSTEIN (1983) have investigated the important case of hierarchically clustered population.

Finite populations: If σ^2 is the typical variance for migration, then (16), (17), and (18) show that the habitat can be treated as infinite only if its typical linear dimension greatly exceeds $\sigma/(2\sqrt{u})$.

MALÉCOT (1951) was the first to formulate and analyze a model for a subdivided finite population. In his *circular stepping-stone model*, n demes, each of which comprises N individuals, form a closed loop; migration is homogeneous. This arrangement might be a mathematical idealization of an atoll; demes around a mountain, lake, or shore of an island; or colonies of amphibians or shallow-water organisms in a large, deep lake or around an island.

MALÉCOT (1951) derived an explicit formula for the probability of identity at equilibrium and deduced from it the limiting cases of panmixia and the unbounded, linear stepping-stone model (see also MALÉCOT 1965, 1975). Much later, MARUYAMA (1969, 1970a, b, c) rederived MALÉCOT's solution. Although theoretically useful (NAGYLAKI 1983), MALÉCOT's solution (a sum of n terms) is too complicated to yield much direct biological insight; for this, approximations are necessary. Approximation of the discrete-time, continuous-space model (NAGYLAKI 1974b) agrees with the more rigorous diffusion approximation (NAGYLAKI 1986), and this simple solution enables one to examine the expected heterozygosity, genetic diversity, and interdeme differentiation of gene frequencies at equilibrium (NAGYLAKI 1986).

MARUYAMA was the first to investigate the rate and pattern of convergence of the circular stepping-stone model. Positing symmetric nearest-neighbor migration and spatial homogeneity, he obtained the exact characteristic equation and found approximations for the eigenvalues and eigenvectors for both strong and weak migration (MARUYAMA 1970d). He confirmed his approximations for the maximal eigenvalue and eigenvector by a diffusion analysis (MARUYAMA 1971a, 1972a). Approximations for all the eigenvalues

and eigenvectors can be derived in the discrete-time, continuous-space model (NAGYLAKI 1974b); these agree with the diffusion limit and enable one to deduce the probability of identity for any spatially homogeneous initial condition (NAGYLAKI 1974b, 1986). MALÉCOT (1975) derived the approximations for the maximal eigenvalue directly from the general discrete model. By Theorem 2.4 and Remark 2.9 of BOUCHER and NAGYLAKI (1988), the assumption of spatial homogeneity does not affect the ultimate rate and pattern of convergence.

To study the effects of dimensionality, MARUYAMA (1969) introduced the model of an abstract *torus*, in which the colonies occupy the product space of d circles. Although he solved this model at equilibrium (MARUYAMA 1969, 1970c, d), his very complicated formula is useful only numerically. MARUYAMA (1972b) has also calculated the asymptotic rate of convergence in some numerical examples. MALÉCOT (1975) deduced the equilibrium solution in a more concise form and obtained some analytic approximations for the rate of convergence.

If the colonies are along a finite *line segment* (MARUYAMA 1970a, b, c, e), the loss of spatial homogeneity greatly increases the difficulty of the analysis. Therefore, even for the equilibrium with symmetric nearest-neighbor migration, MARUYAMA (1970a, b, c) was able to find only rough approximations. For both strong and weak symmetric migration, he obtained also approximations for the maximal eigenvalue and eigenvector (MARUYAMA 1970e, 1971a, 1972a). In the diffusion approximation, FLEMING and SU (1974) deduced explicit formulae for the equilibrium and for all the eigenvalues and eigenvectors.

Only rough approximations are available for a *rectangular habitat* (MARUYAMA 1970a, c, 1971b, 1972b). The general strong-migration limit applies, however, to all finite populations (NAGYLAKI 1980, 1983).

SAWYER and FELSENSTEIN (1983) have studied finite *hierarchically clustered populations.*

DISCUSSION

In this paper, an attempt was made to demonstrate that GUSTAVE MALÉCOT has contributed important and fruitful ideas, methods, models, and results that have permanently transformed theoretical population genetics. By 1948, he had rederived and extended in a lucid, convincing manner many of the classical results of FISHER and WRIGHT, thereby initiating the modern era in population genetics. The first major line of work in modern population genetics was MALÉCOT's formulation and analysis of the stepping-stone model. It was KIMURA who originated and greatly advanced many of the other important lines of modern research.

Why, then, is much of MALÉCOT's work known even now only to a small minority of population geneticists?

First, MALÉCOT usually wrote in French, whereas since FISHER, HALDANE, and WRIGHT, the predominant language of theoretical population genetics has been English. It was not until 1967 that he published a paper in English from which most of his work can be traced. Second, many of his important papers are in journals, such as the *Annals of the University of Lyon*, that are not widely distributed. Third, in most of his papers, MALÉCOT needed and used more mathematics than many population geneticists find palatable. His masterly 1948 book is his most frequently cited work not only because it was translated in 1969, but also because it is more elementary than his major papers.

But do these superficial observations suffice? A fourth point is that MALÉCOT is a theorist's theorist: although he was occasionally stimulated by data, his main interest clearly lay in the development of the theory itself. The desire to develop the theory as an intellectual subdiscipline consistent with known, reasonably idealized biological reality is frequently misperceived as mathematical motivation. It is inevitable and desirable that most theoretical effort should be centered on applications to specific evolutionary problems, to human genetics, and to animal and plant breeding. However, the physical analogy of quantum mechanics and field theory versus their applications to solid state, nuclear, and elementary particle physics demonstrates that symbiotic coevolution of theory and applications is optimal.

Fifth, much of MALÉCOT's research was stimulated by that of WRIGHT. Perhaps partly because of the immensity of WRIGHT's creative accomplishment and the importance and influence of his work (PROVINE 1986), the necessity of MALÉCOT's reformulations and reanalyses is frequently unrecognized. As shown above (and many other examples could be adduced), WRIGHT's formulations were not always clear or complete, his derivations often had logical gaps, and his approximations were sometimes unjustified. These observations refer not to WRIGHT's lack of rigor in the sense of the pure mathematician, for this type of rigor is usually absent even in less original scientific work, but rather to the fact that to a qualified, careful, critical reader who evaluates WRIGHT's work without appeal to external information, his analyses are often unconvincing and the validity of his results sometimes seems uncertain. It is eloquent testimony to both WRIGHT's deep intuition and his remarkable patience with checking special cases numerically (until the middle 1970s on an electromechanical calculator!) that his results, at least when properly restricted and interpreted, are almost invariably correct.

Finally, in modern population genetics, a mathematical model is usually studied as an independent, well-posed entity (*i.e.*, one with acceptable solutions, neither overdetermined nor underdetermined), based on clearly stated biological assumptions, whose analysis may be guided but not replaced by extrinsic biological considerations. (The *interpretation* of the results should, of course, be biological and, as far as possible, intuitive.) Close reading of WRIGHT's work and extensive personal communication with him reveal that he rarely worked in this modern spirit. The first population geneticist to do so consistently was MALÉCOT.

WRIGHT, FISHER, and HALDANE drove many rough trails into the forest. MALÉCOT cleared, widened, and greatly extended some of these trails, significantly facilitating our exploration of the interior. Thus, his rôle in the transition from classical to modern population genetics is a crucial one, and much contemporary theoretical population genetics can be traced back to him, just as he and COTTERMAN taught us to trace the ancestry of genes.

GUSTAVE MALÉCOT's intellectual independence, enthusiasm, and generosity of spirit have been manifest in our extensive correspondence. I am much indebted to him not only for the assistance he thus provided, but also for inspiring my research with his own. I am very grateful to STEWART ETHIER, WARREN EWENS, MOTOO KIMURA, JERRE LEVY, STANLEY SAWYER, STEPHEN STIGLER, and SANDY ZABELL for perceptive comments on the manuscript. I thank MICHEL GILLOIS and ALBERT JACQUARD for useful information and MARC LAVENANT for help with translation. It is a pleasure to thank MITZI NAKATSUKA for careful, beautiful, and rapid typing. This work was supported by National Science Foundation grant BSR-8512844.

LITERATURE CITED

ARZBERGER, P., 1988 Results for generalized regular inbreeding systems. J. Math. Biol. **26:** 535–550.

BARTLETT, M. S., 1947 *Stochastic Processes*. Mimeographed notes of a course given at the University of North Carolina, Chapel Hill, in the fall of 1946.

BARTLETT, M. S., 1949 Some evolutionary stochastic processes. J. R. Stat. Soc. B **11:** 211–229.

BOUCHER, W., 1988 Calculation of the inbreeding coefficient. J. Math. Biol. **26:** 57–64.

BOUCHER, W., and T. NAGYLAKI, 1988 Regular systems of inbreeding. J. Math. Biol. **26:** 121–142.

CANNINGS, C., and E. A. THOMPSON, 1981 *Genealogical and Genetic Structure*. Cambridge University Press, Cambridge.

CAVALLI-SFORZA, L. L., and W. F. BODMER, 1971 *The Genetics of Human Populations*. W. H. Freeman, San Francisco.

COCKERHAM, C. C., 1954 An extension of the concept of partitioning hereditary variance for analysis of covariances among relatives when epistasis is present. Genetics **39:** 859–882.

COCKERHAM, C. C., 1956 Effects of linkage on the covariances between relatives. Genetics **41:** 138–141.

COTTERMAN, C. W., 1940 A calculus for statistico-genetics. Dissertation, Ohio State University, Columbus (pp. 157–272. In: *Genetics and Social Structure*, edited by P. BALLONOFF. Dowden, Hutchinson & Ross, Stroudsburg, Pa., 1974).

COTTERMAN, C. W., 1983 Relationship and probability in Mendelian genetics. Am. J. Med. Genet. **16**: 393–440.

CROW, J. F., and C. DENNISTON, 1988 Inbreeding and variance effective population numbers. Evolution **42**: 482–495.

CROW, J. F., and M. KIMURA, 1956 Some genetic problems in natural populations. Proc. Third Berkeley Symp. Math. Stat. Prob. **4**: 1–22.

CROW, J. F., and M. KIMURA, 1970 *An Introduction to Population Genetics Theory.* Harper & Row, New York.

DARLING, D. A., and A. J. F. SIEGERT, 1953 The first passage problem for a continuous Markov process. Ann. Math. Stat. **24**: 624–639.

DONNELLY, P., 1986 A genealogical approach to variable-population-size models in population genetics. J. Appl. Prob. **23**: 283–296.

DONNELLY, P., and S. TAVARÉ, 1987 The population genealogy of the infinitely-many neutral alleles model. J. Math. Biol. **25**: 381–391.

ETHIER, S. N., and T. NAGYLAKI, 1980 Diffusion approximations of Markov chains with two time scales and applications to population genetics. Adv. Appl. Prob. **12**: 14–49.

EWENS, W. J., 1979 *Mathematical Population Genetics.* Springer, Berlin.

EWENS, W. J., 1989 Population genetics theory—the past and the future. In: *Mathematical and Statistical Developments in Evolutionary Theory,* edited by S. LESSARD. NATO Advanced Study Institutes Series C. D. Reidel, Dordrecht, The Netherlands, in press.

FELDMAN, M. W., 1966 On the offspring number distribution in a genetic population. J. Appl. Prob. **3**: 129–141.

FELLER, W., 1951 Diffusion processes in genetics. Proc. Second Berkeley Symp. Math. Stat. Prob., pp. 227–246.

FELLER, W., 1954 Diffusion processes in one dimension. Trans. Am. Math. Soc. **77**: 1–31.

FELSENSTEIN, J., 1975 A pain in the torus: some difficulties with models of isolation by distance. Am. Nat. **109**: 359–368.

FELSENSTEIN, J., 1981 *Bibliography of Theoretical Population Genetics.* Dowden, Hutchinson & Ross, Stroudsburg, Pa.

FISHER, R. A., 1918 The correlation between relatives on the supposition of Mendelian inheritance. Trans. R. Soc. Edinb. **52**: 399–433.

FISHER, R. A., 1922 On the dominance ratio. Proc. R. Soc. Edinb. **42**: 321–341.

FISHER, R. A., 1930a The distribution of gene ratios for rare mutations. Proc. R. Soc. Edinb. **50**: 204–219.

FISHER, R. A., 1930b *The Genetical Theory of Natural Selection.* Clarendon Press, Oxford.

FLEMING, W. H., AND C.-H. SU, 1974 Some one-dimensional migration models in population genetics theory. Theor. Popul. Biol. **5**: 431–449.

GOLDBERG, S., 1950 On a singular diffusion equation. Dissertation, Cornell University.

HALDANE, J. B. S., 1927 A mathematical theory of natural and artificial selection, Part V: selection and mutation. Proc. Camb. Philos. Soc. **23**: 838–844.

HALDANE, J. B. S., and P. MOSHINSKY, 1939 Inbreeding in Mendelian populations with special reference to human cousin marriage. Ann. Eugen. **9**: 321–340.

HOPPE, F. M., 1987 The sampling theory of neutral alleles and an urn model in population genetics. J. Math. Biol. **25**: 123–159.

HUDSON, R. R., and N. L. KAPLAN, 1988 The coalescent process in models with selection and recombination. Genetics **120**: 831–840.

JACQUARD, A., 1974 *The Genetic Structure of Populations.* Springer, Berlin.

KAPLAN, N. L., T. DARDEN and R. R. HUDSON, 1988 The coalescent process in models with selection. Genetics **120**: 819–829.

KARLIN, S., 1969 *Equilibrium Behavior of Population Genetic Models*

with Non-Random Mating. Gordon and Breach, New York. Originally in J. Appl. Prob. **5**: 231–313, 487–566 (1968).

KEMPTHORNE, O., 1954 The correlation between relatives in a random mating population. Proc. R. Soc. B **143**: 103–113.

KEMPTHORNE, O., 1955a The theoretical values of the correlations between relatives in random mating populations. Genetics **40**: 153–167.

KEMPTHORNE, O., 1955b The correlations between relatives in random mating populations. Cold Spring Harbor Symp. Quant. Biol. **20**: 60–78.

KEMPTHORNE, O., 1957 *An Introduction to Genetic Statistics.* Wiley, New York.

KHINTCHINE, A., 1933 *Asymptotische Gesetze der Wahrscheinlichkeitsrechnung.* Springer, Berlin.

KIMURA, M., 1953 "Stepping-stone" model of population. Annu. Rept. Natl. Inst. Genet. Jpn. **3**: 62–63.

KIMURA, M., 1955 Solution of a process of random genetic drift with a continuous model. Proc. Natl. Acad. Sci. USA **41**: 144–150.

KIMURA, M., 1957 Some problems of stochastic processes in genetics. Ann. Math. Stat. **28**: 882–901.

KIMURA, M., 1962 On the probability of fixation of mutant genes in a population. Genetics **47**: 713–719.

KIMURA, M., 1963 A probability method for treating inbreeding systems, especially with linked genes. Biometrics **19**: 1–17.

KIMURA, M., 1964 Diffusion models in population genetics. J. Appl. Prob. **1**: 177–232.

KIMURA, M., 1983 *The Neutral Theory of Molecular Evolution.* Cambridge University Press, Cambridge.

KIMURA, M., and J. F. CROW, 1963 The measurement of effective population number. Evolution **17**: 279–288.

KIMURA, M., and J. F. CROW, 1964 The number of alleles that can be maintained in a finite population. Genetics **49**: 725–738.

KIMURA, M., and G. H. WEISS, 1964 The stepping stone model of population structure and the decrease of genetic correlation with distance. Genetics **49**: 561–576.

KINGMAN, J. F. C., 1977 Remarks on the spatial distribution of a reproducing population. J. Appl. Prob. **14**: 577–583.

KINGMAN, J. F. C., 1980 *Mathematics of Genetic Diversity.* Society for Industrial and Applied Mathematics, Philadelphia.

KLEBANER, F. C., 1988 Conditions for fixation of an allele in the density-dependent Wright-Fisher models. J. Appl. Prob. **25**: 247–256.

KOLMOGOROV, A., 1931 Über die analytischen Methoden in der Wahrscheinlichkeitsrechnung. Math. Ann. **104**: 415–458.

KOLMOGOROV, A., 1935 Deviations from Hardy's formula in partial isolation. C. R. Acad. Sci. URSS **8**: 129–132.

LAMOTTE, M., 1951 Recherches sur la structure génétique des populations naturelles de *Cepaea nemoralis* L. Bull. Biol. Fr. Belg. Suppl. **35**: 1–238.

LAMOTTE, M., 1959 Polymorphism of natural populations of *Cepaea nemoralis.* Cold Spring Harbor Symp. Quant. Biol. **24**: 65–86.

MALÉCOT, G., 1937 Quelques conséquences de l'hérédité mendélienne. C. R. Acad. Sci. Paris **204**: 619–622.

MALÉCOT, G., 1938a Sur l'analyse des aléatoires et le problème de l'hérédité. C. R. Acad. Sci. Paris **206**: 153–155.

MALÉCOT, G., 1938b Sur les aléatoires mendéliennes et les corrélations de l'hérédité. C. R. Acad. Sci. Paris **206**: 404–406.

MALÉCOT, G., 1939a Théorie mathématique de l'hérédité mendélienne généralisée. Dissertation, Faculté Sciences, University of Paris.

MALÉCOT, G., 1939b Loi de Mendel et homogamie. C. R. Acad. Sci. Paris **208**: 407–409.

MALÉCOT, G., 1939c Les corrélations entre individus apparentés, dans l'hypothèse d'homogamie. C. R. Acad. Sci. Paris **208**: 552–554.

MALÉCOT, G., 1941 Étude mathématique des populations "mendéliennes." Ann. Univ. Lyon Sci. Sec. A **4**: 45–60.

MALÉCOT, G., 1942   Mendélisme et consanguinité. C. R. Acad. Sci. Paris **215**: 313–314.

MALÉCOT, G., 1944   Sur un problème de probabilités en chaîne que pose la génétique. C. R. Acad. Sci. Paris **219**: 379–381.

MALÉCOT, G., 1945   La diffusion des gènes dans une population mendélienne. C. R. Acad. Sci. Paris **221**: 340–342.

MALÉCOT, G., 1946   La consanguinité dans une population limitée. C. R. Acad. Sci. Paris **222**: 841–843.

MALÉCOT, G., 1948   *Les mathématiques de l'hérédité*. Masson, Paris.

MALÉCOT, G., 1949   Les processus stochastiques de la génétique. Coll. Int. Cent. Nat. Rech. Sci. **13**: 121–126.

MALÉCOT, G., 1950   Quelques schémas probabilistes sur la variabilité des populations naturelles. Ann. Univ. Lyon Sci. Sec. A **13**: 37–60.

MALÉCOT, G., 1951   Un traitement stochastique des problèmes linéaires (mutation, linkage, migration) en Génétique de Population. Ann. Univ. Lyon Sci. Sec. A **14**: 79–117.

MALÉCOT, G., 1952   Les processus stochastiques et la méthode des fonctions génératrices ou caractéristiques. Publ. Inst. Stat. Univ. Paris **1**: Fasc. 3, 1–16.

MALÉCOT, G., 1955   The decrease of relationship with distance. Cold Spring Harbor Symp. Quant. Biol. **20**: 52–53.

MALÉCOT, G., 1959   Les modèles stochastiques en génétique de population. Publ. Inst. Stat. Univ. Paris **8**: Fasc. 3, 173–210.

MALÉCOT, G., 1965   Évolution continue des fréquences d'un gène mendélien (dans le cas de migration homogène entre groupes d'effectif fini constant). Ann. Inst. Henri Poincaré B **2**: 137–150.

MALÉCOT, G., 1966   *Probabilités et hérédité*. Presses Universitaires de France, Paris.

MALÉCOT, G., 1967   Identical loci and relationship. Proc. Fifth Berkeley Symp. Math. Stat. Prob. **4**: 317–332.

MALÉCOT, G., 1969   *The Mathematics of Heredity*. W. H. Freeman, San Francisco.

MALÉCOT, G., 1971   Génétique des populations diploïdes naturelles dans le cas d'un seul locus. I. Évolution de la fréquence d'un gène. Étude des variances et des covariances. Ann. Genet. Sel. Anim. **3**: 255–280.

MALÉCOT, G., 1975   Heterozygosity and relationship in regularly subdivided populations. Theor. Popul. Biol. **8**: 212–241.

MALÉCOT, G., 1977   Kinship in the birth and death process of a population subdivided in finite panmictic groups, pp. 147–156 in *Recent Developments in Statistics*, edited by J. R. BARRA, F. BRODEAU, G. ROMIER and B. VAN CUTSEM. North-Holland, Amsterdam.

MALÉCOT, G., 1980   Variability and permanence in molecular genetics, pp. 82–97 in *Vito Volterra Symposium on Mathematical Biology*, edited by C. BARIGOZZI. Springer, Berlin.

MALÉCOT, G., 1981   Évolution, parentés, migrations, pp. 95–119 in *Modèles mathématiques en biologie*, edited by C. CHEVALET and A. MICALI. Springer, Berlin.

MARUYAMA, T., 1969   Genetic correlation in the stepping stone model with non-symmetrical migration rates. J. Appl. Prob. **61**: 463–477.

MARUYAMA, T., 1970a   Effective number of alleles in a subdivided population. Theor. Popul. Biol. **1**: 273–306.

MARUYAMA, T., 1970b   Analysis of population structure. I. One-dimensional stepping stone models of finite length. Ann. Hum. Genet. **34**: 201–219.

MARUYAMA, T., 1970c   Stepping stone models of finite length. Adv. Appl. Prob. **2**: 229–258.

MARUYAMA, T., 1970d   On the rate of decrease of heterozygosity in circular stepping stone models of populations. Theor. Popul. Biol. **1**: 101–119.

MARUYAMA, T., 1970e   Rate of decrease of genetic variability in a subdivided population. Biometrika **57**: 299–311.

MARUYAMA, T., 1971a   The rate of decrease of heterozygosity in a population occupying a circular or a linear habitat. Genetics **67**: 437–454.

MARUYAMA, T., 1971b   Analysis of population structure. II. Two-dimensional stepping stone models of finite length and other geographically structured populations. Ann. Hum. Genet. **35**: 179–196.

MARUYAMA, T., 1972a   The rate of decay of genetic variability in a geographically structured finite population. Math. Biosci. **14**: 325–335.

MARUYAMA, T., 1972b   Rate of decrease of genetic variability in a two-dimensional continuous population of finite size. Genetics **70**: 639–651.

MAYNARD SMITH, J., 1970   Population size, polymorphism, and the rate of non-Darwinian evolution. Am. Nat. **104**: 231–237.

MORAN, P. A. P., 1961   Path coefficients reconsidered. Aust. J. Stat. **3**: 87–93.

MORTON, N. E., 1982   *Outline of Genetic Epidemiology*. S. Karger, Basel.

NAGYLAKI, T., 1974a   The decay of genetic variability in geographically structured populations. Proc. Natl. Acad. Sci. USA **71**: 2932–2936.

NAGYLAKI, T., 1974b   Genetic structure of a population occupying a circular habitat. Genetics **78**: 777–790.

NAGYLAKI, T., 1976a   The decay of genetic variability in geographically structured populations. II. Theor. Popul. Biol. **10**: 70–82.

NAGYLAKI, T., 1976b   The relation between distant individuals in geographically structured populations. Math. Biosci. **28**: 73–80.

NAGYLAKI, T., 1978a   A diffusion model for geographically structured populations. J. Math. Biol. **6**: 375–382.

NAGYLAKI, T., 1978b   The geographical structure of populations, pp. 588–624 in *Studies in Mathematics* **16**: *Studies in Mathematical Biology*, Part II, edited by S. A. LEVIN. Mathematical Association of America, Washington.

NAGYLAKI, T., 1980   The strong-migration limit in geographically structured populations. J. Math. Biol. **9**: 101–114.

NAGYLAKI, Y., 1982a   Assortative mating for a quantitative character. J. Math. Biol. **16**: 57–74.

NAGYLAKI, T., 1982b   Geographical invariance in population genetics. J. Theor. Biol. **99**: 159–172.

NAGYLAKI, T., 1983   The robustness of neutral models of geographical variation. Theor. Popul. Biol. **24**: 268–294.

NAGYLAKI, T., 1985   Homozygosity, effective number of alleles, and interdeme differentiation in subdivided populations. Proc. Natl. Acad. Sci. USA **82**: 8611–8613.

NAGYLAKI, T., 1986   Neutral models of geographical variation, pp. 216–237 in *Stochastic Spatial Processes*, edited by P. TAUTU. Springer, Berlin.

NAGYLAKI, T., 1988a   Gene conversion, linkage, and the evolution of multigene families. Genetics **120**: 291–301.

NAGYLAKI, T., 1988b   The influence of spatial inhomogeneities on neutral models of geographical variation. I. Formulation. Theor. Popul. Biol. **33**: 291–310.

NAGYLAKI, T., and V. BARCILON, 1988   The influence of spatial inhomogeneities on neutral models of geographical variation. II. The semi-infinite linear habitat. Theor. Popul. Biol. **33**: 311–343.

NARAIN, P., 1966   Effect of linkage on homozygosity of a population under mixed selfing and random mating. Genetics **54**: 303–314.

OHTA, T., 1985   A model of duplicative transposition and gene conversion for repetitive DNA families. Genetics **110**: 513–524.

PALM, C., 1943   Intensitätsschwankungen in Fernsprecherverkehr. Ericsson Technics, Stockholm, No. 44.

POLLAK, E., 1977   Effective population numbers and their interrelations, pp. 115–144 in *Proceedings of the Washington State University Conference on Biomathematics and Biostatistics of May*

1974. Department of Pure and Applied Mathematics, Washington State University and Pi Mu Epsilon, Washington Alpha Chapter, Pullman, Wash.

PROVINE, W. B., 1986 *Sewall Wright and Evolutionary Biology.* University of Chicago Press, Chicago.

RUSINEK, R., 1982 Rate of extinction and limiting distribution for a geographically structured population. Soc. Ind. Appl. Math. J. Appl. Math. **42:** 86–93.

SAWYER, S., 1976 Results for the stepping-stone model for migration in population genetics. Ann. Prob. **4:** 699–728.

SAWYER, S., 1977a Asymptotic properties of the equilibrium probability of identity in a geographically structured population. Adv. Appl. Prob. **9:** 268–282.

SAWYER, S., 1977b Rates of consolidation in a selectively neutral migration model. Ann. Prob. **5:** 486–493.

SAWYER, S., 1978 Isotropic random walks in a tree. Z. Wahr. **42:** 279–292.

SAWYER, S., 1979 A limit theorem for patch sizes in a selectively neutral migration model. J. Appl. Prob. **16:** 482–495.

SAWYER, S., and J. FELSENSTEIN, 1981 A continuous migration model with stable demography. J. Math. Biol. **11:** 193–205.

SAWYER, S., and J. FELSENSTEIN, 1983 Isolation by distance in a hierarchically clustered population. J. Appl. Prob. **20:** 1–10.

SCHNELL, F. W., 1963 The covariance between relatives in the presence of linkage, pp. 468–483 in *Statistical Genetics and Plant Breeding,* edited by W. D. HANSON and H. F. ROBINSON. National Academy of Sciences-National Research Council Publication 982, Washington.

SENETA, E., 1974 A note on the balance between random sampling and population size (on the 30th anniversary of G. MALÉCOT's paper). Genetics **77:** 607–610.

SHIGA, T., 1985 Mathematical results on the stepping stone model in population genetics, pp. 267–279 in *Population Genetics and Molecular Evolution,* edited by T. OHTA and K. AOKI. Springer, Berlin.

SHIGA, T., and K. UCHIYAMA, 1986 Stationary states and their stability of the stepping stone model involving mutation and selection. Prob. Theory Rel. Fields **73:** 87–117.

SLATKIN, M., 1985 Gene flow in natural populations. Ann. Rev. Ecol. Syst. **16:** 393–430.

SPITZER, F., 1976 *Principles of Random Walk,* Ed. 2. Springer, Berlin.

SUDBURY, A., 1977 Clumping effects in models of isolation by distance. J. Appl. Prob. **14:** 391–395.

TRUSTRUM, G. B., 1961 The correlations between relatives in a random mating diploid population. Proc. Camb. Philos. Soc. **57:** 315–320.

TUKEY, J. W., 1954 Causation, regression, and path analysis, pp. 35–66 in *Statistics and Mathematics in Biology,* edited by O. KEMPTHORNE, T. A. BANCROFT, J. W. GOWEN and J. L. LUSH. Iowa State College Press, Ames.

VAN AARDE, I. M. R., 1975 The covariance of relatives derived from a random mating population. Theor. Popul. Biol. **8:** 166–183.

WATTERSON, G. A., 1970 On the equivalence of random mating and random union of gametes models in finite, monoecious populations. Theor. Popul. Biol. **1:** 233–250.

WEIR, B. S., AND C. C. COCKERHAM, 1973 Mixed selfing and random mating at two loci. Genet. Res. **21:** 247–262.

WEISS, G. H., and M. KIMURA, 1965 A mathematical analysis of the stepping stone model of genetic correlation. J. Appl. Prob. **2:** 129–149.

WIJSMAN, E. A., and L. L. CAVALLI-SFORZA, 1984 Migration and genetic population structure with special reference to humans. Ann. Rev. Ecol. Syst. **15:** 279–301.

WRIGHT, S., 1921a Correlation and causation. J. Agric. Res. **20:** 557–585.

WRIGHT, S., 1921b Systems of mating. Genetics **6:** 111–178.

WRIGHT, S., 1922a Coefficients of inbreeding and relationship. Am. Nat. **56:** 330–338.

WRIGHT, S., 1922b The effects of inbreeding and crossbreeding on guinea pigs. III. Crosses between highly inbred families, pp. 1–60. Bull. 1121, U. S. Department Agriculture, Washington.

WRIGHT, S., 1929 The evolution of dominance. Am. Nat. **63:** 556–561.

WRIGHT, S., 1931 Evolution in Mendelian populations. Genetics **16:** 97–159.

WRIGHT, S., 1933a Inbreeding and homozygosis. Proc. Natl. Acad. Sci. USA **19:** 411–420.

WRIGHT, S., 1933b Inbreeding and recombination. Proc. Natl. Acad. Sci. USA **19:** 420–433.

WRIGHT, S., 1934 The method of path coefficients. Ann. Math. Stat. **5:** 161–215.

WRIGHT, S., 1937 The distribution of gene frequencies in populations. Proc. Natl. Acad. Sci. USA **23:** 307–320.

WRIGHT, S., 1938a The distribution of gene frequencies under irreversible mutation. Proc. Natl. Acad. Sci. USA **24:** 253–259.

WRIGHT, S., 1938b Size of population and breeding structure in relation to evolution. Science **87:** 430–431.

WRIGHT, S., 1939 *Statistical Genetics in Relation to Evolution.* Actual. Sci. Ind. **802:** Exposés de biométrie et de statistique biologique. XIII, Edited by G. Teissier. Hermann, Paris.

WRIGHT, S., 1943a Isolation by distance. Genetics **28:** 114–138.

WRIGHT, S., 1943b Analysis of local variability of flower color in *Linanthus parryae.* Genetics **28:** 139–156.

WRIGHT, S., 1945 The differential equation of the distribution of gene frequencies. Proc. Natl. Acad. Sci. USA **31:** 382–389.

WRIGHT, S., 1946 Isolation by distance under diverse systems of mating. Genetics **31:** 39–59.

WRIGHT, S., 1948 Genetics of populations, pp. 111–112 in *Encyclopaedia Britannica,* Vol. 10, Ed. 14. Encyclopaedia Britannica, Chicago.

WRIGHT, S., 1951 The genetical structure of populations. Ann. Eugen. **15:** 323–354.

WRIGHT, S., 1968 *Evolution and the Genetics of Populations,* Vol. I. *Genetic and Biometric Foundations.* University of Chicago Press, Chicago.

WRIGHT, S., 1969 *Evolution and the Genetics of Populations,* Vol. II. *The Theory of Gene Frequencies.* University of Chicago Press, Chicago.

WRIGHT, S., 1977 *Evolution and the Genetics of Populations,* Vol. III. *Experimental Results and Evolutionary Deductions.* University of Chicago Press, Chicago.

WRIGHT, S., 1978 *Evolution and the Genetics of Populations,* Vol. IV. *Variability Within and Among Natural Populations.* University of Chicago Press, Chicago.

◦ Fortunes of War ◦

James F. Crow

Genetics Department, University of Wisconsin–Madison, Madison, Wisconsin 53706

DAIGORO MORIWAKI graduated from Tokyo University in 1929 with a degree in zoology, hoping for a career in fisheries science. At that time the Japanese economy was badly depressed and there was no opening in his chosen subject. After two years he gave up the hope and eventually found a position at the Tokyo Prefectural Higher School, later to become a part of Tokyo Metropolitan University. There he sought the advice of his respected Tokyo University professor, NAOHIDE YATSU, who had studied with T. H. MORGAN at Columbia University. At YATSU's suggestion, he asked for guidance from an elder professor at his insitution, YOSHITAKA IMAI. IMAI recommended three specific projects, which MORIWAKI dutifully undertook. One was to induce lethal mutations by radiation in *Drosphila melanogaster*, the second was to investigate the effect of age on crossing over in *Drosphilia virilis*, and the third was to find and study a Drosophila species indigenous to Japan.

Following the third suggestion, MORIWAKI caught an unfamiliar Drosophila in a Tokyo fruit and vegetable market. He immediately started a culture and began collecting and mapping mutants. At about the same time, HIDEO KIKKAWA, a graduate student at the University of Kyoto, also began studying a "new" species. He was a student of TAKU KOMAI, who like YATSU had studied with MORGAN. KIKKAWA's Drosophila stock came from Formosa, now Taiwan, and both his and MORIWAKI's species turned out to be *Drosophila ananassae*.

Actually, MORIWAKI and KIKKAWA were not the first to study this species. As so often happened in early Drosophila genetics, STURTEVANT was first. In 1916 he described 23 new species of Drosophilidae, including one called *Drosophila caribea*, which turned out to have been named *ananassae* in 1858 following its discovery in Indonesia. (*Ananas* means pineapple in several languages; the Japanese word is *ananasu*.). Ironically, *D. ananassae*, chosen to be representative of Japanese Drosophila, is not native to Japan. It is most abundant in tropical areas. MORIWAKI's flies were undoubtedly stowaways on a fruit shipment to Tokyo.

Nevertheless, MORIWAKI and KIKKAWA continued to work on this species, and by 1939 had discovered 117 mutations. All but six had been assigned to linkage groups and most were mapped. *D. ananassae* was more than just another Drosophila species. It had three special features: male crossing over, a high mutation rate, and *bobbed* mutants on both the *Y* and the fourth chromosome (KIKKAWA 1938; MORIWAKI 1940). Linkage data from the Japanese geneticists were used by STURTEVANT and NOVITSKI (1941) to homologize the chromosome arms with those of *melanogaster* and other Drosophila species. In 1938 KIKKAWA changed his emphasis to silkworm genetics and sent all his Drosophila stocks to MORIWAKI in Tokyo. For reviews of this early period, see MORIWAKI and TOBARI (1975); those who read Japanese may refer to MORIWAKI (1988).

With the coming of World War II, research became impossible in many countries and valuable stocks were endangered. One such was the cytoplasmically inherited CO_2 sensitivity in a stock of *D. melanogaster*, discovered by TEISSIER and L'HÉRITIER. In 1939 World War II was beginning and L'HÉRITIER, having survived one war, was pessimistic about his chances in another. So, that year at the International Genetics Congress in Edinburgh he gave his precious stock to H. J. MULLER. Later, L'HÉRITIER was freed from military duties and was able to resume his work. MULLER, who saved the stock and had refrained from working on it, sent the flies back to France on one of the first trans-Atlantic flights, and the now-classical research continued.

On the other side of the world, MORIWAKI was not so fortunate. Concerned that the mutant stocks might be lost, he prepared four replicate sets. He gave one to a friend in Hokkaido University in northern Japan. A second was kept by a biochemist friend in Kyoto. A third went to still another friend in what is now North Korea. The fourth, MORIWAKI himself kept in Tokyo.

The combination of heat, cold, and shortages, to

say nothing of wartime disruption, made stockkeeping almost impossible. For one thing, the necessary ingredients for preparing culture media were often unobtainable. MORIWAKI's own stocks were gradually lost, and he could only hope that at least one of the other three replicates had survived. After the war's end, he learned that the Hokkaido and Kyoto stocks had also been lost. The only hope was that the flies in Korea had survived. Not until September of 1948 was MORIWAKI able to make contact. The stocks had indeed survived the war, but not the transition to a higher technology. One freezing February day the new electric system failed. Had the earlier charcoal burners been retained, the stocks might have survived.

Despite this setback, studies on *D. ananassae* continued after the war. RAY-CHAUDHURI *et al.* (1959) had found a number mutant genes in India. Many of these, and probably a few from MORIWAKI's early studies, were included in the stocks kept and made available by the Zoology Department at the University of Texas at Austin. In the United States, HINTON used these and his own mutant strains, and is responsible for much of the post-war formal genetics and gene mapping. With the establishment of Tokyo Metropolitan University in 1949, MORIWAKI again had an active laboratory and in the mid-1960s began again to report new mutants. Most of the lost ground has now been regained through international cooperation.

Drosophila is exceptional, though not unique, in having no crossing over in the heterogametic sex. *D. ananassae* is the exception to the exception. Male crossing over has never been entirely lost, or perhaps has been regained. Although the rate can be increased by selection, it is still much lower than that in females. There is considerable genetic variability for the property, and both Mendelian and maternally transmitted factors are involved. This species may provide a clue to understanding male meiosis in other Drosophila species. *D. ananassae* has a very high level of inversion polymorphism in natural populations. This is puzzling in view of the male recombination; there is a suggestion that some mechanism restricts exchange within heterozygous inversions during spermatogenesis (HINTON and DOWNS 1975). The high mutability of this species also has chromosomal and extrachromosomal determinants, at least some of which seem also to be concerned with male recombination (TOBARI and MORIWAKI 1983; HINTON 1983).

The species is interesting for comparative studies of ribosomal DNA. The mutation *bobbed* is associated with a reduced number of repeats in ribosomal DNA, and in *melanogaster* is located on the homologous parts of the *X* and *Y* chromosomes. In *ananassae* the mutation is associated with the *Y* and the heterochromatic fourth chromosome (KAUFMANN 1937; KIKKAWA 1938).

HINTON, in addition to his work on mapping, mutation and male crossing over, has found a curious set of optic morphology (*Om*) mutations in *D. ananassae* (HINTON 1984, 1988). These are neomorphic, semidominant, and phenotypically similar to each other. They occur at a high rate at some 25 specific loci, and there are a number of equally specific suppressors. It has been suspected that these are caused by a transposable element with a proclivity for eye morphology loci and this suspicion was confirmed by SHRIMPTON, MONTGOMERY and LANGLEY (1986). Occasionally the *Om* system produces a mutation at other than eye loci, and the finding of one at singed permitted cloning by use of the homologous region from *melanogaster*. The causative element has turned out to be a retrovirus-like transposable element related to *297* and *17.6*, two previously known retroposons (TANDA *et al.* 1988). Further analysis of one of the *Om* loci has shown it to correspond to *Bar* in *melanogaster* (unpublished results of S. TANDA, A. E. SHRIMPTON, C. W. HINTON and C. H. LANGLEY).

World War II had another influence on *D. ananassae*. A postwar resurgence of interest came from its being the only species of Drosophila found in the northern Marshall Islands, the site of some Pacific nuclear tests. It was collected and studied by geneticists from the University of Texas who were observing the effects of radiation on natural populations. Morphologically, *ananassae* is a member of the *melanogaster* species group (BOCK and WHEELER 1972). In addition to a high degree of inversion polymorphism, there is considerable geographical variation in morphology (FUTCH 1966). Two color phases, light and dark, are now regarded as separate species (BOCK and WHEELER 1972), although they occasionally hybridize (FUTCH 1973). Finally, parthenogenetic strains have been reported (FUTCH 1972). There is plenty to study.

It is fitting that this species, with its unusual properties and with interested parties on both sides of the Pacific, be the object of a binational study. This is now assured by a cooperative program sponsored by the U. S. National Science Foundation and the Japan Society for the Promotion of Science. Among the participants are MORIWAKI, TOBARI and MATSUDA in Japan, and LANGLEY and HINTON in the United States.

What of the founders of this work? KIKKAWA became one of Japan's most distinguished scientists. For many years he headed a large and highly productive research laboratory at the University of Osaka. I was privileged to visit Osaka in 1957. At that time Japan was still very poor, and I was astonished at how effectively KIKKAWA and some dozen students could work in an extremely crowded and poorly equipped laboratory. Although most were studying Drosophila, some tackled such diverse creatures as house flies and bacteria. One student, YUKINORI HIROTA, was able to "cure" F[+] strains of *Escherichia coli* by treatment with acridine dyes, making them F[-]. This result had been greeted with skepticism in the United States, but I was able—using picture-drawing and hand-waving as a substitute for a common tongue—to learn HIROTA's procedures. JOSHUA LEDERBERG, following protocols that I brought back from Osaka, immediately verified the results. The technique turned out to be experimentally very useful and helped in understanding the episomal nature of the F factor. This was mentioned as fulfilling the formal paradigm of directed mutation in an earlier *Perspectives* (LEDERBERG 1989). HIROTA was a leading bacterial geneticist until his recent untimely death. KIKKAWA is now retired and living in Hirakata.

MORIWAKI went on to a long career as a researcher, teacher, and administrator. He was President of Tokyo Prefectural Higher School and Director of the National Institute of Genetics in Mishima. He found being Director a taxing, emotion-draining, full-time job, but I always knew where to find him on Sundays. He would be busily doing Drosophila experiments, and I think this was the happiest time of his week. He is now retired, but continues to experiment with his beloved *D. ananassae*.

I should like to thank CLAUDE HINTON, CHARLES LANGLEY and DAVID FUTCH for contributing useful technical comments on this article, and THOMAS NAGYLAKI for noticing some stylistic infelicities. I am especially pleased to acknowledge historical information from three pioneers, DIAGORO MORIWAKI, HIDEO KIKKAWA, and PHILIPPE L'HÉRITIER.

LITERATURE CITED

BOCK, I. R., and M. R. WHEELER, 1972 The *Drosophila melanogaster* species group. Univ. Texas Publ. No. **7212:** 1–102.

FUTCH, D. G., 1966 A study of speciation in South Pacific populations of *Drosophila ananassae*. Univ. Texas Publ. No. **6615:** 79–120.

FUTCH, D. G., 1972 A preliminary note on parthenogenesis in *Drosophila ananassae*. Drosophila Inform. Serv. **48:** 78.

FUTCH, D. G., 1973 On the ethological differentiation of *Drosophila ananassae* and *Drosophila pallidosa* in Samoa. Evolution **27:** 456–467.

HINTON, C. W., 1983 Relations between factors controlling crossing over and mutability in males of *Drosophila ananassae*. Genetics **104:** 95–112.

HINTON, C. W., 1984 Morphogenetically specific mutability in *Drosophila ananassae*. Genetics **106:** 631–653.

HINTON, C. W., 1988 Formal relations between *Om* mutants and their suppressors in *Drosophila ananassae*. Genetics **120:** 1035–1042.

HINTON, C. W., and J. E. DOWNS, 1975 The mitotic, polytene, and meiotic chromosomes of *Drosophila ananassae*. J. Hered. **66:** 353–361.

KAUFMANN, B. P., 1937 Morphology of the chromosomes of *Drosophila ananassae*. Cytologia (Fujii Jubilee Volume), pp. 1043–1055.

KIKKAWA, H., 1938 Studies on the genetics and cytology of *Drosophila ananassae*. Genetica **20:** 458–516.

LEDERBERG, J., 1989 Replica plating and indirect selection of bacterial mutants: isolation of preadaptive mutants in bacteria by sib selection. Genetics **121:** 395–399.

MORIWAKI, D., 1940 Enhanced crossing over in the second chromosome of *Drosophila ananassae*. Jpn. J. Genet. **16:** 37–48.

MORIWAKI, D., 1988 *Note Book of Genetics: My Life with Drosophila* (in Japanese). University of Tokyo Press, Tokyo.

MORIWAKI, D., and Y. N. TOBARI, 1975 *Drosophila ananassae*, pp. 513–535 in *Handbook of Genetics*, Vol 3, edited by R. C. KING. Plenum Press, New York.

RAY-CHAUDHURI, S. P., D. SARKAR, A. S. MUKHERJEE and J. BOSE, 1959 Mutation in *Drosophila ananassae* and their linkage map. Proc. 1st All India Congr. Zool., Pt. 2, Addendum: i–xi.

SHRIMPTON, A. E., E. A. MONTGOMERY and C. H. LANGLEY, 1988 *Om* mutations in *Drosophila ananassae* are linked to insertions of a transposable element. Genetics **114:** 125–135.

STURTEVANT, A. H., 1916 Notes on North American Drosophilidae with descriptions of twenty three new species. Ann. Entomol. Soc. Am. **9:** 323–343.

STURTEVENT, A. H., and E. NOVITSKI, 1941 The homologies of the chromosome elements in the genus Drosophila. Genetics **26:** 517–541.

TANDA, S., A. E. SHRIMPTON, C. L. LING, H. ITAYAMA, H. MATSUBAYASHI, K. SAIGO, Y. N. TOBARI and C. H. LANGLEY, 1988 Retrovirus-like features and site specific insertions of a transposable element, *tom*, in *Drosophila ananassae*. Mol. Gen. Genet. **214:** 405–411.

TOBARI, Y. N., and D. MORIWAKI, 1983 Positive correlation between male recombination and *Minute* mutation frequencies in Drosophila ananassae. Jpn. J. Genet. **58:** 159–163.

August 1989

In Praise of Complexity

Salome Gluecksohn Waelsch

Department of Molecular Genetics, Albert Einstein College of Medicine, Bronx, New York 10461

THE T complex in the mouse has been a favorite target for molecular investigations in recent years, with the result that its area on chromosome *17* has become "one of the most completely analyzed regions of any mammalian chromosome" (LEHRACH 1988). It was 50 years ago last month that GENETICS published a paper by L. C. DUNN and myself that reported detailed genetic and developmental data on mutations at the T locus. This locus had come into the genetical spotlight in 1927 when the dominant mutation T was discovered by a cancer investigator, Madame DOBROVALSKAIA-ZAVADSKAIA, in the Pasteur Laboratory of the Radium Institute in Paris. The shortened tail in heterozygous mice ($T/+$) suggested the name of the mutation, *brachyury*. DOBROVALSKAIA-ZAVADSKAIA also reported the embryonic lethality of homozygotes (T/T). Furthermore, she obtained tailless progeny in outcrosses of short-tailed heterozygotes ($T/+$) to normal-tailed wild mice caught in the laboratory. Remarkably, these wild mice were heterozygous for a recessive t mutation that interacts with T to produce the tailless phenotype (T/t). These tailless heterozygotes bred true when crossed with each other because of the embryonic lethality of both homozygous types, thus constituting the first balanced-lethal system in mammals.

It is strongly to his credit that DUNN's power of intuition and scientific judgment led him to choose the T locus early in its genesis as the main focus of his research activities. Starting in the mid-1930s, DUNN and his colleagues became increasingly impressed by the numerous exceptional and unorthodox aspects of genetic behavior of T-locus mutations and their unwillingness to conform to the expectations of conventional genetics. Rules of Mendelian segregation, of allelism, and of allelic interactions were flaunted, and recombination appeared to be suppressed. DUNN fully realized the potential of this unusual genetic system for the analysis of a number of fundamental problems of gene transmission and expression. He did not share the naive assumption, held at that time by some, of a simple one-to-one relationship between a gene and its phenotype far removed from primary gene action, and he was aware of the great complexities of gene actions and interactions. Speculating about the state of developmental genetics at that time, DUNN (1939) gave credit to GOLDSCHMIDT (1938) for his attempts to deal with developmental effects of genes beyond the level of their transmission or structure. But DUNN felt that, in 1939, developmental genetics had not yet coalesced as a field. This is particularly interesting in view of the close relationship at the beginning of the century between embryology and the emerging science of genetics, as exemplified by the two eminent biologists E. B. WILSON and TH. BOVERI.

The T complex on chromosome *17* includes a range of mutations later discovered to cover about 16 cM (FRISCHAUF 1985). The relevant genes were shown to affect a variety of systems, thus creating a diversity of problems including those of genetic transmission, recombination, gene action, pleiotropy, evolution, genetic control of development and spermatogenesis. Such complexity of effects presented a unique situation as well as opportunity, and raised questions of gene structure, organization and expression, many of which have remained unanswered to this day.

The dominant mutation T causes complete absence of the notochord in homozygous embryos and severe abnormalities of those developmental systems that depend on interaction with the notochord during embryogeny (CHESLEY 1935). It was the causal analysis of these mutational effects that implicated the notochord in normal mechanisms of early mammalian development, analogous to its role in lower vertebrate embryos earlier elucidated by experimental microsurgical procedures.

Our 1939 paper describing the genetic aspects and various effects of mutations at the T locus dealt with the second instance of what was then called a recessive mutation, t^1, causing preimplantation lethality when homozygous. t^1 had been shown earlier to interact with T to produce the tailless phenotype (T/t^1) and to breed true in a balanced-lethal system. The 1939 paper also described the phenomenon of segregation distortion that characterizes males carrying t^1. These regularly transmitted a highly significant excess of t^1 sperm over sperm carrying the wild-type allele. Earlier, DUNN had reported the existence of the recessive mutation t^0 that interacted with T to produce tailless mice (T/t^0). These bred true as a balanced-lethal system because t^0 also was lethal when homozygous. An embryological study of t^0 which I undertook at that time showed it to affect the formation and development of mesoderm in embryos 5 days after fertilization (GLUECKSOHN-SCHOENHEIMER 1940). Since T, t^0 and t^1 failed to recombine with each other, they were considered to be alleles at a single locus. However, even though t^0 and t^1 were lethal when homozygous, the compound t^0/t^1 proved to be viable and the majority of such animals were morphologically normal. Such complementation between supposed alleles raised early questions in DUNN's mind about their allelism and caused him to refer to T as a "complex" locus (DUNN 1954). Eventually, the recessive t "alleles" were shown not to be mutations at a single locus but rather to cover a considerable portion (12–16 cM) of the chromosome and to include closely linked normal and mutant gene sequences held together by inversions with consequent suppression of recombination (FRISCHAUF 1985); they were called t haplotypes. Their widespread distribution in natural populations was discovered and described by DUNN (1964) and is particularly intriguing in view of the earlier mentioned derivation of t^0 and t^1 from wild mice. The evolutionary dynamics of the different haplotypes causing segregation distortion in males and lethality of homozygous embryos has been the subject of much discussion (see, for example, BRUCK 1957 and LEWONTIN and DUNN 1960).

The 1939 paper represented a milestone in the analysis of the T locus, particularly in its relevance to developmental genetics. The identification of three mutations showing no recombination with each other, each affecting the same embryonic elements (notochord, mesoderm and neural tube) and causing early embryonic lethality when homozygous, seemed intriguing in terms of interpretations on both genetic and developmental levels. Because these mutations shared profound effects on early embryogenesis, they seemed for the first time to implicate genes (and, in this case, closely linked genes) in basic mechanisms of vertebrate differentiation. Therefore, the discovery of this mutant system in the mouse not only demonstrated the existence of developmental mechanisms in mammals analogous to those operating in lower animals (see below) but in addition raised the exciting prospect of providing an approach to the identification of specific genes controlling such mechanisms. SPEMANN in his work on embryonic induction in amphibians had totally ignored any role for genes in

early development and instead considered a "vital force" to be instrumental in the action of the "organizer" and the induction of the neural tube by the notochord (cf. HOLTFRETER, as quoted by MOSCONA 1986). As a graduate student in the institute of SPEMANN, I had become acutely conscious of his failure to take into account genetic factors in the interpretations of his experimental results, and this only served to increase my own appreciation of the T locus and its effects as a potential tool in the causal analysis of vertebrate development and its genetic basis. This appeared particularly important at a time when the mammalian embryo had not yet become accessible to the experimental manipulations used in studies of amphibian embryos, and different means of analysis of developmental mechanisms had to be discovered.

The significance of the 1939 paper rests on its demonstration of a genetic system whose complexity has resisted final analysis to this day. On every level of phenotypic expression, mutations in and near the T complex are characterized by unexpected and previously undescribed effects. Developmentally, as mentioned above, inductive interactions in early embryonic stages, specifically between notochord-mesoderm and ectoderm, are affected by various mutations within and near the T complex. As a consequence, more or less severe abnormalities of the axial system (including those of the spine, spinal cord and headfolds) make their appearance and are frequently responsible for the embryonic lethality of homozygotes (GLUECKSOHN-WAELSCH and ERICKSON 1970).

The existence of a genetic basis for embryonic induction and cell-cell interactions, as demonstrated by the developmental analysis of T-complex effects, offers intriguing prospects in various directions, including the chance of finding a molecular basis for the mechanism of embryonic induction. As expressed by J. B. GURDON (1987), "The molecular basis of inducers and the inductive response remains almost totally obscure." Conceivably, a connection might be established between a particular gene sequence in the T-complex region and the effects of its product on neural tube induction, thus providing a clue to the molecular basis of induction.

Obviously, any number of molecules may be candidates for the role of transmitters of inductive signals. Recent studies of embryonic mesoderm induction in amphibians suggest tempting speculations. These involve molecules such as the transforming growth factor TGF-β_2 in the induction process (ROSA et al. 1988), perhaps operating by the modulation of effects of FGF (fibroblast growth factor) in the embryo (KIMELMAN et al. 1988). The latter authors speculate further about the possible role of FGF in mechanisms of signal transmission during gastrulation and neurulation. Growth factors appear to be promising candidates for a prominent role in embryonic induction, and it would be fascinating to explore the possibility that the *T* complex might include DNA sequences that encode growth factors. If this turned out to be the case, it would not only serve to advance our understanding of the molecular basis of embryonic induction, but would also confirm the significant role of the *T* complex in the genetic regulation of mammalian development proposed almost 20 years ago in a *T*-locus review (GLUECKSOHN-WAELSCH and ERICKSON 1970). As stated more recently, present data are "compatible with the possibility that the relevant DNA sequences in the *T*-complex encode regulatory factors concerned with the expression of specific structural genes mapping elsewhere in the genome" (GLUECKSOHN-WAELSCH 1987). The principle of exploiting well defined mutations in a causal analysis of development, as applied for the first time with the *T* complex, was followed by numerous studies of other mutations in the mouse affecting different developmental systems GLUECKSOHN-WAELSCH 1983).

I do not intend to present here an integrated and analytical review of the present status of the *T* complex and its chromosomal neighbors in terms of molecular organization or gene expression; previous reviews include GLUECKSOHN-WAELSCH and ERICKSON (1970), BENNETT (1975), SILVER (1985) and FRISCHAUF (1985). Since the 1939 paper, progress has been particularly impressive on the molecular level of analysis, including the identification and cloning of many segments of the *T* complex and the *t* haplotypes (HERRMANN, BARLOW and LEHRACH 1987).

One of the exceptional phenomena expressed by many recessive *t* mutations (haplotypes) that has been explained is the apparent suppression of recombination between certain *t*-bearing and wild-type chromosomes. It was the failure of recombination that had indicated allelism between *T* and the recessive *t* alleles (DUNN and GLUECKSOHN-SCHOENHEIMER 1939). Later, these *t* haplotypes were shown to actively suppress recombination over a considerable stretch of chromosome *17*. Eventually, chromosome rearrangements such as inversions, suggested by DUNN and GLUECKSOHN-SCHOENHEIMER in 1943, were identified within certain *t* haplotypes, and the absence of recombination could be ascribed to a concrete form of "chromatin mismatching" (SILVER and ARTZT 1981).

The phenomenon of transmission ratio distortion in *t*-carrying males was shown to involve the interaction of "distorter" and "responding" genes (LYON 1984). Male sterility, caused by the interaction of certain *t* haplotypes in viable double heterozygotes, seems to be caused by a minimum of three sterility factors, probably identical to "distorter" genes (LYON 1986). In spite of much analytical progress, details of the mechanisms responsible for the various reproductive abnormalities as well as their biochemical or molecular basis have remained obscure.

The details of phenotypic effects of *T*-complex mutations in heterozygotes and homozygotes have been described exhaustively on various levels and impressive progress has been achieved in the molecular identification of gene sequences included in the *T* complex (BÚCAN *et al.* 1987). Nevertheless, a huge black box filled with unknowns remains between the molecular and phenotypic levels of analysis. Recent approaches inducing point mutations in the *T*-complex region may help to reveal the role of single-base changes in the causation of individual lethal embryonic effects that resemble those described earlier in *t*-haplotype and *T*-complex homozygotes (SHEDLOVSKY, KING and DOVE 1988). Attempting to dissect the *t*-haplotype region by point mutagenesis may reduce the complexity of this area by identifying individual effects. Prior to those studies, there were no indications of direct correlations between singe-base changes in the DNA of the *T* complex and developmental or other effects.

That analytical studies of developmental genetics depend strongly on the choice of proper model systems is demonstrated particularly well by the analysis of homeotic mutations in Drosophila that are able to change the prospective fate of particular cell types. These mutations were used by HADORN (1966) in studies of the genetic basis of cell determination, and particularly by LEWIS (1981) in his brilliant analysis of the *bithorax* gene complex. It was LEWIS who correlated the changes in morphogenesis brought about by these mutations with specific changes in the responsible genes and their organization. LEWIS's classical approach of a developmental geneticist who proceeds from the level of the mutant phenotype back toward the genome has been complemented beautifully by his collaboration with molecular biologists such as D. HOGNESS and W. BENDER. The subsequent identification of specific DNA sequences—homeoboxes—shared by different homeotic genes in Drosophila, and encoding regulatory proteins instrumental in the control of specific developmental genes, has moved Drosophila into the center of interest in developmental genetics. Attempts to extend this flurry of excitement about homeoboxes to the mammalian embryo have had limited success thus far, even though genes containing homeoboxes has been identified in the mouse and have been shown to express spatially restricted patterns during embryogenesis (HOLLAND and HOGAN 1988). As yet, however, it is not possible to assign a decisive role to these genes in normal or mutant developmental mechanisms.

In the intellectual history of genetics, studies of the *T* complex have played a significant role throughout the past 50 years or more. It is one of several prime systems responsible for the emergence of concepts that do not focus on the gene as a single unit acting independently, but that consider the gene a member of a "field of higher order" in which several neighboring functional units may become integrated into one field of action, that is, a domain (GOLDSCHMIDT 1955; PONTECORVO 1958). This would apply in particular to the action of developmental genes. PONTECORVO considered the T locus in the mouse together with homeotic mutants in Drosophila as the "best known examples of such higher fields." He also speculated that MCCLINTOCK's controlling elements in maize might be further examples of "higher fields" and, in support of this, quotes MCCLINTOCK herself: "Controlling elements appear to reflect the presence in the nucleus of highly integrated systems operating to control gene action." Because it is difficult to paraphrase PONTECORVO's writings about the T locus, I would like to quote his own words: ". . . this is probably only a foretaste of what we are likely to find when we pass from the analysis of 'simple' genes like those providing the information for such a minor matter as the mere synthesis of an enzyme, to the genetic organization necessary to carry the information for morphogenetic processes" (PONTECORVO 1958).

Finally, I would like to refer once more to BARBARA MCCLINTOCK, who is quoted as having emphasized in a discussion with students the "hidden complexity" that continues to lurk in the most straightforward-seeming biological systems. It is her view that, following upon the "molecular" revolution in biology, analytical approaches to problems will require patience and must take into account the complexity of organisms (KELLER 1983). This certainly applies to the T complex in the mouse and the problem of eventually clarifying the complexities that characterize the correlation between the molecular identification of gene sequences in this interesting chromosomal region and their far-removed phenotypic expression.

I thank ROBERT P. ERICKSON and SUSAN A. LEWIS for their comments and VIVIAN GRADUS for her untiring help with the preparation of this manuscript.

LITERATURE CITED

BENNETT, D., 1975 The T-locus of the mouse. Cell **6**: 441–454.

BRUCK, D., 1957 Male segregation ratio advantage as a factor in maintaining lethal alleles in wild populations of house mice. Proc. Natl. Acad. Sci. USA **43**: 152–158.

BÚCAN, M., B. G. HERRMANN, A.-M. FRISCHAUF, V. L. BAUTCH, V. BODE, L. M. SILVER, G. R. MARTIN and H. LEHRACH, 1987 Deletion and duplication of DNA sequences is associated with the embryonic lethal phenotype of the t^9 complementation group of the mouse t complex. Genes Dev. **1**: 376–385.

CHESLEY, P., 1935 Development of the short-tailed mutant in the house mouse. J. Exp. Zool. **70**: 429–455.

DOBROVALSKAIA-ZAVADSKAIA, N., 1927 Sur la mortification spontanée de la queue chez la souris nouveau-née et sur l'existence d'un caractère (facteur) héréditaire, non viable. C. R. Soc. Biol. T. **97**: 114–119.

DUNN, L. C., 1939 *A Short History of Genetics.* McGraw-Hill, New York.

DUNN, L. C., 1954 The study of complex loci. Caryologia (Suppl.) **6**: 155–166.

DUNN, L. C., 1964 Abnormalities associated with a chromosome region in the mouse. Science **144**: 260–263.

DUNN, L. C., and S. GLUECKSOHN-SCHOENHEIMER, 1939 The inheritance of taillessness (anury) in the house mouse. II. Taillessness in a second balanced lethal line. Genetics **24**: 587–609.

DUNN, L. C., and S. GLUECKSOHN-SCHOENHEIMER, 1943 Tests for recombination amongst three lethal mutations in the house mouse. Genetics **28**: 29–40.

FRISCHAUF, A.-M., 1985 The T/t complex of the mouse. Trends Genet. **1**: 100–103.

GLUECKSOHN-SCHOENHEIMER, S., 1940 The effect of an early lethal (t^0) in the house mouse. Genetics **25**: 391–400.

GLUECKSOHN-WAELSCH, S., 1983 Genetic control of differentiation. Cold Spring Harbor Conf. Cell Proliferation **10**: 3–13.

GLUECKSOHN-WAELSCH, S., 1987 Regulatory genes in development. Trends Genet. **3**: 123–127.

GLUECKSOHN-WAELSCH, S., and R. P. ERICKSON, 1970 The T-locus of the mouse: implications for mechanisms of development. Current Top. Dev. Biol. **5**: 281–316.

GOLDSCHMIDT, R., 1938 *Physiological Genetics.* McGraw-Hill, New York.

GOLDSCHMIDT, R. B., 1955 *Theoretical Genetics.* University of California Press, Berkeley.

GURDON, J. B., 1987 Embryonic induction—molecular prospects. Development **99**: 285–306.

HADORN, E., 1966 Dynamics of determination, pp. 85–104 in *Major Problems in Developmental Biology,* edited by E. LOCKE. Academic Press, New York.

HERRMANN, B. G., D. P. BARLOW and H. LEHRACH, 1987 A large inverted duplication allows homologous recombination between chromosomes heterozygous for the proximal t complex inversion. Cell **48**: 813–825.

HOLLAND, P. W. H., and B. L. M. HOGAN, 1988 Spatially restricted patterns of expression of the homeobox-containing gene Hox-2.1 during mouse embryogenesis. Development **102**: 159–174.

KELLER, E. F., 1983 *A Feeling for the Organism: The Life and Work of Barbara McClintock.* W. H. Freeman, San Francisco.

KIMELMAN, D., J. A. ABRAHAM, T. HAAPARANTA, T. M. PALISI and M. W. KIRSCHNER, 1988 The presence of fibroblast growth factor in the frog egg: its role as a natural mesoderm inducer. Science **242**: 1053–1056.

LEHRACH, H., 1988 Molecular mapping of the t-complex region of mouse chromosome 17. Mouse Newslet. **82**: 131.

LEWIS, E. B., 1981 Developmental genetics of the bithorax complex in Drosophila, pp. 189–208 in *Developmental Biology Using Purified Genes,* edited by D. D. BROWN and C. F. FOX (ICN-UCLA Symposia on Molecular and Cell Biology, Vol. 23). Academic Press, New York.

LEWONTIN, R. C., and L. C. DUNN, 1960 The evolutionary dynamics of a polymorphism in the house mouse. Genetics **45**: 705–722.

LYON, M. F., 1984 Transmission ratio distortion in mouse t-haplotypes is due to multiple distorter genes acting on a responder locus. Cell **37**: 621–628.

LYON, M. F., 1986 Male sterility of the mouse t-complex is due to homozygosity of the distorter genes. Cell **44**: 357–363.

Moscona, A. A., 1986 Johannes Holtfreter at eighty-five. Cell Differ. **19:** 75–77.

Pontecorvo, G., 1958 *Trends in Genetic Analysis.* Columbia University Press, New York.

Rosa, F., A. B. Roberts, D. Danielpour, L. L. Dart, M. B. Sporn and I. B. Dawid, 1988 Mesoderm induction in amphibians: the role of TGF-β2-like factors. Science **239:** 783–785.

Shedlovsky, A., T. R. King and W. F. Dove, 1988 Saturation germline mutagenesis of the murine *t*-region including a lethal allele at the quaking locus. Proc. Natl. Acad. Sci. USA **85:** 180–184.

Silver, L. M., 1985 Mouse *t* haplotypes. Annu. Rev. Genet. **19:** 179–208.

Silver, L. M., and K. Artzt, 1981 Recombination suppression of mouse *t*-haplotypes due to chromatin mismatching. Nature **290:** 68–70.

M. R. Irwin and
the Beginnings of Immunogenetics

Ray Owen

Division of Biology, California Institute of Technology, Pasadena, California 91125

ABOUT sixty years ago, in the July, 1929 issue of GENETICS, MALCOLM ROBERT IRWIN published his first full-scale research paper, representing the main part of his thesis work at Iowa State. He reported that rats surviving induced infections with Salmonella produced progeny more resistant to the pathogen than the average of the population from which the parents had come, and proposed that the parents had been selected for genetic resistance. Inheritance therefore played a part in the disease susceptibility of their progeny. "This finding," he said in an unpublished autobiographical essay written in 1951, "was contrary to the beliefs of most of the bacteriologists of the time." He had, however, cited a few earlier papers to similar effect, especially a 1921 classic by SEWALL WRIGHT and P. A. LEWIS. "The next step," IRWIN went on to say, "was to apply the technics of immunology to attempt to determine the physiological basis for this natural resistance."

A decade later and just half a century ago, in the September, 1939 issue of GENETICS, IRWIN published "A Genetic Analysis of Species Differences in Columbidae." His emphasis in immunogenetics (a term first used in a paper by IRWIN and L. J. COLE in 1936) had changed from trying to understand the genetic bases of immunity to trying to use immunological reactions to define genes through studies of their antigenic products. Although IRWIN and some of his collaborators at Wisconsin continued to study one of the two arms of immunogenetics—the role of genes in the immune response, as characterized especially by resistance to contagious abortion in dairy cattle—the effort was unrewarding. His summary in the unpublished autobiographical essay written in 1951 was: "Thus in the interaction between host and Br. abortus there is at present no known substance in the blood which may be used as an index of the response to infection of a normal or immunized animal." Effective use of genetics to characterize the immune system was to begin later in that decade, primarily through the insights of people with backgrounds quite different from IRWIN's.

But that is another story. Ours here deals with the other arm of immunogenetics, the gene-to-antigen sequence to which IRWIN's attention was drawn upon his arrival at Madison in 1930. Fresh from postdoctoral work with W. E. CASTLE at the Bussey Institution in 1928–1929 and at the Rockefeller Institute in 1929–1930, IRWIN was the fourth member of the faculty of the Department of Genetics at the University of Wisconsin. L. J. COLE had founded the first genetics department in an American university in 1910; E. W. LINDSTROM had joined in 1919 but left for Iowa State in 1922; R. A. BRINK had come in 1922. IRWIN's appointment was jointly with Bacteriology and the USDA. COLE was interested in the genetics of pigeons and doves; IRWIN had hopes for "the study of gene effects, possibly of the gene itself, by immunological technics." The antigenic relationships of the blood cell of species and hybrids in pigeons and doves proved interesting and potentially profitable; from that time on, IRWIN's main research interests centered in that area. Work in his laboratory soon extended to other birds and to mammals, especially to poultry and dairy cattle.

Defining "the gene itself," or even its effects, by immunological techniques would never in fact have been accomplished without later reinforcement from molecular genetics. Early interest in immunogenetics in this context, as represented by IRWIN and his students, was based on the generally accepted assertion that the cellular antigens were probably immediate products of genes, and could even be the genes themselves. The main reason for this belief was the absence of gene interaction, and of interaction with other developmental or environmental factors, in the determination of cellular antigens as defined by their reactions with antibody reagents. "One gene, one antigen" was an attractive relationship, though it was never precisely stated in quite those words. It came a decade before the common acceptance of the concept of "one gene, one enzyme" and it held a similar hope that in studying an antigen one was learning about a gene. When it came, of course, the gene-enzyme relationship had another more immediate and dynamic realization, a framework for perceiving how genes act.

The promise of immunogenetics that brought it widespread attention at the time, however, was its apparent ability to compare genes among different species, and therefore to illuminate aspects of evolution. Comparative evolutionary genetics had been a compelling interest of biologists for many years. The field was hampered by the recognition that one could not often be sure of the degree to which partially similar phenotypes in different species depended on related genes. Species comparisons were complex and the application of traditional genetic methodology—hybridization, segregation, recombination—was severely limited by barriers to crossing and by hybrid inviability or sterility. If serology could define a gene, then comparative serology could become evolutionary genetics.

The approach was simple, at least in concept. Red blood cells from one species, say the Pearlneck dove, were injected into a rabbit to produce an antiserum reactive with Pearlneck cells. The antiserum could then be tested against the cells of another species, say the Ring dove. When the Ring dove cells reacted they could be said to have antigens, and therefore genes, similar to those of the Pearlneck. But if the antiserum was first "absorbed" with Ring dove cells, removing antibodies that recognized structures shared between the two species, the absorbed "reagent" still reacted with Pearlneck cells and with Pearlneck-Ring dove hybrid cells. These reactions reflected a complex of species differences: antigens characteristic of Pearlneck doves but absent from Ring doves, and expressed as dominant characters, so that the presence of each antigen unfailingly revealed the presence of its controlling gene.

The genetic dissection of the complex of species differences depended on repeated backcrossing to one of the parental species in an interspecific cross. The method of developing stocks that are alike in having the residual genotype of the recurrent backcross parent, but that differ for particular alleles introduced from the other original parent, was to be applied much later by others to other problems, for example dissecting the murine histocompatibility gene complex.

COLE had been interested in a different set of problems, such as, "What was the wild ancestor of the domestic Ring dove, and what did it look like?" Extant Ring doves are blond or white; presumably, their wild ancestors were dark like other wild doves. COLE took some delight in puzzling a museum taxonomist with study skins of dark Ring doves, and receiving the cautious opinion that the skins were from a previously undescribed species—perhaps the long-lost ancestor of Ring doves. The skins were in fact from a stock repeatedly backcrossed to Ring dove, retaining the dark allele introduced by an original cross with a dark dove of a wild species. Part of COLE's pleasure was in suggesting that the substitution of a single allele could create a new species—in the eyes of at least one museum taxonomist. So COLE had at hand not only hybrids between Pearlneck and Ring doves, but also successive generations of backcrosses to Ring doves well suited for IRWIN's purposes. The antiserum to Pearlneck, first absorbed with Ring cells, was then absorbed with the cells of individual backcross hybrids. Segregation of Pearlneck genes in the generations of repeated backcrossing to Ring doves had produced a very diverse population. Different birds had retained different alleles from their Pearlneck ancestor. The complex of species differences had been subdivided into a set of "unit" differences. The unity of a particular difference could be recognized by absorption analysis: the cells of all the backcross hybrids carrying Pearlneck antigen d-1, for example, would remove the antibodies responsible for their common reaction to the anti-d-1 reagent, while a second Pearlneck-specific antigen, d-2, similarly defined, proved to be independent of d-1. A unit difference in serology was shown to depend on a unit difference in inheritance, a confirmation of the "one gene, one antigen" concept and a tool for the study of inherited similarities and differences among species. IRWIN's 1939 paper reported eleven such distinct gene-antigen units distinguishing Pearlneck from Ring doves, two of them only partially defined.

The 1939 paper had been preceded by others by IRWIN, usually with COLE, reporting similar studies with other species. A 1938 paper in the *Journal of Genetics* had resulted in IRWIN's being awarded the Daniel Giraud Elliot Medal. The availability of reagents distinguishing a variety of species promoted the pursuit of answers to a variety of questions. What are the differences between the wild *Columba guinea* and the domestic pigeon *C. livea domestica*? To what extent do the reagents distinguishing Pearlneck from Ring doves recognize similarities with or differences from Senegal doves as well? And so on. (When I took my first genetics course at Wisconsin, in 1937, IRWIN was the teacher. His first lecture was largely a detailed listing, written on the blackboard, of genera and species of birds and the results of crosses among them. My lecture notes have a marginal comment: "If you ever teach Genetics, don't start this way!")

The extension of immunogenetic comparisons from a set of two entities to be distinguished, to a set of three or more related entities, reveals a new dimension. In pairwise combinations, reagents may be developed in either of two ways. One involves reciprocal immunization, A ↔ B. The reagents recognize differences between A and B but provide no basis for recognizing similarities between them. When a third, related entity is included, the reciprocal immunizations A ↔ B, A ↔ C and B ↔ C become possible, and each of these six antisera can be tested against A, B and C. Some of the antibodies produced when A is immunized with B, for example, are likely to cross-react with the related entity C. We suddenly see similarities as well as differences in the set. Equivalent conditions apply to the development of reagents by the second possible approach, immunizing another species. Inject rabbits with cells from dove species A, for example. After absorption with dove species B, only antibodies distinguishing A from B will remain. But a related dove species C is likely to react with only a part of that antibody population. So, for instance, when IRWIN compared three species of doves, he reported that "Senegal shared with Pearlneck all but a part of three of the nine antigenic characters which were peculiar to Pearlneck in contrast to Ring dove." Assuming a simple gene-antigen-antibody relationship, this seemed a step toward describing evolution on a chemically definable basis.

Early in the work, IRWIN (1932) had encountered a disturbing exception to the one-gene, one-antigen concept. An antiserum to cells of a species hybrid, absorbed by cell sof *both* parental species, still contained antibodies reactive with the hybrid. This reaction defined a "hybrid substance" that seemed best explicable as the result of complementation between two or more separate genes contributed by the respective parents. IRWIN had shared with J. B. S. HALDANE the simpler perception of the relation between genes and antigens; in the 1939 paper he quoted HALDANE (1937) as proposing that "The gene is a catalyst making a particular antigen, or the antigen is simply the gene or part of it let loose from its connexion with the chromosome." But in a later reminiscence, IRWIN recalls, "I had believed that cellular antigens might well be more or less direct products of the causative genes. A parallel belief was held by HALDANE, but when told of the hybrid substance, he replied, 'There goes a beautiful theory exploded by a single fact'" (IRWIN 1976).

In retrospect, we can still wonder about the molecular basis of "hybrid substances." Few defined antigens display heterozygous or complementary specificities; an exception may be the still rather mysterious and somewhat controversial "hybrid resistance" phenomenon in the mouse. In certain combinations, parental bone marrow cells grow poorly in irradiated F_1 hybrid hosts, an effect of the "hybrid histocompatability-1" (*Hh-1*) locus, part of the *H-2* complex (CUDKOWICZ and STIMPFLING 1964). IRWIN and HALDANE had no way of knowing at the time about intragenic complementation, or about specificities limited to heteropolymeric molecules composed of two or more polypeptides controlled by separate genes. Antigens like the human M-N-S series illustrate another set of complexities: a multigene complex can give rise to diverse glycophorins, which are in turn glycosylated by transferases controlled by their own, independent sets of multigene complexes. Depending on the reagent used for their detection, the "antigens" may reflect variation in either complex or in both. One or two of us in the lab once wondered whether a "hybrid substance" might sometimes be an artifact resulting from intraspecific differences. We were not sure that the same individuals that had been used initially to create the hybrids were always used to absorb and test the antisera. If a parent of a hybrid contributed antigen X, for example, so that anti-X was present in the antiserum, absorption with blood from doves that lacked X would leave anti-X to react with birds that happened to have it, including particular hybrids and their descendants. The suggestion was not warmly received; IRWIN was confident that he dealt with species characters, not with individual differences within species. There is no real reason to believe that he was wrong, but the issue has not been unambiguously resolved.

However, inherited individual differences within species were shortly to provide a new basis for the emergence of IRWIN's laboratory to world leadership in immunogenetics. The herd of cattle maintained for studies of contagious abortion turned out to have a more fruitful incidental use: immunization of cows with the blood of other cows gave rise to reagents distinguishing a great deal of inherited diversity in cattle (FERGUSON 1941; FERUGSON, STORMONT and IRWIN 1942; STORMONT 1950). The utility of such reagents for defining individuality in dairy cattle and for ascertaining paternity was quickly exploited. This, in turn, generated support for the values of immunogenetics over the whole spectrum from straightforward applications in agriculture to some of the most basic aspects of both genetics and immunology (IRWIN 1974). Similarly, extending these methods to poultry (MCGIBBON 1944; BRILES 1948; BRILES, MCGIBBON and IRWIN 1950), sheep (YCAS 1949; RENDEL, NEIMANN-SORENSEN and IRWIN 1954) and even bison (OWEN, STORMONT and IRWIN 1958) consolidated the Wisconsin laboratory as a world resource for research and training in immunogenetics, especially of farm animals.

There is much more to say about MALCOLM ROBERT IRWIN but those, again, are other stories. He died in Madison in 1987. He, his contributions, the opportunities he gave generations of younger geneticists and his leadership are worth remembering. This issue of GENETICS, on the fiftieth anniversary of his 1939 paper, is a fitting vehicle for remembrance.

LITERATURE CITED

BRILES, W. E., 1948   Induced hemolytic disease in chicks. Genetics **33:** 96–97.

BRILES, W. E., W. H. MCGIBBON and M. R. IRWIN, 1950   On multiple alleles effecting cellular antigens in the chicken. Genetics 35: 633–652.

CUDKOWICZ, G., and J. H. STIMPFLING, 1964   Deficient growth of C57BL marrow cells transplanted into F1 hybrid mice. Immunology **7:** 291–306.

FERGUSON, L. C., 1941   Heritable antigens in the erythrocytes of cattle. J. Immunol. 40: 213–242.

FERGUSON, L. C., C. STORMONT and M. R. IRWIN, 1942   On additional antigens in the erythrocytes of cattle. J. Immunol. **44:** 147–164.

HALDANE, J. B. S., 1937   The biochemistry of the individual, pp. 1–10 in *Perspectives in Biochemistry*, edited by J. NEEDHAM and D. GREEN. University Press, Cambridge.

IRWIN, M. R., 1929   The inheritance of resistance to the Danysz bacillus in the rat. Genetics **14:** 337–365.

IRWIN, M. R., 1932   Dissimilarities between antigenic properties of red blood cells of dove hybrid and parental genera. Proc. Soc. Exptl. Biol. Med. 29: 850–851.

IRWIN, M. R., 1938   Immuno-genetic studies of species relationships in Columbidae. J. Genet. **35:** 351–373.

IRWIN, M. R., 1939   A genetic analysis of species differences in Columbidae. Genetics 24: 709–721.

IRWIN, M. R., 1974   Comments on the early history of immunogenetics. Animal Blood Groups Biochem. Genet. **5:** 65–84.

IRWIN, M. R., 1976   The beginnings of immunogenetics. Immunogenetics **3:** 1–13.

IRWIN, M. R., and L. J. COLE, 1936   Immunogenetic studies of species and of species hybrids in doves, and the separation of species-specific substances in the backcross. J. Exptl. Zool. **73:** 85–108.

MCGIBBON, W. H., 1944   Cellular antigens in species and species hybrids in ducks. Genetics **29:** 407–419.

OWEN, R. D., C. STORMONT and M. R. IRWIN, 1958   Studies on blood groups in the American bison (buffalo). Evolution **12:** 102–110.

RENDEL, J. A., NEIMANN-SORENSEN and M. R. IRWIN, 1954   Evidence for epistatic action of genes for antigenic substances in sheep. Genetics **39:** 396–408.

STORMONT, C., 1950   Additional gene controlled antigenic factors in the bovine erythrocyte. Genetics **35:** 76–94.

WRIGHT, S., and P. A. LEWIS, 1921   Factors in resistance of guinea-pigs to tuberculosis, with special reference to inbreeding and heredity. Am. Nat. **55:** 20–50.

YCAS, M. K. W., 1949   Studies of the development of a normal antibody and of cellular antigens in the blood of sheep. J. Immunol. **61:** 327–347.

October 1989

The Linkage Map of Phage T4

Franklin W. Stahl

Institute of Molecular Biology, University of Oregon, Eugene, Oregon 97403

IN 1964, GENETICS published a pair of papers summarizing T4 linkage data in the form of circular maps. These maps confirmed both the necessity and the adequacy of a circular representation of T4 linkage data, and the phage community enjoyed feelings of both closure and opening. The sense of closure came from the realization that the "T4 problem" was bounded—genetic characterization of the entire chromosome was now a matter of interpolation. The sense of opening was that of founding a new era in transmission genetics, an era of circularity.

The linkage data of *Escherichia coli* had earlier been shown to require a circular representation (JACOB and WOLLMAN 1961) and that representation continued to be adequate as additional data were included (TAYLOR and THOMAN 1964). But *E. coli* may have been unique, or at least unusual. When the map of T4 proved circular, it was a clear case of "1, 2 . . . infinity." We could anticipate that circularity would be common among the prokaryotes.

Prokaryotic circularity is now seen to be almost ubiquitous but does not always have the same source. For *E. coli*, the circular linkage map is a composite of the linkage relations manifested by the known ensemble of Hfr strains, each of which transfers its genes linearly to the F⁻ recipient. These ensembles could be conceived as segments of a hypothetical circular chromosome (JACOB and WOLLMAN 1961). The circularity of the linkage map, however, was a reality independent of the correctness of that interpretation. That a circular chromosome did underlie the map was established later by CAIRNS' (1964) classic (and unique) autoradiograph of an intact *E. coli* chromosome.

T4 may never have a stage in its life cycle in which its chromosome is circular. The circular map is well explained by the model that predicted it (STREISINGER, EDGAR and DENHARDT 1964): individuals in a clone of T4 particles carry terminally redundant chromosomes (MACHATTIE *et al.* 1967) that are individually linear but whose sequences are circular permutations of each other (like a large set of different Hfr proximal segments; THOMAS and RUBENSTEIN 1964).

Because the map constructed from standard phage crosses reflects the average behavior of millions of particles, it shows few signs of the molecular ends of individual members of the population (see MOSIG 1988).

Circularity of the chromosome of the small phage ΦX174 was demonstrated contemporaneously with map circularity of T4 (FEIRS and SINSHEIMER 1962; KLEINSCHMIDT, BURTON and SINSHEIMER 1963). Subsequent genetic analysis (BAKER and TESSMAN 1967; BENBOW *et al.* 1971) revealed that its linkage map, too, was circular.

The linear chromosome of phage λ circularizes upon entering the host cell. It then replicates as a circle, either in the theta or in the sigma form. The chromosome is relinearized and remonomerized upon packaging as a result of cutting at *cos*. The standard linkage map of λ is linear, its ends corresponding to those created by *cos* cutting. The linkage map from lytic crosses shows no sign of the underlying circular state of the intracellular chromosome. However, CAMPBELL (1962) noted that the prophage linkage map offered by CALEF and LICCIARDELLO (1960) was a circular permutation of the map obtained from lytic crosses. On that evidence, and from the genetic maps of specialized λ transducing phages, CAMPBELL proposed that λ had a circular phase and that reciprocal crossing over between circular λ and *E. coli* was the mechanism by which λ established itself as part of the *E. coli* chromosome. I later suggested (STAHL 1967) that recombination between lambdoid phages in nature may occur most frequently between a prophage and a heteroimmune superinfecting phage. Interactions between these circularly permuted states of the phage chromosome would generate recombinants according to the rules of a circular map.

Now, because of the widespread use of circular plasmids for gene cloning, even students of eukaryotes are familiar with circular maps, and everyone's desktop computer knows how to draw them.

Somewhere, there may be a beast with a linear (nonpermuted) chromosome and a circular map that results solely from the habit of engaging in an even number of exchanges in each encounter. Such a circle would be most satisfying—a perfect abstraction, transcending its mundane, linear corporality. The basal body chromosome of Chlamydomonas is a real contender for that honor (HALL, RAMANIS and LUCK 1989).

Linkage maps (*i.e.*, maps based on recombination frequencies) serve several functions. They provide a visual summary of an otherwise daunting set of numbers. They reveal the order of genes on the chromosome that underlies the map and, in so doing, may reveal features of evolutionary or physiological significance. If coupled with the assumption that recombination is uniformly probable along the chromosome, they provide a scalar representation of the chromosome.

There are two approaches to constructing a linkage map, the American and the British. Both approaches aim for a line in which the distances between symbols representing mutant sites are proportional to the mean number of exchanges between the sites. For close markers (but not so close that we are plagued by marker effects), the mean number of exchanges is already proportional to the recombinant frequency, and is conventionally equated with it and defined as map distance. For more distant markers, multiple exchanges between marked sites generate recombinant frequencies that are appreciably less than the mean number of exchanges. The geneticist observes recombinant frequencies, which are generally not additive. To build a map, she must transform those frequencies to distances (*i.e.*, to mean numbers of exchanges), which are additive.

The American approach to such transformations, following STURTEVANT (1913), is saturation genetics: isolate so many mutants that all intervals are either short enough to give recombinant frequencies equal to distance, or are comprised of intervals that are. The distance for a long interval is taken as the sum of the distances of each of the included short intervals. Brute force.

The British approach, following HALDANE (1919), leaves time for Tea. The recombinant frequencies for a number of intervals are measured, but no interval need be so short that its recombinant frequency is equal to its map distance. Instead, an equation (a "mapping function") is created that transforms the set of measured recombinant frequencies into values that are additive. The equation is rigged so that recombinant frequency is set equal to distance for small values, even if none are observed, and approaches ½, the value for random assortment, as distance becomes large. Elegant, making the additional assumption that the rules of interference are invariant throughout the map.

BOB EDGAR's data, which were used to construct the 1964 T4 map, were so abundant that had T4 been like Drosophila, the entire map could have been built in the American way. In Drosophila, interference between exchanges results in recombinant frequencies that are additive even when rather larger. In T4, however, negative interference, both localized and global, produces recombinant frequencies that are nonadditive even when small. Thus, the British approach was in order.

Concocting reasonable mapping functions was fun. STAHL and C. M. STEINBERG (1964) wrote a set of functions suitable for dealing with T4 data involving intervals that were long enough to allow us to ignore localized negative interference. STAHL, EDGAR and J. STEINBERG (1964) adapted those functions to cover the entire range of observed recombinant frequencies. The tested functions contained three or four arbitrarily adjustable parameters. Then, the job of selecting a "best" mapping function became that of finding the sets of parameter values that would best allow each function to transform the measured recombinant frequencies into additive values. The optimized functions were compared and the best became the mapping function of choice. It was used to generate the published map (STAHL, EDGAR and STEINBERG 1964).

A daunting table of data had been reduced to a simple, satisfying figure.

The most striking feature of the map, after its circularity, was the clustering of genes of physiologically related functions–the head genes were close to each other, as were the tail genes, the DNA replication genes, and so on (EPSTEIN *et al.* 1963). That remarkable feature, reminiscent of the operons of *E. coli* (JACOB and MONOD 1961), proved to be a general phenomenon, characteristic of most or all phages subsequently studied. For some of these phages, a force adequate to preserve gene clustering may be the advantage of cotranscription as a basis for coordinate control, as with *E. coli* operons. For T4, however, evidence for operons was lacking–there were no polar mutants indicative of polycistronic transcripts. Indeed, the permuted nature of the chromosome and the shortness of its terminal redundancy hints that the transcription of each gene is independent of promoters more than a gene or so distant (short-range polar mutants being later detected; STAHL *et al.* 1966). What force, then, holds the genes in clusters?

NORMAN HOROWITZ expressed to me the view that genes involved in the same metabolic or developmental pathway arose via tandem duplication followed by functional divergence, and that the rate of gene scrambling by other kinds of events (translocations, inversions) has been too low to hide the evidence of this early history. I haven't heard whether nucleotide sequencing of T4 has supported that view, derived from HOROWITZ (1945), as it could do.

LESLIE BARNETT pointed out to me that R. A. FISHER (1930) had predicted that genes with interacting functions will become linked and remain so if each gene is polymorphic. Because some combinations of alleles are likely to be superior to others, there will be selection for increased linkage between the loci. With such linkage, successful allele combinations can be transmitted intact, suffering minimal disruption by homologous recombination. FISHER's notion was put forth for sexually reproducing eukaryotes, in which genetic recombination is a hazard facing each new generation. For viruses, the argument can be inverted—recombination must be more frequent for them than one might think, judging from the intensity of gene clustering. Some experimental support was obtained for the applicability of FISHER's notion to T4 (STAHL and MURRAY 1966) and lambdologists were driven to the same conclusion (e.g., THOMAS 1964; DOVE 1971).

Contemporaneously with the creation of a definitive linkage map, methods for determining the size of the T4 chromosome became reliable. From the genetic and physical numbers, the probability of recombination per base pair could be calculated. Remarkably, the estimate agreed well with the minimal value for recombination seen by BENZER (1955) in his intensive (and visionary) fine-structure genetic analysis of T4's rII gene. The map had equal success in relating gene sizes to the sizes of their protein products. The T4 map of 1964 remains a valuable guide to the phage chromosome for those who are now engaged in chopping it up and working with the pieces (MOSIG 1988).

The notion of a linkage map has been central to transmission genetics since its discovery (STURTEVANT 1913). A map provides a framework for studies at all levels. New techniques have facilitated the construction of maps and are being applied to human chromosomes. At the gross level, the human map still relies mostly on recombinant frequencies to determine order and distance. At a finer level, however, overlapping cloned restriction fragments in the neighborhood of interesting genes will establish segments of the map in physical units. Ordering these segments with respect to each other will be possible by reference to the linkage map. Continuing effort in restriction fragment mapping, aided by other physical methods (D. WARD, D. COX and R. MYERS, as described in ROBERTS 1989), may eventually yield a densely marked physical map of the human chromosomes. Such a map will establish a framework into which human nucleotide sequence data can be plugged as they become an available by-product of the world's molecular genetic investigations. (S. BRENNER might call this the "British Approach" by contrast to the proposed, boring, brute-force "American Approach" of end-to-end sequencing for its own sake.) Thus, the map will guide and inform the sequencing which, in turn, will propel our understanding of the genetic nature of humankind. What kind of map will guide and inform us in the use of this powerful, new knowledge?

LITERATURE CITED

BAKER, R., and I. TESSMAN, 1967 The circular genetic map of phage S13. Proc. Natl. Acad. Sci. USA **58:** 1438–1445.

BENBOW, R. M., C. A. HUTCHINSON, J. D. FABRICANT and R. L. SINSHEIMER, 1971 Genetic map of bacteriophage ΦX174. J. Virol. **7,** 549–558.

BENZER, S., 1955 Fine structure of a genetic region in bacteriophage. Proc. Natl. Acad. Sci. USA **41:** 344–354.

CAIRNS, J., 1964 The chromosome of *Escherichia coli.* Cold Spring Harbor Symp. Quant. Biol. **28:** 43–46.

CALEF, E., and G. LICCIARDELLO, 1960 Recombination experiments on prophage host relationships. Virology **12:** 81–103.

CAMPBELL, A., 1962 Episomes. Adv. Genet. **11:** 101–145.

DOVE, W. F., 1971 Biological inferences, pp 297–312 in *The Bacteriophage Lambda,* edited by A. D. HERSHEY. Cold Spring Harbor Laboratory, Cold Spring Harbor, NY.

EPSTEIN, R. H., A. BOLLE, C. M. STEINBERG, E. KELLENBERGER, E. BOY DE LA TOUR and R. CHEVALLEY, 1963 Physiological studies of conditional lethal mutants of bacteriophage T4D. Cold Spring Harbor Symp. Quant. Biol. **28:** 375–394.

FIERS, W., and R. L. SINSHEIMER, 1962 The structure of the DNA of the bacteriophage ΦX174. III. Ultracentrifugal analysis for a ring structure. J. Mol. Biol. **5:** 424–434.

FISHER, R. A., 1930 *The Genetical Theory of Natural Selection.* Clarendon Press, Oxford.

HALDANE, J. B. S., 1919 The combination of linkage values, and the calculations of distances between the loci of linked factors. J. Genet. **8:** 299–309.

HALL, J. L., Z. RAMANIS and D. J. L. LUCK, 1989 Basal body/centriolar DNA: molecular genetic studies in *Chlamydomonas.* Cell (in press).

HOROWITZ, N. H., 1945 On the evolution of biochemical syntheses. Proc. Natl. Acad. Sci. USA **31:** 153–157.

JACOB, F., and J. MONOD, 1961 Genetic regulatory mechanisms in the synthesis of proteins. J. Mol. Biol. **3:** 318–356.

JACOB, F., and E. L. WOLLMAN, 1961 *Sexuality and Genetics of Bacteria.* Academic Press, New York.

KLEINSCHMIDT, A. K., A. BURTON and R. L. SINSHEIMER, 1963 Electron microscopy of the replicative form of the DNA of the bacteriophage ΦX174. Science **142:** 961.

MACHATTIE, L. A., D. A. RITCHIE, C. A. THOMAS, JR. and C. C. RICHARDSON, 1967 Terminal repetition in permuted T2 bacteriophage DNA molecules. J. Mol. Biol. **23:** 355–364.

MOSIG, G., 1988 Mapping and map distortions in bacteriophage crosses, pp. 141–167 in *Genetic Recombination,* edited by R. KUCHERLAPATI and G. R. SMITH. American Society for Microbiology, Washington, D.C.

ROBERTS, L., 1989 Genome mapping goal now in reach. Science **244:** 424–425.

STAHL, F. W., 1967 Circular genetic maps. J. Cell. Physiol. **70** (Suppl. 1): 1–12.

STAHL, F. W., R. S. EDGAR and J. STEINBERG, 1964 The linkage map of bacteriophage T4. Genetics **50:** 539–552.

STAHL, F. W., and N. E. MURRAY, 1966   The evolution of gene clusters and genetic circularity in microorganisms. Genetics **53:** 569–576.

STAHL, F. W., N. E. MURRAY, S. NAKATA and J. M. CRASEMANN, 1966   Intergenic *cis-trans* position effects in bacteriophage T4. Genetics **54:** 223–232.

STAHL, F. W., and C. M. STEINBERG, 1964   The theory of formal phage genetics for circular maps. Genetics **50:** 531–538.

STREISINGER, G., R. S. EDGAR and G. H. DENHARDT, 1964   Chromosome structure in phage T4. I. Circularity of the linkage map. Proc. Natl. Acad. Sci. USA **51:** 775–779.

STURTEVANT, A. H., 1913   The linear arrangement of six sex-linked factors in *Drosophila*, as shown by their mode of association. J. Exp. Zool. **14:** 43–59.

TAYLOR, A. L., and M. S. THOMAN, 1964   The genetic map of *Escherichia coli* K-12. Genetics **50:** 659–677.

THOMAS, C. A., JR., and I. RUBENSTEIN, 1964   The arrangement of nucleotide sequences in T2 and T5 bacteriophage DNA molecules. Biophys. J. **4:** 93–106.

THOMAS, R., 1964   On the structure of the genetic segment controlling immunity in temperate bacteriophages. J. Mol. Biol. **8:** 247–253.

November 1989

The Molecular Genetics of Differentiation

Bert Ely* and Lucy Shapiro†

*Department of Biological Sciences, University of South Carolina, Columbia, South Carolina 29208;
and †Department of Developmental Biology, Beckman Center, Stanford University School of Medicine, Stanford, California 94305–5427

HOW can a cell keep track of what it is doing and know what it is supposed to do next? How does it know where to build a particular structure? These questions prompted us to choose *Caulobacter* as a system likely to yield information about fundamental problems in cell differentiation such as how positional information is encoded, how an organism generates asymmetry, and how these events are accomplished within the context of a temporal program. Because the physiology, subcellular architecture and cell cycle of an organism are a single system with intricately bound components, the study of cellular differentiation can only be accomplished in the context of a whole organism. Therefore, it is important to choose an organism that is simple enough to make this integrated approach feasible. Our goal in working with *Caulobacter* was to provide a base of knowledge and technology that would allow the complete molecular dissection of the temporal and spatial control of development in a relatively simple organism.

The unique characteristics of *Caulobacter* that make it a useful organism for the investigation of these questions center on the fact that differentiation results in cell poles that are marked with either a stalk or a flagellum. Therefore, both the bacterium and the investigator always know which end is up. The expression of this cellular asymmetry is easily observed when a cell with only a polar stalk and no flagellum carries out the *de novo* biogenesis of a flagellum at the pole opposite the stalk (Figure 1). Cell division then yields progeny with different morphologies and different developmental programs. One of these cells is stalked like the parent. The other is a swarmer cell which cannot divide until it goes through a differentiation process, ejecting the polar flagellum and assembling a new stalk at the site previously occupied by that flagellum. These changes at the cell poles occur at discrete time intervals during the cell cycle and are independent of environmental fluctuations. Thus, *Caulobacter* undergoes two relatively simple morphogenetic changes during each cell cycle.

In the early 1960s, ROGER STANIER and his students

JEANNE POINDEXTER and JEAN SCHMIDT characterized the biology of the organism. *Caulobacter*, an aquatic bacterium, can be cultured in the laboratory and populations of cells can be easily synchronized by differential centrifugation. Thus, individual cell cycle events are accessible to both biochemical and genetic manipulation without physiological stress. One of the first uses of synchronized cells was the demonstration that flagellin synthesis is temporally controlled (SHAPIRO and MAIZEL 1973). Subsequently, MARY ANN OSLEY in AUSTIN NEWTON's laboratory at Princeton University isolated temperature-sensitive mutants which provided the basis for studies of the timing of the DNA replication and cell division pathways (OSLEY and NEWTON 1977, 1980; NATHAN, OSLEY and NEWTON 1982). This work demonstrated the interdependence of these two pathways during the *Caulobacter* cell cycle and provided a framework for the analysis of developmental events. For instance, the synthesis of flagellar components (OSLEY, SHEFFERY and NEWTON 1977; LAGENAUER and AGABIAN 1978; AGABIAN, EVINGER and PARKER 1979; LOEWY *et al.* 1987) and chemotaxis proteins (GOMES and SHAPIRO 1984) was shown to initiate after the midpoint of DNA replication.

A critical part of our strategy to dissect *Caulobacter*'s temporal and spatial control of development was the establishment of a system for genetic analysis. Accordingly, one of the first objectives of BERT ELY's laboratory at the University of South Carolina was the isolation of a generalized transducing phage which would facilitate exchange of genetic material between *Caulobacter* strains. All of the initial attempts to isolate transducing phage were unsuccessful. However, a breakthrough came with the realization that because tropical fish are shipped in the water they are raised in, local fish stores have water samples from all over the world. Tropical fish tanks proved to be a rich source of *Caulobacter* bacteriophage and a transducing phage was soon found (ELY and JOHNSON 1977). This initial success prompted REID JOHNSON, then an undergraduate, to isolate and characterize a large collec-

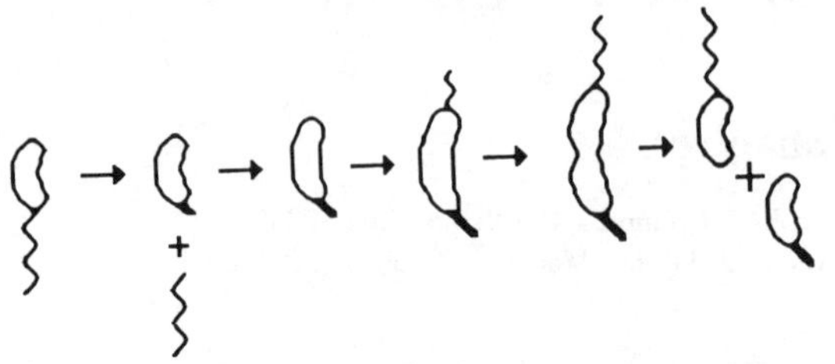

FIGURE 1.— Schematic of the *Caulobacter crescentus* cell cycle.

tion of nutritional and motility mutants which became the basis for all subsequent genetic studies with *Caulobacter* (JOHNSON and ELY 1977, 1979). Other studies led to the development of methods for conjugation (ELY 1979) and transposon mutagenesis (ELY and CROFT 1982) which provided the tools for detailed genetic analyses. Several thousand crosses later, a genetic map was assembled (BARRETT *et al.* 1982a, b) and a workable *Caulobacter* genetic system was available. The utility of this system was demonstrated, in a paper published in GENETICS just five years ago this month, when it was used to determine the map location of 25 flagellar genes which are expressed at precise times in the cell cycle (ELY, CROFT and GERARDOT 1984). This result indicated that the timing of gene expression could not be governed solely by the ordered replication of clustered sets of genes.

Recently, BERT ELY used pulsed field gel electrophoresis of large DNA restriction fragments to construct a physical map of the *Caulobacter* genome (ELY and GERARDOT 1988; ELY and ELY 1989). As a consequence, the effort required to determine the map location of a newly identified gene has been reduced over 100-fold and the location of cloned genes can now be ascertained even when no chromosomal mutation exists. The power of having a coordinated physical and genetic map was demonstrated when a single experiment was used to determine the map position of the origin of DNA replication, bidirectional fork movement, and the rate of *in vivo* replication (DINGWALL and SHAPIRO 1989).

In 1982, the first *Caulobacter* flagellar genes were cloned simultaneously in three different laboratories (OHTA, CHEN and NEWTON 1982; PURUCKER *et al.* 1982; MILHAUSEN *et al.* 1982). Subsequently, PATRICIA SCHOENLEIN in BERT ELY's laboratory developed techniques for the identification of cloned genes by complementation of *Caulobacter* mutants (SCHOENLEIN, GALLMAN and ELY 1988). Thus, virtually any cloned gene could be obtained if mutants are available. In addition, DAVID HODGSON and VIVIAN BELLOFATTO in LUCY SHAPIRO's laboratory at the Albert Einstein College of Medicine made it possible to assay genes with no known product when they constructed a modified Tn5 transposon carrying a promoterless reporter gene (BELLOFATTO, SHAPIRO and HODGSON 1984). Studies using this construct and plasmid complementation experiments allowed the identification

of a positive *trans*-acting hierarchy (BRYAN *et al.* 1984; OHTA *et al.* 1985; CHAMPER *et al.* 1985; CHAMPER, DINGWALL and SHAPIRO 1987). Subsequently, epistasis analysis with cloned flagellar genes established the existence of a complex regulatory network of positive and negative controls that schedules the time of gene expression and demonstrated that the structural genes are expressed in the order of their assembly into the flagellum (XU, DINGWALL and SHAPIRO 1989; NEWTON *et al.* 1989). These observations underscore the need to study differentiation events within the context of the whole organism. Experiments are currently in progress to define the *cis*-acting sequences and their cognate *trans*-acting regulatory factors that specify the time of expression of the flagellar genes. Several of these protein factors have been purified so that biochemical approaches can be used to understand the mechanisms revealed by genetic dissection of the morphogenetic process.

As a consequence of providing a foundation of classical genetics, the developmental processes that result in the unique polarity of *Caulobacter* cells are accessible to molecular genetics. We have the necessary tools to determine how the observed spatial organization is encoded. It is now our task to harness the well developed tools of genetics and biochemistry to discover the mechanisms that decode this positional information. Factors such as cell polarity, sophisticated genetics, defined and easily assayed morphogenesis and the small genome size, all contribute to making *Caulobacter* one of the most accessible organisms available for the study of the molecular basis of cell differentiation.

LITERATURE CITED

AGABIAN, N., M. EVINGER and E. PARKER, 1979 Generation of asymmetry during development. J. Cell Biol. **81**: 123–136.

BARRETT, J. T., R. H. CROFT, D. M. FERBER, C. J. GERARDOT, P. V. SHOENLEIN and B. ELY, 1982a Genetic mapping with Tn5-derived auxotrophs of *Caulobacter crescentus*. J. Bacteriol. **151**: 888–898.

BARRETT, J. T., C. S. RHODES, D. M. FERBER, B. JENKINS, S. A. KUHL and B. ELY, 1982b Construction of a genetic map for *Caulobacter crescentus*. J. Bacteriol. **149**: 889–896.

BELLOFATTO, V., L. SHAPIRO and D. HODGSON, 1984 Generation of a Tn5 promoter probe and its use in the study of gene expression in *Caulobacter crescentus*. Proc. Natl. Acad. Sci. USA **81:** 1035–1039.

BRYAN, R., M. PURUCKER, S. L. GOMES, W. ALEXANDER and L. SHAPIRO, 1984 Analysis of pleiotropic regulation of flagellar and chemotaxis gene expression in *Caulobacter crescentus* by using plasmid complementation. Proc. Natl. Acad. Sci. USA **81:** 1341–1345.

CHAMPER, R., R. BRYAN, S. L. GOMES, M. PURUCKER and L. SHAPIRO, 1985 Temporal and spatial control of flagellar and chemotaxis gene expression during *Caulobacter* cell differentiation. Cold Spring Harbor Symp. Quant. Biol. **50:** 831–840.

CHAMPER, R., A. DINGWALL and L. SHAPIRO, 1987 Cascade regulation of *Caulobacter* flagellar and chemotaxis genes. J. Mol. Biol. **194:** 71–80.

DINGWALL, A., and L. SHAPIRO, 1989 Chromosome replication rate, origin and bidirectionality as determined by pulsed field gel electrophoresis. Proc. Natl. Acad. Sci. USA **86:** 119–123.

ELY, B., 1979 Transfer of drug resistance factors to the dimorphic bacterium *Caulobacter crescentus*. Genetics **91:** 371–379.

ELY, B., and R. H. CROFT, 1982 Transposition mutagenesis in *Caulobacter crescentus*. J. Bacteriol. **149:** 620–625.

ELY, B., R. H. CROFT and C. J. GERARDOT, 1984 Genetic mapping of genes required for motility in *Caulobacter crescentus*. Genetics **108:** 523–532.

ELY, B., and T. ELY, 1989 Use of pulsed field gel electrophoresis to estimate the total number of genes required for motility in *Caulobacter crescentus*. Genetics **123:** (in press).

ELY, B., and C. J. GERARDOT, 1988 Use of pulsed-field-gradient gel electrophoresis to construct a physical map of the *Caulobacter crescentus* genome. Gene **68:** 323–333.

ELY, B., and R. C. JOHNSON, 1977 Generalized transduction in *Caulobacter crescentus*. Genetics **87:** 391–399.

GOMES, S. L., and L. SHAPIRO, 1984 Differential expression and position of chemotaxis methylation protein in *Caulobacter*. J. Mol. Biol. **178:** 551–568.

JOHNSON, R. C., and B. ELY, 1977 Isolation and spontaneously-derived mutants from *Caulobacter crescentus*. Genetics **86:** 25–32.

JOHNSON, R. C., and B. ELY, 1979 Analysis of non-motile mutants of the dimorphic bacterium *Caulobacter crescentus*. J. Bacteriol. **137:** 627–634.

LAGENAUR, C., and N. AGABIAN, 1978 *Caulobacter* flagellar or-

ganelle: synthesis, compartmentation and assembly. J. Bacteriol. **135:** 1062–1069.

LOEWY, Z. G., R. A. BRYAN, S. H. REUTER and L. SHAPIRO, 1987 Control of synthesis and positioning of a *Caulobacter crescentus* flagellar protein. Genes Dev. **1:** 626–635.

MILHAUSEN, M., P. R. GILL, G. PARKER and N. AGABIAN, 1982 Cloning of developmentally regulated flagellin genes from *Caulobacter crescentus* via immunoprecipitation of polyribosomes. Proc. Natl. Acad. Sci. USA **79:** 6847–6851.

NATHAN, P., M. A. OSLEY and A. NEWTON, 1982 Circular organization of the DNA synthetic pathway in *C. crescentus*. J. Bacteriol. **151:** 503–506.

NEWTON, A., N. OHTA, G. RAMAKRISHNAN, D. MULLIN and G. RAYMOND, 1989 Genetic switching in the flagellar gene hierarchy requires negative as well as positive regulation of transcription. Proc. Natl. Acad. Sci. USA **86:** (in press).

OHTA, N., L.-S. CHEN and A. NEWTON, 1982 Isolation and expression of cloned hook protein gene from *Caulobacter crescentus*. Proc. Natl. Acad. Sci. USA **79:** 4863–4867.

OHTA, N., L.-S. CHEN, F. SWANSON and A. NEWTON, 1985 Transcriptional regulation of a periodically controlled flagellar gene operon in *Caulobacter crescentus*. J. Mol. Biol. **186:** 107–115.

OSLEY, M. A., and A. NEWTON, 1977 Mutational analysis of developmental control in *Caulobacter crescentus*. Proc. Natl. Acad. Sci. USA **74:** 124–128.

OSLEY, M. A., and A. NEWTON, 1980 Temporal control and the cell cycle in *Caulobacter crescentus*: roles of DNA chain elongation and completion. J. Mol. Biol. **138:** 109–128.

OSLEY, M. A., M. SHEFFERY and A. NEWTON, 1977 Regulation of flagellin synthesis in the cell cycle of *Caulobacter*: dependence on DNA replication. Cell **12:** 393–400.

PURUCKER, M., R. BRYAN, K. AMEMIYA, B. ELY and L. SHAPIRO, 1982 Isolation of a Caulobacter gene cluster specifying flagellum production by using non-motile Tn5 insertion mutants. Proc. Natl. Acad. Sci. USA **79:** 6797–6801.

SCHOENLEIN, P., L. M. GALLMAN and B. ELY, 1988 Use of transmissable plasmids as cloning vectors in *Caulobacter crescentus*. Gene **70:** 321–329.

SHAPIRO, L., and J. V. MAIZEL, JR., 1973 Synthesis and structure of *Caulobacter crescentus* flagella. J. Bacteriol. **113:** 478–485.

XU, H., A. DINGWALL and L. SHAPIRO, 1989 Negative transcriptional regulation in the *Caulobacter* flagellar hierarchy. Proc. Natl. Acad. Sci. USA **86:** (in press).

See also page 703 in Addenda et Corrigenda.

Intragenic Recombination in Drosophila
The *rosy* Locus

Arthur Chovnick

Molecular and Cell Biology, The University of Connecticut, Storrs, Connecticut 06269-2131

TWENTY-FIVE years ago in GENETICS, my colleagues and I reported, in two papers, results of experiments demonstrating that intragenic recombination occurs in *Drosophila melanogaster,* a representative higher eukaryote. The first paper (CHOVNICK *et al.* 1964) described genetic fine-structure mapping experiments involving an array of fully viable, XDH⁻, rosy eye color mutations representing a single complementation group. Utilizing a selective system to facilitate large-scale sampling, the resolving power of such recombination permitted the elaboration of a linear order of sites within a single gene, quite comparable to that seen in prokaryotes and fungi. The second paper (SCHALET, KERNAGHAN and CHOVNICK 1964) represented an essential "appendix" to the first. Therein we described genetic analysis of an array of mutations induced in the *rosy* region of chromosome *3* and demonstrated that there was only one gene in this region concerned with xanthine dehydrogenase. While the homozygous viable rosy eye color mutations were limited to that gene, the lethal effects seen with certain of the *rosy* mutations were shown to be associated with adjacent vital genes that are functionally and spatially distinct from the *rosy* locus. All of the lethal *rosy* mutations were deletions extending into these vital genes to varying extents.

These papers completed the initial stage of an odyssey that began in my first year in graduate school. I had entered graduate study committed to the pursuit of mechanisms underlying the tissue-specific and temporal control of gene action in development. However, I was diverted from this path in my first year as a graduate student when I read reports on recombination between mutations of the *lozenge* locus (OLIVER 1940; GREEN and GREEN 1949) and other similar genes (see review by LEWIS 1951). These studies involved several different genes, each having multiple mutant alleles, which were subjected to recombination analyses resulting in the recovery of rare recombinants between the mutant alleles. Although invented for use in a broader context (see MCCLINTOCK 1944), the term *pseudoalleles* came to be used to describe

mutations that formerly were considered to be allelic but which subsequently yielded to recombination, and pseudoallelic genes or *complex loci* were expressions used to describe genes whose mutant alleles could be separated by recombination. The use of these expressions reflects the classical conceptual framework within which these cases were interpreted. The classical gene was a unit of function and mutation within which there was no recombination. Recombination occurred only between genes. Hence, the observation of recombination between alleles led to their reclassification as pseudoalleles, members of two separate genetic units in close proximity. Moreover, since mutation of these genetic units produced a similar array of phenotypic effects, it was inferred that these genes were functionally similar or related. An accessory hypothesis (LEWIS 1951) suggested that pseudoallelic genes were instances of gene duplicates in various stages of evolution, and the investigation of such systems was considered to be examining the evolution of new genes and new gene functions. In essence, these studies were interpreted in a fashion entirely consistent with classical notions concerning gene organization.

While LEWIS presented a most persuasive argument for his interpretation of the *bithorax* complex as a cluster of functionally related genes, the interpretation of *lozenge* and other multiply allelic genes on this model seemed open to alternatives. Essentially, multiple functions were inferred purely on the basis of recombination data. In support of the pseudoallelism model was the fact that the mutations fell into a small number of clusters within which recombination seemed not to occur. Yet all of the *lozenge* mutations were recessive, and mutant heteroallelic genotypes were also mutant in phenotype.

These works led me to question the validity of a key feature of the dogma of classical genetics, namely that recombination occurred only between genes and not within a gene. For me, the critical experiment was to examine a single gene with a single, simple mutant effect and with many mutant alleles exhibiting no evidence of complementation or functional complexity. The basic idea was to carry out a recombination study on a scale large enough to identify many separable sites: too many to permit the interpretation of multiple genes and multiple functions. I was convinced that the small number of gene clusters seen, for example, in the *lozenge* case was merely a reflection of inadequate sampling. My Ph.D. mentor, ALLEN FOX, disagreed with this notion, and moreover felt that such a large-scale undertaking would not make a suitable thesis project. Rather, I was directed to a phenotypic analysis of the *lozenge* mutants in the hope that functional distinction among these pseudoalleles would be forthcoming. Such was not the outcome (CHOVNICK and FOX 1953; CHOVNICK and LEFKOWITZ 1956; CHOVNICK, LEFKOWITZ and FOX 1956). Rather, the conclusion of these studies was that these mutations were alleles of a single functional unit.

During the winter of 1953–1954, on my first faculty appointment, I started to collect mutant strains and to construct appropriately marked chromosomes to carry out fine-structure recombination mapping of the *garnet* locus (*g*: 1-44.4), known by a multiple allelic array of noncomplementing eye color mutations. Within a year the first successful intragenic recombinants were recovered. In the absence of a selective procedure, progress was slow. Additionally, these early results were confounded by the recovery of convertants in addition to the crossover products (CHOVNICK 1958, 1961) [see also HEXTER (1958) and CARLSON (1959)]. Although convertants were not seen in prior recombination studies in Drosophila, they were reported in similar studies in fungi (MITCHELL 1955; PRITCHARD 1955) and eventually came to be recognized as an important feature of intragenic recombination (*e.g.*, WHITEHOUSE 1963; HOLLIDAY 1964). Indeed, conversion continues to play a key role in current thinking about recombination mechanisms (*e.g.*, BORTS and HABER 1989; CURTIS *et al.* 1989).

By the fall of 1957, when I was writing the first *garnet* recombination paper (CHOVNICK 1958), I was already contemplating the limitations of my experimental system and the possible alternatives. Several factors were clear to me at this point, not the least of which was that the issue of intragenic recombination was no longer in doubt, at least in prokaryotes and fungi (BENZER 1955; PRITCHARD 1955). I was convinced that the *garnet* work demonstrated that intragenic recombination also occurred in Drosophila. However, this viewpoint was not generally shared with my colleagues in Drosophila research. Given the limited recombination data with only three sites identified at best, and the conversion-like products that looked suspiciously like mutations, additional work seemed necessary to establish this point. Moreover, the origin of the aberrant segregants (*i.e.*, the conver-

sion-like products that resembled reverse mutations) became an issue of considerable interest. I believed that they were recombinational in origin, reflecting extremely tight intragenic mapping (CHOVNICK 1958). A selection system that would permit sampling approaching the scale routinely used in microbial systems was essential for the continued pursuit of these problems. In this context, I began to consider gene-enzyme systems associated with a visible mutant phenotype in the hope that a nutritional selective procedure might be developed. Very few possibilities existed in Drosophila at that time. The report of FORREST, GLASSMAN and MITCHELL (1956) concerning xanthine dehydrogenase and the *rosy* and *maroon-like* genes and the clear evidence of differential gene expression of *rosy* (see review, HADORN 1956) attracted my attention.

In January 1959, I moved to Cold Spring Harbor as Assistant Director of the Biological Laboratory. In this new role I was preoccupied with mastering many administrative responsibilities. Reestablishing a functioning laboratory to continue the *garnet* locus analysis was accomplished only slowly. During this period in 1959, two events provided further encouragement for the xanthine dehydrogenase system. The first was the GLASSMAN and MITCHELL (1959) paper on XDH and the second was a conversation with INGE RASMUSSEN, a postdoctoral fellow in ED LEWIS' laboratory who attended the Cold Spring Harbor Symposium that year. From RASMUSSEN I learned of the construction of compound autosome arm strains in LEWIS' laboratory. Thus, I knew that half-tetrad analysis, essential for the study of conversion, would be possible with the *rosy* locus on chromosome *3*.

Somewhat later, in the fall of 1959, ABE SCHALET joined my research staff. This provided an opportunity to take a new research direction. We initiated work with both *rosy* and *maroon-like*. However, the complementation seen with our first *maroon-like* mutations and the maternal effect associated with *maroon-like* were unfathomed complexities that led me to favor *rosy* as our initial gene of interest. (But we did return to *maroon-like* later: see FINNERTY 1976.) Very early in conversation with SCHALET I emphasized the importance of a selective system for the recombination work. Shortly thereafter, he proposed the flanking-lethal crossover-selector idea that served as the basis for our early fine-structure mapping studies. A pilot experiment mapping the two original rosy mutations (*ry[1]* and *ry[2]*) was successful (SCHALET and CHOVNICK 1960). We then dropped all work on the *garnet* locus in order to mount a factory-like operation on *rosy*. At some point prior to our first reports on the *rosy* locus work, SCHALET stumbled over the WHITTINGHILL (1950) paper which describes lethal-crossover selector systems for the study of radiation-induced crossing over in Drosophila males. At that time, he and I agreed that we simply would acknowledge WHITTINGHILL's priority (SCHALET and CHOVNICK 1960; CHOVNICK *et al.* 1962). The use of the crossover-selector scheme has now come full circle in that we have made use of it in our recent studies of *P*-element transposase-induced male recombination (MCCARRON *et al.* 1989; DUTTAROY *et al.* 1990).

With this beginning, subsequent genetic analysis of *rosy* has focused largely on two topics: gene conversion and its relationship to recombination mechanisms, and gene organization and expression.

In all of the early work on *rosy*, utilizing the lethal-selector system applied to random-strand mapping, conversion products not associated with a single crossover between the flanking lethals were killed. This simplified interpretation of the mapping data and made for easy acceptance of the notion of intragenic crossing over in higher eukaryotes. In 1963 my attention returned to gene conversion when JOHN LUCCHESI mentioned in conversation that *deep orange* (*dor*: 1-0.3) and *rosy* were lethal in double-mutant zygotes (see LUCCHESI 1968). This fact, coupled with the availability of *C(3)L;C(3)R* strains developed by LEWIS (reviewed in HOLM 1976), led me to design a selective system for the study of conversion in half-tetrads utilizing *dor;ry* as a synthetic-lethal combination. DAVID HOLM started graduate work in the spring of 1964 and spent more than a year constructing strains for that first conversion experiment. A cumbersome but effective scheme was constructed and successfully used in one experiment but was never published. Then, in a review article, GLASSMAN (1965) mentioned the discovery of purine selection against XDH⁻ flies, citing a manuscript in preparation. To my knowledge, nothing further on this topic appeared from GLASSMAN's laboratory. However, we seized upon his suggestion and developed the purine selection schemes that were used in all of our subsequent work with both *rosy* and *maroon-like*. The recombination work, entirely consistent with fungal studies, has been reviewed in recent years (HILLIKER and CHOVNICK 1981; HILLIKER, CLARK and CHOVNICK 1988).

The second direction of our genetic studies dealing with gene organization and expression was stimulated by FRANCIS CRICK's "General Model for the Chromosomes of Higher Organisms" (1971). The model was an attempt to relate the huge excess of DNA found in higher organisms relative to prokaryotes to some features of higher-organism chromosomes. Sometime prior to the appearance of this paper, I received a preprint accompanied by a question from CRICK about the location of our *rosy* mutations. Was I able to position them in either a polytene band or interband region? In the context of his paper, the question really asked if I could locate the mutant sites

as lesions of a control or coding region of the gene. The model proposed that the bulk of the DNA (located in the polytene bands) served control functions, in contrast to peptide-coding DNA localized to the interbands. In fact, I had no information other than a linear order of mutations on a genetic map, and some simple phenotypic data. This question served to add a new dimension to our research strategy. With the help of MARGARET MCCARRON, joined shortly thereafter by BILL GELBART and JANARDAN PANDEY, a genetic outline of the organization of the *rosy* locus was developed that offered no evidence for a huge excess of control DNA in contrast to the coding DNA (reviewed in CHOVNICK, GELBART and MCCARRON 1977). This work, supplemented by the efforts of STEVE CLARK, ART HILLIKER and JANIS O'DONNELL (see CHOVNICK *et al.* 1978; HILLIKER *et al.* 1980) attracted the attention of several groups of molecular biologists who tried to clone the *rosy* gene using various state-of-the-art strategies of that time.

The successful cloning of the *rosy* region DNA by BENDER, SPIERER and HOGNESS (1983) and the precise localization of the *rosy* DNA (CLARK *et al.* 1986; COTÉ *et al.* 1986) were factors in the choice of *rosy* for the first *P*-element-mediated transformation experiments (RUBIN and SPRADLING 1982). Our collaboration with WELCOME BENDER and his staff has had a major impact upon the work of my laboratory in recent years (reviewed in DUTTON and CHOVNICK 1988; see also REAUME, CLARK and CHOVNICK 1989). Although somewhat broadened in scope, the odyssey continues with our focus upon such basic genetic mechanisms as recombination and gene expression and the impact of position effects and transposable elements upon these mechanisms.

LITERATURE CITED

BENDER, W., P. SPIERER and D. S. HOGNESS, 1983 Chromosomal walking and jumping to isolate DNA from the *ace* and *rosy* loci and the *bithorax* complex in *Drosophila melanogaster*. J. Mol. Biol. **168:** 17–33.

BENZER, S., 1955 Fine structure of a genetic region in bacteriophage. Proc. Natl. Acad. Sci. USA **41:** 344–354.

BORTS, R. H., and J. E. HABER, 1989 Length and distribution of meiotic gene conversion tracts and crossovers in *Saccharomyces cerevisiae*. Genetics **123:** 69–80.

CARLSON, E. A., 1959 Comparative genetics of complex loci. Quant. Rev. Biol. **34:** 33–67.

CHOVNICK, A., 1958 Aberrant segregation and pseudoallelism at the *garnet* locus in *Drosophila melanogaster*. Proc. Natl. Acad. Sci. USA **44:** 333–337.

CHOVNICK, A., 1961 The *garnet* locus in *Drosophila melanogaster*. I. Pseudoallelism. Genetics **46:** 493–507.

CHOVNICK, A., and A. S. FOX, 1953 Immunogenetic studies of

pseudoallelism in *Drosophila melanogaster*. I. Antigenic effects of the *lozenge* pseudoalleles. Proc. Natl. Acad. Sci. USA **39:** 1035–1043.

CHOVNICK, A., W. GELBART and M. McCARRON, 1977 Organization of the *rosy* locus in *Drosophila melanogaster*. Cell **11:** 1–10.

CHOVNICK, A., and R. J. LEFKOWITZ, 1956 A phenogenetic study of the *lozenge* pseudoalleles in *Drosophila melanogaster*. I. Effects in the development of the tarsal claws in homozygotes. Genetics **41:** 79–92.

CHOVNICK, A., R. J. LEFKOWITZ and A. S. FOX, 1956 A phenogenetic study of the *lozenge* pseudoalleles in *Drosophila melanogaster*. II. Effects on the development of tarsal claws in heterozygotes. Genetics **41:** 589–604.

CHOVNICK, A., A. SCHALET, R. P. KERNAGHAN and J. TALSMA, 1962 The resolving power of genetic fine structure analysis in higher organisms as exemplified by Drosophila. Am. Nat. **46:** 281–296.

CHOVNICK, A., A. SCHALET, R. P. KERNAGHAN and M. KRAUSS, 1964 The *rosy* cistron in *Drosophila melanogaster*: genetic fine structure analysis. Genetics **50:** 1245–1259.

CHOVNICK, A., M. McCARRON, A. HILLIKER, J. O'DONNELL, W. GELBART and S. CLARK, 1978 Gene organization in Drosophila. Cold Spring Harbor Symp. Quant. Biol. **42:** 1011–1021.

CLARK, S. H., M. McCARRON, C. LOVE and A. CHOVNICK, 1986 On the identification of the *rosy* locus DNA in *Drosophila melanogaster*: intragenic recombination mapping of mutations associated with insertions and deletions. Genetics **112:** 755–767.

COTÉ, B., W. BENDER, D. CURTIS and A. CHOVNICK, 1986 Molecular mapping of the *rosy* locus in *Drosophila melanogaster*. Genetics **112:** 769–783.

CRICK, F., 1971 General model for the chromosomes of higher organisms. Nature **234:** 25–27.

CURTIS, D., S. H. CLARK, A. CHOVNICK and W. BENDER, 1989 Molecular analysis of recombination events in Drosophila. Genetics **122:** 653–661.

DUTTAROY, A., M. Y. McCARRON, K. SITARAMAN, G. DOUGHTY and A. CHOVNICK, 1990 The relationship between *P* elements and male recombination in *Drosophila melanogaster*. Genetics **124** (in press).

DUTTON, JR., F. L., and A. CHOVNICK, 1988 Developmental regulation of the *rosy* locus in *Drosophila melanogaster*, pp. 267–316 in *Developmental Biology*, Vol. 5, edited by L. W. BROWDER. Plenum Press, New York.

FINNERTY, V., 1976 Genetic units of Drosophila–simple cistrons, pp. 721–765 in *The Genetics and Biology of Drosophila*, Vol. 16, edited by M. ASHBURNER and E. NOVITSKI. Academic Press, London.

FORREST, H. S., E. GLASSMAN and H. K. MITCHELL, 1956 Conversion of 2-amino-4-hydroxypteridine to isoxanthopterin in *Drosophila melanogaster*. Science **124:** 725–726.

GLASSMAN, E., 1965 Genetic regulation of xanthine dehydrogenase in *Drosophila melanogaster*. Fed. Proc. **24:** 1243–1251.

GLASSMAN, E., and H. K. MITCHELL, 1959 Mutants of *Drosophila melanogaster* deficient in xanthine dehydrogenase. Genetics **44:** 153–162.

GREEN, M. M., and K. C. GREEN, 1949 Crossing over between alleles at the *lozenge* locus in *Drosophila melanogaster*. Proc. Natl. Acad. Sci. USA **35:** 586–591.

HADORN, E., 1956 Patterns of biochemical and developmental biology. Cold Spring Harbor Symp. Quant. Biol. **21:** 363–373.

HEXTER, W. M., 1958 On the nature of the *garnet* locus in *Drosophila melanogaster*. Proc. Natl. Acad. Sci. USA **44:** 768–771.

HILLIKER, A. J., and A. CHOVNICK, 1981 Further observations on intragenic recombination in *Drosophila melanogaster*. Genet. Res. **38:** 281–296.

HILLIKER, A. J., S. H. CLARK and A. CHOVNICK, 1988 Genetic analysis of intragenic recombination in Drosophila, pp. 73–90 in *The Recombination of Genetic Material*, edited by K. B. LOW. Academic Press, San Diego.

HILLIKER, A. J., S. H. CLARK, A. CHOVNICK and W. M. GELBART, 1980 Cytogenetic analysis of the chromosomal region immediately adjacent to the *rosy* locus in *Drosophila melanogaster*. Genetics **95:** 95–110.

HOLLIDAY, R., 1964 A mechanism for gene conversion in fungi. Genet. Res. **5:** 282–304.

HOLM, D. G., 1976 Compound autosomes, pp. 529–561 in *The Genetics and Biology of Drosophila*, Vol. lb, edited by M. ASHBURNER and E. NOVITSKI. Academic Press, London.

LEWIS, E. B., 1951 Pseudoallelism and gene evolution. Cold Spring Harbor Symp. Quant. Biol. **16:** 159–174.

LUCCHESI, J. C., 1968 Synthetic lethality and semi-lethality among functionally related mutants of *Drosophila melanogaster*. Genetics **59:** 37–44.

McCARRON, M. Y., A. DUTTAROY, G. A. DOUGHTY and A. CHOVNICK, 1989 *P* element transposase induces male recombination in *Drosophila melanogaster*. Genet. Res. **54** (in press).

McCLINTOCK, B., 1944 The relation of homozygous deficiencies to mutations and allelic series in maize. Genetics **29:** 478–502.

MITCHELL, M. B., 1955 Aberrant recombination of pyridoxine mutants of Neurospora. Proc. Natl. Acad. Sci. USA **41:** 215–220.

OLIVER, C. P., 1940 A reversion to wild type associated with crossing over in *Drosophila melanogaster*. Proc. Natl. Acad. Sci. USA **26:** 452–454.

PRITCHARD, R. H., 1955 The linear arrangement of a series of alleles of *Aspergillus nidulans*. Heredity **9:** 343–371.

REAUME, A. G., S. H. CLARK and A. CHOVNICK, 1989 Xanthine dehydrogenase is transported to the Drosophila eye. Genetics **123:** 503–509.

RUBIN, G. M., and A. C. SPRADLING, 1982 Genetic transformation of Drosophila with transposable element vectors. Science **218:** 348–353.

SCHALET, A., and A. CHOVNICK, 1960 A crossover-selector system for the study of pseudoallelic recombination in *Drosophila melanogaster*. Drosophila Inform. Serv. **34:** 104–105.

SCHALET, A., R. P. KERNAGHAN and A. CHOVNICK, 1964 Structural and phenotypic definition of the *rosy* cistron in *Drosophila melanogaster*. Genetics **50:** 1261–1268.

WHITEHOUSE, H. L. K., 1963 A theory of crossing-over by means of hybrid deoxyribonucleic acid. Nature **199:** 1034–1040.

WHITTINGHILL, M., 1950 Two crossover-selector systems: new tools in genetics. Science **111:** 377–378.

R. A. Fisher, A Centennial View

James F. Crow

Genetics Department, University of Wisconsin–Madison, Madison, Wisconsin 53706

R. A. FISHER was born 100 years ago on February 17, 1890, in London. He was one of a pair of twin boys, the other being stillborn. What a tragedy that they did not both survive! And I would wish them to have been monozygotic. What would a replicate of FISHER's DNA have produced? Would he have had his brother's extreme nearsightedness? His urbane conversation and graceful prose? His witty and sometimes pointed sarcasm? His unpredictable temper explosions? His social idealism? Above all, his mathematical creativity and his astonishing geometric intuition? And how would two FISHERs have gotten on?

FISHER was an outlier, both scientifically and personally. His scientific work has often been reviewed, and we can expect more in this centennial year. This account is more personal, written by an admirer who knew him less well than some but better than most.

FISHER had an insight into multidimensional geometry that was little short of occult. He could answer questions that completely baffled others. He often arrived at an elegant answer, seemingly with no intermediate steps. Somehow, he found the pearl without opening the oyster. This meant that his papers could not be understood by most mathematicians, with the result that they were often not trusted. Long ago I saw a copy of a FISHER paper that had belonged to a mathematician; in the margin he had scratched "Fisher is fishy." Ultimately, many of FISHER's results were demonstrated in a more orthodox way, often by others.

Although FISHER had a talent for mathematics, his real interest was biology. Nevertheless, he sought and won a maths scholarship at Caius College, Cambridge. He chose mathematics for two reasons. One was that he had seen a mounted, disarticulated codfish skull and envisioned an arduous and futile exercise of learning all the bones. (I, too, was daunted by such a preparation.) The other reason was that he thought that, for a future biologist, "a mathematical technique with biological interests is a rather firmer ground than a biological technique with mathematical interests." His Cambridge tutor said later that he would have been a first class mathematician had he "stuck to the ropes." Yet, FISHER never regarded himself as a mathematician. The title of his biography (BOX 1978) is *R. A. Fisher, the Life of a Scientist*, surely the way he would have wanted it. Nevertheless, FISHER's great mathematical talent was predominant throughout his life.

As a schoolboy, FISHER had eyesight so bad that he was not permitted to read by lamplight and received his instruction, even mathematics, aurally and without visual aids. He developed a remarkable ability to solve problems in his head and acquired the geometrical insights that were so natural to him and so baffling to others. To what extent this was innate ability and to what extent a necessity brought on by poor eyesight, we shall never know. FISHER's development of significance tests for correlation and regression coefficients, for the t distribution, and for the analysis of variance were all done geometrically.

While still a student at Cambridge, he wrote a paper (FISHER 1912) in which he maximized the expression that he later called likelihood. Despite a degree from Cambridge and an evident talent, his next six years (1913–1919) were miserable. He was refused admission to the army. He worked in an office, taught school, and in his spare time tried subsistence farming. Yet, during this period he wrote two famous papers. One (1915) showed how to test the significance of a correlation coefficient, r, and introduced the transformation, $z = \tanh^{-1} r$, in which the distribution of z is nearly normal. The other (1918) reconciled biometry and Mendelism and laid the foundations for quantitative genetics. I have written about this remarkable paper before in this column (CROW 1988). The conclusions have hardly been changed in the 72 years since it was written, although they have been formulated and proved more precisely and rigorously by MALÉCOT (see NAGYLAKI 1989).

Finally, in 1919, FISHER was offered a temporary position to analyze agricultural data at Rothamsted Experimental Station. He accepted, and he stayed. There he developed the statistical procedures and experimental designs that are now universally used.

The early farm-crop influence is reflected in the retention of such words as plots and blocks in analysis of variance and of nitrogen, phosphorus, and potash in textbook explanations of factorial design. The enormous increases in crop yields in the past half century owes a great deal to reliable field testing that used these methods. Fisherian practices spread widely at about the same time that hybrid corn was introduced. Perhaps the inbreeding and hybridization technique should share some of the credit it enjoys with the efficient design of field trials.

FISHER's contributions to statistics are legion, and so well known that I shall mention them only in passing. Small-sample statistics, analysis of variance and covariance, experimental design, and statistical estimation are subjects that he founded. He straightened out the number of degrees of freedom for PEARSON's χ^2 test, he recognized the importance of STUDENT's[1] t test and demonstrated its correctness, and he pointed out the useful properties of the maximum likelihood method. His book *Statistical Methods for Research Workers*, despite being uniformly panned by reviewers, went through 14 editions and was translated into French, German, Italian, Japanese, Spanish and Russian. He was surely the greatest statistician of his time, if not of all time.

Something that is less fully appreciated is that FISHER was the first to employ nonparametric tests involving permutations of the observations. I think it is clear that he regarded randomization as primary, and tests based on normality assumptions as labor-saving approximations. This view is clearly set forth in, of all places, an expository paper on craniometry. Here he described how measurements on two groups of 100 individuals could be written on cards, then shuffled and divided randomly into two sets of 100 each. One could then ask what fraction of such random divisions would lead to a difference between the sets as large as or larger than the observed difference between the two measured groups. If this fraction were small, the groups could be regarded as differing significantly. Then FISHER (1936) wrote: "Actually, the statistician does not carry out this very simple and very tedious process, but his conclusions have no justification beyond the fact that they agree with those which could have been arrived at by this elementary method." One other relevant consideration: FISHER's methods were all devised with a view to minimizing complex computations. I believe that if high speed computers had been available, FISHER would have relied much less on normal distribution theory and much more on robust permutation tests.

This year is the 60th anniversary of another FISHER

tour de force, *The Genetical Theory of Natural Selection*, arguably the deepest and most influential book on evolution since DARWIN. Each rereading of this classic brings something new. The book starts out by contrasting blending and particulate inheritance and emphasizing the remarkable variance-conserving properties of the latter, never before so clearly articulated. FISHER introduced what he called the "Malthusian parameter" as a measure of population increase. This was not new, but what was new was an extension, his "reproductive value." This is a weight to be assigned to each age group in proportion to the contribution of that group to the future population after age stability has been achieved, and thus it has an evolutionary as well as demographic significance. The idea has become popular with demographers (*e.g.*, KEYFITZ 1968). In FISHER's book the central idea was his "Fundamental Theorem of Natural Selection," that the rate of increase of fitness attributable to gene-frequency changes under selection is given by the additive component of the genetic variance. Although a cottage industry has grown up devoted to criticisms, exegeses and proofs, this succinct statement seems to me to capture the essence of the way selection works and to encapsulate a great deal of evolutionary insight in a simple formula.

FISHER not only asked important questions; he found answers. Some of his mathematical tricks were astonishing. He developed an ingenious method for finding the probability of survival of a mutant gene for a specified number of generations. He worked out the partial differential equation for gene-frequency change using a trigonometric transformation that made the variance independent of the allele frequency. He generalized HALDANE's formula, $P = 2s$, for the probability of ultimate fixation of a gene whose heterozygous selective advantage is s; it was further generalized by MALÉCOT (1952) and by KIMURA (1964). He gave the first coherent quantitative theory of sexual selection, mimicry, polymorphism, evolution of recombination rates, and supergenes. He explained why the sex ratio is nearly 1:1, even in polygamous species—one of the best illustrations that natural selection does not necessarily maximize fitness. In doing this he introduced the concept of parental expenditure, thereby precipitating a landslide of ecological literature. Rarely have so many new, and often deep, ideas been put into a single book. Curiously, although FISHER led the way to a quantitative theory of random genetic drift, he never regarded it as having much evolutionary significance. The evolutionary possibilities of random drift were advocated, with quite different emphases, by WRIGHT (1988 and earlier) and KIMURA (1983).

FISHER is never easy reading. The book is far from the explicit formulation and clear exposition that is

---

[1] "STUDENT" was a pseudonym of W. S. GOSSET, whose employers, the Guinness Breweries of Dublin, did not permit him to publish under his own name. Another employee, E. M. SOMERFIELD, published as "ALUMNUS."

the ideal of contemporary population genetics. He was partly poet. He was as much a master of elegant English as of elegant mathematics. But elegance and clarity are not the same. Fisher hardly ever made clear what his assumptions were, when and how he was approximating, and how to get from one equation to the next. I can empathize with GOSSET, who once wrote: "When I come to 'evidently' I know that means two hours hard work at least before I can see why" (BOX 1978, p. 115).

The last five chapters of *The Genetical Theory* are devoted to human society. From his student days FISHER had been an ardent eugenicist, full of idealism and belief that mankind could be persuaded to reproduce so that the hereditary components of health, intelligence, character, and social conscience would increase. A much discussed topic of the time was the rise and fall of civilizations, about which FISHER read a great deal. His idea was that promotion of the gifted and industrious into a higher social class, where they would reproduce less, was a major factor in the decay of civilizations, and he discussed social and economic incentives that might forestall this. He advocated voluntary sterilization of the genetically impaired and family incentive payments proportional to income. As far as I can tell, his eugenic writings have had no lasting influence on either biologists or historians. In his later life Fisher did not write about these subjects, nor did he talk about them (to me at least). I don't think he had changed his mind, but simply tired of trying to get people to take his proposals seriously. At the same time, he was increasingly honored for his statistical and evolutionary work.

FISHER was part of the great trinity that included SEWALL WRIGHT and J. B. S. HALDANE. Together they founded and almost completely dominated the field of population genetics for its first quarter century. Each made important contributions, but in one way FISHER stands apart. HALDANE and WRIGHT formulated a problem and then doggedly ground out the results, come what might. FISHER was more likely to invent a new, neater approach. His work had elegance and grace, and flashes of insight and creativity, along with a touch of genius that can be fully appreciated only by those with mathematical insights deeper than mine.

During all of his active life–at Rothamsted, at University College London, and at Cambridge–FISHER always had genetic experiments going, often in collaboration with friends. He studied dogs, poultry, locusts, butterflies, sorrels, primroses, and especially mice. Many of the animals were kept in his home and he and his family took care of them. The presence of rooms full of mouse cages in the Professor's lodging is said to have been a deterring factor in the selection of his successor at Cambridge. What came out of all

this experimental work was minor, certainly nothing comparable to what came out of his head. Yet, I think FISHER's constant touch with experiments and field observations guided his statistical and evolutionary work along practical lines. His most lasting contributions to experimental genetics are methodological. He showed how to measure linkage when simple backcrosses were impractical. His last paper (1962), lightweight by his standards, was on this subject. He exhaustively classified the gametic output of tetraploids, hexaploids and octoploids and showed how to allow for double reduction. He recognized ascertainment bias in human studies and examined the efficiency of various procedures designed to overcome it. He worked out computation-saving methods of detecting and measuring linkage in human pedigrees. Although his procedures have recently been superseded by computerized methods, his likelihood approach is the basis of most of them.

To FISHER, genetics was transmission genetics, strange as this seems today with the current emphasis on molecular approaches to gene action and development. Intermediate mechanisms were of secondary interest to him. Meiosis, for example, was a black box. In 1947 JOSHUA LEDERBERG and I sat together at the founding meeting of the Biometrics Society at Woods Hole. FISHER was elected president and gave a major address. He presented a model of recombination and interference that, among other things, permitted more than 50% recombination (for which he had some supporting mouse data). We were both taken aback by his not taking account of the four-strand nature of crossing over and exchanged whispered expressions of incredulity. Later, in response to LEDERBERG's question as to why he used a two-strand model, FISHER said: "Young man, it is not a two-strand model, it is a one-strand model." This epitomized FISHER's view of genetics. He developed the point more fully in the published paper and discussion (FISHER 1948). The geneticist's job, he said, is to develop a theory for predicting the frequencies of different genotypes from multiply heterozygous parents.

FISHER placed great emphasis on linkage analysis and chromosome mapping, and much of his mouse work was directed to this end. As soon as he had a formal position in genetics, he extended this interest to human genetics. He played an active role in gathering information on the rapidly increasing number of genetic markers, especially blood groups, with a view to mapping the human genome. Out of this grew his novel three-locus hypothesis for inheritance of the Rhesus factor (FISHER 1947), which at least notationally was a great advance. FISHER loved formal genetics; what a time he would have with human linkage analysis were he still alive, and how he would delight in the powerful computers and the plethora of reliable neutral markers!

FISHER enjoyed conversation and could be utterly charming. He could also be petty, quarrelsome, stubborn and outspoken. He fitted the classical definition of a gentleman: he never insulted anyone unintentionally. He was constantly involved in one or another controversy, often with other distinguished statisticians and geneticists, *e.g.*, JERZY NEYMAN and SEWALL WRIGHT. His sarcastic barbs could be amusing, except to their targets. FISHER was particularly bitter toward KARL PEARSON, who had misunderstood his early work and had treated him with arrogance. He was at has acerbic best (or worst) with PEARSON who, a decade after his death, elicited this: "If peevish intolerance of free opinion in others is a sign of senility, it is one which he had developed at an early age" (FISHER 1950, p. 29.302a).

In his later years FISHER visited the University of Wisconsin several times, mainly because a daughter lived in Madison. He always visited the Genetics Laboratory; we looked forward to his visits and saved problems for him. But it was necessary to engineer his coming and going so that he would not encounter SEWALL WRIGHT in the hallway. Their relationship had deteriorated to the point that neither wanted to see the other.

I shall finish this essay with two personal anecdotes. The first concerns my first meeting FISHER. It was during a statistics course at North Carolina State College in the summer of 1946. He gave an evening lecture to a large audience, composed almost entirely of statisticians, on his three-locus theory of Rh inheritance. This was new to me, and I was entranced. In the question period he was first asked how he did the χ^2 test, to which he gave a curt answer. Clearly it was the genetics that interested him so I asked some genetic questions, which pleased him and which we continued informally after the session was closed. He suggested a glass of beer at a bar across the street. (I then realized for the first time that in poor light Fisher was nearly blind.) This was a time of postwar shortages, and the bar had run out of both beer and wine. There was champagne, however, and we got a bottle, only to be told that North Carolina law prohibited drinking it on the premises. So we repaired to my dormitory room and began, over a shared bottle of champagne, a friendship that lasted through the remainder of his life.

The second anecdote concerns the famous paper of LURIA and DELBRÜCK (1943). I found its argument for the preadaptive nature of evolution of virus resistance in bacteria fully convincing, but thought that the mathematical treatment was shoddy and confusing. Taking advantage of my newly formed acquaintance with FISHER, I asked him how to find the distribution

of mutant cells in an exponentially growing culture. He leaned back in his chair, thought for perhaps a minute, took a scrap of paper, and wrote a generating function. I took the paper and, not understanding it, put it aside to work on later–and then managed to lose it. The solution was published two years later by LEA and COULSON (1949). Unless that scrap of paper turns up, we'll never know whether FISHER was the first to solve this problem.

FISHER died in 1962. He had written several hundred reviews, comments, and letters. His major papers–294 of them–are included in five volumes edited by BENNETT (1971–1974), often with introductory comments and amendments by FISHER himself. The first volume also includes a biography, written by F. YATES and K. MATHER. Those interested in his personal life will enjoy the biography by JOAN FISHER BOX (1978). Written by a loving and admiring daughter, the book is touching as it brings out FISHER's blemishes along with his greatness. It is also scholarly, for BOX took the trouble to understand and explain the difficult conceptual points, especially in statistics.

A large number of people have read an earlier draft of this article and I am grateful for their comments. My greatest debt is to JOAN FISHER BOX and THOMAS NAGYLAKI, who provided numerous improvements in both content and style.

BIBLIOGRAPHY

Books by and about FISHER:

BENNETT, J. H. (Editor), 1971–1974 *Collected Papers of R. A Fisher.* University of Adelaide, Australia.

BENNETT, J. H. (Editor), 1983 *Natural Selection, Heredity, and Eugenics: Including Selected Correspondence of R. A. Fisher with Leonard Darwin and Others.* Clarendon Press, Oxford.

BOX, J. F., 1978 *R. A. Fisher, the Life of a Scientist.* John Wiley & Sons, New York.

FISHER, R. A., 1925–1970 *Statistical Methods for Research Workers.* Oliver and Boyd, Edinburgh. 14th ed. (1971, 1973) Hafner, New York.

FISHER, R. A., 1930 *The Genetical Theory of Natural Selection.* Clarendon Press, Oxford. 2nd ed. (1958) Dover, New York.

FISHER, R. A., 1935–1966 *The Design of Experiments.* Oliver and Boyd, Edinburgh. 8th ed. (1971, 1973) Hafner, New York.

FISHER, R. A., 1949, 1965 *The Theory of Inbreeding.* Oliver and Boyd, Edinburgh.

FISHER, R. A., 1950 *Contributions to Mathematical Statistics.* John Wiley & Sons, New York.

FISHER, R. A., 1956, 1959 *Statistical Method and Scientific Inference.* Oliver and Boyd, Edinburgh. 13th ed. (1973) Hafner, New York.

FISHER, R. A., and F. YATES, 1938–1963 *Statistical Tables for Biological, Agricultural and Medical Research.* Oliver and Boyd, Edinburgh.

Cited articles:

Many of FISHER's papers were published in obscure journals. The best source is the five-volume set, comprising 294 papers, edited by J. H. BENNETT and listed above.

CROW, J. F., 1988 Fifty years ago: the beginnings of population genetics. Genetics **119:** 473–476.

FISHER, R. A., 1912 On an absolute criterion for fitting frequency curves. Messeng. Math. **41:** 155–160.

FISHER, R. A., 1915 Frequency distribution of the values of the correlation coefficients in samples from an indefinitely large population. Biometrika **10:** 507–521.

FISHER, R. A., 1918 The correlation between relatives on the supposition of Mendelian inheritance. Trans. R. Soc. Edinb. **59:** 399–433.

FISHER, R. A., 1936 "The coefficient of racial likeness" and the future of craniometry. J. R. Anthropol. Inst. **66:** 47–63.

FISHER, R. A., 1947 The Rhesus factor: a study in scientific method. Am. Sci. **35:** 95–102, 113.

FISHER, R. A., 1948 A quantitative theory of genetic recombination and chiasma formation. Biometrics **4:** 1–13.

FISHER, R. A., 1962 The detection of sex differences in recombination values using double heterozygotes. J. Theor. Biol. **3:** 509–513.

KEYFITZ, N., 1968 *Introduction to the Mathematics of Population.* Addison-Wesley, Reading, Mass.

KIMURA, M., 1964 Diffusion models in population genetics. J. Appl. Prob. **1:** 177–232.

KIMURA, M., 1983 *The Neutral Theory of Molecular Evolution.* Cambridge University Press, Cambridge.

LEA, D. E., and C. A. COULSON, 1949 The distribution of the numbers of mutants in bacterial populations. J Genet. **49:** 64–285.

LURIA, S. E., and M. DELBRÜCK, 1943 Mutations of bacteria from virus sensitivity to virus resistance. Genetics **28:** 491–511.

MALÉCOT, G., 1952 Les processus stochastiques et la méthode des fonctions génératrices ou caractéristiques. Publ. Inst. Stat. Univ. Paris **1:** Fasc. 3, 1–16.

NAGYLAKI, T., 1989 Gustave Malécot and the transition from classical to modern population genetics. Genetics **122:** 253–268.

WRIGHT, S., 1988 Surfaces of selective value revisited. Am. Nat. **131:** 115–123.

Regulating Tn*10* and IS*10* Transposition

Nancy Kleckner

Harvard University, Department of Biochemistry and Molecular Biology, 7 Divinity Avenue, Cambridge, Massachusetts 02138

TRANSPOSABLE elements are ubiquitous inhabitants of both prokaryotic and eukaryotic genomes. They may be molecular parasites, surviving only because they replicate faster than their hosts; alternatively, they may survive because they confer a selective evolutionary advantage to an individual host, to a host population, or to a particular favorable gene such as antibiotic resistance (for interesting reading see CAMPBELL 1981a, b; ORGEL and CRICK 1980; SAPIENZA and DOOLITTLE 1981; SYVANEN 1984). For bacterial transposons, at least, this final possibility seems particularly simple and attractive. The ability of a gene to spread through a population is greatly enhanced if it can transpose onto and off of transmitting DNA molecules (viruses, plasmids or transforming DNA); transposition of genetic segments in the absence of any element is exceedingly rare. Furthermore, because the transposon remains tightly linked to the favorable gene, selection for and dissemination of that gene necessarily disseminates the transposable element as well.

Regardless of the evolutionary forces involved, stable coexistence of a transposable element with its host requires that a balance be struck between too little transposition and too much. If the element transposes too much, or in an inappropriate way, deleterious effects on the host will counterbalance the advantage conferred by transposition and may cause the host to evolve specific defenses. On the other hand, if the element does not transpose at some minimal level, it cannot maintain itself as an evolutionarily successful unit.

Tn*10* and IS*10*: Tn*10* is a bacterial tetracycline-resistance transposon. It is a composite element because its two ends are inverted repeats of an insertion sequence, in this case IS*10*. While either IS*10* element can transpose individually, IS*10*-Right is fully functional and IS*10*-Left is defective, relying primarily on transposition functions provided by IS*10*-Right. The two IS*10* elements can also cooperate to effect transposition of the entire Tn*10* unit or to generate certain Tn*10*-promoted rearrangements. All of these events

are rare, approximately 1 per 10^3 cell generations for IS*10*, 1 per 10^7 for Tn*10*, and 1 per 10^5 for the rearrangements. All of these events require IS*10*-encoded transposase, which interacts with different pairs of outside and inside IS*10* ends to promote the various events. *In vitro*, Tn*10* and IS*10* transposition also requires a host protein which may be either IHF or HU and which plays an accessory role in the reaction, probably by altering DNA structure. IHF is likely to be the most important host factor *in vivo*.

Tn*10* and IS*10* transpose by a nonreplicative mechanism in which the element is excised from the donor site and inserted at a new target location without any replication of the element except for a small amount of repair synthesis at the very ends. The fate of the donor molecule is not firmly established, but is likely to involve chromosome loss and/or repair of the remaining double-strand gap against another copy of the donor region present on another molecule in the same cell. Loss of a chromosome need not be a lethal event, because bacteria contain more than a single chromosome under most growth conditions.

We describe below the mechanisms by which IS*10*-Right (hereafter called IS*10*) and Tn*10* modulate their transposition activities (Figure 1). Some of these mechanisms are intrinsic to the transposon or insertion sequence itself, while others involve interplay between the transposon and its host. They can all be rationalized as stratagems ensuring that transposition occurs at an appropriate rate and under appropriate circumstances. The existence of these many mechanisms, some of which are quite sophisticated, makes it clear that IS*10* and Tn*10* are evolutionarily successful creatures and that IS*10*, at least, has been with us for a long time. Many of these mechanisms are known or suspected to operate for other IS elements and similar general regulatory strategies are found in many types of transposons. The reader should consult *Mobile DNA* for descriptions of other elements and for a fuller review of Tn*10* and IS*10* with references to the primary literature (KLECKNER 1988).

Features of IS*10* ensuring low levels of transposase expression: The frequency of IS*10* transposition is never very high because the level of transposase

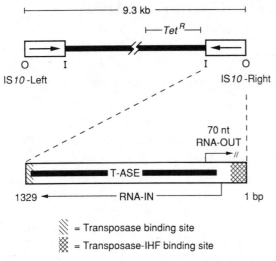

= Transposase binding site

= Transposase-IHF binding site

FIGURE 1.—The structure of Tn*10*.

protein is never very high (RALEIGH and KLECKNER 1986). A single copy of IS*10* in the bacterial chromosome generates fewer than 0.2 molecule per cell per generation as estimated from the level of β-galactosidase in a strain bearing a single-copy transposase/β-galactosidase fusion gene. So little protein is made that polypeptide chains can be detected in enzyme assays only if the cells are broken open so that unassociated fusion-protein monomers can reassemble into active tetramers *in vitro*.

This low level of protein is achieved by a combination of infrequent transcription (0.25 transcript per element per cell generation) and inefficient translation (fewer than 60% of transcripts being translated even once). Transcription is infrequent in part because the transposase gene promoter, pIN, is relatively weak (SIMONS *et al.* 1983), and in part because transcription is confined to a small fraction of the cell cycle (see below). Translation is inefficient primarily because there is no obvious Shine-Dalgarno ribosome binding site consensus sequence; most mutations that increase transposase gene translation bring the sequence closer to consensus (C. JAIN and N. KLECKNER, unpublished results).

Two subtler mechanisms may also contribute to inefficient translation by confining translation initiation on a nascent 5′ mRNA to the first few seconds after transcription is initiated. First, translation is reduced severalfold by fold-back inhibition, in which a region of transposase mRNA about 300 nucleotides (nt) from the 5′ end pairs with and sequesters the ribosome binding site near the start of the message (KITTLE and KLECKNER 1988; J. E. GONZALEZ and R. W. SIMONS, unpublished results). Second, preliminary experiments suggest that failure to initiate translation at the transposase AUG start codon may reduce the stability of the 5′ end of the mRNA (C. JAIN and N. KLECKNER, unpublished results).

Transposition of a single-copy element regulated by *dam* methylation: The most important regulatory mechanism for an IS*10* element present in single copy involves DNA adenine methylation at specific sites in IS*10* (ROBERTS *et al.* 1985; additional discussion in KLECKNER 1988). This mechanism not only reduces the basal level of transposition but also ensures that it occurs specifically in the most appropriate situations. *Escherichia coli* mutants exhibiting increased levels of Tn*10*-promoted rearrangements were isolated and subsequently shown to increase IS*10* transposition more than 100-fold. All of these mutations turn out to be alleles of the *dam* gene whose product, DNA adenine methylase, methylates the N-6 positions of the symmetrical adenines in the sequence 5′GATC. The effects of *dam* mutations are a direct consequence of the absence of methylation at two strategically located GATC sites in IS*10*, one of which overlaps the −10 region of the transposase promoter near the outside end of the element and the second of which occurs within the transposase binding site at the opposite (inside) end of IS*10*.

Because there is normally no fully unmethylated DNA in wild-type *E. coli* strains, and because hemimethylated DNA is generated only transiently upon replication of the transposon, we reasoned that the effects of *dam* mutations must reflect a normal process in which IS*10* is activated by hemimethylation. Additional analysis revealed this to be the case. Furthermore, passage of the replication fork generates two chemically distinguishable hemimethylated IS*10* species, and we found that only one of these is substantially activated for transposition. The ratios of approximate transposition rates for the fully methylated and the two hemimethylated species are 1:12:2,400 (minimum) to 1:12:60,000 (possible). These conclusions were reached largely by direct examination of IS*10* transposition from hemimethylated DNA *in vivo*. Hemimethylated elements were generated *in vivo* by transferring IS*10* from a Dam⁺ host to a Dam⁻ host in an Hfr cross, where one specific strand of the transferred DNA is synthesized in the donor while the complementary strand is synthesized *de novo* in the recipient.

Appropriate variations in the Hfr transfer experiment revealed the basis for these differences. Each of the two hemimethylated versions of the pIN promoter is activated relative to the fully methylated promoter. However, only one of the two hemimethylated inside ends is activated. This *cis* asymmetry ensures that only one of the two hemimethylated elements transposes. The magnitude of activation results in part from the independent effects of methylation on the two determinants and in part from a coupling mechanism: expression of transposase and activation of the inside end are temporally coupled, both GATC sites becoming hemimethylated just as the replication fork passes. In the coupled situation, transposase protein is used more efficiently than it would be were the terminus and promoter activated at independent times.

One important prediction of *dam* regulation is that IS*10* transposition will occur only during a limited period of the cell cycle, immediately after the replication fork passes. Although the IS*10* GATC sites have not yet been examined, recent experiments suggest that a typical GATC site in the *E. coli* chromosome remains hemimethylated for 0.5–4 min, 1–10% of a generation (J. CAMPBELL and N. KLECKNER, unpublished results). Furthermore, during this interval, only one of the two sister chromosomes can generate an IS*10* transposition. This type of regulation should be specifically advantageous to an element like IS*10* that transposes by a nonreplicative mechanism and leaves a hole in the donor chromosome. *dam* regulation should ensure that transposition will never occur unless a second copy of the donor region is present, *i.e.*, on the sister chromatid. Thus, a cell will never die because a donor molecule is not repaired. Furthermore, the likelihood of repair may be increased because a homologous sister-chromatid region is always in the general vicinity of the donor molecule at the time of transposition.

Activation by hemimethylation should also mean that transposition will be transiently induced when IS*10* enters a new host by any mechanism that involves transfer of single-stranded DNA followed by synthesis of the complementary strand in the recipient cell (*i.e.*, conjugal transfer, some types of transformation, or infection by single-stranded DNA phages). This may be particularly important for expediting the dissemination of IS*10* in bacterial populations.

Mechanisms slowing the accumulation of multiple transposon copies: Although IS*10* transposes by a nonreplicative mechanism, the average number of transposons per cell in the population should increase with almost every cycle of transposition. If the gap left behind at the donor site is repaired by interaction with another chromosome, a second copy of the transposon is generated by the restoration process. If the gap is not repaired and the donor chromosome is lost, the average number of transposons per bacterial genome can still increase: if the transposon inserts into a chromosome other than the one that is lost, the number of transposons remains constant while the total number of chromosomes decreases. In either case, the transposon frequency further increases if the moving element inserts ahead of the replication fork in the target chromosome.

If transposition were left unchecked, the average number of transposons per cell would continue to accumulate, and at ever-increasing rates. With more copies, there would be more potential donor elements

and, in addition, the transposase concentration would increase. The cell would eventually explode. For IS*10*, these risks are greatly reduced by diverse mechanisms.

IS10 transposase acts preferentially in cis: cis action is observable in complementation tests: the transposition frequency of an element making its own transposase is much greater than that of an equivalent element provided with the same level of transposase in *trans* (FOSTER *et al.* 1981; N. KLECKNER, unpublished results). As a consequence, increasing the numbers of IS*10* copies no longer increases the effective transposase concentration; each IS*10* element sees only its own transposase.

Formally, failure to observe complementation could result either from an intrinsic failure of the protein to move freely through the cell and/or from coupling of transposase action to transposase expression. In the first case, transposase made by one element would never reach a distant element. In the second case, transposase which reaches an element in *trans* could never act because silent transposons are poor substrates for transposase action. In fact, IS*10* uses both of these mechanisms.

Transposase is indeed intrinsically *cis*-acting. Even when all regulatory mechanisms are experimentally eliminated, transposase made in one location acts preferentially on transposon ends that are located nearby (MORISATO *et al.* 1983). The physical basis for this property is not understood. Perhaps some combination of high nonspecific DNA binding and a finite functional half-life prevents transposase from migrating very far from the site where it first contacts DNA. *cis* action of this type also requires that the transposase mRNA never diffuse very far from the template element. Because the mRNA cannot be separated from the template element until transcription is complete, mRNA localization might be facilitated by translational polarity and/or fold-back inhibition.

In addition, transposase should be effectively *cis*-acting because its action is coupled to its transcription by *dam* regulation. IS*10* elements at different locations in the genome become hemimethylated at different times. Any particular element will be immune to transposase that is made by elements elsewhere in the genome because its inside end will be fully methylated when those transposases are made.

IS10 multicopy inhibition: IS*10* has evolved an entire regulatory process whose sole function is to reduce transposition when the element is present in more than a single copy. IS*10* encodes a *trans*-acting negative regulator of transposase expression whose effectiveness increases with increasing concentration, *i.e.*, with increasing transposon copy number (SIMONS and KLECKNER 1983). The level of this regulator is adjusted so that transposase expression from an element present in single copy is barely affected (SIMONS and

KLECKNER 1983); however, the presence of even two copies results in a threefold inhibition, and 30 copies can inhibit as much as 50-fold (J. MATSUNAGA and R. W. SIMONS, unpublished results). Because transposase is *cis*-acting, any decrease in the level made per copy reduces the frequency of transposition of each copy. Thus, the combination of a *trans*-acting negative regulator and a *cis*-acting transposase means that as the number of IS*10* copies increases, the frequency of transposition per copy decreases. In fact, the overall rate of IS*10* transposition by the ensemble of copies in the cell probably remains essentially constant regardless of the copy number.

This IS*10*-encoded *trans*-acting negative regulator is a 70-nt antisense RNA, RNA-OUT. Its existence was discovered in the course of complementation experiments in which multicopy IS*10* plasmids were tested against transposase-defective Tn*10* derivatives introduced on λ phages. Mysteriously, control experiments demonstrated that wild-type Tn*10* transposed less frequently into cells containing a multicopy IS*10* plasmid than into cells lacking any plasmid. Deletion analysis then demonstrated that this multicopy inhibition was not due to transposase itself. The RNA nature of the inhibitor was revealed by genetic analysis coupled with *in vitro* identification of the responsible promoter, pOUT, located internal to and opposing the transposase gene promoter pIN. The template sequences for RNA-OUT and the transposase mRNA (RNA-IN) overlap for 36 bp. The key evidence that inhibition results from pairing of the two RNAs was the genetic observation that the inhibitory effect conferred by a wild-type plasmid could be titrated by an additional, truncated transposase gene, present in *cis* or in *trans*, expressing the 5′ end of RNA-IN at high levels.

IS*10* antisense control works in a simple and direct way. The region of RNA-IN that is complementary to RNA-OUT includes the ribosome binding site for the transposase gene, and RNA-OUT exerts its effect by preventing ribosome binding to RNA-IN (C. MA and R. W. SIMONS, unpublished results). The paired species is also cleaved by the double-strand-specific RNaseIII, but this cleavage is not required for antisense control (C. C. CASE, E. SIMONS and R. W. SIMONS, unpublished results; see SIMONS and KLECKNER 1988).

Specific features of the antisense system are important for its function. RNA-OUT forms a stem-loop structure, and the 5′ end of the transposase message, RNA-IN, is complementary to the top of the loop. Pairing initiates by interaction at the 5′ terminal sequence GCG, extends through the rest of the loop, and then proceeds by displacement of one strand of the RNA-OUT stem throughout the remaining region of complementarity to the 3′ end of RNA-OUT

(KITTLE *et al.* 1989). The three initial G · C pairs are probably important for nucleation of stable pairing, and initiation at the terminus of RNA-IN permits free rotation of the nascent duplex around the RNA-OUT chain, thus permitting pairing over more than a single turn of the helix. Also, the stem domain of RNA-OUT has several base-pair mismatches while the RNA-IN/RNA-OUT hybrid has perfect complementarity; replacing imperfect matches with perfect ones during pairing may help to drive the strand-displacement reaction in the forward direction.

Biologically, the stem-loop structure of RNA-OUT allows presentation of an exposed single-stranded region (the loop) for pairing initiation in a structure where it is protected from nucleolytic degradation by the stem domain. Mutations in the loop domain alter the rate of antisense pairing *in vitro* but have little effect on stability *in vivo*. In contrast, mutations that reduce intramolecular pairing in the stem domain have little effect on the rate of pairing but drastically reduce the half-life of RNA-OUT inside the cell and are suppressed by compensatory mutations that restore stem pairing (CASE *et al.* 1989). The stem region probably acts to block the progress of exonucleolytic single-strand RNases, which are a major source of single-strand nucleolytic activity in *E. coli*. However, the duplex stem domain is also specifically arranged so as not to be a substrate for RNaseIII: a single-base mutation in RNA-OUT that extends the stem domain pairing up into the loop domain renders the molecule sensitive to that RNase.

As a consequence of these features, RNA-OUT is exceptionally stable; its half-life is more than 40 min as compared with a typical bacterial mRNA half-life of 1–2 min (CASE *et al.* 1989). This stability allows the cell to achieve a high steady-state level of the RNA with a promoter that is only moderately active. Such a mechanism does not permit the level of RNA-OUT to change rapidly, but rapid changes are not necessary for a regulatory process whose role is to reduce risks whose consequences are manifested on an evolutionary time scale. For a contrasting case, read about Col*E1* in SIMONS and KLECKNER (1988).

Mechanisms protecting IS*10* from fortuitous activation by external promoters: An additional set of mechanisms prevents fortuitous activation of the transposase gene by transcripts initiated outside of the element. Because IS*10* inserts randomly in DNA, the element runs a risk of positioning itself immediately adjacent to a strong chromosomal promoter that could direct transcription across the end of the element and through the transposase gene. Such readthrough transcription would disrupt both regulation by *dam* methylation, which depends upon specific activation of pIN, and inhibition by antisense RNA-OUT, which will pair effectively only with target

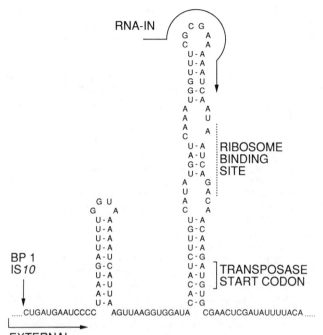

FIGURE 2.—IS*10* transposase expression from readthrough transcripts is blocked by sequestration of translation start signals in a region of secondary structure.

molecules having the precise 5′ end found in wild-type RNA-IN.

The most important IS*10* protection mechanism acts at the level of transposase translation: externally initiated transcripts yield less than 1% as much transposase protein per transcript as do transcripts initiated from pIN (DAVIS, SIMONS and KLECKNER 1985). A portion of this effect is probably due to premature termination of readthrough transcripts before they transverse the transposase gene. However, most inhibition occurs post-transcriptionally. The sequence between the end of IS*10* and the transposase ribosome binding site is such that readthrough transcripts form a strong stem-loop structure, essentially the complement to the RNA-OUT stem-loop, that sequesters the translation-initiation signals (Figure 2). The 5′ end of RNA-IN is at a position corresponding to the top of this loop, and RNA-1N therefore lacks the inhibitory structure.

A second protection mechanism is provided by the fact that transcription initiated outside of the element and across the outside terminus of IS*10* inhibits transposition, even when transposase is provided in *trans* (DAVIS, SIMONS and KLECKNER 1985). This direct inhibition in *cis* is severalfold when transcription is promoted by a fully induced *lac* promoter and is more than sufficient to counteract any small increase in the level of transposase from readthrough transcripts that escape other protection mechanisms.

A third level of protection is provided once again by *dam* methylation. Readthrough transcripts are expressed throughout the cell cycle. However, any residual transposase made from such transcripts will be effective only during that small fraction of the cell cycle when the inside end is activated. The importance of *dam* methylation in this regard is directly observable in IS*10* mutants where the contribution of readthrough transcription is elevated due to reduced translational protection (HUISMAN *et al.* 1989).

A fourth level of protection comes in the form of prevention: insertion of Tn*10* (and thus presumably of IS*10*) is inhibited by transcription of the target region. Transposition into the *E. coli* lactose operon assayed in *Salmonella typhimurium* is tenfold more frequent in the absence of inducer than in its presence; similar effects have been observed in the Salmonella histidine operon (CASADESUS and ROTH 1989). Thus, the probability of risk from external transcription is reduced by the transposon's choice of target sites. This situation should also reduce the probability that Tn*10* or IS*10* will insert into absolutely essential genes or genes that are required for growth at the time of transposition, because both kinds of genes are likely to be actively transcribed.

Tn*10*-specific regulation: Tn*10* poses the same threats to the cell as does IS*10*, although its much lower transposition frequency reduces their extent. The low frequency of transposition is a consequence of the length of the transposon; deletion analysis shows that the rate of Tn*10* transposition increases approximately 40% for every kilobase decrease in transposon length (MORISATO *et al.* 1983). The mechanism for transposition length dependence is not known, but is generally presumed to reflect some aspect of the way in which transposon ends find one another. For example, a complex of transposase protomers might initially bind at one end of the element and then initiate a one-dimensional search for the other end; in this case, length dependence might arise because the complex has a significant chance of getting stuck or otherwise decaying during the search (*e.g.*, WAY and KLECKNER 1985). It could be argued that this transposition length dependence is itself a device for reducing the deleterious effects of the transposon. Perhaps the level of transposition required for Tn*10* to be an evolutionarily successful creature is lower than that required by IS*10*: Tn*10* is presumably maintained because of its linkage to tetracycline resistance, whereas IS*10* maintenance may require the capacity to efficiently generate new types of composite transposable elements by transposition to new locations.

Tn*10* is subject to the same modulation mechanisms as IS*10* except that *dam* methylation operates in an attenuated form (ROBERTS *et al.* 1985). Although transposase expression is *dam*-regulated, the two termini of Tn*10* are both IS*10* outside ends and not *dam*-sensitive inside ends. Preferential transposition of

Tn*10* when the replication fork passes or upon single-stranded entry into a new host should be less dramatic than for IS*10*; furthermore, Tn*10* ends are not protected from outlaw transposase molecules generated by readthrough transcription or by other IS*10* elements.

Questions for the future: Additional features of IS*10* and Tn*10* remain to be discovered. The most important involve the roles of transposition host factors IHF and HU. The bacterial host may use these proteins to communicate with IS*10* regarding the desirability of transposition (HUISMAN *et al.* 1989 and unpublished results; J. KRULL-SUSSMAN and R. W. SIMONS, unpublished results). The outstanding question is: what is the cell trying to say?

A second question is: how does IS*10* manage to make enough transposase molecules to carry out a transposition? Analogies with other systems suggest that numerous molecules (as many as 12) might be needed (GRINDLEY *et al.* 1982; ABDEL-MEGUID *et al.* 1984). Perhaps many cells make some transposase but only a few make enough to produce a transposition. Alternatively, specific mechanisms might ensure that transposase is made in small bursts. In this case, most cells would make no transposase protein, but occasionally a cell would make all of the necessary molecules and would have a very high probability of undergoing transposition. Bursts would be economical and might also minimize potentially damaging abortive events.

Third, is there regulation at the level of transposase itself? IS*10* transposase appears to be rather stable, but is its effective level reduced, or its action modified, by virtue of some functional instability? Furthermore, how are the DNA cleavage activities of the transposon controlled? Interaction with the target site involves cleavage of relatively nonspecific sequences by a pair of staggered nicks located 9 bp apart; what features of the transposition reaction ensure that transposase does not act as a restriction enzyme?

LITERATURE CITED

ABDEL-MEGUID, S. S., N. D. F. GRINDLEY, N. S. TEMPLETON and T. A. STEITZ, 1984 Cleavage of the site-specific recombination protein γδ resolvase: the smaller of two fragments binds DNA specifically. Proc. Natl. Acad. Sci. USA **81:** 2001–2005.

See also page **704** in Addenda et Corrigenda.

CAMPBELL, A., 1981a Evolutionary significance of accessory DNA elements in bacteria. Annu. Rev. Microbiol. **35:** 55–83.

CAMPBELL, A., 1981b Some general questions about movable elements and their implications. Cold Spring Harbor Symp. Quant. Biol. **45:** 1–10.

CASADESUS, J., and J. R. ROTH, 1989 Transcriptional occlusion of transposon targets. Mol. Gen. Genet. **216:** 204–209.

CASE, C. C., S. M. ROELS, P. D. JENSEN, J. LEE, N. KLECKNER and R. W. SIMON, 1989 The unusual stability of the IS*10* antisense RNA is critical for its function and is determined by the structure of its stem-domain. EMBO J. **8:** 4297–4305.

DAVIS, M. A., R. W. SIMONS and N. KLECKNER, 1985 Tn*10* protects itself at two levels against fortuitous activation by external promoters. Cell **43:** 379–387.

FOSTER, T., M. A. DAVIS, K. TAKESHITA, D. E. ROBERTS and N. KLECKNER, 1981 Genetic organization of transposon Tn*10*. Cell **23:** 201–213.

GRINDLEY, N. D. F., M. R. LAUTH, R. G. WELLS, R. J. WITYK, J. J. SALVO and R. R. REED, 1982 Transposon-mediated site-specific recombination: identification of three binding sites for resolvase at the *res* sites of γδ and Tn3. Cell **30:** 19–27.

HUISMAN, O., P. R. ERRADA, L. SIGNON and N. KLECKNER, 1989 Mutational analysis of IS*10*'s outside end. EMBO J. **8:** 2101–2109.

KITTLE, J. D., and N. KLECKNER, 1988 Mechanism of IS*10* antisense RNA pairing in vitro and in vivo, pp. 1–7 in *Antisense RNA and DNA*, edited by D. A. MELTON. Cold Spring Harbor Laboratories, Cold Spring Harbor, N.Y.

KITTLE, J. D., R. W. SIMONS, J. LEE and N. KLECKNER, 1989 Insertion sequence IS*10* anti-sense pairing initiates by an interaction between the 5′ end of the target RNA and a loop in the anti-sense RNA. J. Mol. Biol. **210:** 561–572.

KLECKNER, N., 1988 Transposon Tn*10*, pp. 225–267 in *Mobile DNA*, edited by D. E. BERG and M. M. HOWE. American Society for Microbiology, Washington, D.C.

MORISATO, D., J. C. WAY, H.-J. KIM and N. KLECKNER, 1983 Tn*10* transposase acts preferentially on nearby transposon ends in vivo. Cell **32:** 799–807.

ORGEL, L. E., and F. H. C. CRICK, 1980 Selfish DNA: the ultimate parasite. Nature **284:** 604–606.

RALEIGH, E. A., and N. KLECKNER, 1986 Quantitation of insertion sequence IS*10* transposase gene expression by a method generally applicable to any rarely expressed gene. Proc. Natl. Acad. Sci. USA **83:** 1787–1791.

ROBERTS, D. E., B. C. HOOPES, W. R. McCLURE and N. KLECKNER, 1985 IS*10* transposition is regulated by DNA adenine methylation. Cell **43:** 117–130.

SAPIENZA, C., and W. F. DOOLITTLE, 1981 Genes are things you have whether you want them or not. Cold Spring Harbor Symp. Quant. Biol. **45:** 177–182.

SIMONS, R. W., and N. KLECKNER, 1983 Translational control of IS10 transposition. Cell **34:** 683–691.

SIMONS, R. W., and N. KLECKNER, 1988 Biological regulation by anti-sense RNA in prokaryotes. Annu. Rev. Genet. **22:** 567–600.

SIMONS, R. W., B. HOOPES, W. McCLURE and N. KLECKNER, 1983 Three promoters near the ends of IS10: p-IN, p-OUT and p-III. Cell **34:** 673–682.

SYVANEN, M., 1984 The evolutionary implication of mobile genetic elements. Annu. Rev. Genet. **18:** 271–293.

WAY, J., and N. KLECKNER, 1985 Transposition of plasmid-borne Tn*10* elements does not exhibit simple length-dependence. Genetics **111:** 705–713.

The Foundations of Genetic Fine Structure
A Retrospective from Memory

M. M. Green

Department of Genetics, University of California, Davis, California 95616

THE theory of the gene as formulated by T. H. MORGAN and his associates posited the chromosome to be a linear array of genes, each occupying a fixed position on the chromosome. The frequency of meiotic crossing over between linked genes measured the distance between them. Crossing over was deemed to be intergenic and, with normal disjunction, allelic genes invariably segregated into separate gametes.

The seminal experiments presaging the conclusion that meiotic crossing over is not exclusively intergenic and that allelic genes can segregate into the same gamete originated in 1939 in C. P. (PETE) OLIVER's Drosophila laboratory located in the basement of the Zoology Building at the University of Minnesota. The evidence for intragenic crossing over was simple. From females heteroallelic for mutations at either of two loci, lozenge (lz) eye on the X chromosome and Star (S) eye on chromosome II, phenotypically wild-type progeny were recovered. That the mutant alleles were not simply at different, closely linked loci was indicated by the fact that flies heteroallelic for two different recessive mutations had a mutant phenotype. The reversions to wild type were unique because they were invariably associated with polarized marker exchange. The association of reversion with exchange effectively excluded back mutation as the process involved. But unequal crossing over á la Bar eye could not be excluded because the reciprocal crossover products were not identified. Nevertheless, at the time, intragenic crossing over was a revolutionary concept. It was genetic dogma that the gene was inviolate with respect to crossing over; genetic mapping via meiotic crossing over defined the chromosomal limits of the gene and was intergenic.

The identification of the crossover reciprocal to the wild-type revertant, crucial to a demonstration of equal intragenic crossing over, was a tortuous process at each locus. The task of describing the Star story is best left to ED LEWIS, whose cytogenetic study of this region provided the basis of his doctoral dissertation at the California Institute of Technology (LEWIS 1945). In the narrative that follows I shall describe the lozenge case, for here I have first-hand knowledge. Before doing so, I should emphasize that the demonstrations of intragenic crossing over at the S and lz loci represent contrasting methods of how science happens. In the first case, LEWIS believed that S and its functional allele asteroid (ast, then s^r or Star recessive) occupied separate but contiguous chromosomal sites and therefore should be separable by crossing over. He set out to do this by looking for wild-type recombinants. The lz situation is a classical example of the BATESON-BRIDGES prescription to treasure one's exceptions; the discovery of wild-type recombinants associated with crossing over was serendipitous. The details follow.

In the summer of 1939 I was a graduate student in Zoology at the University of Minnesota, completing an MA thesis under PETE OLIVER's supervision. The Seventh International Congress of Genetics was to convene in Edinburgh at the end of the summer and PETE planned to attend. During his absence, he left me in charge of the lab with a number of tasks. Make the fly medium, clean the vials and bottles, transfer the stocks and, if there was time, find out why homozygous lz females were poorly fertile. (My stipend was $16 per month for the three summer months, which was not very much even for those days. But I was living at home and $16 would pay for trolley fare and lunches. Moreover, because I was making the Drosophila medium, I could eat any left-over bananas.) PETE OLIVER's interests were in X-ray mutagenesis following MULLER's great discovery; PETE was a MULLER student at the University of Texas. His doctoral dissertation had been on the radiation dose-response curve in Drosophila melanogaster and his interest in X-ray mutagenesis had continued. PETE's research philosophy was unambiguous and direct: select a multiple allelic series and go to work. He was particularly interested in two X-ray-induced lz alleles, lz^s (lozenge-spectacle) and lz^g (lozenge-glossy), both in the

X chromosome inversion $\Delta 49$. Each caused poor fertility in homozygous females, although hemizygous males were fully fertile.

So, I undertook the task of finding out why *lozenge* females were poorly fertile. A simple, direct approach was to dissect them to determine the effect of the mutations on internal genitalia. This turned out to be rewarding. Homozygous lz^s and lz^g and heteroallelic lz^s/lz^g were indistinguishable anatomically; all lacked spermathecae and parovariae. I concluded that this was responsible for the reduced fertility and looked no further. [This conclusion is probably wrong. Some 30 years later, in a stock of another allele, lz^{34k}, I found a recessive third-chromosome suppressor. The homozygous suppressor shifts all the phenotypic elements of the lz^{34k} phenotype–eyes, dorsal claws and female fertility–toward wild type. Yet the females lack spermathecae and parovariae (BENDER and GREEN 1960). HARVEY BENDER, then a postdoc, did a histological study of the ovaries of lz^{34k} females with and without the suppressor and concluded that reduced female fertility was associated with the onset of a syndrome causing the oocytes to degenerate. The suppressor delays the onset of the syndrome for several days (BENDER and GREEN 1962). I believe that the entire question of female fertility and lz mutations needs reexamination.]

Subsequent to PETE OLIVER's harrowing return from the Edinburgh Congress, which was marred by the onset of World War II and the torpedoing of ships carrying a number of Congress attendees, a series of experiments was designed to measure the fertility of lz females. The number of eggs, egg hatch, and number of adults were determined for lz^s and lz^g homozygotes and lz^s/lz^g heterozygotes. The order of fertility was $lz^s/lz^g > lz^g/lz^g > lz^s/lz^s$. Such results were not very exciting, but PETE OLIVER found an exception which was. He found occasional lz^+ phenotypes among the progeny of lz^s/lz^g females. Several facts could be established immediately. The lz^+ flies were not contaminants. because they had the appropriate marker genes and the $\Delta 49$ inversion. They were in all probability not back mutations, for no such types were found in the progeny of lz^s or lz^g homozygotes. Crossing over was involved in some way because each exception arose in association with the same unidirectional marker exchange (OLIVER 1940; OLIVER and GREEN 1944). In those days nobody thought of gene conversion as a possibility.

Two crucial points were established directly. The occurrence of the lz^+ flies was not a fluke; they could be recovered regularly from lz^g/lz^s females, always with the same unidirectional marker exchange. In all phenotypic details, including female fertility, the lz^+ flies were wild type. To be sure, crossing over was involved, but was it equal or unequal? The answer

might come from finding the reciprocal crossover product. What would its phenotype be? At the time this was PETE OLIVER's problem. I had a doctoral dissertation to complete, involving mutations at the *vestigial* (*vg*) wing locus and utilizing segmental aneuploidy.

The search for the reciprocal crossover product was fruitless. PETE tested a number of appropriate crossovers involving the outside markers without success. At one point there was great hope that the elusive type had been found, but it turned out to be a mutation of the *glass* (*gl*) locus on the third chromosome.

By the time my doctoral dissertation was completed in 1942, little additional progress had been made. The complementary crossover type was still an unknown. In the interim, PETE OLIVER was occupied with other matters and could spend little time on the lz problem. CHARLES DIGHT, an eccentric physician with an abiding interest in eugenics, had willed to the University of Minnesota funds to establish an Institute for the study of human genetics. PETE OLIVER became the first director of the Dight Institute and was preoccupied with its establishment and with research in human genetics. The organization of the Institute plus the entry of the United States into World War II put the lz problem on the back burner until the war was over. (OLIVER later returned to his roots and joined the faculty of the University of Texas. For many years he was Chairman of the Zoology Department; he is now retired and lives in Austin.)

After completing my dissertation I spent about four years in the U.S. Army. I recall that in the fall of 1945, while waiting in the Philippines for my medical unit to join the occupation army, I mulled over the future–specifically, what Drosophila research to pursue. Among potential research problems that I outlined, the *lozenge* problem was paramount. The issue of the reciprocal crossover product remained unresolved. Was reversion to lz^+ unique to lz^s/lz^g females, or could other heteroallelic combinations generate the same results? This question had been put to OLIVER on more than one occasion but he was reluctant to investigate any other lz alleles until the lz^s-lz^g problem had been solved. Furthermore, these alleles were within the $\Delta 49$ inversion and were therefore useless as testers of other lz alleles carried in chromosomes with the normal sequence.

In the fall of 1946, following discharge from the Army, I joined the Department of Zoology at the University of Missouri. I had spent the summer working in L. J. STADLER's cornfield. The ensuing four-year association with STADLER, one of the real giants of genetics (ROMAN 1988), was a rewarding, exhilarating experience. He provided the intellectual retreading that I needed after four years of military life.

The Zoology Department included a Drosophila

laboratory organized by A. B. GRIFFIN, a Drosophila cytogeneticist from the University of Texas who later moved to The Jackson Laboratory. I returned to Drosophila research and undertook two problems. One was a continuation of the *lz* work; the second was a biochemical study of eye color mutants in Drosophila. For the *lz* problem I turned to the unanswered question, does reversion to wild type occur with any other heteroallelic combinations? I had a number of *lz* mutations, both spontaneous and X-ray-induced, from a number of sources, all in chromosomes with the normal sequence. Phenotypically, these fell into two classes: those essentially like lz^s and those more or less like lz^g. I undertook a systematic study of combinations of lz^g-like with lz^s-like. (I was busy teaching general zoology 14 hours per week and trying to do some biochemistry. Therefore, most of the progeny scoring was done by my wife, an experienced fly-pusher who had completed a Master's degree under PETE OLIVER's guidance.)

This strategy produced mixed results: some heteroallelic females produced wild-type recombinants, others did not. Paralleling the lz^s/lz^g results, lz^{36}/lz^{46} females produced lz^+ progeny associated with polarized crossing over. This was expected because lz^{36} is a phenotypic mimic of lz^s, and lz^{46} of lz^g. In contrast, lz^{36}/lz^{BS} females–lz^{BS} is a lz^g mimic–produced no lz^+ flies among about 6000 progeny when at least five would have been expected. Now we had two questions to answer: why no lz^+, and why still no reciprocal crossover product? There was only one obvious experiment: what happens in lz^{BS}/lz^{46} females? We set up the crosses and, after the first progeny were scored, my wife left for Minneapolis to spend the winter vacation, December 1948, with her family. I remained behind and, being temporarily free of teaching, could score the remaining experiments. Two new results were obtained. First, lz^+ progeny appeared and marker exchange placed lz^{BS} at the same site as lz^{36} despite its phenotypic similarity to lz^g. Second, in two separate vials I saw, stuck in the medium, a male whose phenotype was neither lz^{BS} nor lz^{46} but was identical to lz^s and whose markers were those expected in the hoped-for reciprocal recombinant.

I fished each male out of the medium, hoping that at least one could be bred after drying out. To my disappointment, neither survived. Nonetheless, I was now confident that the long-sought reciprocal crossover had been found. If obtained once, it could be gotten again. Upon repeating the experiment, some 15,000 progeny yielded nine lz^+ and six lz^s-like flies. All had the appropriate marker combination and all six lz^s-like males produced progeny.

The proof that the lz^s-like flies did in fact carry the coupled $lz^{BS} lz^{46}$ mutations on the X chromosome was straightforward. Crossovers between this and a wild-type chromosome should separate the two. When the experiment was done, both lz^{BS} and lz^{46} progeny were recovered with the predicted marker exchange.

The recovery of the coupled $lz^{BS} lz^{46}$ crossover made it clear why all attempts to recover the complementary crossover product among the progeny of lz^g/lz^s females had failed: the recombinants were phenotypically indistinguishable from lz^s. It might be noted that ED LEWIS had a comparable problem identifying the crossover complementary to the wild-type product of *S/ast* females. It turned out that *S +/+ +* and *S ast/+ +* are also phenotypically indistinguishable.

By this time ED NOVITSKI, chromosome engineer par excellence, joined the Missouri Drosophila group as a postdoc. He volunteered to extract lz^g and lz^s from the *Δ49* inversion. (For reasons still not clear, neither mutant could be freed from the inversion by a double crossover.) He exploited the enhanced crossing over in triploid females and thereby succeeded in inserting the mutations into chromosomes of normal sequence (NOVITSKI 1950).

With lz^g in a chromosome of normal sequence, it was now mapped with respect to both lz^{BS} and lz^{46}. To make a long story short, lz^g mapped to a third site (GREEN and GREEN 1949). Eventually, 17 *lz* mutations were mapped and each could be be unambiguously assigned to one of the three identified *lz* sites (GREEN and GREEN 1956). Somewhat later, the mutation lz^k, first described as an *almondex* allele, turned out to be a *lz* allele and mapped to a fourth site (GREEN 1961). The *lz* gene is about 0.1 cM long and is separable into four equidistant, discontinuous sites. Proceeding from telomere to centromere, the four are identified by the mutations lz^{BS}–lz^k–lz^{46}–lz^g.

Ironically, the *lz* locus, the first to reveal the subdivisibility of the gene, has lagged in molecular analysis. The *lz* crossover problem went on the back burner during World War II; *lz* gene structure remains on the back burner. The nature of the phenotypic discontinuity revealed by the four mutation classes is ripe for analysis by modern methods.

The study of intragenic crossing over and genetic fine structure in *D. melanogaster* is a saga of brute-force genetic analysis at a time when selection techniques were not available. The Drosophila research provided the intellectual foundation for the elegant genetic fine structure analysis of the *rII* locus in bacteriophage T4 (BENZER 1955). All told, studies of genetic fine structure forced a rethinking of the concept of the indivisible gene and demonstrated that there is more than one type of gene organization. Gene analysis at the molecular level has reinforced this point of view.

LITERATURE CITED

BENDER, H. A., and M. M. GREEN, 1960 Phenogenetics of the lozenge loci in *Drosophila melanogaster*. I. Effects of a suppressor of lz^{34k}. Genetics **45**: 1563–1566.

BENDER, H. A., and M. M. GREEN, 1962 Phenogenetics of the lozenge loci in *Drosophila melanogaster*. III. Genetically induced pathologies of the ovary. J. Insect Pathol. **4**: 371–380.

BENZER, S., 1955 Fine structure of a genetic region in bacteriophage. Proc. Natl. Acad. Sci. USA **41**: 344–354.

GREEN, M. M., 1961 Phenogenetics of the lozenge loci in *Drosophila melanogaster*. II. Genetics of *lozenge Krivshenko* (lz^k). Genetics **46**: 1169–1176.

GREEN, M. M., and K. C. GREEN, 1949 Crossing over between alleles at the lozenge locus in *Drosophila melanogaster*. Proc. Natl. Acad. Sci. USA **35**: 586–591.

GREEN, M. M., and K. C. GREEN, 1956 A cytogenetic analysis of the lozenge pseudoalleles in Drosophila. Z. Indukt. Abstammungs. Vererbungsl. **87**: 708–721.

LEWIS, E. B., 1945 The relation of repeats to position effect in *Drosophila melanogaster*. Genetics **30**: 137–166.

NOVITSKI, E., 1950 The transfer of genes from small inversions. Genetics **35**: 249–252.

OLIVER, C. P., 1940 A reversion to wild type associated with crossing over in *Drosophila melanogaster*. Proc. Natl. Acad. Sci. USA **26**: 452–454.

OLIVER, C. P., and M. M. GREEN, 1944 Heterosis in compounds of lozenge-alleles of *Drosophila melanogaster*. Genetics **29**: 331–347.

ROMAN, H., 1988 A diamond in the desert. Genetics **119**: 739–741.

May 1990

Studies of Yeast Cytochrome c
How and Why They Started and Why They Continued

Fred Sherman

Department of Biochemistry, University of Rochester Medical School, Rochester, New York 14642

THE *CYC1* and *CYC7* genes in the yeast *Saccharomyces cerevisiae* and their respective gene products, iso-1-cytochrome *c* and iso-2-cytochrome *c*, are among the most thoroughly studied gene-protein systems of eukaryotes. All steps of *CYC1* gene expression have been systematically examined, including transcription, translation, post-translational modification, mitochondrial import and enzymatic functions (Figure 1). These iso-cytochromes *c* have been and are being used to address questions concerning the general principles involved not only in gene expression but also in areas such as mutagenesis, recombination, protein folding and protein stability. Early on, the yeast iso-cytochromes *c* systems played a major role in studies that defined chain terminating codons, nonsense suppressors and initiating codons. This *Perspectives* tells how and why these studies began and why they have continued. It is embarrassing to note that the origin of the first mutant, *cyc1-1*, has not been described previously!

I began investigating yeast cytochrome *c* 30 years ago as a postdoctoral fellow in the laboratory of the late BORIS EPHRUSSI at Gif-sur-Yvette. Previously, I had obtained some experience with ρ^- mitochondrial mutants as a graduate student at Berkeley with ROBERT K. MORTIMER and some experience with yeast genetics as a postdoctoral fellow at Seattle with the late HERSCHEL ROMAN. After arriving in EPHRUSSI's laboratory early in 1960, PIOTR P. SLONIMSKI and I began a study of *pet* mutants–those mutants with mutations in nuclear genes and unable to grow on media having a nonfermentable carbon compound as a sole energy source (SHERMAN and SLONIMSKI 1964). These *PET* nuclear genes encode essential components of mitochondria but are distinct from the ρ^+ determinant that was eventually shown to correspond to mitochondrial DNA. Before starting this study, I collected mutants that were already demonstrated or suspected to have nuclear defects. For this purpose, I contacted D. PITTMAN, M. OGUR, D. C. HAWTHORNE and R. K. MORTIMER, who constituted the majority of yeast geneticists at that time. One of the strains, 662.8, obtained from M. OGUR, was a challenging genetic mess. The strain contained a mixture of haploid and diploid cells and, as desired, did not grow on nonfermentable substrates. Genetic analysis revealed that the strain contained two mutations: *pet4-1*, which prevented growth on the nonfermentable substrates, and *cyc1-1*, which did not block growth on nonfermentable substrates but which did cause a 95% diminution of cytochrome *c*. Thus, the *cyc1-1* mutation was uncovered only because it was fortuitously in the same strain with *pet4* and because the cytochrome spectra of the meiotic segregants were systematically examined. At that time, it was indeed puzzling why the *cyc1-1* mutation was carried in the strain. A further puzzle was that the *cyc1-1* mutation also conferred sensitivity to UV light and to hypertonic media (SHERMAN, TABER and CAMPBELL 1965), phenotypes eventually shown to be due to the deletion of an approximately 12-kb segment that encompassed the *RAD7* and *OSM1* loci as well as *CYC1* (SINGH and SHERMAN 1978; STILES, FRIEDMAN and SHERMAN 1981). Some five years later, a second deletion (*cyc1-237*) with the same seemingly pleiotropic phenotypes was unexpectedly uncovered among segregants. The origin of this type of deletion was not understood until LIEBMAN, SINGH and SHERMAN (1979) noted that certain laboratory strains spontaneously gave rise to high frequencies of deletions encompassing the *CYC1*, *OSM1* and *RAD7* genes and that these deletions are flanked by Ty1 elements (STILES, FRIEDMAN and SHERMAN 1981; LIEBMAN, SHALIT and PICOLOGLOUS 1981). Thus, *cyc1-1*, the first mutant deficient in cytochrome *c*, was uncovered because of the rare occurrence of a spontaneous deletion in a strain containing an unrelated *pet* mutation.

Finding a cytochrome *c* yeast mutant was of considerable importance in 1960. At that time, when DNA sequencing was in the realm of science fiction, information on gene structure was inferred from mutationally altered proteins. Early in 1960 only three proteins

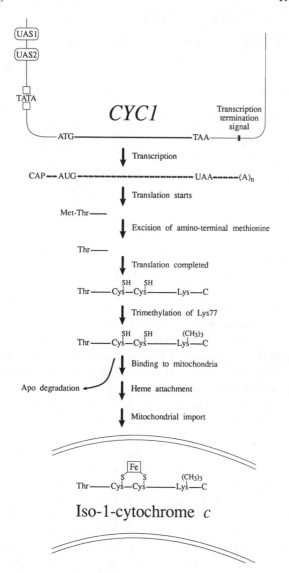

ATG ———————————————— TAA

Iso-1-cytochrome c

FIGURE 1.—All steps leading from the *CYG1* gene to the formation of iso-1-cytochrome c have been investigated, including: transcription initiation (GUARENTE 1987) and termination (RUSSO and SHERMAN 1989); translation initiation (SHERMAN and STEWART 1982) and termination (SHERMAN, ONO and STEWART 1979); excision of amino-terminal methionine (SHERMAN, STEWART and TSUN-ASAWA 1985); trimethylation of lysine 77 (FROST and PAIK 1990); degradation of apo-iso-1-cytochrome c (DUMONT et al. 1990); and heme attachment and mitochondrial import (DUMONT, ERNST and SHERMAN 1988).

were amenable to mutational analysis: tryptophan synthetase from *Escherichia coli* (YANOFSKY, HELSINKI and MALING 1962), lysozyme from bacteriophage T4 (STREISINGER et al. 1966) and coat protein from tobacco mosaic virus (TSUGITA and FRAENKEL-CONRAT 1963). Cytochrome c was one of the few proteins that could be easily purified. Its low molecular weight allowed ready diagnosis of altered sequences by peptide mapping and amino acid compositional analysis. Furthermore, the segment of 12 amino acids encompassing the heme group was already sequenced

(TUPPY 1958) and entire cytochromes c were being sequenced in several laboratories. Thus, investigating cytochrome c appeared to be an ideal project, especially because yeast had the advantage of being a eukaryotic microorganism with a well defined genetic system.

The *cyc1-1* mutant contained a minor form of a chromatographically distinct cytochrome c. After arriving at the University of Rochester late in 1960, I initiated experiments that led to the characterization of two forms of cytochrome c in yeast, iso-1-cytochrome c and iso-2-cytochrome c (SHERMAN, TABER and CAMPBELL 1965). A similar study was carried out at Gif-sur-Yvette (SLONIMSKI et al. 1965). (Only recently has the biological relevance of two iso-forms been suggested: see below.) In Rochester, a major effort was made to devise methods to detect mutants deficient in cytochrome c. The first study involved low temperature ($-196°$) spectroscopic examination of approximately 14,800 clones derived from mutagenized cultures; this first systematic screen uncovered *cyc1-2*, the second mutation at the *CYC1* locus, as well as mutations of the *CYC2* and *CYC3* loci (SHERMAN 1964). The identification of altered forms of iso-1-cytochrome from revertants of this *cyc1-2* mutant was critical for establishing in 1966 that the *CYC1* gene encodes the primary structure of iso-1-cytochrome c (SHERMAN et al. 1966). The *CYC3* gene was shown 23 years after that initial screen to encode heme lyase, the enzyme catalyzing the covalent attachment of the heme group to the iso-cytochromes c (DUMONT, ERNST and SHERMAN 1987). The *CYC2* gene has only recently been cloned, sequenced, and shown to encode a mitochondrial protein required for normal mitochondrial import of cytochrome c (J. B. SCHLICHTER, M. E. DUMONT and F. SHERMAN, unpublished results).

After it was established that *CYC1* encodes iso-1-cytochrome c, and after the amino acid sequence of iso-1-cytochrome c was reported by NARITA et al. (1963), numerous *cyc1* mutations were identified, their sites were determined by deletion mapping and, in collaboration with J. STEWART, their DNA sequences were deduced from the amino acid alterations in revertant proteins (SHERMAN and STEWART 1971, 1978). During the course of experiments that spanned more than two decades, STEWART analyzed over 3000 altered forms of iso-1-cytochromes c. These early studies covered diverse topics, including nonsense codons and their suppressors, the initiation of translation, mutagenesis, and recombination. Long before the existence of site-directed mutagenesis, specific sequences were generated by recombination between *cyc1* mutations *in vivo* (SHERMAN and STEWART 1975, 1982). Also, early in 1970, we attempted to isolate altered forms of revertant proteins that could be used to deduce the DNA sequence of the *CYC1* gene. The sequence of 44 bp at the 5' translated region of the gene was deduced from altered iso-1-cytochromes *c* encoded by revertants of frameshift and initiator mutations (SHERMAN and STEWART 1973; STEWART and SHERMAN 1974).

The development of recombinant DNA procedures in the mid-1970s obviously eliminated the critical need for altered protein sequences to deduce sequences. However, prior to the reports of DNA transformation by yeast in *E. coli* (STRUHL, CAMERON and DAVIS 1976) and of yeast itself (HINNEN, HICKS and FINK 1978), the only practical procedure for identifying a yeast DNA clone was by hybridization to nucleic acid probes. Other than the tRNA and rRNA genes, *CYC1* was the only yeast gene with at least a partially known DNA sequence. With a knowledge of the 44-bp 5'-untranslated sequence, SZOSTAK *et al.* (1977) and MONTGOMERY *et al.* (1978) synthesized oligonucleotides that were used to identify a clone containing the *CYC1* gene (MONTGOMERY *et al.* 1978; SMITH *et al.* 1979; STILES *et al.* 1981). The availability of the cloned *CYC1* gene and, soon after, the *CYC7* gene encoding iso-2-cytochrome *c* (MONTGOMERY *et al.* 1980) stimulated investigations of transcriptional regulation in numerous laboratories, including those of M. SMITH, L. GUARENTE, B. HALL and R. ZITOMER, as well as my own. A detailed analysis of the promoter region, primarily by GUARENTE and co-workers, has revealed TATA elements and the upstream activation sites UAS1 and UAS2 (GUARENTE 1987). These upstream regions were instrumental for identifying and isolating proteins required for *CYC1* transcription, including HAP1, which activates UAS1, and HAP2 and HAP3, which activate UAS2 (GUARENTE 1987). Furthermore, the transcription termination region, originally identified with the *cyc1-512* mutant obtained *in vivo* (ZARET and SHERMAN 1982), has been systematically investigated for mRNA cleavage (BUTLER and PLATT 1988) and termination properties (RUSSO and SHERMAN 1989).

Recently, provocative findings have surfaced concerning the post-translational modification, heme attachment, mitochondrial import, and structure, stability and folding of the iso-cytochromes *c*. The three-dimensional structures of iso-1-cytochrome *c* (LOUIE, HUTCHEON and BRAYER 1988) and iso-2-cytochrome *c* (G. D. BRAYER, unpublished results) have been determined, allowing better interpretations of the altered forms (HAMPSEY, DAS and SHERMAN 1988). The ability to transform yeast directly with synthetic oligonucleotides (MOERSCHELL, TSUNASAWA and SHERMAN 1988) has permitted the convenient generation of large numbers of altered iso-1-cytochromes *c*, each present as a single copy at the normal chromosomal site. These studies are revealing a role for protein stability in the post-translational regulation of the iso-

cytochromes *c*. Apparently, partially repressed yeast uses both differential transcription (LAZ, PIETRAS and SHERMAN 1984) and differential stability (DUMONT *et al.* 1990) of the apo-cytochromes *c* as regulatory mechanisms for maintaining elevated proportions of iso-2-cytochrome *c*. It is satisfying to feel that we have just begun to exploit this beautiful iso-cytochromes *c* system, even though it started 30 years ago.

LITERATURE CITED

BUTLER, J. S., and T. PLATT, 1988   RNA processing generates the mature 3' end of yeast *CYC1* messenger RNA *in vitro*. Science **242:** 1270–1274.

DUMONT, M. E., J. F. ERNST and F. SHERMAN, 1987   Identification and sequence of the gene encoding cytochrome *c* heme lyase in the yeast *Saccharomyces cerevisiae*. EMBO J. **6:** 235–241.

DUMONT, M. E., J. F. ERNST and F. SHERMAN, 1988   Coupling of heme attachment to import of cytochrome *c* into yeast mitochondria: studies with heme lyase deficient mitochondria and altered apocytochromes *c*. J. Biol. Chem. **263:** 15928–15937.

DUMONT, M. E., A. J. MATHEWS, B. T. NALL, S. B. BAIM, D. C. EUSTICE and F. SHERMAN, 1990   Differential stability of two apo-isocytochromes *c* in the yeast *Saccharomyces cerevisiae*. J. Biol. Chem. **265:** 2733–2739.

FROST, B., and W. K. PAIK, 1990   cytochrome *c* methylation, pp. 60–77 in *Protein Methylation*, edited by W. K. PAIK and S. KIM. CRC Press, Boca Raton, Fla.

GUARENTE, L., 1987   Regulatory proteins in yeast. Annu. Rev. Genet. **21:** 425–452.

HAMPSEY, D. M., G. DAS and F. SHERMAN, 1988   Yeast iso-1-cytochrome *c*: genetic analysis of structure-function relationships. FEBS Lett. **231:** 275–283.

HINNEN, A., J. B. HICKS and G. R. FINK, 1978   Transformation of yeast. Proc. Natl. Acad. Sci. USA **75:** 1929–1933.

LAZ, T. M., D. F. PIETRAS and F. SHERMAN, 1984   Differential regulation of the duplicated iso-cytochrome *c* genes in yeast. Proc. Natl. Acad. Sci. USA **81:** 4475–4479.

LIEBMAN, S. W., P. SHALIT and S. PICOLOGLOUS, 1981   Ty elements are involved in the formation of deletions in *DEL1* strains of *Saccharomyces cerevisiae*. Cell **26:** 401–409.

LIEBMAN, S. W., A. SINGH and F. SHERMAN, 1979   A mutator affecting the region of the iso-1-cytochrome *c* gene in yeast. Genetics **92:** 783–802.

LOUIE, G. V., W. L. B. HUTCHEON and G. D. BRAYER, 1988   Yeast iso-1-cytochrome *c*: a 2.8 Å resolution three-dimensional structure determination. J. Mol. Biol. **199:** 295–314.

MOERSCHELL, R. P., S. TSUNASAWA and F. SHERMAN, 1988   Transformation of yeast with synthetic oligonucleotides. Proc. Natl. Acad. Sci. USA **85:** 524–528.

MONTGOMERY, D. L., B. D. HALL, S. GILLAM and M. SMITH, 1978   Identification and isolation of the yeast cytochrome *c* gene. Cell **14:** 673–680.

MONTGOMERY, D. L., D. W. LEUNG, M. SMITH, P. SHALIT, G. FAYE and B. D. HALL, 1980   Isolation and sequence of the gene coding for iso-2-cytochrome *c*. Proc. Natl. Acad. Sci. USA **77:** 541–545.

NARITA, K., K. TITANI, Y. YAOI and H. MURAKAMI, 1963   The complete amino acid sequence in baker's yeast cytochrome *c*. Biochim. Biophys. Acta **77:** 688–690.

RUSSO, P., and F. SHERMAN, 1989   Transcription termtnates near the poly(A) site in the *CYC1* gene of the yeast *Saccharomyces cerevisiae*. Proc. Natl. Acad. Sci. USA **86:** 8348–8352.

SHERMAN, F., 1964 Mutants of yeast deficient in cytochrome *c*. Genetics **49:** 39–48.

SHERMAN, F., B. ONO and J. W. STEWART, 1979 Use of the iso-1-cytochrome *c* system for investigating nonsense mutants and suppressors in yeast, pp. 133–153 in *Nonsense Mutations and tRNA Suppressors*, edited by J. E. CELLIS and J. D. SMITH. Academic Press, London.

SHERMAN, F., and P. P. SLONIMSKI, 1964 Respiration-deficient mutants of yeast. II. Biochemistry. Biochim. Biophys. Acta **90:** 1–15.

SHERMAN, F., and J. W. STEWART, 1971 Genetics and biosynthesis of cytochrome *c*. Annu. Rev. Genet. **5:** 257–296.

SHERMAN, F., and J. W. STEWART, 1973 Mutations at the end of the iso-1-cytochrome *c* gene of yeast, pp. 56–86 in *The Biochemistry of Gene Expression in Higher Organisms*, edited by J. K. POLLAK and J. W. LEE. Australian and New Zealand Book Co., Sydney.

SHERMAN, F., and J. W. STEWART, 1975 The use of iso-1-cytochrome *c* mutants of yeast for elucidating the nucleotide sequences that govern initiation of translation, pp. 175–191 in *Organization and Expression of the Eukaryotic Genome. Biochemical Mechanisms of Differentiation in Prokaryotes and Eukaryotes*, Vol. 38, edited by G. BERNARDI and F. GROS. Proceedings of the 10th FEBS Meetings. North Holland/American Elsevier, New York.

SHERMAN, F., and J. W. STEWART, 1978 The genetic control of yeast iso-1 and iso-2 cytochrome *c* after 15 years, pp. 273–316 in *Biochemistry and Genetics of Yeast. Pure and Applied Aspects*, edited by M. BACILA, B. L. HORECKER and A. O. M. STOPPANI. Academic Press, New York.

SHERMAN, F., and J. W. STEWART, 1982 Mutations altering initiation of translation of yeast iso-1-cytochrome *c*: contrast between the eukaryotic and prokaryotic process, pp. 301–333 in *Molecular Biology of Yeast Saccharomyces: Metabolism and Gene Expression*, edited by J. N. STRATHERN, E. W. JONES and J. R. BROACH. Cold Spring Harbor Laboratory, Cold Spring Harbor, N.Y.

SHERMAN, F., J. W. STEWART and S. TSUNASAWA, 1985 Methionine or not methionine at the beginning of a protein. BioEssays **3:** 27–31.

SHERMAN, F., H. TABER and W. CAMPBELL, 1965 Genetic determination of iso-cytochromes *c* in yeast. J. Mol. Biol. **13:** 21–39.

SHERMAN, F., J. W. STEWART, E. MARGOLIASH, J. PARKER and W. CAMPBELL, 1966 The structural gene for yeast cytochrome *c*. Proc. Natl. Acad. Sci. USA **55:** 1498–1504.

SINGH, A., and F. SHERMAN, 1978 Deletions of the iso-1-cytochrome *c* and adjacent genes of yeast: discovery of the *OSM1* gene controlling osmotic sensitivity. Genetics **89:** 653–665.

SLONIMSKI, P. P., R. ACHER, G. PÉRÉ, A. SELS and M. SOMLO, 1965 Éléments du système respiratoire et leur régulation: cytochromes et iso-cytochromes, pp. 435–461 in *Colloques Internationaux du Centre National de la Recherche Scientifique, No. 124, Mécanismes de Régulation des Activities Cellulaires chez les Micro-organismes*, edited by M. JACQUES and C. SENEZ. CNRS, Paris.

SMITH, M., D. W. LEUNG, S. GILLAM, R. ASTELL, D. L. MONTGOMERY and B. D. HALL, 1979 Sequence of the gene for iso-1-cytochrome *c* in *Saccharomyces cerevisiae*. Cell **16:** 753–761.

STEWART, J. W., and F. SHERMAN, 1974 Yeast frameshift mutations identified by sequence changes in iso-1-cytochrome *c*, pp. 102–127 in *Molecular and Environmental Aspects of Mutagenesis*, edited by L. PRAKASH, F. SHERMAN, M. W. MILLER, C. W. LAWRENCE and H. W. TABER. Charles C Thomas, Springfield, Ill.

STILES, J. I., L. R. FRIEDMAN and F. SHERMAN, 1981 Studies on transposable elements in yeast. II. Deletions, duplications and transpositions of the COR segment that encompasses the structural gene of yeast iso-1-cytochrome *c*. Cold Spring Harbor Symp. Quant. Biol. **45:** 602–607.

STILES, J. I., J. W. SZOSTAK, A. T. YOUNG, R. WU, S. CONSAUL and F. SHERMAN, 1981 DNA sequence of a mutation in the leader region of the yeast iso-1-cytochrome *c* mRNA. Cell **25:** 277–284.

STREISINGER, G., Y. OKADA, J. EMRICH, J. NEWTON, A. TSUGITA, E. TERZAGHI and M. INOUYE, 1966 Frameshift mutations and the genetic code. Cold Spring Harbor Symp. Quant. Biol. **31:** 77–84.

STRUHL, K., J. R. CAMERON and R. W. DAVIS, 1976 Functional genetic expression of eukaryotic DNA in *Escherichia coli*. Proc. Natl. Acad. Sci. USA **73:** 1471–1475.

SZOSTAK, J. W., J. I. STILES, C. P. BAHL and R. WU, 1977 Specific binding of a synthetic oligonucleotide to yeast cytochrome *c* mRNA. Nature **265:** 61–63.

TSUGITA, A., and H. FRAENKEL-CONRAT, 1963 Contributions from TMV studies to the problem of genetic information transfer and coding, pp. 477–520 in *Molecular Genetics, Part I*, edited by J. H. TAYLOR. Academic Press, New York.

TUPPY, H., 1958 Über die Artspezifität der Proteinstrukur, pp. 66–67 in *Symposium on Protein Structure*, edited by A. NEUBERGER. Wiley, New York.

YANOFSKY, C., D. H. HELINSKI and B. D. MALING, 1962 The effects of mutation on the composition and properties of the A protein of *Escherichia coli* tryptophan synthetase. Cold Spring Harbor Symp. Quant. Biol. **26:** 11–23.

ZARET, K. S., and F. SHERMAN, 1982 DNA sequence required for efficient transcription termination in yeast. Cell **28:** 563–573.

See also page 706 in Addenda et Corrigenda.

L. C. Dunn and Mouse Genetic Mapping

Mary F. Lyon

M. R. C. Radiobiology Unit, Chilton, Didcot, Oxon OX11 ORD, United Kingdom

THE year 1990 marks the 70th anniversary of the beginning of systematic mapping of the mouse genome. The first detection of linkage between two genes in the mouse, and also the first in any vertebrate, had occurred five years earlier, when HALDANE and his colleagues (1915) described the linkage of the coat color genes for *albinism* and *pink-eyed dilution*. However, it was not till 1920 that L. C. DUNN (1920a) published a paper on a systematic search for linkage among various coat color genes.

This was just one of many major contributions made by DUNN which laid foundations for the present highly detailed knowledge of the mouse genetic map. This map in turn makes the mouse now one of the key experimental organisms in genetics, particularly in relation to present efforts to elucidate the structure and function of the human genome. In the same year, DUNN (1920b) published what must have been the first paper on comparative mapping, in which he compared the linkage of *albinism* and *pink-eye* in mice and rats and investigated in detail factors, such as age and sex, which affect recombination between these genes in the mouse. Later, DUNN was involved in the development of inbred strains of mice, which are now very important in the mapping of DNA and protein variants. He was also one of the founders of the mouse Nomenclature Committee and of *Mouse News Letter*, which have provided the underlying framework for the databases which are now essential to successful mapping. In yet another contribution, DUNN was one of the first to use wild mice in genetic research (WAELSCH 1989). The wealth of genetic variation in wild mice, including species and subspecies closely related to laboratory mice, has led to the present most widely used mapping method, the interspecific back-cross (AVNER *et al.* 1988). DUNN's particular interest in wild mice was the insight they provided into understanding the *t*-complex on mouse chromosome *17* (WAELSCH 1989). The pioneering work of DUNN and his colleagues on this fascinating genetic variant has led to much recent molecular mapping, to the proximal half of chromosome *17* being now the most intensively mapped region of the mouse genome, and to

the cloning of a gene of major importance in vertebrate development (HERRMANN *et al.* 1990).

Progress in mouse genetic mapping has always been exponential (EICHER 1981), with the number of mapped genes doubling approximately every seven years. Thus, from our present vantage, the pace of advance in the early years appears slow. The first 50 years were spent in defining linkage groups. New genes were tested against all known genes or linkage groups, as in DUNN's (1920a) paper on independent genes. GRÜNEBERG's (1943, 1952) reference work of this time included tables showing which of these "tests for independent segregation" had already been completed. Also during this time, the statistical and theoretical backgrounds for the estimation of linkage or independence were much improved. In his 1920 papers DUNN used no statistics, but later FISHER (1946) published the maximum likelihood method for estimating recombination fractions, now the standard method. The detection of linkage between genes was put on a more rational basis by CARTER and FALCONER (1951), who put forward the concept of the "swept radius" or length of the genetic maps scanned in any given test for linkage, and thereby enabled the development of more rationally designed stocks for detecting linkage.

During the first 40 years or so, the genes mapped were mainly those producing some visible phenotypic effect, such as changes in coat color or texture, or in the skeleton or behavior. The work used "linkage testing stocks" of the type developed by CARTER and FALCONER. In the 1920s and 1930s much work went into the development of inbred strains (FESTING 1979; MORSE 1978, 1981). DUNN was the founder of the 129 strain, now widely used, but the great value of inbred strains in mapping studies was to emerge much later. The first biochemical genetic variant in inbred strains was found in 1941 (F. H. J. FIGGE and L. C. STRONG, quoted by MORSE 1981) and in the 1960s and 1970s emphasis shifted to the mapping of enzyme and other protein variants. It was then that the immense value of the inbred strains as a source of genetic variation became clear. Strains were typed for a wealth of variants and RODERICK and his colleagues (RODER-ICK, STAATS and WOMACK 1981; RODERICK and GUIDI 1989) developed an extensive database of the alleles carried at particular loci in inbred strains. RODERICK and GUIDI (1989) provide a table of data on 338 loci in 246 strains, derived from a larger database at The Jackson Laboratory containing information on 426 loci in 569 strains. A breakthrough occurred when BAILEY (1971) developed the concept of recombinant inbred strains, subsequently developed further by TAYLOR (1978) for use in genetic mapping. In this method, two inbred strains with known genetic characteristics are crossed. The F_2 offspring are then paired at random and their offspring are mated brother × sister for 20 or more generations to form a new set of strains, the recombinant inbred or RI strains. In the formation of the new strains, genetically linked characters will tend to stay together and the number of cases of separation of two linked traits will depend on the recombination between them. Hence, if the set of recombinant inbred strains is typed, one can detect which traits are linked and the approximate recombination frequency between them. As a database of typed traits builds up, a given set of RI strains becomes steadily more powerful for linkage detection (TAYLOR 1989).

The study of biochemical variants led to increasing interest not only in inbred strains but also in wild mice. DUNN (DUNN and MORGAN 1952) had first used wild mice to search for new forms of the *t*-complex. He indeed found a range of different *t*-haplotypes and concluded that they are maintained as polymorphisms in the wild as a result of their abnormally high transmission from heterozygous males (DUNN and MORGAN 1952; DUNN 1957, 1964). Wild mice were then found to provide a rich source of biochemical genetic variation (CHAPMAN 1978) and numerous inbred strains were developed from various subspecies and species (BONHOMME and GUÉNET 1989). Another type of variation found among wild mice, and of key importance in genetic mapping, was karyotypic variation. For the first 50 years of mapping, mouse linkage groups could not be assigned to chromosomes. Many induced chromosome aberrations, mainly reciprocal translocations, had been studied (SEARLE 1989) and, following the pioneering work of SNELL (1946), had been shown to involve particular linkage groups. However, mouse chromosomes were not cytogenetically distinguishable until, in 1971, techniques for chromosome banding made possible the identification of individual chromosomes (MILLER and MILLER 1975). Knowledge of which linkage groups were associated with particular chromosome aberrations then enabled the assignment of linkage groups to chromosomes. The aberrations used included not only the induced reciprocal translocations, but also Robertsonian translocations found in wild mice, especially in

Mus poschiavinus in certain alpine valleys where some populations had up to nine pairs of Robertsonians (GROPP and WINKING 1981).

Thus, in 1972 the linkage map appeared for the first time with the linkage groups assigned to chromosomes (GREEN 1972). Mapping then entered a new phase involving the precise location of genes, both in terms of their recombination with other genes and in their physical location with respect to chromosome G-bands. A recent advance in methodology has again involved the use of wild mice. GUÉNET and his colleagues (AVNER *et al.* 1988) showed that, if subspecies or closely related species of mice are compared, restriction fragment length variants (RFLVs) can be found for nearly all probes with the use of only one or two retriction enzymes. Thus, if laboratory mice are crossed with a wild species, usually *Mus spretus*, and the F_1 female is backcrossed to the laboratory strain (in a so-called interspecific backcross), all genes or other DNA markers can be mapped by their RFLVs. If DNA from individual backcross animals is stored, successive markers can be mapped, so that a panel of DNA from backcross animals becomes a resource which yields more detailed information as time progresses. DNA from animals with recombination within a certain interval can be used for further and finer mapping within that interval, thus enabling "homing in" on a region of interest as, for instance, in attempts to clone a gene. DUNN's interest in the *t*-complex has led to recent work which provides an interesting example of the use that can be made of a collection of rare recombinants in the region of interest. The *t*-complex is now known to involve a variant region of chromosome *17* (SILVER 1985; FRISCHAUF 1989; LYON 1990), which was first recognized by an interaction with the mutant gene for *brachyury, T.* Heterozygotes of *T* with wild type are short-tailed, whereas *T/t* heterozygotes are tailless. In mice heterozygous for a *t*-complex and a wild-type chromosome *17*, recombination is suppressed over the region occupied by the *t*-complex as a result of four inversions carried in the *t*-complex (HAMMER, SCHIMENTI and SILVER 1989). However, rare recombinants are found. These recombinants have been kept and used to provide evidence for the genetic basis of the transmission ratio distortion and male sterility which are other features of the *t*-complex (LYON 1984, 1986). Further use of these rare recombinants has enabled the ordering on the chromosome of numerous DNA markers derived by microdissection of the proximal region of chromosome *17* (FOX *et al.* 1985; FRISCHAUF 1989). Together with cloned genes and DNA markers from other sources, there are now over 100 markers on chromosome *17*, mainly in the proximal region (VIN-CEK *et al.* 1989). About 20 megabase pairs in three segments have been mapped by pulsed-field gel electrophoresis (BARLOW and LEHRACH 1989). In turn this has facilitated the detection of candidate genes for the *distorter* and *responder* genes (RAPPOLD *et al.* 1987; SCHIMENTI *et al.* 1988) thought to be responsible for the transmission ratio distortion and male sterility, and also has led to the cloning of the *brachyury* gene (HERRMANN *et al.* 1990). The cloning of this gene is a major step forward because it plays a crutical role in the development of vertebrates. It is thought to be important in mesoderm formation and homozygotes fail to develop the notochord and the entire posterior part of the body.

With the detailed knowledge of comparative mapping now available, it should be possible to map the human homolog of *brachyury* very quickly. Although comparative mapping began at the same time as systematic mapping of the mouse itself with DUNN's paper on linkage in mice and rats, progress was relatively slow during the subsequent 50 years. Mapping was then largely restricted to markers with visible phenotypes and it was difficult to be sure of the homologies of particular syndromes. For instance, the mouse has many known genes for short tail or for polydactyly. Which of these might be the homolog of a gene with a similar effect in another species? With the use of protein variants, and even more when DNA markers became a standard tool for mapping, the determination of homologies could be made with much more confidence. Comparative mapping has since proceeded very rapidly, particularly in the comparison of mouse and human gene maps. The human homologies of nearly half the length of the mouse recombination map are now known (NADEAU 1989; SEARLE *et al.* 1989; LALLEY *et al.* 1989). Each mouse chromosome has homologies with from two to seven human chromosomes, and the known length of conserved segments ranges from <1 cM to >30 cM. Similarly, each human chromosome has homologies with up to six mouse chromosomes. So far, for instance, all known homologs of genes on human *17* are on mouse chromosome *11*, but mouse *11* has homologies with five other human chromosomes (BUCHBERG *et al.* 1989). Knowledge of homologies is not only valuable in making chromosome assignments in other species, it is also important in identifying mouse homologs of human syndromes. Many such homologs of human syndromes are now known, particularly for those diseases in which the underlying protein or DNA defect is known. Some syndromes are clearly similar in man and mouse. Examples include the testicular feminization syndrome, due to a mutation in the androgen receptor (LYON, CATTANACH and CHARLTON 1981), and the hemoglobin mutants, in which comparable molecular changes produce comparable physiological effects (PETERS *et al.* 1985). In other cases the phenotypes of homologous mouse and human genetic defects may be rather different. The mouse mutant *mdx*, with a lesion in the dystrophin

gene *Dmd* (RYDER-COOK *et al.* 1988), has a much milder syndrome than is seen in Duchenne muscular dystrophy resulting from dystrophin defects in man. Similarly, the mouse gene *small-eye* (*Sey*) is apparently homologous with the aniridia defect of the Wilmsaniridia syndrome in man, but has a rather different effect (GLASER and HOUSMAN 1989; HOGAN *et al.* 1986). In these cases, knowledge that the mouse gene was appropriately located was important in finding the homology, and further homologous syndromes will no doubt be identified in this way in the future.

With the wealth of information now available on the mouse map, the importance of coordinated and widely available databases becomes clear. Here DUNN was once again a pioneer. Fifty years ago, in 1939, with GRÜNBERG and SNELL, DUNN founded the first Nomenclature Committee for the mouse, and produced the first gene list (DUNN, GRÜNEBERG and SNELL 1940). Ten years later, in 1949, DUNN, together with SALOME GLUECKSOHN-SCHOENHEIMER (now WAELSCH), edited the first edition of *Mouse News Letter* (now *Mouse Genome*) (SEARLE 1974). Both the Nomenclature Committee and *Mouse News Letter* have continued ever since. The Nomenclature Committee not only promulgates rules for genetic nomenclature but also promotes the dissemination of gene lists and maps with *Mouse News Letter* as its main organ of publication, and has sponsored the production of works of reference giving not only mapping data but also data on the necessary resources such as inbred strains, RI strains and wild strains (GREEN 1981; LYON and SEARLE 1989). The database underlying the mouse map was for many years maintained by M. C. GREEN (1966) and more recently by DAVISSON and RODERICK and their colleagues (DAVISSON, RODERICK and DOOLITTLE 1989). With the exponential growth of information, in the near future the maps are likely to become too detailed to be published regularly on paper, and there will be a move toward electronic publication. Already The Jackson Laboratory makes available on-line the set of databases known as Gbase, including a list of loci, mapping data, and lists of inbred strains and their variants (DAVISSON *et al.* 1989).

Indeed, in the future the previously exponential rate of increase in mapped genes may be surpassed. With the use of interspecific backcrosses, suitable RFLVs for mapping will be available for almost all genes. In addition, there will be anonymous DNA markers generated by microdissection, chromosome sorting and other means. However, in view of the wealth of RFLVs for known genes, anonymous DNAs will be relatively less important than in human genetic mapping. Other variants for mapping will be generated by induced mutagenesis. This may either use conventional agents such as chemicals or radiation, with mutants being collected from known loci or

regions (RINCHIK *et al.* 1986, 1990; RINCHIK, CARPEN-
TER and SELBY 1990; RUSSELL, MONTGOMERY and
RAYNER 1982; RUSSELL *et al.* 1979; HITOTSUMACHI,
CARPENTER and RUSSELL 1985; SHEDLOVSKY *et al.*
1986; KING *et al.* 1989), or may involve insertional
mutagenesis, with the advantage that the mutations
will be tagged and thus cloning will be facilitated
(GRIDLEY, SORIANO and JAENISCH 1987). Directed
mutagenesis by homologous recombination will obviously be an important tool (CAPECCHI 1989). It is
probable that the wheel will come full circle and that
mutants with visible phenotypes will again become
important, either as homologs of human syndromes
or as genes with major roles in development.

For the first time, the true length in centimorgans
of the mouse genome should become known. For this,
convenient markers of centromeres and telomeres are
needed and will surely become available. A problem
is that this length may well be that, not of the laboratory mouse genome but of the F$_1$ between *Mus spretus*
and the laboratory mouse. Already, one small inversion has been found which differentiates these two
genomes (HAMMER, SCHIMENTI and SILVER 1989) and
there may well be others. Indeed, there may be differences among strains in small inversions or recombination hot spots, so that details of map lengths may
vary from strain to strain. Insight will also be gained
into chromosome structure and the genetic content
of light and dark G-bands (BICKMORE and SUMNER
1989). At present there is strong variation in the
density of markers on the map, from about 20 markers
per 10 cM in some regions to fewer than one per 20
cM in others. Does this reflect real differences in the
density of genes in different regions or variations in
chiasma frequency, or is it merely an artifact of incomplete knowledge?

Thus, it is clear that the mouse has a key role in
relation to the human genome mapping project. On
the one hand it is by far the best mapped experimental
vertebrate, and indeed ranks among the best mapped
higher organisms. On the other hand there is detailed
knowledge of the comparative mapping of the mouse
and human genomes. The mouse is also an excellent
organism, in both techniques and resources, for experimental manipulation and analysis of the genome.
This means that the mouse will be of fundamental
importance in elucidating the genetic basis of mammalian development and will be equally valuable in
understanding the genetic basis of human disease.

LITERATURE CITED

AVNER, P., L. AMAR, L. DANDOLO and J.-L. GUÉNET,
1988 Genetic analysis of the mouse using interspecific crosses.
Trends Genet. **4:** 18–23.

BAILEY, D. W., 1971 Recombinant inbred strains: an aid to finding
identity, linkage, and function of histocompatibility and other
genes. Transplantation **11:** 325–327.

BARLOW, D. P., and H. LEHRACH, 1989 Pulsed field gel mapping
of the mouse *t*-complex: implications for chromosome restriction mapping. Mouse News Lett. **85:** 81.

BICKMORE, W. A., and A. T. SUMNER, 1989 Mammalian chromosome banding–an expression of genome organization.
Trends Genet. **5:** 144–148.

BONHOMME, F., and J.-L. GUÉNET, 1989 The wild house mouse
and its relatives, pp. 649–662 in *Genetic Variants and Strains of
the Laboratory Mouse*, Second Edition, edited by M. F. LYON
and A. G. SEARLE. Oxford University Press.

BUCHBERG, A. M., E. BROWNELL, S. NAGATA, N. A. JENKINS and
N. G. COPELAND, 1989 A comprehensive genetic map of
murine chromosome *11* reveals extensive linkage conservation
between mouse and human. Genetics **122:** 153–161.

CAPECCHI, M. R., 1989 The new mouse genetics: altering the
genome by gene targeting. Trends Genet. **5:** 70–76.

CARTER, T. C., and D. S. FALCONER, 1951 Stocks for detecting
linkage in the mouse, and the theory of their design. J. Genet.
50: 307–323.

CHAPMAN, V. M., 1978 Biochemical polymorphisms in wild mice,
pp. 555–568 in *Origins of Inbred Mice*, edited by H. C. MORSE.
Academic Press, New York.

DAVISSON, M. T., T. H. RODERICK and D. P. DOOLITTLE,
1989 Recombination percentages and chromosomal assignments, pp. 432–505 in *Genetic Variants and Strains of the
Laboratory Mouse*, Second Edition, edited by M. F. LYON and
A. G. SEARLE. Oxford University Press.

DAVISSON, M. T., T. H. RODERICK, D. P. DOOLITTLE, A. L. HILL-
YARD and J. N. GUIDI, 1989 Gbase, a genomic database of
the mouse. Mouse News Lett. **85:** 83.

DUNN, L. C., 1920a Independent genes in mice. Genetics **5:** 344–
361.

DUNN, L. C., 1920b Linkage in mice and rats. Genetics **5:** 325–
343.

DUNN, L. C., 1957 Evidence of evolutionary forces leading to the
spread of lethal genes in wild populations of house mice. Proc.
Natl. Acad. Sci. USA **43:** 158–163.

DUNN, L. C., 1964 Abnormalities associated with a chromosome
region in the mouse. Science **144:** 260–263.

DUNN, L. C., and W. C. MORGAN, 1952 A mutable locus in wild
populations of house mice. Am. Nat. **86:** 321–323.

DUNN, L. C., H. GRÜNEBERG and G. D. SNELL, 1940 Report of
the Committee on Mouse Genetics Nomenclature. J. Hered.
31: 505–506.

EICHER, E. M., 1981 Foundations for the future: formal genetics
of the mouse. Prog. Clin. Biol. Res. **45:** 207–249.

FESTING, M. F. W., 1979 *Inbred Strains in Biomedical Research.*
Macmillan, London.

FISHER, R. A., 1946 A system of scoring linkage data with special
reference to the pied factors in mice. Am. Nat. **80:** 568–578.

FOX, H. S., G. R. MARTIN, M. F. LYON, B. HERRMANN, A.-M.
FRISCHAUF, H. LEHRACH and L. M. SILVER, 1985 Molecular
probes define different regions of the mouse *t* complex. Cell
40: 63–69.

FRISCHAUF, A.-M., 1989 Map of the t-complex, pp. 428–432 in
Genetic Variants and Strains of the Laboratory Mouse, Second
Edition, edited by M. E. LYON and A. G. SEARLE. Oxford
University Press.

GLASER, T., and D. E. HOUSMAN, 1989 The small eye mouse (Sey), an animal model of aniridia (AN2). Cytogenet. Cell Genet. **51:** 1005.

GREEN, M. C., 1966 Mutant genes and linkages, pp. 87–150 in *Biology of the Laboratory Mouse*, Second Edition, edited by E. L. GREEN. McGraw-Hill, New York.

GREEN, M. C., 1972 Linkage map of the mouse. Mouse News Lett. **47:** 16.

GREEN, M. C. (Editor), 1981 *Genetic Variants and Strains of the Laboratory Mouse.* Gustav Fischer, Stuttgart.

GRIDLEY, T., P. SORIANO and R. JAENISCH, 1987 Insertional mutagenesis in mice. Trends Genet. **3:** 162–166.

GROPP, A., and H. WINKING, 1981 Robertsonian translocations: cytology, meiosis, segregation patterns and biological consequences of heterozygosity, pp. 141–181 in *Biology of the House Mouse*, edited by R. J. BERRY. Academic Press, London,

GRÜNEBERG, H., 1943 *The Genetics of the Mouse.* Cambridge University Press.

GRÜNEBERG, H., 1952 *The Genetics of the Mouse*, Second Edition. Martinus Nijhoff, The Hague.

HALDANE, J. B. S., A. D. SPRUNT and N. M. HALDANE, 1915 Reduplication in mice. J. Genet. **5:** 133–135.

HAMMER, M. F., J. SCHIMENTI and L. M. SILVER, 1989 Evolution of mouse chromosome 17 and the origin of inversions associated with *t* haplotypes. Proc. Natl. Acad. Sci. USA **86:** 3261–3265.

HERRMANN, B. G., S. LABEIT, A. POUSTKA, T. R. KING and H. LEHRACH, 1990 Cloning of the *T* gene required in mesoderm formation in the mouse. Nature **343:** 617–622.

HITOTSUMACHI, S., D. A. CARPENTER and W. L. RUSSELL, 1985 Dose repetition increases the mutagenic effectiveness of *N*-ethyl-*N*-nitrosourea in mouse spermatogonia. Proc. Natl. Acad. Sci. USA **82:** 6619–6621.

HOGAN, B. L. M., G. HORSBURGH, J. COHEN, C. M. HETHERINGTON, G. FISHER and M. F. LYON, 1986 *Small eyes (Sey)*: a homozygous lethal mutation on chromosome 2 which affects the differentiation of both lens and nasal placodes in the mouse. J. Embryol. Exp. Morphol. **97:** 95–110.

KING, T. R., W. F. DOVE, B. HERRMANN, A. R. MOSER and A. SHEDLOVSKY, 1989 Mapping to molecular resolution in the *T* to *H-2* region of the mouse genome with a nested set of recombinants. Proc. Natl. Acad. Sci. USA **86:** 222–226.

LALLEY, P. A., M. T. DAVISSON, J. A. M. GRAVES, S. J. O'BRIEN, J. E. WOMACK, T. H. RODERICK, N. CREAU-GOLDBERG, A. L. HILLYARD, D. P. DOOLITTLE and J. A. ROGERS, 1989 Report of the committee on comparative mapping. Cytogenet. Cell Genet. **51:** 503–523.

LYON, M. F., 1984 Transmission ratio distortion in mouse *t*-haplotypes is due to multiple distorter genes acting on a responder locus. Cell **37:** 621–628.

LYON, M. F., 1986 Male sterility of the mouse *t*-complex is due to homozygosity of the distorter genes. Cell **44:** 347–363.

LYON, M. F., 1990 The genetic basis of transmission ratio distortion and male sterility due to the *t* complex. Am. Nat. (in press).

LYON, M. F., and A. G. SEARLE (Editors), 1989 *Genetic Variants and Strains of the Laboratory Mouse*, Second Edition. Oxford University Press.

LYON, M. F., B. M. CATTANACH and H. M. CHARLTON, 1981 Genes affecting sex differentiation in mammals, pp. 329–386 in *Mechanisms of Sex Differentiation in Animals and Man*, edited by C. R. AUSTIN and R. G. EDWARDS. Academic Press, London.

MILLER, O. J., and D. A. MILLER, 1975 Cytogenetics of the mouse. Annu. Rev. Genet. **9:** 285–303.

MORSE, H. C., III, 1978 Introduction, pp. 3–21 in *Origins of Inbred Mice*, edited by H. C. MORSE. Academic Press, New York.

MORSE, H. C., III, 1981 The laboratory mouse–a historical perspective, pp. 1–16 in *The Mouse in Biomedical Research*, Vol. I, edited by H. L. FOSTER, J. D. SMALL and J. G. FOX. Academic Press, New York.

NADEAU, J. H., 1989 Maps of linkage and synteny homologies between mouse and man. Trends Genet. **5:** 82–86.

PETERS, J., S. J. ANDREWS, J. F. LOUTIT and J. B. CLEGG, 1985 A mouse β-globin mutant that is an exact model of hemoglobin Rainier in man. Genetics **110:** 709–721.

RAPPOLD, G. A., L. STUBBS, S. LABIET, R. B. CRKVENJAKOV and H. LEHRACH, 1987 Identification of a testis-specific gene from the mouse t-complex next to a CpG-rich island. EMBO J. **6:** 1975–1980.

RINCHIK, E. M., D. A. CARPENTER and P. B. SELBY, 1990 A strategy for fine-structure functional analysis of a 6- to 11-centimorgan region of mouse chromosome 7 by high-efficiency mutagenesis. Proc. Natl. Acad. Sci. USA **87:** 896–900.

RINCHIK, E. M., L. B. RUSSELL, N. G. COPELAND and N. A. JENKINS, 1986 Molecular genetic analysis of the *dilute-short ear* (*d-se*) region of the mouse. Genetics **112:** 321–342.

RINCHIK, E. M., J. W. BANGHAM, P. R. HUNSICKER, N. L. A. CACHEIRO, B. S. KWON, I. J. JACKSON and L. B. RUSSELL, 1990 Genetic and molecular analysis of chlorambucil-induced germ-line mutations in the mouse. Proc. Natl. Acad. Sci. USA **87:** 1416–1420.

RODERICK, T. H., and J. N. GUIDI, 1989 Strain distribution of polymorphic variants, pp. 663–772 in *Genetic Variants and Strains of the Laboratory Mouse*, Second Edition, edited by M. F. LYON and A. G. SEARLE. Oxford University Press.

RODERICK, T. H., J. STAATS and J. WOMACK, 1981 Strain distribution of polymorphic variants, pp. 377–396 in *Genetic Variants and Strains of the Laboratory Mouse*, edited by M. C. GREEN. Gustav Fischer, Stuttgart.

RUSSELL, L. B., C. S. MONTGOMERY and G. D. RAYNER, 1982 Analysis of the albino-locus region of the mouse. IV. Characterization of 34 deficiencies. Genetics **100:** 427–453.

RUSSELL, W. L., E. M. KELLY, P. R. HUNSICKER, J. W. BANGHAM, S. C. MADDUX and E. L. PHIPPS, 1979 Specific-locus test shows ethylnitrosourea to be the most potent mutagen in the mouse. Proc. Natl. Acad. Sci. USA **76:** 5818–5819.

RYDER-COOK, A. S., P. SICINSKI, K. THOMAS, K. E. DAVIES, R. G. WORTON, E. A. BARNARD, M. G. DARLISON and P. J. BARNARD, 1988 Localization of the *mdx* mutation within the mouse dystrophin gene. EMBO J. **7:** 3017–3021.

SCHIMENTI, J., J. A. CEBRA-THOMAS, C. L. DECKER, S. D. ISLAM, S. H. PILDER and L. M. SILVER, 1988 A candidate gene family for the mouse *t complex responder* (*Tcr*) locus responsible for haploid effects on sperm function. Cell **55:** 71–78.

SEARLE, A. G., 1974 The origins of *Mouse News Letter*. Mouse News Lett. **50:** 5–6.

SEARLE, A. G., 1989 Numerical variants and structural rearrangements, pp. 582–616 in *Genetic Variants and Strains of the Laboratory Mouse*, Second Edition, edited by M. F. LYON and A. G. SEARLE. Oxford University Press.

SEARLE, A. G., J. PETERS, M. F. LYON, J. G. HALL, E. P. EVANS, J. H. EDWARDS and V. J. BUCKLE, 1989 Chromosome maps of man and mouse, IV. Ann. Hum. Genet. **53:** 89–140.

SHEDLOVSKY, A., J. L. GUÉNET, L. L. JOHNSON and W. F. DOVE, 1986 Induction of recessive lethal mutations in the *T/t–H-2* region of the mouse genome by a point mutagen. Genet. Res. **47:** 135–142.

SILVER, L. M., 1985 Mouse *t* haplotypes. Annu. Rev. Genet. **19:** 179–208.

SNELL, G. D., 1946 An analysis of translocations in the mouse. Genetics **31:** 157–180.

TAYLOR, B. A., 1978 Recombinant inbred strains: use in gene mapping, pp. 423–438 in *Origins of Inbred Mice*, edited by H. C. MORSE. Academic Press, New York.

TAYLOR, B. A., 1989 Recombinant inbred strains, pp. 773–796 in *Genetic Variants and Strains of the Laboratory Mouse*, Second Edition, edited by M. F. LYON and A. G. SEARLE. Oxford University Press.

VINCEK, V., H. KAWAGUCHI, K. MIZUNO, Z. ZALESKA-RUTCZYNSKA, M. KASAHARA, J. FOREJT, F. FIGUEROA and J. KLEIN, 1989 Linkage map of mouse chromosome 17: localization of 27 new DNA markers. Genomics 5: 773–786.

WAELSCH, S. G., 1989 In praise of complexity. Genetics 122: 721–725.

July 1990

The Role of Similarity and Difference in Fungal Mating

Robert L. Metzenberg

Department of Physiological Chemistry, University of Wisconsin–Madison, Madison, Wisconsin 53706

THE notion of alleles, introduced by JOHANNSEN in 1909, has been one of the most useful concepts in genetics. The *Glossary of Genetics and Cytogenetics* (RIEGER, MICHAELIS and GREEN 1976) defines it in part as "one of two or more alternate forms of a gene occupying the same locus on a particular chromosome or linkage structure and differing from other alleles of that locus at one or more mutational sites. . . Members of a set of alleles are mutually exclusive genetic markers and arise by gene mutation. Their activity is concerned with the same biochemical and developmental process." Implicit here is the idea that alleles of a gene are more similar than they are different–often being identical except at a single nucleotide base pair–and that the different alleles obviously arose by a few mutations from a single ancestral form. Indeed, until the coalescence of genetics and biochemistry allowed a gene to be thought of as a hereditary unit encoding a polypeptide, the very existence of a gene could only be inferred by the identification of two or more alleles that gave distinguishable phenotypes.

Some recent work on cloned DNA of the mating type regions of several filamentous fungi has challenged our understanding of what is meant by "alleles." The finding is simple. The determinants of mating type in any species have long been considered as textbook examples of two or more alternate alleles in organisms with a single mating type locus (bipolar), or in organisms with mating type determinants at two unlinked loci (tetrapolar). Surprisingly, these "alleles" have often turned out to be detectably similar neither in DNA sequence nor in the proteins for which they code, and possibly are not even of common origin. The word *idiomorph* has been suggested for these very different forms to avoid giving the impression that, like classical alleles, they differ only by a few mutations (METZENBERG and GLASS 1990; STABEN and YANOFSKY 1990; GLASS, GROTELUESCHEN and METZENBERG 1990). The phenomenon has turned up in filamentous Ascomycetes such as members of the genera *Neurospora* and *Gelasinospora* (GLASS *et al.* 1988; N. L.

GLASS, R. L. METZENBERG and N. B. RAJU, unpublished results), in *Cochliobolus heterostrophus* (B. G. TURGEON and O. C. YODER, personal communication), in the basidiomycete *Schizophyllum commune*, a wood-rotting fungus (GIASSON *et al.* 1989; R. C. ULLRICH, L. GIASSON, C. P. NOVOTNY, C. A. SPECHT and M. M. STANKIS, personal communication), in *Coprinus cinereus* (CASSELTON *et al.* 1989; L. A. CASSELTON, personal communication; G. MAY and P. J. PUKKILA, personal communication), in a limited degree in the smut fungus *Ustilago maydis* (SCHULZ *et al.* 1990; J. W. KRONSTAD, personal communication) and in the budding yeasts of the genus *Saccharomyces* (HERSKOWITZ 1988) and in the fission yeast *Schizosaccharomyces pombe* (KELLY *et al.* 1988). The expression of idiomorphs in these yeasts and the switching from one functional idiomorph to the other in a single haploid cell lineage have been intensively studied. In this *Perspectives* I will limit discussion to the filamentous fungi. The heterothallic species of these fungi, unlike heterothallic yeasts, do not carry any unexpressed copies of an idiomorph. Therefore, they cannot switch mating type by inserting previously silent information into a functional mating type locus.

At least superficially, the mating systems of the heterothallic ascomycetes *Neurospora crassa* and *Cochliobolus heterostrophus* are simpler than those of the tetrapolar higher fungi. These bipolar fungi, which are haploid except for a fleeting diploid phase between caryogamy and meiosis, carry only a single mating type idiomorph in each haploid genome. In *N. crassa* they are designated *A* (5.3 kbp) GLASS, GROTELUESCHEN and METZENBERG 1990) or *a* (3.2 kbp) (STABEN and YANOFSKY 1990); in *C. heterostrophus* they are *MAT1-1* or *MAT1-2* (each 1.3 kbp) B. G. TURGEON and O. C. YODER, personal communication). In the case of *N. crassa*, the two idiomorphs each appear to code for a single protein, although the protein-coding region is a minor fraction of the total region of dissimilarity. Analysis of mutations of the *A* idiomorph showed that integrity of the amino-terminal portion of the inferred protein is necessary for function, but that a portion of the carboxyl end can be removed without visible consequence. The coding regions of the two idiomorphs in *N. crassa* are transcribed from opposite strands and are located near the opposite ends of their idiomorphs. In both *N. crassa* and *C. heterostrophus*, the regions of dissimilarity are flanked by regions in which the DNA sequence between the two mating types is identical or nearly so, the transitions between dissimilarity and identity being very sharp. If we imaging homologs being paired at meiosis, the chromatids bearing the mating type loci would be paired along their entire length– of the order of 10^4 kbp–except for a bubble corresponding to the two idiomorphs. Even if such a bubble does form, its existence would leave many questions unanswered. Some of the most important actions of the mating type idiomorphs are programmed to occur when nuclei of the two mating types are in a common cytoplasm, but before caryogamy and therefore before any such bubble could exist. The same is true of the tetrapolar fungi, but in a way that is even more striking.

The tetrapolar mating type systems of the higher fungi are remarkably complex. However, they tend to follow a discernible pattern for which the well studied wood-rotting basidiomycete *Schizophyllum commune* can be taken as the prototype (see RAPER 1966). Each haploid isolate of this organism has information for mating type encoded into two regions, *A* and *B*, on separate chromosomes. For two fusant hyphae to be compatible–that is, to undergo cross-migration of nuclei into one another's cytoplasm and to undergo conjugate division of paired nuclei, to form clamp-connections typical of dicaryons between successive cell compartments and, finally, to form fruiting bodies and undergo caryogamy followed by meiosis–the genetic information of the two potential mates must be both nonidentical in their *A* regions and nonidentical in their *B* regions. Individual aspects of this developmental sequence are under control of one region or the other (see RAPER 1983). For example, nuclear migration is indifferent to the information in the *A* region but requires nonidentity in the *B* regions of the two fusants. Formation of clamp cells requires nonidentity of the two strains in the *A* region but does not require any special heteromorphism in the *B* region, although fusion to give true clamp connections requires nonidentity in the *B* region as well. Full compatibility and production of sexual progeny requires heteromorphism at both loci, for example, A_xB_x and A_yB_y.

At first glance, the requirement for difference might seem like a modest extension of the old homily that opposites attract. A riddle becomes apparent when we consider how many "opposites" there are and ponder what we mean by opposites. While the exact numbers in nature are not known, there may be as many as 288 kinds of cross-compatible, self-incompatible *A* regions; the corresponding number for *B* regions is 81. Thus, any strain would be able to mate productively with tens of thousands of different genotypic strains but not with itself. Classical experiments in which heterozygous diploids were mated with haploids showed that what is needed for compatibility is a difference at both *A* and *B* between two strains, not the absence of sameness. For example, A_xB_x will, of course, mate normally with A_yB_y, but it will also mate productively with the diploids A_xB_x/A_yB_y or A_xB_y/A_yB_x. More recent experiments in which heterozygosity of one fusant was produced by transformation with cloned DNA rather than by diploidization of a heterocaryon have given the same result. Therefore, differences between nuclei must act to turn on sexual differentiation rather than identities acting to turn it off. This principle should be contrasted with that operating in the systems of idiomorph-like gene sequences giving rise to self-sterility in higher plants (NASRALLAH *et al.* 1987; MCCLURE *et al.* 1989); in these systems, the absence of identity is necessary for fertility (LEWIS 1979).

The large number of non-identical *A* and *B* factors results in part from the fact that both the *A* region and the *B* region are themselves genetically complex, consisting of loosely linked regions called $A\alpha$ and $A\beta$, and $B\alpha$ and $B\beta$, respectively. For *Schizophyllum commune*, the number of different versions of these in nature has been estimated as 9, 32, 9 and 9, respectively (KOLTIN, STAMBERG and LEMKE 1972). All that is necessary for *A*-factor compatibility is for two potential mates to be different at $A\alpha$ or at $A\beta$ (being different at both of them not seeming to interfere with compatibility); hence, the potential $9 \times 32 = 288$ kinds of *A*-factor. Likewise, difference at either $B\alpha$ or $B\beta$ is sufficient for *B*-factor compatibility, and this leads to $9 \times 9 = 81$ kinds of *B*-factor.

Most of us automatically try to visualize biological specificity in terms of complementary surfaces, such as lock and key. Here, though, we are faced with the ridiculous picture of a lock that works with many different keys, but not with one made in the same factory as the lock! Nevertheless, it is profitable to push the faulty analogy one step further and ask whether *any* random key will work as long as it matches the lock badly. A classical genetic approach has been to prepare heterocaryons that are compatible for one factor but not for the other, *e.g.*, one consisting of A_xB_x plus A_xB_y. If change of any random sort were sufficient to create a new specificity, then classical mutagenesis of such a strain should readily give rise to fully compatible combinations of the type A_zB_x plus A_xB_y. From these, it should be possible to prepare *incompatible* heterocaryons of the general composition

A_zB_x plus A_zB_y. Despite a number of attempts, no new mating type specificities meeting the description of A_z have been described in either *S. commune* or *C. cinereus*. In the corn smut *Ustilago maydis*, conceptually analogous experiments have given a similar answer. *In vitro* mutagenesis adding a few codons or removing anywhere from one to about 60 codons has produced inactive genes, not new specifities (SCHULZ *et al.* 1990). While production of new specificities in nature obviously has occurred in each of these organisms, it is probably not a facile process.

Nevertheless, in both *Coprinus* and *Schizophyllum*, spontaneous or induced mutations in heterocaryons of the general form A_xB_x plus A_xB_y do produce new kinds of fertile derivatives, which take the form $A_{mut}B_x$ plus A_xB_y (DAY 1963; RAPER, BOYD and RAPER 1965). A mutant form of A is not, however, a close mimic of the various natural specificities. Instead, it is self-compatible, so that constructs like $A_{mut}B_x$ plus $A_{mut}B_y$ behave much like a compatible dicaryon. Analogous B_{mut} strains can be produced by mutagenesis (PARAG 1962; KOLTIN *et al.* 1979). Monocaryotic strains of the general form $A_{mut}B_{mut}$ have most, but not all, of the properties of dicaryons and are self-fertile. This self-fertility is dominant: it is not abolished by the simultaneous presence of a normal, self-sterile form of the gene. However, the self-fertile strain is not a perfect mimic of a normal dicaryon. In an ordinary dicaryon between two self-sterile forms, monocaryon functions—for example the production of oidia in *C. cinereus*—are turned off (reviewed in CASSELTON *et al.* 1989). In self-fertile mutants, the monocaryon functions continue in the dicaryophase, but can be turned off if a normal self-sterile version of the same gene is present. In other words, inappropriate continuation of monocaryon functions is recessive. These rather peculiar results can be summed up as follows: (1) *In vitro* mutagenesis shows that it is very easy to produce strains which are sterile in crosses to dissimilar strains. Thus, most mutations do not result in new mating type specificities. (2) Classical *in vivo* mutagenesis shows that it is quite feasible to produce strains which are self-fertile; however, monocaryon functions fail to be turned off normally in such mutants. (3) Classical mutagenesis shows that it is very difficult, if not imposible, with a single round of mutagenesis and selection, to produce new mating types which are fertile with others but self-sterile; see, however, RAPER, BOYD and RAPER (1965) for a single fairly close approach to a new mating type by two rounds of mutagenesis and selection. This empirical set of rules also describes quite satisfactorily some observations made on the phyletically very distant slime mold *Physarum polycephalum* (GORMAN, DOVE and SHAIBE 1979). These rules, therefore, are likely to reflect an underlying mechanism of considerable biological generality,

one for which we do not yet have any molecular explanation. I will touch upon our fragmentary but rapidly growing knowledge of the DNA sequence and proteins encoded in the mating type genes of the tetrapolar fungi *S. commune*, *C. cinereus* and *U. maydis*, and then I will present a highly tentative model to explain the interaction of dissimilar gene products in the tetrapolar systems.

Three forms of the $A\alpha$ region of *S. commune*, $A\alpha 1$, $A\alpha 3$ and $A\alpha 4$, have been cloned and about 3.4, 2.9 and 1.25 kbp of these have been sequenced. None of these DNAs cross-hybridizes to either of the other two, nor to strains carrying a variety of other compatibility factors. $A\alpha 1$ and $A\alpha 4$ have no detectable similarity in DNA sequence and are therefore clearly idiomorphs by the definition given above (GIASSON *et al.* 1989; R. C. ULLRICH, L. GIASSON, C. P. NOVOTNY, C. A. SPECHT and M. M. STANKIS, personal communication). However, $A\alpha 3$ and $A\alpha 4$ show substantial similarity at the 5' ends of their large open reading frames; 51 of the first 114 amino acids are the same. For convenience, I will also call these idiomorphs, though obviously the distinction between idiomorphs and homologous alleles becomes arbitrary when regions exist that show some relatedness. It is not known whether there is any similarity between the $A\alpha$ and the $A\beta$ regions at the level of sequence analysis, or between these and the $B\alpha$ and the $B\beta$ regions; clearly they are not sufficiently similar for the DNA sequences to cross-hybridize.

In the case of *C. cinereus*, the $A\alpha$ and $A\beta$ regions are much more closely linked than in *S. commune*, so that it has been possible to clone both of them from successive overlap of cosmids (CASSELTON *et al.* 1989; L. A. CASSELTON, personal communication; G. MAY and P. J. PUKKILA, personal communication). There appears to be no cross-hybridization between $A\alpha$ and $A\beta$ DNA sequences isolated from a single strain, nor between either of these and DNA from strains with at least some other specificities. Therefore it is likely that different $A\alpha$ forms should be thought of as idiomorphs rather than homologous alleles, and the same is probably true of different $A\beta$ forms. Whether subtle similarities will show up when sequence information is analyzed remains to be seen.

The situation in the tetrapolar basidiomycete *U. maydis* is somewhat different from that in the two species discussed above. Neither of the two regions concerned with mating type, here called a and b, is complex in the sense of having α and β subregions. Only two forms are known at the a locus (ROWELL and DeVAY 1954; BANUETT and HERSKOWITZ 1989), but some 18 forms have been identified at the b locus and about 25 are thought to exist (PUHALLA 1970). The region that includes the b locus has been cloned (KRONSTAD and LEONG, 1989; SCHULZ *et al.* 1990) and, unlike the previously discussed examples, functionally different forms of the region cross-hybridize freely. Some seven of these, b_1, b_2, b_3 (b_H?), b_4, b_5 (b_J), b_6 (b_K) and b_7 (b_L) have been cloned and sequenced (SCHULZ et al. 1990; J. W. KRONSTAD, personal communication). The essence of the findings is that all of these appear to code for a protein of 410 amino acids; of the first 110 amino acids proceeding from the amino terminus, 40 are identical in all seven forms of b that have been investigated; among the next 130 amino acids, there are substantial invariant sequences interrupted by islands of high variability; while the final 170 amino acids are almost completely invariant. Thus there are still striking differences in the structure of different forms but much more constancy than is seen in the foregoing examples. Nevertheless this variability must be enough to provoke the reaction of nonidentity necessary for specifying the mating type and developmental specificity. SCHULZ et al. (1990) have found that even small in-frame insertions anywhere in the amino-terminal portion eliminate biological activity but that, as with the A idiomorph of N. crassa, a considerable portion of the carboxyl terminus is not necessary for function. They have proposed in one type of model that heterodimers of composition $b_x b_y$ exert their effects by forming domains involving the amino terminus and that these domains bind target regions of DNA.

A provisional model of idiomorph interaction in mating-type heterocaryons or dicaryons should deal with the following facts. (1) In the dicaryon, a normal idiomorph, acting alone, can turn off purely monocaryotic functions like formation of oidia in C. cinereus. (2) Major differences between the structures of two idiomorph-encoded proteins are usually necessary to elicit a biological effect. Many kinds of major differences—but not random ones readily produced by a single mutation—will satisfy this need. (3) Nevertheless, mutation can convert a normal self-sterile, cross-fertile idiomorph to one that is self-fertile, and this self-fertility is dominant. At the same time, these mutations to self-fertility destroy the ability to turn off monocaryon functions during dicaryophase, but this failure is recessive to the functioning of a normal idiomorph if both are present.

Here is one attempt. (It will be obvious that the model should be taken illustratively, not literally, and not overly seriously.) Imagine that different self-sterile, cross-fertile idiomorphs encode rather thin, flat proteins with the general shape of equilateral parallelograms (rhombi), the length of the sides being always the same but the angles beween them being characteristic of each idiomorph (see Figure 1, A and B). These associate randomly to form tetramers. The requirement for turning off monocaryon functions during dicaryophase is that the tetramer lie in a single

plane. It is easy to see that any tetramer made from a single kind of parallelogram will meet this requirement. I have shown the monomers as always presenting the same face to the viewer, but they could as well alternate, so that two present the front face and two the rear.

The requirement for turning on dicaryon functions is simply that the tetramer not lie in a single plane, but take on a three-dimensional shape. Figure 1C shows that any tetramer made of two kinds of equilateral parallelogram seamed along the edges will buckle out of the plane of the paper, giving a saddle-shaped structure. This is true whether the tetramer contains two monomers of each idiomorph or three of one and one of the other. One can imagine that certain pairs of idiomorphs, in which the monomers were of extremely dissimilar shape, would give an overly deep saddle with two of each monomer but a more conventional saddle shape at ratios of either 3:1 or 1:3 (not shown). Dicaryons formed by the growing together of two such idiomorphic strains on petri plates might show two regions of typical dicaryotic morphology with a region of monocaryotic morphology between them.

Finally, mutation of an idiomorph, such that it codes for a protein taking the shape of a general quadrilateral polygon with three sides equal as in the ancestral parallelogram but the fourth side longer or shorter than the rest, results in a monomer that obligately forms a nonplanar puckered or saddle-shaped tetramer (Figure 1D). An idiomorph coding for such a quadrilateral, designated above as A_{mut} or B_{mut}, would be expected to be dominant in its self-fertility. In addition, it would be unable to turn off monocaryon functions because it could never form a planar tetramer. This property would, however, be expected to be recessive to the presence of a normal idiomorph which could contribute parallelograms allowing the formation of some planar tetramers. The difficulty or near impossibility of creating new self-sterile, cross-fertile idiomorphs by mutation and the relative ease of creating new self-fertile idiomorphs can also be rationalized by this model: conversion of a parallelogram monomer to a nonparallelogram monomer requires only a change in the length of one side, with the four angles taking the geometrically necessary values; the conversion of one parallelogram to another requires changes in all four angles without changing the length of any side. Because the area within the perimeter is protein and not empty space, this will require multiple, precise adjustment of amino acids, which will happen only very rarely by mutation.

This model, like others that have come before it, depends on the formation of a heteromeric aggregate; see PRÉVOST (1962), RAPER (1966), KUHN and PARAG (1972) and SCHULZ et al. (1990) for examples.

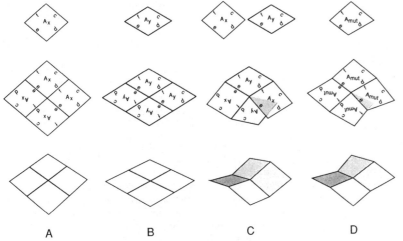

A B C D

FIGURE 1.—Model for interaction between like and unlike idiomorphs and between self-compatible mutant idiomorphs. **A.** Top: a monomer of the protein coded by the A_x idiomorph; c, d, e and f designate different edges. Middle: homotetramer of A_x. Bottom: the same, viewed in perspective. **B.** Protein coded by the A_y idiomorph. **C.** A mixture of monomers coded by A_x and A_y give rise to a saddle-shaped tetramer. **D.** A homotetramer coded by the A_{mut} idiomorph gives rise to a shape very much like that in C.

Whether or not this particular model has any merit, biologists interested in fungi will continue to find a challenge in understanding the origin of widely dissimilar idiomorphs. Did the idiomorphs arise within a single lineage over a very long time by conventional mutation? Or did they arise by some sort of hypermutability over a somewhat shorter period of time? Or might they have been acquired still more recently by horizontal transmission from other, perhaps unrelated organisms? We cannot now answer any of these questions. However, we can compare the putative protein sequences from mating type idiomorphs of some very distantly related fungi. In the case of *N. crassa*, the putative protein encoded by the *A* idiomorph has significant similarity with the *MATα1* idiomorph of *S. cerevisiae*, while the protein encoded by the *a* idiomorph of *N. crassa* has a comparable degree of similarity with the *mat-M_c* idiomorph of *S. pombe* (GLASS, GROTELUESCHEN and METZENBERG 1990; STABEN and YANOFSKY 1990). In contrast, the idiomorphs of *C. heterostrophus* have no detectable resemblance to any of these (B. G. TURGEON and O. C. YODER, personal communication). Even where a significant resemblance is detected, it could be due to homology (common origin) or to convergent evolution from independent origins. We may hope, as more of these idiomorphs are cloned, sequenced and analyzed for similarities, that the history of these interesting proteins will become more clear.

I am grateful to LORNA CASSELTON, LUC GIASSON, JAMES KRONSTAD, GEORGIANA MAY, CHARLES NOVOTNY, PATRICIA PUKKILA, CHARLES SPECHT, MARY STANKIS, B. GILLIAN TURGEON, ROBERT ULLRICH and OLEN YODER for letting me use their unpublished findings; and to LINDA CLIPSON for working her wizardry at graphics.

LITERATURE CITED

BANUETT, F., and I. HERSKOWITZ, 1989 Different *a* alleles of *Ustilago maydis* are necessary for maintenance of filamentous growth but not for meiosis. Proc. Natl. Acad. Sci. USA **86:** 5878–5882.

CASSELTON, L. A., E. S. MUTASA, A. TYMON, F. M. MELLON, P. F. R. LITTLE, S. TAYLOR, J. BERNHAGEN and R. STRATMANN, 1989 The molecular analysis of basidiomycete mating type genes, pp. 139–148 in *Proceedings of the EMBO-Alko Workshop on Molecular Biology of Filamentous Fungi*, Vol. 6, edited by H. NAVALAINEN and M. PENTTILÄ. Foundation for Biotechnical and Industrial Fermentation Research, Helsinki.

DAY, P. R., 1963 Mutations affecting the *A* mating-type locus in *Coprinus lagopus*. Genet. Res. **4:** 55–64.

GIASSON, L., C. A. SPECHT, C. MILGRIM, C. P. NOVOTNY and R. C. ULLRICH, 1989 Cloning and comparison of the *Aα* mating-type alleles of the basidiomycete *Schizophyllum commune*. Mol. Gen. Genet. **218:** 72–77.

GLASS, N. L., J. GROTELUESCHEN and R. L. METZENBERG, 1990 The *Neurospora crassa A* mating type region. Proc. Natl. Acad. Sci. USA **87:** (in press).

GLASS, N. L., S. J. VOLLMER, C. STABEN, J. GROTELUESCHEN and R. L. METZENBERG, 1988 DNAs of the two mating-type alleles of *Neurospora crassa* are highly dissimilar. Science **241:** 570–573.

GORMAN, J. A., W. F. DOVE and E. SHAIBE, 1979 Mutations affecting the initiation of plasmodial development in *Physarum polycephalum*. Dev. Genet. **1:** 47–60.

HERSKOWITZ, I., 1988 Life cycle of the budding yeast *Saccharomyces cerevisiae*. Microbiol. Rev. **52:** 536–553.

JOHANNSEN, W., 1909 *Elemente der Exacten Erblichkeitslehre*. Fischer, Jena.

KELLY, M., J. BURKE, M. SMITH, A. KLAR and D. BEACH, 1988 Four mating-type genes control sexual differentiation in the fission yeast. EMBO J. **7:** 1537–1547.

KOLTIN, Y., J. STAMBERG, N. BAWNIK, A. TAMARKIN and R. WERCZBERGER, 1979 Mutational analysis of natural alleles in and affecting the *B* incompatibility factor of Schizophyllum. Genetics **93:** 383–391.

KOLTIN, Y., J. STAMBERG and P. A. LEMKE, 1972 Genetic structure and evolution of the incompatibility factors in higher fungi. Bacteriol. Rev. **36:** 156–171.

KRONSTAD, J. W., and S. A. LEONG, 1989 Isolation of two alleles of the *b* locus of *Ustilago maydis*. Proc. Natl. Acad. Sci. USA **86:** 978–982.

KUHN, J., and Y. PARAG, 1972 Protein-subunit aggregation model for self-incompatibility in higher fungi. J. Theor. Biol. **35:** 77–91.

LEWIS, D., 1979 Genetic versatility of incompatibility in plants. N.Z. J. Bot. **17:** 639–644.

MCCLURE, B. A., V. HARING, P. R. EBERT, M. A. ANDERSON, R. J. SIMPSON, F. SAKIYAMA and A. E. CLARKE, 1989 Style self-incompatibility gene products of *Nicotiana alata* are ribonucleases. Nature **342:** 955–957.

METZENBERG, R. L., and N. L. GLASS, 1990 Mating type and mating strategies in *Neurospora*. BioEssays **12:** 53–59.

NASRALLAH, J. B., T.-H. KAO, C.-H. CHEN, M. L. GOLDBERG and M. E. NASRALLAH, 1987 Amino-acid sequence of glycoproteins encoded by three alleles of the S locus of *Brassica oleracea*. Nature **326:** 617–619.

PARAG, Y., 1962 Mutations in the *B* incompatibility factor of *Schizophyllum commune*. Proc. Natl. Acad. Sci. USA **48:** 743–750.

PRÉVOST, G., 1962 Étude génétique d'un Basidiomycete: *Coprinus radiatus*. Ph.D. thesis, Université de Paris, Paris.

PUHALLA, J. E., 1970 Genetic studies of the *b* incompatibility locus of *Ustilago maydis*. Genet. Res. **16:** 229–232.

RAPER, C. A., 1983 Controls for development and differentiation of the dikaryon in Basidiomycetes, pp. 195–238 in *Secondary Metabolism and Differentiation in Fungi*, edited by J. W. BENNETT and A. CIEGLER. Marcel Dekker, New York.

RAPER, J. R., 1966 *Genetics of Sexuality in Higher Fungi*. Ronald Press, New York.

RAPER, J. R., D. H. BOYD and C. A. RAPER, 1965 Primary and secondary mutations at the incompatibility loci in *Schizophyllum commune*. Proc. Natl. Acad. Sci. USA **53:** 1324–1332.

RIEGER, R., A. MICHAELIS and M. M. GREEN, 1976 *Glossary of Genetics and Cytogenetics*, Fourth Edition. Springer-Verlag, Berlin.

ROWELL, J. B. and J. E. DEVAY, 1954 Genetics of *Ustilago zeae* in relation to basic problems of its pathogenicity. Phytopathology **45:** 356–362.

SCHULZ, B., F. BANUETT, M. DAHL, R. SCHLESINGER, W. SCHÄFER, T. MARTIN, I. HERSKOWITZ and R. KAHMANN, 1990 The *b* alleles of U. maydis, whose combinations program pathogenic development, code for polypeptides containing a homeodomain-related motif. Cell **60:** 295–306.

STABEN, C., and C. YANOFSKY, 1990 The *Neurospora crassa a* mating type region. Proc. Natl. Acad. Sci. USA **87:** (in press).

Mapping Functions

James F. Crow

Genetics Department, University of Wisconsin–Madison, Madison, Wisconsin 53706

IT is said that R. A. FISHER, on first meeting the MORGAN group of Drosophila geneticists, asked, "Why don't you people ever do a proper mapping experiment?" This, to the group that invented linkage maps, seems like asking Shakespeare or Shaw why he never learned to use the English language. I don't know whether the anecdote is true, but if it is, one can easily guess that FISHER had three things in mind.[1] First, the MORGAN group paid little attention to estimating statistical errors. Second, they never did the kind of balanced experiment that FISHER advocated, i.e., using two matings in which the heterozygous parents are in opposite linkage phases, so that viability differences cancel (although MULLER thought of it). Third, they ordinarily made no distinction between the percent of recombination and map distance.

The Drosophila group did experiments involving large numbers under fairly standardized environmental conditions, which reduced statistical errors. But the mutant phenotypes were almost always less viable than wild type. When viability differences were large, the experimenters made arbitrary corrections, or devised special tricks. For example, they could keep deleterious recessives heterozygous and identify genotypes by progeny tests, although this was extremely laborious. A serviceable alternative, if interactions were small, was BRIDGES' procedure of alternating mutant and wild-type alleles along the chromosome. Finally, the strategy was to build up the map by combining distances between adjacent genes, and as the map became more dense, undetected double crossovers were decreasingly important. So FISHER's refinements, although they might have improved efficiency, made little difference in the long run.

FRANK STAHL (1989) referred to these two approaches as the American and the British. The American style was to use brute force, collecting so many mutant genes that the intervals between adjacent pairs were small. The cunning British used a mapping function to correct for undetected multiple crossovers.

Thus, fewer markers were needed and the lesser effort "leaves time for tea."

Balanced experiments to correct for interactions among viability factors are particularly neat. Suppose two matings are made in equal numbers, (1) $AB/ab \times ab/ab$ and (2) $Ab/aB \times ab/ab$, and let R_1, N_1, R_2 and N_2 be the expected proportion of recombinants and nonrecombinants in the two experiments. Suppose further that the viability of $Ab + aB$ phenotypes is v relative that that of $AB + ab$. Then the expected ratio of recombinants, r, to nonrecombinants, $1 - r$, in the combined experiments is $\sqrt{R_1 v R_2 / N_1 N_2 v}$ and the viability factor, v, cancels out regardless of interactions. Equating the corresponding function of the observed proportions, $\sqrt{R_1 R_2 / N_1 N_2}$, to $r/(1 - r)$ gives a consistent estimate of r. A simple formula for the variance of r is available (FISHER 1949a, p. 221ff). The two matings also permit direct estimates of the viabilities. Extension to three factors is straightforward, but four balanced matings are required. Such an experiment was carried out in mice by MARGARET WALLACE (see FISHER 1949b). In a way the result was an anticlimax, because there were no detectable viability differences. Such experiments have not been the practice in Drosophila. One reason is that most Drosophila mapping experiments involve multiple markers, and the number of matings required for a balanced experiment doubles with each added marker.

The MORGAN school and its successors throughout the Drosophila world have not made use of mapping functions. The group was, of course, keenly aware that there were multiple exchanges and that the proportion of recombinants was not linear with map distance when the distances were large; and MULLER had defined coincidence and interference. In the early days, before the map became dense, corrections for undetected multiple crossovers would have been useful. HALDANE's (1919) pioneering paper was ignored, however.

Following HALDANE's procedure, let r be the pro-

---

[1] I would enjoy hearing from anyone who can offer any information as to the truth of this story.

portion of recombinants and m the map distance in morgans. His formula is then

$$\frac{dr}{dm} = 1 - 2cr \qquad (1)$$

in which c is the coincidence, (actual double crossovers)/(number expected with no interference). Incidentally, this paper also added to the vocabulary of genetics: here HALDANE proposed "that the unit of distance in a chromosome . . . be termed a 'morgan,' on the analogy of the ohm, volt, etc. Morgan's unit of distance is therefore a centimorgan."

HALDANE noted that when $c = 0$, as is true for closely linked genes, then

$$r = m \qquad (2)$$

and recombination percent and map distance are the same. He also noted that as the distance increases, c approaches 1. When $c = 1$, we get the well known HALDANE mapping function

$$r = \tfrac{1}{2}(1 - e^{-2m}). \qquad (3)$$

It is not fair to HALDANE to say that he thought of this as a realistic mapping function, for in this paper he showed that the already quite extensive Drosophila data fell between the curves given by (2) and (3). A possible reason for the nonuse of mapping functions may be that the function that HALDANE found to best fit the data was a very complicated one, with no theoretical underpinning.

Not for a quarter century (KOSAMBI 1944) did a formula appear that caught on. A natural extension of constant c in Equation 2 is to let it be a function of r. KOSAMBI took the simplest and very reasonable next step, making $c \propto r$. Letting $c = 2r$, which gives the correct values at $r = 0$ and 1, leads immediately to the widely used KOSAMBI mapping function

$$r = \tfrac{1}{2}\tanh 2m. \qquad (4)$$

This formula fits most data fairly well, or at least well enough for most purposes. I think one reason for its popularity is that tables of hyperbolic functions have long been readily available, and in precomputer days they saved a great deal of tedious calculation. Furthermore, the addition rule for adding recombination values follows from the ordinary rules of hyperbolic functions

$$r_{12} = \frac{r_1 + r_2}{1 + 4r_1r_2}. \qquad (5)$$

Devising different mapping functions has provided diversion, if not gainful employment, for a number of mathematically inclined geneticists. Most of the earlier work in this area has been reviewed by BAILEY (1961). Equation 1 has natural extensions in several direc-

tions, of which I shall mention three. FELSENSTEIN (1979) assumed that c increases linearly with r, but takes a value K when $r = 0$. This has the advantage of permitting "map expansion" ($K < 0$) and "negative interference" ($K > 1$). Like the KOSAMBI function it has a simple addition rule, analogous to (5). Its flexibility, which may be desirable for some situations, can be undesirable for routine mapping in higher eukaryotes if one wants $c = 0$ for short distances; in this case the FELSENSTEIN and KOSAMBI formulas are the same. For a lucid and entertaining discussion of mapping functions in prokaryotes and references to earlier work, see STAHL (1989).

A second, and natural, extension is to let c be proportional to a higher power of $2r$. CARTER and FALCONER (1951) assumed that $c = (2r)^3$ and preferred this for mouse data. A more elaborate formula by RAO et al. (1977) includes the KOSAMBI and CARTER-FALCONER formulas as special cases. It has one adjustable parameter and, when this is chosen optimally, the function gives a very good fit to data on human chiasma frequencies.

PASCOE and MORTON (1987) found that the formula of RAO et al. gave a better fit to the Drosophila data than any of the others that I have mentioned. They noted, however, that a simpler formula assuming $c = (2r)^2$ gave essentially the same results. The integrated form is given as Equation 3 in their paper. Given that the data lie between the equation with $c = 2r$ and $c = (2r)^3$, then, as PASCOE and MORTON implied, it requires no great intellectual leap to think of $(2r)^2$. In fact I had used this in an elementary textbook (see curve C on p. 68 of CROW 1983).

The analysis of PASCOE and MORTON (1987) is reassuring in that the best fitting formulas are the same for data based on human chiasma frequencies as for recombination data in Drosophila. Furthermore, the high interference over the range 0–15 cm in the mouse (KING et al. 1989) is consistent with $c = (2r)^2$, although the data are insufficient to distinguish between this and the CARTER-FALCONER function.

In contrast to these more or less empirical functions, there are those that depend on specific, more mechanistic assumptions. One such is the model of FISHER (1948) and OWEN (1950), in which exchanges start at some point, say the centromere, with an assumed probability distribution, and subsequent exchanges depend on this and on an interference function. One feature of this model is that it permits greater than 50% recombination for certain map distances. Some mouse data support this, but the question warrants further investigation.

All of these functions overpredict the number of triple and higher crossovers, suggesting higher-order interference not accounted for in theories developed from three-locus models. This is strikingly evident in

7-point and 9-point crosses in Drosophila (PASCOE and MORTON 1987). Furthermore, it is to be expected that there are telomere and centromere effects as well as local differences in coincidence, so that no global mapping function can be correct everywhere. An approach based on chiasma distributions has been advocated by GOLDGAR, FAIN and KIMBERLING (1989). Chiasmata serve two functions. One is extending the evolutionary advantages of recombination to genes on the same chromosome. The other is mechanical, regularizing meiosis by reducing nondisjunction. These functions may call for different numbers and distributions of chiasmata, and the existing values may be some sort of compromise between conflicting optima. In any event, the chiasma distribution is far from random, and taking this into account may well provide a better approach to mapping.

The increasing practicality of human multipoint mapping, foreshadowed by BOTSTEIN et al. (1980) and involving increasingly effective computer routines (LANDER and GREEN 1987; LATHROP and LALOUEL 1988), raises anew the question of mapping functions. To write likelihood equations, one must make some assumption about interference. It is not clear (to me, at least) how much practical difference the specific interference assumption makes (see for example LATHROP et al. 1985 and PASCOE and MORTON 1987). In any case it is comforting that the simple formula based on $c = (2r)^2$ works well in those circumstances in which the data are sufficient to test it, and it can be built into computer routines. To quote GOLDGAR, FAIN and KIMBERLING (1989), "Given the enormous resources now being devoted to mapping and sequencing the entire human genome, methods which produce even a modest increase in efficiency are of value."

During the long period when human linkage studies were making very little progress for want of sufficient markers, the mouse map was progressing steadily. The pioneering role of J. B. S. HALDANE and L. C. DUNN in getting this started, and the progress and improved methodology in the ensuing years, was reviewed in this column two months ago (LYON 1990). Detailed comparative mapping of murine and human genes, now at hand, offers exciting prospects.

Linkage maps are a step toward physical maps. But they are more. However detailed the physical map, down to knowing the nucleotide sequence, we require linkage information in many species for the study of transmission genetics and for analyzing phenotypes whose molecular basis is not known. Human genetics, specifically, calls for ever better means of predicting the gametic output of persons of specified genotype.

For this, chromosome maps and interference functions will continue to be needed.

LITERATURE CITED

BAILEY, N. T. J., 1961 Introduction to the Mathematical Theory of Genetic Linkage. Clarendon Press, Oxford.

BOTSTEIN, D., R. L. WHITE, M. H. SKOLNICK and R. W. DAVIS, 1980 Construction of a genetic linkage map in man using restriction fragment length polymorphisms. Am. J. Hum. Genet. 32: 314–331.

CARTER, T. C., and D. C. FALCONER, 1951 Stocks for detecting linkage in the mouse and the theory of their design. J. Genet. 50: 307–323.

CROW, J. F., 1983 Genetics Notes, Ed. 8. Burgess, Minneapolis.

FELSENSTEIN, J., 1979 A mathematically tractable family of genetic mapping functions with different amounts of interference. Genetics 91: 769–775.

FISHER, R. A., 1948 A quantitative theory of genetic recombination and chiasma formation. Biometrics 4: 1–9.

FISHER, R. A., 1949a The Design of Experiments, Ed. 5. Oliver & Boyd, London.

FISHER, R. A., 1949b Note on the test of significance for differential viability in frequency data from a complete three-point cross. Heredity 3: 215–219.

GOLDGAR, D. E., P. R. FAIN and W. J. KIMBERLING, 1989 Chiasma-based models of multilocus recombination: increased power for exclusion mapping and gene ordering. Genomics 5: 283–290.

HALDANE, J. B. S., 1919 The combination of linkage values, and the calculation of distance between the loci of linked factors. J. Genet. 8: 299–309.

KING, T. R., W. F. DOVE, B. HERRMANN, A. R. MOSER and A. SHEDLOVSKY, 1989 Mapping to molecular resolution in the T to H-2 region of the mouse genome with a nested set of meiotic recombinants. Proc. Natl. Acad. Sci. USA 86: 222–226.

KOSAMBI, D. D., 1944 The estimation of map distance from recombination values. Ann. Eugen. 12: 172–175.

LANDER, E. S., and P. GREEN, 1987 Construction of multilocus genetic linkage maps in humans. Proc. Natl. Acad. Sci. USA 84: 2263–2367.

LATHROP, G. M., and J.-M. LALOUEL, 1988 Efficient computations in multilocus linkage analysis. Am. J. Hum. Genet. 42: 498–505.

LATHROP, G. M., J.-M. LALOUEL, C. JULIER and J. OTT, 1985 Multilocus linkage analysis in humans: detection of linkage and estimation of recombination. Am. J. Hum. Genet. 37: 482–498.

LYON, M. F., 1990 L. C. Dunn and mouse genetic mapping. Genetics 125: 231–236.

OWEN, A. R. G., 1950 The theory of genetical recombination. Adv. Genet. 3: 117–157.

PASCOE, L., and N. E. MORTON, 1987 The use of map functions in multipoint mapping. Am. J. Hum. Genet. 40: 174–183.

RAO, D. C., N. E. MORTON, J. LINDSTEN, M. HULTÉN and S. YEE, 1977 A mapping function for man. Hum. Hered. 27: 99–104.

STAHL, F., 1989 The linkage map of T4. Genetics 123: 245–248.

"Joy of the Worm"

○ ○

—W. SHAKESPEARE, *Antony and Cleopatra*, Act V, Sc. II

H. Robert Horvitz* and John E. Sulston†

*Howard Hughes Medical Institute, Department of Biology, Massachusetts Institute of Technology, Cambridge, Massachusetts 02139; and †Medical Research Council Laboratory of Molecular Biology, Cambridge CB2 2QH, England

IT has been ten years since we published in GENETICS a paper describing the isolation and genetic characterization of cell lineage mutants of the nematode *Caenorhabditis elegans* (HORVITZ and SULSTON 1980). We have reviewed elsewhere what has been learned from the study of these and other mutants abnormal in the pattern of cell divisions and cell fates that characterizes *C. elegans* development (HORVITZ 1988, 1990). Here we wish to reflect upon the days of our initial experiments, and to recall our excitement, our visions and our qualms as we elucidated the nematode cell lineage and began exploring methods for its genetic analysis.

In the beginning there was SYDNEY BRENNER (see HODGKIN 1989). It was BRENNER who selected *Caenorhabditis* for the study of developmental genetics. In 1963, BRENNER wrote to MAX PERUTZ, the head of the Medical Research Council Laboratory of Molecular Biology in Cambridge, England, " . . . we propose to identify every cell in the worm and trace lineages. We shall also investigate the constancy of development and study its genetic control by looking for mutants" (cited by BRENNER 1988).

BRENNER was particularly interested in the development of the nervous system and in 1970 he hired one of us (SULSTON) to analyze the neurochemistry of *C. elegans*. SULSTON joined BRENNER's group after a postdoctoral stint with LESLIE ORGEL working on prebiotic chemistry and hoping to discover the basis of the origin of life. SULSTON used the technique of Feulgen-staining to examine nuclei within the nervous system of nematodes of different developmental stages. He noticed that the number of neurons along the ventral cord was 15 in young larvae and 57 in older animals. Now, anyone familiar with nematode biology knew nematodes were eutelic, *i.e.*, constant in cell number after hatching; as an invertebrate zoology text blithely stated (see p. 245 of BORRADAILE *et al.* 1961), ". . . in the embryo all cell division soon ceases except for that seen in the reproductive cells. Growth consists of vacuolation and extension of the cells already present." Fortunately, in one example of what has proved to be an important regular infusion of inexperts into the *C. elegans* field, SULSTON was unaware of this fact and was happy to pursue his presumably impossible observation.

SULSTON decided to try to discover how 15 cells become 57. He took advantage of the fact that ROGER FREEDMAN and SIMON PICKVANCE, two other members of BRENNER's laboratory, had found that a light microscope equipped with Nomarski differential interference contrast optics allowed individual nuclei to be observed in living *C. elegans* embryos. SULSTON placed young *C. elegans* larvae on a glass microscope slide supporting a thin pad of agar with a dab of bacteria (nematode food), which both allowed the larvae to grow and attracted them (thereby preventing them from crawling away). He dropped a coverslip over the nematodes and observed them through the microscope using Nomarski optics. Every nucleus could be seen within a living animal. So SULSTON watched an animal, waiting to see which of the 15 cells would divide to generate the 42 new ones. None of them did. Instead, ten new cells spontaneously appeared within the ventral cord. Now the inexpert was taken aback. It was one matter to discover that older nematodes have more neurons than do young nematodes, but quite another to discover that cells could be generated spontaneously, without mitosis, meiosis or any other known biological phenomenon.

So SULSTON watched some more. It proved easy to see development proceed by observing a cell and following what it did. It was much harder to study development backward in time, for example to identify the source of the spontaneously appearing ventral cord cells. One had to guess a possible origin for a cell and observe the candidate precursor cell to see if the guess was correct. The solution to the source of the ten new cells came when SULSTON realized that these cells were squeezing into the ventral cord from nearby positions out of the plane of focus; the rapid migration and distortion of the cells made it appear that at one moment there was no cell while only shortly later a cell came into view.

Watching the ten new cells proved quite interesting. In contrast to the ventral cord cells present in the newly hatched larva, these cells divided! Observing that first cell division within a living animal was truly exhilarating, not only in itself but also because it meant that in principle one could determine the whole lineage. Strikingly, each of the ten cells, as well as two other cells slightly removed from the central region of the ventral cord, divided according to the same pattern and produced six descendants, five of which were neural and one of which was non-neural. Four of the 50 neural descendants migrated out of this central region and another four died (revealing the phenomenon of programmed cell death in *C. elegans* development). These events completely accounted for the origin of the 42 postembryonic neural cells. SULSTON determined the entire development of the ventral cord over a single weekend.

How did the stereotyped division pattern expressed by all of these precursor cells relate to the specific nerve cell types generated? To answer this question required knowing precisely what type of neuron each of the descendant cells became. This in turn required waiting until Monday when JOHN WHITE returned from sailing. WHITE had been analyzing the neuroanatomy of *C. elegans*, and from the equivalent of 20,000 serial sections of each of a number of individual animals he was eventually able to describe the complete connectivity of the animal's 302-celled nervous system (WHITE *et al.* 1986). However, at this earlier time WHITE had studied primarily the ventral cord, and only WHITE knew the results of these studies. He took SULSTON's lineage data and sat down to compare the relative positions of the newly generated and preexisting cells with the positions of the seven types of motor neurons present in the adult ventral cord. WHITE soon returned with the conclusion that cells homologous in lineage history differentiated into neurons of the same type. For example, the anterior daughter of the posterior daughter of the anterior daughter of each of the precursor cells (each P.apa cell, for short) became a specific neuron type known as a dorsal AS neuron. WHITE's studies of ventral

nerve cord anatomy were published together with SULSTON's studies of ventral nerve cord development (WHITE *et al.* 1976; SULSTON 1976). These observations established both the invariance and the striking relationship between lineage history and cell fate that characterize much of *C. elegans* development.

For years afterward, we were reminded of the excitement over these cell assignments by a red stain on the ceiling of the division's seminar room. WHITE had won a bet with BRENNER over a detailed aspect of the assignments and the stake, a bottle of wine, was produced at group meeting. In the absence of a corkscrew, the bottle was opened by injecting pressurized Freon from an ozone-destroying microscope duster through the cork via a hypodermic needle. The consequences were geyser-like. Sadly, the gloss of refurbishment has now obscured this moment of history.

In 1974, just prior to the shower of wine, the second of us (HORVITZ) entered the scene. A new postdoctoral fellow fresh from the molecular biology laboratory of JAMES WATSON and WALLY GILBERT, HORVITZ had been studying phage T4-induced modifications of *Escherichia coli* RNA polymerase with the belief that this training would somehow lead him into the world of neurobiology. Initially, HORVITZ was rather skeptical about the worth of watching cells divide: he wanted to do hard science, with radioactivity, gels and molecules, and he had to be convinced that what his eyes could see directly provided scientific information as reliable as what his eyes could see when they viewed the output of a scintillation counter. The thrill of directly watching development and the elegance and intriguing nature of the cell lineage diagrams that resulted—coupled with the potential for experimental intervention—soon dissuaded him of his parochial view.

HORVITZ decided to begin his foray into nematodes and behavioral systems by focusing on muscle. It was clear from the anatomy that just as the older animal had more neurons than did the younger animal, it also had more muscle cells: some of the somatic muscle cells used for locomotion and all of the vulval muscle cells used for egg laying were added after hatching. The origin of the new somatic muscles proved easy to determine, as a large blast cell (now called M) present in the newly hatched animal divided during the first larval stage to generate 18 cells located within the four longitudinal bands of muscle. However, the origin of the vulval muscles, which appeared much later, proved elusive. Again, observing development backward in time was not possible.

The two of us had different theories. HORVITZ, based on the principle from classical embryology that muscle derives from the mesoderm, suggested that somehow the M cell descendants generate the vulval muscles, despite the fact that these cells were located quite far from the vulva and did not look like blast cells. SULSTON, by contrast, noted that the vulval muscles differentiated in the region of the gonad from cells very similar to gonadal cells in morphology, and suggested that the somatic gonad would prove to be the source of the vulval muscles. So one day a race began, with each of us starting on a different track. SULSTON followed the gonadal cell lineages while HORVITZ stared at the 18 M cell descendants. SULSTON's gonadal lineage proliferated, generating more and more potential vulval muscle precursor cells, while the M descendants did nothing. Two of HORVITZ's 18 cells withdrew their candidacies, differentiating into non-muscle cells known as coelomocytes. Then, two of the 16 remaining descendants of M, one on each side of the animal, started to move. They migrated from the posterior region of the animal to positions directly flanking the developing gonad, which was still being observed by SULSTON. These two cells grew and then divided, each generating eight descendants, which then differentiated into four vulval and four uterine muscles.

Classical embryology had won, and the race to the vulval muscles was soon followed by the elucidation of the complete postembryonic cell lineages of *C. elegans* (SULSTON and HORVITZ 1977; KIMBLE and HIRSH 1979). But although classical notions of development had in this case led to the correct prediction, their absolute generality failed later, as the study of the embryonic lineage (SULSTON *et al.* 1983) revealed that a number of cells transgress their presumptive embryonic developmental boundaries. For example, certain neurons derive from embryonic mesoderm and certain muscles derive from embryonic ectoderm. Generalities often have exceptions in biology.

By determining the *C. elegans* postembryonic cell lineages, we had described many of the problems of developmental biology at the level of single cells. The issue now became how to proceed from description to mechanism. We discussed two general approaches. First, there were the classical methods of experimental embryology, in which various bits and pieces of developing organisms were removed and/or transplanted. With this direction in mind, JOHN WHITE began pursuing a conceptually similar approach based upon modern technology, namely a laser microbeam. WHITE, who received his basic training in physics, is a tinkerer; he loves to design and implement new technologies and he is extraordinarily good at doing so. One of his most recent contributions is the confocal microscope (WHITE, AMOS and FORDHAM 1987). WHITE designed a system that allowed him to focus a laser beam inside an animal being viewed with Nomarski optics, and he found he could kill single cells in living animals in this way. (WHITE also found he could destroy expensive microscope objectives, as HORVITZ discovered after returning from lunch one day to continue some cell lineage studies; his micro-

scope no longer worked, and the reason proved to be that WHITE had borrowed, and melted, the objective.) The technique of laser microsurgery could be used to define the functions of individual cells, either in the mature organism or during development (WHITE and HORVITZ 1979; SULSTON and WHITE 1980). Such experiments have helped reveal that cell interactions play a major role during *C. elegans* development, and that the invariance of normal development to a significant degree reflects the invariance of cell interactions.

The second possible approach toward the analysis of cell lineage was genetics. BRENNER (1974) had already established *C. elegans* as a genetic system. The disadvantage, and the advantage, of using genetics for the study of cell lineage was that it was entirely exploratory. In our pessimistic moments we feared that it would be impossible to isolate cell lineage mutants: any mutation that perturbed one cell division might well perturb so many divisions as to lead to an uninterpretable lethality (at least at that point, prior to the elucidation of the embryonic cell lineage). Furthermore, we suspected that even if we found mutants abnormal in specific postembryonic cell divisions, very few would be interesting. After all, one could easily imagine that leaky mutations in any housekeeping gene would cause a defect in the set of cells most sensitive to decreases in the activity of that gene. How could such mutations be distinguished from those in important developmental control genes?

With these concerns in mind, the rationale we offered in our first discussion of *C. elegans* cell lineage mutants, at an MRC joint worm-fly group meeting in March of 1976, was that mutations offered a useful complement to the laser: each could destroy the functions of particular cells, and the pleiotropies that resulted using the two methodologies were likely to be very different. Nonetheless, what we really hoped was that mutations that perturbed cell lineage would lead us to interesting genes. Unlike the laser, which could reveal the developmental functions of cells but go no further, mutations in principle could lead to an understanding of the genes and molecules that specified development.

The problem was how to begin. Because we did not even know if cell lineage mutants could exist, we hardly could know what phenotypes to seek. As described in the GENETICS paper published ten years ago this month (HORVITZ and SULSTON 1980), we divided the problem into two parts: first deciding what methods to use to identify mutants defective in cell lineage (the direct observation of lineages in living animals would be prohibitively slow) and then deciding what mutant phenotypes to examine using these methods. Our methods were based on the idea that animals abnormal in the number of cells of a particular type might well be abnormal in cell lineage. So we looked at fixed and stained mutant strains by techniques that allowed the visualization of individual cells, such as Feulgen-staining (which could be used to observe nuclei in the ventral nerve cord and the vulva) and formaldehyde-induced fluorescence (which revealed dopaminergic neurons). Only after seeing anatomical abnormalities did we use Nomarski optics to determine if these abnormalities reflected cell lineage defects. These methods require the establishment of mutant strains, as opposed to allowing the direct screening of living individuals. We did not have the confidence to attempt the more powerful approach of examining the cellular anatomy of living individuals using Nomarski optics, and it was not until later that ED HEDGECOCK proved that this method could be highly efficient and successful (HEDGECOCK and THOMSON 1982).

Our choice of mutant phenotypes to be examined was dictated by our desire to have some logical rationale but not to limit ourselves given our ignorance. For this reason, we examined mutants with behavioral or morphological abnormalities that we suspected might be consequences of cell lineage defects, and we also examined at random worms derived from mutagenized parents or grandparents. For example, we thought that defects in the behavior of egg laying could reflect defects in postembryonic cell lineages. One of the major consequences of the postembryonic cell divisions is sexual maturation. Not surprisingly, the young larva and the adult face many of the same biological challenges and need many of the same cells. However, only the adult must reproduce. For the *C. elegans* hermaphrodite, this means that only the adult needs the cells necessary for egg laying and copulation, namely the cells of the vulva, the vulval and uterine muscles, and the neurons that innervate these muscles. We knew that egg laying is not essential for either viability or fertility, so that homozygous egg-laying defective strains could be established. (Animals that cannot lay eggs are nonetheless fertile because the *C. elegans* hermaphrodite is internally self-fertilizing, and fertilized eggs can develop and hatch *in utero*.) It was very easy to recognize mutants defective in egg laying, either as animals severely bloated with retained eggs or as "bags of worms" formed when internally hatched larvae consume the body of their mother-father but remain (transiently) trapped within its cuticle. We hoped that among mutants defective in the vulval cells, the sex muscles or the sex neurons would be some that were abnormal in the lineages that generate these cells.

We also examined mutants with other behavioral or morphological abnormalities that we thought might be caused by defects in cell lineage. For example, BRENNER (1974) had isolated many mutants with locomotory defects, and it seemed likely that some of these would have defects in the postembryonic lineages that generate the ventral cord motor neurons.

Similarly, BRENNER had also isolated, but not described in print, three mutants with abnormal ventral growths. He had suspected these growths to be supernumerary vulva-like structures, and we confirmed his suspicion by determining the cell lineages of these mutants and finding that extra cells underwent vulval cell division patterns.

Finally, because we really had no idea what mutant phenotypes to anticipate, we screened at random the F_1 and F_2 progeny of mutagenized hermaphrodites. We placed single animals on Petri plates and used the anatomical techniques described above to examine some of the progeny while saving the unfixed, unstained and living siblings to establish mutant strains. This clonal mutant hunt allowed us to isolate cell lineage mutants that were sterile as homozygotes and thus could not have been isolated in either of our other two screens.

These initial experiments led to the identification of 24 cell lineage mutants that defined 14 genes. Three simple attributes of these mutants were very exciting to us. First and foremost, cell lineage mutants existed. Second, many of these mutants could be established as homozygous viable strains. Third, some appeared to be null mutants in which the activities of particular genes were completely eliminated. These observations proved that we could indeed find mutants abnormal in specific cell lineages and established that different genes function in different cell lineages, suggesting that it could be possible to define the set of genes that specifically controls any particular cell division.

A fourth and completely unexpected feature that intrigued us was that most of our cell lineage mutants could be considered to be homeotic at the level of single cells. Specifically, the abnormal phenotypes of most of these mutants result from transformations in cell fates, with particular cells expressing not their own fates (as recognized by patterns of cell division and by the types of descendant cells generated) but rather fates normally expressed by other cells. Genes defined by such mutants seemed likely to function in specifying cell fates and seemed to be excellent candidates for playing important roles in controlling development.

Now, ten years after we described the first *C. elegans* cell lineage mutants, the numbers of *C. elegans* cell lineage mutants, genes and researchers continue to increase dramatically. Specific cell lineage genes have been shown to have specific and distinct functions in generating cellular diversity during development. Although confusing at first, genes with broadly pleiotropic effects have proved easier to understand than genes specific for single cell divisions. For example, we were able to conclude that *lin-17* acts to make certain sister cells different from each other because mutations in this gene cause a variety of blast cells to produce identical instead of different daughters (STERNBERG and HORVITZ 1988), and that *lin-14* and the other heterochronic genes control developmental timing because they perturb the relative time of expression of multiple cell lineages as well as of other developmental events (AMBROS and HORVITZ 1984). Similarly, other genes act to make certain daughter cells different from their mother cells (CHALFIE, HORVITZ and SULSTON 1981), while still others play fundamental roles in controlling cell-cell interactions (GREENWALD, STERNBERG and HORVITZ 1983; KENYON 1986; PRIESS, SCHNABEL and SCHNABEL 1987; AUSTIN and KIMBLE 1987).

The study of the genetic control of vulval development has identified a network of about 50 interacting genes that regulate the three rounds of cell division that constitute the vulval cell lineages. These genes control the generation of the six potential vulval precursor cells, the actions of two distinct pathways of intercellular signalling that determine which of three alternative fates will be expressed by each vulval precursor cell, and the expression of the fates of these cells once these fates have been determined (FERGUSON, STERNBERG and HORVITZ 1987; STERNBERG and HORVITZ 1989; R. HORVITZ, P. STERNBERG, I. GREENWALD and colleagues, work in progress).

The molecular characterization of *C. elegans* cell lineage genes is progressing at an ever increasing rate, in part as a consequence of the availability of a nearly complete physical map of the *C. elegans* genome (COULSON *et al.* 1988). The physical map allows a gene to be cloned simply by knowing its position on the genetic map and using previously cloned DNA from the region to rescue the mutant phenotype in germline transformation experiments (FIRE 1986; WAY and CHALFIE 1988). Some cell lineage genes encode familiar types of proteins, and the presumed functions of these genes in controlling such processes as cell-cell interactions and gene expression can readily account for their roles in specifying cell lineage. For example, the gene *unc-86*, identified in our first genetic study, causes certain daughter cells to express characteristics different from those of their mother cells (CHALFIE, HORVITZ and SULSTON 1981). *unc-86* also controls the differentiation of certain nondividing cells (DESAI *et al.* 1988). Together, these observations indicate that *unc-86* regulates the expression of novel cell-type-specific traits. The molecular analysis of *unc-86* revealed a mechanistic basis for its action: *unc-86* encodes a protein with a homeodomain and extended similarity to a variety of mammalian transcription factors (FINNEY, RUVKUN and HORVITZ 1988). Thus, *unc-86* presumably acts by controlling the transcription of cell-type-specific genes, which in turn causes the expression of cell-type-specific characteristics. The class of transcription factors defined by *unc-86*, known as the POU proteins (for *p*ituitary, *o*ctamer-binding

and *unc-86*) (HERR *et al.* 1988), seems likely to regulate development not only in *C. elegans* but in many other organisms as well.

Other genes involved in the generation of cellular diversity during development also have proved to have molecular structures that are interpretable in the context of their mutant phenotypes. For example, the gene *lin-12* was discovered on the basis of its effects on the vulval cell lineages and found to control the fates not only of the vulval cells but also of many other cell types with fates regulated by cell-cell interactions (GREENWALD, STERNBERG and HORVITZ 1983; FERGUSON and HORVITZ 1985). Thus, *lin-12* seemed likely to function in intercellular signalling. The DNA sequence of *lin-12* showed that this gene encodes a transmembrane protein in the same family as the LDL receptor and the *Drosophila Notch* protein (GREENWALD 1985; YOCHEM, WESTON and GREENWALD 1988), and genetic mosaic analysis indicated that the *lin-12* protein is probably the receptor in a system of inductive signalling (SEYDOUX and GREENWALD 1989).

Not surprisingly, some cell lineage genes encode proteins that are novel in sequence (*e.g.*, RUVKUN *et al.* 1989; KIM and HORVITZ 1990). These genes promise to reveal new types of proteins that play regulatory roles in development.

The initial goals of BRENNER—to identify every cell in the worm, to trace lineages and investigate the constancy of development, and to discover mutants—have certainly been fulfilled. Furthermore, we now know a lot about genes that can mutate to perturb the *C. elegans* cell lineage. Studies of *C. elegans* cell lineage genes have revealed that neither the most pessimistic nor the most simplistic view of the genetic control of cell lineage is valid: on the one hand, every gene that affects a particular cell division is not required for all other cell divisions; on the other hand, the hypothesis of one gene, one cell division clearly is untenable. Rather, each cell division appears to be controlled by a number of genes, and many of these genes control other cell divisions as well. How specific combinations of these genes interact to cause the expression of distinct cell fates remains to be elucidated. Today's dream is to identify every gene that controls the worm's cell lineage, and to determine at a molecular level how these genes specify the development of *C. elegans*.

We thank JOHN WHITE and the members of the HORVITZ laboratory for comments concerning the manuscript. We thank our many colleagues in the community of *C. elegans* researchers for collaboration and support over the years.

LITERATURE CITED

AMBROS, V., and H. R. HORVITZ, 1984 Heterochronic mutants of the nematode *Caenorhabditis elegans.* Science **226:** 409–416.
AUSTIN, J., and J. KIMBLE, 1987 *glp-1* is required in the germ line

for regulation of the decision between mitosis and meiosis in *Caenorhabditis elegans*. Cell **51**: 589–599.

BORRADAILE, L. A., F. A. POTTS, L. E. S. EASTHAM and J. T. SAUNDERS, 1961 The minor acoelomate phyla, pp. 228–265 in *The Invertebrata*, Fourth Edition, edited by G. A. KERKUT. Cambridge University Press, Cambridge, England.

BRENNER, S., 1974 The genetics of *Caenorhabditis elegans*. Genetics **77**: 71–94.

BRENNER, S., 1988 Foreword, pp. ix–xiii in *The Nematode Caenorhabditis elegans*, edited by W. WOOD and the Community of *C. elegans* Researchers. Cold Spring Harbor Laboratory, Cold Spring Harbor, N.Y.

CHALFIE, M., H. R. HORVITZ and J. E. SULSTON, 1981 Mutations that lead to reiterations in the cell lineages of *C. elegans*. Cell **24**: 59–69.

COULSON, A., R. WATERSTON, J. KIFF, J. SULSTON and Y. KOHARA, 1988 Genome linking with yeast artificial chromosomes. Nature **335**: 184–186.

DESAI, C., G. GARRIGA, S. MCINTIRE and H. R. HORVITZ, 1988 A genetic pathway for the development of the *Caenorhabditis elegans* HSN motor neurons. Nature **336**: 638–646.

FERGUSON, E., and H. R. HORVITZ, 1985 Identification and characterization of 22 genes that affect the vulval cell lineages of *Caenorhabditis elegans*. Genetics **110**: 17–72.

FERGUSON, E. L., P. W. STERNBERG and H. R. HORVITZ, 1987 A genetic pathway for the specification of the vulval cell lineages of *Caenorhabditis elegans*. Nature **326**: 259–267.

FINNEY, M., G. RUVKUN and H. R. HORVITZ, 1988 The C. elegans cell lineage and differentiation gene *unc-86* encodes a protein with a homeodomain and extended similarity to transcription factors. Cell **55**: 757–769.

FIRE, A., 1986 Integrative transformation of *Caenorhabditis elegans*. EMBO J. **5**: 2673–2680.

GREENWALD, I., 1985 *lin-12*, a nematode homeotic gene, is homologous to a set of mammalian proteins that includes epidermal growth factor. Cell **43**: 583–590.

GREENWALD, I. S., P. W. STERNBERG and H. R. HORVITZ, 1983 The *lin-12* locus specifies cell fates in *Caenorhabditis elegans*. Cell **34**: 435–444.

HEDGECOCK, E. M., and J. N. THOMSON, 1982 A gene required for nuclear and mitochondrial attachment in the nematode *Caenorhabditis elegans*. Cell **30**: 321–330.

HERR, W., R. STURM, R. CLERC, L. CORCORAN, D. BALTIMORE, P. SHARP, H. INGRAHAM, M. ROSENFELD, M. FINNEY, G. RUVKUN and H. R. HORVITZ, 1988 The POU domain: a large conserved region in the mammalian *pit-1, oct-1, oct-2,* and *Caenorhabditis elegans unc-86* gene products. Genes Dev. **2**: 1513–1516.

HODGKIN, J., 1989 Early worms. Genetics **121**: 1–3.

HORVITZ, H. R., 1988 Genetics of cell lineage, pp. 157–190 in *The Nematode Caenorhabditis elegans*, edited by W. WOOD and the Community of *C. elegans* Researchers. Cold Spring Harbor Laboratory, Cold Spring Harbor, N.Y.

HORVITZ, H. R., 1990 Genetic control of *Caenorhabditis elegans* cell lineage. Harvey Lect. **84**: 65–77.

HORVITZ, H. R., and J. E. SULSTON, 1980 Isolation and genetic characterization of cell-lineage mutants of the nematode *Caenorhabditis elegans*. Genetics **96**: 435–454.

KENYON, C., 1986 A gene involved in the development of the posterior body region of *Caenorhabditis elegans*. Cell **46**: 477–487.

KIM, S., and H. R. HORVITZ, 1990 The *Caenorhabditis elegans* gene *lin-10* is broadly expressed while required specifically for the determination of vulval cell fates. Genes Dev. **4**: 357–371.

KIMBLE, J., and D. HIRSH, 1979 The post-embryonic cell lineages of the hermaphrodite and male gonads in *Caenorhabditis elegans*. Dev. Biol. **70**: 396–417.

PRIESS, J., H. SCHNABEL and R. SCHNABEL, 1987 The *glp-1* locus and cellular interactions in early *Caenorhabditis elegans* embryos. Cell **51**: 601–611.

RUVKUN, G., V. AMBROS, A. COULSON, R. WATERSTON, J. SULSTON and H. R. HORVITZ, 1989 Molecular genetics of the *Caenorhabditis elegans* heterochronic gene *lin-14*. Genetics **121**: 501–516.

SEYDOUX, G., and I. GREENWALD, 1989 Cell autonomy of *lin-12* function in a cell fate decision in *C. elegans*. Cell **57**: 1237–1245.

STERNBERG, P. W., and H. R. HORVITZ, 1988 *lin-17* mutations of *Caenorhabditis elegans* disrupt certain asymmetric cell divisions. Dev. Biol. **130**: 67–73.

STERNBERG, P. W., and H. R. HORVITZ, 1989 The combined action of two intercellular signaling pathways specifies three cell fates during vulval induction in *C. elegans*. Cell **58**: 679–693.

SULSTON, J. E., 1976 Post-embryonic development in the ventral cord of *Caenorhabditis elegans*. Philos. Trans. R. Soc. Lond. B Biol. Sci. **275**: 287–297.

SULSTON, J. E., and H. R. HORVITZ, 1977 Post-embryonic cell lineages of the nematode, *Caenorhabditis elegans*. Dev. Biol. **56**: 110–156.

SULSTON, J. E., and J. G. WHITE, 1980 Regulation and cell autonomy during postembryonic development of *Caenorhabditis elegans*. Dev. Biol. **78**: 577–597.

SULSTON, J. E., E. SCHIERENBERG, J. G. WHITE and J. N. THOMSON, 1983 The embryonic cell lineage of the nematode *Caenorhabditis elegans*. Dev. Biol. **100**: 64–119.

WAY, J., and M. CHALFIE, 1988 *mec-3*, a homeobox-containing gene that specifies differentiation of the touch receptor neurons in *C. elegans*. Cell **54**: 5–16.

WHITE, J. G., and H. R. HORVITZ, 1979 Laser microbeam techniques in biological research. Electro-Optical Systems Design **11**: 23–24.

WHITE, J. G., W. B. AMOS and M. FORDHAM, 1987 An evaluation of confocal versus conventional imaging of biological structures by fluorescence light microscopy. J. Cell Biol. **105**: 41–48.

WHITE, J. G., E. SOUTHGATE, J. N. THOMSON and S. BRENNER, 1976 The structure of the ventral nerve cord of *Caenorhabditis elegans*. Philos. Trans. R. Soc. Lond. B Biol. Sci. **275**: 327–348.

WHITE, J. G., E. SOUTHGATE, J. N. THOMSON and S. BRENNER, 1986 The structure of the nervous system of *Caenorhabditis elegans*. Philos. Trans. R. Soc. Lond. B Biol. Sci. **314**: 1–340.

YOCHEM, J., K. WESTON and I. GREENWALD, 1988 *C. elegans lin-12* gene encodes a transmembrane protein similar to *Drosophila Notch* and yeast cell cycle gene products. Nature **335**: 547–550.

November 1990

Genes and Development
Molecular and Logical Themes

Sydney Brenner,* **William F. Dove,**[†,1] **Ira Herskowitz,**[‡] **and René Thomas**[§]

*Medical Research Council, Molecular Genetics Unit, Hills Road, Cambridge CB2 2QH, England;
†McArdle Laboratory for Cancer Research, University of Wisconsin–Madison, Madison, Wisconsin 53706;
‡Department of Biochemistry and Biophysics, School of Medicine, University of California, San Francisco, California 94143;
and §Laboratoire de Génétique, Université Libre de Bruxelles, 67, rue des Chevaux 1640 Rhode-St-Genèse, Belgium

"INFLUENTIAL ideas are always simple," said HERSHEY (1970). The operon model of JACOB and MONOD (1961a) introduced the idea of the control unit for gene expression–a regulatory protein and its DNA target. The regulatory protein can respond to one or more effectors; the target controls the initiation step for the transcription of sequences joined to it. And, or course, there can be multiple targets. In bacteria, each target can control one or many separate genes, whereas in eukaryotes each target usually controls a single gene. Thus, the concept of the operon as a mechanism of regulation transcends prokaryotes and provides a simple, universal mechanism for coordinate regulation of gene expression.

Whole organisms contain multiple control units. For example, the bacteriophage λ utilizes an ensemble of control units to mediate the choice between lysogeny and lytic viral growth and to drive the succession of stages in gene expression characteristic of viral multiplication. A chain of control units can be either open (a cascade) or closed (a loop).

Do control units of the sort described for microbial gene regulation play a universal role in development? The proponents of the operon idea noted ways in which control loops could maintain alternative stable patterns of gene expression (JACOB and MONOD 1961b). Indeed, phage λ can display just such a pair of stable regulatory states (EISEN et al. 1970; NEUBAUER and CALEF 1970). This gives flesh to the abstract notion of epigenetic determination raised by DELBRÜCK (1949). But does development involve regulatory proteins of the conceptual class revealed by the analysis of prokaryotic operons?

Many different experimental systems are being employed to study aspects of development and may provide answers to the following questions. How do bacteria, such as *Caulobacter crescentus* and *Bacillus subtilis*, coordinate their complex morphogenetic programs? How do unicellular eukaryotes, such as yeast, manage to exhibit three different cell types? And, of course, how do multicellular eukaryotes do all of the above and a lot more?

Genetic analysis played a major role in uncovering the operon mechanism: mutations affecting the regulatory proteins and the target sites had striking and informative effects. Amphibia, marine invertebrates and avian vertebrates have their own strong points for the study of development, so that one asks whether genetic analysis can play a role in answering the questions posed above. To what extent is the *modus operandi* of molecular genetics–identification of the important molecular players by isolation of defective mutants–a sufficient approach?

A number of investigators accustomed to the study of gene regulation in microbes have been involved in studying development directly with metazoons. A group of such biologists joined together, *autour de* FRANÇOIS JACOB, in May, 1990, at the Fondation Les Treilles in Provence, France, to discuss their experiences and prospects. This essay explores four themes on which there was extensive conversation: the strengths and limitations of the operon paradigm; the dialogue between gene action and morphogenesis; the formal logical elements of complex biological systems; and "back to the bench," challenges for developmental genetics in the 1990s.

The operon paradigm and its limitations: MARK PTASHNE presented a scheme, supported by considerable experimental evidence, in which the molecular mechanism of action of regulatory proteins in eukaryotes, including higher organisms, could constitute a

[1] To whom correspondence and requests for reprints should be addressed.

reenactment of the same molecular principles discovered initially in the regulation of bacteriophage λ. In outline, the following molecular modules could be defined as sufficient and necessary:

- A DNA-binding domain that recognizes a short sequence of DNA, usually about 5–8 nucleotides, which provides the address.
- A dimerizing domain that allows the protein to form homodimers with itself or heterodimers with another recognition protein to enhance both selectivity and affinity.
- A patch for direct or indirect interaction with another protein that itself has a patch interacting with the transcriptional machinery.
- Patches for interaction with other sets of proteins of the same type. This feature allows action at a distance, from several addresses, which in higher organisms are not confined to a few dozen base pairs at the 5′ ends of the genes. There are even effects from paired homologs. The network of interactions permits the assembly of a complex regulatory agglomerate ("regglomerate") with many different components. The specificity rules for interaction may be quite relaxed (LIN *et al.* 1990). All of this can be, and has been, tested by experiments of the kind done most extensively with the GAL4 regulator of yeast, by artificially joining different domains (BRENT and PTASHNE 1985).

A good example of formation of heterodimers to create a new regulatory protein comes from yeast, where the regulator a1/α2 is formed by association of a1 and α2 polypeptides (GOUTTE and JOHNSON 1988). A spectacular example of this combinatorial association has been described by SCHULZ *et al.* (1990).

The howls of protest were generally of two types:

The molecular mechanism: If the operon paradigm is confined exclusively to the control of transcription initiation, then it is not enough, even for λ, where we also have control by antitermination (*N* and *Q*) and by protein stability (*N* and *cII*). In higher organisms, splicing is regulated; TOM CLINE explicated its role in the mechanism of sex determination in Drosophila (SALZ *et al.* 1989). There are also likely to be mechanisms at other levels, such as messenger lifetime or even translation, as discussed by JONATHAN HODGKIN. One can also imagine that the regulating molecule could be made of RNA rather than protein. If the operon paradigm of genetic regulation merely implies that somewhere, in DNA or RNA, nucleotide sequences in a particular gene provide a specific address for protein to assemble a regulatory apparatus, there would be few objections.

How might such regulation occur in cellular development? This concerns programming and signaling. In prokaryotes and yeast, regulation is mostly coupled to outside environmental variation. Thus, the induction

of λ by UV or of β-galactosidase by lactose involves chains of initial events until the λ repressor is proteolyzed or the *lac* repressor dissociates from its operator. These are "ready to go" systems that require a trigger, and triggers often have induction pathways. IRA HERSKOWITZ pointed out that there is, in fact, the equivalent of an outside environment in higher organisms; it is not the world, but other cells. So there may be many "ready to go" systems in development requiring triggers provided by other cells either as molecules or by cell contact. The induction pathways are very complicated and include receptors, G proteins, protein kinases, internal messengers and so on; and their final acts could be phosphorylation or dephosphorylation, or other chemical alterations of the regglomerate. The intercellular signaling system of Myxococcus, discussed below, illustrates the intimate environment.

HERSKOWITZ summarized the yeast situation (see HERSOKWITZ 1989a). Haploid yeast cells (either **a** or α) are partially differentiated: they have receptors on their surface and they produce the mating factors. When prospective mating partners approach each other they signal their presence with these factors, thereby inducing the final differentiation into cells competent for mating. The mating factors are differentiation signals that induce the expression of various genes involved in mating (such as for cell fusion *per se*). There is a good argument that the mating pathway in yeast culminates by regulating the activity of a transcriptional activator protein, STE12, which might well be activated by phosphorylation.

For more solipsistic acts of development, transcription could be timed and located, not by "ready to go" systems but by the stepwise accumulation, substitution or modification of the components of the regglomerate. These might be called "go when ready" systems, so that each control state not only does something to the cell by altering the transcription pattern, but prepares for the next control state, reached by reiteration of the same mechanism. The cascade of *Bacillus subtilis* transcription factors, discussed below, illustrates successive steps of "readiness."

Because both "ready to go" and "go when ready" systems operate in development, perhaps this is the only way to maintain a self-consistent organization in development. It seems that development could not involve dead reckoning in a purely solipsistic system.

The operon paradigm survives, but with numerous twists.

The dialogue between gene action and morphogenesis: Embryogenesis involves processes that are visibly complex in both space and time. Gastrulation reaches levels of complexity that baffle the imagination of those comfortable with the one-dimensional character of chromosomes, genes, and polypeptides.

Are developmental genes qualitatively distinct in their complexity (WAELSCH 1989)?

A reduction of this issue of developmental complexity is to ask how one-dimensional genes and their polypeptide products can give rise to three-dimensional patterns. In *Caulobacter crescentus*, the products of certain flagellar (*fla*) and chemotaxis (*che*) genes are specifically directed to the swarmer cell in the polarized division process. Two mechanisms were discussed by LUCILLE SHAPIRO. The methylated chemotactic protein encoded by the *mcp* gene carries a carboxy-terminal segment that is necessary and sufficient for segregation to the swarmer cell. By contrast, the gene (*flaK*) encoding the flagellar hook protein directs its transcript selectively to the swarmer cell. Fusions of the *flaK* promoter alone to the marker polypeptide neomycin phosphotransferase can direct the marker antigen to the swarmer cell. In this case, the problem of gene product segregation is replaced by a problem in selective transcription. The issue becomes whether the swarmer cell contains a distinct transcription factor for the *flaK* promoter, or a distinct chromosomal template in which the *flaK* gene is active, or both.

The patterns of successive cell divisions can engender three-dimensional arrays of distinct cell types by these and perhaps other mechanisms. In this reduction of the problem of multidimensionality, the issue becomes the determination of cell division pattern. *Saccharomyces cerevisiae* displays two distinct patterns of bud formation: axial in haploid **a** or α cells and polar in **a**/α diploid cells (J. CHANT and I. HERSKOWITZ, unpublished results). HERSKOWITZ summarized a mutational analysis indicating that the axial pattern requires the action of five genes, two of which are unnecessary for the polar pattern. For at least three of these pattern-determining genes, null alleles are fully viable. Thus, the cell division patterns of *S. cerevisiae* seem to be completely dispensable in the laboratory; the prospects for an extensive genetic analysis are correspondingly large!

The nematode *C. elegans* illustrates the importance of cell division patterns in metazoan development (see HORVITZ and SULSTON 1990). BILL WOOD summarized the three early cleavage divisions by which the anterior/posterior, dorsal/ventral and left/right assymetries are established in this species. He has begun to describe mutants affected in left-right asymmetry.

Spatial morphogenesis is but one aspect of embryogenesis. How does the morphology of a particular stage lead to the patterns of gene expression that generate the next stage? PATRICK STRAGIER gave several illustrations, from studies of the sporulation process in *B. subtilis*, of particular morphogenetic steps that activate new patterns of gene expression (STRAGIER and LOSICK 1990). The proteolytic activation of the late-acting transcription factor σ^E requires the formation of the asymmetric septum that divides the forespore from the mother cell. Three layers of morphogenetic control play a role in elaborating active transcription factor σ^K in the mother cell. Firstly, genetic rearrangement deletes an interrupting sequence from the coding region for σ^K. For reasons not yet known, this rearrangement occurs only in the terminal mother cell compartment. Secondly, the transcription of the rearranged gene for σ^K depends on a factor that is present only in the mother cell. Finally, the σ^K product is activated by a protease that depends on the formation of the forespore compartment for activation. The developmental companion to σ^K is the forespore-specific transcription factor σ^G. Its synthesis is coupled to morphogenesis by its dependence upon a set of DNA-binding proteins that fail to act unless an intact forespore membrane is formed. A mutant described by STRAGIER exhibits a perforated forespore membrane and fails to synthesize σ^G even though the DNA-binding regulators of σ^G have been synthesized. Thus, the cascade of transcription factors that drives the sporulation process in *B. subtilis* is thoroughly coupled to morphogenesis in the developing system.

DALE KAISER gave examples of factors that act between cells to promote development of the microbe *Myxococcus xanthus*. Unlike the solitary sporulation habit of *B. subtilis*, *M. xanthus* sporulates in clusters of approximately 10^5 cells. Mutants with nonautonomous defects in sporulation identify four stages of interaction, A, B, C, and D. The gene product of the *csgC* gene that acts at the final stage, C, is a 17-kD protein tightly associated with the cell membrane. This protein, C factor, can be solubilized and can act to rescue the sporulation of stage-C mutants. Interestingly, nonmotile mutants affected in any of six motility loci of *M. xanthus* mimic the sporulation defect of stage-C mutants and can be rescued by solutions of C factor. But paradoxically, normal amounts of C factor are produced by these nonsporulating motility mutants. KIM and KAISER (1990) have shown that these nonmotile mutants become competent to sporulate when they are aligned within fine grooves on agar surfaces. Thus, the successful transfer of C factor requires intimate cell alignment, which normally depends on the motile behavior of the bacterium. The notion of "microenvironment" is appropriate to the C-factor interaction in *M. xanthus*, just as it is to the action of the *Steel* gene in murine hematopoiesis.

The richness of analysis of these issues in the development of Drosophila was conveyed by SPYROS ARTAVANIS-TSAKONAS, SEYMOUR BENZER, TOM CLINE, ANTONIO GARCÍA-BELLIDO, DAVE HOGNESS, FOTIS KAFATOS and RUTH LEHMANN, but we lack the space to describe their observations. However, certain of these issues have recently been summarized (HARTLEY and WHITE 1990).

Formal logical circuits: The concept of operon is generative; not only is it sufficient to cover the diverse situations that prompted its discovery, but it helps in imagining new situations that it may also cover. An amplification of the operon paradigm prolongs and extends it rather than replacing it; the paradigm uses the elements of the operon and similar elements as building blocks for ever more elaborate networks. As developed by RENÉ THOMAS, the individual wheels of these nets are feedback loops (THOMAS and D'ARI 1990). According to this view, the elementary principles governing regulatory nets are the following.

- Any regulatory net can be decomposed into a well-defined set of simple feedback loops that usually interact with each other.
- A feedback loop is either positive (each element in the loop exerting a positive influence on its own later development) or negative (each element exerting a negative influence on its own later expression).
- Whether a loop is positive or negative depends only on the even versus odd parity of the number of negative control units.
- Negative feedback loops generate homeostasis with or without periodicity. Whereas a negative control unit reduces expression without influencing gene dosage effects, a negative loop not only attenuates expression but also tends to abolish gene dosage effects.
- Positive feedback loops (that is, direct or indirect autocatalysis) generate multiple alternative steady states; m independent positive loops can generate up to 3^m steady states, 2^m of which can be stable (that is, m binary choices).

A number of illustrations of these principles were heard in conversations at Les Treilles.

A negative feedback loop can abolish gene dosage effects. Thus, SHAPIRO observed that when the *Hook* operon of Caulobacter is cloned in a multicopy plasmid, there is no gene dosage effect. And the negative loop involving the λ *cro* gene presumably results in the levels of products of *cII*, *O* and *P* being relatively insensitive to the number of gene copies. In the absence of such regulation, the rate of synthesis of these products (which is already sufficient for replication when there is a single copy of the λ chromosome) would be over 100 times higher after 20 min. Such levels are probably unnecessary for O and P and toxic with regard to cII.

A positive feedback loop may associate with a choice. The detailed mechanisms vary from case to case but the principle is the same: positive autocontrol by the λ *cI* gene (PTASHNE); positive autocontrol by various σ factors in *B. subtilis* (STRAGIER); induced synthesis of receptor and mating factor by the yeast mating factors so that, by positive reinforcement, **a** and α cells are indeed making a commitment to differentiation and a commitment to each other (HERSKOWITZ); a positive control loop involving the *Sx1* gene in sex determination in Drosophila (CLINE); and a positive control loop of the C-factor gene in Myxococcus (KAISER). THOMAS suggested that a fruitful avenue for cloning developmental regulatory genes is to screen for activities that have a positive effect on their own expression level, directly or indirectly.

Chains of control units are also an important feature of the networks involved in development. Primary sex determination in Drosophila and Caenorhabditis involves multiple regulators acting in series, as summarized by HODGKIN (see HODGKIN 1990). In contrast, ANNE MCLAREN noted the apparent simplicity of primary male determination in mammals by a positive regulator [see MCLAREN (1990) and references cited therein]. But λ regulation was also simple at first glance.

The genetic analysis of development: Three topics were intensively discussed.

The saturation genetics approach: One of the fundamental genetic strategies for identifying the components of a process, whether it be biosynthesis of histidine or mating ability of yeast, is to isolate mutants defective in the process and then figure out what the wild-type genes do. A variation on this scheme has been used to study sex determination in multicellular organisms (fruit flies, nematodes, mammals), in which mutants are identified that are transformed from one sex into the other. Assuming that the logistics of such an extensive mutant hunt can be worked out, can this "saturation genetics approach" identify all of the important molecular protagonists?

The simple answer is that many important genes and proteins have been identified in this way, including several that fill the bill of being regulatory proteins of the type conceived by JACOB and MONOD. These include the regulatory proteins encoded by the yeast mating-type locus, the cascade of regulatory proteins in early Drosophila development (*bicoid, hunchback, ftz,* etc.) (INGHAM 1988), and the regulators responsible for sex determination in nematodes and fruit flies (*her-1, tra-1,* etc., in nematodes; *Sxl, dsx,* etc., in fruit flies) (HODGKIN 1990). The discovery of these proteins by genetic methods represents a tremendous advance in understanding the programming of development, but is it complete? We are sensitive to the issue of whether the tools that we use to study the process may perturb the process or introduce a bias in our view of the process.

Essentiality and redundancy: Genetic analysis may give an incomplete or distorted view by failing to identify important genes through the isolation of mutants: a gene might be essential or functionally redundant. The essentiality issue was dramatized by HER-SKOWITZ with an example from cell-type determination in yeast. It is clear that the mating-type locus determines whether a yeast cell is **a** or α (HERSKOWITZ 1989b). The α1 protein coded by the α mating-type allele activates transcription of α-specific genes, and the α2 protein turns off transcription of the **a**-specific genes in these cells. Genetic analysis, however, failed to reveal that both the α1 and α2 proteins work in conjunction with a general transcription factor, MCM1 (KELEHER, GOUTTE and JOHNSON 1988; BENDER and SPRAGUE 1987). As noted earlier, α1 stimulates transcription by assisting MCM1 protein and α2 inhibits transcription by blocking the function of MCM1. These relationships were discovered not by isolating mutants defective in *MCM1*–we now know that inactivation of this gene leads to cell inviability (PASSMORE *et al.* 1988)–but instead by good old biochemistry: α1 binds to DNA only in the presence of MCM1 (BENDER and SPRAGUE 1987) and α2 binds to DNA more strongly with MCM1 (KELEHER, GOUTTE and JOHNSON 1988).

There are many genes identified in fruit flies, nematodes, mice and other organisms in which the canonical mutation is leaky and in which null alleles cause inviability. In fact, *MCM1* was originally identified genetically in this way (PASSMORE *et al.* 1988). Although genetic analysis can identify important genes such as *MCM1* of yeast and *daughterless* of Drosophila (CLINE 1983), special mutations of these genes that allow viability but confer a mutant phenotype are obviously much rarer than mutations that simply inactivate genes. The flip side to this coin is that some viable mutations turn out to affect essential genes, as exemplified by the recently identified lethal alleles at the murine *quaking* locus discussed by BILL DOVE (SHEDLOVSKY, KING and DOVE 1988). When BENZER discussed some of the more than 100 genes known to affect eye development in Drosophila, GARCÍA-BELLIDO pointed out that, for the vast majority of these genes, null alleles are lethal. BARBARA MEYER developed this theme in depth for sex determination in *C. elegans*. The control gene *xol-1* (*XO lethal*) is vital for dosage compensation (for review see HODGKIN 1990).

Redundancy strikes fear in the hearts of geneticists. KOREN has drawn a cartoon in which a monster is looming over one couple while they are conversing with another couple. They know the monster is there and explain, "We deal with it by talking about it." BOB HORVITZ described at least three different types of functional redundancy, and he and GERRY FINK gave examples of these from nematodes and Arabidopsis. He characterized them as redundancies of genes, of pathways and of cells. MCLAREN noted the analogy to the principle of "double assurance" from experimental embryology.

Many examples are now known in which there are duplicate genes, or else two genes that code for proteins with similar amino acid sequences and similar functions. There are even examples in nematodes and yeast in which genes are triply redundant: three *ACE* genes in nematodes (RAND and RUSSELL 1984) and three *CLN* genes in yeast (RICHARDSON *et al.* 1989). In these cases, certain mutant phenotypes are observed only in triply mutant strains!

Arabidopsis provides a good example of redundant pathways. FINK described recent studies indicating that it has two independent pathways for tryptophan biosynthesis (BERLYN, LAST and FINK 1989). Inactivation of any of three genes in one of the pathways causes a leaky tryptophan requirement, apparently because the other pathway can provide some tryptophan. It appears that the second pathway is located in the chloroplast. FINK suggested that the two pathways may be regulated differently, one, for example, being specialized for a stress response and used to synthesize various protective products.

Nematodes provide an example of redundancy at the cellular level. A particularly valuable experimental approach in nematodes is cell ablation with a laser microbeam followed by analysis of behavior. This technique provides a preview of the phenotype that might be exhibited by mutants defective for the functions of the ablated cells. HORVITZ described studies of the excitation of certain intestinal cells by neighboring neurons called AVL and DVB. Although ablation of either neuron has no phenotype, ablation of both causes a mutant phenotype, defective defecation. Thus, genetic analysis of either the AVL or DVB cell type must be performed in a strain defective in the reciprocal neuron.

Given functional redundancy, is it ever possible to obtain mutants defective in such a function? It is indeed and, as described by HORVITZ, functional redundancy provides one explanation for a puzzling type of mutant that has cropped up in nematodes. These carry mutations that have an observable phenotype (such as altered body shape or movement) but which then exhibit no phenotype when the original mutation is converted to a null. A tidy explanation is that the affected gene is a member of a multigene family and that the original mutation is analogous to a dominant negative mutation, one that creates an abnormal protein that inhibits the proteins encoded by the other, redundant loci (PARK and HORVITZ 1986). In cases where one gene of a multigene family has been cloned, such dominant negative versions can be designed *in vitro* and then introduced into the genome, where overproduction is likely to cause a mutant phenotype (HERSKOWITZ 1987).

HODGKIN described mutants of nematodes that can be used to reveal the inhibitory effects of a mutant product on a wild-type product. In *smg* mutants (HODGKIN *et al.* 1989), it appears that certain transcripts are more stable than in wild-type strains (R. PULAK and P. ANDERSON, unpublished results). The striking finding is that some truncated polypeptides (resulting from nonsense mutations) become dominant in a smg^- background. Even amber mutations, which are expected to be well-behaved losses of function, can become dominant-negatives if the amber fragment is sufficiently long.

JANET ROSSANT described the new era of gene knock-out in mouse genetics: it is now possible to use a mouse gene mutated *in vitro* to inactivate the wild-type gene, by first modifying cells in culture and then deriving a mouse with the mutation in its germ line. That is the good news. Now the bad news: sometimes the mutant has no overt phenotype! One explanation for this disappointing result is functional redundancy. A strategy to contend with this difficulty is to begin another mutant hunt using the silent mutant as the starting strain. This approach has been used successfully in yeast, nematodes, and fruit flies, but of course it has no guarantee of success and can be quite cumbersome.

For the mouse, the tools for genetic analysis are under active development. ROSSANT discussed enhancer-trap protocols and DOVE summarized point mutagenesis by ENU, each of which very efficiently generates mutants on the basis of phenotype (GOSSLER *et al.*, 1989; MCDONALD *et al.* 1990). JACOB raised the conundrum that patterns in the expression of *lacZ* insertions do not match classical embryological lineages. PETER GOODFELLOW noted the difficulties of identifying sex-determining elements by analyzing translocation chromosomes. GYORGY GEORGIEV explored the development of transfection assays for genes controlling metastatic cell behavior. The new genetic tools in mice may soon participate as partners comparable to transplantation and cell culture analysis of the neural crest as summarized by NICOLE LE DOUARIN.

Identifying interacting components: Along with saturation genetics and gene knock-outs using cloned genes, another important genetic strategy for the nineties is the identification of interacting components. At least four different schemes were discussed in the formal sessions and during the unforgettable Provençal meals. The central idea is to use one mutant strain as a springboard to identify another gene, one that is functionally related in some way to the original gene. The standard fantasy is that the two gene products physically interact (the "geneticist's immunoprecipitate"). But this should not be assumed *a priori* to be the case.

The first method, described by HOGNESS, involves identifying interacting components through mutations that are nonallelic noncomplementers. These present themselves as genetic anomalies in which mutations at two separate loci are recessive to their corresponding wild-type alleles but whose double heterozygote exhibits a mutant phenotype. Mutations of this sort have been interpreted to affect components of a multisubunit structure, for example of the mitotic apparatus (HAYS *et al.* 1989).

A classical method to identify interacting components, and one that remains powerful, is to identify modifier mutations. These are mutations distinct from the initial mutation that cause the original phenotype to be relieved (a suppressor mutation) or exacerbated (an enhancer mutation). GARCÍA-BELLIDO is analyzing the morphogenesis of the Drosophila wing. He has classified the 30 genes known to be involved into five synergy groups. Combinations of two mutations from the same synergy group give an enhanced phenotype. DOVE mentioned that the dominant allele *Min*, causing multiple intestinal adenomas in the mouse (MOSER, PITOT and DOVE 1990), responds to dominant suppressor alleles carried by particular mouse strains. ARTAVANIS-TSAKONIS described the use of this approach to identify genes that interact with the Drosophila *Notch* gene. He created a situation in which a certain *Notch* heterozygote was inviable and identified numerous revertants to viability. In so doing, he found mutations in several known genes and in a previously unidentified gene, *deltex* (XU and ARTAVANIS-TSAKONIS 1990).

HERSKOWITZ described the strategy of searching for high-copy-number plasmids carrying one gene that can compensate for a mutation in another gene. This technique has been used profitably in fission and budding yeast to identify genes whose products interact with the cdc2/CDC28 protein kinase (HAYLES *et al.* 1986; HADWIGER *et al.* 1989). In these cases, high-copy-number plasmids were identified that could suppress the growth defect of thermosensitive mutants at semipermissive temperature. One mechanism for this suppression is expected to be by mass action, providing more of one interacting component for association, and this strategy ought to identify proteins that bind to mutated target sites. Other mechanisms for high-copy-number suppression can also be imagined. For example, increased gene dosage might enable the synthesis of sufficient product to bypass a defect in expression of that gene. Although the technique of high-copy-number plasmid suppression is currently available only for microbial systems, it might be worthwhile to develop an analog for nematodes, fruit flies or mice.

The prototype has recently been described for a potentially powerful new method for identifying interacting components. Dubbed by the group the protein interaction trap, this method is based on the two-domain structure of the yeast transcriptional activator protein GAL4–one (D) the DNA-binding domain and the other (A) necessary for transcriptional activation (BRENT and PTASHNE 1985). FIELDS and SONG (1989) have exploited the fact that these two domains must be physically associated in order to function. They have shown that the two domains can be brought together with two hybrid proteins, D/P_1 and A/P_2, where P_1 and P_2 are protein segments that associate with each other. FIELDS and SONG suggest that it is in principle possible to use this as a screening method. For example, a protein segment of interest (P_3) could be attached to the GAL4 DNA-binding domain to form D/P_3. Then a library of hybrid proteins (A/P_i), formed by joining the GAL4 activation domain to random coding segments, could be examined for one that can associate with the DNA-binding domain. Although not yet implemented, this scheme presents exciting possibilities. The regglomerate may be dissected in this way.

Concluding remarks: SYDNEY BRENNER gave the following overview in the opening conversation.

Biology is concerned just as much with particular implementations as with general principles. GUNTHER STENT long ago put forward the idea that development was a trivial problem because, given the JACOB-MONOD model of gene regulation, all development could be reduced to that paradigm. It was simply a matter of turning on the right genes in the right places at the right times. Of course, while absolutely true this is also absolutely vacuous. The paradigm does not tell us how to make a mouse but only how to make a switch. The real answers must surely be in the detail. It is also a mistake to think that general principles float about in the cosmos waiting for God or Nature or even the NIH to pluck them out and embed them in the real world. But I can hear a complaint: we cannot accept that everything exists separately in unique worlds, and what is true of λ should be true of lambs. However, there is a global constraint, and that is the connectedness by descent of all present living systems and the impossibility in evolution of going back to the drawing board once a certain level of complexity has been reached. Thus, anything successful that appears in evolution will be retained and elaborated as organisms advance in complexity and will be found over and over not as the instantiation of a general principle, but only thorough the continuity of utility.

A skeptic might at this stage ask what is meant by the terms complex and simple. The answer is, it depends. Thus, from the point of view of amino acids, λ repressor is a complex piece of machinery; but from the point of view of *Escherichia coli*, it is part of a simple switch. Biological systems have a hierarchical structure, and a poem at one level is an expletive at

another. The same relativity applies to the words primitive and advanced. There is a view that *E. coli* is primitive and we are advanced. That is true from the point of view of function and action. But it is not true from the point of view of genome structure. Here it is *E. coli* that is streamlined and sophisticated, whereas it is our genome that has preserved a far more primitive condition.

A paradigm is a fancy word for an example, but it has come to mean more than that today. It carries the more distinctive flavor of a canonical case, something we all have to follow. But the operon paradigm should have no statutory requirements; it is a classical example and one which we will find, perhaps in more baroque contexts, as we disentangle the regulatory switches of higher organisms.

We thank JONATHAN HODGKIN for helpful comments. We are deeply grateful to ANNETTE GRUNER SCHLUMBERGER for sharing with us the spirit of the Fondation Les Treilles. Additional support came from the U.S.-Western Europe Cooperative Program of the National Science Foundation.

LITERATURE CITED

BENDER, S., and G. F. SPRAGUE, JR., 1987 MATα1 protein, a yeast transcription activator, binds synergistically with a second protein to a set of cell-type-specific genes. Cell **60:** 681–691.

BERLYN, M. B., R. L. LAST and G. R. FINK, 1989 A gene encoding the tryptophan synthase β subunit of *Arabidopsis thaliana*. Proc. Natl. Acad. Sci. USA **86:** 4604–4608.

BRENT, R., and M. PTASHNE, 1985 A eukaryotic transcriptional activator bearing the DNA specificity of a prokaryotic repressor. Cell **43:** 729–736.

CLINE, T. W., 1983 The interaction between daughterless and sex-lethal in triploids: a lethal sex-transforming maternal effect linking sex determination and dosage compensation in Drosophila melanogaster. Dev. Biol. **95:** 260–274.

DELBRÜCK, M., 1949 Pp. 33–35 in *Symposium sur Unités Biologiques Donées de Continuité Génétique*. Publications Centre National de la Recherche Scientifique, Paris.

EISEN, H., P. BRACHET, L. PEREIRA DA SILVA and F. JACOB, 1970 Regulation of repressor expression in λ. Proc. Natl. Acad. Sci. USA **66:** 855–862.

FIELDS, S., and O.-X. SONG, 1989 A novel genetic system to detect protein-protein interactions. Nature **340:** 245–246.

GOSSLER, A., A. L. JOYNER, J. ROSSANT and W. C. SKARNES, 1989 Mouse embryonic stem cells and reporter constructs to detect developmentally regulated genes. Science **244:** 463–465.

GOUTTE, C., and A. D. JOHNSON, 1988 a1 protein alters the DNA binding specificity of α2 repressor. Cell **52:** 875–882.

HADWIGER, J. A., C. WITTENBERG, M. E. RICHARDSON, M. DE BARRO LOPES and S. I. REED, 1989 A family of cyclin homologs that control the G_1 phase in yeast. Proc. Natl. Acad. Sci. USA **86:** 6255–6259.

HARTLEY, D., and R. WHITE, 1990 *Drosophila* in Crete: a flying visit. Trends Genet. **6:** 199–201.

HAYLES, J., D. H. BEACH, B. DURKACZ and P. M. NURSE, 1986 The fission yeast cell cycle control gene *cdc2*: isolation of a sequence *suc1+* that suppresses *cdc2−* mutant function. Mol. Gen. Genet. **202:** 291–293.

HAYS, T. S., R. DEURING, B. ROBERTSON, M. PROUT and M. T. FULLER, 1989 Interacting proteins identified by genetic interactions: a missense mutation in α-tubulin fails to complement alleles of the testis-specific β-tubulin gene of *Drosophila melanogaster*. Mol. Cell. Biol. **9:** 875–884.

HERSHEY, A. D., 1970 Genes and hereditary characteristics. Nature **226:** 697–700.

HERSKOWITZ, I., 1987 Functional inactivation of genes by dominant negative mutations. Nature **329:** 219–222.

HERSKOWITZ, I., 1989a Life cycle of the budding yeast *Saccharomyces cerevisiae*. Microbiol. Rev. **52:** 536–553.

HERSKOWITZ, I., 1989b A regulatory heirarchy for cell specialization in yeast. Nature **342:** 749–757.

HODGKIN, J., 1990 Sex determination compared in *Drosophila* and *Caenorhabditis*. Nature **344:** 721–728.

HODGKIN, J., A. PAPP, R. PULAK, V. AMBROS and P. ANDERSON, 1989 A new kind of informational suppression in the nematode *Caenorhabditis elegans*. Genetics **123:** 301–313.

HORVITZ, H. R., and J. E. SULSTON, 1990 Joy of the worm. Genetics **126:** 287–292.

INGHAM, P. W., 1988 The molecular genetics of embryonic pattern formation in *Drosophila*. Nature **335:** 25–34.

JACOB, F., and J. MONOD, 1961a Genetic regulatory mechanisms in the synthesis of proteins. J. Mol. Biol. **3:** 318–356.

JACOB, F., and J. MONOD, 1961b On the regulation of gene activity. Cold Spring Harbor Symp. Quant. Biol. **26:** 193–211.

KELEHER, C. A., C. GOUTTE and A. D. JOHNSON, 1988 The yeast cell-type-specific repressor α2 acts cooperatively with a non-cell-type-specific protein. Cell **53:** 927–936.

KIM, S. K., and D. KAISER, 1990 Cell alignment required in differentiation of *Myxococcus xanthus*. Science **249:** 926–928.

LIN, Y.-S., M. CAREY, M. PTASHNE and M. R. GREEN, 1990 How different eukaryotic transcriptional activators can cooperate promiscuously. Nature **345:** 359–361.

McDONALD, J. D., V. C. BODE, W. F. DOVE and A. SHEDLOVSKY, 1990 Pah[hph-5]: a mouse mutant deficient in phenylalanine hydroxylase. Proc. Natl. Acad. Sci. USA **87:** 1965–1967.

McLAREN, A., 1990 What makes a man a man? Nature **346:** 216–217.

MOSER, A. R., H. C. PITOT and W. F. DOVE, 1990 A dominant mutation that predisposes to multiple intestinal neoplasia in the mouse. Science **247:** 322–324.

NEUBAUER, Z., and E. CALEF, 1970 Immunity phase-shift in defective lysogens: non-mutational hereditary change of early regulation of λ prophage. J. Mol. Biol. **51:** 1–13.

PARK, E. C., and H. R. HORVITZ, 1986 Mutations with dominant effects on the behavior and morphology of the nematode *Caenorhabditis elegans*. Genetics **113:** 821–852.

PASSMORE, S., G. T. MAINE, R. ELBLE, C. CHRIST and B.-K. TYE, 1988 *Saccharomyces cerevisiae* protein involved in plasmid maintenance is necessary for mating of *MATα* cells. J. Mol. Biol. **204:** 593–606.

RAND, J. B., and R. L. RUSSELL, 1984 Choline acetyltransferase-deficient mutants of the nematode *Caenorhabditis elegans*. Genetics **106:** 227–248.

RICHARDSON, H. E., C. WITTENBERG, F. CROSS and S. I. REED, 1989 An essential G1 function for cyclin-like proteins in yeast. Cell **59:** 1127–1133.

SALZ, H. K., E. M. MAINE, L. N. KEYES, M. E. SAMUELS, T. W. CLINE and P. SCHEDL, 1989 The *Drosophila* female-specific sex-determination gene, *sex-lethal*, has stage-, tissue-, and sex-specific RNAs suggesting multiple modes of regulation. Genes Dev. **3:** 708–719.

SCHULZ, B., F. BANUETT, M. DAHL, R. SCHLESINGER, W. SCHÄFER, T. MARTIN, I. HERSKOWITZ and R. KAHMANN, 1990 The *b* alleles of U. maydis, whose combinations program pathogenic development, code for polypeptides containing a homeodomain-related motif. Cell **60:** 295–306.

SHEDLOVSKY, A., T. R. KING and W. F. DOVE, 1988 Saturation germ line mutagenesis of the murine *t* region including a lethal allele at the quaking locus. Proc. Natl. Acad. Sci. USA **85:** 180–184.

STRAGIER, P., and R. LOSICK, 1990 Cascades of sigma factors revisited. Mol. Microbiol. (in press).

THOMAS, R., and R. D'ARI, 1990 *Biological Feedback*. CRC Press, Boca Raton, Fla.

WAELSCH, S. G., 1989 In praise of complexity. Genetics **122:** 721–725.

XU, T., and S. ARTAVANIS-TSAKONAS, 1990 *deltex*, a locus interacting with the neurogenic genes, *Notch, Delta* and *mastermind* in *Drosophila melanogaster*. Genetics **126:** 665–677.

December 1990

Sixty Years of Mystery

Allan C. Spradling and Gary H. Karpen

Howard Hughes Medical Institute Research Laboratories, Department of Embryology,
Carnegie Institution of Washington 115 West University Parkway, Baltimore, Maryland 21210

NO induced mutations fascinated H. J. MULLER more than the five *white-mottled* strains (w^{m1}-w^{m5}) recovered among the progeny of X-ray-treated flies (MULLER 1930). Radiation treatment was providing unprecedented opportunities to systematically mutate genes and rearrange chromosomes in *Drosophila melanogaster*. Most induced mutations behaved like previously studied spontaneous lesions. In contrast, the variegated strains displayed novel and perplexing properties. Each individual from these strains showed variable expression of the *white* gene among the hundreds of ommatidia in the compound eyes. This suggested that the gene was "eversporting," *i.e.*, that it underwent frequent genetic changes during eye development like previously described mutable genes in maize and *Drosophila virilis*. However, unlike mutable genes, germinal changes in the *white-mottled* strains occurred very rarely, no reversions to a stable state appearing after more than 50 generations (MULLER 1930).

Several additional properties distinguished the lesions in the eversporting strains from simple gene mutations. Linkage analysis showed that all the mottled strains had undergone chromosome rearrangements. Furthermore, the w^{m1} strain also showed variable expression of *Notch*, a gene separated from *white* by 1.5 map units. Effects on the two genes were coupled in some way because flies with strong *white* mottling usually had notched wings while weakly mottled flies did not. Existing theory seemed inadequate to explain these "peculiar manoeuvers of some portion of chromatin larger than a gene which has been displaced from its original position" (MULLER 1930).

MULLER's "eversporting displacements" displayed an unusual susceptibility to modification. The w^{m1} strain immediately gave rise to strongly and weakly mottled derivatives. As reported in GENETICS (GOWEN and GAY 1934), addition of a Y chromosome was shown to suppress variegating rearrangements and removal of the Y to enhance them. Presumably, MULLER's dark-eyed w^{m1} lines contained an extra Y chromosome. Subsequently, it was shown that altering the dosage of heterochromatin on other chromosomes also modified variegation. Temperature altered mottling in an unexpected direction: unlike most familiar chemical reactions, variegation was increased at low temperature. However, the discovery that variegation could be predictably modified only increased the mystery surrounding the mechanisms that produced such lesions.

JACK SCHULTZ, one of MORGAN's last graduate students at Columbia, maintained an interest in variegation over much of his career. He was one of the first to apply the new technique of polytene chromosome analysis to eversporting strains. SCHULTZ (1936) found that rearrangements producing variegated effects always involved breakage within heterochromatic ("inert") regions. The unusual effects on gene expression therefore appeared to result from placing genes abnormally close to the centric heterochromatic regions. Furthermore, phenotypic instability was paralleled by variation in the banding pattern near the rearrangement breakpoint among individual salivary gland cells (CASPERSSON and SCHULTZ 1938). MILISLAV DEMEREC (1941) carefully studied rearrangements involving genes in the *Notch* region and established that both phenotypic and cytogenetic variegation could affect multiple genes and polytene chromosome bands, but in a polar manner that always seemed to "spread" from the heterochromatin.

In 1937, SCHULTZ described the appearance of a third-chromosome genetic modifier that "exercises a dominant maternal effect for the suppression of variegation" (MORGAN, BRIDGES and SCHULTZ 1937). It soon became apparent that variegating rearrangements were sensitive to changes in genomic elements besides the major heterochromatic blocks. In an attempt at a more systematic study of background influences, SCHULTZ induced a large number of dominant suppressors (*Suvar*) and enhancers (*Evar*) of w^{m4} variegation (MORGAN, SCHULTZ and CURRY 1941). This collection included an unusual group of autosomal modifiers "deficient for regions within the sections ordinarily called euchromatic." SCHULTZ believed that these modifiers corresponded to deletions of "interstitial" heterochromatin and could be used to map and study such domains (MORGAN and SCHULTZ 1942). The realization that variegation could be influenced in *trans* by the activity of "normal" euchromatic genes dawned slowly. SPOFFORD (1967) used recombination to map precisely the first *Suvar* to a specific locus on *2L*.

Direct proof that variegation was caused by a position effect required that the gene be separated intact from its association with heterochromatin. Several investigators showed that variegation could be alleviated by secondary rearrangements, but the reinversion study of *In(1)roughest³* reported by ED NOVITSKI (1961) was probably the most elegant. However, the possibility remained that these reversions might have resulted from secondary mutations, and many of the so-called reversions could be demonstrated to still variegate under appropriate conditions. The Russians N. B. DUBININ and B. N. SIDOROV (1935) and I. B. PANSHIN (1935) reported beautiful experiments in which variegating genes were cleanly separated from the inducing rearrangement by recombination. The "variegating" allele then behaved like a normal, wild-type gene when present on an unrearranged chromosome; conversely, a wild-type allele from a normal-sequence chromosome variegated when recombined onto the rearranged homolog. These studies also eliminated a role for structural heterozygosity between homologs, a component of some early models. Final acceptance of these proofs followed analogous studies on a variegating *white* rearrangement by BURKE JUDD (1955).

Forays into understanding the relationship between development and variegation began as early as 1930 with MULLER who, aided by THEODOSIUS DOBZHANSKY's dissecting skills, discovered that the original w^m rearrangements were associated with mottled pigmentation of the testis sheath as well as in the eye. More detailed studies revealed that, for a given rearrangement, different larval and adult tissues and even bristle cells in different regions of the notum (NOUJDIN 1936) could vary widely in the probability of expressing the variegated phenotype and in the type of variegation (fine grain or large patches). The idea that expression of the variegated phenotype was influenced by events occurring many cell divisions prior to final action of the gene was hinted at by studies of S. Y. CHEN (1948), SCHULTZ (1956) and others who determined that *white* mottling could be altered by temperature shifts applied not only during the time of eye differentiation (pupariation) but also early in development (blastoderm to hatching). These temperature-sensitive periods were later confirmed by correlating the size of variegating patches with the size of marked clones induced at specific times in development. Surprisingly, variegation could even be modified prior to fertilization. The parental source of the rearrangement and the genetic constitution (*i.e.*, presence or absence of a *Y* chromosome) of the parent were found to greatly influence the extent of $In(1)scute^8$ (sc^8) variegation in the progeny both phenotypically (NOUJDIN 1944) and cytogenetically (PROKOFYEVA-BELGOVSKAYA 1947).

As with most genetic phenomena, interesting exceptions appeared almost immediately that complicated the "rules" established by the properties of most variegating rearrangements. MULLER (1930) reported the appearance of rearrangements that displayed a dominant eye color variegation (*Plum*, later called *brown-dominant* or bw^V). Most other variegating genes behaved as recessives in the presence of a wild-type allele on the normal sequence homolog. Although bw^V rearrangements displayed many similarities to recessive variegation (association with heterochromatic breakpoints, *Y* suppressibility), attempts to force *bw* into the prevailing view of variegation were generally unsuccessful. Another exception was "reverse" position effects exhibited by normally heterochromatic genes such as *light* (*lt*) (SCHULTZ and DOBZHANSKY 1934), *cubitus interruptus* (*ci*) (DUBININ and SIDOROV 1934) and, in *Drosophila virilis*, *peach* (BAKER 1953). Variegation occurred when these heterochromatic genes were moved to distal euchromatin (HESSLER 1958); *lt* variegation was enhanced (instead of suppressed) by an extra *Y* chromosome.

By the end of the 1930s the phenomenology of position-effect variegation was clear. It was less certain whether heterochromatic rearrangements in organisms other than Drosophila produced variegation. DAVID CATCHESIDE's (1939) discovery of a rearrangement that exerted a position effect on the *P* locus in *Oenothera blandina* supported the view that these effects were more widespread. However, the underlying mechanisms responsible for position-effect variegation remained obscure. DEMEREC (1941) summarized the possible explanations in terms that have hardly changed: "This instability may be due either to a reversible chemical change in the gene or may be caused by a reversible suppression of the activity of the gene." Arguments between these two views comprise much of the subsequent history of research on this subject.

SCHULTZ's observations of variegating rearrangements in polytene chromosomes convinced him that genic material had been lost, possibly due to a change in replication within those cells whose expression was weakened (MORGAN, BRIDGES and SCHULTZ 1936). SCHULTZ took ultraviolet pictures of variegating chromosomes in TORBJÖRN CASPERSSON's laboratory in Stockholm and thought he had detected at least one example where the absorbance of a band had changed, although it showed an increase instead of the expected loss (CASPERSSON and SCHULTZ 1938). However, P. A. COLE and E. SUTTON (1941) were unable to confirm the findings.

The alternative view, that variegation suppressed gene activity, was bolstered by other cytogenetic studies. A. A. PROKOFYEVA-BELGOVSKAYA (1939) noted striking variation between individual salivary gland cells in the appearance of the polytene chromosome regions that contained variegating genes. Whereas SCHULTZ thought the affected regions had been lost in some cells, she interpreted these changes as a transformation of the bands to a heterochromatic state. The cytological analysis of heterochromatin was inherently subjective; these different interpretations were never resolved. The difficulties were underscored by PROKOFYEVA-BELGOVSKAYA's 1937 GENETICS publication describing the detailed structure of the Y chromosome in salivary gland cells, but other cytologists have been unable to detect this chromosome.

The many similarities between position-effect variegation and mutable genes in maize led BARBARA McCLINTOCK (1950, 1951) to postulate a close relationship between the two phenomena. Like Drosophila variegation, maize controlling elements were linked to heterochromatin because cytogenetic and irradiation studies suggested that they derived from rearranged heterochromatin regions. The suppression of Ds-induced mottling by an extra dose of Ac appeared similar to the suppression of variegation by an extra Y chromosome. This view generated little interest among workers studying position-effect variegation.

The volume of literature devoted to position effects decreased substantially between 1950 and the late 1970s despite a seminal review by E. B. LEWIS (1950) that introduced the problem to a new generation of students. Nevertheless, each new fact learned about heterochromatin stimulated new approaches to understanding the mechanism of variegation. The discovery that heterochromatin replicated late in the cell cycle led J. HEBERT TAYLOR (1964) to resurrect a relationship between replication and position-effect

variegation. The finding that the copy number of DNA sequences within heterochromatic regions was drastically reduced within polytene salivary gland cells (GALL, COHEN and POLAN 1971; HENNIG and MEER 1971) also suggested that changes in replication might lead to underrepresentation of variegating genes. WARGENT and HARTMANN-GOLDSTEIN (1974) found that incorporation of thymidine into a variegating region was not synchronized with its normal counterpart. Late replication and slightly reduced DNA content were detected in some salivary gland cells within a variegating region under enhanced conditions (ANANIEV and GVOZDEV 1974). The limited copy-number changes observed in these and subsequent studies (HENIKOFF 1981; KORNHER and KAUFMAN 1986) called into question whether changed DNA content was relevant to variegated gene expression.

Finally, molecular studies using cloned genes revealed that both of DEMEREC's proposed mechanisms, gene inactivation and gene loss, could be produced by juxtaposition with heterochromatin. The copy number of the *rosy* gene within the variegating rearrangement $ry^{ps11187}$ was shown to remain unchanged despite a sevenfold reduction in enzyme activity (RUSHLOW, BENDER and CHOVNICK 1984). In this case, position-effect variegation affects gene activity rather than copy number. However, studies of the sc^8 junction in the minichromosome $Dp(1;f)1187$ yielded a different result (KARPEN and SPRADLING 1990). Euchromatic sequences spanning more than 100 kb adjacent to the breakpoint were underrepresented as much as 39-fold in larval salivary glands. The degree of underrepresentation varied among individual cells and was suppressed by a Y chromosome. Reduced gene copy number might therefore be sufficient to explain the *yellow* variegation associated with this rearrangement, although an independent effect on transcription could not be ruled out.

Because many different heterochromatic breaks can induce mottling, inducing sequences must be dispersed within the heterochromatin of all the chromosomes. Several factors have complicated searches for specific inducing sequences. In particular, the quantity as well as the quality of specific *cis*-regulatory sequences may influence the nature of induced variegation. For example, retrotransposons were found at the breakpoints of three inversions variegating for *white*, including w^{m4} (TARTOF, HOBBS and JONES 1984). X-ray-induced revertants were obtained that still retained the transposon sequences, suggesting that variegation was induced by sequences located within heterochromatin some distance from the breakpoint. However, the apparent revertants of w^{m4} still exhibited mottling in the presence of strong variegation enhancers, indicating that the strength of variegation was related to the quantity of heterochromatin adjacent to the breakpoint (REUTER, WOLFF and FRIEDE 1985).

Some recent progress in our understanding of the molecular nature of *cis* sequences involved in variegation has been generated by studies of the "exceptional" variegating systems. The molecular cloning of the *bw* locus (HENIKOFF and DREESEN 1989) and a deletion analysis of a rearrangement that causes variegation of a transformed copy of *brown* suggested that sequences close to or within the gene, as well as somatic pairing between homologues, are essential components of *bw* dominant variegation (HENIKOFF 1990). The *lt* gene is embedded in a region rich in repetitive sequences (DEVLIN, BINGHAM and WAKIMOTO 1990). This unusual organization may underlie the reverse position effects observed in lt^V rearrangements. Recently, genes inserted into telomeric heterochromatin via *P* element transformation have been observed to undergo *Y*-suppressible position effects (G. KARPEN and A. M. SPRADLING, unpublished observations). Variegation-inducing sequences may be easier to localize within the relatively small blocks of heterochromatin at telomeres.

The proteins encoded by some modifier loci have been characterized recently. TOM GRIGLIATTI, GÜNTER REUTER and KEN TARTOF have systematically screened for loci that dominantly enhance or suppress w^{m4} variegation (see SINCLAIR, MOTTUS and GRIGLIATTI 1983; REUTER *et al.* 1990; LOCKE, KOTARSKI and TARTOF 1988). These studies have identified many new loci with strong effects on variegation and suggest that at least 50 such loci exist within the Drosophila genome. Variegation is sensitive to the dosage of many of these loci. Most commonly, a single dose suppresses variegation while three doses enhance; however, the reverse situation holds for a few other genes. Some of the genes mutate to lethality or female sterility, suggesting that they play a role in development. REUTER *et al.* (1990) recently cloned *Suvar(3)7* and showed that it encodes a putative DNA-binding protein containing several predicted zinc fingers. Another locus, *Suvar(2)5*, may encode the C1A9 heterochromatin-binding protein (see EISSENBERG 1989). Further study of modifier loci should provide a wealth of important information on variegation, heterochromatin, and the developmental control of chromosomal functions.

Although we have learned that variegating rearrangements can suppress gene activity and sometimes are associated with sequence underrepresentation, the task remains of elucidating the molecular mechanisms that produce these changes. A detailed heterochromatinization model has been formulated (ZUCKERKANDL 1974; SINCLAIR, MOTTUS and GRIGLIATTI 1983; LOCKE, KOTARSKI and TARTOF 1988). Chromosome compaction was postulated to initiate at specific sequences within centric DNA and spread until termination sequences were encountered, due to the formation of a large complex of proteins. Rearrangements placing euchromatic sequences within such a domain would become partially heterochromatinized as the protein complex assembled along its length. Enhancer and suppressor loci were postulated to encode structural proteins of the complex or modifiers of such proteins. Presumably, the *Y* chromosome suppresses variegation by titrating these heterochromatin-binding proteins, reducing the tendency of heterochromatin to spread across the breakpoint.

Recent progress in understanding variegation at the molecular level has encouraged some workers to conclude that the heterochromatization model is essentially correct and that position-effect variegation can now join the mainstream of molecular biology (EISSENBERG 1989). Unfortunately, such optimism seems premature. Several properties of variegation are not simply explained by spreading domains of heterochromatin. Why should a heterochromatin complex move a variable distance along euchromatin in different cells, but after some point in development faithfully maintain its position through multiple cell cycles? How can parental source effects be explained by maternal heterochromatin titrating binding proteins during oogenesis, when heterochromatin is severely underrepresented in nurse cells? Critical tests of the model will be difficult to accomplish. For example, even if modifier loci are shown to encode proteins that bind heterochromatic DNA, it would be necessary to show that such proteins actually mediate heterochromatin formation in a manner that can spread along a chromosome region.

There are alternatives to spreading domains of heterochromatin. The strong similarities between position-effect variegation and mutable genes were noted by MULLER, but the germinal stability of genes affected by variegating rearrangements differentiated these two phenomena. This objection carries little weight since the discovery that transposable elements can be subject to different regulation in somatic and germline cells. KARPEN and SPRADLING (1990) suggested that transposable elements located within heterochromatin might induce position-effect variegation in somatic cells by transposing into juxtaposed euchromatin. The relevant mobile elements would have to transpose predominantly locally and conservatively to explain the spreading effect; multiple rounds of cell division may be required to invade hundreds of kilobases of DNA. Transposons are known to suppress the transcription of genes near their site of residence and this suppression is subject to modification by genomic suppressor loci (SPANA, HARRISON and CORCES 1988). Furthermore, transposons can catalyze imprecise excisions that would lead to the observed reductions in sequence copy number. Transposons encode regulators of their own activity; the modifying effects of added heterochromatin would result from altering the dosage of heterochromatic transposons and their genes. Transposon regulatory proteins could be inherited maternally to account for parental source effects. In this model it is easy to understand why gene inactivation would be stochastic but relatively stable, because a covalent change (an inserted element) would be responsible.

Position-effect variegation has now fascinated several successive generations of geneticists. This phenomenon should remind us that very basic aspects of chromosome structure and function remain poorly ⁓understood. Although 60 years of research have still not solved the problem, systems have been developed that should facilitate an understanding of position-effect variegation at the molecular level. The continued interest of geneticists speaks to the striking nature of the phenomenon and suggests that, when the solution does emerge, it will have been worth waiting for.

LITERATURE CITED

ANAVIEV, E. V., and V. A. GVOZDEV, 1974   Changed pattern of transcription and replication in polytene chromosomes of Drosophila melanogaster resulting from eu-heterochromatin rearrangement. Chromosoma 45: 173–191.

BAKER, W. K., 1953   V-type position effects of a gene in Drosophila virilis normally located in heterochromatin. Genetics 38: 328–344.

CASPERSSON, T., and J. SCHULTZ, 1938   Nucleic acid metabolism of the chromosomes in relation to gene reproduction. Nature 142: 294–295.

CATCHESIDE, D. B., 1939   A position effect in Oenothera. J. Genet. 38: 345–352.

CHEN, S.-Y., 1948   Action de la temperature sur trois mutants a panachure de Drosophila melanogaster: w^{258-18}, w^{m5}, et z. Bull. Biol. Fr. Belg. 82: 114–129.

COLE, P. A., and E. SUTTON, 1941   The absorption of ultraviolet radiation by bands of the salivary gland polytene chromosomes of Drosophila melanogaster. Cold Spring Harbor Symp. Quant. Biol. 9: 66–70.

DEMEREC, M., 1941   The nature of changes in the white-Notch region of the X chromosome of Drosophila melanogaster. Proc. 7th Int. Congr. Genet., pp. 99–103.

DEVLIN, R. H., B. BINGHAM and B. WAKIMOTO, 1990   The organization and expression of the light gene, a heterochromatic gene of Drosophila melanogaster. Genetics 125: 129–140.

DUBININ, N. P., and B. N. SIDOROV, 1934   Relationship between the effect of a gene and its position in the system. Am. Nat. 68: 377–381.

DUBININ, N. P., and B. N. SIDOROV, 1935   The position effect of the hairy gene. Biol. Zh. 4: 555–568.

EISSENBERG, J. C., 1989   Position effect variegation in Drosophila: towards a genetics of chromatin assembly. BioEssays 11: 14–17.

GALL, J. G., E. H. COHEN and M. L. POLAN, 1971   Repetitive DNA sequences in Drosophila. Chromosoma 33: 319–344.

GOWEN, J. W., and E. H. GAY, 1934   Chromosome constitution and behavior in eversporting and mottling in Drosophila melanogaster. Genetics 19: 189–208.

HENIKOFF, S., 1981   Position-effect variegation and chromosome structure of a heat shock puff in Drosophila. Chromosoma 83: 381–393.

HENIKOFF, S., 1990   Position-effect variegation after 60 years. Trends Genet. 6: (in press).

HENIKOFF, S., and T. D. DREESEN, 1989   Trans-inactivation of the Drosophila brown gene: evidence for transcriptional repression and somatic pairing dependence. Proc. Natl. Acad. Sci. USA 86: 6704–6708.

HENNIG, W., and B. MEER, 1971   Reduced polyteny of ribosomal RNA cistrons in giant chromosomes of Drosophila hydei. Nature New Biol. 233: 70–72.

HESSLER, A. Y., 1958   V-type position effects at the light locus in Drosophila melanogaster. Genetics 43: 395–403.

JUDD, B. H., 1955   Direct proof of a variegated-type position effect at the white locus in Drosophila melanogaster. Genetics 40: 739–744.

KARPEN, G. H., and A. C. SPRADLING, 1990   Reduced DNA polytenization of a minichromosome region undergoing position-effect variegation in Drosophila. Cell 63: 97–107.

KORNHER, J. S., and S. A. KAUFMAN, 1986   Variegated expression of the Sgs-4 locus in Drosophila melanogaster. Chromosoma 94: 205–216.

LEWIS, E. B., 1950   The phenomenon of position effect. Adv. Genet. 3: 73–115.

LOCKE, J., M. A. KOTARSKI and K. D. TARTOF, 1988   Dosage-dependent modifiers of position effect variegation in Drosophila and a mass action model that explains their effect. Genetics 120: 181–198.

MCCLINTOCK, B., 1950   The origin and behavior of mutable loci in maize. Proc. Natl. Acad. Sci. USA 36: 344–355.

MCCLINTOCK, B., 1951   Chromosome organization and genic expression. Cold Spring Harbor Symp. Quant. Biol. 16: 13–47.

MORGAN, T. H., C. B. BRIDGES and J. SCHULTZ, 1936   Constitution of the germinal material in relation to heredity. Yearbook Carnegie Inst. 35: 289–297.

MORGAN, T. H., C. B. BRIDGES and J. SCHULTZ, 1937   Constitution of the germinal material in relation to heredity. Yearbook Carnegie Inst. 36: 298–305.

MORGAN, T. H., and J. SCHULTZ, 1942   Investigations on the constitution of the germinal material in relation to heredity. Yearbook Carnegie Inst. 41: 242–245.

MORGAN, T. H., J. SCHULTZ and V. CURRY, 1941   Investigations on the constitution of the germinal material in relation to heredity. Yearbook Carnegie Inst. 40: 282–287.

MULLER, H. J., 1930   Types of visible variations induced by X-rays in Drosophila. J. Genet. 22: 299–334.

NOUJDIN, N. I., 1936   Genetic analysis of certain problems of the physiology of development of Drosophila melanogaster. Biol. Zh. (Mosk.) 4: 571–624.

NOUJDIN, N. I., 1944   The regularities of the influence of heterochromatin on mosaicism. Zh. Obshch. Biol. 5: 357–388.

NOVITSKI, W., 1961   The regular reinversion of the roughest[3] inversion. Genetics 46: 711–717.

PANSHIN, I. B., 1935   New evidence for the position effect hypothesis. C. R. Acad. Sci. USSR 4: 85–88.

PROKOFYEVA-BELGOVSKAYA, A. A., 1937   Structure of the Y-chromosome in salivary gland's cells of Drosophila melanogaster. Genetics 22: 94–104.

PROKOFYEVA-BELGOVSKAYA, A. A., 1939   Cytological mechanism of variegation and chromosomal rearrangements. C. R. Acad. Sci. USSR 22: 274–277.

PROKOFYEVA-BELGOVSKAYA, A. A., 1974   Heterochromatization as a change of chromosome cycle. J. Genet. 48: 80–98.

REUTER, G., I. WOLFF and B. FRIEDE, 1985   Functional properties of the heterochromatic sequences inducing w^{m4} position-effect variegation in *Drosophila melanogaster*. Chromosoma **93:** 132–139.

REUTER, G., M. GIARRE, J. PARAH, J. GAUSZ, A. SPIERER and P. SPIERER, 1990 Dependence of position-effect variegation in Drosophila on dose of a gene encoding an unusual zinc-finger protein. Nature **344:** 219–225.

RUSHLOW, C. A., W. BENDER and A. CHOVNICK, 1984 Studies on the mechanism of heterochromatic position effect at the *rosy* locus of *Drosophila melanogaster*. Genetics **108:** 603–615.

SCHULTZ, J., 1936 Variegation in Drosophila and the inert chromosome regions. Proc. Natl. Acad. Sci. USA **22:** 27–33.

SCHULTZ, J., 1956 The relationship of heterochromatic chromosome regions to the nucleic acids of the cell. Cold Spring Harbor Symp. Quant. Biol. **21:** 307–328.

SCHULTZ, J., and T. DOBZHANSKY, 1934 The relation of a dominant eye color in *Drosophila melanogaster* to the associated chromosome rearrangement. Genetics **19:** 344–364.

SINCLAIR, D. A. R., R. C. MOTTUS and T. A. GRIGLIATTI, 1983 Genes which suppress position-effect variegation in *Dro-sophila melanogaster* are clustered. Mol. Gen. Genet. **191:** 326–333.

SPANA, C., D. A. HARRISON and V. G. CORCES, 1988 The *Drosophila melanogaster suppressor of Hairy-wing* protein binds to specific sequences of the gypsy retrotransposon. Genes Dev. **2:** 1414–1423.

SPOFFORD, J. B., 1967 Single-locus modification of position-effect variegation in *Drosophila melanogaster*: I. *white* variegation. Genetics **57:** 751–766.

TARTOF, K. D., C. HOBBS and M. JONES, 1984 A structural basis for variegating position effects. Cell **37:** 869–878.

TAYLOR, J. H., 1964 Regulation of DNA replication and variegation-type position-effect. Cytogenetics of cells in culture. Symp. Int. Soc. Cell Biol. **3:** 175–183.

WARGENT, J. M., and I. J. HARTMANN-GOLDSTEIN, 1974 Replication behavior and morphology of a rearranged chromosome region in Drosophila. Chromosomes Today **5:** 109–116.

ZUCKERKANDL, E., 1974 Recherches sur les propriétés et l'activité biologique de la chromatine. Biochimie **56:** 937–954.

Our Diamond Birthday Anniversary

James F. Crow

Genetics Department, University of Wisconsin–Madison, Madison, Wisconsin 53706

GENETICS is 75 years old. Volume 1, number 1 was dated January, 1916 and with this issue the journal begins its 76th year. At this ripe age, the journal shows none of the telltale signs of senescence; it is still in the growth phase. Although the science of genetics has changed enormously–has indeed been revolutionized–the important features of GENETICS have remained intact. It is still, as it was in 1916, "a periodical record of investigations bearing on heredity and variation." The relationship between GENETICS and the Genetics Society of America has always been close, although the journal did not become the official organ of the Society until 1963.

The very first article was pure sterling; I can't imagine a better beginning. It was C. B. BRIDGES' classic, "Nondisjunction as proof of the chromosome theory of heredity." Here he showed that each genetic misbehavior was accompanied by a cytologically visible chromosome error, clinching the argument for the chromosomal basis of heredity. It is hard now to understand why this idea was so slow to be universally accepted. There were still skeptics in 1916, but BRIDGES' study left no room for doubt. What a way to launch a new journal!

Before discussing other pioneering articles, I'll give some statistics. The original number of subscribers was 270. The present mailing list is about 5000. The journal began with 6 issues per year. This was adhered to, with occasional extra numbers to shorten the backlog, until 1960 when the present monthly schedule was adopted. The original price was $6 per year, and this continued until 1951 when, with considerable reluctance, the Editorial Board raised it to $8. The journal originally gave each author 100 free reprints with covers. This was later reduced to 50 without covers, and by 1953 none was free. The first volume had 627 pages. In contrast, the three volumes in 1990 totaled 3022 pages.

Papers were long in those early days. In the first issue the journal announced that "shorter" articles were preferred: "Length of contributions to GENETICS will not be arbitrarily limited, but articles of less than 50 pages may be expected to appear more promptly than those of greater length." Nevertheless, several articles exceeding 50 pages appeared in early volumes. The entire September issue the first year was devoted to a 128-page article by H. S. JENNINGS on the genetics of the rhizopod *Difflugia corona*. The November issue of Volume 2 was devoted to a 105-page article by E. M. EAST on self-sterility mechanisms. DAVENPORT's article on human stature in July, 1917 ran to 77 pages. (Incidentally, JENNINGS, EAST, and DAVENPORT were all members of the Editorial Board.) And BRIDGES' blockbuster took 109 pages and was divided between the first two issues. The journal soon became more strict and, by 1953, only 20 pages were permitted. I should note, for those making comparisons to the present, that a page in those days had about 500 words, about 60% of the current number.

The original Editorial Board was an eminent group, all prominent researchers: WILLIAM E. CASTLE (mammalian genetics), EDWIN G. CONKLIN (cell lineages), CHARLES B. DAVENPORT (human genetics), BRADLEY M. DAVIS (Oenothera), EDWARD M. EAST (plant genetics), R. A. EMERSON (maize), H. S. JENNINGS (protozoa), T. H. MORGAN (Drosophila) and RAYMOND PEARL (poultry breeding and human demography). The founding editor was GEORGE H. SHULL. The new journal was his passion and he gave it minute and loving attention. Long after his retirement, subsequent editors were made aware of his continued interest. They frequently heard from him regarding what he took to be lapses in the editing process. In particular, an asterisk was to be used specifically to designate support for unusual composition or illustration costs from the Galton and Mendel Fund *and for no other purpose*. Violation of this latter clause guaranteed a prompt reprimand from SHULL.

SHULL was a pioneer in plant breeding. He first realized the great importance of heterosis when he observed hybrid sunflowers that were twice as tall as their parents. He was already involved in inbreeding and hybridization of a number of plants. Most noteworthy, of course, was maize. He quickly discovered the useful properties—high yield and uniformity—of hybrids between inbred lines. This led him to become the founder of what has turned out to be the outstanding practical application of genetics, hybrid corn. SHULL also coined the word "heterosis." By the time he became editor of GENETICS, his greatest work had been done. The journal took a great deal of his time and he published relatively little after accepting the editorship, which he held until 1926.

The earlier articles in GENETICS were not always in English. RICHARD GOLDSCHMIDT wrote two in German (July, 1916 and January, 1917). The second was particularly foolish, arguing against chromosome maps in Drosophila. Crossing over, GOLDSCHMIDT said, was an artifact caused by the chromosomes breaking into small pieces during interphase and later reassembling. This was promptly answered by STURTEVANT in the same volume (May, 1917). The early issues contained much more raw data than is now customary. Several times these involved large foldouts. A Drosophila pedigree in the BRIDGES paper was of a size that would rarely be found now, even in a human genetics article. Colored pictures also appeared in the first volume, in an article by R. R. HYDE in the November issue discussing the six alleles then known at the Drosophila *white* eye locus.

The famous lead article by BRIDGES did much more than clinch the chromosomal basis of heredity, which by this time was old hat to many, especially the MORGAN group. It was based on his doctoral thesis, a detailed study of nondisjunction in *Drosophila ampelophila* (as *D. melanogaster* was then called). The exceptions, which BRIDGES set such store by, proved immediately that the X chromosomes and not the Y determine the sex. The frequency, phenotype, and synapsis and segregation patterns of different nondisjunctional types—XO, XXY, XYY, XXX—were studied quantitatively and in great detail. These, along with triploid females, triploid intersexes (flies with two X chromosomes and three sets of autosomes), and female haploid tissue in mosaics, led BRIDGES to his genic balance theory of sex determination. Characteristic of his careful observation and his ability to recognize the significance of exceptions, was his finding that heterozygous females sometimes produced a nondisjunctional gamete with one crossover and one noncrossover chromosome. This offered for the first time genetic evidence for the four-strand nature of crossing

over. BRIDGES also used genetic evidence—missing markers and locally reduced recombination—to prove the existence of a deletion and determine its extent. And in the course of this research he uncovered more than a dozen new mutations.

BRIDGES was orphaned at age two and lived with his grandmother. He was sent to a small district school "when convenient." At age 14 he had missed so much that he failed the high school entrance examination and had to study two more years before being admitted. He finally graduated at age 20, but made up for lost time by finishing Columbia University in three years. He was hard pressed for funds. Scholarships helped, but he worked at various odd jobs, did tutoring and sold encyclopedias. He received his Ph.D. with MORGAN and was paid thereafter by the Carnegie Institution of Washington while working at Columbia and Caltech. Throughout his life he was underpaid and was the only one of MORGAN's group never to have a professorial position. I have often wondered if, in those less permissive days, his well known promiscuity might have limited his consideration for academic jobs.

BRIDGES continued to do great work. More than anyone else he was responsible for the collection and standardization of linkage data and the construction of chromosome maps. He was a founder and the major organizer of "Drosophila Information Service." He was the person who most successfully exploited the salivary gland chromosomes, and his cytological maps quickly became standard. He and H. J. MULLER did not always get on too well, although each respected the other, and there is a sad story to relate. In 1938 BRIDGES wrote to MULLER to suggest that they forget their differences and collaborate, blending his cytological skills with MULLER's genetic inventiveness. But BRIDGES died unexpectedly in 1938 when he was only 49. MULLER's friendly reply arrived a few days too late and BRIDGES never saw it.

There were other noteworthy articles in the early volumes of GENETICS. Two papers by EAST (March and July, 1916) set forth with great clarity the theoretical consequences and the experimental evidence for independent additive Mendelian factors for quantitative traits, especially in Nicotiana. D. F. JONES published an influential paper in September, 1917 arguing for dominance of linked genes as an alternative to overdominance in explaining heterosis. JONES also introduced four-way crosses so that the seeds could be grown on hybrid plants, thus greatly increasing the yield and reducing the cost of seed with no appreciable change in the yield of field plantings. He succeeded SHULL as editor of GENETICS from 1926 to 1936. (Some years later, when I had just finished graduate school and had been pronounced fully educated, he was introduced to me as "Mr. Jones, who is interested in genetics," whereupon I proceeded to explain the subject to him. He was a quick study, I needn't say and, I happily add, completely forgiving of my presumption.) In January, 1917 R. A. EMERSON published an article on variegated pericarp in maize, a forerunner of later work on transposable elements by MCCLINTOCK and BRINK. In September, 1918 MULLER published a pioneering paper in which he pointed out that lethal mutations are probably much more frequent than visibles, explained the enforced heterozygosis of a balanced lethal system in Drosophila, and discussed how such systems could be used in genetic research and stock-keeping.

The first issue of GENETICS included an article that is noteworthy, not so much for its content as for its author. HARVEY CUSHING, the famous Boston surgeon, reported an enormous pedigree of dominantly inherited symphalangism (stiff finger joints). The third article in the first issue–there were only three– was a numerical study of inbreeding by JENNINGS. It attracted considerable interest at the time, but was of little lasting value because it was soon subsumed under WRIGHT's inbreeding and relationship algorithms. Another early article, the one by DAVENPORT on human stature and body measurements, is interesting mainly for reaching a wrong conclusion. DAVENPORT believed that the genetic factors controlling body parts, such as arm and leg length, are largely independent of each other and that total size is the resultant of a number of such independent parts. This led WRIGHT (July, 1918), who disagreed with this interpretation, to examine some existing data on rabbits and to demonstrate the much greater influence of general size factors. An implication of WRIGHT's analysis here and later is that hybrids and F_2s between divergent strains have more harmonious body parts than if these were developmentally independent. This kind of analysis became important in dispelling fears, growing out of such ideas as DAVENPORT's, that segregants from crosses between human races of different sizes would have mismatches between different body parts. WRIGHT's paper is also noteworthy as an early example of subdividing the total variance into meaningful components, and it foreshadowed the kind of correlation analysis that characterized his later work.

By 1950 genetic research was invaded by microbes and molecules, and a new era had begun. In that year graduate students at the University of California in Berkeley, undoubtedly with the kindly guidance of then-editor CURT STERN, prepared an index of the first 35 volumes. It is a convenient way to see who and what dominated the contents of the journal in the days when classical genetics was paramount. One question that immediately arises is: who published the most papers? The two most prolific authors were SEWALL WRIGHT (29 articles) and THEODOSIUS DOBZHANSKY (32). In contrast, among those of comparable influence, STURTEVANT published 16, BRIDGES 10, MULLER 10, STADLER 3, and MORGAN only a biography (of BRIDGES). DOBZHANSKY's prolificacy in this period is especially impressive because his first article did not appear until 1930. He was one of the reasons for founding a new journal, *Evolution*, in 1947. And, to nobody's surprise, the first article in the new journal was by him. A second budding off from GENETICS occurred in 1949 with the first issue of *The American Journal of Human Genetics*. In this instance the leading figure was MULLER.

The first issue of GENETICS included a photograph and biography of GREGOR MENDEL. This started a trend. The first issues of succeeding volumes honored GALTON, DARWIN, DEVRIES, KÖLREUTER and WEISMANN; LAMARCK didn't make it until Volume 29. This fine custom has continued. The first issue of the most recent volume included an obituary of HERSCHEL ROMAN.

Finally, why did I entitle this article "*Our* Diamond Birthday Anniversary"? Because we share it. GENETICS and I were both expected in January, 1916. I arrived on schedule, but GENETICS was late; the first issue, although dated January, was mailed on March 10.

February 1991

Haldane's Solution
of the Luria-Delbrück Distribution

Sahotra Sarkar

Boston Center for the Philosophy and History of Science, Boston University, 745 Commonwealth Avenue, Boston, Massachusetts 02215

IN the 1940s it was still controversial whether bacterial mutants, such as those resistant to a particular phage, arose spontaneously (that is, at random) during the growth of a bacterial culture or in response to the presence of phage in the environment (SARKAR 1991). In order to answer this question, LURIA and DELBRÜCK (1943) devised their famous "fluctuation test." Several bacteria of the same genotype are allowed to grow for many generations in separate test tubes. The contents of these tubes are then separately inoculated onto plates containing phage. Sensitive bacteria die on the plates while resistant ones flourish and produce visible colonies. The number of such colonies, then, is equal to the number of resistant cells present in the generation of bacteria first plated.

Suppose that the resistant bacteria arose through spontaneous mutations during the growth of the bacteria in each of the tubes prior to plating. If there is always a small finite probability of mutation, mutations would occur very early in a few tubes and many mutant cells would be present in a generation much later because of exponential growth of the mutants through ordinary cell division (assuming back-mutations are negligible). In many other tubes there would be no mutations at all or only one in the last few generations. The distribution of mutants observed after plating would reflect this fact and would show considerable variance. Suppose, however, that mutations arose only because of some interaction between the bacteria and the phage. Then, in each of the plates, the only mutants observed would be those produced during the last generation, that is, after plating. The probability of a large number of mutants so produced in only a few tubes is low, and the distribution of observed mutants would have much lower variance than in the former case. This insight into the highly differing variances expected under the two possibilities of mutagenesis lies at the core of the fluctuation test.

The distribution of the number of mutants in the former case has since been routinely called the Luria-Delbrück distribution (SARKAR 1990). In the latter case, it becomes the familiar Poisson distribution with a mean and variance equal to the product of the probability of mutation of a bacterium and the number of bacteria. LURIA and DELBRÜCK's insight was not completely new. As LEDERBERG (1989) has pointed out, YANG and BRUCE WHITE (1934) had made a similar point while studying the resistance of *Vibrio cholerae* to cholera phage. However, LURIA and DELBRÜCK were the first to develop the insight systematically. In order to apply this test to their cultures, they had to investigate the theoretical properties of the Luria-Delbrück distribution. They managed to derive approximate expressions for the mean and the variance of the distribution but, citing "considerable mathematical difficulties," could not devise a way to compute the distribution itself.

Not surprisingly, LURIA and DELBRÜCK's results attracted the attention of J. B. S. HALDANE, then Weldon Professor of Biometry at University College, London. HALDANE found LURIA and DELBRÜCK's conclusion about mutagenesis convincing but set out to "improve" their statistical treatment. What he provided, in the process, was a combinatorial method for obtaining approximate but explicit expressions for the distribution. The results were recorded in a handwritten manuscript, "The Statistical Theory of Bacterial Mutations." HALDANE sent the manuscript to DELBRÜCK in 1946. It was read by LURIA, HERSHEY and others, and DELBRÜCK gave a talk based on it during the Phage Course at Cold Spring Harbor. It was attended, DELBRÜCK (1946) observed, "by those who took the phage course this year and by a few outsiders, mostly people to whom algebra is more strange than Chinese." DELBRÜCK also had the manuscript typed by a student and both the original and the typed copy were returned to HALDANE. He further circulated a copy to a few individuals, including LEDERBERG, who wrote to HALDANE trying (unsuccessfully) to enlist the latter's help for some related statistical problems (LEDERBERG 1946). This was the only exposure that the manuscript enjoyed. Though HALDANE's was the first solution of the Luria-Delbrück distribution, he never published it; possible reasons for this will be discussed below. The original manuscript is currently preserved in the archives of University College Library among a large collection of HALDANE's papers "rediscovered" there in the early 1980s.

The purpose of this article is to present HALDANE's main results with just enough detail to indicate how they may be obtained. Details of the method and its relation to subsequent work on the Luria-Delbrück distribution will be published separately. Besides their obvious historical interest, HALDANE's calculations are interesting for three other reasons. (i) Ever since the publication of the results of CAIRNS, OVERBAUGH and MILLER (1988) suggesting the possibility of directed mutagenesis in bacteria, the power and limitations of fluctuation analysis have once again become a matter of controversy (see SARKAR 1991 for a review). (ii) No closed analytic solution of the Luria-Delbrück distribution yet exists and, surprisingly, HALDANE's approximate method of calculation comes closest. (iii) It turns out that HALDANE, with his usual prescience, noted some difficulties (including deviations due to various factors) with the use of the distribution (and, consequently, fluctuation analysis) which would only resurface later. In describing HALDANE's results, some trivial algebraic errors have been corrected; any remaining errors are likely to be mine, not his. Some of HALDANE's mathematical claims were left without proof. These have been checked.

In passing it should be noted that R. A. FISHER, too, might have solved the Luria-Delbrück distribution in 1946. CROW (1990) notes that he was convinced by LURIA and DELBRÜCK's experiments but found their mathematical treatment "shoddy and confusing." In 1946 he approached FISHER with the problem. FISHER "leaned back in his chair, thought for perhaps a minute, took a scrap of paper, and wrote a generating function." CROW, not immediately understanding the result, set the paper aside to work on later but lost it along with interest in the problem. Unless that scrap of paper is rediscovered it is improbable that FISHER's possible solution will ever be brought to light.

HALDANE'S RESULTS

Assume, initially, that all the bacteria have grown from a single genotype and that divisions are synchronous, that there are no deaths and no back-mutation, and that mutation occurs only during cell division with only one of the resultant cells being mutant. These are the conditions of an "ideal" experiment. HALDANE treated this case first before studying the effect of four different factors on the resulting distribution. Let n be the number of cell generations after which phage is added. Then $N = 2^n$ is the number of bacteria in a culture. Let m be the probability of mutation during a division, x the number of mutants in a culture of $N = 2^n$ bacteria, and P_x the probability of finding just x mutants. Let $g = mN/2$.

HALDANE argues that, for a successful experiment, N must be so chosen that $g \approx 1$. If it is much smaller, virtually all cultures will contain no mutants. If it is much larger, the number of mutants will be practically uncountable. Now, P_0 is the probability that no mutants are present, that is, no mutations have occurred in $N - 1$ divisions. Thus, for $g \approx 1$,

$$P_0 = (1 - m)^{N-1}$$
$$= e^{-2g}[1 + 2g(1 - g)N^{-1} + O(N^{-2})] \approx e^{-2g}$$

where $O(N^{-2})$ means neglected terms of order N^{-2} or less. When no mutations occurred during the first $n - 2$ generations and one mutation occurred in the last $(n - 1)$ generation, exactly one mutant is present. Thus

$$P_1 = (1 - m)^{N-2}(mN/2)$$
$$= ge^{-2g}[1 + 2g(2 - g)N^{-1} + O(N^{-2})] \approx ge^{-2g}.$$

When $x > 1$, all the different ways in which x mutants could have arisen have to be considered. For $x = 2$, either one mutation occurred two generations ago, or two occurred one generation ago. Thus

$$P_2 = (1 - m)^{N-4}(mN/4) + (1 - m)^{N-3}m^2(N/2)(N/2 - 1)$$
$$= (1/2)e^{-2g}\{g[1 + 2g(4 - g)N^{-1}]$$
$$+ g^2[1 - 2(2 - 3g + g^2)N^{-1}] + O(N^{-2})\}$$
$$\approx [g(1 + g)/2]e^{-2g}.$$

HALDANE observes that the number of ways corresponds to all partitions of x into powers of 2 (including $1 = 2^0$). The number of such partitions is the coefficient of t^x in the expansion of $1/[(1 - t)(1 - t^2) \cdot (1 - t^4) \dots]$ in increasing powers of t. Each partition corresponds to a different way of generating x mutants.

HALDANE considers the case $x = 5$ in detail. There are four possible partitions of 5: $1(2^2) + 1(2^0)$; $2(2^1) + 1(2^0)$; $1(2^1) + 3(2^0)$; and $5(2^0)$ (see Figure 1). For each of these mutually exclusive cases, the probability has to be computed and then summed to obtain P_5. Consider the third partition, $1(2^1) + 3(2^0)$. One mutation occurred during the $N/4$ divisions two generations

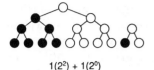

$1(2^2) + 1(2^0)$

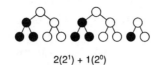

$2(2^1) + 1(2^0)$

Form 1

Form 2

FIGURE 2.—The two forms of the terminal section of pedigrees when cell division is asynchronous. In form 1, both cells (after the first division) have undergone further division; in form 2, only one has.

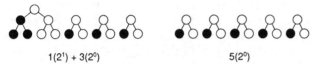

$1(2^1) + 3(2^0)$

$5(2^0)$

FIGURE 1.—Mutant pedigrees corresponding to partitions of 5 into powers of 2. Black circles represent mutants; white circles, nonmutants. Each of the four figures represents a possible set of pedigrees where only the part of the pedigree relevant to the mutation is shown. The numbers inside parentheses represent the type of mutation classified by when it occurred; the power of 2 is the number of generations ago that the mutation occurred. The numbers outside parentheses are the numbers of such mutations.

ago; its probability is $mN/4$. The other three took place in the nonmutant cells during the last $N/2$ divisions; their probability is $(1/3!)m^3(N/2 - 1)(N/2 - 2)(N/2 - 3)$. Thus the total probability associated with this partition is

$$(1 - m)^{N-6}(mN/24)m^3(N/2 - 1)(N/2 - 2)(N/2 - 3)$$

$$= (1/12)g^4 e^{-2g}[1 - 2(6 - 6g + g^2)N^{-1} + O(N^{-2})].$$

Computing probabilities for the other partitions in this fashion,

$$P_5 = (g^5 + 10g^4 + 15g^3 + 30g^2)e^{-2g}/5! + O(N^{-1}).$$

In general, according to HALDANE, a partition of x into $\Sigma_{i=0,k}a(i)2^i$ gives rise to a term $e^{-2g}g^{\Sigma a(i)}/\prod_{i=0,k}a(i)2^{ia(i)}$. These values are accurate only when N is infinite. Consequently, HALDANE notes, the moments of the distribution of x cannot be obtained in this manner because, as N goes to infinity, the moments diverge. For finite N, however, HALDANE calculates the moments by deriving recursion relations for the change of the moments with n (the number of generations). This gives the following expressions for the mean (k_1), the variance (k_2) and the third moment (k_3):

$$k_1 = g(\log N)/(\log 2) + O(N^{-1}),$$

$$k_2 = gN + O(N^{-1}),$$

$$k_3 = gN^2/2 + O(N^{-1}).$$

HALDANE observes that these results show that the mutation rate, m, cannot be reliably obtained from the mean. If values of x are obtained from s populations of N, the variance of the mean is $1/s$ times the variance of x and, therefore, extremely large (when N/s is large, as is usual).

HALDANE next gives a systematic treatment of the effects on these results of deviations from the conditions of the ideal experiment. Four cases are considered. *First*, he considers the effect of plating only a fraction of the total population, gives expressions for P_x in this case and calculates the moments of the distribution. As previously, he shows that the mean does not give a reliable measure of the mutation rate. *Second*, he considers nonsynchronous divisions. He notes that P_0 and P_1 are unaffected because, in the formation of N bacteria, exactly $N - 1$ divisions must have taken place and the calculation of these two numbers depends on nothing else. P_2, however, is diminished. This is so because the terminal sections of the pedigrees have one of the two forms indicated in Figure 2. Let there be a instances of the first form and b instances of the second. Then $N = 4a + 3b$. Now, from the first form there can be 2 related mutants present if either (but not both) of the products of the first division is a mutant. From the second form, however, the cell that undergoes further division must be mutant to produce 2 related mutants. Nonrelated mutants can occur as before. Hence, approximately,

$$P_2 = [m(a + b/2) + (m^2/2)(N/2)^2](1 - m)^N + O(N^{-1})$$

$$\approx g[(2a + b)/(4a + 3b) + g/2]e^{-2g}.$$

This number is smaller than the case when divisions are synchronous; $(2a + b)/(4a + 3b)$ would be replaced by $1/2$. However, a similar analysis shows that P_3 increases. The general effect is that the distribution becomes smoother, that is, the variance decreases.

Third, HALDANE considers the effect of the death of some bacteria. Let h be the probability that a bacterium dies before it divides and assume that this is constant. If divisions are synchronous, $N = 2^n(1 - h)^n$. The average number of last divisions is $N/2(1 - h)$. Consequently P_0, P_1, etc., all turn out to be smaller than before and the distribution once again becomes smoother. *Fourth*, HALDANE argues that mutants must have a lower growth rate than nonmutants in the original medium because their frequencies are so low. This can happen because of a lower fitness or a back-mutation rate greater than the forward rate, though this latter possibility would have only a negligible effect on P_x when x is small. Let the average growth rate of mutants be q times that of the normal ($q \leq 1$). Suppose that 2^n bacteria would have resulted in the absence of any mutation. If $x = 0$ or 1, the actual number (N) of bacteria would be unaffected. P_0 will thus be unaltered. However,

$$P_1 = (1 + q/2)ge^{-2g} + O(N^{-1})$$

because only a fraction q of mutants which would otherwise have divided will actually have done so. Thus P_1 will be slightly increased. Similar results hold for the other P^x. In either of these last two situations, Haldane observes, it can be shown that the moments are finite.

DISCUSSION

At the time that HALDANE completed these calculations no solutions of the Luria-Delbrück distribution, approximate or otherwise, were available. Though his correspondence suggests that he ultimately wanted to publish the results, other work, especially in human genetics, as well as departmental reorganization after the War seems to have taken precedence. Meanwhile, in 1948, C. A. COULSON submitted to the *Journal of Genetics*, of which HALDANE was editor, a paper by COULSON and D. E. LEA entitled "The Distribution of the Number of Mutants in Bacterial Populations." LEA, who had collaborated earlier with HALDANE on a mathematical approach to chromosomal rearrangements (LEA and HALDANE 1947), had unexpectedly died in June, 1947. LEA and COULSON had not been able to provide a closed analytic solution of the Luria-Delbrück distribution but, treating the problem using differential equations, had developed an explicit procedure that permitted accurate numerical calculation of the distribution, though only under the conditions of the ideal experiment. HALDANE agreed to print the paper and apparently wanted only to add an appendix containing the argument about asynchronous divisions outlined above (COULSON 1948). However, COULSON was in a hurry and HALDANE appears not to have had time to write this appendix. The paper by LEA and COULSON (1949) was published without it and HALDANE never returned to the problem. Given his general tendency to treat the solution of theoretical problems only to the extent of their numerical evaluation (with a hope of eventually connecting the theory with experiment), HALDANE probably felt that his method had been superseded by that of LEA and COULSON or, at least, that there was not enough important novelty in his method to make it worth pursuing, especially given the wide variety of his interests. In any case, LEA and COULSON's paper has since routinely been considered the first solution

of the Luria-Delbrück distribution (SARKAR 1991).

However, HALDANE's method permits writing closed analytic (though only approximate) expressions for P_x, which no other method does to date. Moreover, the combinatorial argument used to obtain these values is elegant and simple, which adds didactic value to this treatment. It is also the only combinatorial treatment of what is essentially a combinatorial problem. Further, no one seems to have discussed the effect of asynchronous division in such explicit detail. The effect of deaths seems also to have been largely ignored. Differential growth rates and the effect of sampling were first treated by ARMITAGE (1952) who gave a much more rigorous treatment of the problem than did LEA and COULSON (1949). ARMITAGE also treated phenotypic lag, the one major confounding factor ignored by HALDANE. That this would cause a problem had already been noticed by DELBRÜCK (1946) in the letter to HALDANE which accompanied the returned manuscript. MANDELBROT (1974) attempted to explain why the various moments of the distribution diverged in the way they did. He also provided an analytic form for the Laplace transform of the Luria-Delbrück distribution, though this is of hardly any use in computation.

STEWART, GORDON and LEVIN (1990) have provided the most extensive procedure to date for the numerical calculation of the Luria-Delbrück distribution under a wide variety of "nonideal" conditions. W. T. MA, G. VH. SANDRI and S. SARKAR (unpublished results) have provided the simplest and most efficient procedure for calculating the Luria-Delbrück distribution and also a new integral representation. Virtually all the new concerns treated comprehensively by STEWART, GORDON and LEVIN (1990) are strikingly present in HALDANE's original attempt. Most importantly, he had first seen that the effect of these other factors would decrease the variance of the distribution. Such a shift alone, therefore, does not demonstrate the occurrence of any directed mutations in bacteria and it is precisely this point, and claims that the late-appearing mutants follow a Poisson distribution and seem to be under genetic control, which lie at the core of the current controversy about directed mutations that began with the publication of the experimental results of the CAIRNS group in 1988 (SARKAR 1990). As in so many other areas, HALDANE had shown remarkable prescience.

Thanks are due to JOHN CAIRNS and FRANK STEWART for comments on an earlier draft of this paper. Moreover, this paper would not have been possible without the assistance of G. FURLONG and the staff of the archives of University College Library, London, R. D. HARVEY, Archivist, John Innes Institute, Norwich, the archival staff of the National Library of Scotland, and the encouragement of JOHN MAYNARD SMITH, GRAEME MITCHISON and NAOMI MITCHISON. The work reported here was supported by an archival research grant from the American Philosophical Society. TRACY

LUBAS prepared the diagrams. It is a pleasure to acknowledge these debts. This is Contribution No. BTBG 90-4 from the Boston Theoretical Biology Group.

LITERATURE CITED

ARMITAGE, P., 1952 The statistical theory of bacterial populations subject to mutation. J. R. Stat. Soc. B **14:** 1–40.

CAIRNS, J., J. OVERBAUGH and S. MILLER, 1988 The origin of mutants. Nature **335:** 142–145.

COULSON, C. A., 1948 Letter to J. B. S. Haldane, 12/14/48. Haldane Archives, National Library of Scotland.

CROW, J. F., 1990 R. A. Fisher, a centennial view. Genetics **124:** 207–211.

DELBRÜCK, M., 1946 Letter to J. B. S. Haldane, 8/20/46. Haldane Papers, University College Library, London.

LEA, D. E., and A. C. COULSON, 1949 The distribution of the numbers of mutants in bacterial populations. J. Genet. **49:** 264–285.

LEA, D. E., and J. B. S. HALDANE, 1947 A mathematical theory of chromosomal rearrangements. J. Genet. **48:** 1–10.

LEDERBERG, J., 1946 Letter to J. B. S. Haldane, 10/12/46. Genetical Society Papers. John Innes Institution, Norwich.

LEDERBERG, J., 1989 Replica plating and indirect selection of bacterial mutants: isolation of preadaptive mutants in bacteria by sib selection. Genetics **121:** 395–399.

LURIA, S. E., and M. DELBRÜCK, 1943 Mutations of bacteria from virus sensitivity to virus resistance. Genetics **28:** 491–511.

MANDELBROT, B., 1974 A population birth-and-mutation process. I. Explicit distributions for the number of mutants in an old culture of bacteria. J. Appl. Prob. **11:** 437–444.

SARKAR, S., 1990 On the possibility of directed mutagenesis in bacteria: statistical analyses and reductionist strategies, pp. 111–124 in *PSA–1990*, Vol. 1, edited by A. FINE, M. FORBES and L. WESSELS. Philosophy of Science Association, East Lansing, Mich.

SARKAR, S., 1991 Lamarck contre Darwin, reduction versus statistics–conceptual aspects of the directed mutagenesis in bacteria controversy, in *Organism and the Origin of Self*, edited by A. I. TAUBER. Kluwer, Dordrecht (in press).

STEWART, F., D. GORDON and B. LEVIN, 1990 Fluctuation analysis: the probability distribution of the number of mutants under different conditions. Genetics **124:** 175–185.

YANG, Y. N., and P. BRUCE WHITE, 1934 Rough variation in *V. cholerae* and its relation to cholera-phage. J. Pathol. Bacteriol. **38:** 187–200.

April 1991

Fifty Years Ago
The Neurospora Revolution

Norman H. Horowitz

Biology Division, California Institute of Technology, Pasadena, California 91125

THIS year marks the fiftieth anniversary of the publication of one of the pivotal works of modern biology, the first Neurospora paper of BEADLE and TATUM (1941). This brief paper, revolutionary in both its methods and its findings, changed the genetic landscape for all time. Where previously there existed only scattered observations (albeit with some acute insights) on the relation between genetics and biochemistry, this paper established biochemical genetics as an experimental science, one in which progress would no longer be limited by the rarity of mutants with biochemically knowable phenotypes, but where such mutants would be generated at will and where findings could be repeated and hypotheses explored, as in other experimental sciences. This paper was the first in a series of fundamental advances in chemical genetics that by 1953 had bridged the gap between genetics and biochemistry and ushered in the age of molecular biology.

I have explained in a recent memoir of BEADLE (HOROWITZ 1990) how the Neurospora investigation arose from his earlier study of the genetics of eye-color synthesis in Drosophila with BORIS EPHRUSSI, and I will not repeat this history here.

The methodological innovations of the BEADLE-TATUM paper were twofold. First, the authors introduced what was for most geneticists a new kind of experimental organism–a microorganism that was ideally suited for classical genetic studies but which differed from the classical organisms in that it grew readily on a medium of defined chemical composition. It was actually superior in some ways to the usual experimental species because the entire meiotic tetrad could be recovered and cultured. This novel creature was the filamentous ascomycete *Neurospora crassa*. (*Neurospora sitophila* was also used in the early studies, but was abandoned before long in favor of *N. crassa*.) It is well known that the investigations that led to the development of molecular genetics largely employed microorganisms, but it should be pointed out that the Neurospora discoveries first described in the 1941 paper were crucial for making bacteria genetically useful.

BEADLE had learned of Neurospora at a lecture by B. O. DODGE given at Cornell University in 1930, when the former was a graduate student. DODGE, a mycologist at the New York Botanical Garden, was a strong advocate of Neurospora as a genetic organism. It was he who found that the ascospores–the products of meiosis–required heat shock to induce germination. (He had made this discovery originally in Ascobolus, by accident, after setting down some plates of ascospores in a sterilizing oven that he thought was turned off.) This finding made Neurospora available for genetic studies, and DODGE worked out the basic genetics of the organism. Among other things, he investigated the inheritance of mating type, albinism, and other monogenic characters. He showed that the eight ascospores of an ascus display a perfect Mendelian ratio (4:4). By isolating and culturing the ascospores in the linear order in which they occur in the ascus, he discovered the patterns of first- and second-division segregations. DODGE also understood the benefits that haploidy offered for genetic studies. When combined with the other features of Neurospora, it convinced him that this ascomycete was the ideal genetic organism. He frequently pointed this out to his friend T. H. MORGAN, arguing that it was actually superior to Drosophila (ROBBINS 1962).

As its second methodological innovation, the BEADLE-TATUM paper introduced a procedure for recovering an important class of lethal mutations, namely those blocking the synthesis of essential biological substances. These were expressed in the organism as new nutritional requirements. These mutations were crucial for understanding the biochemistry of gene action. They displayed in a most convincing manner the central importance of genes in biochem-

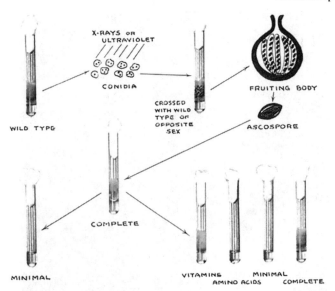

FIGURE 1.—BEADLE's lantern slide explaining the procedure for isolating biochemical mutants of Neurospora.

istry and ended forever the idea that the role of the genes in metabolism was somehow a subordinate one. Genetics, which before the Neurospora revolution had been notably isolated from the physical sciences, now found itself in the mainstream of biochemistry. Or, more correctly, genetics and biochemistry were now seen to be different aspects of the same thing.

A diagram of the BEADLE-TATUM procedure is shown in Figure 1. This figure is reproduced from a lantern slide drawn and lettered by BEADLE, one of a set that he used in lectures in the 1940s. As the slide suggests, BEADLE favored the word "sex" rather than "mating type" in his writing and speaking about Neurospora. It should be noted that the test tube labeled "vitamins" also contained nucleic acid components.

The essential character of the substances whose syntheses were affected in the Neurospora mutants—amino acids, purines, pyrimidines, vitamins—suggested that similar mutations should occur in other microbial species. This proved to be the case. In the first important extension of the Neurospora findings, GRAY and TATUM (1944) showed that "biochemical mutations" could be induced in bacteria. This result solved a fundamental difficulty that had long prevented progress toward a genetics of bacteria–that is, the lack of suitable markers–and led directly to the demonstration of genetic recombination in *Escherichia coli* by TATUM's student JOSHUA LEDERBERG. Biochemical mutations were induced later in yeast and other microorganisms. Modern microbial genetics is to a large extent based on mutations of the type first described by BEADLE and TATUM in their 1941 paper and on temperature-sensitive alleles of these and other essential genes. The discovery of temperature-sensitive mutants followed directly from the 1941 paper, as will be shown later.

Aside from its revolutionary methods, the BEADLE-TATUM paper was remarkable for the results it reported. It described three X-ray-induced mutants that grew on "complete medium" (a complex, undefined mixture containing yeast extract), but that failed to grow on "minimal medium" (a mixture consisting of the minimal nutrients capable of supporting the growth of wild-type Neurospora). The presumption was that the mutations expressed in these cultures affected genes needed for the production of growth-essential compounds present in complete, but not minimal, medium. A systematic search revealed that each of the mutants required a different substance. The three substances were pyridoxine, thiamine and *p*-aminobenzoic acid, and the inability to synthesize them was eventually shown, in every case, to be inherited as a single-gene defect. (The 1941 paper reported on the genetics of only the "pyridoxineless" mutant.) The thiamine-requiring mutant was found to respond to the thiazole moiety of thiamine by itself, implying that the mutant could synthesize the pyrimidine half of the molecule and showing that genes were limited in the range of their individual chemical effects.

The fact that the first three mutants found by BEADLE and TATUM were vitamin auxotrophs reflects, at least in part, the relatively high frequency of such mutants recovered by their method of mutant selection. [See BEADLE and TATUM (1945), Table 5, for a listing of all Neurospora mutants identified and cited in the literature up to that time.] In this method, ascospore descendants of irradiated conidia were isolated and cultured separately (see Figure 1), a procedure that recovers even mutants with trace requirements. The mass selection procedures that came later are biased against such mutants because of cross-feeding.

The pyridoxineless mutant, No. 299, is of special interest. This was the first mutant found by BEADLE and TATUM, and it was one of the few that were recovered in *N. sitophila*. It was, so to speak, the breakthrough mutant, the one that vindicated their ideas about a new kind of genetics. But its importance did not end there. Soon after the 1941 paper was published, BEADLE received a letter from an acquaintance at the Merck Research Laboratory requesting a culture of No. 299 for the purpose of developing an assay method for pyridoxine. BEADLE sent a transfer, as he invariably did once a mutant had been referred to in print. BEADLE firmly believed that this policy was in the best interest of science, a belief that was certainly confirmed in this case because, in the course of their investigation, the Merck group discovered that No. 299 would grow without pyridoxine if the pH of minimal medium was raised to 6 from its normal value of 5 (STOKES, FOSTER and WOODWARD 1943).

I recall first hearing of this unexpected result at an

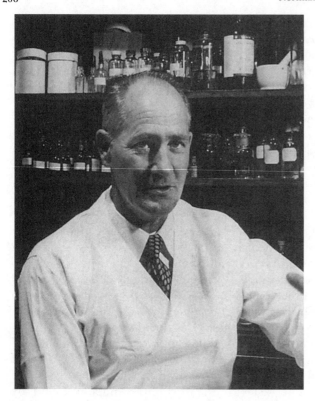

GEORGE BEADLE

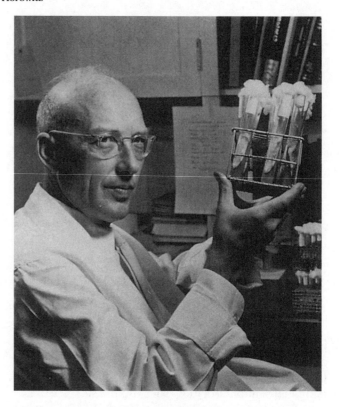

EDWARD TATUM

afternoon tea-break in the BEADLE lab at Stanford University. In the ensuing discussion, it was decided to learn if other environmental variables–temperature, in particular–might also affect the phenotype of mutants in a specific way. The mutant hunt that ran more or less continuously in the lab was accordingly modified to include an incubation step at 35° in addition to the usual one at 25°. Soon the first temperature-sensitive mutants were found. The first published description of one of these was by MITCHELL and HOULAHAN (1946). These mutants turned out to be very important–arguably more important than the nonconditional auxotrophs. By modifying the gene in such a way that its activity was abolished in only part of the organism's normal temperature range, temperature-sensitive mutants were essentially unselected. That is, mutants which in the ordinary course of events would be lost because of the impermeability, instability, or unavailability for any other reason of the genetic end-product, can be recovered as temperature-sensitive alleles. Regarding them in the light of present-day knowledge, we can see that any gene whose end-product is a protein should be recoverable as a temperature-sensitive mutant. This attribute made them useful in an early test of the one gene-one enzyme hypothesis (HOROWITZ 1948, 1950; HOROWITZ and LEUPOLD 1951). The utility of temperature-sensitive mutants for problems of this kind was rediscovered years later by EDGAR,

who has written a perceptive essay on the rediscovery (EDGAR 1966).

In another, and different, early application, a temperature-sensitive mutant of *E. coli* was used to demonstrate that genes determine the molecular properties, as well as the presence or absence, of enzymes (MAAS and DAVIS 1952).

The Neurospora mutants, as everyone knows, opened a new approach to the study of biosynthetic pathways, the cumulative results of which led to the one gene-one enzyme theory (BEADLE 1945). This theory had already been foreshadowed in the first paragraph of the 1941 paper, where the authors suggest the possibility that genes may act "by determining the specificities of enzymes" with the further possibility of "simple one-to-one relations" between genes and chemical reactions. These ideas doubtless grew out of the authors' earlier work on Drosophila eye colors. In his Nobel lecture, BEADLE, in an oft-quoted passage referring to one gene-one enzyme, said, "In this long, roundabout way, first in Drosophila and then in Neurospora, we had rediscovered what GARROD had seen so clearly so many years before" (BEADLE 1959; GARROD 1909). BEADLE was without doubt sincere in this characteristically generous remark, but was he right? And if he was right, does this diminish the importance of the BEADLE-TATUM accomplishment? The answer to both questions is, I think, "No."

In a penetrating discussion of the first question,

SCRIVER and CHILDS (1989) raise the question of whether, at this date, we can actually know what was in GARROD's mind when he wrote his great works on human hereditary disease. These authors show that GARROD's understanding of genetics appears not to have extended beyond 1910 (he lived until 1936). They suggest that "His words could have meant one thing to him when he uttered them and something else to us who are tempted to freight them with contemporary significance." They conclude that GARROD could hardly have had BEADLE's "one gene-one enzyme" idea in mind. It is hard to disagree with them when one considers the state of genetics and biochemistry at the time. The year 1909, when GARROD's famous book was published, was the same year that JOHANNSEN introduced the word *gene* into the language. The chromosome theory of inheritance was still in the future. Biochemistry was also in an embryonic state. In a monograph published in 1914, W. M. BAYLISS considered it necessary to defend the idea that enzymes could be assumed to be definite chemical compounds, "at all events until stronger evidence has been brought to the contrary." The one thing that seemed clear was that enzymes were not proteins (BAYLISS 1914). This question was not settled until SUMNER crystallized urease in 1926.

The same considerations must apply with equal or greater force to the most prescient of all writings about genes and enzymes, those of the French geneticist LUCIEN CUÉNOT. In 1903, CUÉNOT discussed his celebrated experiments on the inheritance of coat color in mice in terms of *mnémons* (genes), enzymes, and a chromogen (see WAGNER 1989). Sadly, CUÉNOT gave up genetics and discouraged his students from entering the field; see BURIAN, GAYON and ZALLEN (1988).

There were, of course, later antecedents of the one gene-one enzyme principle in the writings of WRIGHT, HALDANE and others, where unfamiliarity with modern science does not enter in. But while these works were correct in deducing that genes must act through their effects on enzymes (and other proteins), none of them succeeded in persuading geneticists of the classical era that a direct relation between genes and proteins was real and important and was, in fact, the key to understanding the organization of living matter. According to STURTEVANT (1965), geneticists were disinclined to accept simple ideas of gene action because they were convinced that development was too complex a process to be explained by any simple theory. Not long before he died, STURTEVANT told me that especially E. B. WILSON's position on gene action had carried much weight. WILSON, a cytologist, was one of the most influential figures in American biology. Although he died in 1939, the third edition of his monumental book, *The Cell in Development and Heredity*, published in 1925, is still in print. Usually very clearheaded, Wilson took what can only be described as an exceedingly murky view when, regarding the role of the genes, he wrote:

In what sense can the chromosomes be considered as agents of determination? By many writers they have been treated as the actual and even as the exclusive "bearers of heredity"; numerous citations from the literature of the subject might be offered to show how often they have been treated as central, governing factors of heredity and development, to which all else is subsidiary . . . Many writers, while avoiding this particular usage, have referred to the chromosomes or their components [WILSON rarely used the word "gene"] as "determiners" of corresponding characters; but this term, too, is becoming obsolete save as a convenient descriptive device. The whole tendency of modern investigation has been toward a different and more rational conception which recognizes the fact that the egg is a reaction-system . . . and that (to cite an earlier statement) "the whole germinal complex is directly or indirectly involved in the production of every character" (WILSON 1925).

In an obvious and not very interesting sense, the foregoing statement is correct; but in another and much more important one, it is altogether wrong. With the Neurospora revolution, musings of this sort on the nature of gene action faded away. The evidence for a one-to-one relation between genes and enzymes (actually proteins, later modified to polypeptides) now became clear, abundant and undeniable. The individual gene in some way determined the specific enzyme, although it was not yet seen how. The efforts of the pre-Neurospora workers to understand gene action had been made with systems often not suited for both biochemical and genetic studies. BEADLE and TATUM changed this by founding a new science based on an organism and an experimental protocol designed to be maximally useful for the purposes of biochemical genetics. In doing so, they transformed biology, and that is the reason we remember this fiftieth anniversary.

LITERATURE CITED

BAYLISS, W. M., 1914 *The Nature of Enzyme Action*, pp. 33, 36. Longmans, Green & Co., London.

BEADLE, G. W., 1945 Biochemical genetics. Chem. Rev. **37:** 15–96.

BEADLE, G. W., 1959 Genes and chemical reactions in Neurospora. Science **129:** 1715–1719.

BEADLE, G. W., and E. L. TATUM, 1941 Genetic control of biochemical reactions in *Neurospora*. Proc. Natl. Acad. Sci. USA **27:** 499–506.

BEADLE, G. W., and E. L. TATUM, 1945 Neurospora. II. Methods of producing and detecting mutations concerned with nutritional requirements. Am. J. Bot. **32:** 678–686.

BURIAN, R. M., J. GAYON and D. ZALLEN, 1988 The singular fate of genetics in the history of French biology, 1900–1940. J. Hist. Biol. **3:** 357–402.

EDGAR, R. S., 1966 Conditional lethals, pp. 166–170 in *Phage and the Origins of Molecular Biology*, edited by J. CAIRNS, G. S. STENT and J. D. Watson. Cold Spring Harbor Laboratory, Cold Spring Harbor, N.Y.

Garrod, A. E., 1909 *Inborn Errors of Metabolism.* Frowde, Hodder & Stoughton, London.

Gray, C. H., and E. L. Tatum, 1944 X-ray induced growth factor requirements in bacteria. Proc. Natl. Acad. Sci. USA **30:** 404–410.

Horowitz, N. H., 1948 The one gene-one enzyme hypothesis. Genetics **33:** 612–613.

Horowitz, N. H., 1950 Biochemical genetics of Neurospora. Adv. Genet. **3:** 33–71.

Horowitz, N. H., 1990 George Wells Beadle (1903–1989). Genetics **124:** 1–6.

Horowitz, N. H., and U. Leupold, 1951 Some recent studies bearing on the one gene-one enzyme hypothesis. Cold Spring Harbor Symp. Quant. Biol. **16:** 65–74.

Maas, W. K., and B. D. Davis, 1952 Production of an altered pantothenate-synthesizing enzyme by a temperature-sensitive mutant of *Escherichia coli.* Proc. Natl. Acad. Sci. USA **38:** 785–797.

Mitchell, H. K., and M. B. Houlahan, 1946 Neurospora. IV. A temperature-sensitive, riboflavinless mutant. Am. J. Bot. **33:** 31–35.

Robbins, W. J., 1962 Bernard Ogilvie Dodge. Biogr. Mem. Natl. Acad. Sci. USA **36:** 85–124.

Scriver, C. R., and B. Childs, 1989 *Garrod's Inborn Factors in Disease.* Oxford University Press, New York.

Stokes, J. L., J. W. Foster and C. R. Woodward, Jr., 1943 Synthesis of pyridoxin by a "pyridoxinless" x-ray mutant of *Neurospora sitophila.* Arch. Biochem. **2:** 235–245.

Sturtevant, A. H., 1965 *A History of Genetics,* p. 101. Harper & Row, New York.

Wagner, R. P., 1989 On the origins of the gene-enzyme hypothesis. J. Hered. **80:** 503–504.

Wilson, E. B., 1925 *The Cell in Development and Heredity,* 3rd edition, pp.975–976. Macmillan, New York.

Tomato Paste
A Concentrated Review of Genetic Highlights
from the Beginnings to the Advent of Molecular Genetics

Charles M. Rick

Department of Vegetable Crops, University of California, Davis, California 95616

THE following attributes account for the popularity of the tomato (*Lycopersicon esculentum*) for genetic research.

1. It is a basic diploid with minimal DNA duplication.

2. Its 12 chromosomes are highly differentiated and distinguishable.

3. The genome is replete with conventional and molecular markers and has well developed linkage maps.

4. The plant structure allows detection of a vast array of hereditary modification.

5. Related, intercrossable species afford a great wealth of readily accessible germplasm.

6. Excellent stock collections are maintained by the National Plant Germplasm System and the Tomato Genetics Resource Center.

7. The tomato is naturally self-pollinated, yet flowers are easily manipulated to yield large quantities of hybrid seed.

8. Tomato cells are readily cultured, hybridized, and whole plants regenerated therefrom.

9. The plants can be easily cultured in a wide range of environmental conditions; the tomato is amenable to sexual and asexual propagation.

10. The tomato offers the advantages of its edible crop status; much mutual benefit results from frequent exchanges between applied and basic research. You can study tomatoes and eat them too!

11. Recent developments reveal the tomato to be ideal for research in certain aspects of molecular genetics (RICK and YODER 1988). The maize *Ac* and *Ds* transposable elements have been incorporated into the tomato, where they actively transpose. Insertional mutagenesis may provide a means for cloning desired genes. Tomato has been transformed with DNA determining economic traits, including the delta endotoxin of *Bacillus thuringiensis* (which confers insect resistance), the capsid protein of tobacco mosaic virus (TMV) (which protects against infection by TMV), resistance to the herbicide glyphosate, and, via antisense RNA, reduced synthesis of polygalacturonase (which affects fruit firmness and disease susceptibility). Restriction fragment length polymorphism (RFLP) traits have been employed to greatly elucidate the genetics of several quantitative traits. These and other exciting developments were expedited by the pioneer studies of tomato genetics, the key events of which constitute the substance of this article.

The tomato was one of the many organisms investigated in the rash of genetic studies shortly after the "rediscovery" of MENDEL's work. The first publication was that of HALSTED, OWEN and SHAW (1905) on five distinctive morphological traits: dwarf plant habit, potato leaf, peach (fuzzy) fruits, yellow fruit flesh and colorless fruit epidermis. Although they ascertained dominance relations, it remained for PRICE and DRINKARD (1908) to demonstrate monogenic inheritance for these traits, in addition to lutescent foliage and pyriform fruit shape.

In the next three decades tomato investigations were sporadic and lagged far behind those in maize. Linkage studies trace back to D. F. JONES (1917), better known for his contributions to inbreeding and heterosis in maize, who reinterpreted data of HEDRICK and BOOTH (1907) on the cosegregation of dwarfness (*d*) and elongate fruit shape (*o*) as the consequence of linkage between them. E. W. LINDSTROM, whose major research was also in maize, followed with an intensive study of linkage on chromosome *2*, utilizing JONES' markers in addition to *p* and *s*. He also investigated autopolyploidy and radium-induced mutation, and described the first tomato haploid.

WINKLER (1909) reported the first autotetraploid

tomato, a somaclonal variant from tomato callus tissue developed at the region of grafting between tomato and *Solanum nigrum*. J. W. LESLEY (1928) reported and intensively studied the first known autotriploid. In the progeny of his triploid, LESLEY obtained the first tomato primary trisomics and, via the standard trisomic-ratio method, assigned four markers to their respective chromosomes. In subsequent years LESLEY and his wife MARGARET MANN LESLEY made many other important contributions to tomato genetics and cytogenetics.

Other pioneers of this period were J. W. MAC-ARTHUR and his student L. BUTLER. Their specialties were linkage and quantitative inheritance. Remarkable in both careers was their location in the Department of Zoology at the University of Toronto. Their research in tomato genetics was probably tolerated there because they concurrently investigated the genetics of mice (and muskrat ecology!).

In the 1940s and 1950s tomato genetics experienced a great expansion as a result of concurrent synergistic events. Until that time the tomato was regarded as poor material for chromosome cytology; only the tiny somatic and meiotic metaphase chromosomes seemed workable, but useful only for counts and extent of pairing. It is to BARBARA MCCLINTOCK that we owe an appreciation of the potential of the pachytene stage in tomato. Always active and scientifically curious, MCCLINTOCK applied her masterful techniques to demonstrate the potentialities of tomato cytogenetics. Her suggestions prompted S. W. BROWN (1949) to pursue the subject and reveal that the greatly extended chromosomes at this stage display good morphological differentiation into euchromatic and heterochromatic regions and that each arm terminates in a detectable telomere. Also significant was his observation that the contraction process after pachytene occurs primarily in euchromatin, the visible elements at metaphase being mostly heterochromatic. BROWN's student D. W. BARTON (1950) continued the research, providing the first descriptions and measurements for the identification of each of the 12 bivalents.

No account of this period would be complete without reference to the massive contributions of HANS STUBBE, for many years Director of the Institut für Kulturpflanzenforschung at Gatersleben, East Germany. Already renowned as successor to ERWIN BAUR as the world's authority on *Antirrhinum* genetics, STUBBE established an extensive program in the genetics and breeding of the cultivated tomato and the closely related wild species *Lycopersicon pimpinellifolium*. The large resources of this center and its professional staff were dedicated to various aspects of these subjects as well as the biochemistry and physiology of the tomato. As by-products of a search for agriculturally useful mutations induced by X-rays, about 300 monogenic mutants were induced in the former and 200 in the latter species. He documented the phenotypes and inheritance of all these mutants in a series of highly useful publications of the Institute. Eventually many of the mutants became well known as important linkage markers or genetic variants for a wide range of morphophysiological investigations. To mention examples, three of the *esculentum* mutants (*flc, not, sit*) tend to overwilt when drought-stressed. This phenomenon owes to aberrant stomate behavior caused by deficiency of abscisic acid. Also it is to the great credit of STUBBE that these mutants were freely exchanged internationally. He also conducted an elaborate investigation of the effects of grafts between 25 of these mutant strains and their isogenic normals, presumably to test claims by the LYSENKO group of graft-induced heritable changes. From 2,455 surviving grafts, some 30,000 first- and second-generation progeny were grown without detecting evidence of induced heritable changes (STUBBE 1954). Another experiment (STUBBE 1971) demonstrated that, by a program of induced mutation and selection, the fruit size of *L. pimpinellifolium* (~1 g) could be progressively increased within a few generations to approximate that of *L. esculentum* (150 g) and, similarly, fruit size of the latter could be diminished almost to the dimensions of the former.

Remarkable as these contributions were, it is all the more astonishing that they were accomplished behind the former "iron curtain." It is a credit to his personal courage that STUBBE could thus proceed in direct contradiction of the then prevailing LYSENKO dogma of graft hybridization and other aspects of the inheritance of acquired characters.

My role in this period was that of the lucky guy who happened to blunder onto the scene at the right time. Although I had experimented briefly with tomato genetics as a new graduate student under E. M. EAST, it was not until the late summer of 1942, after moving to my present position in Davis, that I delved into the subject in earnest. This renewed interest traces to a fertile suggestion by a fellow Department member, JOHN MACGILLIVRAY, that it might prove interesting to probe the causes of infertility of the so-called "bull" (unfruitful) plants commonly seen in tomato plantings. My first reaction was that this was a stupid, silly idea, but about a month later it dawned on me that such a survey might indeed be worthwhile. A few forays into nearby fields, then approaching harvest, revealed an unexpected wealth of genetic and cytological variation. By the end of that season we had acquired a series of male-sterile mutants in the three principal cultivars of that period, an array of meiotic and floral structural defects (all of which proved to be monogenic recessives), haploids, triploids (comprising two-thirds of the unfruitful plants), and tetraploids (RICK

1945). I was totally hooked and off to the races! In the next year 8 of the 12 primary trisomics, as well as other aneuploids, were identified morphologically in the progeny derived from the wealth of seeds in fruits naturally set on the triploids.

The timing of these events could not have been better. I teamed with BARTON for an attack on the primary trisomics; he identified the extra chromosomes in each trisomic type while I conducted genetic tests to identify the associated linkage groups (RICK and BARTON 1954). The acquisition of mutants from STUBBE and others provided the desired markers to populate the linkage maps; in fact, we had such a large array of mutants that we could afford to be selective, using only those with traits well expressed in early seedling stages. The program was also expedited by the establishment of the Tomato Genetics Cooperative (TGC) by BARTON and A. BURDICK in 1949 and administered at Davis for the following 32 years. The exchange of genetic stocks and information fostered by the TGC greatly facilitated and coordinated efforts to explore the genetic genome. Rules were adopted for systematization of tomato genetics and its nomenclature. We benefited in no small measure by the advice of M. M. GREEN and others with experience in genetically more advanced organisms.

The next great asset to tomato genetics was the arrival on the scene of GURDEV S. KHUSH. Having just completed his Ph.D. under G. L. STEBBINS (to my regret, not me, as so many assume), KHUSH joined our group at Davis, where his cytological skills provided a real shot in the arm for most of the 1960s. We embarked on a program of radiation-induced chromosomal changes that generated haploids, monosomics and trisomics of secondary, tertiary, telosomic and compensating types. Cytogenetic investigations of these aneuploids afforded localization of markers to all euchromatic arms and provided stocks for many other purposes and utilized in a wide variety of investigations.

In another phase of the project we induced deficiencies, irradiating normal (wild-type) pollen with fast neutrons to be applied to stigmas of various recessive marker stocks. Recessive progeny were selected for cytological study in the standard "pseudodominant" system used so effectively for cytological mapping in Drosophila. We chose to irradiate pollen rather than somatic tissue in order to avoid chimeral situations. The choice proved fortunate for another reason of which we were unaware at the time: recovery of deficiencies that would not survive gametogenesis. Because growth of angiosperm pollen tubes is presumably determined by the tube nucleus, defective sperm nuclei of irradiated mature pollen can be delivered at fertilization. The heterozygous deficiencies thereby generated were beautifully delineated at pachytene by

KHUSH's expertise, infinite patience and diligence. In this fashion we localized many markers in the complement, thereby matching the cytological and genetic maps (KHUSH and RICK 1968). In contrast to maize, disappointingly, none of the many cytologically detectable euchromatin deficiencies were transmitted through either male or female gametogenesis, thereby precluding establishing stocks of any of them. The only locus (ra) for which deficiencies were transmitted proved to reside in the proximal heterochromatin of 9L (KHUSH, RICK and ROBINSON 1964). The possibility could not be discounted that this marker is situated in a tiny enclave of euchromatic within an otherwise heterochromatic zone. Monosomics were also generated, but only for chromosomes 5, 11 and 12, leading to the conclusion that the imbalance of monosomy can exceed the tolerance of sporophytes, again in contrast to maize, in which all monosomics are viable. This extreme sensitivity to deficiency served to reinforce the concept (RICK 1971) that the tomato is essentially a basic diploid with little duplication of DNA in its complement.

The events of this early period were reflected in rapid progress in mapping the genome. When BUTLER (1952) published an early summary, linkage had been detected for 35 markers. By 1956, 45 were situated to their loci among 56 allocated to their respective chromosomes. A summary in 1963 revealed 86 loci for 136 allocated markers. These categories reached 190 of 258 markers in 1975. About 70% of these determinations were made by our team at Davis. Thus, by the end of the 1960s, the framework of the tomato genome had been established.

The prime development of the 1970s was the application of electrophoretic characters to resolve problems in the genome. At the 1968 International Congress of Genetics in Montreal, DICK LEWONTIN encouraged me to approach these problems by means of isozyme markers, research then in its early days. The suggestion proved timely and eventually fruitful. In this effort we were assisted greatly by R. W. ALLARD and his student ALEX KAHLER, who were already proficient in electrophoretic techniques and applying them to the population genetics of barley and other plants.

Our preliminary effort was a survey of the nature of enzyme variation in representative cultivated L. esculentum and its wild var. cerasiforme. We were disappointed at the lack of variation, virtually nil in the former and only sporadic in the latter, and these mostly in the native Andean area. One bonus of this otherwise rather uninteresting situation was the discovery that older cultivated tomato stocks and var. cerasiforme from Mesoamerica have identical genotypes, thus supporting JENKINS' (1948) hypothesis that the former were products of the latter's domestication. Undoubtedly the many bottlenecks experienced by the predominantly self-pollinating var. *cerasiforme* during its migrations from the Andes to Mesoamerica (the generally accepted area of domestication) account for this extreme genetic uniformity.

These results stimulated us to turn our attention to the related wild species. Fortunately, the very closely related currant tomato (*L. pimpinellifolium*) proved to be rich in isozyme variation (RICK, FOBES and HOLLE 1977). Because *L. esculentum* and *L. pimpinellifolium* are conspecific according to genetic criteria (reciprocally crossable, homosequential chromosomes, highly fertile F₁ hybrids, and normal inheritance), inheritance patterns of electrophoretic banding pattern differences in crosses between these species resolved loci *vs.* alleles (hence allozymes). These markers were quickly mapped in tests against standard linkage markers, thereby enriching the array of useful markers and adding another handy mapping technique. We eventually adopted the LA716 accession of *Lycopersicon pennellii* (also homosequential with *L. esculentum*) as a key parent for linkage tests. This stock has the advantage of a self-pollinating pure line, in contrast to the strict allogamy and consequent extreme polymorphy of all other accessions of the species (RICK and TANKSLEY 1981). Additionally, alleles of LA716 and standard *L. esculentum* differ at 20 loci among 10 of the 12 chromosomes. A single cross between LA716 and any tomato line will therefore provide a linkage survey of about 70% of the genome. Such crosses have consequently become standard for linkage screening of new mutants.

In the meantime, allozyme surveys were made of various other *Lycopersicon* species. Extensive collections were made of these species in their native regions in a fashion appropriate for determining various population parameters. It was thereby possible to ascertain the comparative extent of genetic variation within and between populations. The data also permit estimates of outcrossing and analysis of mating systems. Among the tomato species, the situation varies from strict autogamy through intermediate, facultative types to obligate allogamy enforced by self-incompatibility. Major differences in these parameters exist even within several of the species, the autogamous groups always being geographically peripheral to the central, vastly more variable groups (RICK 1983). These findings have considerable bearing on evolution in the genus, on utilization of the wild species for tomato improvement, and on germplasm preservation.

Allozyme mapping has also been applied to investigations of quantitative traits. Analysis of cosegregation of these molecular markers with metric traits in interspecific hybrids has been particularly instructive. Thus, research on the potential insect antibiotic 2-tridecanone in hybrids of *L. esculentum* × *Lycopersicon hirsutum* f. *glabratum* revealed complex determination by genes at a minimum of five loci (ZAMIR *et al.* 1984), thereby providing valuable (if not discouraging) information to breeders. In another study, by TANKSLEY, MEDINA-FILHO and RICK (1982), the nature of inheritance of four quantitative traits was investigated in the *esculentum-pennellii* hybrid in cosegregation with 13 allozymic loci. A single backcross to *esculentum* progeny afforded a wealth of information: the minimum number of quantitative loci (QTL) could be estimated; the positive or negative effect of wild alleles could be detected; as anticipated, the trait with the best +/− balance exhibited the greatest degree of transgressive segregation; epistatic interactions could be detected between allozymic loci and QTLs; and pairwise tests of allozymic loci detected interactions between QTLs, sometimes revealing the existence of QTLs not ascertained by tests for epistatic interactions. The merits of molecular markers for simultaneous analysis of metric traits were thereby demonstrated, and foundations were laid for recent sophisticated mapping of QTLs with RFLP markers.

Tomato genetics has benefited greatly from interactions with applied research; in fact, I would be remiss not to cite mutual advantages of exchanges with workers in tomato breeding both in public agencies and private firms. Many valuable spontaneous mutants have been discovered and transmitted and important observations made by several members of my Department, Cooperative Extension, and many workers in private industry.

A by-product of tomato genetics research was the establishment at Davis of the Tomato Genetics Resource Center. As stocks of mutants and cytological deviants accumulated and more collections of wild species were made, it behooved us to take measures to preserve this material. With support from various public agencies and the tomato industry, it has been possible to perform the standard functions of this service of germplasm collections: acquisition, maintenance, evaluation, utilization, distribution and relevant research.

Tomato genetics has clearly become a very active field of research. The record proves that the tomato species offer unique advantages for certain investigations. The groundwork studies on the nature of the tomato genome paved the way for molecular genetic studies, some already completed and many others in progress. In conclusion, if I may be allowed a metaphor, if *Arabidopsis* is the *Drosophila* of plant genetics, then the tomato has become the mouse.

The editorial advice of R. T. CHETELAT and M. M. GREEN is gratefully acknowledged.

LITERATURE CITED

BARTON, D. W., 1950 Pachytene morphology of the tomato chromosome complement. Am. J. Bot. **37:** 639–643.

BROWN, S. W., 1949 The structure and meiotic behavior of the differentiated chromosomes of the tomato. Genetics **34:** 437–461.

BUTLER, L., 1952 The linkage map of the tomato. J. Hered. **43:** 25–25.

HALSTED, B. D., E. J. OWEN and J. K. SHAW, 1905 Experiments with tomatoes. New Jersey Agric. Exp. Stn. Annu. Rep. **26:** 447–477.

HEDRICK, U. P., and N. O. BOOTH, 1907 Mendelian characters in tomatoes. Proc. Am. Soc. Hortic. Sci. **5:** 19–24.

JENKINS, J. A., 1948 The origin of the cultivated tomato. Econ. Bot. **2:** 379–392.

JONES, D. F., 1917 Linkage in *Lycopersicum*. Am. Nat. **51:** 608–621.

KHUSH, G. S., and C. M. RICK, 1968 Cytogenetic analysis of the tomato genome by means of induced deficiencies. Chromosoma **23:** 452–484.

KHUSH, G. S., C. M. RICK and R. W. ROBINSON, 1964 Genetic activity in a heterochromatic chromosome segment of the tomato. Science **145:** 1432–1434.

LESLEY, J. W., 1928 A cytological and genetical study of progenies of triploid tomatoes. Genetics **13:** 1–43.

PRICE, H. L., and A. W. DRINKARD, JR., 1908 Inheritance in tomato hybrids. Va. Agric. Exp. Stn. Bull. **177:** 1–53.

RICK, C. M., 1945 A survey of cytogenetic causes of unfruitfulness in the tomato. Genetics **30:** 347–362.

RICK, C. M., 1971 Some cytogenetic features of the genome in diploid plant species. Stadler Genet. Symp. **2:** 153–174.

RICK, C. M., 1983 Evolution of mating systems: evidence from allozyme variation, pp. 215–221 in *Genetics: New Frontiers* (Proceedings VX International Congress of Genetics), Vol. 4, edited by V. L. CHAPRA, B. C. JOSHI, R. P. SHARMA and H. C. BANSAL. Bowker, Epping, Essex.

RICK, C. M., and D. W. BARTON, 1954 Cytological and genetical identification of the primary trisomics of the tomato. Genetics **39:** 640–666.

RICK, C. M., J. F. FOBES and M. HOLLE, 1977 Genetic variation in *Lycopersicon pimpinellifolium*: evidence of evolutionary change in mating systems. Plant Syst. Evol. **127:** 139–170.

RICK, C. M., and S. D. TANKSLEY, 1981 Genetic variation in *Solanum pennellii*: comparisons with two other sympatric species. Plant Syst. Evol. **139:** 11–45.

RICK, C. M., and J. I. YODER, 1988 Classical and molecular genetics of tomato: highlights and perspectives. Annu. Rev. Genet. **22:** 281–300.

STUBBE, H., 1954 Über die vegetative Hybridisierung von Pflanzen. Kulturpflanze **2:** 185–236.

STUBBE, H., 1971 Weitere evolutionsgenetische Untersuchungen in der Gattung *Lycopersicon*. Biol. Zentralbl. **90:** 545–559.

TANSKLEY, S. D., H. MEDINA-FILHO and C. M. RICK, 1982 Use of naturally-occurring enzyme variation to detect and map genes controlling quantitative traits in an interspecific backcross of tomato. Heredity **49:** 11–25.

WINKLER, H., 1909 Über die Nachkommenschaft der *Solanum*-Pfropfbastarde und die Chromosomenzahlen ihrer Keimzellen. Z. Bot. **2:** 1–38.

ZAMIR, D., T. S. BEN-DAVID, J. RUDICH and J. A. JUVIK, 1984 Frequency distributions and linkage relationships of 2-tridecanone in interspecific segregating generations of tomato. Euphytica **33:** 481–488.

Impact of the Douglas-Hawthorne Model as a Paradigm for Elucidating Cellular Regulatory Mechanisms in Fungi

Yasuji Oshima

Department of Biotechnology, Faculty of Engineering, Osaka University, Suita-shi, Osaka 565, Japan

IN 1966, the first concrete genetic model of gene regulation in *Saccharomyces cerevisiae* was proposed for genes of the galactose pathway enzymes by H. C. DOUGLAS and D. C. HAWTHORNE at the University of Washington. Since then, the *GAL* system has been studied intensively as a major paradigm for the mechanism of fungal gene regulation and has provided much information. My colleagues and I in Osaka started with this model and refined it into a subsequent model by genetic analysis. In parallel, we carried out a study on a system for phosphatase regulation, also in *S. cerevisiae*. This *Perspective* describes how the Douglas-Hawthorne model attracted our attention and how it stimulated the elucidation of mechanisms of cellular regulation in yeast. During the past 25 years, these studies have led to an analysis of the function of cyclic AMP in yeast and its connection with the yeast homolog of the *ras* oncogene.

Galactose pathway enzymes and the Douglas-Hawthorne model: Galactose coordinately induces the activity of several enzymes involved in galactose utilization. This action was later shown to be at the level of mRNA synthesis. Between 1954 and the mid-1960s, DOUGLAS and HAWTHORNE and their colleagues identified three tightly linked genes on *S. cerevisiae* chromosome *II* encoding the enzymes of the Leloir pathway, *GAL1* (galactokinase), *GAL7* (galactose-1-phosphate uridyltransferase) and *GAL10* (uridine diphosphoglucose 4-epimerase), and also identified *GAL2* (encoding a specific galactose transport protein) and *GAL5* (controlling the phosphoglucomutase activity); but the order *GAL7–GAL10–GAL1* on chromosome *II* was not known until 1971 (BASSEL and MORTIMER 1971). Two principal regulatory genes for coordinate regulation of the *GAL* system, *GAL4* and *GAL80*, were also identified early in their studies. *GAL4*, a positive regulatory gene, was identified by isolating recessive mutations that caused a simultaneous block in the syntheses of all the enzymes of the Leloir pathway (DOUGLAS and HAWTHORNE 1964). *GAL80*, a negative regulatory gene, was identified by recessive mutations, *i* (now *gal80*), at a locus separate from *GAL4*, which conferred constitutive synthesis of the enzymes of the galactose pathway. The *i* mutations were isolated by DOUGLAS and PELROY (1963) as suppressor mutations for a peculiar phenomenon, long-term adaptation to galactose utilization, studied in *S. chevalieri* (synonymous with *S. cerevisiae*) since the pioneering genetic study of WINGE and ROBERTS (1948), and shown to be due to the *gal3* mutation. A group of *cis*-dominant constitutive mutations at the *GAL4* locus, named *C* (subsequently named *GAL81*, and now *GAL4ᶜ*) were also isolated as suppressors of *gal3*. These mutant phenotypes of the *GAL* regulatory genes are summarized in Table 1.

It was not known whether the *GAL4* and *GAL80* genes encode proteins until the isolation of suppressible (nonsense) mutations (DOUGLAS and HAWTHORNE 1972). The fact that these genes also contribute to the regulation of *MEL1*, which encodes α-galactosidase, was not shown until later (KEW and DOUGLAS 1976). However, in 1966 DOUGLAS and HAWTHORNE proposed a model in which the *GAL80* gene produces a repressor that regulates the expression of *GAL4* by interacting at a controlling site for *GAL4* (the *GAL81* site) in the absence of galactose. In the presence of galactose, the repressor is inactivated by its interaction with galactose and the *GAL4* gene is expressed to produce a diffusible intermediary. This in turn exerts positive control over the expression of the three linked genes coding for the enzymes of the Leloir pathway and possibly also *GAL2*, specific for the galactose transport system. Thus, the Douglas-Hawthorne model was analogous to that of the *lac*

TABLE 1

Phenotypes of mutants with mutations in the GAL and PHO regulatory genes

Category of gene product	System bearing the mutation[a]		Phenotype
	GAL	PHO	
Positive factor	gal4	pho4	Unable to synthesize enzymes in the relevant regulon
	GAL4^c(GAL81)	PHO4^c(PHO82)	cis-Dominant constitutive synthesis of the enzymes
Negative factor	gal80	pho80	Constitutive synthesis of the enzymes
	GAL80^s		Dominant noninducibility of the enzymes
		pho85	Constitutive synthesis of the enzymes; unable to activate PHO80 protein
Mediator	gal3		Long-term adaptation to galactose utilization
		pho81	Unable to synthesize the enzymes of the PHO regulon
Transcriptional factor[b]	gal11		Reduced transcription of genes for the enzymes of the Leloir pathway
		gfr10(pho2)	Unable to transcribe some of the genes in the PHO regulon

[a] Mutations in lower-case letters are recessive, while those in upper-case are dominant.

[b] The GAL11 and GRF10 proteins are also important or essential for the transcription of a wide variety of other genes.

operon proposed for *Escherichia coli* by JACOB and MONOD (1961), and implied that the *GAL81* site plays essentially the same role as the *lac* operator. In the bacterial system, the adjacent structural genes code directly for the enzymes involved in lactose utilization. In contrast, in the yeast system the adjacent gene *GAL4* codes for a regulatory protein, an intermediary between *GAL80* and the structural genes for the enzymes. Because the model proposed that *GAL80* encodes a repressor of *GAL4* transcription, a dominant, super-repressible, galactose-negative mutation at the *GAL80* locus would be expected, as in the bacterial system. Such mutations, designated *i^s* or *GAL80^s*, were indeed isolated and found to be *trans*-dominant over the wild-type and mutant alleles of *GAL80* (DOUGLAS and HAWTHORNE 1972). With these observations, the Douglas-Hawthorne model was widely accepted as the most plausible mechanism for regulation of the *GAL* system in yeast. The model did not specify whether the *GAL4* protein controls mRNA transcription or some subsequent step in the synthesis of active enzymes.

Revision of the model: Enzyme regulation is important in fermentation industries in order to increase the accumulation of metabolites such as amino acids and nucleic acid bases, and for the heightened production of enzymes. Therefore, my colleagues and I became interested in the regulation of gene expression in yeast. With this ultimate aim, I began genetic studies on regulatory mechanisms in *Saccharomyces* in 1955 when I was a graduate student at Osaka University. I first chose to study a system for adaptive synthesis of α-glucosidase, namely maltose fermentation, because I thought that the findings might have direct application to alcoholic fermentation. I continued this study at the Research Laboratories of Suntory Ltd., where I worked for the next 11 years. However, I soon realized that this system was not suitable for basic studies of gene regulation because determining the

enzyme activities of large numbers of tetrad segregants was laborious and inaccurate. At that time, I used the indirect method with Durham fermentation tubes for assaying enzyme activity. In addition to these disadvantages, there were other methodological difficulties in the enzyme assay. Moreover, as α-glucosidase synthesis is controlled by polymeric genes, various independent *mal$^-$* mutant genes complemented each other (OSHIMA 1967).

During this initial period of my studies, from 1963 to 1965, I had the opportunity to work as a postdoctoral research fellow in the laboratory of C. C. LINDEGREN at Southern Illinois University. Throughout the period from 1955 to the early 1970s, I examined several other enzyme systems, such as those for α-methylglucoside and galactose fermentation, and those in the biosynthetic pathways for various amino acids. In 1970 I gained a position at Osaka University and AKIO TOH-E came from the University of Tokyo to join my laboratory. Following his suggestion, I finally concluded that phosphatase would be one of the best systems for studying gene regulation in *S. cerevisiae*. The phosphatase system is suitable for four reasons. The acid phosphatase activity of each colony on a plate is easily detected by specific staining because the enzyme is localized on the cell surface. Enzyme synthesis is regulated in response to a simple effector, inorganic phosphate (P$_i$). The same regulatory system (with minor differences) also controls the synthesis of alkaline phosphatase, which is located entirely within the cell envelope and whose activity is also easily detectable in colonies by specific staining after permeabilizing the cells to the substrate. And there is a 500-fold difference between the repressed and derepressed levels of acid phosphatase activity.

With this advantageous system, we were able to isolate various mutants deficient in or constitutive for synthesis of repressible acid and alkaline phosphatases. We then analyzed these mutant genes and found that

at least four, *PHO2*, *PHO80*, *PHO81* and *PHO85*, plus
the gene cluster *pho82-PHO4*, all participate at the
transcriptional level in regulating the structural genes
for repressible acid phosphatase (*PHO5*), repressible
alkaline phosphatase (*PHO8*), and the other genes of
the phosphatase family, in response to the presence
or absence of P$_i$ in the medium; for reviews, see
OSHIMA (1982) and YOSHIDA *et al.* (1987). (*PHO2* was
shown not to be directly concerned with *PHO8* transcription.)

We found close similarities between the *PHO* system
and the *GAL* system (Table 1): *pho82-PHO4* corresponds to *gal81-GAL4* and the *PHO80* and *PHO85*
genes correspond to *GAL80*. The *PHO81* gene was
inferred to be the regulatory gene farthest from the
phosphatase structural genes because mutations in
PHO81 were hypostatic to mutations in the other
regulatory genes. Recent observations suggest that
PHO81 (YOSHIDA, OGAWA and OSHIMA 1989) and
GAL3 (BHAT, OH and HOPPER 1990) have similar
functions because they are probably concerned with
the conversions of P$_i$ and galactose, respectively, to
active effector or co-effector.

Soon after starting the more detailed analyses of
the *PHO* system, we found several discrepancies with
the model for *GAL* proposed by DOUGLAS and HAW-
THORNE. First, when cells of a temperature-sensitive
pho80 mutant were cultivated in high P$_i$ medium at
permissive (low) temperature and then transferred to
restrictive (high) temperature, they abruptly increased
acid phosphatase activity (Y. UEDA, A. TOH-E and Y.
OSHIMA, unpublished results). This increase occurred
sooner than expected if *PHO4* protein needed to be
synthesized first. Second, yeast cells grown at pH 3.0
in low-phosphate medium had no acid phosphatase
activity (TOH-E, KOBAYASHI and OSHIMA 1978). These
cells produced acid phosphatase activity by *de novo*
synthesis of the enzyme immediately after shift-up to
pH 4.0 or higher. A temperature-shift experiment
with a temperature-sensitive *pho81* mutant, coupled
with a pH shift, suggested that the functions of the
PHO81 and *PHO80* genes are necessary simultaneously, not sequentially, for expression of *PHO5*; it was
later claimed that this phenomenon is due to instability
of acid phosphatase at the lower pH (BOSTIAN, LEMIRE
and HALVORSON 1982). Third, fine-structure mapping of the *PHO4* gene by meiotic recombination
showed that the *PHO82* mutant alleles mapped *within*
the *PHO4* locus (TOH-E, INOUYE and OSHIMA 1981);
because of the development of base-sequencing techniques, this and a similar map of the *GAL81* and *gal4*
mutant alleles (MATSUMOTO *et al.* 1980) may be the
last fine-structure maps of yeast genes constructed by
meiotic recombination. Fourth, doubly heterozygous
diploids (*PHO82 PHO4/pho82⁺ pho4*) were found to
possess widely different activities when grown under

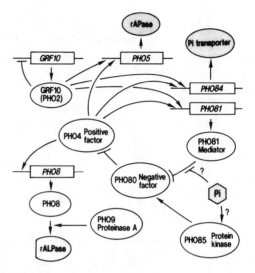

FIGURE 1.—The regulatory circuit for the phosphatase genes.
The protein factors, enzymes, and enzyme precursors in the regulatory circuit are shown in open ovals, and the genes under regulation by these proteins are shown in boxes. The factors in the
shaded hexagon and ovals, P$_i$, rAPase (repressible acid phosphatase;
EC 3.1.3.2) and rALPase (repressible alkaline phosphatase; EC
3.1.3.1), are the input signals and outputs of the regulatory circuit,
respectively. The regulatory factor, for which the corresponding
gene is not shown, is produced constitutively, or its regulation is
unknown. The arrows in the regulatory circuit indicate positive or
stimulating function of the factors, and the bars indicate repressive
or inhibitory functions. The PHO9 (PEP4) protein, proteinase A,
is needed for processing the PHO8 polypeptide.

repressing conditions, depending on the combination
of the *PHO82* and *pho4* mutant alleles (TOH-E, INOUYE
and OSHIMA 1981). These observations could not be
explained by the Douglas-Hawthorne galactose
model, so we speculated that the *PHO* regulatory
genes function in a different way. We proposed that
the PHO4 protein is synthesized constitutively but
that its activity is modulated by its interaction with
the PHO80 protein (and also with the PHO85 protein) at a site in the PHO4 protein encoded by *PHO82*
(OSHIMA 1982); Figure 1 gives recent details.

Assuming that the *GAL4* gene is expressed constitutively, the observed data for the *gal4*, *GAL81* and
gal80 mutants are consistent with a mechanism similar
to our model for the *PHO* system. In this mechanism,
the *GAL81* mutation does not delineate an operator
region contiguous to *GAL4*, but rather lies within the
GAL4 gene and defines the affinity site in the GAL4
protein at which the GAL80 protein acts. Because our
proposal for the *PHO* system was hardly acceptable as
a critique of the Douglas-Hawthorne model without
any direct evidence, we examined this possibility in
the *GAL* system.

I had worked on the *GAL* system during my graduate study, but that had been 20 years earlier, so we
were not familiar with the system. However, we isolated *gal4* and *gal80* mutants with thermolabile products by following a scheme for mutant isolation based

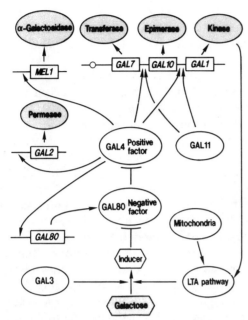

FIGURE 2.—The regulatory circuit for the genes encoding galactose pathway enzymes. The long-term adaptation (LTA) pathway is characteristic of respiratory-competent *gal3* mutant cells. This pathway requires mitochondrial function for the onset of galactose adaptation. The other symbols are as in the phosphatase circuit shown in Figure 1.

on the toxicity of galactose-1-phosphate in *gal7* and *gal10* mutants. A kinetic study of galactokinase synthesis with these mutants strongly suggested constitutive expression of *GAL4* (MATSUMOTO, TOH-E and OSHIMA 1978). This finding was supported by the semi-dominance of the *GAL81* mutation (MATSUMOTO *et al.* 1980), by detecting *GAL4* mRNA with a wheat germ *in vitro* translation system (PERLMAN and HOPPER 1979) and, finally, by Northern blots of *GAL4* mRNA (LAUGHON and GESTELAND 1982).

The conclusion that the *GAL81* mutation sites are in the protein-coding region was supported by a meiotic fine-structure map of *GAL4* with various *gal4* and *GAL81* mutant alleles, some of which were susceptible to nonsense suppressors (MATSUMOTO *et al.* 1980). The *GAL81* region was mapped at almost the center of the *GAL4* locus in a narrow segment (not more than 4% of the total *GAL4* map) that contained two nonsense alleles, *gal4-62* and *gal4-69*. However, more recent physical mapping shows that the *gal4-62* site is in codon 851 of the *GAL4* open reading frame (JOHNSTON, SALMERON and DINCHER 1987), which has 881 codons. We indeed see the unreliability of map positions determined by recombinational analysis!

From the above and other findings, I proposed in 1982 a revised model for the regulation of the *GAL* genes, along with the *PHO* system (OSHIMA 1982). An updated form of this model is given in Figure 2. The *GAL4* gene encodes a protein that activates transcription of the *GAL1*, *GAL2*, *GAL7*, *GAL10* and *MEL1* genes by binding to specific sites located in regions

upstream of these genes. *GAL4* is expressed constitutively and produces a constant amount of protein. In the absence of galactose, the GAL80 protein binds to the GAL4 protein, preventing the latter from activating transcription of the five *GAL* and *MEL1* genes. The presence of inducer inhibits the function of the GAL80 protein or dissociates it from the GAL4 protein, allowing the latter to activate transcription of the various target genes. Although no conclusive evidence was available at that time, I thought that the GAL80 protein might dissociate from the GAL4 protein in the presence of inducer, because synchronous mating experiments (PERLMAN and HOPPER 1979) showed that preexisting *GAL4* activity is promptly blocked by introducing the *GAL80^s* product. [It has recently been suggested that galactose may activate transcription by causing a conformational change in the GAL4-GAL80 complex rather than by leading to dissociation of GAL80 from GAL4 (CHASMAN and KORNBERG 1990).] I did not know the function of *GAL3* at that time, but recent studies suggest that it may be concerned with transformation of galactose into an unidentified active inducer molecule (BHAT, OH and HOPPER 1990). Several other mechanisms have been postulated for regulating the *GAL* and *PHO* systems, but none is consistent with the genetic data. The revised model has been examined critically by molecular analyses in the laboratories of TOSHIO FUKASAWA, JAMES HOPPER, MARK JOHNSTON, STEPHEN A. JOHNSTON, ROGER D. KORNBERG, MARK PTASHNE and others and has been generally supported, as reviewed by JOHNSTON (1987).

Positive and negative regulatory factors: The essential difference between the Douglas-Hawthorne model and the revised model is that the former proposes a protein-DNA interaction between *GAL80* and *GAL4*, and the latter a protein-protein interaction. Thus, the GAL80 protein is a regulatory protein of a category different from repressors in bacterial systems, which function by binding to specific DNA sequences. I therefore named the GAL80 protein a negative factor or negative regulator; this type of regulatory protein was termed a primary repressor by JOHNSTON (1987). The same is true for the PHO80 protein in the *PHO* system (Table 1). [A subunit structure of the negative factor composed of PHO80 and PHO85 proteins was suggested in the model, but now it is known that the PHO85 protein activates the PHO80 protein (TOH-E *et al.* 1988).] By extension of this idea, the protein encoded by *GAL4* and the PHO4 protein in the *PHO* system were named positive factors or positive regulators [or primary activators (JOHNSTON 1987).

Positive and negative factors have both been detected in various other regulatory systems in fungi examined so far (JOHNSTON 1987). Conceivably, most fungal genes are controlled by a similar mechanism, although some systems may have only positive or only negative factors. In addition to the positive and negative factors, the regulatory systems for general control of amino acid biosynthesis in *S. cerevisiae* (HINNEBUSCH 1988) and the system for phosphatase regulation in *Neurospora crassa* (METZENBERG 1979) seem to contain a gene (or genes) similar to *PHO81* of *S. cerevisiae*, which I have termed a mediator because its product mediates signals between the effector and the negative factor. The *PHO2* gene (now named *GRF10*), with wide specificity, is also indispensable for *PHO5* transcription. This gene might be autoregulated (YOSHIDA *et al.* 1989) but is not concerned with signal transduction (YOSHIDA, OGAWA and OSHIMA 1989). A similar regulatory gene, *GAL11*, has been identified in the *GAL* system (NOGI and FUKASAWA 1980) and suggested to mediate the activation functions of two different *trans*-acting factors, GAL4 and a second protein which has a variety of names (general regulatory factor I, repressor-activator site binding protein 1, and translation upstream factor) (NISHIZAWA *et al.* 1990). Of these, the positive factors have been the main object of recent studies, with interest in their specific binding to the UASs (upstream activating sequences) in the 5′ upstream regulatory regions [GINIGER, VARNUM and PTASHNE (1985) and BRAM, LUE and KORNBERG (1986) for the *GAL* system; VOGEL, HÖRZ and HINNEN (1989) and HAYASHI and OSHIMA (1991) for the *PHO* system], in the mechanism of transcriptional activation (PTASHNE 1988) and in the mechanism of modulation by negative factors (MYLIN, BHAT and HOPPER 1989).

Key regulators of *GAL* and *PHO* systems controlled by regulatory loops: Although the *GAL4* (LAUGHON and GESTELAND 1982) and *PHO4* (YOSHIDA *et al.* 1989) genes are both transcribed constitutively, their protein products participate in a regulatory loop that controls their activity. In particular, transcription of the *GAL80* gene is controlled by the *GAL* regulatory system: high-level transcription of *GAL80* requires GAL4, and galactose leads to a fivefold or greater increase in transcription of the *GAL80* gene (SHIMADA and FUKASAWA 1985; IGARASHI *et al.* 1987). Thus, the *GAL4* and *GAL80* genes participate in a regulatory loop (a closed regulatory circuit) in which the *GAL4* and *GAL80* genes are coupled by protein-protein and protein-DNA interactions (Figure 2). Key regulators of the *PHO* system also participate in a regulatory loop (Figure 1). In this case, *PHO80* transcription is constitutive (TOH-E and SHIMAUCHI 1986) but transcription of the mediator gene, *PHO81*, is enhanced by PHO4 (YOSHIDA *et al.* 1987; YOSHIDA, OGAWA and OSHIMA 1989). Because PHO81 inhibits PHO80, the net effect of this regulatory loop is to reinforce an inducing signal: active PHO4 leads to

further activation of PHO4. In contrast, the regulatory loop in the *GAL* system may serve to restrain induction, because active GAL4 stimulates synthesis of an inhibitor. These regulatory loops thus may serve to either amplify or restrain molecular signals.

A similar regulatory loop was observed for quinic acid catabolism in *N. crassa* (GILES *et al.* 1985), in which expression of various genes encoding enzymes for catabolism of quinic acid is under the control of qa-1F+ protein, analogous to GAL4 and PHO4, and a repressor gene, *qa-1S+*, similar to *GAL80* and *PHO80*. Transcription of both *qa-1F+* and *qa-1S+* is controlled by the qa-1F+ protein and increases 40- to 50-fold upon induction with quinic acid.

Expansion of the model: Enzymes of the galactose pathway are also under the control of carbon catabolite repression, and several other genes responsible for this control have been identified since the model shown in Figure 2 was developed. Characterization of these genes indicated that signals due to the presence or absence of glucose in the medium are conveyed to the genes for galactose pathway enzymes through three or more separate circuits overlapping the galactose circuit (MATSUMOTO, YOSHIMATSU and OSHIMA 1983) (for review, see JOHNSTON 1987). Some of the circuits are specific for the *GAL* system; others are also involved in glucose repression of invertase synthesis. The detailed mechanisms of these circuits are the subjects of intensive study at present (WEST *et al.* 1987; FLICK and JOHNSTON 1990). Because cyclic AMP plays an essential role in catabolite repression in *E. coli*, we sought to determine whether it plays a similar role in yeast. To address this problem, we first isolated mutants that can transport cyclic AMP into cells (MATSUMOTO *et al.* 1982b) and also mutants that are unable to synthesize cyclic AMP (MATSUMOTO *et al.* 1983). These studies showed that there was no correlation between the amount of intracellular cyclic AMP and catabolite repression of the *GAL* system and thus that yeast differs from bacteria in the mechanism of catabolite repression.

Having established that cyclic AMP is not responsible for carbon catabolite repression in the *GAL* system, we wondered what physiological roles are played by cyclic AMP in yeast. Our mutants provided an experimental approach to addressing this question, and led to the discovery of a cyclic AMP cascade in *S. cerevisiae* (MATSUMOTO *et al.* 1982a; MATSUMOTO, UNO and ISHIKAWA 1983a,b). This cascade proved to be involved in another pathway of signal transduction similar to that of higher eukaryotic cells; it plays a role in the control of the cell division cycle. Moreover, this cAMP cascade has been shown to be connected to the function of the yeast analogues of the *ras* oncogenes (for review, see GIBBS and MARSHALL 1989). These discoveries led to the elucidation of the role of cAMP-dependent and cAMP-independent protein kinases in cellular regulation in yeast.

The yeast cell has several regulatory systems that govern its behavior. For example, there must be mechanisms that couple a cell's position in the cell division cycle to its physiological state: cells in the resting state generally cannot synthesize enzymes. Such complex regulatory systems will probably involve regulatory circuits analogous to those for galactose and phosphate utilization. In the *GAL* and *PHO* systems, we have seen an interplay of different types of interactions: between proteins and DNA and between proteins and small molecules, as proposed in the original Douglas-Hawthorne model, and between regulatory proteins, as brought to light by our studies. The Douglas-Hawthorne model was an important first step in developing a comprehensive understanding of the mechanism of cellular regulation, a search that continues with vigor.

I thank IRA HERSKOWITZ for his comments and suggestions on the manuscript.

LITERATURE CITED

BASSEL, J., and R. MORTIMER, 1971 Genetic order of the galactose structural genes in *Saccharomyces cerevisiae*. J. Bacteriol. **108:** 179–183.

BHAT, P. J., D. OH and J. E. HOPPER, 1990 Analysis of the *GAL3* signal transduction pathway activating *GAL4* protein-dependent transcription in *Saccharomyces cerevisiae*. Genetics **125:** 281–291.

BOSTIAN, K. A., J. M. LEMIRE and H. O. HALVORSON, 1982 Synthesis of repressible acid phosphatase in *Saccharomyces cerevisiae* under conditions of enzyme instability. Mol. Cell. Biol. **2:** 1–10.

BRAM, R. J., N. F. LUE and R. D. KORNBERG, 1986 A *GAL* family of upstream activating sequences in yeast: roles in both induction and repression of transcription. EMBO J. **5:** 603–608.

CHASMAN, D. I., and R. D. KORNBERG, 1990 GAL4 protein: purification, association with GAL80 protein, and conserved domain structure. Mol. Cell. Biol. **10:** 2916–2923.

DOUGLAS, H. C., and D. C. HAWTHORNE, 1964 Enzymatic expression and genetic linkage of genes controlling galactose utilization in Saccharomyces. Genetics **49:** 837–844.

DOUGLAS, H. C., and D. C. HAWTHORNE, 1966 Regulation of genes controlling synthesis of the galactose pathway enzymes in yeast. Genetics **54:** 911–916.

DOUGLAS, H. C., and D. C. HAWTHORNE, 1972 Uninducible mutants in the *gali* locus of *Saccharomyces cerevisiae*. J. Bacteriol. **109:** 1139–1143.

DOUGLAS, H. C., and G. PELROY, 1963 A gene controlling inducibility of the galactose pathway enzymes in Saccharomyces. Biochim. Biophys. Acta **68:** 155–156.

FLICK, J. S., and M. JOHNSTON, 1990 Two systems of glucose repression of the *GAL1* promoter in *Saccharomyces cerevisiae*. Mol. Cell. Biol. **10:** 4757–4769.

GIBBS, J. B., and M. S. MARSHALL, 1989 The *ras* oncogene—an important regulatory element in lower eucaryotic organisms. Microbiol. Rev. **53:** 171–185.

GILES, N. H., M. E. CASE, J. BAUM, R. GEEVER, L. HUIET, V. PATEL and B. TYLER, 1985 Gene organization and regulation in the *qa* (quinic acid) gene cluster of *Neurospora crassa*. Microbiol. Rev. **49:** 338–358.

GINIGER, E., S. M. VARNUM and M. PTASHNE, 1985 Specific DNA binding of GAL4, a positive regulatory protein of yeast. Cell **40:** 767–774.

HAYASHI, N., and Y. OSHIMA, 1991 Specific *cis*-acting sequence for *PHO8* expression interacts with PHO4 protein, a positive regulatory factor, in *Saccharomyces cerevisiae*. Mol. Cell. Biol. **11:** 785–794.

HINNEBUSCH, A. G., 1988 Mechanisms of gene regulation in the general control of amino acid biosynthesis in *Saccharomyces cerevisiae*. Microbiol. Rev. **52:** 248–273.

IGARASHI, M., T. SEGAWA, Y. NOGI, Y. SUZUKI and T. FUKASAWA, 1987 Autogenous regulation of the *Saccharomyces cerevisiae* regulatory gene *GAL80*. Mol. Gen. Genet. **207:** 273–279.

JACOB, F., and J. MONOD, 1961 Genetic regulatory mechanisms in the synthesis of proteins. J. Mol. Biol. **3:** 318–356.

JOHNSTON, M., 1987 A model fungal gene regulatory mechanism: the *GAL* genes of *Saccharomyces cerevisiae*. Microbiol. Rev. **51:** 458–476.

JOHNSTON, S. A., J. M. SALMERON, JR. and S. S. DINCHER, 1987 Interaction of positive and negative regulatory proteins in the galactose regulon of yeast. Cell **50:** 143–146.

KEW, O. M., and H. C. DOUGLAS, 1976 Genetic co-regulation of galactose and melibiose utilization in *Saccharomyces*. J. Bacteriol. **125:** 33–41.

LAUGHON, A., and R. F. GESTELAND, 1982 Isolation and preliminary characterization of the *GAL4* gene, a positive regulator of transcription in yeast. Proc. Natl. Acad. Sci. USA **79:** 6827–6831.

MATSUMOTO, K., A. TOH-E and Y. OSHIMA, 1978 Genetic control of galactokinase synthesis in *Saccharomyces cerevisiae*: evidence for constitutive expression of the positive regulatory gene *gal4*. J. Bacteriol. **134:** 446–457.

MATSUMOTO, K., I. UNO and T. ISHIKAWA, 1983a Initiation of meiosis in yeast mutants defective in adenylate cyclase and CYCLIC AMP DEPENDENT PROTEIN KINASE. CELL **32:** 417–424.

MATSUMOTO, K., I. UNO and T. ISHIKAWA, 1983b Control of cell division in *Saccharomyces cerevisiae* mutants defective in adenylate cyclase and cyclic AMP dependent protein kinase. Exp. Cell. Res. **146:** 151–162.

MATSUMOTO, K., T. YOSHIMATSU and Y. OSHIMA, 1983 Recessive mutations conferring resistance to carbon catabolite repression of galactokinase synthesis in *Saccharomyces cerevisiae*. J. Bacteriol. **153:** 1405–1414.

MATSUMOTO, K., Y. ADACHI, A. TOH-E and Y. OSHIMA, 1980 Function of positive regulatory gene *gal4* in the synthesis of galactose pathway enzymes in *Saccharomyces cerevisiae*: evidence that the *GAL81* region codes for part of the *gal4* protein. J. Bacteriol. **141:** 508–527.

MATSUMOTO, K., I. UNO, Y. OSHIMA and T. ISHIKAWA, 1982a Isolation and Characterization of Yeast *Saccharomyces cerevisiae* mutants deficient in adenylate cyclase and cyclic AMP dependent protein kinase. Proc. Natl. Acad. Sci. USA **79:** 2355–2360.

MATSUMOTO, K., I. UNO, A. TOH-E, T. ISHIKAWA and Y. OSHIMA, 1982b Cyclic AMP may not be involved in catabolite repression in *Saccharomyces cerevisiae*: evidence from mutants capable of utilizing it as an adenine source. J. Bacteriol. **150:** 277–285.

MATSUMOTO, K., I. UNO, T. ISHIKAWA and Y. OSHIMA, 1983 Cyclic AMP may not be involved in catabolite repression in *Saccharomyces cerevisiae*: evidence from mutants unable to synthesize it. J. Bacteriol. **156:** 898–900.

METZENBERG, R. L., 1979 Implications of some genetic control mechanisms in *Neurospora*. Microbiol. Rev. **43:** 361–383.

MYLIN, L. M., J. P. BHAT and J. E. HOPPER, 1989 Regulated phosphorylation and dephosphorylation of GAL4, a transcriptional activator. Genes Dev. **3:** 1157–1165.

NISHIZAWA, M., Y. SUZUKI, Y. NOGI, K. MATSUMOTO and T. FUKASAWA, 1990 Yeast Gal11 protein mediates the transcriptional activation signal of two different transacting factors, Gal4 and general regulatory factor I/repressor/activator site binding protein 1/translation upstream factor. Proc. Natl. Acad. Sci. USA **87:** 5373–5377.

NOGI, Y., and T. FUKASAWA, 1980 A novel mutation that affects utilization of galactose in *Saccharomyces cerevisiae*. Curr. Genet. **2:** 115–120.

OSHIMA, Y., 1967 The inter-cistronic complementation of the polymeric genes for maltose fermentation in *Saccharomyces*. J. Ferment. Technol. **46:** 550–565.

OSHIMA, Y., 1982 Regulatory circuits for gene expression: the metabolism of galactose and phosphate, pp. 159–180 in *The Molecular Biology of the Yeast Saccharomyces: Metabolism and Gene Expression*, edited by J. N. STRATHERN, E. W. JONES and J. R. BROACH. Cold Spring Harbor Laboratory Press, Cold Spring Harbor, N.Y.

PERLMAN, D., and J. E. HOPPER, 1979 Constitutive synthesis of the GAL4 protein, a galactose pathway regulator in *Saccharomyces cerevisiae*. Cell **16:** 89–95.

PTASHNE, M., 1988 How eukaryotic transcriptional activators work. Nature **335:** 683–689.

SHIMADA, H., and T. FUKASAWA, 1985 Controlled transcription of the yeast regulatory gene *GAL80*. Gene **39:** 1–9.

TOH-E, A., S. INOUYE and Y. OSHIMA, 1981 Structure and function of the *PHO82-pho4* locus controlling the synthesis of repressible acid phosphatase of *Saccharomyces cerevisiae*. J. Bacteriol. **145:** 221–232.

TOH-E, A., S. KOBAYASHI and Y. OSHIMA, 1978 Disturbance of the machinery for the gene expression by acidic pH in the repressible acid phosphatase system of *Saccharomyces cerevisiae*. Mol. Gen. Genet. **162:** 139–149.

TOH-E, A., and T. SHIMAUCHI, 1986 Cloning and sequencing of the *PHO80* gene and *CEN15* of *Saccharomyces cerevisiae*. Yeast **2:** 129–139.

TOH-E, A., K. TANAKA, Y. UESONO and R. B. WICKNER, 1988 PHO85, a negative regulator of the *PHO* system, is a homolog of the protein kinase gene, *CDC28*. Mol. Gen. Genet. **214:** 162–164.

VOGEL, K., W. HÖRZ and A. HINNEN, 1989 The two positively acting regulatory proteins PHO2 and PHO4 physically interact with *PHO5* upstream activation regions. Mol. Cell. Biol. **9:** 2050–2057.

WEST, JR., R. W., S. CHEN, H. PUTZ, G. BUTLER and M. BANERJEE, 1987 *GAL1-GAL10* divergent promoter region of *Saccharomyces cerevisiae* contains negative control elements in addition to functionally separate and possibly overlapping upstream activating sequences. Genes Dev. **1:** 1118–1131.

WINGE, Ö., and C. ROBERTS, 1948 Inheritance of enzymatic characters in yeast, and the phenomenon of long-term adaptation. C. R. Trav. Lab. Carlsberg Ser. Physiol. **24:** 135–263.

YOSHIDA, K., N. OGAWA and Y. OSHIMA, 1989 Function of the *PHO* regulatory genes for repressible acid phosphatase synthesis in *Saccharomyces cerevisiae*. Mol. Gen. Genet. **217:** 40–46.

YOSHIDA, K., Z. KUROMITSU, N. OGAWA, K. OGAWA and Y. OSHIMA, 1987 Regulatory circuit for phosphatase synthesis in *Saccharomyces cerevisiae*, pp. 49–55 in *Phosphate Metabolism and Cellular Regulation in Microorganisms*, edited by A. TORRIANI-GORINI, F. G. ROTHMAN, S. SILVER, A. WRIGHT and E. YAGIL. American Society for Microbiology, Washington, D.C.

YOSHIDA, K., Z. KUROMITSU, N. OGAWA and Y. OSHIMA, 1989 Mode of expression of the positive regulatory genes *PHO2* and *PHO4* of the phosphatase regulon in *Saccharomyces cerevisiae*. Mol. Gen. Genet. **217:** 31–39.

See also page 706 in Addenda et Corrigenda.

The Regulation of Arginine Biosynthesis
Its Contribution to Understanding
the Control of Gene Expression

Werner K. Maas

Department of Microbiology, New York University Medical Center, 550 First Avenue, New York, New York 10016

IN the 1950s there occurred a fundamental change in the outlook of biologists on the regulation of biochemical processes. Certain studies on the regulation of arginine synthesis in *Escherichia coli* played a role in bringing about this change and the present article is an account of these studies. Because I started to work on the regulation of arginine biosynthesis in the mid-1950s, the story told here will be of a somewhat personal nature.

What was the nature of the fundamental change that occurred in the 1950s? To answer this question I shall first describe the general picture of the regulation of biochemical pathways and of gene expression that was in vogue before the change. Regulation of biochemical pathways belonged at that time in the domain of biochemists, whereas regulation of gene expression belonged in the domain of geneticists, and there was little interchange of ideas between the two. In regard to biochemical pathways, regulation was thought to be somehow built into the chemical structures of enzymes and their substrates and products. Rates of reactions were thought to be controlled by affinities of substrates for their enzymes and by inhibition by products formed during a reaction. These concepts seemed to be implicit in the thinking of biochemists and very little was said explicitly about regulation in textbooks published at that time, such as in the excellent book by FRUTON and SIMMONDS (1953).

In regard to the control of gene expression, the thinking of geneticists was very much influenced by the one gene, one enzyme hypothesis of BEADLE and TATUM, which in a general form stated that a gene determines a specific protein molecule. Little was known about how a gene determines a protein molecule and even less about how this gene activity was

controlled. Again, this lack of concrete ideas was reflected in then current textbooks of genetics. An exception to the lack of specific information was the work on adaptive enzymes, which at that time was carried out mainly by JACQUES MONOD and his co-workers at the Pasteur Institute in Paris. It was shown that for these enzymes, such as β-galactosidase, the substrate or an analog of the substrate was required to bring about synthesis of the enzyme and that this "induction" was controlled by a specific gene. Constitutive mutants were isolated in which the "inducer" was no longer required for enzyme synthesis. MONOD's interpretation of the findings was that the inducer somehow molded the information into an enzyme-forming system to produce a specific enzyme. In a constitutive mutant, a specific gene gave rise to an internal inducer, whereas in the wild type, this gene was inactive and the inducer had to be supplied externally. This picture of gene control, like that of the control of enzymatic reactions, involves chemical information contained in the substrate, which brings about regulation of, in one case, enzymatic reactions and, in the other case, the synthesis of enzymes. The thinking behind these concepts was based largely on then current concepts of interactions between proteins and low molecular substrates and also on template mechanisms, such as that invoked for the synthesis of antibodies. The latter was developed largely by HAUROWITZ (1952) and has been referred to as the HAUROWITZ-PAULING or "direct template" theory (BURNET 1959). It holds that antibody molecules have their specificity determined by being synthesized against a template of the antigen molecules themselves.

The big change in thinking about regulation was the realization that there is no direct chemical relationship between the regulating substance and the

This article is dedicated to the memory of LEO SZILARD.

protein whose production is regulated by this substance. Instead, the response to the regulating substance is mediated by the products of genes whose only function is the regulation of gene expression. This view was expressed by LEDERBERG (1956) during the discussion of a lecture by MONOD (1956) in which the latter had stated that "the 'S' substance (a common precursor) might be capable of giving rise to several different enzymes, depending on the nature of the inducer with which it reacted." LEDERBERG's response was, "Dr. MONOD asked whether the inducer carries the information needed for the specification of the enzyme. One permissible view holds that the enzyme, or its critical surface, is directly molded on the inducing substrate. The alternative, which I prefer, is that all the specifications are already inherent in the genetic constitution of the cell. The inducer signals a regulatory system to accelerate the synthesis of the corresponding enzyme protein." This notion of specific regulatory gene products (presumably proteins) was novel to biochemists and had a profound effect on subsequent research in biochemistry. It brought biochemists together with geneticists and it did much to create the field of molecular biology, in which guidance was provided mainly by the results of genetic experiments. I have tried to formulate this change in an article written for a Lipmann Symposium (MAAS 1974) by saying, "It has become clear that during evolution, mechanisms previously considered unlikely, can become established in living cells, as long as they give the organism a selective advantage over its competitors. The cell is no longer considered as a chemical machine, but as a *cybernetic* chemical machine."

The source of these novel ideas was the discovery of end-product repression in biosynthetic pathways, including that of arginine. These end products could control the synthesis of enzymes whose substrates bore little structural similarity to the end product.

Discovery of the repression of arginine biosynthesis: To make it easier for the reader to follow the text, the pathway of arginine biosynthesis in *E. coli* is shown in Figure 1. The first studies were carried out by HENRY VOGEL (1953). He noticed that in an arginine-requiring mutant blocked before *N*-acetylornithine (Figure 1), the level of acetylornithinase (Figure 1, step 5) was higher in cells grown with acetylornithine than in cells grown with arginine. He subsequently extended these studies by growing the cells on mixed supplements of arginine and acetylornithine, in order to distinguish between induction by acetylornithine or inhibition by arginine as an explanation for his observations. In 1957, in a paper given at the McCollum Pratt Symposium (VOGEL 1957), he presented data showing that his observed effects were due to inhibition by arginine. He coined the term

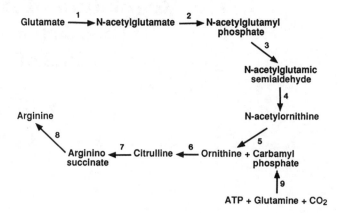

FIGURE 1.—The biosynthesis of arginine. The reaction steps shown are controlled by the arginine repressor. The enzymes catalyzing these reactions are, in order of the steps: 1, *N*-acetylglutamate synthase; 2, *N*-acetylglutamate kinase; 3, *N*-acetylglutamyl-phosphate reductase; 4, *N*-acetylornithine transaminase; 5, *N*-acetyl ornithinase; 6, ornithine carbamoyl transferase; 7, argininosuccinate synthetase; 8, argininosuccinase; 9, carbamoylphosphate synthetase.

"enzyme repression" to describe this phenomenon. The substance inhibiting enzyme synthesis was named a "repressor." (The alternative spelling "repressor" has since been accepted, whereas "promotor" has not.)

My own involvement with the regulation of arginine biosynthesis began in 1955 and was unrelated to VOGEL's work. At that time I was interested in how genes control the production of enzymes. In 1952 I had shown that in a temperature-sensitive mutant of *E. coli* blocked in the synthesis of pantothenic acid, the enzyme catalyzing the conditionally blocked reaction was more heat-labile than the corresponding enzyme in the wild type (MAAS and DAVIS 1952). The results showed that an altered protein was produced as a result of mutation and that a gene could therefore control the structure of its protein product.

After a stay in LIPMANN's laboratory in 1953 and 1954, I returned to New York University to continue the study of gene-enzyme relationships. I looked for mutants of a known gene in which the *rate* of enzyme synthesis was altered. To do this, I screened revertants from completely blocked mutants that could grow without the required growth factor at 37° but could not at 25° (cold-sensitive mutants). One of the strains from which I obtained such mutants was an arginine auxotroph blocked between ornithine and citrulline (Figure 1, step 6) and unable to make the enzyme ornithine transcarbamoyltransferase (OTCase). From this strain the desired revertants were obtained. OTCase was produced when the cells were grown at 37° but not at 25°. At 25° the mutant had to be grown with arginine, but at 37° it grew in a minimal medium without arginine. The surprise came when the cells were grown at 37° with arginine: no OTCase was produced. Subsequently, inhibition of OTCase formation by arginine was found in the wild-type strain as well, at both 37° and 25°. It was shown that the inhibition was specific for arginine. Growth with citrulline did not inhibit OTCase synthesis, whereas growth with arginine did (MAAS 1956). Presumable citrulline is converted to arginine too slowly to establish the arginine concentration required for full repression. In this roundabout way I had serendipitously discovered that end-product repression of OTCase was a general phenomenon and had nothing to do with the cold-sensitive mutations.

By 1957 it was thus established that arginine could repress the formation of at least two enzymes in its biosynthetic pathway. Both enzymes catalyzed reactions before the last step in the pathway. It seemed most probable that this repression was not due to arginine alone and that other components must be involved. The most obvious way to look for such components was to isolate mutants in which OTCase formation was not repressed by arginine. I shall describe such mutants after first considering the impact of the arginine studies on the then current ideas about the regulation of enzyme formation.

A unified hypothesis for the regulation of enzyme synthesis: In 1957, enzyme induction and enzyme repression were two different ways in which the formation of an enzyme could be controlled. At that time the notion was prevalent that the primary mechanism for the two types of control should be the same. This view was especially propounded by MONOD. It is curious today to see this insistence on a unitary mechanism. The reason may be that, at the time, our thinking was much influenced by the then fashionable concept of the "Unity of Biochemistry." I stated this view during the discussion of a paper I presented in 1957 (MAAS and GORINI 1958): "I think that most people feel the distinction between adaptive (*i.e.*, inducible) and constitutive (*i.e.*, biosynthetic) enzymes is an artificial one. In the case of constitutive enzymes the inducer is always present, whereas in the case of adaptive enzymes it ·is ordinarily not present. Alternatively, it is possible that adaptive enzyme formation is due to the inhibition of a feed-back inhibitor normally present, and that inducers act by preventing the action of such feed-back inhibitors."

On the basis of his studies on the induction of β-galactosidase, MONOD at first believed strongly in induction as the primary mechanism (positive and "instructive" control). The story of how he changed his mind and how the work on arginine regulation contributed to his conversion to a hypothesis involving negative control has been told several times (JUDSON 1970; SCHAFFNER 1974; BROCK 1990). Nevertheless, I shall give my personal account of this history and of the seminal role played by LEO SZILARD in the exchange of ideas.

I had already demonstrated (MAAS 1956) that the substrate ornithine was not required for the synthesis of OTCase and concluded, "here the substrate may not function as an inducer for enzyme formation." At that time LUIGI GORINI, who was a visiting investigator in our pharmacology department at New York University, joined me in investigating the kinetics of OTCase formation. Following a discussion with NOVICK and SZILARD, we decided to study OTCase synthesis in a chemostat, a device for constant growth devised by NOVICK and SZILARD (1950). For our studies we used a mutant blocked before ornithine and we grew it in a chemostat with arginine limiting the growth rate. Under these conditions OTCase was produced at a high "derepressed" rate, yet its substrate ornithine was not present in the bacteria (GORINI and MAAS 1957).

In April, 1957 I attended the Federation Meetings in Chicago and stayed at the Quadrangle Club where SZILARD was also staying. I met him during breakfast and told him about the synthesis of OTCase in the absence of a substrate. Yet the kinetics of enzyme synthesis were like those observed during the induction of β-galactosidase. On the basis of a unitary hypothesis, one had to conclude that induction was a removal of repression and that the inducer acted secondarily in counteracting a repressor. SZILARD was impressed with this idea and said that it could explain some findings on β-galactosidase formation that MILTON WEINER had made in their laboratory. We had more discussions during breakfast on subsequent days and at the end SZILARD was ready to publish a paper. I felt reluctant because we had no experimental evidence in an inducible system but SZILARD did publish a theoretical paper (SZILARD 1960).

Early in 1958, SZILARD presented the unitary hypothesis we had formulated in Chicago at a seminar at the Pasteur Institute in Paris. At that time, ARTHUR PARDEE in MONOD's laboratory had just begun to carry out experiments to study the expression of the inducibility gene for β-galactosidase formation following transfer of this gene during matings (later known as the PARDEE-JACOB-MONOD or "Pajamo" experiment or, in a lighter vein, the "Pajama" experiment). The thinking of MONOD at that time was still in favor of an "internal inducer" hypothesis but it appears that SZILARD's seminar and the subsequent discussion had a strong influence in convincing him of the validity of the "removal of repressor" hypothesis to explain β-galactosidase induction. To quote from MONOD's Nobel lecture, "Why not suppose, then, since the existence of repressible systems and their extreme generality were now proven, that induction could be effected by an anti-repressor, rather than repression by an anti-inducer? This is precisely the thesis that LEO SZILARD, while passing through Paris, happened to propose to us during a seminar. We had only recently obtained the first results of the injection ('Pajama') experiment, and we were still not sure about its interpretation. I saw that our preliminary observations confirmed SZILARD's penetrating intuition, and when he had finished his presentation, my doubts about the theory of the 'double bluff' (induction equals removal of repression) had been removed . . ." (MONOD 1966). The results of the completed experiments did indeed establish the validity of the "removal of repressor" model as originally postulated from results with the repression of OTCase. It is interesting that the belief in a unitary mechanism had such a strong influence on the willingness of MONOD and others to accept the interpretation of the inducer as an anti-repressor. Nowadays, and for good reasons, our attitude has become much more flexible because both primary negative actions and primary positive actions have been found in the control of enzyme synthesis.

Isolation and properties of derepressed (argR⁻) mutants: In order to study components other than arginine required for repression, I started to look for derepressed mutants in 1957. Canavanine, an analog of arginine, was found to inhibit growth by competing for arginine in protein synthesis (SCHWARTZ and MAAS 1960). It seemed reasonable to suppose that mutants resistant to canavanine might be derepressed because they would produce more arginine than the repressible wild type and thus overcome inhibition by canavanine.

At that time our wild-type strain was *E. coli* W. We isolated many canavanine-resistant mutants but they all turned out to be defective in the uptake of canavanine, arginine and other basic amino acids (SCHWARTZ, MAAS and SIMON 1959). These mutants started us on further investigations of permeases for basic amino acids.

During the summer of 1959 I worked in JACOB's laboratory at the Pasteur Institute in Paris and again I looked for canavanine-resistant mutants, this time starting with *E. coli* K12. The first mutants I isolated were derepressed for OTCase. Later they were shown to be derepressed also for other enzymes of the arginine pathway. I named the gene that had mutated *argR*. I supposed that *argR* controlled the production of an "aporepressor," arginine being the "corepressor." After my return to New York University in the fall, I mapped the *argR* gene as well as several genes of the arginine biosynthetic pathway. The results of these studies were presented at the 1961 Cold Spring Harbor Symposium (MAAS 1961). At the same meeting, GORINI presented his work on *argR* mutants which he had isolated by another, more complicated method (GORINI, GUNDERSEN and BURGER 1961). The Operon Model was also described at this meeting by JACOB and MONOD (1961). One of the unusual features of the arginine system was that, in contrast to the

genes of other biosynthetic pathways (tryptophan, histidine), its genes were not next to each other but were scattered over the chromosome, yet were all controlled by the same regulator gene. It was shown that the tryptophan genes and the histidine genes were united in single operons, but the arginine genes were present in several operons. A. J. CLARK and I, in a paper demonstrating the dominance of repressibility over nonrepressibility in diploids (MAAS and CLARK 1964), introduced the term "regulon" to describe the situation of the arginine genes. This paper established clearly that the control of the arginine pathway is negative via a repressor, the product of the gene *argR*.

The nature of the arginine repressor and its targets: In 1961 the general outline of how the synthesis of enzymes is regulated had been established, thanks largely to genetic experiments, and now it became necessary to fill in details in different systems. For example, the chemical nature of repressors was not known, and it was also not known whether they worked at the level of transcription or translation or even post-translationally (MAAS and McFALL 1964). These questions were answered during the 1960s and 1970s for many systems, including the arginine system. It was shown that repressors are proteins and that they act at the level of transcription. Their targets, the operator sites, are short, specific DNA sequences located close to the promoters of the regulated genes. In the case of arginine, the question was raised whether arginine or a derivative of arginine is the corepressor. After considerable efforts it was shown that arginine itself is the corepressor. The developments that occurred in the study of arginine regulation in prokaryotes up to 1985 have been reviewed by CUNIN et al. (1986).

Since then, the *argR* gene of *E. coli* K12 has been cloned and sequenced and the arginine repressor protein has been isolated and its interactions with its operator sites analyzed (LIM et al. 1987). Several unusual features distinguish the arginine repressor from other repressors. It appears to be a hexamer, whereas other repressors are either dimers or tetramers. Its target site consists of two 18-bp palindromic sequences (ARG boxes) located near each other within the promoter region of each gene of the arginine regulon. Recently, co-crystals of the repressor protein with synthetic ARG boxes have been obtained by JOACHIMIAK in SIGLER's laboratory at Yale University and are being subjected to X-ray diffraction analysis. Studies on the interaction of the arginine repressor with its operator sites have thus reached the level of atomic resolution.

Another feature of the arginine system is of general interest. It had already been noted in 1961 by GORINI that the regulation of arginine synthesis is different in *E. coli* B and *E. coli* K12 (ENNIS and GORINI 1961).

During growth in the absence of added arginine, endogenously produced arginine brings about the same degree of repression of the arginine enzymes (about 90%) in both strains. With added arginine, the arginine enzymes of *E. coli* K12 are totally repressed, whereas the arginine enzymes of *E. coli* B are only about 80% repressed. Later, this difference was shown by JACOBY and GORINI (1967) and by us (KADNER and MAAS 1971) to be due to different *argR* alleles in the two strains. Recently, DONGBIN LIM in our laboratory has cloned and sequenced the *argR* gene of *E. coli* B and has isolated the arginine repressor from this strain (LIM *et al.* 1988). The B repressor differs by one amino acid from the K12 repressor but some of its properties, such as solubility, are quite different. The question is, how could the difference between the two repressors account for the observed difference in the regulation of enzyme synthesis by arginine?

We have now found a partial answer to this question. It should be recalled that the active repressor consists of the ArgR protein (aporepressor) and arginine (corepressor). The degree of repression is therefore determined by the concentrations of repressor protein and arginine. Limiting either can lead to derepression. The formation of the K12 repressor is autoregulated (LIM *et al.* 1987) and there is presumptive evidence that this is also true for the B repressor. In fact, it appears that autoregulation by the B repressor is so strong that the repressor concentration can become limiting for repression, so that derepression of OTCase and other arginine enzymes may ensue. When the operator and promoter sites of the B repressor are removed and replaced by the potent *tac* promoter, which does not have the *argR* operator sites, the addition of arginine brings about complete repression, as it does with the K12 *argR* gene. After induction with the inducer IPTG, presumably more repressor protein is produced with the *tac* promoter than with the normal *argR* promoter.

These findings raise an interesting question. Why should a wild-type strain of *E. coli* increase the level of arginine-forming enzymes when it is supplied with external arginine? So far I have no clear answer for this paradoxical situation, but the persistence of *E. coli* B in nature suggests that there must be a selective advantage for B-type regulation of arginine biosynthesis in the ecological niche occupied by *E. coli* B. If we do find an answer, we may uncover new principles that apply to the regulation of gene expression in general. Thus, even after 35 years of investigation, the regulation of arginine biosynthesis raises challenging questions for future research.

The author is grateful for continuous supported since 1958 by Public Health Service Grant GM-06048 from the National Institute for General Medical Sciences for studies on the regulation of arginine biosynthesis.

LITERATURE CITED

BROCK, T. D., 1990 *The Emergence of Bacterial Genetics*, Chapter 10. Cold Spring Harbor Laboratory, Cold Spring Harbor, N.Y.

BURNET, M., 1959 *The Clonal Selection Theory of Acquired Immunity*, pp. 50–51. Vanderbilt University Press, Nashville, Tenn.

CUNIN, R., N. GLANSDORFF, A. PIERARD and V. STALON, 1986 Biosynthesis and metabolism of arginine in bacteria. Microbiol. Rev. **50:** 314–352.

ENNIS, H. L., and L. GORINI, 1961 Control of arginine biosynthesis in strains of *Escherichia coli* not repressible by arginine. J. Mol. Biol. **3:** 439–446.

FRUTON, J. S., and S. SIMMONDS, 1953 *General Biochemistry*. John Wiley & Sons, New York.

GORINI, L., W. GUNDERSEN and M. BURGER, 1961 Genetics of regulation of enzyme synthesis in the arginine biosynthetic pathway of *Escherichia coli*. Cold Spring Harbor Symp. Quant. Biol. **26:** 173–182.

GORINI, L., and W. K. MAAS, 1957 The potential for the formation of a biosynthetic enzyme in *Escherichia coli*. Biochim. Biophys. Acta **25:** 208–209.

HAUROWITZ, F., 1952 The mechanism of the immunological response. Biol. Rev. **27:** 247–280.

JACOB, F., and J. MONOD, 1961 On the regulation of gene activity. Cold Spring Harbor Symp. Quant. Biol. **26:** 193–211.

JACOBY, G. A., and L. GORINI, 1967 Genetics of control of the arginine pathway in *Escherichia coli* B and K. J. Mol. Biol. **24:** 41–50.

JUDSON, H. F., 1970 *The Eighth Day of Creation*, Chapter 7. Simon & Schuster, New York.

KADNER, R. J., and W. K. MAAS, 1971 Regulatory gene mutations affecting arginine biosynthesis in *Escherichia coli*. Mol. Gen. Genet. **111:** 1–14.

LEDERBERG, J., 1956 Comments on gene-enzyme relationships, pp. 161–162 in *Enzymes: Units of Biological Structure and Function*, edited by O. H. GAEBLER. Academic Press, New York.

LIM, D., J. D. OPPENHEIM, T. ECKHARDT and W. K. MAAS, 1987 Nucleotide sequence of the *argR* gene of *Escherichia coli* K-12 and isolation of its product, the arginine repressor. Proc. Natl. Acad. Sci. USA **84:** 6697–6701.

LIM, D., J. OPPENHEIM, T. ECKHARDT and W. K. MAAS, 1988 The unitary hypothesis for the repression mechanism of arginine biosynthesis in *E. coli* B and *E. coli* K12 revisited after 18 years, pp. 55–63 in *Gene Expression and Regulation: The Legacy of Luigi Gorini*, edited by M. BISSELL, G. DEHO, G. SIRONI and A. TORRIANI. Excerpta Medica, New York.

MAAS, W. K., 1956 Regulation of arginine biosynthesis in *Escherichia coli*. Biol. Bull. **111:** 319.

MAAS, W. K., 1961 Studies on repression of arginine biosynthesis in *Escherichia coli*. Cold Spring Harbor Symp. Quant. Biol. **26:** 183–191.

MAAS, W. K., 1974 Some thoughts on the regulation of arginine biosynthesis and its relation to biochemistry, pp 399–403 in *Lippmann Symposium: Energy, Biosynthesis and Regulation in Molecular Biology*, edited by D. RICHTER. Walter de Gruyter, New York.

MAAS, W. K., and A. J. CLARK, 1964 Studies on the mechanism of repression of arginine biosynthesis in *Escherichia coli*. II. Dominance of repressibility in diploids. J. Mol. Biol. **8:** 365–370.

MAAS, W. K., and B. D. DAVIS, 1952 Production of an altered pantothenate-synthesizing enzyme by a temperature-sensitive mutant of *Escherichia coli*. Proc. Natl. Acad. Sci. USA **38:** 785–797.

MAAS, W. K., and L. GORINI, 1958 Negative feed-back control of the formation of biosynthetic enzymes, pp. 151–158 in *Physiological Adaptation*, edited by C. L. PROSSER. American Physiological Society, Washington, D.C.

Maas, W. K., and E. McFall, 1964   Genetic aspects of metabolic control. Annu. Rev. Microbiol. **18:** 95–110.

Monod, J., 1956   Remarks on the mechanism of enzyme induction, p. 26 in *Enzymes: Units of Biological Structure and Function,* edited by O. H. Gaebler. Academic Press, New York.

Monod, J., 1966   From enzymatic adaptation to allosteric transitions. Science **154:** 475–483.

Novick, A., and L. Szilard, 1950   Description of the chemostat. Science **112:** 715–716.

Schaffner, K. F., 1974   Logic of discovery and justification in regulatory genetics. Stud. Hist. Philos. Sci. **4:** 349–385.

Schwartz, J. H., and W. K. Maas, 1960   Analysis of the inhibition of growth produced by canavanine in *Escherichia coli.* J. Bacteriol. **79:** 794–799.

Schwartz, J. H., W. K. Maas and E. J. Simon, 1959   An impaired concentrating mechanism for amino acids in mutants of *Escherichia coli* resistant to L-canavanine and D-serine. Biochim. Biophys. Acta **32:** 582–583.

Szilard, L., 1960   The control of the formation of specific proteins in bacteria and in animal cells. Proc. Natl. Acad. Sci. USA **46:** 277–291.

Vogel, H. J., 1953   On growth-limiting utilization of α-N-acetyl-L-ornithine. Proc. 6th Int. Congr. Microbiol. (Rome) **1:** 269–271.

Vogel, H. J., 1957   Repression and induction as control mechanisms of enzyme biogenesis: the "adaptive" formation of acetylornithinase, pp 276–289 in *The Chemical Basis of Heredity,* edited by W. D. McElroy and B. Glass. The Johns Hopkins Press, Baltimore.

Twenty-five Years Ago in *Genetics*
Electrophoresis in the Development
of Evolutionary Genetics—Milestone or Millstone?

○ ○

R. C. Lewontin

Museum of Comparative Zoology, Harvard University, Cambridge, Massachusetts 02138

WHEN I entered TH. DOBZHANSKY's laboratory as a graduate student in 1951, the problematic of population genetics was the description and explanation of genetic variation within and between populations. That remains its problematic 40 years later in 1991. What has changed is our ability to characterize variation at the genic and nucleotide level and, linked to the ability to give detailed descriptions of variation, the development of a theory of population genetics that takes into account the full implication of historical ancestries in real populations.

In the 1950s and before, observations of genetic variation were confined to two sorts of data. On the one hand, some morphological variation was a consequence of the segregation of alleles at single loci in classical Mendelian fashion and these could be studied either by direct observation of phenotypes in nature or, if there was complete dominance of one allele, by test crosses in species that could be bred. The blood group and hemoglobin polymorphisms in humans (BOYD 1950; ALLISON 1955), shell markings in snails (LAMOTTE 1951; CAIN and SHEPPARD 1954), wing patterns in Lepidoptera (FORD 1953), and rare recessive mutations in Drosophila were the materials of such studies. Although they provided individual model systems for the study of evolution in action, it was not clear how general a picture of genetic variation they represented. Moreover, it was notoriously difficult to establish differential fitness for different genotypes and up to the present no convincing selective story has been given either for snail shells or human blood groups.

In contrast, it was possible to measure large fitness differences between genotypes when whole chromo-

somes were the unit of observation. There were extensive studies by DOBZHANSKY and his school of inversion polymorphism in Drosophila (summarized in LEWONTIN *et al.* 1981). But the largest single form of data was on the fitness distributions of whole chromosome homozygotes and heterozygotes in Drosophila using some variant of MULLER's *ClB* technique [see LEWONTIN (1974) for a summary]. There was universal agreement that genomes totally homozygous for one or more chromosomes were on the average lower in viability and fecundity than were random heterozygotes. The problem was that the observations could not be interpreted at the gene level. Was the inbreeding effect the consequence of a few nearly recessive deleterious alleles carried by each genome as a consequence of the constant rain of mutations, or was it the consequence of homozygosity at very large numbers of loci that were normally heterozygous, held in heterozygous state in natural populations by some form of balancing selection?

This same problem was at issue in corn breeding. The entire hybrid corn industry depended on the fact that *some* inbred lines, when crossed, produced hybrids with higher yields than the open-pollinated population from which the lines were drawn. Was this because heterozygotes at individual loci gave higher yields than either homozygote (overdominance) or was it simply the effect of covering the effect of partly dominant deleterious genes? If the former, then the inbred-hybrid method was optimal for producing high-yielding corn. If the latter, then a program of selection would be best. Whether in studies of natural populations or in agricultural genetics, the problems could not be solved because no method existed for identifying genotypes at individual segregating loci unless allelic differences at single loci led to clearly distinguishable phenotype classes. So it was impossible

This is emphatically not meant to be a review of the immense literature on the subject, but a commentary on salient points. Thus, the literature actually cited is spotty, unsystematic, and in some ways unrepresentative of the vast corpus of knowledge in the field.

to describe the genetic variation for the genome as a whole in populations, nor to make inferences about the effects of single allelic substitutions. Yet, these were the very data that population genetic theory demanded for making causal explanations.

Needless to say, nothing could be asserted about the genetic differences *between* species either. Under the circumstances, it is not surprising that evolutionary geneticists were divided into opposing schools with more or less uncompromising views of the truth. DOBZHANSKY and his followers belonged to what he called the "balance" school (DOBZHANSKY 1955), holding that every individual in a sexually reproducing population was heterozygous at most or all of its loci. DOBZHANSKY's opponents were derogatorily called by him the "classical" school, whose most influential spokesman was H. J. MULLER, a school that believed nearly all loci to be essentially homozygous, with rare deleterious mutations segregating to produce a "genetic load" (MULLER 1950). Population genetics seemed doomed to a perpetual struggle between alternative interpretations of great masses of inevitably ambiguous data.

All the while, molecular and biochemical genetics was developing a picture of the relationship between genes and proteins that could provide a way out. Putting aside redundant nucleotide substitution at silent sites, a point mutation in a coding sequence would result in an amino acid substitution in a coded protein and, in principle at least, that substitution could be detected unambiguously by the analysis of the protein. In practice, however, the application of this knowledge to population genetics seemed hopeless. No on could seriously propose the amino acid sequencing, by the laborious chemical methods available, of even one protein from hundreds of single individuals sampled from a population, nor would single individuals provide nearly enough purified protein for the analysis. What was required was some technique that would be sensitive enough to amino acid sequence variation to detect that variation in single individuals as small as Drosophila and be applicable to large population samples with reasonable effort. In 1966 two laboratories, one in Chicago and one in London, independently published experimental results that apparently solved the problem (HARRIS 1966; HUBBY and LEWONTIN 1966; LEWONTIN and HUBBY 1966), initiating 20 years of intensive investigation of protein variation in natural populations by hundreds of laboratories. (The latter two papers were published in GENETICS 25 years ago this month.)

The method introduced by HARRIS, HUBBY and LEWONTIN was gel electrophoresis of proteins. It was already well known that single enzyme species could be visualized in unpurified extracts from single individuals by cytochemical staining, and that single amino acid substitutions could change the pI of a protein sufficiently that it would move at a detectably different rate in a charge field. As a consequence, electrophoretic variation in proteins was already known to exist. A survey of the literature by SHAW (1965) found 16 different enzymes in 20 species of organisms from flagellates to mammals for which evidence of electrophoretic variation existed. It remained only to adapt this method to large-scale surveys of individual genomes from natural populations and to demonstrate that any electrophoretic differences observed did indeed mendelize.

The first results were startling. Of 18 proteins (loci) surveyed by LEWONTIN and HUBBY in five natural populations of *Drosophila pseudoobscura*, an average of 30% were polymorphic (*i.e.*, had more than one allele present at a frequency greater than 1%) within populations and the average heterozygosity was 11.5%. For the human population studied by HARRIS, the comparable values were 30% polymorphic and 9.9% heterozygosity. The extraordinarily high genetic variation seemed, on the face of it, to support definitively the views of DOBZHANSKY and WALLACE on the ubiquity of genetic variation segregating within species.

The publication of these results in 1966 had an immediate effect on experimental population genetics and research on species comparisons. Here was a technique that could be learned easily by any moderately competent person, that was relatively cheap as compared with most physiological and biochemical methods, that gave instant gratification by revealing before one's eyes the heritable variation in unambiguously scoreable characters, and most important, could be applied to *any* organism whether or not the organism could be genetically manipulated, artificially crossed, or even cultivated in the laboratory or greenhouse. It is little wonder that there was a virtual explosion of electrophoretic investigations. A comprehensive literature search made by NEVO, BEILES and BEN-SHLOMO (1984) 18 years after the first experiments were published, found studies of intraspecific variation in 1111 species, with an average of 23 loci and 200 individuals per species examined. The range of organisms that have been studied to date includes bacteria, fungi, vascular and nonvascular plants, many phyla of invertebrates, especially insects and mollusks, and vertebrates from fish to humans. While this immense collective body of work is sometimes derisively referred to as the "find 'em and grind 'em" school of population genetics, it established a general fact about genetic variation that could not have been otherwise determined. A typical species population for most organisms is polymorphic for about 1/3 of its loci that code for enzymes and other soluble proteins, and an average individual is heterozygous (or, for haploid organisms, has a probability of nonidentity with another individual) at about 10% of its loci. Of course, there are differences among species. A few, like the cheetah, are virtually completely monomorphic. Fossorial animals as different as moles and mole crickets have very low variation. Vertebrates are somewhat less variable than invertebrates, probably because of their generally smaller population sizes, with average polymorphisms of about 25% and heterozygosity of 7%, but the difference from invertebrates is not large.

In addition to the purely population genetic applications, gel electrophoresis became a widely used tool for species comparisons. Morphological differences between species involve unknown numbers of genes and, to some extent, are not genetic but a consequence of different developmental environments. Electrophoretic phenotypes ("electromorphs") are discrete differences, almost certain to be a consequence of single gene differences, and are immune to developmental variation. As a result, a widespread and often uncritical use was made of electromorphic characters for systematics. It is not always appreciated that two indistinguishable electromorphs may result from two different amino acid sequences so that false convergences will appear in phylogenies, and that the order of mobility of electrophoretic variants from fast to slow does not correspond to an ordering of successive amino acid substitutions, so that there is no rationale for ordering character states in an evolutionary sequence, as there may be for morphological characters. When phylogenetic reconstruction based on electromorphs disagrees with a phylogeny based on morphology, there is no *a priori* reason for preferring one or the other. On the other hand, electrophoresis has been a powerful device for discriminating populations whose specific or subspecific status is in doubt and for detecting hybrid zones between differentiated populations. The boundaries between geographically contiguous species can be found and complex patterns of related species biogeography can be resolved, as for example in Mus (SELANDER, HUNT and YANG 1969).

From the publication of the first results of electrophoretic surveys of variation in 1966, the problem of the explanation of the variation became primary. Is the large amount of standing genetic variation in populations a consequence of some form of variation-preserving natural selection, such as overdominance or frequency dependent selection, or is the variation simply what one would expect from the random accumulation of selectively neutral mutations reaching intermediate frequencies by genetic drift in finite populations accompanied by some small migration between populations? If the former were the case, then the protein variation seen is the stuff of adaptive evolution and is the proper object of genetic studies of evolution by natural selection. If, on the other

hand, the latter is true, then the observed variation is more or less irrelevant to adaptive evolution, at least in the ecological conditions prevailing at present. Then, to the extent that the protein variation is the actual precursor of species differentiation, it would simply be a stage in nonselective neutral divergence between species. The struggle between these two views of genetic variation was evident from the beginning of electrophoretic studies. LEWONTIN and HUBBY, already in 1966, pointed out the immense genetic load that would exist in a population with 10% heterozygosity if it were maintained by simple overdominant selection, even very weak selection. Various more complex selective schemes were immediately proposed to meet the difficulty (KING 1967; MILKMAN 1967; SVED, REED and BODMER 1967). On the other hand, a theory of selectively neutral evolution of protein differences between species was proposed by KIMURA (1968) and KING and JUKES (1969), and it was KIMURA's view that electrophoretic polymorphism was simply a stage in this neutral evolution of species differences (KIMURA and OHTA 1971). Thus, the old struggle between those who saw natural selection as the preserver of variation and those who saw it as essentially a purifying process, was transferred to the domain of electrophoretic polymorphism. Although no one could now deny that there was indeed a great deal of genetic variation in natural populations, the assumption that this variation was unselected made the observations perfectly compatible with a view that when selection *did* occur, it was purifying in nature.

The question was, would the immense body of information from electrophoresis resolve the issue? The electrophoretic variation provided two categories of data that could be brought to bear: *static* data and *functional* data. By static data, I mean the observed frequency distributions of electromorphic variants within and between populations. By functional data, I mean observations on physiological and fitness differences among electromorphs, including correlations between electromorph frequencies and ecological variables.

The simplest form of static data is the gross proportion of loci polymorphic and the average heterozygosity. While heterozygosity *might* have turned out to be so low or so high as to exclude one or another hypothesis, it turns out, in fact, to be just in the range that makes the interpretation totally ambiguous. See LEWONTIN (1974) for a detailed discussion of this problem.

It might have been, however, that heterozygosity was grossly overestimated or underestimated because of artifacts of the technique. On the one hand, the loci surveyed were those coding for soluble proteins (mostly enzymes) or enzymes that could easily be freed from their association with subcellular particles. Insoluble structural proteins like lens, muscle, and membrane proteins might be highly monomorphic. Unfortunately, the methods available to study these require their denaturation and charge saturation so that only size variation could be observed electrophoretically. To the present, we do not know how variable in amino acid sequence such proteins are. On the other hand, gel electrophoresis, depending upon charge changes as it does, might not have been able to detect all amino acid substitutions. Only about 1/4 of all random code changes that lead to an amino acid substitution results in a change from one charge class to another. So, loci found to be monomorphic might easily have been polymorphic, and a serious underestimate of genetic variation would have resulted. As pointed out by JOHNSON (1974), the usual conditions of electrophoresis were just those that provide the least sensitivity to charge differences. To investigate this question, SINGH, LEWONTIN and FELTON (1976) developed the system of sequential gel electrophoresis that uses various pH values and buffer systems to detect hidden electrophoretic variation, and RAMSHAW, COYNE and LEWONTIN (1979) used the sequential system to calibrate electrophoresis on a sample of proteins with known amino acid substitutions. The result of these experiments were that sequential electrophoresis could detect about 85% of all amino acid substitutions at different positions in the polypeptide chain. Application of the method to a variety of proteins (COYNE and FELTON 1977; KEITH 1983; KEITH et al. 1985) gave a clear result. Loci that had been revealed as polymorphic originally by electrophoresis increased in their observed heterozygosity by the discovery of new alleles and in some cases the increase of the number of alleles was dramatic (from 8 to 27 in xanthine dehydrogenase). But loci previously classified as monomorphic remained monomorphic. The result is that the estimate of average polymorphism did not change, and the average heterozygosity over all loci increased only slightly. The data remained ambiguous.

A second consequence of the introduction of sequential electrophoresis was that a few extremely rich data sets became available so that more sophisticated tests of neutrality or selection could be applied to the static frequency distribution of alleles within and between populations. Tests for the operation of selection like those of EWENS (1972) and WATTERSON (1977) are most powerful when applied to multiple allelic loci. When these tests were applied to the extremely polymorphic loci studied by KEITH, loci that had identical frequency distributions in two populations separated by 300 miles, again the results were ambiguous. Even the richest available static data set on electrophoretic variability lacks the statistical power to discriminate unambiguously between selection and neu-

trality in large populations with a small amount of migration.

When we turn to functional data, the situation is not much better. The earliest attempts to find fitness differences between electromorphs by population cage selection experiments seemed to show very large fitness effects (e.g., BERGER 1971). But these effects turned out to be the result of linked fitness modifiers and when large samples of independently derived electromorphs were tested using replicated large populations in laboratory culture, differences in fitness were found to be extremely small or nondetectable (YAMAZAKI 1971; ARNASON 1982) as might have been expected. There has been considerable success in demonstrating enzyme kinetic differences and differences in total enzyme activity for numerous polymorphic enzymes as, for example, in a variety of human polymorphic enzymes (see review in HARRIS 1980), lactate dehydrogenase in fish (POWERS, DIMICHELE and PLACE 1983) and a variety of enzymes in Drosophila (LAURIE-AHLBERG et al. 1982). But it has been rather more difficult to relate these differences consistently to fitness differences, and especially when exogenously provided substrates like alcohol or starch are involved, there is great sensitivity of fitness estimates to the exact conditions of the experiment. At this point, the only case of convincing fitness differences in nature is for alcohol dehydrogenase in D. melanogaster where a combination of consistent altitudinal and latitudinal clines, laboratory selection experiments, and kinetic data come together. Good evidence of some selection on electromorphs is the observation of strong linkage disequilibrium between loci within inversions and of these loci with the inversion karyotype, maintained over very long evolutionary time (PRAKASH and LEWONTIN 1968). However, no such disequilibria are observed in the absence of the extreme recombination suppression created by inversions, so epistatic fitness interactions between loci cannot be large.

Attempts to understand protein polymorphisms by studies of comparative heterozygosity are suggestive but not compelling. So, enzymes in the glycolytic pathway in Drosophila are less variable than other enzymes (KOJIMA, GILLESPIE and TOBARI 1970) and weak correlations between the degree of heterozygosity of a species and aspects of its ecology have been found for various environmental factors (NEVO, BEILES and BEN-SHLOMO 1984). Because loci differ markedly in their heterozygosity, the standard error of average heterozygosity for a species is very large and results are very sensitive to the sample of loci studied. On the order of 100 loci per species would be needed before ecological correlations would be convincing, although there are extreme cases, like the absence of heterozygosity in fossorial mammals and insects. Attempts to predict heterozygosity from evolutionary plasticity have proved disappointing. Thus the morphologically conservative horseshoe crab, Limulus, often thought of as a phylogenetic "relic," is no less heterozygous than the mouse (SELANDER *et al.* 1970). If Limulus is morphologically conservative in its evolution, it is not a general lack of genetic variation that is the cause.

The question raised in the subtitle of this commentary is whether electrophoresis has been a milestone or a millstone in the development of evolutionary genetics. It has been a milestone, literally, because it marked the first stage in a new path of evolutionary genetics, a path that was so ostentatiously announced in the title of HUBBY and LEWONTIN's paper, "A molecular approach to the study of genetic heterozygosity in natural populations." Molecular biology and evolutionary biology are in constant danger of diverging totally, both in the problems with which they are concerned, that is, the "how" as against the "why," and as scientific communities ignorant and disdainful of each other's methods and concepts. The introduction of electrophoresis in evolutionary studies went some way toward impeding that separation and led naturally to an important second stage, the introduction of DNA sequence studies into population genetics.

Electrophoresis was also a milestone in that it provided for the first time the possibility of including virtually any organism in the study of evolutionary variation on the basis of a common denominator across species. It thus broke the monopoly of a few genetically manipulable forms like Drosophila, mouse and corn as subjects for general genetic and evolutionary studies. As a consequence, it has been possible, by the collective work of large numbers of investigators, to characterize the genetic potential for evolutionary change for organisms in general.

The immense outpouring of data on genetic variation has also been a millstone around our necks. Its first effect was a considerable depauperization of the diversity of empirical work in evolutionary genetics. Within a few years experiments on fitness variation in natural and laboratory populations, selection experiments on morphological and physiological traits, studies of developmental regulation and flexibility in an evolutionary context, work on chromosomal variation, studies of segregation distortion in natural populations–all of the rich diversity of evolutionary genetic investigation–nearly disappeared from the literature of our subject as one investigator after another discovered the joys of electrophoresis. But the problems raised by those earlier studies have not been solved. They have only disappeared from our collective consciousness. Nor are they likely to reappear now, as the ever more seductive offspring of electrophoresis, DNA sequencing, becomes the mode.

The second reason that electrophoresis is a fardel that we bear is that the result it has generated is so rich and so general, yet not, in itself, rich enough to solve the riddle of its own existence. So, ironically, the methods introduced to break the old impasse of evolutionary genetics has created a new and more frustrating impasse precisely because the data are so tantalizingly clear-cut and universal.

Those of us who now study DNA sequence variation believe that at this level we will resolve the problems generated by electrophoretic studies and that finally, because the structure of the observation of DNA sequences is qualitatively different from observations of amino acid variation, that the ambiguities will disappear. But that is another story, and anyway it is somewhat reminiscent of one that I remember telling before, about 25 years ago.

LITERATURE CITED

ALLISON, A. C., 1955 Aspects of polymorphism in man. Cold Spring Harbor Symp. Quant. Biol. **20:** 239–255.

ARNASON, E., 1982 An experimental study of neutrality at the malic dehydrogenase and esterase-5 loci in *Drosophila pseudoobscura*. Hereditas **96:** 13–27.

BERGER, E. M., 1971 A temporal survey of allelic variation in natural and laboratory populations of *D. melanogaster*. Genetics **67:** 121–136.

BOYD, W. C., 1950 *Genetics and the Races of Man*. Little Brown, Boston.

CAIN, A. J., and P. M. SHEPPARD, 1950 Selection in the polymorphic land snail, *Cepaea nemoralis*. Heredity **4:** 275–294.

COYNE, J. A., and A. A. FELTON, 1977 Genetic heterogeneity at two alcohol dehydrogenase loci in *Drosophila pseudoobscura* and *Drosophila persimilis*. Genetics **87:** 285–304.

DOBZHANSKY, TH., 1955 A review of some fundamental concepts and problems of population genetics. Cold Spring Harbor Symp. Quant. Biol. **20:** 1–15.

EWENS, W. J., 1972 The sampling theory of selectively neutral alleles. Theor. Popul. Biol. **3:** 87–112.

FORD, E. B., 1953 The genetics of polymorphism in the Lepidoptera. Adv. Genet. **5:** 43–88.

HARRIS, H., 1966 Enzyme polymorphism in man. Proc. R. Soc. Ser. B **164:** 298–310.

HARRIS, H., 1980 *The Principles of Human Biochemical Genetics*. Elsevier/North Holland, Amsterdam.

HUBBY, J. L., and R. C. LEWONTIN, 1966 A molecular approach to the study of genetic heterozygosity in natural populations. I. The number of alleles at different loci in *Drosophila pseudoobscura*. Genetics **54:** 577–594.

JOHNSON, G. B., 1974 On the estimation of the effective number of alleles from electrophoretic data. Genetics **78:** 771–776.

KEITH, T. P., 1983 Frequency distribution of esterase-5 alleles in populations of *Drosophila pseudoobscura*. Genetics **105:** 135–155.

KEITH, T. P., L. D. BROOKS, R. C. LEWONTIN, J. C. MARTINEZ and D. R. RIGBY, 1985 Nearly identical allelic distributions of xanthine dehydrogenase in two populations of *Drosophila pseudoobscura*. Mol. Biol. Evol. **2:** 206–216.

KIMURA, M., 1968 Evolutionary rate at the molecular level. Nature **217:** 624–626.

KIMURA, M., and T. OHTA, 1971 Protein polymorphism as a phase of molecular evolution. Nature **229:** 467–469.

KING, J. L., 1967 Continuously distributed factors affecting fitness. Genetics **55**: 483–492.

KING, J. L., and T. H. JUKES, 1969 Non-Darwinian evolution: random fixation of selectively neutral mutations. Science **164**: 788–798.

KOJIMA, K., J. GILLESPIE and Y. N. TOBARI, 1970 A profile of Drosophila species enzymes assayed by electrophoresis. I. Number of alleles, heterozygosities and linkage disequilibrium in glucose-metabolizing systems and some other enzymes. Biochem. Genet. **4**: 627–637.

LAMOTTE, M., 1951 Recherches sur la structure génétique des populations naturelles de *Cepaea nemoralis* (L.). Bull. Biol. Fr. Belg. Suppl. **35**: 1–238.

LAURIE-AHLBERG, C. C., A. N. WILTON, J. W. CURTSINGER and T. H. EMIGH, 1982 Naturally occurring enzyme activity variation in *Drosophila melanogaster*. I. Sources of variation for 23 enzymes. Genetics **102**: 191–206.

LEWONTIN, R. C., 1974 *The Genetic Basis of Evolutionary Change.* Columbia University Press, New York.

LEWONTIN, R. C., and J. L. HUBBY, 1966 A molecular approach to the study of genetic heterozygosity in natural populations. II. Amount of variation and degree of heterozygosity in natural populations of *Drosophila pseudoobscura*. Genetics **54**: 595–609.

LEWONTIN, R. C., J. A. MOORE, W. PROVINE and B. WALLACE, 1981 *Dobzhansky's Genetics of Natural Populations.* Columbia University Press, New York.

MILKMAN, R. D., 1967 Heterosis as a major cause of heterozygosity in nature. Genetics **55**: 493–495.

MULLER, H. J., 1950 Our load of mutations. Am. J. Hum. Genet. **2**: 111–176.

NEVO, E., A. BEILES and R. BEN-SHLOMO, 1984 The evolutionary significance of genetic diversity: ecological, demographic and life history correlates. Lect. Notes Biomath. **53**: 13–213.

POWERS, D. A., L. DIMICHELE and A. R. PLACE, 1983 The use of enzyme kinetics to predict differences in cellular metabolism, developmental rate, and swimming performance between LDH-β genotypes of the fish, *Fundulus heteroclitus*. Isozymes **10**: 147–170.

PRAKASH, S., and R. C. LEWONTIN, 1968 A molecular approach to the study of genic heterozygosity. III. Direct evidence of coadaptation in gene arrangements of Drosophila. Proc. Natl. Acad. Sci. USA **59**: 398–405.

RAMSHAW, J. A. M., J. A. COYNE and R. C. LEWONTIN, 1978 The sensitivity of gel electrophoresis as a detector of genetic variation. Genetics **93**: 1019–1037.

SELANDER, R. K., W. A. HUNT and S. Y. YANG, 1969 Protein polymorphism and genetic heterozygosity in two European subspecies of the house mouse. Evolution **23**: 379–390.

SELANDER, R. K., S. Y. YANG, R. C. LEWONTIN and W. E. JOHNSON, 1970 Genetic variation in the horseshoe crab (*Limulus polyphemus*), a phylogenetic "relic." Evolution **24**: 402–414.

SHAW, C. R., 1965 Electrophoretic variation in enzymes. Science **149**: 936–943.

SINGH, R. S., R. C. LEWONTIN and A. A. FELTON, 1976 Genetic heterogeneity within electromorphic alleles of xanthine dehydrogenase in *Drosophila pseudoobscura*. Genetics **84**: 609–629.

SVED, J. A., T. E. REED and W. F. BODMER, 1967 The number of balanced polymorphisms that can be maintained in a natural population. Genetics **55**: 469–481.

WATTERSON, G. A., 1977 Heterosis or neutrality? Genetics **85**: 789–874.

YAMAZAKI, T., 1971 Measurement of fitness at the esterase-5 locus in *Drosophila pseudoobscura*. Genetics **67**: 579–603.

Alfred Henry Sturtevant and Crosses between
Drosophila melanogaster and *Drosophila simulans*

William B. Provine

Section of Ecology and Systematics and Department of History, Cornell University, Ithaca, New York 14850

WHEN SEWALL WRIGHT wrote a recommendation for H. J. MULLER in the late 1930s, he described MULLER as perhaps the greatest living geneticist. WRIGHT later expressed this evaluation in conversation on many occasions. But when it came to the relationships among genetics, evolution and systematics, WRIGHT's clear candidate for honors in the MORGAN group was A. H. STURTEVANT.

From his student days on, STURTEVANT had been an avid taxonomist of Drosophila and its close relatives. When WRIGHT first met STURTEVANT during the summer of 1912 at Cold Spring Harbor, STURTEVANT spent much of his time collecting wild Drosophila (PROVINE 1986). In 1916 STURTEVANT published a paper on North American Drosophilidae in which he described 23 new species, including *D. saltans, virilis, robusta* and *affinis*.

STURTEVANT was also keenly interested in speciation and mechanisms of evolution generally. I have argued elsewhere (PROVINE 1981) that he was probably the author of the first document outlining the ambitious "genetics of natural populations" series carried out by THEODOSIUS DOBZHANSKY and his co-workers.

One of the first published manifestations of STURTEVANT's larger interests in the interactions of genetics, systematics and speciation came with his discovery that *Drosophila melanogaster* was really two species instead of one. STURTEVANT collected *melanogaster* everywhere he went, especially from his own home town of Kushla, Alabama, and brought them back to the laboratory at Columbia. Males from one Kushla stock were bred by Mr. A. M. BROWN (whom I suppose to be a Columbia undergraduate working in the Fly Room) with females from other mutant laboratory stocks. These matings produced only sterile female offspring. STURTEVANT was fascinated by this unexpected result. He immediately asked his friend, the cytogeneticist C. W. METZ, to send him more wild-trapped *D. melanogaster* from Lakeland, Florida. From these flies, about half of the males produced the same strange results when bred with laboratory females. STURTEVANT gave the flies to C. B. BRIDGES, who quickly discovered a consistent and substantial difference between the male genitalia of the unusual flies and the existing laboratory stocks of *melanogaster*.

STURTEVANT named the new species *Drosophila simulans* Sturtevant and published the description immediately saying, "Since it is evidently a distinct species that has hitherto been overlooked, and since it will certainly be extensively discussed in genetic literature in the future, the following name and description are presented" (STURTEVANT 1919, p. 153).

Why would a new species of Drosophila be "extensively discussed"? STURTEVANT's belief was that an understanding of differences between closely related species would give the greatest insight into the process of speciation. Until the crossing of *melanogaster* and *simulans*, no two species of Drosophila had ever been known to cross. The beauty of this new species was that it could cross with *melanogaster*, the most studied and best understood species. Here was an opportunity to examine species differences with an exciting set of experimental possibilities. Within less than a year, STURTEVANT prepared for publication a series of three important papers under the title, "Genetic studies on *Drosophila simulans*" (STURTEVANT 1920, 1921a,b).

From STURTEVANT's perspective, *simulans* had the major advantage of producing hybrids with *melanogaster*. But there were also two disadvantages. First, all the hybrids were sterile. No progeny testing beyond the F_1 generation was possible. Second, "since the two parent species are extremely similar and probably have identical chromosome groups, the data that are to be obtained from the study do not throw as much light as might be wished on many of the problems concerning the nature of the specific differences found in the genus Drosophila." Added STURTEVANT, "Nevertheless, the investigation has led to interesting results bearing on such subjects as interspecific sterility, parallel mutations, chromosome maps, and sex determination" (STURTEVANT 1920, p. 488).

By early 1920, STURTEVANT maintained in the laboratory stocks of simulans from Florida, New Hampshire, New York, Minnesota, Virginia, Georgia, Alabama, Costa Rica, Panama and Brazil. Why, with the breeding of melanogaster in laboratories all over the United States, was simulans not discovered and named earlier? STURTEVANT noted that a case of unisexual broods reported by QUACKENBUSH (1910) was almost certainly produced by a cross of melanogaster and simulans. QUACKENBUSH thought the case was important because it might shed light upon the problem of sex determination, but he guessed nothing about another species being involved. (Incidentally, QUACKENBUSH did this work at Columbia when STURTEVANT was an undergraduate.) My own guess is that such matings between melanogaster and simulans had been observed but attributed to bad media, X-linked lethals, or something of the sort. STURTEVANT always valued exceptions and the unexpected.

The three papers, "Genetic studies on Drosophila simulans," bore the subtitles, "I. Introduction. Hybrids with Drosophila melanogaster," "II. Sex-linked group of genes" and "III. Autosomal genes. General discussion." The easiest cross was between melanogaster females and simulans males. Only sterile female offspring were produced, bearing the expected female sex-linked characters. STURTEVANT also crossed XXY melanogaster females with simulans males, producing the usual daughters but also sons with sex-linked genes from the father (Y egg from mother, fertilized by X sperm). The reciprocal mating of simulans females with melanogaster males produced males with the usual sex-linked characters, and a very occasional female (which STURTEVANT could not explain). Mating XXY simulans females with melanogaster males produced regular sons and females with sex-linked characters only from their mothers (XX eggs and Y sperm).

When STURTEVANT compared these matings, he discovered that identical chromosome complements (e.g., in reciprocal F_1 females) fared differently depending upon the cytoplasm of the mother. Thus he concluded that species differences pointed clearly to cytoplasmic differences as well as chromosomal genes. This was a very important observation. In addition, STURTEVANT observed that sexual selection was a powerful factor in preventing crossing between melanogaster and simulans in nature. Females were far more likely to mate with males of their own species (although males were ready to mate with females of either species). "Sexual selection, then, is one means whereby the two species are kept from crossing." But, STURTEVANT added, this barrier would "probably be ineffective if fertile hybrids were produced when cross-mating does occur" (STURTEVANT 1920, p. 499).

Complete sterility of the hybrids was a sadness to STURTEVANT. "It had been hoped, had the hybrids been fertile, that the genetic make-up of simulans could be studied through the hybrids. This hope disappeared when the hybrids were found to be sterile, so the problem had to be attacked in another way,— namely, by studying the genetics of pure simulans" (STURTEVANT 1921a, p. 43). STURTEVANT did a neat little trick here. He simply examined hybrid females with chromosome complements from both melanogaster and simulans. If two similar X-linked recessive mutations from the two species produced a recessive phenotype, they were allelic, and if the dominant phenotype appeared, then the two mutations were not allelic. Of six X-linked mutations tested, five were allelic in the two species. Clearly, the two species were very closely related. Oh, how STURTEVANT wanted to see the F_2 generation of the cross between simulans and melanogaster!

In the third paper of the series, STURTEVANT used the same technique as in the previous paper but focussed upon the autosomal genes of simulans and their relationships with the autosomal genes of melanogaster and other species of Drosophila. Two of four third-chromosome recessive mutations in simulans were allelic with recessives in melanogaster; none of four recessive mutations on the second chromosome, however, had corresponding alleles in melanogaster. The linkage groups were very similar (but he had no mutations on the fourth chromosome to work with). From these data and cytological examination, STURTEVANT concluded that the chromosome groups were in fact physically similar. In each of the linkage groups, the order of the mutations appeared to be the same (this conclusion would soon change).

In this set of three papers, STURTEVANT had proved that two closely related species had newly recurring mutations that were allelic and thus probably identical. He claimed that this was the first demonstration of parallel mutations in two distinct species (STURTEVANT 1921b, p. 205–206) and I see no historical evidence to the contrary.

Clearly simulans and melanogaster were two species. Hybrids between them always had only rudimentary sex organs and no hybrids were fertile. Where were the hereditary differences that made them into good species? One place where such differences definitely existed, according to STURTEVANT's evidence, was the cytoplasm. He suggested another extremely interesting possibility in a summary section titled "Complemental Genes" (STURTEVANT 1921b, p. 200–201). Pointing to "the extraordinary variability that has been observed in the F_2 generation of many species crosses," STURTEVANT argued that many of the genes in a species had their greatest phenotypic effect when in the presence of the genes of another closely related species. "Such genes are perhaps to be thought of as having arisen by mutation and having been perpetuated through chance. Since they do not produce any significant effect in the genetic complex in which they arose, they are not eliminated by natural selection, and some of them will sooner or later happen to be incorporated into the race" (STURTEVANT 1921b, p. 200).

Random genetic drift (of course STURTEVANT did not have the name, which was yet to be invented) was perhaps a key to understanding species differences! This was precisely the argument given by SEWALL WRIGHT in the years 1929–1932, but I for one had never appreciated STURTEVANT's suggestion in this paper. (WRIGHT's copy of the paper is checked on the front as having been read; there are no marginal checks or comments.)

While this paper was in press, STURTEVANT discovered that one of his conclusions required revision. He had found two more mutant genes on the third chromosome of *simulans* that were allelic with two known genes in *melanogaster*. Crossover frequencies showed clearly that identical loci were not in the same sequence. STURTEVANT reviewed the evidence for a translocation, the explanation favored by BRIDGES and WEINSTEIN, then offered his own suggestion: "the simple inversion of a section of a normal chromosome."

Such an accident seems not unlikely to occur at the stage of crossing over. If we suppose a chromosome to occasionally have a "buckle" at a crossing over point, it is conceivable that crossing over might be followed by fusion of the broken ends in such a way as to bring about an inversion of a section of the chromosome (STURTEVANT 1921c, p. 236).

So inversions were also possible factors in species differences. First-generation crosses between *simulans* and *melanogaster*, under STURTEVANT's analytical eye, yielded a cascade of important insights into species differences.

STURTEVANT continued his work on *simulans* during the 1920s. A brief report of this research can be found in each *Year Book of the Carnegie Institution of Washington*. STURTEVANT and PLUNKETT (1926) published further evidence indicating that the third chromosomes in *simulans* and *melanogaster* differed by an inversion. Three years later, STURTEVANT (1929) published his major summary paper on the genetics of *Drosophila simulans*. He described newly discovered

mutations, but little of interpretive interest had changed in the meantime.

Because he had done just about all that he considered interesting and possible on the crossing of *simulans* and *melanogaster*, STURTEVANT turned his attention to other problems. As he had stated earlier, STURTEVANT wanted the hybrids to be fertile so that progeny testing for later generations would be possible. Thus, when he wrote his famous three little "Essays on Evolution" (STURTEVANT 1937, 1938a,b), he neither mentioned nor cited any of his work on the crossing of *simulans* and *melanogaster*, not even in the last one, subtitled "On the origin of interspecific sterility." Instead, he talked about the differences between races A and B of *Drosophila pseudoobscura*, arguing that interspecific sterility was probably a product of the occurrences of inversions and small translocations between populations, thus introducing a loss of fertility in hybrids. Under natural selection (on the argument of FISHER), any tendency not to blunder into producing sterile hybrids by cross-mating would be amplified by natural selection, leading to complete isolation of the species.

As I have argued earlier (PROVINE 1981), STURTEVANT probably gave up the *simulans-melanogaster* crossing because the hybrids were completely sterile. LANCEFIELD's discovery of the two races of *D. pseudoobscura*, which could produce some F_2 and backcross hybrid offspring, offered much greater possibility for genetic analysis than with the *simulans-melanogaster* crosses.

But STURTEVANT also believed that something crucial was missing from the *pseudoobscura* case. He did not believe the two races A and B were different species. There were no certain taxonomic markers, such as the male genitalia differences between *melanogaster* and *simulans*. Thus, for STURTEVANT, elucidating the differences between these two races was not as significant as doing the same for two different species. When DOBZHANSKY and EPLING (1944) renamed the races A and B as *D. pseudoobscura* and *D. persimilis*, STURTEVANT (1944) sharply disagreed with their classification. Whether or not DOBZHANSKY and EPLING were justified in their classification, STURTEVANT was right that finding out more about the differences between *simulans* and *melanogaster* was crucially important to understanding more about speciation. Yet it was also true that STURTEVANT had reached an impasse because of the total sterility of the hybrids.

This is the end of the story of STURTEVANT's work on the crossing of *simulans* and *melanogaster*, but it is really only the beginning of what has become a very lively and complicated story that continues to unfold at the present day. Only the barest outline is possible here.

Soon after STURTEVANT published his three papers on the crosses between *melanogaster* and *simulans* in 1921, the Swedish geneticist GERT BONNIER, who was keenly interested in the whole issue of speciation in Drosophila, began to work on the *melanogaster-simulans* hybrids. He believed that the differences between the two species could not be fully understood by STURTEVANT's genetical approach:

As it appears to me necessary for the purpose of gaining a deeper insight into the question, investigations of a physiological, microchemical and anatomical nature on the relations between the two species . . . may be made . . . I hope that these studies will only be precursory to others of the same nature . . . The question of the interspecific relations between melanogaster and simulans appears to me of such import for a great part of the problem of heredity research, that I believe it to be worth while to attack this question from several different points of view (BONNIER 1924, p. 58).

BONNIER's histological study of the hybrids, based upon only a few individuals, clearly did not impress STURTEVANT (1929, p. 9), but did open this general approach to the study of the cross and led to a series of investigations in the 1930s.

Primary among these were the studies of JULIUS KERKIS of the Laboratory of Genetics, USSR Academy of Sciences in Leningrad. During the 1930s, KERKIS conducted a series of investigations of the influence of temperature on the hybrids (KERKIS 1933a), development of gonads in the hybrids (KERKIS 1933b) and chromosome conjugation in the hybrids using the giant salivary chromosomes (KERKIS 1936, 1937). Independently, KLAUS PÄTAU, of the Max Planck Institute in Berlin-Dahlem (later of the University of Wisconsin), reached conclusions similar to those of KERKIS' 1936 paper (PÄTAU 1935).

In 1933, JACK SCHULTZ and THEODOSIUS DOBZHANSKY published their results from crossing *D. simulans* males with *D. melanogaster* triploid females. They saw no way at the time to produce recombinants using this cross.

Enter MULLER again. MULLER was always trying to find techniques that could accomplish the apparently impossible. What STURTEVANT wanted was the recombinant types that normally appear only when the hybrids are fertile. MULLER and PONTECORVO (1940a,b; 1942) and PONTECORVO (1943a,b) figured out a way to produce these genotypes by crossing triploid *melanogaster* females (which often produce gametes with extra chromosomes) with irradiated *simulans* males (which sometimes produce sperms with missing chromosomes). This technique enabled them to produce, for example, a fly with a third chromosome from *simulans* and one from *melanogaster*, but with all other chromosomes from *melanogaster*. MULLER and PONTECORVO concluded that all genetic factors causing

hybrid sterility between *simulans* and *melanogaster* were on the chromosomes. They also found that the sterility factors were found throughout the genome; moreover, the factors were highly interactive. They concluded that even these closely related species differed by a large number of genes that affected fertility.

The final conclusion of MULLER and PONTECORVO (1942) is worth quoting in full, as PATTERSON and STONE (1952, p. 388) already noted and quoted:

The fact that even these minor chromosomes exhibit so many gene differences indicates that the reaction systems producing the similar phenotypes of apparently closely related species may be highly divergent. Hybrid sterility is but one expression of this cryptic divergence, which need not in itself have had a selective value.

This conclusion is notable not only for its challenge to future students of speciation (species differences being very complex genetically) but also because it raises again the thesis that species differences may have come about by random genetic drift of genes that have little or no selective value.

The status of hybrids in the genus *Drosophila* was covered in detail by PATTERSON and STONE (1952, Chapter 9). The hope of understanding the *simulans-melanogaster* cross has never died. A combination of molecular biology and new discoveries of genes that rescue the classes of hybrids that always died in STURTEVANT's crosses has renewed interest in this historically important species cross.

In 1979 WATANABE discovered a gene in *simulans* that rescued the lethal hybrids, and in 1987 HUTTER and ASHBURNER discovered a gene in *melanogaster* that accomplished the same lethal hybrid rescue (see also HUTTER, ROOTE and ASHBURNER 1990 for a more detailed account of this gene). WATANABE and HUTTER and ASHBURNER suggest that, because a single gene is found to rescue the lethal hybrids, studying hybrid rescue loci may elucidate the genetic basis of speciation. MULLER's belief was that a great many genetic factors were involved with speciation of *D. melanogaster* and *D. simulans*, and that studying one locus would reveal rather little.

COYNE, who has also been working on the genetic basis of sterility between closely related species of Drosophila (COYNE 1985; COYNE and ORR 1989), including *simulans-melanogaster* hybrids, thinks that MULLER's thesis deserves very careful consideration before being rejected (J. A. COYNE, personal communication). His hunch stems from the focus of MULLER and PONTECORVO upon the sterility of the hybrids rather than upon the rescue of lethal classes of hybrids. If the genes for lethal hybrid rescue had been found in 1940, I suspect that MULLER would not have changed his opinion, based as it was upon recombinants rather than flies hybrid for each chromosome pair. Time will tell the outcome of this important difference of opinion about genetic differences and speciation.

STURTEVANT believed in 1921 that understanding the genetic differences between *melanogaster* and *simulans* would not only elucidate the genetic basis of sterility but also yield insights into mechanisms of speciation. For 70 years his belief has stimulated a steady flow of important research that still exhibits great vitality.

An excellent recent analysis and overview of the *simulans-melanogaster* hybrids, complete with detailed bibliography, can be found in ASHBURNER (1989, pp. 1178–1190).

LITERATURE CITED

ASHBURNER, M., 1989 *Drosophila: A Laboratory Handbook.* Cold Spring Harbor Laboratory, Cold Spring Harbor, N.Y.

BONNIER, G., 1924 Contributions to the knowledge of intra- and inter-specific relationships in Drosophila. Acta Zool. **5:** 1–122.

COYNE, J. A., 1985 Genetic studies of three sibling species of Drosophila with relationship to theories of speciation. Genet. Res. **46:** 169–192.

COYNE, J. A., and H. A. ORR, 1989 Patterns of speciation in Drosophila. Evolution **43:** 362–381.

DOBZHANSKY, TH., and C. EPLING, 1944 Contributions to the genetics, taxonomy and ecology of *Drosophila pseudoobscura* and its relatives. Carnegie Inst. Wash. Publ. **554:** 1–183.

HUTTER, P., and M. ASHBURNER, 1987 Genetic rescue of inviable hybrids between *Drosophila melanogaster* and its sibling species. Nature **327:** 331–333.

HUTTER, P., J. ROOTE and M. ASHBURNER, 1990 A genetic basis for the inviability of hybrids between sibling species of Drosophila. Genetics **124:** 909–920.

KERKIS, J., 1933a Einfluss der Temperatur auf die Entwicklung der Hybriden von *Drosophila melanogaster* × *Drosophila simulans*. Wilhelm Roux' Arch. Entwicklungmech. Org. **130:** 1–10.

KERKIS, J., 1933b Development of gonads in hybrids between *Drosophila melanogaster* and *Drosophila simulans*. J. Exp. Zool. **66:** 477–509.

KERKIS, J., 1936 Chromosome conjugation in hybrids between *Drosophila melanogaster* and *Drosophila simulans*. Am. Nat. **70:** 81–96.

KERKIS, J., 1937 The causes of imperfect conjugation of chromosomes in hybrids of *Drosophila melanogaster* and *Drosophila simulans*. Bull. Acad. Sci. USSR 459–468.

MULLER, H. J., and G. PONTECORVO, 1940a Recombinants between Drosophila species the F₁ hybrids of which are sterile. Nature **146:** 199.

MULLER, H. J., and G. PONTECORVO, 1940b The artificial mixing of incompatible germ plasms in Drosophila. Science **92:** 418.

MULLER, H. J., and G. PONTECORVO, 1942 Recessive genes causing interspecific sterility and other disharmonies between *Drosophila melanogaster* and *simulans*. Genetics **27:** 157.

PÄTAU, K., 1935 Chromosomenmorphologie bei *Drosophila melanogaster* und *Drosophila simulans* und ihre genetische Bedeutung. Naturwissenschaften **23:** 537–543.

PATTERSON, J. T., and W. S. STONE, 1952 *Evolution in the Genus Drosophila.* Macmillan, New York.

PONTECORVO, G., 1943a Hybrid sterility in artificially produced recombinants between *Drosophila melanogaster* and *D. simulans*. Proc. R. Soc. Edinb. Sect. B **61:** 385–397.

PONTECORVO, G., 1943b Viability interactions between chromosomes of *Drosophila melanogaster* and *Drosophila simulans*. J. Genet. **45:** 51–66.

PROVINE, W. B., 1981 Origins of the Genetics of Natural Populations series, pp. 5–83 in *Dobzhansky's Genetics of Natural Populations*, edited by R. C. LEWONTIN, J. A. MOORE, W. B. PROVINE and B. WALLACE. Columbia University Press, New York.

PROVINE, W. B., 1986 *Sewall Wright and Evolutionary Biology.* University of Chicago Press, Chicago.

QUACKENBUSH, L. S., 1910 Unisexual broods of Drosophila. Science **32:** 183–185.

SCHULTZ, J., and TH. DOBZHANSKY, 1933 Triploid hybrids between *Drosophila melanogaster* and *Drosophila simulans*. J. Exp. Zool. **65:** 73–82.

STURTEVANT, A. H., 1916 Notes on North American Drosophilidae with descriptions of twenty-three new species. Ann. Entomol. Soc. Am. **9:** 323–343.

STURTEVANT, A. H., 1919 A new species closely resembling *Drosophila melanogaster*. Psyche **26:** 153–155.

STURTEVANT, A. H., 1920 Genetic studies with *Drosophila simulans*. I. Introduction. Hybrids with *Drosophila melanogaster*. Genetics **5:** 488–500.

STURTEVANT, A. H., 1921a Genetic studies on *Drosophila simulans*. II. Sex-linked group of genes. Genetics **6:** 43–64.

STURTEVANT, A. H., 1921b Genetics studies on *Drosophila simulans*. III. Autosomal genes. General discussion. Genetics **6:** 179–207.

STURTEVANT, A. H., 1921c A case of rearrangement of genes in Drosophila. Proc. Natl. Acad. Sci. USA **7:** 235–237.

STURTEVANT, A. H., 1929 The genetics of *Drosophila simulans*. Carnegie Inst. Wash. Publ. **399:** 1–62.

STURTEVANT, A. H., 1937 Essays on evolution. I. On the effects of selection on mutation rate. Q. Rev. Biol. **12:** 464–467.

STURTEVANT, A. H., 1938a Essays on evolution. II. On the effects of selection on social insects. Q. Rev. Biol. **13:** 74–76.

STURTEVANT, A. H., 1938b Essays on evolution. III. On the origin of interspecific sterility. Q. Rev. Biol. **13:** 333–335.

STURTEVANT, A. H., 1944 *Drosophila pseudoobscura.* Ecology **25:** 476–477.

STURTEVANT, A. H., and C. R. PLUNKETT, 1926 Sequence of corresponding third-chromosome genes in *Drosophila melanogaster* and *D. simulans*. Biol. Bull. **50:** 56–60.

WATANABE, T. K., 1979 A gene that rescues the lethal hybrids between *Drosophila melanogaster* and *D. simulans*. Jpn. J. Genet. **54:** 325–331.

The Gene (H. J. Muller 1947)

Joshua Lederberg

The Rockefeller University, New York, New York 10021

"THE Gene" was H. J. MULLER's Pilgrim Trust lecture, delivered before the Royal Society of London on November 1, 1945. World War II was barely over, but sea travel was still hazardous. A storm had dislodged a number of floating mines, and the transit to port of SS *Queen Mary* was something of an adventure (CARLSON 1981). Published in 1947, "The Gene" is the finest exposition of the state of development of genetics at the very dawn of its turning molecular in the decade spanned by AVERY, MACLEOD and McCARTY (1944) and WATSON and CRICK (1953). The explosive transition was of course closely linked to contemporaneous history: the burgeoning commitment to scientific research, now strongly supported by government in a style inherited from wartime experience. I will be reviewing this paper in a retrospective mood: "now" (as opposed to "today") will mean 1945. The contrast of 1945 with 1991 gives us a chance to reflect how much we have learned in 46 years, and how much was anticipated. It is especially instructive to reread this work in company with DU-BOS's *The Bacterial Cell* (1945), a noted microbiologist's synthesis that almost converges with "The Gene."

MULLER's leading argument is whether there is "even such a thing as genetic material at all, as distinct from other constituents of living matter." He responds that the simplest observation of the developmental life cycle points to some conserved invariant that persists from fertilization, through embryonic development and the formation of gametes, returning to the fertilized egg. This is then complicated by the requirement for accurate duplication of that invariant, whatever it may be, under its own influence. Discrete mutations are then further evidence of correspondingly discrete particles as the material basis of inheritance. However, the knowledge of chromosomes now enables an appeal to much more direct pragmatic evidence, if not yet of the material composition of the gene, at least of its cytological location. Most of the genetic research during 1900–1945 was indeed devoted to chromosome mechanics; today we view Mendelian ratios less as a fundamental law of biology than of the idiosyncrasies of chromosome partition in material carefully chosen for the avoidance of particularities like meiotic drive, nondisjunction, gene conversion or paternal imprinting.

MULLER turns to the chemical composition of chromosomes as predominantly "nucleoprotein, a compound of protein with nucleic acid, [as] was shown in analyses of sperm chromosomes by MIESCHER, 1897." The reference is to a compilation of MIESCHER's work for the previous 30 years. MULLER remarks that "only recently has it become reasonably certain–through the analogous finding in viruses–that it is really this major component rather than some elusive accompaniment of it which constitutes the genetic material itself." Protein, rather than monotonous nucleic acid, is presumably the information-bearer; however, "nucleic acid also exists in highly polymerized form . . . as may be very significant."

Much of MULLER's own research had concerned mutagenesis, including that induced by X-rays. Again, the gene is a particle with highly circumscribed locality. Mutation can alter one allele and leave its homologous partner "lying but a fraction of a micron away . . . undisturbed." "Blindness and molar indeterminacy" characterize mutation. How this can lead to constructive evolution is usually through the action of natural selection on ensembles of mutations each with small effect, and therefore unlikely to be disastrous. MULLER reaches hard to extract useful hints on the chemistry of the gene from X-ray mutagenesis. At least it is internally nonrepetitive or "aperiodic" (per SCHRÖDINGER; but most molecules are), on the feeble argument that mutation is a discrete event, not a protracted instability that might speak for continued internal reshuffling.

News of chemical mutagenesis was just trickling in, especially of the war gas, mustard (AUERBACH, ROBSON and CARR 1947). These studies were inspired by similarities between mustard gas burns and radiation damage. MULLER was aware of the mustard gas work at the time of his lecture, but military restrictions prevented his mentioning it (CROW 1990). MULLER also recited more dubious claims from Caltech of antibody-induced mutations in Neurospora (EMERSON 1944) which, together with PAULING and CAMPBELL's (1942) claims for antibody synthesis by protein folding *in vitro*, have been consigned to oblivion. Alkylation mutagenesis remains a lively research topic today and, indeed, "These . . . experiments constitute the first decided break in the impasse that had developed in studies directed toward the chemistry of the mutation process." Nevertheless, genetic chemistry has contributed more to the rather intricate and still problematical mechanism of mutagenesis than the converse (DRAKE 1989).

Historically, the validation of chemical mutagenesis seems long overdue, considering that almost every molecule is suspect today. This can be attributed in part to the tediousness of methods, requiring elaborate statistical validation, before bacterial systems were developed. Furthermore, few of MULLER's contemporaries were intellectually positioned to be able to marry concepts from genetics and chemistry; MULLER was by no means a sophisticated chemist, but used an aggressive and insightful imagination in borrowing from the insights of other disciplines.

The new horizon of chemical mutagenesis offered no obstacle as yet to the concept of evolutionary indeterminacy. Despite effects on "the frequency of gene mutation in general, . . . each individual mutation remains a chance and uncontrollable event, from the macroscopic standpoint." This has remained genetic orthodoxy to the present day, bolstered by revulsion about the criminal excesses of the Lysenkoist counter-doctrine. It deserves reexamination in the light of the intricacies of DNA conformation and its secondary structure, which are indisputably coupled to regulated gene expression (DAVIS 1989; LEDERBERG 1989). MULLER's consideration of heterochromatin position effect as a *cis*-acting influence of chromatin coiling on gene expression is a harbinger of today's second look.

Despite the molar indeterminacy of evolution, and the disruptive "bad" consequence of most mutations, "the Maxwell demon of natural selection. . . brings order out of mutation's chaos despite itself." MULLER could not yet know of the plethora of phenotypically silent mutations in DNA which today support a much greater role of mutation pressure and genetic drift in evolution (KIMURA 1991).

MULLER then turns to nonchromosomal genes.

Chloroplasts are the best worked out; but animal cells can do without them. Uniparental inheritance constrains the diversification of chloroplast genomes, and their limited content suggests they have a correspondingly small role in evolution. The chloroplast probably "had a common ancestry with the chromosomal genes, dating back to the period before the latter had become organized into typical nuclear chromosomes." This conjecture was voiced on the brink of a new and successful cycle of evolutionary attribution of chloroplasts to endosymbiotic cyanobacteria (LEDERBERG 1952; MARGULIS 1981). LINDEGREN and SPIEGELMAN's yeast "cytogenes" are also mentioned, but with cautious reservations about the "links of the evidence" for the regular production of self-reproducing replicas from a chromosomal gene. This caution was amply vindicated. However, proviruses, from lambda to HIV today, securely occupy that niche. Some exceptional instances of gene amplification may follow a similar pattern (STARK *et al.* 1989).

For nonchromosomal genes in animal cells, MULLER attends to DARLINGTON and ALTENBURG's speculations about plasmagenes and viroids. These had some support from SONNEBORN's work on kappa in Paramecium, and this is extensively discussed. But while "The Gene" was in press, SONNEBORN revised his prior formulation of a chromosomal origin of kappa, and MULLER footnotes this. The polemics about such particles being viruses, symbionts or genes were the immediate stimulant for the overarching concept of plasmids (LEDERBERG 1952), which has largely dissolved the controversy.

Gene duplication within the chromosome is uncontroversial. After subsequent divergent mutation, "the germ plasm becomes not merely more compound but more complex and . . . the possibilities of organizational complexity for the body in general should rise also."

MULLER was the first high peer in genetics to enunciate that "virus particles . . . which fulfil the definition of genes in being self-determining in their reproduction and capable of transmitting their mutations, are composed of . . . nothing but nucleoprotein." He finds appealing DELBRÜCK's early ideas (1941) about polypeptide template-directed assembly "by means of a resonance . . . at peptide links . . . followed up by a finishing up of the peptide connections, and associated undoing of the" bonding of the old and new chains. To be sure, there is no evidence that gene synthesis involves peptide links; and protamines are too simple. However, some kind of steric complementarity might pertain between basic proteins and acid DNA. By 1953, WATSON and CRICK would model DNA-DNA complementarity as the core of modern molecular genetics. In 1947, chromosome synapsis was a possible clue to recognitional mechanisms in gene duplication, though MULLER is quick to emphasize that karyological synapsis involves forces over microscopically visible distances. Especially perplexing (then and today) is meiosis in Neurospora, where "the chromosomes come into contact while still in a condensed, closely coiled condition . . ." MULLER's response here is an invocation of temporal vibrations, a premonition of holography, better left without further comment, though similar ideas still recur in neurobiological speculation. Many aspects of synapsis, and the example of Neurospora's ability to scan for duplicated segments (SELKER 1990), remain a challenging mystery today.

Akin to virus replication is pneumococcal transformation. MULLER's endorsement was an important testimonial for geneticists of that decade:

> In my opinion, the most probable interpretation of these virus and Pneumococcus results then becomes that of actual entrance of the foreign genetic material already there, by a process essentially of the type of crossing over, though on a more minute scale . . . that is, there were, in effect, still viable bacterial "chromosomes" or parts of chromosomes floating free in the medium used. These might, in my opinion, have penetrated the capsuleless bacteria and in part at least taken root there, perhaps after having undergone a kind of crossing over with the chromosomes of the host. In view of the transfer of only a part of the genetic material at a time, at least in the viruses, a method appears to be provided whereby the gene constitution of these forms can be analyzed, much as in the cross-breeding test on higher organisms. However, unlike what has so far been possible in higher organisms, viable chromosome threads could also be obtained from these lower forms for *in vitro* observation, chemical analysis, and determination of the genetic effects of treatment.

This emboldened me to posit a close analogy to the newly discovered phenomenon of genetic exchange in bacteria (LEDERBERG 1947). But he could not yet accept that the transforming activity had been proven to be pure DNA (contra "nucleoprotein"). PHOEBUS LEVENE had laid the groundwork of DNA chemical structure with the elucidation of the constituent deoxyribonucleotides and their linkage through phosphotriester bonds. But the model closest to hand was that of a monotonous tetranucleotide, which left little room for genetic informational variety. MULLER left several hints that larger polymers might alter our perceptions, but he had no platform for more detailed chemical modeling or experiment.

How do genes work? MULLER cautions against too facile a depiction of the gene or its primary product as an enzyme. I translate his two arguments: that the known primary gene product is another gene, and this has properties not shared by known enzymes; and that developmental pathways will almost always show pleiotropic complications, *viz.* several genes affecting one enzyme even if this is not seen in initial surveys ("new methods will be needed before the primary gene products can be identified"). I shared this skepticism about the ultimate rigor of the "one-gene:one-

47 P ROY SOC LOND B BIO 134				
ABOLINS L	EXP CELL RE		3	1	52
ANDERSON TF	BOTAN REV		15	464	49
BEADLE GW	ANN R BIOCH	R	17	727	48
"	ANN R PHYSL	R	10	17	48
"	FORTSCH CH		5	300	48
BLUMEL J	P NAS US		34	561	48
BROWN GB	ANN R BIOCH	R	22	141	53
BURT NS	BLOOD		6	906	51
CHAYEN J	NATURE		171	472	53
COULSON CA	T FARAD SOC		48	777	52
DAVIDSON JN	ANN R BIOCH	R	18	155	49
DEVI P	NATURE	L	160	503	47
ESSRIG IM	N ENG J MED	R	240	15	49
FRANKEL OH	HEREDITY		4	103	50
GULLAND JM	COLD S HARB		12	95	47
HARRISON JA	ANN R MICRO		1	19	47
HERSHEY AD	ADV GENETIC		5	89	53
HOFFMANN.H	Z NATURFO B		6	63	51
HOROWITZ NH	ADV GENETIC	R	3	33	50
HUSKINS CL	AM NATURAL		81	401	47
"	NATURE		161	80	48
JEHLE H	P NAS US		36	238	50
"	SCIENCE	M	111	454	50
KNIGHT CA	ADV VIRUS R	R	2	153	54
LANHAM UN	AM NATURAL		86	213	52
LAVELLE A	ANAT REC		119	305	54
LEDERBER.J	COLD S HARB		16	413	51
"	GENETICS		32	505	47
"	PHYSIOL REV	R	32	403	52
LEWIS EB	ADV GENETIC		3	73	50
LILLIE RS	AM NATURAL		82	5	48
LWOFF A	ANN IN PAST		78	711	50
MAZIA D	P NAS US		40	521	54
MEDAWAR PB	BIOL REV	R	22	360	47
MULLER HJ	AM J HU GEN		2	111	50
PONTECOR.G	ADV ENZYMOL		13	121	52
"	ADV GENETIC		5	141	53
"	SYM SOC EXP		6	218	52
ROPER JA	NATURE	L	166	956	50
SCHMITT FO	ANN R PHYSL	R	10	1	48
SPARROW AH	AM J BOTANY		34	439	47
SPIEGELM.S	COLD S HARB		12	211	47
"	SYM SOC EXP		2	286	48
STONE WS	P NAS US		33	59	47
VOGT M	Z INDUKT AB		83	324	50
WATSON JD	COLD S HARB		18	123	53
WITKIN EM	"		12	256	47
ZINDER ND	J BACT		64	679	52

FIGURE 1.—*Science Citation Index* to MULLER (1947) for the years 1947–1954 (reprinted from the *Science Citation Index® 1945–54 Cumulation* with permission of the Institute for Scientific Information® (ISI®), ©Copyright 1991). The most recent recorded citation is in ROBERT H. HAYNES' (1989) presidential address to the International Congress of Genetics.

enzyme" theory, to the irritation of BEADLE and HOROWITZ (LEDERBERG 1956). In retrospect, it was an indispensable heuristic, and complications like the intervention of mRNA, RNA splicing and editing, and post-translational modifications could be left for later historical superimposition on the initial skeleton of colinearity of DNA with protein.

MULLER was among the first to extrapolate from basic scientific knowledge of genetic mutation and evolution to their human implications. Mutational disorder will eventually afflict the human genome as a result of the blunting of natural selection by culture; but this process will take centuries and we have time to educate ourselves in countermeasures of genetic hygiene. His estimate of one lethal equivalent as the genetic load of recessive mutation in the contemporary human still stands.

Meanwhile, we should be cautious about exposure to X-rays and to "special chemicals." It is curious that he makes no reference here to nuclear explosions. Fallout was yet to enter the lexicon (after the H-bomb tests), and even then MULLER was concerned that its effects might be exaggerated in contrast to other radiation hazards, and in ways that might erode nuclear deterrence of Soviet aggression (CARLSON 1981).

Horrified by the "terrible Nazi perversion of genetics," he believes that "any conscious guidance over our own genetic processes" be deferred for voluntary concern, understanding, and better developed social consciousness. Many psychological traits, in particular, are attributed to "training or by largely unwitting conditioning." But eventually social wisdom should allow "the self-reproduction of the gene and the self-reproduction of intelligence [to] reinforce one another in an ascending curve."

It will illustrate the impact of this article to list the citations that appeared in 1947–1954 (Figure 1).

LITERATURE CITED

AUERBACH, C., J. M. ROBSON and J. G. CARR, 1947 The chemical production of mutations. Science **105:** 243–247.

AVERY, O. T., C. M. MACLEOD and M. MCCARTY, 1944 Studies on the chemical nature of the substance inducing transformation of pneumococcal types. J. Exp. Med. **79:** 137–158.

CARLSON, E. A., 1981 *Genes, Radiation, and Society. The Life and Work of H. J. Muller.* Cornell University Press, Ithaca, N.Y.

CROW, J. F., 1990 H. J. Muller, scientist and humanist. Wis. Acad. Rev. **36**(3): 19–22.

DAVIS, B. D., 1989 Transcriptional bias: a non-Lamarckian mechanism for substrate-induced mutations. Proc. Natl. Acad. Sci. USA **86:** 5005–5009.

DELBRUCK, M., 1941 A theory of autocatalytic synthesis of polypeptides and its application to the problem of chromosome reproduction. Cold Spring Harbor Symp. Quant. Biol. **9:** 122–126.

DRAKE, J. W., 1989 Mechanisms of mutagenesis. Environ. Mol. Mutagen. **14**(16): 11–15.

DUBOS, R. J., 1945 *The Bacterial Cell.* Harvard University Press, Cambridge, Mass.

EMERSON, S., 1944 The induction of mutation by antibodies. Proc. Natl. Acad. Sci. USA **30:** 179–183.

HAYNES, R. H., 1989 Genetics and the unity of biology. Genome **31:** 1–7.

KIMURA, M., 1991 Recent development of the neutral theory viewed from the Wrightian tradition of theoretical population genetics. Proc. Natl. Acad. Sci. USA **88:** 5969–5973.

LEDERBERG, J., 1947 Gene recombination and linked segregations in *Escherichia coli.* Genetics **32:** 505–525.

LEDERBERG, J., 1952 Cell genetics and hereditary symbiosis. Physiol. Rev. **32:** 403–430.

LEDERBERG, J., 1956 Comments on gene-enzyme relationship, in *Enzymes: Units of Biological Structure and Function* (Ford Hospital International Symposia), edited by O. H. GAEBLER. Academic Press, New York.

LEDERBERG, J., 1989 Replica plating and indirect selection of bacterial mutants: isolation of preadaptive mutants in in bacteria by sib selection. Genetics **121:** 395–399.

MARGULIS, L., 1981 *Symbiosis in Cell Evolution.* Freeman Press, San Francisco.

MULLER, H. J., 1947 The gene. Proc. R. Soc. Lond. B **134:** 1–37.

PAULING, L., and D. H. CAMPBELL,, 1942 The manufacture of antibodies *in vitro.* J. Exp. Med. **76:** 211–220.

SELKER, E. U., 1990 Premeiotic instability of repeated sequences in *Neurospora crassa.* Annu. Rev. Genet. **24:** 579–613.

STARK, G. R., M. DEBATISSE, E. GIULOTTO and G. M. WAHL, 1989 Recent progress in understanding mechanisms of mammalian DNA amplification. Cell **57:** 901–908.

WATSON, J. D., and F. H. C. CRICK, 1953 Molecular structure of nucleic acids. A structure for deoxyribose nucleic acid. Nature **171:** 737–738.

Qualitative and Quantitative Genetic Studies
of *Arabidopsis thaliana*

Bruce Griffing and Randall L. Scholl

The Arabidopsis Biological Resource Center at O.S.U., College of Biological Sciences, Ohio State University, Columbus, Ohio 43210

GENETIC research involving *Arabidopsis thaliana* dates back to the 1940s. A renewed interest has developed recently, however, due to recognition of the unique genomic properties of Arabidopsis, which make it an ideal system for molecular studies of flowering plants. This interest has increased to such a point that the international community of Arabidopsis geneticists organized a formal *Arabidopsis thaliana* Genome Research Project (MEYEROWITZ *et al.* 1990). Their overall goal is "to understand the physiology, biochemistry, and growth and developmental processes of a flowering plant at the molecular level, using Arabidopsis as an experimental model system."

The plan for this project predicts, with some assurance, that "recent progress in the area of genome mapping and of sequencing of specific genes amply demonstrate that Arabidopsis will be as useful to plant biology, and possibly to higher eukaryotes, as *E. coli* has been to microbiology in particular and to biology in general." This is heady stuff to be focused on a small, useless (*i.e.*, noncommercial) plant, but it indicates that many plant biologists worldwide have confidence that Arabidopsis is becoming the system of choice for flowering plants.

There have been many reviews of Arabidopsis genetic research over the years, including eight since 1985. Hence a similar review will not be presented but rather a different perspective will be given, with a different orientation of past work and future prognoses. Here, Arabidopsis research is partitioned into a dichotomy based on the complexity of the genetic systems. The two categories are *qualitative* and *quantitative* systems. The qualitative studies deal with genes of sufficiently large effect to be manipulated individually. The quantitative genetic studies deal with variables controlled by genes at many loci which are, characteristically, strongly influenced by environmental fluctuations. Such a classification is somewhat arbitrary, and under certain conditions one system may

be converted into the other. Nevertheless, it is a useful classification for what follows.

At present, qualitative genes are the targets of molecular geneticists and quantitative genes have been largely ignored. Recently, however, interest in molecular analyses of quantitative systems and molecular approaches to plant improvement has increased. This is because essentially all important agronomic traits are controlled by quantitative systems, and the quantitative genes must be located in order to clone and manipulate them. How Arabidopsis might be used to help solve this complex problem will be discussed in the last section.

We shall present a brief account of qualitative studies and then a somewhat more detailed account of those quantitative studies that relate to arguments to be made regarding strategies for the molecular analysis of quantitative genes. The objectives of this perspective are to point out characteristics of Arabidopsis that make it ideally suited for qualitative and quantitative genetic analyses, and to present progress in these areas; to outline procedures for cloning qualitative genes and progress to date; and to suggest a procedure for cloning quantitative genes.

We also wish to recognize the contributions of one of the pioneers of Arabidopsis research, JOHN LANGRIDGE, whose initiatives provide the basis for the overall theme of this perspective.

Qualitative genetics: Qualitative genetic studies are concerned with the induction, isolation, location and developmental study of individual mutations of large effect. Characteristics of Arabidopsis that facilitate qualitative studies are a rapid generation time (about 5 weeks), small plant size, many seeds per plant, many self-fertilized but cross-compatible ecotypes collected worldwide, a low chromosome number ($n = 5$), and ease of isolating mutants.

Studies with Arabidopsis ultimately trace back to the life-long efforts of FREDERICK LAIBACH who became Professor of Botany at the University of Frankfurt am Main, Germany. He was an enthusiastic promoter of Arabidopsis for the study of plant biology (LAIBACH 1943). According to RÉDEI (1974), however, Arabidopsis genetics was formally initiated by two graduate students, ERNA REINHOLZ (a student of LAIBACH in Germany) and LANGRIDGE (a student of DAVID CATCHESIDE in Australia). The following discussion centers on developments from these two initiatives.

REINHOLZ (1947) worked out details for producing mutants by seed irradiation. This and other mutagenic procedures generated hundreds of mutants and led to traditional qualitative studies. The kinds of mutants isolated and studied included morphological mutants affecting all plant parts, developmental (including homeotic) mutants, physiological (including phytohormonal) mutants, and biochemical (including conditional lethal, herbicide-resistant, and photorespiratory) mutants. Mutant descriptions are found in all Arabidopsis reviews, but those especially devoted to mutant descriptions are MCKELVIE (1962); KOORNNEEF *et al.* (1983), MEYEROWITZ and PRUITT (1984), ESTELLE and SOMERVILLE (1986) and KOORNNEEF (1987). Tremendous effort has been expended to assign about 200 qualitative mutations to the five chromosomes. This mapping is proceeding rapidly, the latest report being KOORNNEEF (1987).

As MEYEROWITZ (1987) pointed out, this approach to qualitative genetics is not unique to Arabidopsis but has been used with considerable success in other experimentally useful plants, such as maize and tomato. The properties of Arabidopsis permit these studies to be accomplished more quickly and efficiently, but no new techniques are introduced which are applicable only to Arabidopsis.

We turn now to the LANGRIDGE initiative, which did introduce a technique unique to Arabidopsis. In his graduate studies, LANGRIDGE wanted to extend the BEADLE-TATUM analytical procedure from Neurospora to flowering plants. This required growing plants aseptically on well defined media through their entire life cycle. He searched the literature and discovered *A. thaliana* as described by LAIBACH in 1943. This plant proved ideal. Although LAIBACH had indicated that aseptic culture of Arabidopsis was possible, he gave no procedural details. Thus, it was up to LANGRIDGE to develop procedures using standard test tubes and other containers suitable for large numbers of plants. These procedures were set out in his Ph.D. dissertation (1955a) and published in 1957, opening a new dimension for Arabidopsis research which was not available with any other flowering plant.

LANGRIDGE's first paper (1955b) reported the discovery of the first auxotrophic mutant in flowering plants. LANGRIDGE's dream of extending the BEADLE-TATUM technique to flowering plants had come true. This mutant involved thiamine synthesis, and it is interesting to note that the second mutant reported by BEADLE-TATUM was also a thiamine auxotroph. Although an auxotrophic mutation in a flowering plant was of considerable interest, probably of more general interest were the pictures of a plant flowering in a test tube and of a Petri dish containing 45 plants! During the late 1950s, LANGRIDGE used the aseptic culture method to study mutants and a variety of other phenomena in Arabidopsis. Thus, the beginnings of aseptic culture techniques were established, and this novel approach has been utilized in much Arabidopsis research involving the isolation of mutants by special screening methods and in studies of their nutritional requirements. As discussed in the next section, it has also been used in a novel way in quantitative genetic research.

Quantitative genetics: Quantitative genetic analyses deal with traits that are jointly determined by genes at many loci and are usually strongly influenced by environmental fluctuations. Only those quantitative studies combining the LANGRIDGE culture procedures with growth of plants in controlled environments will be considered here. These studies are unique to Arabidopsis and demonstrate its remarkable utility for quantitative studies in a flowering plant. This class of experimental procedures will be integrated with the molecular approach in the last section.

In the late 1950s and early 1960s the excellent Canberra phytotron facilities (developed by the Division of Plant Industry, CSIRO) became operational. It soon became apparent that Arabidopsis culture is ideal for such a facility for several reasons. First, test-tube culture permits many plants (at least 1000) to be grown in a single growth cabinet. Second, rapid plant growth results in rapid experiments (15–20 days), which ensures economy of cabinet use and minimizes the probability of cabinet breakdown during an experiment.

Furthermore, test-tube culture ensures that each plant receives the same quantity of a defined nutrient medium. Growing a single plant in each tube eliminates competition between plants for limited nutrients. These two properties of test-tube culture minimize environmental variation and thereby reduce the number of plants required for measuring a quantitative variable. Growth cabinets also provide controlled and reproducible climates, producing exact and reproducible plant responses for many environmental variables.

The remainder of this section briefly reviews Arabidopsis studies conducted in the Canberra phytotron. They are directly attributable to LANGRIDGE or his colleagues.

In the late 1950s, BONNER (1957) suggested the

possibility of a "chemical cure of climatic lesions" for sensitive crop plants. LANGRIDGE and GRIFFING (1959) put this hypothesis to test by growing 43 ecotypes of Arabidopsis at different temperature regimens. Eight ecotypes showed high temperature sensitivity and three of these were cured by appropriate supplements. Hence, the hypothesis was corroborated.

A quantitative design was added to the procedures for most of the remaining phytotron studies. This not only permitted estimation of genetic parameters associated with different environmental regimes, but also provided opportunities to explore genotype-environmental interactions.

The first such study (GRIFFING and LANGRIDGE 1963) compared phenotypic stability of an inbreeding species, Arabidopsis, with that of an outbreeding species, Drosophila. The study involved two parts. First, growth response was characterized at six different temperature regimens for each of 38 Arabidopsis ecotypes. Second, a quantitative genetic analysis was conducted with a diallel of five ecotypes and all possible hybrids grown at the six temperature regimens. The heterotic responses of Arabidopsis closely paralleled those of Drosophila reared in similar environmental conditions, the differences being only in degree. About 5000 plants were included. In practical terms, Arabidopsis is the only plant that could be used for such a comprehensive study. Therefore, it is not surprising that SEWALL WRIGHT (1977) described this work as "probably the most thoroughly controlled study of heterosis that has been made with a self-fertilizing plant."

An even more massive study was conducted by PEDERSON (1968), who grew 10 ecotypes, 15 F_2s and 15 double crosses at three different levels of four environmental variables (temperature, light intensity, moisture stress and nutrient concentration). This involved over 8,600 plants!

Another novel use of Arabidopsis culture was made by BROCK (1970). He was interested in detecting variation in quantitatively inherited traits induced by thermal neutrons and gamma irradiation. This required comparing genotypic variation in irradiated and unirradiated populations. He pointed out that culturing Arabidopsis in growth cabinets controlled the environmental component of variation so well that small differences in genotypic variation were detectable.

In 1971, GRIFFING and ZSIROS examined the role of heterosis in the total stimulus pattern. Two ecotypes and their hybrid progeny were grown in different but quantitatively related environmental regimens. These included three temperatures, two nutritional levels and two planting densities (one and two plants per tube), and plants were harvested at four times. Different forms of heterosis were identified as

dependent on temperature regimes, nutrient levels, biotic environments, and developmental times. This type of experiment illustrates how the complexities of heterosis can be dissected into more meaningful parts.

More recently, GRIFFING (1989) conducted a similarly designed experiment involving competition induced by including more than one plant per tube, in order to test a genetic theory specifically designed to accommodate competition between plants. The Arabidopsis model system provided a successful test.

It is clear from the above that Arabidopsis culture in controlled-environment facilities provides a procedure that remains unique to this flowering plant. The system allows almost complete control over all major facets of plant growth: through appropriate genetic design, the genetic facet of plant growth is controlled; with test-tube culture, the composition and quantity of nutrients available to each plant is controlled; and using growth cabinets, the physical environment in which the plant grows is controlled. Thus, Arabidopsis culture in the phytotron facilitates the dissection of a *quantitative* variable into *qualitative* subunits that may be detected by linkage studies, leading to the cloning and characterization of quantitative genes.

Molecular genetics: According to the *Arabidopsis thaliana* Genome Research Project, the immediate goal of molecular geneticists working with Arabidopsis is "identification and characterization of the structure, function and regulation of Arabidopsis genes." The first step is to clone genes, notably the developmentally important ones. However, this represents a substantial challenge and requires unique approaches. Arabidopsis, and the genetic techniques developed for it, lend themselves well.

For molecular genetic studies, the primary advantage of Arabidopsis over other flowering plants is the physical properties of its genome. That it has the smallest known genome among flowering plants was suggested as early as 1961 by SPARROW and EVANS and confirmed in MEYEROWITZ's laboratory (LEUTWILER, HOUGH-EVANS and MEYEROWITZ 1984; PRUITT and MEYEROWITZ 1986). The reasons for a small genome include little repetitive DNA and, in some cases, simpler gene families.

BOWMAN, YANOFSKY and MEYEROWITZ (1988) suggested that there are essentially four approaches to cloning genes. These are use of a heterologous probe derived from a cloned gene from another organism, differential screening of genomic clones with cDNA synthesized from RNA isolated from various tissues, shotgun cloning, and chromosome walking. Methods of cloning that rely only on the identification of an interesting phenotype, utilizing either walking or shotgun approaches, are being developed in Arabidopsis. Chromosome walking can be applied to a mutant that is characterized by its phenotype and map position.

Although chromosome walking can be applied to other plant species, its most efficient use would be with Arabidopsis because of the small genome. The procedure requires dense restriction fragment length polymorphism (RFLP) maps which are now under construction, the marker total for these maps being about 300.

The development of yeast artificial chromosome (YAC) libraries, with very large insert sizes, should greatly enhance the efficiency of cloning Arabidopsis genes (GRILL and SOMERVILLE 1991). Once a gene has been associated with a RFLP marker, it should be found within one or a few YAC-sized steps. It is also feasible to develop a complete physical map of overlapping YAC clones within a few years. Then mapping a mutation should place it within a small set of YAC clones.

Another approach to gene cloning in Arabidopsis is random tagging of genes. Several methods are possible, the one already developed being insertion of T-DNA by Agrobacterium transformation (FELDMANN *et al.* 1989). Thousands of tagged lines have been identified and several genes have been cloned and characterized. Yet another cloning method being developed uses subtractive hybridization procedures with deletion mutants (STRAUS and AUSUBEL 1990).

These approaches have moved Arabidopsis to the forefront of plant molecular biology and biotechnology. Any or all of them may be possible with other plant species. However, the special properties of Arabidopsis make it the clear choice for such research. Aseptic growth now represents a major tool for efficiently isolating interesting mutants in Arabidopsis. Hence, the contributions of pioneers in this field, especially LANGRIDGE's development of the genetic system, should be remembered as Arabidopsis emerges as a model for genetical research with flowering plants.

Synthesis: Consider now the actual and potential results from applying molecular analyses to the qualitative and quantitative genetics of Arabidopsis.

Qualitative genetics: Several cloning methods have been applied. The *Arabidopsis thaliana* Genome Research Project Report reveals that about 60 qualitative genes have been cloned. Thus, the Project is well underway with this class of genes. While problems remain in isolating and characterizing qualitative genes, including the development of gene replacement techniques and more efficient expression systems, progress toward the major goal is rapid.

Quantitative genetics: No quantitative genes have been cloned, so that the following discussion is purely speculative. Let us assume that chromosome walking is the most plausible method. In this case, the first step is to map quantitative trait loci (QTLs) to their approximate chromosomal positions.

Attempts to map QTLs go back to the early 1920s, with marginal success. However, a recent resurgence of interest has developed among molecular geneticists interested in plant improvement. For example, PATTERSON *et al.* (1988) reported on the use of a complete RFLP tomato linkage map to locate 15 QTLs to their approximate chromosomal positions. However, with present techniques available for tomato, the final step, exactly pinpointing the location of these genes so that they can be cloned, remains elusive. This problem holds for all agronomic crops.

Because of its unique genomic properties, a way may exist to clone quantitative genes in Arabidopsis. The procedure with the greatest chance of success would be as follows. First, grow all plants in a regime using test-tube culture in growth cabinets, thus minimizing environmental variation and enhancing dissection of the quantitative system into individual genes. Next, roughly locate the quantitative genes of larger effect using a dense RFLP map. Then chromosome-walk with YAC clones to pinpoint their locations. Applying techniques such as complementation testing, identify and clone the quantitative gene. Lastly, use molecular techniques to characterize the genes and their main functions and interactions.

Finally, the practical aspect of Arabidopsis would be realized by making DNA probes of quantitative genes and using them to locate homologous genes in any agronomic crop. For example, heterosis could be examined. In the section on quantitative genetic systems, we suggested that heterosis in Arabidopsis was similar to that in a crossbreeding species. Therefore, assuming that Arabidopsis heterosis is of a general type, it could be subjected to molecular analysis in Arabidopsis and then, through appropriate DNA probing, the analyses could be transferred to any agronomic crop. We also suggested that heterosis could be dissected into more meaningful parts. In this case, its molecular analyses in Arabidopsis could provide the means for similar analyses in crop species. In this way, the molecular basis of heterosis, which has been so elusive in the past, may finally come to be understood.

LITERATURE CITED

BONNER, J., 1957 The chemical cure of climatic lesions. Engng. Sci. Mag. **20:** 28–30.

BOWMAN, J. L., M. F. YANOFSKY and E. M. MEYEROWITZ, 1988 *Arabidopsis thaliana:* a review, pp. 57–87 in *Oxford Survey of Plant Molecular and Cell Biology,* Vol. 5, edited by B. J. MIFLIN. Oxford University Press, New York.

BROCK, R. D., 1970 Mutations in quantitatively inherited traits induced by neutron irradiation. Radiat. Bot. **10:** 209–223.

ESTELLE, M. A., and C. R. SOMERVILLE, 1986 The mutants of Arabidopsis. Trends Genet. **2:** 89–93.

FELDMANN, K. A., M. D. MARKS, M. L. CHRISTIANSON and R. S. QUATRANO, 1989 A dwarf mutant of Arabidopsis generated by T-DNA insertion mutagenesis. Science **243:** 1351–1354.

GRIFFING, B., 1989   Genetic analysis of plant mixtures. Genetics **122:** 943–956.

GRIFFING, B., and J. LANGRIDGE, 1963   Phenotypic stability of growth in the self-fertilized species, *Arabidopsis thaliana*, pp. 368–394 in *Statistical Genetics and Plant Breeding*, edited by W. D. HANSON and H. F. ROBINSON. National Research Council Publ. No. 982, National Academy of Science, Washington, D.C.

GRIFFING, B., and E. ZSIROS, 1971   Heterosis associated with genotype-environmental interactions. Genetics **68:** 443–455.

GRILL, E., and C. SOMERVILLE, 1991   Construction and characterization of a yeast artificial chromosome library of Arabidopsis which is suitable for chromosome walking. Mol. Gen. Genet. **226:** 484–490.

KOORNNEEF M., 1987   Linkage map of *Arabidopsis thaliana* (2n = 10), pp. 742–745 in *Genetic Maps 1987: A Compilation of Linkage and Restriction Maps of Genetically Studied Organisms*, edited by S. J. O'BRIEN. Cold Spring Harbor Laboratory, Cold Spring Harbor, N.Y.

KOORNNEEF, M., J. VAN EDEN, C. J. HANHART, P. STAM, F. J. BRAAKSMA and W. J. FEENSTRA, 1983   Linkage map of *Arabidopsis thaliana*. J. Hered. **74:** 265–272.

LAIBACH, F., 1943   *Arabidopsis thaliana* (L.) Heynh. als Objekt für genetische und entwicklungsphysiologische Untersuchungen. Bot. Archiv. **44:** 439–455.

LANGRIDGE, J., 1955a   Mutation studies of *Arabidopsis thaliana* grown in aseptic culture. Ph.D. thesis, University of Adelaide, Adelaide.

LANGRIDGE, J., 1955b   Biochemical mutations in the crucifer *Arabidopsis thaliana* (L.) Heynh. Nature **176:** 260–261.

LANGRIDGE, J., 1957   The aseptic culture of *Arabidopsis thaliana* (L.) Heynh. Aust. J. Biol. Sci. **10:** 243–252.

LANGRIDGE, J., and B. GRIFFING, 1959   A study of high temperature lesions in *Arabidopsis thaliana*. Aust. J. Biol. Sci. **12:** 117–135.

LEUTWILER, L. S., B. R. HOUGH-EVANS, and E. M. MEYEROWITZ, 1984   The DNA of *Arabidopsis thaliana*. Mol. Gen. Genet. **194:** 15–23.

MCKELVIE, A. D., 1962   A list of mutant genes in *Arabidopsis thaliana* (L.) Heynh. Radiat. Bot. **3:** 105–123.

MEYEROWITZ, E. M., 1987   *Arabidopsis thaliana*. Annu. Rev. Genet. **21:** 93–111.

MEYEROWITZ, E. M., and R. E. PRUITT, 1984   *Genetic Variations of Arabidopsis thaliana*. California Institute of Technology, Pasadena.

MEYEROWITZ, E. M., C. DEAN, R. B. FLAVELL, H. M. GOODMAN, M. KOORNNEEF, W. J. PEACOCK, Y. SHIMURA, C. SOMERVILLE and M. VAN MONTAGU, 1990   A long range plan for the multinational coordinated *Arabidopsis thaliana* genome research project. Publ. 90–80, National Science Foundation, Washington, D.C.

PATTERSON, A. H., E. S. LANDER, J. D. HEWITT, S. PETERSON, S. E. LINCOLN and S. D. TANKSLEY, 1988   Resolution of quantitative traits into Mendelian factors by using a complete linkage map of restriction fragment length polymorphisms. Nature **335:** 721–726.

PEDERSON, D. G., 1968   Environmental stress, heterozygote advantage and genotype-environment interaction in *Arabidopsis*. Heredity **23:** 127–138.

PRUITT, R. E., and E. M. MEYEROWITZ, 1986   Characterization of the genome of *Arabidopsis thaliana*. J. Mol. Biol. **187:** 169–183.

RÉDEI, G. P., 1974   *Arabidopsis thaliana*, pp. 151–180 in *Handbook of Genetics*, edited by R. C. KING. Plenum, New York.

REINHOLZ, E., 1947   Auslösung von Röntgenmutationen bei *Arabidopsis thaliana* (L.) Heynh. und ihre Bedeutung für die Pflanzenzuchtung und Evolutionstheorie. Field Inform. Agency Tech. Rep. **1006:** 1–70.

SPARROW, A. H., and H. J. EVANS, 1961   Nuclear factors affecting radiosensitivity. I. The influence of nuclear size and structure, chromosome complement, and DNA content. Brookhaven Symp. Biol. **14:** 76–100.

STRAUS, D., and F. M. AUSUBEL, 1990   Genomic subtraction for cloning DNA corresponding to deletion mutations. Proc. Natl. Acad. Sci. USA **87:** 1889–1893.

WRIGHT, S., 1977   *Evolution and the Genetics of Populations, Vol. 3. Experimental Results and Evolutionary Deductions*, p. 20. University of Chicago Press, Chicago.

December 1991

Twenty-five Years of Cell Cycle Genetics

Leland H. Hartwell

Department of Genetics, University of Washington, Seattle, Washington 98195

IN the last few years, a unified view of the eukaryotic cell cycle has arisen that had its origins in several diverse areas of research including the activation of amphibian oocytes, protein synthesis in cleavage-stage embryos, histone phosphorylation, and yeast genetics. My own involvement began with a genetic analysis of essential functions in the yeast *Saccharomyces cerevisiae* that soon focused on the control of the cell cycle. The historical development of my concepts about the cell cycle, related here, is likely to result in a different perspective from that of those who began their work with maturation promoting factor, cyclins, H1-kinase or even the yeast *Schizosaccharomyces pombe*; hopefully, we would all arrive at a similar current picture. Other recent reviews emphasize the developments of the last few years in greater detail (DUNPHY and NEWPORT 1988; HARTWELL and WEINERT 1989; MINSHULL *et al.* 1989; MURRAY and KIRSCHNER 1989a; LEWIN 1990; NURSE 1990; ENOCH and NURSE 1991; MALLER 1991).

Detecting cell cycle mutants: Although a few cell division cycle (*cdc*) mutants of *S. cerevisiae* were first recognized among a larger collection of temperature-sensitive lethal mutants in 1967 (HARTWELL 1967), the application of time-lapse photomicroscopy in 1970 (HARTWELL, CULOTTI and REID 1970) resulted in the rapid identification of many such mutants. Temperature-sensitive *cdc* mutants were defined as mutants that arrested division at a unique stage of the cell cycle regardless of their stage at the time they were shifted from permissive to restrictive temperature. The detection of *cdc* mutants was aided in *S. cerevisiae* by the observation that all of the cells with the same *cdc* mutation arrested division with the same parent-bud morphology at the restrictive temperature.

About 10% of all temperature-sensitive mutants of *S. cerevisiae* were *cdc* mutants, suggesting that there may be as many as 500 genes with stage-specific functions in the eukaryotic cell (HARTWELL *et al.* 1973).

However, the number of *CDC* genes that could be found easily by analyzing temperature-sensitive mutants plateaued at around 70, a result that probably reflects the difficulty of obtaining temperature-sensitive alleles of many gene products and the fact that many genes are present in redundant copies. Through the advent of new approaches, many new *CDC* genes are currently being identified in a variety of organisms, especially *S. cerevisiae, S. pombe, Aspergillus nidulans* and *Drosophila melanogaster*, and it is likely that several hundred will be known within the next few years.

Dependent order of events: The phenotypes of the *cdc* mutants revealed a fundamental fact about the control of the cell cycle, namely that the execution of late events in the cell cycle depended on the prior completion of early events (HARTWELL *et al.* 1974; NURSE, THURIAUX and NASMYTH 1976), a condition that defines a *dependent pathway* or *dependent events*. Although more than one pathway of events was evident, most of the mutant phenotypes could be explained by a relatively small number of pathways. For example, most of the mutants with defects in spindle morphogenesis, DNA replication, chromosome segregation or nuclear division are organized into a single dependent pathway. The functions executed by the heat-sensitive *cdc* gene products were ordered with respect to the functions inhibited by stage-specific inhibitors (HEREFORD and HARTWELL 1974; HARTWELL 1976; WOOD and HARTWELL 1982) or with respect to cold-sensitive *cdc* gene products (MOIR and BOTSTEIN 1982); these studies revealed that the dependent order of cell cycle events was a result of an underlying order of gene product function. The view of the yeast cell cycle generated by these observations was that of a cascade of events whose order was invariant because late functions could not occur until preceding early functions had been completed. Less comprehensive studies with stage-specific inhibitors and with mutants of metazoan somatic cells were consistent with this view.

Contrasting embryonic cell divisions: The cell divisions of the early Xenopus embryo presented a striking contrast to this view of a cascade of dependent events. Mitosis does not depend on DNA replication as it does in many other cells because inhibition of DNA synthesis does not prevent nuclear division (KIMELMAN, KIRSCHNER and SCHERSON 1987; RAFF and GLOVER 1988). Moreover, inhibition of mitosis does not prevent successive rounds of DNA replication (KIMELMAN, KIRSCHNER and SCHERSON 1987) as it does in many other cells. The early embryos of Drosophila (RAFF and GLOVER 1988) and sea urchins (NISHIOKA, BALCZON and SCHATTEN 1984) display a similar uncoupling of cell cycle events. Furthermore, the activated but enucleated Xenopus egg exhibits contractions with the same periodicity as the divisions of a nucleated egg, suggesting the presence of a cytoplasmic clock that controls cell divisions (HARA, TYDEMAN and KIRSCHNER 1980).

The unified view: How were these differences to be reconciled? On the one hand the cell cycle of yeast and most other eukaryotic cells appeared to be a cascade of events, each succeeding event depending on the former (the domino model), while the cell cycle of the Xenopus embryo seemed to be a number of independent events possibly controlled by a central clock (the clock model) (MURRAY and KIRSCHNER 1989a).

Despite these striking apparent differences in how cell cycles could be controlled, certain observations hinted that the two cell cycles might share elements of both models. For example, in Xenopus (NEWPORT and DASSO 1989) the control of the cell cycle changes during development: at later stages, mitosis comes to depend on the completion of DNA replication. Thus, the two types of cell cycle organization can exist within a single organism, a fact which suggests that the two modes may not be fundamentally different. Furthermore, one *cdc* mutant of yeast displays periodic behavior, suggesting the presence of a cell cycle clock (HARTWELL 1971); *cdc4* mutants arrest the nuclear cycle at the restrictive temperature but continue multiple rounds of budding with a periodicity similar to the interval between normal cell cycles. Hence, yeast seems to have a clock as well as a cascade of events.

Recent work has suggested a synthesis of these two models. The cell cycle of all cells is now thought to be driven by a protein kinase that exhibits cyclic behavior and is the biochemical basis of the "clock" evident in both Xenopus and yeast. In some embryonic cell cycles this clock activates successive events in turn and the events do not depend on one another. In the cell cycles of most other eukaryotic cells, the same kinase activates events in the cell cycle but, in addition,

control circuits are present which prevent late events from occurring until early events have been completed. I will consider the evidence for the kinase clock first and then the evidence for the control circuits that enforce dependent pathways.

The clock: The genetic analysis of the clock began with the identification of mutants in genes that occupied a central role in cell cycle control. One gene, *CDC28*, identified the first function (termed "Start") in the sequence of dependent events in the *S. cerevisiae* mitotic cell cycle (HEREFORD and HARTWELL 1974). *CDC28* was necessary to activate two independent pathways, one leading to bud emergence and cytokinesis and the other to DNA replication and nuclear division (HARTWELL *et al.* 1974). In addition to occupying the first step in the cycle, it was also the focus for cell cycle control both by pheromones (HEREFORD and HARTWELL 1974) and by nutrients (JOHNSTON, PRINGLE and HARTWELL 1977).

A central control gene in *S. pombe* was identified as the *CDC2* gene. Attention was focused on this gene in *S. pombe* because it was essential for mitosis and because certain alleles altered cell size at mitosis (NURSE and THURIAUX 1980). Like the *CDC28* gene of *S. cerevisiae*, it appeared to be involved in the integration of growth and division. However, dramatic differences between the apparent functions of *CDC28* of *S. cerevisiae* and *CDC2* of *S. pombe* initially obscured their relationship. *CDC28* was essential in G1 while *CDC2* was essential in G2. However, once again certain facts hinted that these apparent differences might not be fundamental. The *CDC2* gene of *pombe* did affect G1 when cells were emerging from stationary phase (NURSE and BISSETT 1981) and one specific allele of the *CDC28* gene of *cerevisiae* was reported to arrest in G2 (PIGGOTT, RAI and CARTER 1982).

Three other lines of research ultimately proved to be related to these two control genes of the yeasts. Fertilized or otherwise activated eggs of Xenopus contained a cytoplasmic factor, maturation promoting factor, that could stimulate unactivated eggs to mature and begin cleavage divisions. This activity appeared periodically in cleaving eggs at about the time of mitosis (GERHARDT, WU and KIRSCHNER 1984). Another protein, cyclin, was observed to be destroyed and resynthesized in cleavage embryos of marine invertebrates with the periodicity of the cell cycle and it was guessed that this protein might be related to the maturation promoting factor (EVANS *et al.* 1983). In addition, studies of protein phosphorylation during the cell cycle of mammalian cells showed that several proteins, including histone H1, were phosphorylated at mitosis, and this led to a search for the histone H1 kinase.

In what must be one of the most unifying discoveries in cell biology, biochemical studies demonstrated that the *CDC28* gene product of *S. cerevisiae*, the *CDC2* gene product of *S. pombe*, and the maturation promoting activity of Xenopus were all related serine-threonine protein kinases (NURSE 1990); genetic studies have shown that the kinases from *S. pombe*, *S. cerevisiae* and humans are functionally homologous (BEACH, DURKACZ and NURSE 1982; BOOHER and BEACH 1986; LEE and NURSE 1987). The active kinase is composed of the p34 gene product (*CDC2pombe/ CDC28cerevisiae* protein) and a cyclin protein. I will refer to this kinase activity as the *CDC2/CDC28* kinase. Elegant experiments of MURRAY and KIRSCHNER (1989b), using cell free extracts from Xenopus oocytes that undergo cyclic DNA replication and mitosis *in vitro*, demonstrated that cyclin synthesis is necessary and sufficient to drive successive cell cycles. Hence the Xenopus oscillator is due in part to the periodic synthesis and degradation of cyclin coupled with the activation and inactivation of the *CDC2/CDC28* kinase.

A great deal of research activity focused on the *CDC2/CDC28* kinase family is revealing considerable complexity. Many members of the family have been identified (for example, four in *S. cerevisiae*) (REED, HADWIGER and LORINCZ 1985; COURCHESNE, KUNISAWA and THORNER 1989; ELION, GRISAFI and FINK 1990; LEVIN *et al.* 1990) and it is unclear at the present time how many kinases of this family are involved in controlling the cell cycle in any one organism. Furthermore, the cyclins also constitute a large family, seven being known in *S. cerevisiae* (HADWIGER *et al.* 1989; SURANA *et al.* 1991). With numerous kinases and cyclins, the possibilities for different combinations are enormous. The complexity of the system is greater still because several proteins control the activity of the kinase by phosphorylation and dephosphorylation (NURSE 1990; MALLER 1991). In addition, both the synthesis and the activity of the cyclins are controlled (CHANG and HERSKOWITZ 1990; ELION, GRISAFI and FINK 1990; CROSS and TINKELENBERG 1991; DIRICK and NASMYTH 1991). One of the central questions to be addressed is how many different steps in the cell cycle are controlled by a member of the *CDC2/CDC28* kinase family. At the present time we know that the *CDC28* product of *S. cerevisiae* and the *CDC2* product of *S. pombe* are required both in early G1, at Start, and at Mitosis; three cyclins function in *S. cerevisiae* G1 (RICHARDSON *et al.* 1989) and four in G2 (SURANA *et al.* 1991). In Xenopus, distinct kinases are required for DNA replication on the one hand and for mitosis on the other (FANG and NEWPORT 1991).

Checkpoints: Now, if we accept the idea that all cells employ the same *CDC2/CDC28* kinase to activate key steps of the cell cycle, then it appears as if all cell cycles are basically the same. However, there remains the issue of why in some cases late events depend on

early events and in other cases they do not.

Insight into this paradox has come primarily from studies on the dependence of mitosis upon prior DNA replication (or upon the repair of DNA damage). In some cases this dependence has been overcome by fusing cells at different stages, by adding inhibitors, or by mutations. Fusing M phase mammalian cells with G1 cells causes the G1 nuclear membrane to break down and chromosomes of the G1 cell to condense, suggesting that replication is not necessary for mitosis but rather that the cytoplasm of the cell must reach a "mitotic" state (RAO and JOHNSON 1970). Adding caffeine causes mammalian cells to enter mitosis prior to completing DNA replication (SCHLEGEL and PARDEE 1986). The *tsBN2* mutation of mouse cells (NISHIMOTO *et al.* 1981), the *bimE7* mutation of Aspergillus (OSMANI *et al.* 1988), or eliminating the *RAD9* gene of *S. cerevisiae* (WEINERT and HARTWELL 1988) or the *wee1* and *mik1* genes of *S. pombe* (LUNDGREN *et al.* 1991) allows cells to enter mitosis without first completing DNA replication. These results demonstrate that the dependence of mitosis upon prior DNA replication is not intrinsic to the mitotic apparatus but rather is due to an extrinsic control mechanism. It is likely that the dependent relations between many events of the cell cycle are due to similar controls (HARTWELL and WEINERT 1989). We have termed these control points in the cell cycle "checkpoints" and we think of them as signal transduction pathways that generate an inhibitory signal in response to delayed upstream events and target this signal to the next downstream event.

We can now reconcile the domino and clock models of the cell cycle. All cell cycles may be run by the *CDC2/CDC28* kinase oscillator; in addition to this, somatic cells and eukaryotic microorganisms have checkpoint controls that feed forward to the next event to ensure that it does not occur if the previous event has not been completed. The early embryonic cell cycles of Xenopus and Drosophila appear to lack some checkpoint controls; these are imposed later in development. Recent work has shown that one of these control circuits is, in fact, present in the early Xenopus embryo even though it is cryptic. Injection of an inhibitor of DNA replication will inhibit mitosis only if a large amount of DNA is also injected, suggesting that the lack of dependence observed in the early embryo is explained by the fact that there is not enough DNA in the large egg cell to create a sufficiently strong signal (DASSO and NEWPORT 1990).

One of the important issues for the immediate future is to determine how many such checkpoints there are in the eukaryotic cell cycle. The phenotypes of cell cycle mutants indicate that there are many dependent steps in the cell cycle. Some of these may be simply due to the fact that the upstream event provides an essential substrate for the downstream event. Others may be due to checkpoint controls extrinsic to the events themselves. These possibilities can be resolved by genetic analysis. If a loss-of-function mutation in one gene can relieve the dependence of certain cell cycle events, then it is clear that a checkpoint exists. Recently, mutants that relieve the dependence of budding or DNA replication on completion of the previous mitosis have been found in *S. cerevisiae* (LI and MURRAY 1991; HOYT, TOTIS and ROBERTS 1991).

Another important question is whether the control circuits are really extrinsic to the events that are being controlled. Although the *RAD9* gene is dispensable for the yeast cell cycle, other mutations that relieve the dependence of mitosis on DNA replication are lethal. Is this because it is essential to have such control or because the components that mediate the control also perform other essential functions?

Finally, it will be important to determine the signals and targets of these signal transduction pathways. There is evidence that at least some of these controls act on the *CDC2/CDC28* kinase. Certain mutations in the *CDC2* gene of *S. pombe*, or in genes that control the activity of the *CDC2* kinase, relieve the dependence of mitosis upon prior DNA replication (ENOCH and NURSE 1990; LUNDGREN *et al.* 1991). Moreover, inhibiting DNA replication in cycling Xenopus extracts (with added excess DNA) inhibits mitosis and concomitantly prevents activation of MPF kinase (DASSO and NEWPORT 1990). Whether the *CDC2/CDC28* kinase controls other steps in the cell cycle in addition to Start and Mitosis and whether all of the checkpoints target the *CDC2/CDC28* kinase are also issues to be resolved in the future.

Fidelity: In addition to understanding how any biological process works, it is also of interest to understand how its precision is achieved. The fidelity of mitotic chromosome transmission in *S. cerevisiae* is quite high; cells lose or gain a particular chromosome only about once in 10^5 divisions (ESPOSITO and BRUSCHI 1982; HARTWELL *et al.* 1982; WHITTAKER *et al.* 1988). This accuracy can be compromised by perturbations in the activity of essential components of the mitotic machinery. If essential components are rate limiting for progress or are supplied in excess of other components, then dramatic increases in the rate of chromosome loss often result (HARTWELL and SMITH 1985).

Checkpoints are likely to be another important component in mitotic fidelity. Indeed, I presume that the advantage conferred by a more accurate mitosis motivated the evolution of checkpoints. Loss of the *RAD9* checkpoint decreases mitotic fidelity 10–20-fold in an unperturbed cell (WEINERT and HARTWELL 1990) and has a much greater effect if the cell is experiencing

DNA damage or defects in DNA replication. Similar effects on mitotic fidelity were found for the loss of another checkpoint control (LI and MURRAY 1991). The high fidelity of the *S. cerevisiae* cell cycle may be due to many such checkpoints that delay the cell cycle whenever intrinsic errors are made in order to permit repair of these errors.

If it is true that checkpoints exist to ensure the high fidelity of mitosis, we might wonder how the early embryos of Drosophila and Xenopus came to dispense with these controls. One would think that errors during early embryonic divisions would be especially devastating. We have suggested that some early embryos have dispensed with these controls because their developmental strategies require very rapid and synchronous mitotic divisions. Checkpoints act antagonistically to these needs because they delay division to permit repair and they do so only in the subset of cells that have experienced a perturbation to the normal process.

Is there any way for these embryos to avoid the mitotic errors that would occur in the absence of cell cycle checkpoints? One method would be to wait until the early divisions are complete, survey the nuclei, and discard those that are abnormal. This idea is not as far-fetched as it may seem because it is clear that organisms can detect the number of *X* chromosomes in a nucleus, as well as autosomal aneuploidy; furthermore, embryos can develop normally after surgical removal of many nuclei. There is evidence that Drosophila embryos discard abnormal nuclei. Nuclei that have failed to separate completely from neighboring nuclei (SULLIVAN, MINDEN and ALBERTS 1990) or nuclei with a chromosome that is lagging on the metaphase plate because it is abnormally large (W. SULLIVAN, personal communication) frequently are removed from the surface of the Drosophila embryo and segregated to the interior yolk mass. An important goal for the future will be to determine how widespread among organisms is the absence of checkpoints during early embryonic divisions and what mechanisms, if any, exist for discarding abnormal nuclei.

Finally, it is almost certain that cell cycle work will inform human disease research. Intense research is currently focused on identifying oncogenes and tumor suppressor genes and in finding out how their products impinge upon the expression or activity of the *CDC2/CDC28* kinase. Furthermore, an important component in the origin of cancer is likely to be found in changes in the fidelity of mitosis that permit rapid evolution of malignant cells; the changes that lead to this infidelity may be found in perturbations to the checkpoints of the cell cycle.

I thank LISA KADYK, WENDY RAYMOND and TODD SEELEY for their comments on the manuscript. My research has been supported by the National Institutes of Health, the National Science Foundation, the American Business Foundation for Cancer Research and I am currently an American Cancer Society Research Professor.

LITERATURE CITED

BEACH, D., B. DURKACZ and P. NURSE, 1982 Functionally homologous cell cycle control genes in budding and fission yeast. Nature **300:** 706–709.

BOOHER, R., and D. BEACH, 1986 Site-specific mutagenesis of *cdc2+*, a cell cycle control gene of the fission yeast *Schizosaccharomyces pombe*. Mol. Cell. Biol. **10:** 3523–3530.

CHANG, F., and I. HERSKOWITZ, 1990 Identification of an effector for cell-cycle arrest by a negative growth factor of yeast: *FAR1* is an inhibitor of a G1 cyclin, *CLN2*. Cell **63:** 999–1011.

COURCHESNE, W. E., R. KUNISAWA and J. THORNER, 1989 A putative protein kinase overcomes pheromone-induced arrest of cell cycling in *S. cerevisiae*. Cell **58:** 1107–1119.

CROSS, F. R., and A. H. TINKELENBERG, 1991 A potential positive feedback loop controlling *CLN1* and *CLN2* gene expression at the start of the yeast cell cycle. Cell **65:** 875–883.

DASSO, M., and J. W. NEWPORT, 1990 Completion of DNA replication is monitored by a feedback system that controls the initiation of mitosis *in vitro*: studies in Xenopus. Cell **61:** 811–823.

DIRICK, L., and K. NASMYTH, 1991 Positive feedback in the activation of G1 cyclins in yeast. Nature **351:** 754–757.

DUNPHY, W. G., and J. W. NEWPORT, 1988 Unraveling of mitotic control mechanisms. Cell **55:** 925–928.

ELION, E. A., P. L. GRISAFI and G. R. FINK, 1990 *FUS3* encodes a *cdc2+/CDC28*-related kinase required for the transition from mitosis to conjugation. Cell **60:** 649–664.

ENOCH, T., and P. NURSE, 1990 Mutation of fission yeast cell cycle control genes abolishes dependence of mitosis on DNA replication. Cell **60:** 665–673.

ENOCH, T., and P. NURSE, 1991 Coupling M phase and S phase: controls maintaining the dependence of mitosis on chromosome replication. Cell **65:** 921–923.

ESPOSITO, M. S., and C. V. BRUSCHI, 1982 Molecular mechanisms of DNA recombination: testing mitotic and meiotic models. Rec. Adv. Yeast Mol. Biol. **1:** 242–253.

EVANS, T., E. T. ROSETHAL, J. YOUNGBLOM, D. DISTEL and T. HUNT, 1983 Cyclin: a protein specified by maternal mRNA in sea urchin eggs that is destroyed at each cleavage division. Cell 33: 389–396.

FANG, F., and J. W. NEWPORT, 1991 Evidence that the G1-S and G2-M transitions are controlled by different *cdc2* proteins in higher eukaryotes. Cell **66:** 731–742.

GERHARDT, J., M. WU and M. KIRSCHNER, 1984 Cell cycle dynamics of an M-phase-specific cytoplasmic factor in *Xenopus laevis* oocytes and eggs. J. Cell Biol. **98:** 1247–1255.

HADWIGER, J. A., C. WITTENBERG, H. E. RICHARDSON, M. DE BANOS LOPES and S. I. REED, 1989 A family of cyclin homologs that control the G1 phase in yeast. Proc. Natl. Acad. Sci. USA **86:** 6255–6259.

HARA, K., P. TYDEMAN and M. KIRSCHNER, 1980 A cytoplasmic clock with the same period as the division cycle in Xenopus eggs. Proc. Natl. Acad. Sci. USA **77:** 462–466.

HARTWELL, L. H., 1967 Macromolecule synthesis in temperature-sensitive mutants of yeast. J. Bacteriol. **93:** 1662–1670.

HARTWELL, L. H., 1971 Genetic control of the cell division cycle in yeast. II. Genes controlling DNA replication and its initiation. J. Mol. Biol. **59:** 183–194.

HARTWELL, L. H., 1976 Sequential function of gene products relative to DNA synthesis in the yeast cell cycle. J. Mol. Biol. **104:** 803–817.

HARTWELL, L. H., J. CULOTTI and B. REID, 1970 Genetic control

of the cell division cycle in yeast. I. Detection of mutants. Proc. Natl. Acad. Sci. USA 66: 352–359.

HARTWELL, L. H., and D. SMITH, 1985 Altered fidelity of mitotic chromosome transmission in cell cycle mutants of *S. cerevisiae*. Genetics 110: 381–395.

HARTWELL, L. H., and T. A. WEINERT, 1989 Checkpoints: controls that ensure the order of cell cycle events. Science **246:** 629–634.

HARTWELL, L. H., R. K. MORTIMER, J. CULOTTI and M. CULOTTI, 1973 Genetic control of the cell division cycle in yeast. V. Genetic analysis of mutants. Genetics **74:** 267–286.

HARTWELL, L. H., J. CULOTTI, J. R. PRINGLE and B. J. REID, 1974 Genetic control of the cell division cycle in yeast. Science **183:** 46–51.

HARTWELL, L. H., S. K. DUTCHER, J. S. WOOD and B. GARVIK, 1982 The fidelity of mitotic chromosome reproduction in *S. cerevisiae*. Rec. Adv. Yeast Mol. Biol. **1:** 28–38.

HEREFORD, L. M., and L. H. HARTWELL, 1974 Sequential gene function in the initiation of *Saccharomyces cerevisiae* DNA synthesis. J. Mol. Biol. **84:** 445–461.

HOYT, M. A., L. TOTIS and B. T. ROBERTS, 1991 *Saccharomyces cerevisiae* genes required for cell cycle arrest in response to loss of microtubule function. Cell **66:** 507–517.

JOHNSTON, G. C., J. R. PRINGLE and L. H. HARTWELL, 1977 Coordination of growth with cell division in the yeast *Saccharomyces cerevisiae*. Exp. Cell Res. **105:** 79–98.

KIMELMAN, D., M. KIRSCHNER and T. SCHERSON, 1987 The events of the midblastula transition in Xenopus are regulated by changes in the cell cycle. Cell **48:** 399–407.

LEE, M. G., and P. NURSE, 1987 Complementation used to clone a human homolog of the fission yeast cell cycle control gene *cdc2+*. Nature **327:** 31–35.

LEVIN, D. E., F. O. FIELDS, R. KUNISAWA, J. M. BISHOP and J. THORNER, 1990 A candidate protein kinase C gene, *PKC1*, is required for the *S. cerevisiae* cell cycle. Cell **62:** 213–224.

LEWIN, B., 1990 Driving the cell cycle: M phase kinase, its partners, and substrates. Cell **61:** 743–752.

LI, R., and A. W. MURRAY, 1991 Feedback control of mitosis in budding yeast. Cell **66:** 519–531.

LUNDGREN, K., N. WALWORTH, R. BOOHER, M. DEMBSKI, M. KIRSCHNER and D. BEACH, 1991 *mik1* and *wee1* cooperate in the inhibitory tyrosine phosphorylation of *cdc2p*. Cell **64:** 1111–1122.

MALLER, J. L., 1991 Mitotic control. Curr. Opin. Cell Biol. **3:** 269–275.

MINSHULL, J., J. PINES, R. GOLSTEYN, N. STANDART, S. MACKIE, A. COLMAN, J. BLOW, J. V. RUDERMAN, M. WU and T. HUNT, 1989 The role of cyclin synthesis, modification and destruction in the control of cell division. J. Cell Sci. Suppl. **12:** 77–97.

MOIR, D., and D. BOTSTEIN, 1982 Determination of the order of gene function in the yeast nuclear division pathway using *cs* and *ts* mutants. Genetics **100:** 565–577.

MURRAY, A. W., and M. W. KIRSCHNER, 1989a Dominoes and clocks: the union of two views of cell cycle regulation. Science **246:** 614–621.

MURRAY, A. W., and M. W. KIRSCHNER, 1989b Cyclin synthesis drives the early embryonic cell cycle. Nature **339:** 275–280.

NEWPORT, J., and M. DASSO, 1989 A functional link between DNA replication and mitosis. J. Cell Sci. Suppl. **12:** 149–160.

NISHIMOTO, T., R. ISHIDA, K. AJIRO, S. YAMAMOTO and T. TAKAHASHI, 1981 The synthesis of protein(s) for chromosome condensation may be regulated by a post-transcriptional mechanism. J. Cell. Physiol. **109:** 299–308.

NISHIOKA, D., R. BALCZON and G. SCHATTEN, 1984 Relationship between DNA synthesis and mitotic events in fertilized sea urchin eggs. Cell Biol. Int. Rep. **8:** 337–346.

NURSE, P., 1990   Universal control mechanism regulating onset of
M-phase. Nature **344:** 503–508.

NURSE, P., and Y. BISSETT, 1981   Cell cycle gene required in G1
for commitment to cell division and in G2 for control of mitosis
in fission yeast. Nature **292:** 558–560.

NURSE, P., and P. THURIAUX, 1980   Regulatory genes controlling
mitosis in the fission yeast *Schizosaccharomyces pombe*. Genetics
96: 627–637.

NURSE, P., P. THURIAUX and K. NASMYTH, 1976   Genetic control
of the cell division cycle in the fission yeast *Schizosaccharomyces
pombe*. Mol. Gen. Genet. **146:** 167–178.

OSMANI, S. A., D. B. ENGLE, J. H. DOONAN and N. R. MORRIS,
1988   Spindle formation and chromatin condensation in cells
blocked at interphase by mutation of a negative cell cycle
control gene. Cell **52:** 241–251.

PIGGOTT, J. R., R. RAI and B. L. A. CARTER, 1982   A bifunctional
gene product involved in two phases of the yeast cell cycle.
Nature **298:** 391–393.

RAFF, J. W., and D. M. GLOVER, 1988   Nuclear and cytoplasmic
mitotic cycles continues in Drosophila embryos in which DNA
synthesis is inhibited with aphidicolin. J. Cell Biol. **107:** 2009–
2019.

RAO, P. N., and R. T. JOHNSON, 1970   Mammalian cell fusion:
studies on the regulation of DNA synthesis and mitosis. Nature
225: 159–164.

REED, S. I., J. A. HADWIGER and A. T. LORINCZ, 1985   Protein
kinase activity associated with the product of the yeast cell
division cycle gene *CDC28*. Proc. Natl. Acad. Sci. USA **82:**
4055–4059.

RICHARDSON, H. E., C. WITTENBERG, F. CROSS and S. I. REED,
1989   An essential G1 function for cyclin-like proteins in yeast.
Cell **59:** 1127–1133.

SCHLEGEL, R., and A. PARDEE, 1986   Caffeine-induced uncoupling
of mitosis from the completion of DNA replication in mammalian cells. Science **232:** 1264–1266.

SULLIVAN, W., J. MINDEN and B. ALBERTS, 1990   daughterless-
abo-like, a Drosophila maternal-effect mutation that exhibits
abnormal centrosome separation during the late blastoderm
divisions. Development **110:** 311–323.

SURANA, U., H. ROBITSCH, C. PRICE, T. SCHUSTER, I. FITCH, A. B.
FUTCHER and K. NASMYTH, 1991   The role of *CDC28* and
cyclins during mitosis in the budding yeast *S. cerevisiae*. Cell **65:**
145–161.

WEINERT, T. A., and L. H. HARTWELL, 1988   The *RAD9* gene
controls the cell cycle response to DNA damage in *Saccharomyces cerevisiae*. Science **241:** 317–322.

WEINERT, T. A., and L. H. HARTWELL, 1990   Characterization of
RAD9 of *Saccharomyces cerevisiae* and evidence that its function
acts posttranslationally in cell cycle arrest after DNA damage.
Mol. Cell. Biol. **10:** 6554–6564.

WHITTAKER, S. G., B. M. ROCKMILL, A. E. BLECHL, D. H. MALONEY,
M. A. RESNICK and S. FOGEL, 1988   The detection of mitotic
and meiotic aneuploidy in yeast using a gene dosage selection
system. Mol. Gen. Genet. **215:** 10–18.

WOOD, J. S., and L. H. HARTWELL, 1982   A dependent pathway
of gene functions leading to chromosome segregation in *S.
cerevisiae*. J. Cell. Biol. **94:** 718–726.

Centennial
J. B. S. Haldane, 1892–1964

James F. Crow

Genetics Department, University of Wisconsin–Madison, Madison, Wisconsin 53706

REMARKABLY, three years, 1889–1892, saw the birth of six men who dominated genetics in its pre-molecular days: C. B. BRIDGES, 1889; SEWALL WRIGHT, 1889; R. A. FISHER, 1890; H. J. MULLER, 1890; A. H. STURTEVANT, 1891; and J. B. S. HALDANE, 1892.

By far the most broadly knowledgeable of these pioneers was HALDANE, "probably the most erudite biologist of his generation, and perhaps of the century" (WHITE 1965). Yet, whereas each of the others is known for at least one path-breaking accomplishment, HALDANE is not. Why? I think the answer lies in the very breadth of his knowledge and interest. He did too many things, he had too many distractions, he was too eclectic, he was too interested in the work of others, and he was too open-minded to push specific ideas. His name is now regularly associated with only two phenomena, HALDANE's rule for interspecies hybrids and the BRIGGS-HALDANE equations for enzyme kinetics. Yet, his influence was felt throughout genetics and considerably beyond.

JOHN BURDON SANDERSON HALDANE was the son of a distinguished physiologist, JOHN SCOTT HALDANE. He actively aided his father in his respiratory experiments, frequently as an experimental subject, and being mathematically precocious, often did calculations and derivations. He was educated at Eton, which he hated, and Oxford, which he loved. He studied maths and won a prize, then switched to classics and graduated with a first in "greats." He never ceased to enjoy quoting poetry in Greek, Latin and the several other languages in which he was fluent. In his sixties in India, he complained that it was no longer easy to learn a new language. He had no graduate degree in science; if you know as much as HALDANE you don't need one. As a student he intended to follow in his father's footsteps and go on to graduate work in physiology, but World War I intervened and he spent four and half years as a bombing officer in the Black Watch. Amazingly, despite being injured twice, he found the whole bloody experience exciting, even exhilarating.

Returning to Oxford in 1919 he became a fellow in physiology. In 1923 he became a reader in biochemistry at Cambridge under F. GOWLAND HOPKINS. After 10 years he moved to University College, London, remaining until 1957. He then migrated to India, first to the Indian Statistical Institute in Calcutta and eventually to Bhubaneswar, Orissa. Changes of locale were usually precipitated by a disagreement, followed by a characteristic Haldanian denunciation and a highly public resignation. In particular, his move to India was the result of increasing dissatisfaction with England, and the Suez crisis in particular. He seized the opportunity to say that he could not continue to live in a criminal police state dominated by a foreign power. He also said that he was increasingly uncomfortable with not being able to understand all the latest technology, particularly electronics, and preferred to move to a country whose technology he could fully understand.

Associating with HALDANE was always stimulating, but not easy. His students admired him, but feared his unpredictability. He could be excessively friendly, but also prickly. He was often insulting, but claimed to be impartial by insulting everyone. Yet he enjoyed conversation and could be completely charming. CLARK (1969) called him a "cuddly cactus."

Biology, especially genetics: In 1901, when HALDANE was 8 years old, his father took him to hear a lecture by DARBISHIRE on the new Mendelian theory. He found it "interesting, but difficult," and his interest in the subject never ceased. A decade later he found evidence for reduplication (as linkage was then called) in some of DARBISHIRE's mouse data. He was advised by PUNNETT not to publish until he did experiments of his own, which he started with a friend A. D. SPRUNT and his gifted younger sister, NAOMI (MIT-

CHISON). They soon confirmed the results, but not until HALDANE was in the battlefield. The paper, I suppose the most important science article ever written in a front-line trench, was finally published in 1915. SPRUNT had already been killed. HALDANE always regretted not publishing the work sooner, for he would then have been contemporaneous with MORGAN.

HALDANE soon developed a much deeper insight into linkage, and was the first to derive a mapping function. The widely used KOSAMBI formula is a particular solution of HALDANE's differential equation. Later, he demonstrated interference by chiasma distribution and measured linkage in polyploids, finding the values roughly the same as in diploids. He also contributed substantially to the theory of polyploid segregation.

During the early twenties he formulated the empirical generalization, now known as HALDANE's rule, that in interspecies hybrids if one sex has reduced viability or fertility, it is the heterogametic sex. He changed his mind at least once about the explanation and the genetic basis is still in dispute, as attested by a flurry of recent articles–see, for example, COYNE and ORR (1989), FRANK (1991), and HURST and POMIANKOWSKI (1991).

As a physiologist and biochemist he quantified his father's theories about blood pH and alkaline reserve. He followed his usual practice of experimenting on himself and found that drinking ammonium chloride gave symptoms of severe acid poisoning. Ammonium chloride turned out to be an effective treatment for babies whose fits were caused by excess blood alkalinity. As a result of his experiments on respiration he learned the trick for which he later became famous. This was to speak, harmonica-like, while inhaling as well as while exhaling–amusing, but sometimes exasperating to those who might have wished to interrupt his continuous flow of words. Another consequence of his knowledge of respiratory physiology was his subsequent life-saving wartime work, again with himself and friends as guinea pigs, on life at high pressures, such as were encountered in submarines and escapes therefrom.

Also during this period he did fundamental work on enzymology, culminating in a classic book (HALDANE 1930). It was reprinted in the last year of his life. The most important result was the BRIGGS-HALDANE relationship which added realism and specificity to the MICHAELIS-MENTON equation. The form of the equation remained the same, but the MICHAELIS constant, K_m, now became a ratio of different velocity constants and no longer a simple dissociation constant. Somewhat later HALDANE, in his association with the John Innes Horticulural Institution, instigated several studies on the biochemistry of flower colors, in some

ways anticipating modern biochemical genetics. He organized human enzymatic pathways in a highly influential book *New Paths in Genetics* (HALDANE 1942). Among a number of original touches in this book, he purloined the words *cis* and *trans* from chemistry and introduced them in their now-familiar genetic context.

As a human geneticist, HALDANE, along with FISHER, pioneered in developing methods for segregation and linkage analysis. He was the first to measure a human recombination value, that between hemophilia and color-blindness. He worked out the equilibrium relationship between mutation and selection and used this to measure the rate of mutation of the hemophilia gene. Remarkably, he discovered that the male rate is an order of magnitude higher than that in females. This was doubted at the time, but is now abundantly confirmed. This led to the idea, for which there is now strong evidence, that neutral molecular evolution in primates is male-driven (MIYATA *et al.* 1990).

HALDANE was a prophet ahead of his time in suggesting that abnormal hemoglobins were maintained at high frequency by heterozygote resistance to malaria. He also noticed the polymorphism at the *Rh* locus in Europeans and their derivatives, when the equilibrium should be unstable. He argued for infectious disease as a major selective factor in human evolution.

Finally, I should mention one of HALDANE's most influential thoughts. As early as 1924 he foretold the current heterotrophic theory of the origin of life. (He and OPARIN apparently arrived at this independently.) HALDANE was much impressed by MULLER's analogizing viruses and genes. He noted that the primitive atmosphere contained little or no oxygen, hence more UV impinged on the earth. To quote: "Now, when ultraviolet light acts on a mixture of water, carbon dioxide, and ammonia, a vast variety of organic substances are made, including sugars and apparently some of the materials from which proteins are built up ... In this present world such substances, if left about, decay–that is to say, they are destroyed by microorganisms. But before the origin of life they must have accumulated till the primitive oceans reached the consistency of hot dilute soup. Today an organism must trust to luck, skill, or strength to obtain its food. The first precursors of life found food available in considerable quantities, and had no competitors in the struggle for existence."

Evolution theory: HALDANE's best known work is his mathematical work in evolution. He, along with WRIGHT and FISHER, founded the subject of population genetics. In a series of papers starting in 1924 he made a systematic study of the kinetics of selection. His tables giving the rate of change of gene frequencies under selection are found in one textbook after another. He showed the relationship between intensity of selection and the change in a quantitative trait, fundamental to selection of such traits. His paper on metastable equilibrium anticipated much of WRIGHT's work. A striking result was his calculating, as early as 1927, that the probability of ultimate fixation of a new mutation with heterozygous selective advantage s is 2s, a relationship later extended by FISHER, MA-LÉCOT, and especially KIMURA who used it in developing his neutral theory. HALDANE also discussed the evolution of cooperation and of altruism by what is now called kin selection. In this context I recall a famous retort attributed to him. He was asked if he would follow the biblical injunction and lay down his life for his brother. He answered that he would not, but he would consider it for two brothers. Simple kin-selection arithmetic!

HALDANE's most famous papers are "The effect of variation on fitness" and "The cost of natural selection." In the first he showed that the impact of mutation on the population is given by the mutation rate, not by the severity of effect of the individual mutations. This principle, now called mutation load, has been greatly extended and used for quantifying the impact of mutation on the population, for analyzing the effect of inbreeding in the human population, and for developing ideas about the evolutionary advantages of diploidy and sexual reproduction. The second paper showed that the amount of selection required to fix a gene depends on its initial frequency rather than the selection coefficient. This was used by KI-MURA in his initial argument for neutral molecular evolution. These two papers are vintage HALDANE. Both show that a factor that might be thought to be essential for the calculations, the selective intensity, cancels out in such a way as to permit a very strong conclusion without knowing this difficult-to-measure quantity.

I hope I have mentioned enough things to show not only the influence of HALDANE in the past, but the continuing influence of his ideas in current research. The best way to flesh out this skimpy account is to read HALDANE himself. DRONAMRAJU (1990) has assembled many of his best genetical papers.

HALDANE, polymath and curmudgeon: HALDANE's life was a mosaic of contrasts. His erudition and memory were legend. He could (and would) quote endlessly from western classics and Hindu mystics. He could remember mathematical formulas and bibliographic references, which greatly speeded up his paper writing. He carried a pad of paper with him and used spare minutes, such as on train rides, to work on problems or write articles. Sometimes he trusted his memory too far, and minor errors in formulas and bibliographies attest to this. Also, his multitudinous

activities and travels sometimes kept him from reading proof, with troublesome but usually only minor consequences. The most amusing is in his classic, *The Causes of Evolution*, in which all his papers are attributed to his wife.

HALDANE often mentioned one deficiency; he was tone deaf. He said that the only way in which he could recognize "God Save the Queen" was by seeing people standing up. He also said, with typical Haldanian absence of false modesty, that this was good; if he had not had a tin ear he would have wasted time listening to music and would have done less research. The world would be the loser.

HALDANE was one of the best popular science writers. In addition to his books, he wrote hundreds of essays. Almost 400 were written for one publication, the *Daily Worker*, during his Communist period. HAL-DANE had a superb gift for writing simply, yet without losing the essential meaning. His prose style had the terseness and economy of HEMINGWAY with a vocabulary of Basic English. And it was punctuated with witty and quotable epigrams. He also wrote some charming books for children, and at the other extreme, science fiction. His articles are notable not only for their number but for the astonishing variety of subjects. To mention a few: air raid protection, quantum mechanics, animal behavior, dialectics, economics, ecological cycles, astronomy, biochemistry, blood groups, chemical warfare, embryology, on being the right size, bee communication, nuclear energy (he discussed bombs in 1939), relativity, origin of life, origin of the universe, underwater survival, statistics, demography, the taste of oxygen under high pressure, kidney function, effects of hot baths, human races, and heterostyly. In addition to hundreds of popular articles he wrote one on how to write a popular article.

HALDANE must have been a reporter's dream. He could be counted on to answer any question no matter how far out. Not only was he informed on almost any subject, he had an opinion on it, and was uninhibitedly outspoken. Often outlandish, brutally honest, unexpected, irreverent and witty, he was always quotable. And he enjoyed being a character. I'm sure that if he were alive today he would enjoy the stories about himself, and the way they improve with age; indeed, he would be abetting the improvement process.

He was the perfect discussant at a scientific meeting or seminar. (A contemporary rival for this distinction was H. J. MULLER.) Although he could be cutting, much more often his role was to find something interesting about the paper, something that the author had not thought of. His vast knowledge let him see connections with other work that most mortals would miss. Young scientists learned that their work was more important than they had realized. I should like to add that he was remarkably generous regarding some of my work, which was derivative from his. He played a similarly constructive role for the *Journal of Genetics*, which he edited for many years. His book reviews often displayed HALDANE's unique combination of knowledge, wit and irreverence.

HALDANE also loved to argue. He could be stubborn. He was a Rock of Gibraltar with a voice. There weren't many who could argue with him on equal terms, but he delighted in those who could. During part of World War II he and FISHER were both located at Rothamsted, and their endless arguments are legend. Any subject would do. How I would like to have listened in!

HALDANE was unselfish, especially in citing the work of others and in helping his students and other young scientists, often spending his own money. At the same time he was in constant rebellion against any and all regulations. Every molehill was made into a mountain, and every molecule into a molehill. What others would regard as necessary rules for keeping the machinery oiled or as petty annoyances easier to put up with than to make a fuss over were for him matters of high principle. In most cases his rebellion against rules had little reforming effect and only made life miserable for those, usually low in the pecking order, who were responsible for administering them. And, what a waste of his enormous talents it was.

A low point in HALDANE's genetic career occurred during LYSENKO's powerful and tragic influence over Soviet genetics. HALDANE must have realized that LYSENKO's claims were nonsense. Yet his loyalty to the Communist cause, and perhaps his excessive open-mindedness, led him to equivocate, to find some things in LYSENKO's experiments that might be correct, and to avoid any outright disagreement. Later HALDANE dropped out of the Communist Party and had very little to say about LYSENKO, but the period before this is not a point of light in his life.

HALDANE was extreme in his reckless disregard for his own health and safety. His war work on surviving at high under-water pressures led to convulsions which produced a back injury that pained him the rest of his life. In 1961 he visited Ceylon and, characteristically, while searching for ancient artifacts broke his leg (Figure 1). "This has seriously diminished my capacity for work," he wrote. That year he was to receive the Kimber Award from the National Academy of Sciences. The injury prevented his making the trip, but despite this and despite the fact that acceptance speeches were not customary, he wrote one, which I quote, courtesy of ERNST MAYR. It's classic HALDANE.

In thanking the Academy for the honor bestowed on me, I should first like to say that, although I have been awarded several other medals in the past, I have always felt that I would have been still prouder if one or two names had been omitted from the list of my predecessors. For the first time

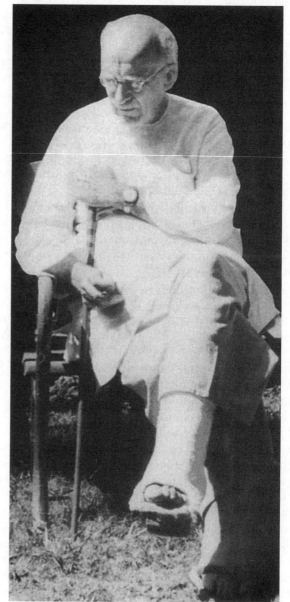

FIGURE 1.—HALDANE (his leg having been broken in Ceylon) is pictured in Calcutta in 1961.

in my experience this is not so today. I am proud to be classed with each one of the previous recipients of the Kimber Medal.

He then went on to describe a number of his recent experiments in India.

He also mentioned as "stop press news" his latest discovery, that the expectations of FISHER's cumulant statistics in a sample are equal to the corresponding parameters in the population. A significant intellectual feat, no doubt, but hardly HALDANE's most lasting achievement.

In the fall of 1963 he gave a series of lectures at the University of Wisconsin after his outspoken revolutionary views prevented this in another state. He was at his charming best. In particular, after a highly laudatory introduction by SEWALL WRIGHT in which many of HALDANE's accomplishments were cited, he began with a correction, saying that the introduction would have been more accurate if "WRIGHT" were substituted for "HALDANE." He already had the early symptoms of the cancer that was soon to kill him, but he made no mention of it and none of us knew it.

On returning to England for an operation he wrote a remarkable bit of doggerel, entitled (after W. H. AUDEN) "Cancer is a funny thing." Great poetry it wasn't, but there were wit and rhymes worthy of OGDEN NASH. The first two lines go

> I wish I had the voice of Homer
> To sing of rectal carcinoma.

At this time the late PHILIP DALY was starting a project for future generations of filming scientists who had made great accomplishments (including SEWALL WRIGHT and LINUS PAULING). He had the daring idea of asking HALDANE to write his own obituary, which HALDANE accepted with relish. It reads, in part:

I am going to begin with a boast. I believe that I am one of the most influential people living today, although I haven't got a scrap of power. Let me explain. In 1932 I was the first person to estimate the rate of mutation of a human gene.

It was read on the BBC after his death a few months later. According to DALY, HALDANE originally wrote "*the* most influential person" but thought better of it later.

I find it interesting to think about the similarities and differences between HALDANE and his great contemporary, both friend and rival, FISHER. HALDANE was much more learned and could remember almost everything. His mind, I think, was like that of most other people, except enormously magnified. FISHER, in contrast, had a touch of genius, a kind of mathematical magic. Their differences were qualitative, not quantitative. WRIGHT had less mathematical training than HALDANE, yet solved more difficult problems. KIMURA also has a special gift and extended the work of all three. There is a great difference in style, however, between HALDANE and the three others. He never argued for any particular hypothesis. He was open-minded to a fault. Here lies another HALDANE contradiction: he was completely undogmatic in science, while being highly dogmatic about almost everything else.

How does one sum up the life of such a person? Did he live up to his expectations? Did his breadth of accomplishment make up for his not having developed a few subjects more fully and founding a school? Were his popular writings and political activities as important as the science that he might have done with the extra time? According to WHITE (1965), "The tragedy of his life was that the breadth of his interests and activities precluded the long concentration of effort needed to develop a distinct new field of biology. This fact is certainly connected with [his] openness of mind . . . He was possibly too much interested in the work of others to bother greatly in what directions his own was tending . . . In the history of genetics he will remain a great, sympathetic and yet deeply tragic figure."

I am not so sure. Can a life that full be tragic? Might his breadth not make up for the scatter? Did he not enjoy facing intellectual challenges in many areas? How could a life so interesting to others not be exciting to live? His life was one of almost continuous conflict and petty warfare, but I believe he actually enjoyed it. We are all unique; but the adjective seems to have been invented for HALDANE. The world is enriched by his having been here, and I for one would not want him to have lived his life differently.

I should like to acknowledge my indebtedness to the HALDANE biography by RONALD W. CLARK. Most of the personal details are from this source. I have gotten additional information from SAHOTRA SARKAR. No serious scientific biography of HALDANE exists, but SARKAR is working on one, and I eagerly await it. Finally, I am indebted to KRISHNA DRONAMRAJU for many personal incidents about HALDANE and for supplying the photograph in Figure 1.

LITERATURE CITED

Books by HALDANE:

I have listed only the most biological of HALDANE's, 23 books and none of his articles. Nearly complete scientific bibliographies are given by CLARK (1969) and DRONAMRAJU (1985, 1990). As far as I know, no one has undertaken the daunting task of compiling a list of *all* his writings.

HALDANE, J. B. S., 1930 *Enzymes.* Longmans, Green & Co., London. Reprinted 1965 by MIT Press, Cambridge, Mass.

HALDANE, J. B. S., 1932 *The Causes of Evolution.* Harper & Brothers, New York & London. Reprinted 1990, with an introduction and afterword by E. G. LEIGH, by Princeton University Press, Princeton, N.J.

HALDANE, J. B. S., 1932 *The Inequality of Man and Other Essays.* Chatto & Windus, London.

HALDANE, J. B. S., 1939 *Heredity and Politics.* W. W. Norton, New York.

HALDANE, J. B. S., 1939 *The Marxist Philosophy and the Sciences.* Random House, New York.

HALDANE, J. B. S., 1942 *New Paths in Genetics.* Harper & Brothers, New York.

HALDANE, J. B. S., 1954 *The Biochemistry of Genetics.* Macmillan, New York.

Books about HALDANE:

CLARK, R. W., 1969 *JBS: The Life and Work of J. B. S. Haldane.* Coward-McCann, New York.

DRONAMRAJU, K. R., (Editor), 1968 *Haldane and Modern Biology.* Johns Hopkins Press, Baltimore.

DRONAMRAJU, K. R., 1985 *Haldane: The Life and Work of J. B. S. Haldane with Special Reference to India.* Aberdeen University Press, Aberdeen.

DRONAMRAJU, K. R., (Editor), 1990 *Selected Genetic Papers of J. B. S. Haldane.* Garland Publishing, Inc., New York. This includes 46 of his genetics papers. All quotes in my article not otherwise identified are from papers in this book.

Additional literature cited:

COYNE, J. A., and H. A. ORR, 1989   Two rules of speciation, pp. 180–207 in *Speciation and Its Consequences*, edited by D. OTTE and J. A. ENDLER. Sinauer, Sunderland, Mass.

FRANK, S. A., 1991   Divergence of meiotic drive-suppression systems as an explanation for sex-biased hybrid sterility and inviability. Evolution **45:** 262–267.

HURST, L. D., and A. POMIANKOWSKI, 1991   Causes of sex ratio bias may account for unisexual sterility in hybrids: a new explanation of HALDANE's rule and related phenomena. Genetics **128:** 841–858.

MIYATA, T., K. KUMA, N. IWABE, H. HAYASHIDA and T. YASUNAGA, 1990   Different rates of evolution of autosome-, X chromosome-, and Y chromosome-linked genes: hypothesis of male-driven molecular evolution, pp. 341–357 in *Population Biology of Genes and Molecules,* edited by N. TAKAHATA and J. F. CROW. Baifukan, Tokyo.

WHITE, M. J. D., 1965   J. B. S. HALDANE. Genetics **52:** 1–7.

Erwin Schrödinger
and the Hornless Cattle Problem

James F. Crow

Genetics Department, University of Wisconsin–Madison, Madison, Wisconsin 53706

ERWIN SCHRÖDINGER was a Nobel Prize winning physicist, the founder of wave mechanics. He was also fascinated by genetics and in 1944 published a remarkable book, *What Is Life?* Fewer than 100 pages long, it was influential out of all proportion to its size. "No doubt molecular biology would have developed without 'What Is Life?,' but it would have been at a slower pace, and without some of its brightest stars" (MOORE 1989).

KRISHNA DRONAMRAJU has called my attention to a small but interesting episode in SCHRÖDINGER's life. In early 1945 he wrote two letters to J. B. S. HALDANE about the "hornless cattle problem." In these letters he defined the following quantities: p = the proportion with horns, q = the proportion of heterozygous hornless, r = the proportion of homozygous hornless, $p + q + r = 1$. He found it useful to introduce the variables x and y, where $x = r + q/2$ and $y = r + q$.

Using the subscript 1 to stand for the next generation, the recurrence equations are

$$x_1 = x(1 + y)/2y \tag{1}$$
$$y_1 = x(1 + y - x)/y \tag{2}$$

SCHRÖDINGER went on to say that he couldn't solve the problem (it is still not solved), although he had found an approximate solution for the value of x after n generations. But here's the rub: nowhere in the letters does SCHRÖDINGER mention what the genetic problem is; he gives only the equations. Given the answer, can you guess the question? I won't spoil your fun by telling you now. If you are impatient, jump to the end of this article.

SCHRÖDINGER was born in Vienna on August 12, 1887. His father was in the oilcloth business, but I don't think his heart was in it, for he spent a great deal of time on his hobbies. He wrote several articles on plant breeding and was a great devotee of Italian painting. ERWIN was his only child and was tutored at home during his early years; undoubtedly, he learned

a great deal from his informed and articulate father. It goes without saying that young SCHRÖDINGER excelled in mathematics and physics, but he also had a love for poetry and drama and a continuing interest in philosophy. He knew several languages in addition to German, and gave lectures in English, French, Spanish or German, adapting the language to the audience. Rereading *What Is Life?* after 45 years, I am once again impressed by the fluent, graceful English, by a feigned naiveté that is somehow charming, and by his subtle, low-key wit.

In 1921 SCHRÖDINGER moved to Zurich, accepting the position formerly held by EINSTEIN. He then moved to Berlin in 1927, this time replacing the retiring MAX PLANCK. The years from 1926 to 1928 were his scientific zenith. He wrote six famous papers that founded wave mechanics. Although he was not Jewish, he found Nazi Germany most distressing and moved to Oxford in 1933. He had barely arrived there when he received the Nobel Prize, shared with DIRAC. A few years later, he returned to his native Austria just in time for its annexation by the Nazis and moved again, probably just in time. This time he went to Dublin. President EAMON DE VALERA planned to establish an Institute for Advanced Studies and SCHRÖDINGER became Director of the School of Theoretical Physics. President DE VALERA, himself a mathematician, regularly took part in SCHRÖDINGER's informal discussions. (It's been a long time since an American president has had time and interest to work on a mathematical problem. We might have to go back to THOMAS JEFFERSON who, while he was Vice-President, used his recently learned calculus to design a better plow; and while he was President he took off half a day to make a model.) Retiring in 1956, SCHRÖDINGER returned to his native Vienna and died there in 1961.

In 1926 WERNER HEISENBERG developed the radically new method of matrix mechanics to formulate quantum theory. Soon after, SCHRÖDINGER wrote a series of papers with a wave formulation, called wave mechanics. By 1928 he realized that the two descriptions were logically equivalent, and the modern subject of quantum mechanics was unified in close to its present form. The wave theory is regarded as one of the most beautiful in physics. According to MOORE (1989), by 1960 more than 100,000 papers had been based on the SCHRÖDINGER equation. Although SCHRÖDINGER's Nobel Prize was given for wave mechanics, that is only one contribution. His scope of interest included almost the whole of theoretical physics. He was impressed with how much we owe to the Greeks and wrote a book on this subject. Altogether, he authored eight nontechnical books, two technical books on physics, a volume of poems and more than 150 papers. Many more details of SCHRÖDINGER's work are given by SCOTT (1967) and MOORE (1989).

Geneticists–at least those with long memories–know SCHRÖDINGER best for his little book *What Is Life?* I can't think of another popular book written by an outsider that had such an influence on a field. Everybody seems to have read it. JIM WATSON is quoted (JUDSON 1979) as saying this book was the decisive influence in leading him to the study of the gene. MAURICE WILKINS read it too. So did JOSHUA LEDERBERG. So did SEYMOUR BENZER. So did FRANCIS CRICK, although he was less effusive: ". . . it's a book written by a physicist who doesn't know any chemistry. But . . . it suggested that biological problems could be *thought* about, in physical terms–and thus it gave the impression that exciting things in this field were not far off" (JUDSON 1979, p. 109). The book had the salutary effect of attracting physical scientists to genetics, and molecular genetics was the beneficiary. Physicists brought the view, foreign to most biologists of the time, that the basic mysteries of biology *could* be understood, provided that one found the appropriate system. SCHRÖDINGER's book was based mainly on the work of MAX DELBRÜCK; it brought DELBRÜCK to attention and inspired others to work with him. Furthermore, the book awakened English-speaking geneticists to the research of TIMOFÉEFF-RESSOVSKY.

What specifically attracted all these people, later to be leaders in molecular biology? Perhaps it was SCHRÖDINGER's characterization of the gene as an "aperiodic crystal." Perhaps it was his view of the chromosome as a message written in code. Perhaps it was his statement that life "feeds on negative entropy." Perhaps it was his notion that quantum indeterminacy at the gene level is converted by cell multiplication into molar determinacy. Perhaps it was his emphasis on the stability of the gene and its ability to perpetuate order. Perhaps it was his faith that the all too obvious difficulties of interpreting life by physical principles need not imply that some super-physical law is required, although some new physical laws might be.

Along with GUNTHER STENT (1966), I don't know why the book had such an impact, but I *do* know what most impressed me at the time, enough to look up the original work. SCHRÖDINGER, following DELBRÜCK (TIMOFÉEFF-RESSOVSKY, ZIMMER and DELBRÜCK 1935), placed great emphasis on the stability of the gene and its resistance to the effects of thermal accidents. He noted that in this theory the stability (time until mutation) is $t = \tau e^{W/kT}$, in which W is the threshold energy difference, T is temperature, and k and τ are constants (k is BOLTZMAN's constant and τ is of order 10^{-13} or 10^{-14} sec). Four facts were said to fit this idea very well: mutation rates vary considerably, as expected with even very small changes in energy threshold; mutation rates have a rather high temperature coefficient, as expected with a high threshold energy; mutable genes are less influenced by temperature than are more stable ones, again as expected because they would have a lower activation energy; and X-ray-induced mutation rates do not correlate with spontaneous rates, once more as expected, because the amount of energy imparted by the radiation is so great as to erase any distinctions among lower thresholds. It all seemed very neat.

This is a far cry from current chemical concepts of mutagenesis, and DELBRÜCK's early ideas turned out to be far off the track. The stability of the gene is now explained by its complementary internal structure and various error-preventing and error-correcting enzymes. The measured temperature coefficients are not those of the gene itself, but of the associated enzymes. In fact, DNA alone has a low temperature coefficient. Many mutations, especially the mutable ones, are probably caused by transposable elements. Nevertheless, DELBRÜCK's ideas had great appeal at the time. For thoughtful recent appraisal, see SARKAR (1991).

SCHRÖDINGER clearly has a place in the origins of molecular biology, not comparable to his enormous contributions to physics but historically significant all the same. He wrote a great deal about the nature of scientific knowledge and scientific research. All these writings have SCHRÖDINGER's characteristic depth and charm, but they are not easy reading for a biologist. His philosophy was a different animal. He was impressed and puzzled by the human body's functioning as a mechanism and yet being under the control of the mind, as was SEWALL WRIGHT (1964). He was religious, but not in a conventional Western way. His views were based on ancient Hindu mysticism. I'll leave comments on this to others more sympathetic and better qualified to judge. Those who would like to know more about SCHRÖDINGER's science, his philosophy, and his ceaseless search for broader aspects of reality than science could provide, along with his personal life and numerous love affairs, will find an engaging account in MOORE (1989).

What Is Life? is based on three public lectures given in Dublin in February, 1943. SCHRÖDINGER was a popular speaker and each lecture had to be repeated to accommodate the overflow crowd. He planned to publish the book in Ireland, but after being set in type it was rejected; his imprudent denial of individual souls was too much for the priesthood. He also incurred the opprobrium of H. J. MULLER (1946), who charged from the opposite direction. MULLER approved of most of the book, although he thought that SCHRÖDINGER had missed, or insufficiently emphasized, the gene's property of unlimited replication not only of itself but of its variants, a favorite MULLER idea. He also remarked that SCHRÖDINGER had learned his genetics from too few sources and therefore had not realized how far back some of his ideas could be traced (here MULLER was tooting his own horn). But MULLER reserved his strongest statements for the last chapter of the book where SCHRÖDINGER used "his foregoing conceptions as the means of projecting his boat on the sea of straight old-fashioned mysticism . . . If the collaboration of the physicist in the attack on biological questions finally leads to his concluding that 'I am God Almighty' and that the ancient Hindus were on the right track after all, his help should become suspect." I am sure that CRICK would agree.

HALDANE's and SCHRÖDINGER's shared interests were not only in science and mathematics. HALDANE also had a broad knowledge of Hindu philosophy and religion, although I don't think his own philosophical views would have permitted him to go along with SCHRÖDINGER's Vedanta metaphysics.

Let's get back to the hornless cattle problem. SCHRÖDINGER introduced an approximation that amounts to assuming HARDY-WEINBERG proportions and treated the process as continuous in time. The rate of change of x with respect to generation number n is then

$$\frac{dx}{dn} = \frac{(1-x)^2}{2[1+(1-x)]}$$

which integrates to

$$n = 2[(1-x_n)^{-1} - \ln(1-x_n) - (1-x_0)^{-1} + \ln(1-x_0)].$$

For $x_0 = 0.5$ and $x_n = 0.95$, the time n is 40.6

generations. The exact answer is that, after 40 generations, $x_{40} = 0.9516$. Actually, the simple asymptotic approximation $1 - x_n \approx 2/n$ does very well, giving $x_{40} = 0.9500$.

SCHRÖDINGER concludes his letter to HALDANE by saying, "Well, I wonder whether I have told you *anything* new! At any rate it has given me great pleasure to work the problem out–though I know you wanted something better."

Now what is the question to which this is the answer? Here is one situation that SCHRÖDINGER's equations describe. Suppose a breeder wants to get rid of his dangerous horned cattle. He can't afford not to breed each cow, but he can easily afford to discard some bulls, so each generation he mates only hornless bulls. This leads directly to Equations 1 and 2, in which x is the frequency of the dominant allele for hornlessness and y is the frequency of the hornless phenotype.

HALDANE had an interest in various selection problems, and selection on only one sex was one of them. He noted that selection at half the intensity in both sexes is very nearly equivalent to full intensity in one. In this case, eliminating half the horned individuals of each sex for 40 generations gives $x_{40} = 0.9510$. SCHRÖDINGER's heavy-handed game was hardly worth the candle.

I am indebted to KRISHNA DRONAMRAJU for bringing the SCHRÖDINGER letters to my attention and to TOM NAGYLAKI and SAHOTRA SARKAR for help in writing this article.

LITERATURE CITED

JUDSON, H. F., 1979 *The Eighth Day of Creation.* Simon & Schuster, New York.

MOORE, W., 1989 *Schrödinger, Life and Thought.* Cambridge University Press, Cambridge.

MULLER, H. J., 1946 A physicist stands amazed at genetics. J. Hered. **37:** 90–92.

SARKAR, S., 1991 *What Is Life* revisited. BioScience **41:** 631–634.

SCHRÖDINGER, E., 1944 *What Is Life?* Cambridge University Press, Cambridge.

SCOTT, W. T., 1967 *Erwin Schrödinger. An Introduction to His Writings.* University of Massachusetts Press, Amherst, Mass.

STENT, G. S., 1966 Introduction: waiting for the paradox, pp. 3–8 in *Phage and the Origins of Molecular Biology,* edited by J. CAIRNS, G. S. STENT and J. D. WATSON. Cold Spring Harbor Laboratory, Cold Spring Harbor, N.Y.

TIMOFÉEFF-RESSOVSKY, N. W., K. G. ZIMMER and M. DELBRÜCK, 1935 Über die Natur der Genmutation und der Genstruktur. Nachr. Ges. Wiss. Göttingen, Fachgr. 6, N.F. 1, **13:** 190–245.

WRIGHT, S., 1964 Biology and the philosophy of science. Monist **48:** 265–290.

March 1992

Twenty-five Years Ago in *Genetics*
Identical Triplets

James F. Crow

Genetics Department, University of Wisconsin–Madison, Madison, Wisconsin 53706

THE March, 1967 issue of GENETICS contained three articles, independently written yet remarkably similar (SVED, REED and BODMER 1967; KING 1967; MILKMAN 1967). Although the three articles differed in style, length and approach, their essential message was the same. What point were they making? Why this curious concatenation in a single issue of GENETICS? Before discussing this, a bit of background.

The decade preceding these papers had been one of heated controversy in the genetics community. Many geneticists, led by H. J. MULLER, were concerned about the human mutation rate and the possibility that radiation and chemicals might be causing substantial harm to our descendants. MULLER (1950), following HALDANE (1937), pointed out that the cumulative impact of deleterious mutations over all future generations, measured as reduced fitness, is independent of individual mutation effects; for mutations with any appreciable dominance it is simply the total number of new mutations per zygote. The proportion by which fitness (or other attribute of interest) is reduced by recurrent mutation is now called the mutation load. In MULLER's words, each mutation, irrespective of how harmful it is, leads in the long run to one "genetic death," *i.e.*, a pre-reproductive death or failure to reproduce. (In a growing population this number must be appropriately increased.) Estimates of spontaneous mutation rates current at the time would place the mutation load at about 10%, although MULLER thought it might be as much as twice this value. He used this principle to argue that any increase in the human mutation rate would cause a proportional increase in the mutation load. His impassioned advocacy, supported by others, was responsible for initiating radiation protection standards widely adopted throughout much of the world, followed later by testing of chemicals for mutagenic activity.

Geneticists had long recognized the possibility that at some loci a heterozygote may be more fit than either of its component homozygotes, and this led to considerable discussion of the importance of such loci for hybrid vigor and for the high fitness of randomly mating populations compared to inbred derivatives. It had been recognized since FISHER (1922, 1930) and HALDANE (1937) that each overdominant locus makes a disproportionately large contribution to the population variance, and that even a small proportion of such loci could be of major importance. This view was carried further by LERNER (1954). Taking a lead from SCHMALHAUSEN (1949), LERNER was interested in developmental buffering that produced not only high fitness, but phenotypic constancy despite genetic variability. He argued that "heterozygosity *per se* rather than the genic contents of the individual is the important consideration" (LERNER 1954, p. 67).

DOBZHANSKY (1955) made this idea more explicit. The finding by his associates VETUKHIV (1953) and BRNCIC (1954) that interpopulation hybrids were more fit than progeny of intrapopulation crosses led him to conclude, at first reluctantly, then enthusiastically (LEWONTIN 1981), that overdominance is of the essence. He then formulated the "balance" hypothesis (DOBZHANSKY 1955) whereby the typical individual is heterozygous at a major fraction of its loci (*e.g.*, WALLACE and DOBZHANSKY 1959, p. 164). He contrasted this to the "classical" hypothesis, which he attributed to MULLER, that overdominant loci are at best a tiny minority and that most loci in most individuals are homozygous except for a small proportion of recurrent harmful mutations. What would ordinarily be a scientific argument became politicized because, on the balance hypothesis, the HALDANE-MULLER mutation load principle is not applicable. MULLER, in particular, thought that acceptance of the DOBZHANSKY view would result in a relaxation of radiation protection standards. Words flew and tempers flared. The word "classical" was used to imply out-of-date-

262

ness, while the classicists retorted that the standard alternative to classical was "romantic."

According to LEWONTIN (1981), DOBZHANSKY "devoted a large part of his remaining scientific work to an unsuccessful attempt to demonstrate the generally superior fitness of genic heterozygotes." Those who would like to read DOBZHANSKY's series of papers on this and many other subjects, and see why he had such an enormous influence, will find them reprinted along with a thoughtful appraisal in LEWONTIN et al. (1981). Yet it was clear at the time that the actual amount of heterozygosity could not be answered by the genetic methods of the day. It was a molecular question and would require molecular methods not yet available.

Into this vacuum stepped LEWONTIN and HUBBY (1966). Various workers had done electrophoretic studies of isozymes and reported considerable variation. But LEWONTIN and HUBBY measured the variability quantitatively and showed that the average Drosophila pseudoobscura was heterozygous at about 12% of the loci tested. Similar results for the human species were reported by HARRIS (1966). Furthermore, the method was expected to detect only about a third of the variants, so that heterozygosity could be as much as ⅓, with the majority of loci segregating two or more alleles in the population. Thus, it looked as if DOBZHANSKY had been correct about the amount of heterozygosity. The great variability dramatized the meaninglessness of characterizing any species by a single genotype.

LEWONTIN and HUBBY (1966) pointed out that if a large fraction of loci were overdominant, there would be an enormous number of deleterious homozygotes and these would result in a large decrease in fitness—the "segregation" or "balanced" load. Calculations based on their data and assuming independent effects on fitness led to an absurdly large segregation load, if the loci were indeed overdominant.

The triplets, whose 25th birthday anniversary we celebrate, were stimulated by the LEWONTIN and HUBBY paper. Each group had the same idea at about the same time, although the juxtaposition of the papers in the journal was by arrangement. They were directed to showing how such a seemingly large load could be accommodated. The essential arguments (SVED, REED and BODMER 1967; KING 1967; MILKMAN 1967) were the same, although KING's was the most explicit: if the genotypes in a population are lined up in order of fitness potential (in this case number of heterozygous loci) and a fixed fraction, the least fit, are removed by selection (truncation selection), then multiple homozygotes are eliminated preferentially, and the load is much less than if individual homozygous loci were eliminated independently. Geneticists could once again breathe easily; the implica-

tions of the LEWONTIN-HUBBY findings weren't so dreadful after all.

But these papers did not show that selection operated in this way; only that if it did, the segregation load could be reduced to manageable proportions. Did nature imitate animal breeders and practice truncation selection? It seemed doubtful. Equally important, the isozyme data told nothing about selection; all they did was measure the amount of variability. By themselves they offered no support for overdominance. The allelic forms might simply be "classical," but very weakly selected or even neutral, and this was suggested by several people.

So the LEWONTIN-HUBBY and HARRIS discovery didn't solve the load problem (LEWONTIN 1991). What it did do was to seduce an enormous number of researchers into dropping whatever they had been working on and start running gels. The problem of how genetic variability is maintained was not really solved, it was simply abandoned as the new user-friendly techniques led people to work on more tractable projects. Most workers preferred a research problem that promised a clean-cut answer, rather than a more important problem that was difficult and might lead to inconclusive results. Within a few years more than a thousand species had been studied, with many loci in each; for documentation of this overkill, see NEVO (1984). Curiously, the 35% heterozygosity expected with better techniques hasn't appeared; the increase from this source has been negated by the finding of more monomorphic loci. NEVO gives heterozygosity values of 9% for invertebrates, 6% for vertebrates and 7% for plants. This is perhaps more than MULLER might have expected (I don't know what he actually thought), but is considerably less than DOBZHANSKY believed.

Over time, the belief in ubiquitous overdominance has largely disappeared as contrary evidence from several sources has accumulated (see CROW 1987), but the relative importance of different variability-maintaining mechanisms is still not sorted out. For an engaging personalized historical review by one of the main participants and a discussion of early experimental results that are still hard to explain, see WALLACE (1991).

A year after the three papers and 13 years after DOBZHANSKY's bomb, KIMURA (1968) dropped another by introducing the neutral theory, which was immediately followed by an independent presentation of the same idea by KING and JUKES (1969). KIMURA and OHTA (1971) soon suggested that most polymorphism was simply a transitory snapshot of neutral evolution. The classical-balance argument was immediately replaced by a no less vehement neutralist-selectionist debate.

There is now very little discussion of the segregation

load; it has been replaced as a problem by the mutation load. This is the result of experiments by MUKAI *et al.* (1972 and earlier) showing that the rate of occurrence of deleterious mutations in *Drosophila melanogaster* is of the order of one per zygote, and may be higher because the procedure gives a minimum rather than a most-likely estimate. If this is correct for the human species, the HALDANE-MULLER principle would seem to say that we should have become extinct long ago.

But the kind of reasoning used by SVED *et al.*, KING, and MILKMAN can equally well be applied to harmful mutations. Doubts as to whether nature truncates have largely been dispelled by MILKMAN's (1978) discovery that a crude approximation to truncation selection, quasi-truncation, is almost as effective as precise truncation in eliminating harmful mutations in bunches (see also CROW and KIMURA 1979). It is unlikely that nature truncates exactly, but it is quite likely that in density-regulated populations truncation is approximated well enough by quasi-truncation to have similar load-reducing properties.

Mutation load theory has other uses (*pace* GILLESPIE 1991). A curious by-product is a new theory for the value of sexual reproduction (for a review, see KONDRASHOV 1988). KING formulated the mutation load as the total zygotic mutation rate divided by the difference in number of mutations per individual between those eliminated by selection and those before selection (see KONDRASHOV and CROW 1988). Once again the triplets get into the act. Mutations can be eliminated in bunches by synergism, of which truncation selection is an extreme form. But an asexual species cannot do this; without recombination, mutations must be eliminated in the same genotypic combinations in which they occurred (KIMURA and MARUYAMA 1966). Thus the mutation load problem is much greater for asexual species. Do asexual species have a lower rate of mutation than their sexual counterparts? Comparative data on genomic deleterious mutation rates among multicellular eukaryotes are lacking, in contrast to microbes (DRAKE 1991) where roughly half of all mutations are likely to be deleterious.

As I mentioned earlier, before the molecular revolution there were a number of important unsolved problems in genetics and evolution. They were left unsolved largely because of the lure of other problems for which molecular methods provided definitive answers. Nevertheless, the old problems are still with us. Happily, some are now being addressed, and a combination of classical and molecular methods should bring a new level of understanding.

A question that has long suffered benign neglect is the total human *deleterious* mutation rate. Our society spends considerable resources testing potential envi-

ronmental mutagens, although often only because they are potential carcinogens. But surely spontaneous mutations are a far greater hazard to future generations. Direct measurement in mammals doesn't appear feasible at present. If we accept the pseudogene evolution rate in recent human ancestry as a direct measure of the mutation rate (KIMURA 1983) and multiply the rate per nucleotide pair per generation by the diploid number of nucleotide pairs, 6×10^9, we obtain roughly 10^2 for the zygotic mutation rate. SVED *et al.*, KING, and MILKMAN told us how truncation selection can eliminate deleterious genotypes (and mutations) efficiently. They helped us to understand how a species with a zygotic mutation rate greater than one can survive. But even the most optimistic efficiency of truncation selection can hardly eliminate mutations occurring at $\sim 10^2$ times this rate.

Most of these mutations must be effectively neutral, but how many are deleterious, to be eliminated only at some cost? Presumably the human rate is no less than that of Drosophila. Our reproductive rate is relatively low (although still too high in much of the world). Quasi-truncation selection may have operated in the past to keep mutations in check, but hardly does so at present. Can we count on future environmental improvements to offset mutational deterioration? If MULLER were still alive and were aware of MUKAI's results, he would be expressing great concern for our genetic future. And he might be right. But first we need to answer the question: what is the genomic rate of deleterious mutations?

I am happy to acknowledge the help of ALEX KONDRASHOV, RAYLA TEMIN and ROGER MILKMAN in improving both the accuracy and and clarity of the presentation.

LITERATURE CITED

BRNCIC, D., 1954 Heterosis and integration of the genotype in geographic populations of *Drosophila pseudoobscura*. Genetics **39**: 77–88.

CROW, J. F., 1987 Muller, Dobzhansky, and overdominance. J. Hist. Biol. **20**: 351–380.

CROW, J. F., and M. KIMURA, 1979 Efficiency of truncation selection. Proc. Natl. Acad. Sci. USA **76**: 396–399.

DOBZHANSKY, TH., 1955 A review of some fundamental concepts and problems of population genetics. Cold Spring Harbor Symp. Quant. Biol. **20**: 1–15.

DRAKE, J. W., 1991 A constant rate of spontaneous mutation in DNA-based microbes. Proc. Natl. Acad. Sci. USA **88**: 7160–7164.

FISHER, R. A., 1922 On the dominance ratio. Proc. R. Soc. Edinb. **52**: 321–341.

FISHER, R. A., 1930 *The Genetical Theory of Natural Selection.* Clarendon Press, Oxford. Second edition, 1958. Dover Press, New York.

GILLESPIE, J. H., 1991 The burden of genetic load. Science **254**: 1049.

HALDANE, J. B. S., 1937 The effect of variation on fitness. Am. Nat. **71**: 337–349.

HARRIS, H., 1966 Enzyme polymorphism in man. Proc. R. Soc. Lond. Ser. B **164**: 298–310.

KIMURA, M., 1968 Evolutionary rate at the molecular level. Nature **217**: 624–626.

KIMURA, M., 1983 *The Neutral Theory of Molecular Evolution.* Cambridge University Press, Cambridge.

KIMURA, M., and T. MARUYAMA, 1966 The mutation load with epistatic gene interactions in fitness. Genetics **54**: 1337–1351.

KIMURA, M., and T. OHTA, 1971 Protein polymorphism as a phase of molecular evolution. Nature **229**: 467–469.

KING, J. L., 1967 Continuously distributed factors affecting fitness. Genetics **55**: 483–492.

KING, J. L., and T. H. JUKES, 1969 Non-Darwinian evolution: random fixation of selectively neutral mutations. Science **164**: 788–798.

KONDRASHOV, A. S., 1988 Deleterious mutations and the evolution of sexual reproduction. Nature **336**: 435–440.

KONDRASHOV, A. S., and J. F. CROW, 1988 King's formula for the mutation load with epistasis. Genetics **120**: 853–856.

LERNER, I. M., 1954 *Genetic Homeostasis.* Wiley, New York.

LEWONTIN, R. C., 1981 The scientific work of Th. Dobzhansky, pp. 93–119 in *Dobzhansky's Genetics of Natural Populations I–XLIII.* Columbia University Press, New York.

LEWONTIN, R. C., 1991 Twenty-five years ago in GENETICS. Electrophoresis in the development of evolutionary genetics: milestone or millstone? Genetics **128**: 657–662.

LEWONTIN, R. C., and J. L. HUBBY, 1966 A molecular approach to the study of genetic heterozygosity in natural populations. II. Amount of variation and degree of heterozygosity in natural populations of *Drosophila pseudoobscura.* Genetics **54**: 595–609.

LEWONTIN, R. C., J. A. MOORE, W. B. PROVINE and B. WALLACE, 1981 *Dobzhansky's Genetics of Natural Populations I–XLIII.* Columbia University Press, New York.

MILKMAN, R., 1967 Heterosis as a major cause of heterozygosity in nature. Genetics **55**: 493–495.

MILKMAN, R., 1978 Selection differentials and selection coefficients. Genetics **88**: 391–403.

MUKAI, T., S. I. CHIGUSA, L. E. METTLER and J. F. CROW, 1972 Mutation rate and dominance of genes affecting viability in *Drosophila melanogaster.* Genetics **72**: 335–355.

MULLER, H. J., 1950 Our load of mutations. Am. J. Hum. Genet. **2**: 111–176.

NEVO, E., 1984 The evolutionary significance of genetic diversity: ecological, demographic and life history correlates. Lect. Notes Biomath. **53**: 13–213.

SCHMALHAUSEN, I. I., 1949 *Factors of Evolution.* Blakiston, Philadelphia.

SVED, J. A., T. E. REED and W. F. BODMER, 1967 The number of balanced polymorphisms that can be maintained in a natural population. Genetics **55**: 469–481.

VETUKHIV, M. A., 1953 Viability of hybrids between local populations of *Drosophila pseudoobscura.* Proc. Natl. Acad. Sci. USA **39**: 30–34.

WALLACE, B., 1991 *Fifty Years of Genetic Load. An Odyssey.* Cornell University Press, Ithaca, N.Y.

WALLACE, B., and TH. DOBZHANSKY, 1959 *Radiation, Genes, and Man.* Henry Holt, New York.

Neurospora
The Organism behind the Molecular Revolution

David D. Perkins

Department of Biological Sciences, Stanford University, Stanford, California 94305–5020

UNDER the title "Fifty Years Ago: The Neurospora Revolution," HOROWITZ (1991) has celebrated an anniversary of the epochal 1941 paper of BEADLE and TATUM, which reported the first mutants with biochemically defined nutritional requirements. HOROWITZ's account and others (HOROWITZ 1973, 1985, 1990; LEDERBERG 1990) have focused on the people who were involved, the genesis of their ideas, and the role of the 1941 results in transforming biology. The present essay will be concerned mainly with the research organism that was so important to the success of the initial experiments. Neurospora possesses a combination of features that made it an ideal choice not only for accomplishing the original objectives set by BEADLE and TATUM but also for a continuing succession of contributions, including many in areas that transgress the bounds of biochemical genetics and molecular biology. I shall begin by outlining the story of Neurospora prior to BEADLE and TATUM and then go on to sketch its subsequent history. The previous accounts have stressed biochemical genetics and molecular biology. I shall consider other aspects as well, focusing first on genetics, continuing with a summary of research accomplishments of all sorts, and concluding with a consideration of the potential usefulness of Neurospora for population studies.

The vegetative phase of Neurospora was described and used for experiments by French microbiologists nearly 100 years before BEADLE and TATUM (PAYEN 1843; MONTAGNE 1843). In the warm, humid summer of 1842, bread from bakeries in Paris was spoiled by massive growth of an orange mold. A commission was set up by the minister of war to investigate the cause of the infestation and to make recommendations. The commission's report (PAYEN 1843) includes a colored plate which shows colonies, mycelia, conidiophores and conidia of the "champignons rouges du pain." An experiment in photobiology is described. Colonies grown in the light quickly became bright orange. Colonies grown in the dark, however, remained white for more than 8 days, but the white colonies developed orange pigment within 2 hr when they were brought into the light. Thermal tolerance was also studied (see PAYEN 1848, 1859). These results were cited by PASTEUR (1862) in reporting his own experiments on the survival of mold spores, which helped to refute theories of spontaneous generation.

The next experimental study of Neurospora began in Indonesia during Dutch colonial times. In marketplaces of East Java, bright orange cakes are displayed. These consist of Neurospora grown on soybean or peanut solids from which oil and protein for curd have been pressed. The Javanese inoculate the solids with conidia to create an appetizing and highly nutritious food called oncham, which has a mushroom-like taste (WENT 1901a; SHURTLEFF and AOYAGI 1979; HO 1986). Producing oncham is a cottage industry which has probably gone on for centuries and which continues today.

A Dutch plant physiologist, F. A. F. C. WENT, was stationed at the famous Buitzenjorg (now Bogor) Botanic Gardens in Java at the turn of the century. WENT was attracted by the orange oncham fungus and started experimenting with it. He was frustrated because humidity in Java is so great that the organism grew through the cotton plugs of his culture tubes. WENT (1904) also found Neurospora in Surinam, where he noted that the fungus was used to process cassava meal in preparation of an indigenous alcoholic beverage. Back home in Utrecht, he described the oncham fungus and its culture (WENT 1901a) and used it for a series of studies on the effects of various substrates on enzymes such as trehalase, invertase and tyrosinase (WENT 1901b). WENT (1904) also studied the effect of light on carotenoid production. With knowledge of WENT's work, PRINGSHEIM (1909) included Neurospora in a study of oxidases, and KUNKEL

(1913, 1914) used it in studies of chemical toxicity. All these observations were made using the vegetative phase of the organism and the asexually produced powdery conidia (vegetative spores).

The association of Neurospora with heat and fire must have been known from the earliest times. We now know that the sexually produced heat-tolerant ascospores remain dormant until exposed to heat. Heat activation of ascospores explains the occurrence of Neurospora both in bakery infestations and on burned vegetation. Numerous records going back over a century describe large orange areas following volcanic eruptions in tropical areas. In New Guinea, tribesmen traditionally set hillsides on fire to flush game, and Neurospora bloomed following the burns. In Brazil, MÖLLER (1901) described an orange fungus growing on burned vegetation (and on maize bread). A typically ascomycete sexual phase appeared in his cultures, and the sexual fruiting bodies (perithecia) and ascospores were later identified as Neurospora. In Japan, Neurospora made a dramatic appearance following the great Tokyo earthquake and fire of 1923. Within a few days, burned and scorched trees became festooned with orange. Mycologists in two laboratories cultured the organism. KITAZIMA (1925) observed perithecia in his cultures, and going back to the source, discovered that perithecia were present under the bark of trees in the Temple of Shiba. Orange progeny were obtained from single ascospores. TOKUGAWA and EMOTO (1924) studied survival of the fungus following exposure to moist and dry heat, and identified the orange pigment as a carotenoid.

Neurospora is commonly seen following agricultural burning in warm, moist climates. Sugar cane appears to be an ideal substrate. Ascospores are no doubt activated by burning in the fields and by heating in the mill. Bales of bagasse (fiber from which the sap has been pressed) become orange. In Australia, solids from refinery filters are spread on fields as fertilizer. Large orange colonies develop on this filter mud. Honey bees can be seen visiting the colonies and filling their pollen baskets with the brightly colored conidia (SHAW and ROBERTSON 1980).

The modern history of Neurospora begins in the mid-1920s with material from sugar cane bagasse. The key person was BERNARD DODGE. Like BEADLE, DODGE had grown up on a farm. He worked for years as a school teacher and managed to complete his bachelor's degree only at age 39. He published his first paper at the age of 40 and was already past 50 when he began to work with Neurospora (ROBBINS 1962). Prior to the Neurospora work, DODGE was the first to discover heat activation of ascospores (1912) and to describe mating types in ascomycetes (1920), both in Ascobolus.

About the time KITAZIMA was examining his orange fungus in Japan, CHARLES THOM, a colleague of DODGE's at the Department of Agriculture mycology and pathology laboratory in Arlington, Virginia, was studying cultures of orange mold from sugar cane bagasse in Louisiana. THOM was of the opinion that the orange fungus, then called Monilia sitophila, lacked a sexual stage. However, C. L. SHEAR, the head of the laboratory, found perithecia in one of THOM's plates. The material was given to DODGE for analysis. The success of DODGE's experimental crosses kindled his enthusiasm, and Neurospora became his main lifelong interest.

DODGE's first Neurospora paper, with SHEAR in 1927, goes far beyond the conventional taxonomic descriptions of genus and species. Cultures of the orange fungus had been obtained from many sources. Isolates were assigned to the new genus Neurospora on the basis of their grooved ascospores. (Prior to 1927, the vegetative stage had successively been called Oidium aurantiacum, Penicillium sitophilum and Monilia sitophila.) DODGE showed that the cultures included three species which were set off from one another by their crossing behavior. Hybrid perithecia from crosses between different species developed slowly and were unproductive or poorly fertile. Although a conventional morphologically based taxonomic species description was provided for each species, crossing behavior was implicitly taken into consideration and used to assign strains to the designated species. This innovation contrasted with the purely morphological criteria then used by mycologists and clearly anticipated the idea of biological species long before the concept was formalized.

Two species with eight-spored asci, Neurospora crassa and Neurospora sitophila, were shown to be heterothallic: individual haploid cultures from single ascospores were unable to enter the sexual cycle. They fell into two mating types, defined because crosses could occur only between strains of opposite mating type.

DODGE carried out the first tetrad analysis with N. crassa, showing that the mating types segregated 4:4 in individual asci. The asci were obtained as groups of eight ascospores that had been spontaneously ejected from the perithecia. The Neurospora ascospores were activated by heat, as in Ascobolus. In contrast to the eight-spored species, isolates of Neurospora tetrasperma, with four-spored asci, appeared to be homothallic. Cultures from single ascospores were usually self-fertile. A few self-sterile progeny were produced, however, that behaved as though they were heterothallic. DODGE (1927) was shortly to describe the cytological basis of this "pseudohomothallic" behavior of N. tetrasperma, showing that individual ascospores were usually (but not always) heterokar-

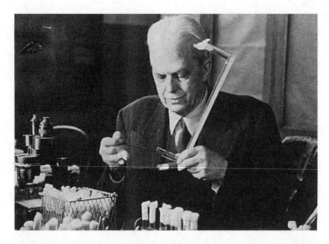

B. O. DODGE

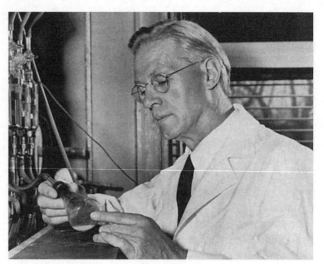

CARL C. LINDEGREN

yons that contained haploid nuclei of opposite mating types.

DODGE lost no time in communicating his enthusiasm. At Columbia University, he urged T. H. MORGAN and the Drosophila group to use Neurospora. He traveled to Cornell for a seminar. Among the graduate students in the audience were GEORGE BEADLE and BARBARA MCCLINTOCK. BEADLE (1966) later recalled how the students, familiar with then-recent results of E. G. ANDERSON using Drosophila attached-X half-tetrads, were able to point out to DODGE how the second-division segregations he described in Neurospora could be explained by crossing over between chromatids at the four-strand stage.

DODGE soon moved to a job as plant pathologist at the New York Botanical Garden. In addition to his official duties, he managed to continue experiments with Neurospora. These included pioneering work on interspecies crosses and on mutations affecting ascus development. He was intrigued by heterokaryons and obtained combinations of strains that showed heterokaryotic vigor (DODGE 1942). In the next 30 years he published nearly 50 papers on the genetics, cytology, morphology and life cycle of Neurospora.

DODGE's enthusiasm resulted indirectly in the recruitment of CARL LINDEGREN, who did the most significant genetic work with Neurospora prior to BEADLE and TATUM. In 1928, LINDEGREN moved to California from Wisconsin, where he had obtained a Master's degree in Plant Pathology. He visited T. H. MORGAN to inquire about continuing graduate work at the California Institute of Technology, where MORGAN had come with his Drosophila group to head the new Biology Division. LINDEGREN found MORGAN using dissecting needles in an attempt to isolate Neurospora ascospores from an agar plate (see LINDEGREN 1973). MORGAN suggested that LINDEGREN work with Neurospora. Following a visit to DODGE, LINDEGREN chose the species N. crassa as best suited for genetic work. He developed highly fertile wild-type strains,

identified mutants that could be used as markers and discovered the first linkages. The linked genes provided confirming proof that crossing over occurred at the four-strand stage. Genetic maps were constructed for two linkage groups using mating type, centromeres, and morphological mutants. But at about the time BEADLE and TATUM were turning from Drosophila to Neurospora, LINDEGREN abandoned Neurospora to begin work on Saccharomyces. His last Neurospora paper (LINDEGREN and LINDEGREN 1942), written with his life-long collaborator GERTRUDE LINDEGREN, was submitted just as the Stanford workers were about to obtain their first biochemical mutant. LINDEGREN's Neurospora papers are listed in BACHMANN and STRICKLAND (1965).

Neurospora was used for several other investigations during the decade before 1941. I first heard of it in a plant physiology course taught by DAVID GODDARD, who used N. tetrasperma in studies of ascospore activation and dormancy (GODDARD 1935, 1939). BUTLER, ROBBINS and DODGE (1941) demonstrated that biotin was the sole growth factor requirement. In England, WHITEHOUSE (1942) subjected LINDEGREN's tetrad data to a detailed analysis and went on to produce his own five-point map of the mating-type chromosome of N. sitophila. It was DODGE and LINDEGREN, however, who developed the genetics of Neurospora during the 1930s and made the organism known to geneticists. The accumulated information enabled DODGE (1939) to assert: "The fungi in their reproduction and inheritance follow exactly the same laws that govern these activities in higher plants and animals."

Additional information regarding early history can be found in the introductory sections of SHEAR and DODGE (1927), MOREAU-FROMENT (1956), and PERKINS and BARRY (1977), and in essays by RYAN and OLIVE (1961), TATUM (1961), LEDERBERG (1990), SRB (1973), CATCHESIDE (1973) and LINDEGREN (1973).

Three genetics textbooks published in 1939 (STURTEVANT and BEADLE, SINNOTT and DUNN, AND WADDINGTON) included accounts of Neurospora in the context of recombination and sex determination, with diagrams showing the relation of crossing over to second division segregation in the linear ascus.

In February 1941, BEADLE wrote to DODGE regarding stocks. His letter begins "Dr. Tatum and I are interested in doing some work on the nutrition of Neurospora with the eventual aim of determining whether the requirements might be dependent on genetic constitution." Eight months later, their paper reporting success in obtaining nutritional mutants was submitted to the *Proceedings of the National Academy of Science*.

Obtaining the first biochemical mutants and proposing the one-gene one-enzyme hypothesis were only two of many advances in which Neurospora played a pioneering role. The problems for which it has since been used are extremely diverse, often ranging far afield from the biochemical genetics that first made it famous. For example, Neurospora soon made fundamental contributions to understanding the mechanism of recombination. It was also used to resolve the great confusion existing at that time about fungal chromosomes and their behavior in meiosis.

In 1944, BARBARA MCCLINTOCK visited Stanford University at BEADLE's invitation; KELLER (1983, pp. 113–118) describes the visit. MCCLINTOCK's long experience with maize enabled her to show convincingly that the chromosomes of Neurospora and their behavior in the ascus were typically eukaryotic. Using simple light microscopy, she went far beyond the original objective of determining the chromosome number. She outlined the details of meiosis and described the seven chromosomes. The smallest Neurospora chromosomes are now known each to have a 1C DNA content less than that of *Escherichia coli*. She showed that they were nevertheless individually recognizable by their distinctive morphology at pachytene (MCCLINTOCK 1945; for photographs comparing Neurospora and maize pachytene chromosomes see Figure 6 in PERKINS 1979). She went on to describe pachytene pairing in a translocation heterozygote and to record the ascus types that resulted from different modes of segregation when the translocation was heterozygous. At the end of her two-month stay in California there was no longer any question: it was clear that fungal chromosome cytology, like fungal genetics, is basically similar to that of plants and animals.

The 1941 paper of BEADLE and TATUM opened up exciting possibilities just at a time when war was diverting funds from pure to applied research and when young scientists were moving either into applied research or into the military. BEADLE's success in keeping his group intact and in obtaining support

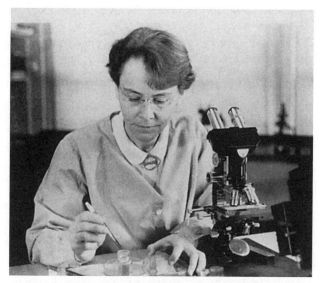

BARBARA MCCLINTOCK

testifies to his confidence in the importance of the research and his persuasiveness as to its value. (There was then no National Science Foundation and no program of external research support by the National Institutes of Health. BEADLE turned to the Rockefeller Foundation and the Nutrition Foundation, and to pharmaceutical firms. See BEADLE 1974; KAY 1989.)

Not everyone was persuaded. HOROWITZ (1979) describes how some geneticists continued to resist the idea that individual enzymes were specified by single genes. And BEADLE (1974) recalls a wartime visit by the mycologist, CHARLES THOM. After being shown some of the striking morphological mutants that were known to segregate as single-gene differences, THOM took BEADLE aside and advised him "What you need is a good mycologist. Those cultures you call mutants are not mutants at all. They are contaminants!"

At the war's end in 1945, the Neurospora work had progressed substantially and was widely known. (When I returned to Columbia University from the army, DOBZHANSKY told me that the two highlights in biology during the war had been HUXLEY's book *Evolution the Modern Synthesis* and BEADLE and TATUM's Neurospora mutants.) Students were attracted to Neurospora. So also were established scientists who had previously been working on other organisms: D. G. CATCHESIDE, STERLING EMERSON, NORMAN GILES, HERSCHEL MITCHELL, FRANCIS RYAN and MOGENS WESTERGAARD. During this period, Neurospora also provided the first introduction to research for numerous individuals who were later to become known for their work with other organisms. Among those whose careers began in this way were EDWARD ADELBERG, BRUCE AMES, AUGUST DOERMANN, NAOMI FRANKLIN, LEONARD HERZENBERG, DAVID HOGNESS, BRUCE HOLLOWAY, ESTHER LEDERBERG, JOSHUA LEDERBERG, NOREEN MURRAY, NOBORU SUEOKA and CHARLES

YANOFSKY; see, for example, RYAN and LEDERBERG (1946).

The Neurospora approach was soon extended to other fungi such as Ophiostoma and Ustilago. GUIDO PONTECORVO, who had previously worked on Drosophila with H. J. MULLER, began his program with *Aspergillus nidulans*. Genetic work flourished on Podospora, Sordaria, Ascobolus, Coprinus and Schizophyllum. Biochemical mutants were obtained in Schizosaccharomyces, Chlamydomonas and even in a flowering plant, Arabidopsis (LANGRIDGE 1955).

Application of the Neurospora approach to bacteria was not long delayed. Auxotrophic mutants of *E. coli* were obtained by CHARLES GRAY (a Stanford undergraduate) and TATUM (1944), and independently by ROEPKE, LIBBY and SMALL (1944). These made possible the 1946 demonstration of recombination in *E. coli* and opened the way for the explosive development of bacterial genetics.

Saccharomyces was a relatively slow starter. Heterothallism with two mating types was discovered by CARL and GERTRUDE LINDEGREN only in 1943. The first induced auxotrophic mutations and the first linkages were reported in 1949. Eleven workers attended the first yeast conference in 1961 (VON BORSTEL 1963), compared to 92 participants at a Neurospora conference held the same year (DE SERRES 1962). (Attendance at international yeast meetings now exceeds 1000!)

Advantageous features of Neurospora that were recognized as novel and noteworthy in the 1940s are now largely taken for granted because the same features are shared in various combinations by many other organisms that have since come into common use. Neurospora differed in important ways from the animals and plants used by most geneticists in 1941. It was haploid. All four products of individual meioses could be recovered, and in such a way that centromeres were readily mapped. Heterokaryons could be formed. Nutritional requirements were defined and simple. Stocks could be preserved in suspended animation, effectively conferring immortality on individual strains. In addition, growth was rapid, generation time short and fecundity high. Propagules suitable for plating were produced abundantly. Pure cultures could readily be obtained and tested for auxotrophic mutations.

Neurospora ascospores are large enough to permit manual isolation without a micromanipulator. Workers were initially intrigued by the ability to map centromeres, and genetic analysis was mostly done at first by laboriously dissecting the spores from linear asci in serial order. With time, it was realized that ordered ascus analysis is rarely necessary and that for most purposes random ascospores provide the needed information with far less effort (see PERKINS 1953).

When entire asci are needed for such purposes as studying interference, obtaining double mutants, or identifying chromosome rearrangements, it was found that unordered asci, shot from the perithecium as octets, can easily be obtained in large numbers (STRICKLAND 1960). Addition of a centromere marker made these unordered groups essentially as informative as intact asci (*e.g.*, PERKINS *et al.* 1986).

Neurospora conidia are a boon for transferring, plating, transforming, preserving stocks and sampling wild populations. These powdery vegetative spores are potentially hazardous as airborne contaminants, however. Laboratory practices were quickly developed that minimized the risk. It was found that if simple precautions are taken, there is no reason why Neurospora cannot coexist in the same laboratory with bacteria, yeast or slowly growing microorganisms.

The rapid linear growth of Neurospora (which can exceed 4 mm/hr) is a great advantage for many purposes, but for platings it was necessary to develop appropriate media containing colonializing agents such as sorbose (TATUM, BARRATT and CUTTER 1949) or to use genetic variants with restricted growth, such as the conditional colonial mutant *cot-1*.

Reliable and economic methods were developed for maintaining permanent stocks in suspended animation in silica gel, by lyophilization, or by freezing. These methods (WILSON 1986) enable the Fungal Genetics Stock Center (1990) to carry over 7000 Neurospora strains, with no need for periodic serial transfers.

Along with successes, Neurospora workers inevitably experienced frustrations and disappointments. It was initially hoped that new mutations might reveal previously undiscovered essential metabolites, but none were found. (A prospective new amino acid, tentatively named neurosporin, proved to be a crystalline mixture of isoleucine, valine and leucine; see KAY 1989). An elegant scheme to use heterokaryons for quantitative studies of dominance (BEADLE and COONRADT 1944) proved impractical because many laboratory stocks were heterokaryon incompatible, but this finding opened up the study of vegetative incompatibility and led to the finding that genes responsible for this incompatibility are numerous and are highly polymorphic in natural populations.

Recombinant DNA research with Neurospora was initially impeded by regulatory guidelines that first denied permission to proceed, then required that a disabling mutant be built into recipient strains. After permission was granted, it was found that genes introduced by transformation were poorly recovered from crosses, although they remained stably integrated in the chromosomes during vegetative growth. The poor sexual transmission proved to be due to RIP (repeat-induced point mutation), a process that mutates duplicate genes during the sexual phase (see below and SELKER 1990). RIP was then shown to provide an effective means of achieving targeted gene mutation, an asset which more than compensated for the inconvenience of poor transmission.

Inevitably, other organisms sometimes proved to be superior to Neurospora for particular purposes. For example, bioassays using induced auxotrophs were first developed in Neurospora during the war years, but bacteria proved to be so much faster for bioassay that Neurospora was not used to any extent.

Beginning in the 1950s, Neurospora played a central role in studies of recombination, providing the first proof of gene conversion (MITCHELL 1955) and revealing its main features (see below). Targeted regulation of local recombination frequencies by *rec* genes that are unlinked or nonadjacent was discovered in Neurospora (CATCHESIDE, JESSUP and SMITH 1964). Random ascospores of Neurospora continue to be the main source of information on recombination control of this type. Other fungi proved to be superior for recombination studies that required tetrads, however. Conversion frequencies were found to be much higher in yeast and Ascobolus than in Neurospora, while Sordaria and Ascobolus both had the advantage of numerous viable, readily scorable, autonomously expressed ascospore mutants. Neurospora was still a major source of information on gene conversion in the early 1960s when molecular models for eukaryotic conversion and crossing over were proposed by HOLLIDAY and by WHITEHOUSE and HASTINGS. However, by the mid-1970s, when the more detailed Aviemore model was put forward by MESELSON and RADDING, the most extensive and most critical data came from asci of Saccharomyces, Sordaria and Ascobolus. As a result of this trend, one geneticist whose interests focused almost exclusively on recombination models asked me bluntly in 1984 what I had been doing since the demise of Neurospora!

In fact, the change of emphasis away from recombination may have been a blessing in disguise for Neurospora genetics. In my own laboratory, it resulted in attention being given to other problems which might otherwise have been neglected. Chief among these was the study of chromosome rearrangements (see PERKINS 1979). Because deficiency ascospores remain unpigmented while nondeficiency spores are black, Neurospora proved ideal for detecting and diagnosing rearrangements. Meiotic mutants were examined cytologically and genetically, together with other mutants affected in development of the sexual phase. I also began to collect and analyze Neurospora from natural populations. This led, among other things, to the discovery of Spore killer elements, which bear a striking formal resemblance in their behavior to Segregation distorter in Drosophila, the

t-complex of mice, and *gamete eliminator* in tomato.

Far from being defunct, Neurospora continues to be a superb research organism. At the present time, it is used as the primary research object in about 70 laboratories in North America and 25 laboratories in 16 countries abroad. It remains the microorganism of choice for numerous specific problems. The knowledge and the genetic resources that have been acquired during 65 years are invaluable assets. But the most important factor responsible for its wide use is probably an exceptionally happy combination of traits that makes it suitable for research on problems spanning the entire range from molecules to populations.

The versatility of the organism is illustrated by the examples gathered below. Many of the contributions that will be cited were pioneered using Neurospora. Some of the advances were the first for filamentous fungi, others for the fungal kingdom, and others for all eukaryotes. However, the object in citing them is not to stress priority but to illustrate the variety of research areas to which Neurospora has contributed significantly. The list is far from complete. For example, no attempt has been made to cover the extensive work on specific enzymes or pathways, or on novel biochemical mutants; for documentation of many of these see PERKINS *et al.* (1982).

Nutritional mutants were used for many purposes. Intermediate steps in biosynthetic pathways were determined. By 1944, at least seven different genes had been identified that were involved in the synthesis of arginine (SRB and HOROWITZ 1944). [For early work on biosynthesis, see the reviews by HOROWITZ (1950) and by VOGEL and BONNER (1959).] In contrast to what is often the situation in bacteria, genes concerned with successive steps of the same biosynthetic pathway were shown not to be clustered but to be scattered through the genome (for review see HOROWITZ 1950). An apparent exception, the *aro* cluster-gene (GROSS and FEIN 1960), proved to make a single protein product with segments that specify five separate enzymatic activities (GAERTNER and COLE 1977).

The first conditional biochemical mutants were identified (STOKES, FOSTER and WOODWARD 1943; MITCHELL and HOULAHAN 1946). Temperature-sensitive mutants were used for testing the one-gene one-enzyme hypothesis (HOROWITZ and LEUPOLD 1951). Different alleles at a locus were shown to produce forms of an enzyme with qualitatively different properties (HOROWITZ and FLING 1953). Some mutant strains that lacked a specific enzymatic activity were shown to produce a protein that cross-reacted with antibody against the enzyme (SUSKIND, YANOFSKY and BONNER 1955).

Complementation of allelic mutations was demonstrated, first between nuclei in heterokaryons (FINCHAM and PATEMAN 1957; GILES, PARTRIDGE and NELSON 1957), then between the protein products *in vitro* (WOODWARD 1959; for review see FINCHAM 1966).

Translational suppression was analyzed for the first time at the molecular level (YANOFSKY 1956). Perhaps the best understood mechanism of metabolic suppression was described, involving suppression of *arg-2* by *pyr-3d* and *pyr-3a* by *arg-12ˢ* (DAVIS 1967; REISSIG, ISSALY and ISSALY 1967). These studies entailed the discovery of two genes for one enzyme, one gene for two enzyme activities, and duplicate enzyme activities for two pathways.

Proof was obtained for the channeling of pathway-specific enzymes in separate pools (WILLIAMS, BERNHARDT and DAVIS 1971). Compartmentation of metabolic pools and pathways within vacuoles, cytosol and mitochondria was established and studied in detail (WEISS 1973) (for reviews see DAVIS 1986; DAVIS and WEISS 1988).

Unlinked genes concerned with the same pathway were shown to be coordinately controlled (GROSS 1965). Crosspathway (general) control of amino acid biosynthetic enzymes was discovered (CARSIOTIS and LACY 1965; CARSIOTIS, JONES and WESSELING 1974). Convincing evidence for positive control was provided for the first time in eukaryotes in a pioneering study of the regulation of sulfur metabolism (MARZLUF and METZENBERG 1968); sulfur regulation in eukaryotes has since been analyzed most fully in Neurospora (for review see FU *et al.* 1990). A hierarchy of regulatory elements involved in phosphate metabolism was identified and, on the basis of genetic evidence, the novel concept was proposed that regulation is not limited to interactions between regulatory complexes and the DNA sequences of succeeding elements in the regulatory cascade, but that it also involves direct interaction between the protein products of regulatory genes (METZENBERG and CHIA 1979) (for review see METZENBERG 1979).

Mutants with a wide spectrum of altered vegetative morphologies were obtained and analyzed (*e.g.*, GARNJOBST and TATUM 1967) and biochemical defects were identified in some of them (for review see MISHRA 1977). The morphological mutant *crisp-1* (one of LINDEGREN's first markers) was shown to lack adenylate cyclase activity (TERENZI, FLAWIA and TORRES 1974). (The important regulatory signal cyclic AMP is therefore absent and must be dispensable in Neurospora, unlike Saccharomyces.) The process of conidiation was studied in wild type and in mutants (SPRINGER and YANOFSKY 1989). Genes with greatly elevated expression during conidial differentiation, identified by BERLIN and YANOFSKY (1985), were used in studying regulation (*e.g.*, ROBERTS and YANOFSKY 1989).

Mutants affected in development of the sexual cycle were examined (for review see RAJU 1992b). One of these (RAJU 1986) appears to be the Neurospora counterpart of the *polymitotic* mutant in maize, which BEADLE described and studied early in his career.

Electrodes were successfully inserted into Neurospora hyphal cells (SLAYMAN and SLAYMAN 1962). Electrophysiological studies showed that glucose transport is driven by a transmembrane proton gradient (SLAYMAN 1970; for review see SLAYMAN 1987); unlike animal cells, the plasma membrane potential is maintained primarily by proton flux rather than by potassium and sodium fluxes (SLAYMAN 1965). Other transport systems were shown to be driven by a proton-cotransport mechanism (SLAYMAN and SLAYMAN 1974). Mutant strains were obtained that can be grown indefinitely as protoplasts, without a cell wall (EMERSON 1963; SELITRENNIKOFF, LILLEY and ZUCKER 1981). These were used to isolate and characterize plasma membranes, to

prepare plasma membrane vesicles and to demonstrate that membrane ATPase is a proton pump (SCARBOROUGH 1975; for review see SCARBOROUGH 1978).

Kinetic and genetic studies of amino acid transport (by GABRIEL LESTER, DAVID STADLER, MARTIN PALL, GIB DEBUSK, and WILLIAM THWAITES and LAKSHMI PENDYALA) identified several transport systems with broad substrate specificities, unlike the highly specific "permeases" of bacteria but resembling the broad-specificity systems of mammalian cells, which had been based on kinetic evidence alone. Four major amino acid uptake systems were characterized, distinct from those in yeast (for review see PALL 1970).

Maternal transmission was demonstrated for a class of non-Mendelian respiratory defects (MITCHELL, MITCHELL and TISSIÈRES 1953). A non-Mendelian cytochrome defect was transferred between vegetative strains by injecting mitochondria (DIACUMAKOS, GARNJOBST and TATUM 1965). Mitochondria were shown to increase in number by division of preexisting mitochondria rather than being formed *de novo* (LUCK 1963). DNA was isolated from mitochondria for the first time (LUCK and REICH 1964). Progeny were shown to receive mitochondrial DNA only from the maternal parent, in both interspecific and intraspecific crosses (REICH and LUCK 1966; MANNELLA, PITTENGER and LAMBOWITZ 1979). A cyanide-insensitive alternative oxidase was identified for the first time in fungi (LAMBOWITZ and SLAYMAN 1971).

The first sequencing of a nucleic acid from mitochondria (HECKMAN *et al.* 1978) revealed unique features of initiator tRNA that foreshadowed the discovery of numerous unexpected features of mitochondrial genomes (for review see BREITENBERGER and RAJBHANDARY 1985). A protein-coding gene was shown to be located within an intron of another mitochondrial gene (BURKE and RAJBHANDARY 1982), extending a discovery in yeast to the filamentous fungi. Self-splicing of a mitochondrial intron was first demonstrated (GARRIGA and LAMBOWITZ 1984) and the first mutants were found that are affected in the splicing of mitochondrial RNA (MANNELLA *et al.* 1979). Reverse transcriptase was first shown to be present in mitochondria (AKINS, KELLEY and LAMBOWITZ 1986; KUIPER and LAMBOWITZ 1988). Tyrosyl-tRNA synthetase was shown to play an essential role in splicing (AKINS and LAMBOWITZ 1987).

Several key discoveries concern the mechanisms responsible for the import into mitochondria of polypeptides that are synthesized on cytoplasmic ribosomes. Pools of completed polypeptides were shown to be present in the cytoplasm (HALLERMAYER, ZIMMERMAN and NEUPERT 1977). Different mitochondrial receptors were indicated to be responsible for the import of different precursor polypeptides (ZIMMERMAN, HENNIG and NEUPERT 1981). The first sequence was obtained for the precursor of a nuclear-coded protein of the mitochondrial inner membrane or matrix (VIEBROCK, PERZ and SEBALD 1982). Contact sites functioning in import were demonstrated between inner and outer mitochondrial membranes (SCHLEYER and NEUPERT 1985). A processing protease responsible for cleaving targeting sequences in the mitochondrial matrix was purified (HAWLITSCHEK *et al.* 1988).

Mitochondrial plasmids were found, with sequences unrelated to those of mitochondrial DNA (COLLINS *et al.* 1981). Strains were discovered that became senescent following integration of plasmids into the mitochondrial DNA (RIECK, GRIFFITHS and BERTRAND 1982; for review see BERTRAND and GRIFFITHS 1989). Horizontal transfer of mitochondrial plasmids was shown to occur, independently of mitochondrial DNA (MAY and TAYLOR 1989; GRIFFITHS *et al.* 1990; COLLINS and SAVILLE 1990).

The first circadian rhythm in fungi was discovered, manifested as periodic conidiation that provided a permanent record as bands were formed along a growth continuum (PITTENDRIGH *et al.* 1959). Mutations were obtained that affect the free-running period length of the circadian clock (FELDMAN and HOYLE 1973). Clock-controlled genes were identified that are transcribed only at specific times in the circadian day (LOROS, DENOME and DUNLAP 1989). For reviews see FELDMAN and DUNLAP (1983), LAKIN-THOMAS, COTÉ and BRODY (1990) and DUNLAP (1990).

Resetting the circadian clock was shown to be mediated by a blue-light photoreceptor (SARGENT and BRIGGS 1967). Other effects of blue light were studied, including the induction of carotenogenesis, formation of protoperithecia, and phototropism of perithecial beaks (for review see DEGLI-INNOCENTI and RUSSO 1984). Mutants were identified that are blind to photoinduction (HARDING and TURNER 1981).

Heterokaryons (for review see DAVIS 1966) were used, first to study dominance and complementation, then to transfer mitochondria, plasmids and transposable elements, to rescue and maintain lethal or deleterious mutations, to map deficiencies, and to determine mutation frequencies.

Use of Neurospora heterokaryons led to the discovery of vegetative (heterokaryon) incompatibility (for review see PERKINS 1988). It was found that the mating type locus functions vegetatively as a heterokaryon incompatibility locus (BEADLE and COONRADT 1944; SANSOME 1945). Other genes controlling the formation of stable heterokaryons (*het* genes) were identified and mapped (GARNJOBST 1953). Microinjection of incompatible cytoplasm or extracts was shown to be lethal to recipient cells (WILSON, GARNJOBST and TATUM 1961). Partial diploids heterozygous for a *het* locus were obtained and shown to be highly abnormal (NEWMEYER and TAYLOR 1967; PERKINS 1975). An unlinked suppressor was discovered that neutralizes the vegetative incompatibility function of the mating type genes but not their mating function (NEWMEYER 1970). Polymorphic *het* genes were found to be so numerous that they effectively preclude formation of heterokaryons in natural populations of *N. crassa* (MYLYK 1976).

The mating type genes *A* and *a* were cloned, sequenced, and shown to be present in a single copy per genome, with characteristics quite unlike those of the mating type genes of yeast. Although *A* and *a* occupy precisely the same locus, their DNA sequences were found to contain no recognizable homology (GLASS *et al.* 1988) (for reviews see METZENBERG and GLASS 1990; GLASS and STABEN 1990). Mutations had earlier been obtained that inactivate the mating type genes (GRIFFITHS and DELANGE 1978). Genes were identified that are transcribed preferentially during sexual development, and cloned sequences of these mating-specific genes were used to obtain, by RIP and gene disruption, mutant strains in which sexual development is impaired (M. A. NELSON

and R. L. METZENBERG, unpublished results). Attraction of trichogynes to cells of opposite mating type was shown to be mediated by a diffusible mating-type specific pheromone (BISTIS 1983).

Cytological techniques were perfected and details of meiosis and ascus development and of chromosome morphology and behavior were examined by light microscopy, both in wild type and in mutants (for reviews see RAJU 1980, 1992b). Synaptonemal-complex karyotypes were obtained by reconstructing meiotic prophase nuclei from thin sections (GILLIES 1972). Recombination nodules were shown to be correlated with reciprocal crossing over events at pachytene and to exhibit positive interference (GILLIES 1972, 1979; BOJKO 1989). Synaptic adjustment of the synaptonemal complex was shown to occur in inversion heterozygotes (BOJKO 1990). Neurospora was the first filamentous fungus for which intact DNA molecules from entire individual chromosomes were separated electrophoretically, extending the maximum chromosome length that was then physically resolvable (ORBACH *et al.* 1988).

Tetrad analysis using a long multiply marked chromosome arm showed that meiotic crossing over and interference closely resemble those in Drosophila and *Zea mays* (PERKINS 1962).

The first definitive proof of gene conversion was accomplished in Neurospora (MITCHELL 1955). Important characteristics of conversion were delineated, especially by MARY MITCHELL, MARY CASE, NOREEN MURRAY and DAVID STADLER; see FINCHAM, DAY and RADFORD (1979).

Genes were discovered that dramatically control the frequency of recombination at unlinked or nonadjacent target sites (CATCHESIDE, JESSUP and SMITH 1964), with recombination reduced by dominant alleles at the controlling loci (for review see CATCHESIDE 1975).

N. crassa was the first fungus to have all linkage groups mapped genetically (BARRATT *et al.* 1954) and assigned to cytologically distinguished chromosomes (for review see PERKINS and BARRY 1977). Tester strains that incorporate translocations were devised and greatly speeded linkage detection and mapping (PERKINS *et al.* 1969). Genes at nearly 700 loci and breakpoints of more than 300 rearrangements have been mapped (PERKINS *et al.* 1982; PERKINS 1990; PERKINS and BARRY 1977; and D. D. PERKINS, unpublished results). The conventional maps have been complemented using restriction fragment length polymorphisms (METZENBERG *et al.* 1984, 1985; METZENBERG and GROTELUESCHEN 1990) and random amplified polymorphic DNA markers (RAPD mapping) (WILLIAMS *et al.* 1991).

Genes specifying 5S RNA were shown to be dispersed through the genome in single copies (FREE, RICE and METZENBERG 1979; SELKER *et al.* 1981). Telomeres were cloned and shown to have a DNA sequence identical to that in *Homo sapiens* (SCHECHTMAN 1987, 1990). Random breaks in ribosomal DNA sequences of the nucleolus organizer region were shown to acquire telomere sequences *de novo* (BUTLER 1991).

Following MCCLINTOCK (1945), chromosome rearrangements of various types were identified and put to many uses (for review see PERKINS and BARRY 1977). Because ascospores that contain deficiencies fail to darken, frequencies of ejected asci with different numbers of black and nonblack spores could be used to distinguish different rearrangement types (PERKINS 1974). Genetic analysis of insertional translocations has been more thorough than in other organisms (see, for example, PERKINS 1972). Numerous quasiterminal rearrangements with chromosome segments translocated to telomeres or subtelomere regions were also studied. Insertional and terminal rearrangements were shown to generate partial-diploid progeny (DE SERRES 1957; ST. LAWRENCE 1959; NEWMEYER and TAYLOR 1967). The duplications obtained as segmental aneuploids from insertional and terminal rearrangements proved useful for mapping (PERKINS 1975) and for studying vegetative incompatibility (NEWMEYER 1970; PERKINS 1975), instability (NEWMEYER and GALEAZZI 1977), and dominance and dosage of regulatory genes (e.g., METZENBERG and CHIA 1979). Partial-diploid progeny from crosses heterozygous for terminal rearrangements were found to revert frequently to euploid condition, usually by loss of the translocated segment.

Heterokaryons were used to recover and characterize recessive lethal mutations (ATWOOD and MUKAI 1953; DE SERRES and OSTERBIND 1962), to determine the frequency of recessive mutation for loci throughout the genome (DE SERRES and MALLING 1971; STADLER and CRANE 1979), and to study mutagenesis, DNA repair, and dose-rate effects (STADLER and MOYER 1981; STADLER 1983; STADLER and MACLEOD 1984). The spectra of mutational lesions were examined for different mutagens and genotypes (e.g., DE SERRES and BROCKMAN 1991; KINSEY and HUNG 1981).

An excision-repair mutant was obtained that shows increased sensitivity solely to UV, the first example of its type in eukaryotes (ISHII, NAKAMURA and INOUE 1991). A subset of mutagen-sensitive mutants was shown to be abnormally sensitive to histidine and hydroxyurea, and to cause chromosome instability (SCHROEDER 1986); this includes members of two epistasis groups (KÄFER 1983). Many mutants of this subset were found to have abnormal deoxyribonucleotide triphosphate pools (SRIVASTAVA and SCHROEDER 1989). Histidine and hydroxyurea were shown to cause chromosome instability in the absence of any mutation causing mutagen sensitivity (NEWMEYER, SCHROEDER and GALEAZZI 1978; SCHROEDER 1986), and histidine was found to cause breaks or nicks in DNA (HOWARD and BAKER 1988).

An endo-exonuclease of Neurospora was characterized and shown to be immunochemically related both to the RecC polypeptide of E. coli and to an endo-exonuclease that is deficient in the rad52 mutant of Saccharomyces (FRASER, KOA and CHOW 1990).

The first DNA-mediated transformation in a sexual fungus was achieved in Neurospora (N. C. MISHRA, SZABO and TATUM 1973). [Aspergillus niger had been transformed earlier by SEN, NANDI and A. K. MISHRA (1969).] The prototrophic character, putatively due to transformation, was poorly transmitted through crosses (N. C. MISHRA and TATUM 1973), behavior now attributable to RIP but then a cause for skepticism. With the advent of DNA technology and efficient transformation methods (CASE et al. 1979), integration of transforming DNA was found to be primarily nonhomologous. [For a review see FINCHAM (1989).]

Inactivation of duplicated DNA sequences was found to occur premeiotically during the period of proliferation between fertilization and fusion of nuclei (SELKER et al. 1987; for review see SELKER 1990). This phenomenon, termed repeat-induced point mutation (RIP), was shown to involve methylation and C to T mutation in both copies of duplicated sequences. RIP can be used to achieve targeted gene inactivation following transformation. [Premeiotic inactivation of duplicated segments has since been shown to occur in other fungi; for review see SELKER (1990).] Independently, BUTLER and METZENBERG (1989) found that the number of ribosomal DNA repeats in the nucleolus organizer region undergoes change during the same premeiotic period that is subject to RIP.

An active transposable element was identified, the first to be characterized molecularly in filamentous fungi (KINSEY and HELBER 1989). This LINE-like element was shown to be transmitted from one nucleus to another in heterokaryons (KINSEY 1990).

Methods were devised for sampling natural populations, and wild-collected strains were analyzed (PERKINS, TURNER and BARRY 1976; for review see PERKINS and TURNER 1988). Discrete orange colonies found on burned vegetation in warm, moist climates were shown usually to represent pure haploid clones of Neurospora from different ascospores. Fertility in crosses to standard reference strains was shown to be a convenient and reliable criterion for determining the species of wild-collected isolates. New heterothallic species were described. Homothallic Neurospora species, devoid of conidia, were also discovered (see FREDERICK, UECKER and BENJAMIN 1969).

Genetic polymorphisms at the protein level were shown to be abundant in natural populations of heterothallic species (SPIETH 1975), not a foregone conclusion for a haploid organism. Numerous vegetative incompatibility loci were identified and shown to be polymorphic (MYLYK 1975, 1976). Wild populations were shown to carry a load of phase-specific recessive mutations that adversely affect meiosis and the sexual diplophase (LESLIE and RAJU 1985). The nonselective abortion of asci in crosses between inbred strains of a normally outbreeding species provided an example of inbreeding depression in fungi (RAJU, PERKINS and NEWMEYER 1987).

Chromosomal elements ("Spore killers") were discovered that show meiotic drive, resulting in the death of meiotic products that do not contain the element. Recombination was shown to be blocked in the chromosomal region that contains the killer element, reminiscent of SD in Drosophila and the t-complex in mice (TURNER and PERKINS 1979; for review see TURNER and PERKINS 1991).

Length mutations in mitochondrial DNA were studied in different N. crassa populations (TAYLOR, SMOLICH and MAY 1986) and were used to construct a phylogenetic tree for four different species (TAYLOR and NATVIG 1989). Mitochondrial plasmid DNAs were also compared in different populations and species (NATVIG, MAY and TAYLOR 1984).

Clearly, Neurospora research has till now been concerned mostly with genetic, cellular and molecular mechanisms. Relatively little attention has been paid to evolutionary biology, or to population genetics, which has been based since its beginnings almost exclusively on plants and animals while the fungal kingdom has been largely ignored. Yet the fungi offer certain advantages for studying populations, not least of which is haploidy during the vegetative stage. Imagine what could be done if it were possible to sample animal or plant populations by obtaining individual sperm or pollen grains and growing them up into immortal haploid or homozygous individuals. The equivalent of this is accomplished routinely in Neurospora, where orange haploid colonies that originated from single ascospores are readily sampled in the wild, propagated in the laboratory, and maintained as permanent viable stocks in suspended animation. Some 4000 strains are already available that have been obtained in this way from populations in many parts of the world. What has been learned from them so far suggests that Neurospora can perhaps become for the population genetics of haploid organisms what Drosophila has been for diploids (for review see PERKINS and TURNER 1988).

As with Drosophila, attention in the laboratory has been focussed primarily on one Neurospora species, *N. crassa*, but other species have also come into use. The known Neurospora species range from highly outbred to highly inbred. Some are heterothallic and cross-fertilizing, others are homothallic and self-fertilizing. One species, *N. tetrasperma*, does not fall into either category and has been termed pseudohomothallic. Like its counterparts in other genera, it represents a breeding system that is based on heterokaryosis and is therefore unique to the fungi. *N. tetrasperma* normally perpetuates itself as a self-fertile heterokaryon containing haploid nuclei of both mating types. Most conidia and ascospores are heterokaryotic, producing self-fertile cultures that behave as though they were homothallic. A minority of the spores are homokaryotic, however, resulting in self-sterile, functionally heterothallic cultures. The species is therefore predominantly inbred, but it retains the capacity for outbreeding as a ready option (RAJU 1992a). This diversity of life styles in the various Neurospora species shows promise for comparative studies.

After many years of asking "how" questions about the way that Neurospora functions, we should now be in a strong position to ask "why" questions about adaptations, populations and evolutionary origins. Research on molecular, cellular and genetic mechanisms is certain to continue. It remains to be seen whether the promise of Neurospora for population genetics will be fulfilled.

Sixty-five years have passed since SHEAR and DODGE named and described Neurospora, and 50 years since BEADLE and TATUM thrust it into prominence. In 1952, DODGE felt that he would soon be able to assert, "The old red bread-mold has at last come into its own." Developments since then have taken his favorite

organism far beyond what he could have imagined. Neurospora continues to be a source of innovations and surprises.

This essay is dedicated to the memory of B. O. DODGE on the 120th anniversary of his birth. The summary of research contributions benefited from discussion with numerous colleagues. Their comments are much appreciated. I am indebted to the Library of the New York Botanical Garden, Bronx, New York, for the photograph of DODGE, to HERSCHEL ROMAN for that of LINDEGREN, and to MARJORIE M. BHAVNANI for the 1947 photograph of McCLINTOCK. Work on Neurospora in my laboratory has been supported since 1956 by grant AI 01462 from the National Institutes of Health.

LITERATURE CITED

AKINS, R. A., R. L. KELLEY and A. M. LAMBOWITZ, 1986 Mitochondrial plasmids of Neurospora: integration into mitochondrial DNA and evidence for reverse transcription in mitochondria. Cell **47:** 505–516.

AKINS, R. A., and A. M. LAMBOWITZ, 1987 A protein required for splicing group I introns in Neurospora mitochondria is mitochondrial tyrosyl-tRNA synthetase or a derivative thereof. Cell **50:** 331–345.

ATWOOD, K. C., and F. MUKAI, 1953 Indispensable gene functions in Neurospora. Proc. Natl. Acad. Sci. USA **39:** 1027–1035.

BACHMANN, B. J., and N. W. STRICKLAND, 1965 *Neurospora Bibliography and Index.* Yale University Press, New Haven, Conn.

BARRATT, R. W., D. NEWMEYER, D. D. PERKINS and L. GARNJOBST, 1954 Map construction in *Neurospora crassa.* Adv. Genet. **6:** 1–93.

BEADLE, G. W., 1966 Biochemical genetics: some recollections, pp. 23–32 in *Phage and the Origins of Molecular Biology,* edited by J. CAIRNS, G. S. STENT and J. D. WATSON. Cold Spring Harbor Laboratory, Cold Spring Harbor, N.Y.

BEADLE, G. W., 1974 Recollections. Annu. Rev. Bioch. **43:** 1–13.

BEADLE, G. W., and V. L. COONRADT, 1944 Heterocaryosis in *Neurospora crassa.* Genetics **29:** 291–308.

BEADLE, G. W., and E. L. TATUM, 1941 Genetic control of biochemical reactions in Neurospora. Proc. Natl. Acad. Sci. USA **27:** 499–506.

BERLIN, V., and C. YANOFSKY, 1985 Isolation and characterization of genes differentially expressed during conidiation of *Neurospora crassa.* Mol. Cell. Biol. **5:** 849–855.

BERTRAND, N., and A. J. F. GRIFFITHS, 1989 Linear plasmids that integrate into mitochondrial DNA in Neurospora. Genome **31:** 155–159.

BISTIS, G. N., 1983 Evidence for diffusible, mating-type-specific trichogyne attractants in *Neurospora crassa.* Exp. Mycol. **7:** 292–295.

BOJKO, M., 1989 Two kinds of "recombination nodules" in *Neurospora crassa.* Genome **32:** 309–317.

BOJKO, M., 1990 Synaptic adjustment of inversion loops in *Neurospora crassa.* Genetics **124:** 593–598.

BREITENBERGER, C. A., and U. L. RAJBHANDARY, 1985 Some highlights of mitochondrial research based on analyses of *Neurospora crassa* mitochondrial DNA. Trends Biochem. Sci. **10:** 478–483.

BURKE, J. M., and U. L. RAJBHANDARY, 1982 Intron within the large rRNA gene of *N. crassa* mitochondria: a long open reading frame and a consensus sequence possibly important in splicing. Cell **31:** 509–520.

BUTLER, D. K., 1991 Recombination and chromosome breakage in the nucleolus organizer region of Neurospora crassa. Ph.D. Thesis, University of Wisconsin, Madison.

BUTLER, D. K., and R. L. METZENBERG, 1989 Premeiotic change

of nucleolus organizer size in Neurospora. Genetics **122:** 783–791.

BUTLER, E. T., W. J. ROBBINS and B. O. DODGE, 1941 Biotin and the growth of Neurospora. Science **94:** 262–263.

CARSIOTIS, M., R. F. JONES and A. C. WESSELING, 1974 Cross-pathway regulation: histidine-mediated control of histidine, tryptophan, and arginine biosynthetic enzymes in *Neurospora crassa.* J. Bacteriol. **119:** 893–898.

CARSIOTIS, M., and A. M. LACY, 1965 Increased activity of tryptophan biosynthetic enzymes in histidine mutants of *Neurospora crassa.* J. Bacteriol. **89:** 1472–1477.

CASE, M. E., M. SCHWEIZER, S. R. KUSHNER and N. H. GILES, 1979 Efficient transformation of *Neurospora crassa* by utilizing hybrid plasmid DNA. Proc. Natl. Acad. Sci. USA **76:** 5259–5263.

CATCHESIDE, D. G., 1973 *Neurospora crassa* and genetics. Neurospora Newsl. **20:** 6–8.

CATCHESIDE, D. G., 1975 Regulation of genetic recombination in *Neurospora crassa*, pp. 301–312 in *The Eukaryote Chromosome*, edited by W. J. PEACOCK and R. D. BROCK. Australian National University Press, Canberra.

CATCHESIDE, D. G., A. P. JESSUP and B. R. SMITH, 1964 Genetic controls of allelic recombination in Neurospora. Nature **202:** 1242–1243.

COLLINS, R. A., and B. J. SAVILLE, 1990 Independent transfer of mitochondrial chromosomes and plasmids during unstable vegetative fusion in Neurospora. Nature **345:** 177–179.

COLLINS, R. A., L. L. STOHL, M. D. COLE and A. M. LAMBOWITZ, 1981 Characterization of a novel plasmid DNA found in mitochondria of *N. crassa.* Cell **24:** 443–452.

DAVIS, R. H., 1966 Mechanisms of inheritance. 2. Heterokaryosis, pp. 567–588 in *The Fungi: An Advanced Treatise*, Vol. 2, edited by G. C. AINSWORTH and A. S. SUSSMAN. Academic Press, New York.

DAVIS, R. H., 1967 Channeling in Neurospora metabolism, pp. 303–322 in *Organizational Biosynthesis*, edited by H. J. VOGEL, J. O. LAMPEN and V. BRYSON. Academic Press, New York.

DAVIS, R. H., 1986 Compartmental and regulatory mechanisms in the arginine pathways of *Neurospora crassa* and *Saccharomyces cerevisiae.* Microbiol. Rev. **50:** 280–313.

DAVIS, R. H., and R. L. WEISS, 1988 Novel mechanisms controlling arginine metabolism in Neurospora. Trends Biochem. Sci. **31:** 101–104.

DEGLI-INNOCENTI, F., and V. E. A. RUSSO, 1984 Genetic analysis of the blue light-induced responses in *Neurospora crassa*, pp. 213–219 in *Blue Light Effects in Biological Systems*, edited by H. SENGER. Springer Verlag, Berlin.

DE SERRES, F. J., 1957 A genetic analysis of an insertional translocation involving the *ad-3* region in *Neurospora crassa.* Genetics **42:** 366–367 (Abstr.)

DE SERRES, F. J. (Editor), 1962 *Neurospora Information Conference* (National Research Council Publication 950). National Academy of Science, Washington, D.C.

DE SERRES, F. J., and H. E. BROCKMAN, 1991 Qualitative differences in the spectra of genetic damage in 2-aminopurine-induced *ad-3* mutants between nucleotide excision-repair-proficient and -deficient strains of *Neurospora crassa.* Mutat. Res. **251:** 41–58.

DE SERRES, F. J., and H. V. MALLING, 1971 Measurement of recessive lethal damage over the entire genome and at two specific loci in the *ad-3* region of a two-component heterokaryon of *Neurospora crassa*, pp. 311–342 in *Chemical Mutagens*, Vol. 2, edited by A. HOLLAENDER. Plenum, New York.

DE SERRES, F. J., and R. S. OSTERBIND, 1962 Estimation of the relative frequencies of the X-ray-induced viable and recessive lethal mutations in the *ad-3* region of *Neurospora crassa.* Genetics **47:** 793–796.

DIACUMAKOS, E. G., L. GARNJOBST and E. L. TATUM, 1965 A

cytoplasmic character in *Neurospora crassa*: the role of nuclei and mitochondria. J. Cell Biol. **26:** 427–443.

DODGE, B. O., 1927 Nuclear phenomena associated with heterothallism and homothallism in the ascomycete Neurospora. J. Agric. Res. **35:** 289–305.

DODGE, B. O., 1939 Some problems in the genetics of fungi. Science **90:** 379–385.

DODGE, B. O., 1942 Heterocaryotic vigor in Neurospora. Bull. Torrey Bot. Club **69:** 1–74.

DODGE, B. O., 1952 The fungi come into their own. Mycologia **44:** 273–291.

DUNLAP, J. C., 1990 Closely watched clocks. Trends Genet. **6:** 159–165.

EMERSON, S., 1963 Slime, a plasmodioid variant in *Neurospora crassa.* Genetica **34:** 162–182.

FELDMAN, J. F., and J. C. DUNLAP, 1983 *Neurospora crassa*: a unique system for studying circadian rhythms. Photochem. Photobiol. Rev. **7:** 319–368.

FELDMAN, J. F., and M. N. HOYLE, 1973 Isolation of circadian clock mutants of *Neurospora crassa.* Genetics **75:** 605–613.

FINCHAM, J. R. S., 1966 *Genetic Complementation*. W. A. Benjamin, New York.

FINCHAM, J. R. S., 1989 Transformation in fungi. Microbiol. Rev. **53:** 148–170.

FINCHAM, J. R. S., P. R. DAY and A. RADFORD, 1979 *Fungal Genetics*, Ed. 4. Blackwell, Oxford.

FINCHAM, J. R. S., and J. A. PATEMAN, 1957 Formation of an enzyme through complementary action of mutant "alleles" in separate nuclei in a heterocaryon. Nature **179:** 741–742.

FRASER, M. J., H. KOA and T. Y.-K. CHOW, 1990 Neurospora endo-exonuclease is immunochemically related to the *recC* gene product of *Escherichia coli.* J. Bacteriol. **172:** 507–510.

FREDERICK, L., F. A. UECKER and C. R. BENJAMIN, 1969 A new species of Neurospora from the soil of West Pakistan. Mycologia **61:** 1077–1084.

FREE, S. J., P. W. RICE and R. L. METZENBERG, 1979 Arrangement of the genes coding for ribosomal ribonucleic acid in *Neurospora crassa.* J. Bacteriol. **137:** 1219–1226.

FU, Y.-H., H.-J. LEE, J. L. YOUNG, G. JARAI and G. A. MARZLUF, 1990 Nitrogen and sulfur regulatory circuits of Neurospora, pp. 319–335 in *Developmental Biology*, edited by E. H. DAVIDSON, J. V. RUDERMAN and J. W. POSAKONY. Wiley-Liss, New York.

Fungal Genetics Stock Center, 1990 *Catalog of Strains*. (Supplement to Fungal Genet. Newsl. **37**.)

GAERTNER, F. H., and K. W. COLE, 1977 A cluster-gene: evidence for one gene, one polypeptide, five enzymes. Biochem. Biophys. Res. Commun. **75:** 259–264.

GARNJOBST, L., 1953 Genetic control of heterocaryosis in *Neurospora crassa.* Am. J. Bot. **40:** 607–614.

GARNJOBST, L., and E. L. TATUM, 1967 A survey of new morphological mutants in *Neurospora crassa.* Genetics **57:** 579–604.

GARRIGA, G., and A. M. LAMBOWITZ, 1984 RNA splicing in Neurospora mitochondria: self-splicing of a mitochondrial intron *in vitro.* Cell **39:** 631–641.

GILES, N. H., C. W. H. PARTRIDGE and N. J. NELSON, 1957 The genetic control of adenylosuccinase in *Neurospora crassa.* Proc. Natl. Acad. Sci. USA **43:** 305–317.

GILLIES, C. B., 1972 Reconstruction of the *Neurospora crassa* pachytene karyotype from serial sections of synaptonemal complexes. Chromosoma **36:** 119–130.

GILLIES, C. B., 1979 The relationship between synaptinemal complexes, recombination nodules and crossing over in *Neurospora crassa* bivalents and translocation quadrivalents. Genetics **91:** 1–17.

GLASS, N. L., and C. STABEN, 1990 Genetic control of mating in *Neurospora crassa.* Semin. Dev. Biol. **1:** 177–184

GLASS, N. L., S. J. VOLLMER, C. STABEN, J. GROTELUESCHEN, R. L.

METZENBERG and C. YANOFSKY, 1988 DNAs of the two mating-type alleles of *Neurospora crassa* are highly dissimilar. Science **241**: 570–573.

GODDARD, D. R., 1935 The reversible heat activation inducing germination and increased respiration in the ascospores of *Neurospora tetrasperma*. J. Gen. Physiol. **19**: 45–60.

GODDARD, D. R., 1939 The reversible heat activation of respiration in Neurospora. Cold Spring Harbor Symp. Quant. Biol. **7**: 362–376.

GRAY, C. H., and E. L. TATUM, 1944 X-ray induced growth factor requirements in bacteria. Proc. Natl. Acad. Sci. USA **30**: 404–410.

GRIFFITHS, A. J. F., and A. M. DELANGE, 1978 Mutations of the *a* mating-type gene in *Neurospora crassa*. Genetics **88**: 239–254.

GRIFFITHS, A. J. F., S. R. KRAUS, R. BARTON, D. A. COURT, C. J. MEYERS and H. BERTRAND, 1990 Hetrokaryotic transmission of senescence plasmid DNA in Neurospora. Curr. Genet. **17**: 139–145.

GROSS, S. R., 1965 The regulation of synthesis of leucine biosynthetic enzymes in Neurospora. Proc. Nat. Acad. Sci. USA **54**: 1538–1546.

GROSS, S. R., and A. FEIN, 1960 Linkage and function in Neurospora. Genetics **45**: 885–904.

HALLERMAYER, G., R. ZIMMERMAN and W. NEUPERT, 1977 Kinetic studies on the transport of cytoplasmically synthesized proteins into the mitochondria in intact cells of *Neurospora crassa*. Eur. J. Biochem. **81**: 523–532.

HARDING, R. W., and R. V. TURNER, 1981 Photoregulation of the carotenoid biosynthetic pathway in albino and white collar mutants of *Neurospora crassa*. Pl•nt Physiol. **68**: 745–749.

HAWLITSHECK, G., H. SCHNEIDER, B. SCHMIDT, M. TROPSCHUG, F.-U. HARTL and W. NEUPERT, 1988 Mitochondrial protein import: identification of processing peptidase and of PEP, a processing enhancing protein. Cell **53**: 795–806.

HECKMAN, J. E., L. I. HECKER, S. D. SCHWARTZBACH, W. E. BARNETT, B. BAUMSTARK and U. L. RAJBHANDARY, 1978 Structure and function of initiator methionine tRNA from the mitochondria of *Neurospora crassa*. Cell **13**: 83–95.

HO, C. C., 1986 Identity and characteristics of *Neurospora intermedia* responsible for oncom fermentation in Indonesia. Food Microbiol. **3**: 115–132.

HOROWITZ, N. H., 1950 Biochemical genetics of Neurospora. Adv. Genet. **3**: 33–71.

HOROWITZ, N. H., 1973 Neurospora and the beginnings of molecular genetics. Neurospora Newsl. **20**: 4–6.

HOROWITZ, N. H., 1979 Genetics and the synthesis of proteins. Ann. NY Acad. Sci. **325**: 253–266.

HOROWITZ, N. H., 1985 The origins of molecular genetics: one gene, one enzyme. BioEssays **3**: 37–39.

HOROWITZ, N. H., 1990 George Wells Beadle. Biogr. Mem. Natl. Acad. Sci. **59**: 26–52.

HOROWITZ, N. H., 1991 Fifty years ago: the Neurospora revolution. Genetics **127**: 631–635.

HOROWITZ, N. H., and M. FLING, 1953 Genetic determination of tyrosinase thermostability in Neurospora. Genetics **38**: 360–374.

HOROWITZ, N. H., and U. LEUPOLD, 1951 Some recent studies bearing on the one gene-one enzyme hypothesis. Cold Spring Harbor Symp. Quant. Biol. **16**: 65–74.

HOWARD, C. A., and T. I. BAKER, 1988 Relationship of histidine to DNA damage and stress induced responses in mutagen sensitive mutants of *Neurospora crassa*. Curr. Genet. **13**: 391–399.

ISHII, C., K. NAKAMURA and H. INOUE, 1991 A novel phenotype of an excision-repair mutant in *Neurospora crassa*: mutagen sensitivity of the *mus-18* mutant is specific to UV. Mol. Gen. Genet. **228**: 33–39.

KÄFER, E., 1983 Epistatic grouping of DNA repair-deficient mutants in Neurospora: comparative analysis of two *uvs-3* alleles and *uvs-6*, and their *mus* double mutant strains. Genetics **105**: 19–33.

KAY, L. E., 1989 Selling pure science in wartime: the biochemical genetics of G. W. Beadle. J. Hist. Biol. **22**: 73–101.

KELLER, E. F., 1983 *A Feeling for the Organism. The Life and Work of Barbara McClintock.* Freeman, San Francisco.

KINSEY, J. A., 1990 *Tad*, a LINE-like transposable element of Neurospora, can transpose between nuclei in heterokaryons. Genetics **126**: 317–323.

KINSEY, J. A., and J. HELBER, 1989 Isolation of a transposable element from *Neurospora crassa*. Proc. Natl. Acad. Sci. USA **86**: 1929–1933.

KINSEY, J. A., and B.-S. T. HUNG, 1981 Mutation at the *am* locus of *Neurospora crassa*. Genetics **99**: 405–414.

KITAZIMA, K., 1925 On the fungus luxuriantly grown on the bark of the trees injured by the great fire of Tokyo on Sept. 1, 1923. Ann. Phytopathol. Soc. Jpn. **1**: 15–19.

KUIPER, M. T. R., and A. M. LAMBOWITZ, 1988 A novel reverse transcriptase activity associated with mitochondrial plasmids of Neurospora. Cell **55**: 693–704.

KUNKEL, L. O., 1913 The influence of starch, peptone, and sugars on the toxicity of various nitrates to *Monilia sitophila* (Mont.) Sacc. Bull. Torrey Bot. Club **40**: 625–639.

KUNKEL, L. O., 1914 Physical and chemical factors influencing the toxicity of inorganic salts to *Monilia sitophila* (Mont.) Sacc. Bull. Torrey Bot. Club **41**: 265–293.

LAKIN-THOMAS, P. L., G. G. COTÉ and S. BRODY, 1990 Circadian rhythms in *Neurospora crassa*: biochemistry and genetics. Crit. Rev. Microbiol. **17**: 365–416.

LAMBOWITZ, A. M., and C. W. SLAYMAN, 1971 Cyanide-resistant respiration in *Neurospora crassa*. J. Bacteriol. **108**: 1087–1096.

LANGRIDGE, J., 1955 Biochemical mutations in the crucifer *Arabidopsis thaliana* (L.) Heynh. Nature **176**: 260.

LEDERBERG, J., 1990 Edward Lawrie Tatum. Biogr. Mem. Natl. Acad. Sci. **59**: 356–386.

LESLIE, J. F., and N. B. RAJU, 1985 Recessive mutants from natural populations of *Neurospora crassa* that are expressed in the sexual diplophase. Genetics **111**: 759–777.

LINDEGREN, C. C., 1973 Reminiscences of B. O. Dodge and the beginnings of Neurospora genetics. Neurospora Newsl. **20**: 13–14.

LINDEGREN, C. C., and G. LINDEGREN, 1942 Locally specific patterns of chromatid and chromosome interference in Neurospora. Genetics **27**: 1–24.

LOROS, J. J., S. A. DENOME and J. C. DUNLAP, 1989 Molecular cloning of genes under control of the circadian clock in Neurospora. Science **243**: 385–388.

LUCK, D. J. L., 1963 Genesis of mitochondria in *Neurospora crassa*. Proc. Natl. Acad. Sci. USA **49**: 233–240.

LUCK, D. J. L., and E. REICH, 1964 DNA in mitochondria of *Neurospora crassa*. Proc. Natl. Acad. Sci. USA **52**: 931–938.

MANNELLA, C. A., T. H. PITTENGER and A. M. LAMBOWITZ, 1979 Transmission of mitochondrial deoxyribonucleic acid in *Neurospora crassa* sexual crosses. J. Bacteriol. **137**: 1449–1451.

MANNELLA, C. A., R. A. COLLINS, M. R. GREEN and A. M. LAMBOWITZ, 1979 Defective splicing of mitochondrial rRNA in cytochrome-deficient nuclear mutants of *Neurospora crassa*. Proc. Natl. Acad. Sci. USA **76**: 2635–2639.

MARZLUF, G. A., and R. L. METZENBERG, 1968 Positive control by the *cys-3* locus in regulation of sulfur metabolism in Neurospora. J. Mol. Biol. **33**: 423–437.

MAY, G., and J. W. TAYLOR, 1989 Independent transfer of mitochondrial plasmids in *Neurospora crassa*. Nature **339**: 320–322.

MCCLINTOCK, B., 1945 Neurospora. I. Preliminary observations of the chromosomes of *Neurospora crassa*. Am. J. Bot. **32**: 671–678.

METZENBERG, R. L., 1979 Implications of some genetic control mechanisms in Neurospora. Microbiol. Rev. **43**: 361–383.

METZENBERG, R. L., and W. CHIA, 1979 Genetic control of phosphorus assimilation in *Neurospora crassa*: dose-dependent dominance and recessiveness in constitutive mutants. Genetics **93**: 625–643.

METZENBERG, R. L., and N. L. GLASS, 1990 Mating type and mating strategies in Neurospora. BioEssays **12**: 53–59.

METZENBERG, R. L., and J. GROTELUESCHEN, 1990 *Neurospora crassa* restriction polymorphism map, pp. 3.22–3.29 in *Genetic Maps*, Ed. 5, edited by S. J. O'BRIEN. Cold Spring Harbor Laboratory, Cold Spring Harbor, N.Y.

METZENBERG, R. L., J. N. STEVENS, E. U. SELKER and E. MORZYCKA-WROBLEWSKA, 1984 A method for finding the genetic map position of cloned DNA fragments. Neurospora Newsl. **31**: 35–39.

METZENBERG, R. L., J. N. STEVENS, E. U. SELKER and E. MORZYCKA-WROBLEWSKA, 1985 Identification and chromosomal distribution of 5S RNA genes in *Neurospora crassa*. Proc. Natl. Acad. Sci. USA **82**: 2067–2071.

MISHRA, N. C., 1977 Genetics and biochemistry of morphogenesis in Neurospora. Adv. Genet. **19**: 341–405.

MISHRA, N. C., G. SZABO and E. L. TATUM, 1973 Nucleic acid induced genetic changes in Neurospora, pp. 259–268 in *The Role of RNA in Reproduction and Development*, edited by M. C. NIU and S. J. SEGAL. Elsevier/North Holland, Amsterdam.

MISHRA, N. C., and E. L. TATUM, 1973 Non-mendelian inheritance of DNA-induced inositol independence in Neurospora. Proc. Natl. Acad. Sci. USA **70**: 3875–3879.

MITCHELL, H. K., and M. B. HOULAHAN, 1946 Neurospora. IV. A temperature-senstivie, riboflavinless mutant. Am. J. Bot. **33**: 31–35.

MITCHELL, M. B., 1955 Aberrant recombination of pyridoxine mutants of Neurospora. Proc. Natl. Acad. Sci. USA **41**: 215–220.

MITCHELL, M. B., H. K. MITCHELL and A. TISSIÈRES, 1953 Mendelian and non-Mendelian factors affecting the cytochrome system in *Neurospora crassa*. Proc. Natl. Acad. Sci. USA **39**: 601–613.

MÖLLER, A., 1901 Phycomyceten und Ascomyceten. Untersuchungen aus Brasilien, pp. 1–319 in *Botanische Mittheilungen aus den Tropen*, Vol. 9, edited by A. F. A. SCHIMPER. Fischer, Jena.

MONTAGNE, C., 1843 Quatrième centurie de plantes cellulaires exotiques nouvelles. Ann. Sci. Nat. Bot. 2e Ser. **20**: 352–379 (+ one plate).

MOREAU-FROMENT, M., 1956 Les Neurospora. Bull. Soc. Bot. Fr. **103**: 678–738.

MYLYK, O. M., 1975 Heterokaryon incompatibility genes in *Neurospora crassa* detected using duplication-producing chromosome rearrangements. Genetics **80**: 107–124.

MYLYK, O. M., 1976 Heteromorphism for heterokaryon incompatibility genes in natural populations of *Neurospora crassa*. Genetics **83**: 275–284.

NATVIG, D. O., G. MAY and J. W. TAYLOR, 1984 Distribution and evolutionary significance of mitochondrial plasmids in Neurospora spp. J. Bacteriol. **159**: 288–293.

NEWMEYER, D., 1970 A suppressor of the heterokaryon-incompatibility associated with mating type in *Neurospora crassa*. Can. J. Genet. Cytol. **12**: 914–926.

NEWMEYER, D., and D. R. GALEAZZI, 1977 The instability of Neurospora duplication *Dp(IL→IR)H4250* and its genetic control. Genetics **85**: 461–487.

NEWMEYER, D., A. L. SCHROEDER and D. R. GALEAZZI, 1978 An apparent connection between histidine, recombination and repair in Neurospora. Genetics **89**: 271–279.

NEWMEYER, D., and C. W. TAYLOR, 1967 A pericentric inversion in Neurospora, with unstable duplication progeny. Genetics **56**: 771–791.

ORBACH, M. J., D. VOLLRATH, R. W. DAVIS and C. YANOFSKY, 1988 An electrophoretic karyotype of *Neurospora crassa*. Mol. Cell. Biol. **8**: 1469–1473.

PALL, M. L., 1970 Amino acid transport in *Neurospora crassa*. III. Acidic amino acid transport. Biochim. Biophys. Acta **211**: 513–520.

PASTEUR, L., 1862 L'influence de la température sur la fécundité des spores de Mucédinées. Compt. Rend. Acad. Sci. **52**: 16–19.

PAYEN, A. (rapporteur), 1843 Extrait d'un rapport adressé à M. Le Maréchal Duc de Dalmatie, Ministre de la Guerre, Président du Conseil, sur une altération extraordinaire du pain de munition. Ann. Chim. Phys. 3e Ser. **9**: 5–21 (+ one plate).

PAYEN, A., 1848 Températures qui peuvent supporter les sporules de l'*Oidium aurantiacum* sans perdre leur faculté végétative. Compt. Rend. Acad. Sci. **27**: 4–5.

PAYEN, A., 1859 Untitled discussion following remarks of M. Milne Edwards rejecting spontaneous generation of animalcules. Compt. Rend. Acad. Sci. **48**: 29–30.

PERKINS, D. D., 1953 The detection of linkage in tetrad analysis. Genetics **38**: 187–197.

PERKINS, D. D., 1962 Crossing-over and interference in a multiply-marked chromosome arm of Neurospora. Genetics **47**: 1253–1274.

PERKINS, D. D., 1972 An insertional translocation in Neurospora that generates duplications heterozygous for mating type. Genetics **71**: 25–51.

PERKINS, D. D., 1974 The manifestation of chromosome rearrangements in unordered asci of Neurospora. Genetics **77**: 459–489.

PERKINS, D. D., 1975 The use of duplication-generating rearrangements for studying heterokaryon incompatibility genes in Neurospora. Genetics **80**: 87–105.

PERKINS, D. D., 1979 Neurospora as an object for cytogenetic research. Stadler Genet. Symp. **11**: 145–164.

PERKINS, D. D., 1988 Main features of vegetative incompatibility in Neurospora. Fungal Genet. Newsl. **35**: 44–46.

PERKINS, D. D., 1990 *Neurospora crassa* genetic maps, June 1989. Genet. Maps **5**: 3.9–3.18.

PERKINS, D. D., and E. G. BARRY, 1977 The cytogenetics of Neurospora. Adv. Genet. **19**: 133–285.

PERKINS, D. D., and B. C. TURNER, 1988 Neurospora from natural populations: toward the population biology of a haploid eukaryote. Exp. Mycol. **12**: 91–131.

PERKINS, D. D., B. C. TURNER and E. G. BARRY, 1976 Strains of Neurospora collected from nature. Evolution **30**: 281–313.

PERKINS, D. D., D. NEWMEYER, C. W. TAYLOR and D. C. BENNETT, 1969 New markers and map sequences in *Neurospora crassa*, with a description of mapping by duplication coverage and of multiple translocation stocks for testing linkage. Genetica **40**: 247–278.

PERKINS, D. D., A. RADFORD, D. NEWMEYER and M. BJÖRKMAN, 1982 Chromosomal loci of *Neurospora crassa*. Microbiol. Rev. **46**: 426–570.

PERKINS, D. D., N. B. RAJU, V. C. POLLARD, J. L. CAMPBELL and A. M. RICHMAN, 1986 Use of Neurospora Spore killer strains to obtain centromere linkage data without dissecting asci. Can. J. Genet. Cytol. **28**: 971–981.

PITTENDRIGH, C. S., V. G. BRUCE, N. S. ROSENSWEIG and M. L. RUBIN, 1959 A biological clock in Neurospora. Nature **184**: 169–170.

PRINGSHEIM, H., 1909 Studien über den Gehalt verschiedener Pilzpresssäfte an Oxydasen. Hoppe-Seylor's Z. Physiol. Chem. **62**: 386–389.

RAJU, N. B., 1980 Meiosis and ascospore genesis in Neurospora. Eur. J. Cell Biol. **23:** 208–223.

RAJU, N. B., 1986 Postmeiotic mitoses without chromosome replication in a mutagen-sensitive Neurospora mutant. Exp. Mycol. **10:** 243–251.

RAJU, N. B., 1992a Functional heterothallism resulting from homokaryotic conidia and ascospores in *Neurospora tetrasperma*. Mycol. Res. **96:** (in press).

RAJU, N. B., 1992b Genetic control of the sexual cycle in Neurospora. Mycol. Res. **96:** (in press).

RAJU, N. B., D. D. PERKINS and D. NEWMEYER, 1987 Genetically determined nonselective abortion of entire asci in *Neurospora crassa*. Can. J. Bot. **65:** 1539–1549.

REICH, E., and D. J. L. LUCK, 1966 Replication and inheritance of mitochondrial DNA. Proc. Nat. Acad. Sci. USA **55:** 1600–1608.

REISSIG, J. L., A. S. ISSALY and I. M. ISSALY, 1967 Arginine-pyrimidine pathways in microorganisms. Natl. Cancer Inst. Monogr. **27:** 259–271.

RIECK, A., A. J. F. GRIFFITHS and H. BERTRAND, 1982 Mitochondrial variants of *Neurospora intermedia* from nature. Can. J. Genet. Cytol. **24:** 741–759.

ROBBINS, W. J., 1962 Bernard Ogilvie Dodge. Biogr. Mem. Natl. Acad. Sci. **36:** 85–124.

ROBERTS, A. N., and C. YANOFSKY, 1989 Genes expressed during conidiation in *Neurospora crassa*: characterization of *con-8*. Nucleic Acids Res. **17:** 197–214.

ROEPKE, R. R., R. L. LIBBY and M. H. SMALL, 1944 Mutation or variation of *E. coli* with respect to growth requirements. J. Bacteriol. **48:** 401–419.

RYAN, F. J., and J. LEDERBERG, 1946 Reverse-mutation and adaptation in leucineless Neurospora. Proc. Natl. Acad. Sci. USA **32:** 163–173.

RYAN, F. J., and L. S. OLIVE, 1961 The importance of B. O. Dodge's work for the genetics of fungi. Bull. Torrey Bot. Club **88:** 118:120.

SANSOME, E. R., 1945 Heterokaryosis and the mating-type factors in Neurospora. Nature **156:** 47.

SARGENT, M. L., and W. R. BRIGGS, 1967 The effects of light on a circadian rhythm of conidiation in Neurospora. Plant Physiol. **42:** 1504–1510.

SCARBOROUGH, G. A., 1975 Isolation and characterization of *Neurospora crassa* plasma membranes. J. Biol. Chem. **250:** 1106–1111.

SCARBOROUGH, G. A., 1978 The Neurospora plasma membrane: a new experimental system for investigating eukaryote surface membrane structure and function. Methods Cell Biol. **20:** 117–133.

SCHECHTMAN, M. G., 1987 Isolation of telomere DNA from *Neurospora crassa*. Mol. Cell. Biol. **7:** 3168–3177.

SCHECHTMAN, M. G., 1990 Characterization of telomere DNA from *Neurospora crassa*. Gene **88:** 159–165.

SCHLEYER, M., and W. NEUPERT, 1985 Transport of proteins into mitochondria: translocational intermediates spanning contact sites between outer and inner membranes. Cell **43:** 339–350.

SCHROEDER, A. L., 1986 Chromosome instability in mutagen sensitive mutants of Neurospora. Curr. Genet. **10:** 381–387.

SELITRENNIKOFF, C. P., B. L. LILLEY and R. ZUCKER, 1981 Formation and regeneration of protoplasts derived from a temperature-sensitive osmotic strain of *Neurospora crassa*. Exp. Mycol. **5:** 155–161.

SELKER, E. U., 1990 Premeiotic instability of repeated sequences in *Neurospora crassa*. Annu. Rev. Genet. **24:** 579–613.

SELKER, E. U., C. YANOFSKY, K. DRIFTMIER, R. L. METZENBERG, B. ALZNER-DEWEERD and U. L. RAJBHANDARY, 1981 Dispersed 5S RNA genes in *N. crassa*: structure, expression and evolution. Cell **24:** 819–828.

SELKER, E. U., E. B. CAMBARERI, B. C. JENSEN and K. R. HAACK,

1987 Rearrangement of duplicated DNA in specialized cells of Neurospora. Cell **51:** 741–752.

SEN, K., P. NANDI and A. K. MISHRA, 1969 Transformation of nutritionally deficient mutants of *Aspergillus niger*. J. Gen. Microbiol **55:** 195–200.

SHAW, D. E., and D. F. ROBERTSON, 1980 Collection of Neurospora by honeybees. Trans. Br. Mycol. Soc. **74:** 459–464.

SHEAR, C. L., and B. O. DODGE, 1927 Life histories and heterothallism of the red bread-mold fungi of the *Monilia sitophila* group. J. Agric. Res. **34:** 1019–1042.

SHURTLEFF, W., and A. AOYAGI, 1979 Oncham or ontjam. Appendix H, pp. 205–214 in *The Book of Tempeh*, Professional Edition. Harper & Row, New York.

SLAYMAN, C. L., 1965 Electrical properties of *Neurospora crassa*: respiration and the intercellular potential. J. Gen. Physiol. **49:** 93–116.

SLAYMAN, C. L., 1970 Movement of ions and electrogenesis in microorganisms. Am. Zool. **10:** 377–392.

SLAYMAN, C. L., 1987 The plasma membrane ATPase of Neurospora: a protein-pumping electroenzyme. J. Bioenerg. Biomembr. **19:** 1–20.

SLAYMAN, C. L., and C. W. SLAYMAN, 1962 Measurement of membrane potentials in Neurospora. Science **136:** 876–877.

SLAYMAN, C. L., and C. W. SLAYMAN, 1974 Depolarization of the plasma membrane of Neurospora during active transport of glucose: evidence for a proton-dependent cotransport system. Proc. Natl. Acad. Sci. USA **71:** 1935–1939.

SPIETH, P. T., 1975 Population genetics of allozyme variation in *Neurospora intermedia*. Genetics **80:** 785–805.

SPRINGER, M. L., and C. YANOFSKY, 1989 A morphological and genetic analysis of conidiophore development in *Neurospora crassa*. Genes Dev. **3:** 559–571.

SRB, A. M., 1973 Beadle and Neurospora, some recollections. Neurospora Newsl. **20:** 8–9.

SRB, A. M., and N. H. HOROWITZ, 1944 The ornithine cycle in Neurospora and its genetic control. J. Biol. Chem. **154:** 129–139.

SRIVASTAVA, V., and A. L. SCHROEDER, 1989 Deoxyribonucleoside triphosphate pools in mutagen sensitive mutants of *Neurospora crassa*. Biochem. Biophys. Res. Commun. **162:** 583–590.

ST. LAWRENCE, P., 1959 Gene conversion at the *nic-2* locus of *Neurospora crassa* in crosses between strains with normal chromosomes and a strain carrying a translocation at the locus. Genetics **44:** 532.

STADLER, D. R., 1983 Repair and mutation following UV damage in heterokaryons of Neurospora. Mol. Gen. Genet. **190:** 227–232.

STADLER, D. R., and E. CRANE, 1979 Analysis of lethal events induced by ultraviolet in a heterokaryon of Neurospora. Mol. Gen. Genet. **171:** 59–68.

STADLER, D. R., and H. MACLEOD, 1984 A dose-rate effect in UV mutagenesis in Neurospora. Mutat. Res. **127:** 39–47.

STADLER, D. R., and R. MOYER, 1981 Induced repair of genetic damage in Neurospora. Genetics **98:** 763–774.

STOKES, J. L., J. W. FOSTER and C. R. WOODWARD, JR., 1943 Synthesis of pyridoxin by a "pyridoxinless" X-ray mutant of *Neurospora sitophila*. Arch. Biochem. **2:** 235–245.

STRICKLAND, W. N., 1960 A rapid method for obtaining unordered Neurospora tetrads. J. Gen. Microbiol. **22:** 583–588.

SUSKIND, S. R., C. YANOFSKY and D. M. BONNER, 1955 Allelic strains of Neurospora lacking tryptophan synthetase: a preliminary immunochemical characterization. Proc. Natl. Acad. Sci. USA **8:** 577–582.

TATUM, E. L., 1961 Contributions of Bernard O. Dodge to biochemical genetics. Bull. Torrey Bot. Club **88:** 115–118.

TATUM, E. L., R. W. BARRATT and V. M. CUTTER, 1949 Chemical

induction of colonial paramorphs in Neurospora and Syncephalastrum. Science **109**: 509–511.

TAYLOR, J. W., and D. O. NATVIG, 1989 Mitochondrial DNA and evolution of heterothallic and pseudohomothallic Neurospora species. Mycol. Res. **93**: 257–272.

TAYLOR, J. W., B. D. SMOLICH and G. MAY, 1986 Evolution and mitochondrial DNA in *Neurospora crassa*. Evolution **40**: 716–739.

TERENZI, H. F., M. M. FLAWIA and H. N. TORRES, 1974 A *Neurospora crassa* morphological mutant showing reduced adenylate cyclase activity. Biochem. Biophys. Res. Commun. **58**: 990–996.

TOKUGAWA, Y., and Y. EMOTO, 1924 Über einen Kurz nach der letzten feuersbrunst plötzlich entwickelten Schimmelpilz. Jpn. J. Bot. **2**: 175–88.

TURNER, B. C., and D. D. PERKINS, 1979 Spore killer, a chromosomal factor in Neurospora that kills meiotic products not containing it. Genetics **93**: 587–606.

TURNER, B. C., and D. D. PERKINS, 1991 Meiotic drive in Neurospora and other fungi. Am. Nat. **137**: 416–429.

VIEBROCK, A., A. PERZ and W. SEBALD, 1982 The imported preprotein of the proteolipid subunit of the mitochondrial ATP synthase from *Neurospora crassa*. Molecular cloning and sequencing of the mRNA. EMBO J. **1**: 565–571.

VOGEL, H. J., and D. M. BONNER, 1959 The use of mutants in the study of metabolism, pp. 1–32 in *Encyclopedia of Plant Physiology*, Vol. 2, edited by W. RUHLAND. Springer, Heidelberg.

VON BORSTEL, R. C., 1963 Carbondale yeast genetics conference. Microb. Genet. Bull. **19** (Suppl.): 1–21.

WEISS, R. L., 1973 Intracellular localization of ornithine and arginine pools in Neurospora. J. Biol. Chem. **248**: 5409–5413.

WENT, F. A. F. C., 1901a *Monilia sitophila* (Mont.) Sacc., ein technischer Pilz Javas. Zentralbl. Bakteriol. Abt. II, **7**: 544–550, 591–598.

WENT, F. A. F. C., 1901b Über den Einfluss der Nahrung auf die Enzymbildung durch *Monilia sitophila* (Mont.) Sacc. Jahrb. Wiss. Bot. **36**: 611–664.

WENT, F. A. F. C., 1904 Über den Einfluss des Lichtes auf die Entstehung des Carotins und auf die Zersetzung der Enzyme. Rec. Trav. Bot. Neerl. **1**: 106–119.

WHITEHOUSE, H. L. K., 1942 Crossing-over in Neurospora. New Phytol. **41**: 23–62.

WILLIAMS, L. G., S. A. BERNHARDT and R. H. DAVIS, 1971 Evidence for two discrete carbamyl phosphate pools in Neurospora. J. Biol. Chem. **246**: 973–978.

WILLIAMS, J. G. K., A. R. KUBELIK, J. A. RAFALSKI and S. V. TINGEY, 1991 Genetic analysis with RAPD markers, pp. 431–439 in *More Gene Manipulations in Fungi*, edited by J. W. BENNETT and L. L. LASURE. Academic Press, Orlando, Fla.

WILSON, C., 1986 FGSC culture preservation methods. Fungal Genet. Newsl. **33**: 47–48.

WILSON, J. F., L. GARNJOBST and E. L. TATUM, 1961 Heterokaryon incompatibility in *Neurospora crassa*-micro-injection studies. Am. J. Bot. **48**: 299–305.

WOODWARD, D. O., 1959 Enzyme complementation *in vitro* between adenylosuccinaseless mutants of *Neurospora crassa*. Proc. Natl. Acad. Sci. USA **45**: 846–850.

YANOFSKY, C., 1956 Gene interactions in enzyme synthesis, pp. 147–160 in *Enzymes: Units of Biological Structure and Function*, edited by O. H. GAEBLER. Academic Press, New York.

ZIMMERMAN, R., B. HENNIG and W. NEUPERT, 1981 Different transport pathways of individual precursor proteins in mitochondria. Eur. J. Biochem. **116**: 455–460.

Looking for the Homunculus in Drosophila

Alan Garen

Department of Molecular Biophysics and Biochemistry, Yale University, New Haven, Connecticut 06511

BY 1965 it was evident that the reductionist approach of molecular biology to complex biological phenomena was proving remarkably effective, at least as applied to bacteria and their viruses. The basic mechanisms underlying the genetic control of cellular processes seemed sufficiently well understood for JACQUES MONOD to proclaim that what is true for *Escherichia coli* is true for elephants. Such magisterial confidence in a future as yet uncharted was bolstered by the elegant simplicity and generality of the operon model of gene regulation and expression, derived mainly from studies of β-galactosidase synthesis in *E. coli*. Nevertheless, the obstacles facing anyone hoping to achieve a comparable understanding of developmental processes in higher organisms were daunting. I recall the humbling impact of viewing a time-lapse film on early Drosophila development. The kaleidoscopic cascade of coordinated changes in cell number, movement, morphology and function, compressed into a brief span of 24 hr, seemed beyond the scope of molecular dissection with techniques then available. What was needed as a first step into the field was a conceptual framework for transforming such enormous phenomenological complexity into experimentally manageable problems.

I can trace my beginnings as a developmental biologist back to the summer of 1965 when I had the good fortune of attending a lecture at Yale by ERNST HADORN, a pioneer in reestablishing the vital link between genetics and development that had been forged earlier by THOMAS HUNT MORGAN but surprisingly neglected afterward. Focusing on Drosophila, the geneticists' favorite eucaryotic organism, HADORN (and also DONALD POULSON at Yale and EDWARD LEWIS at Cal Tech) used mutants to identify several key genes involved in development and to characterize the mutant phenotypes. These early studies demonstrated the value of mutants as starting material for dissection of complex developmental processes, and provided insights into the developmental roles of individual genes which would serve as valuable guides for subsequent molecular studies.

In HADORN's lecture I learned about a basic aspect of Drosophila development, namely that early in embryogenesis two separate developmental pathways are established, one for larval structures and another for imaginal (adult) structures (HADORN 1965). The imaginal pathway involves an initial stage of cell proliferation during which separate populations of undifferentiated imaginal cells are generated within the imaginal discs; each disc subsequently differentiates during the pupal stage into a particular adult structure. HADORN and his students at the University of Zurich had succeeded in culturing undifferentiated imaginal cells *in vivo*, using the abdomens of adult flies as incubators, for extended periods spanning virtually an unlimited number of cell divisions. When the cultured imaginal cells were transplanted back into a larval host, the transplanted cells usually differentiated according to their original fate; for example, cultured wing disc cells differentiated into wing structures, similarly cultured eye disc cells differentiated into eye structures, and so forth. This result was a revelation for me: it provided a powerful simplifying concept of development by demonstrating a clear operational distinction between the programming of cells for specific developmental fates, called determination, and the expression of the program, called differentiation. Furthermore, imaginal cell determination was shown to be a stable heritable state, which was a puzzling finding because determination presumably has an epigenetic rather than a primary genetic basis. HADORN's seminal achievement in developing reliable and accessible methods for culturing and assaying specifically determined imaginal cells provided an opening for entering the field, and helped to define as a clear if distant goal the elucidation of the genetic and molecular basis of determination.

Given the sophisticated level of Drosophila genetics, in contrast to the limited options available at that time for molecular studies of complex biological systems, we chose as a first project to search for mutants affecting imaginal determination. One important class of such mutants was already known, namely the homeotic class which exhibits striking imaginal transformations, for example an antenna to leg transformation in *antennapedia* or a haltere to wing transformation in *bithorax*. The homeotic mutants, in common with most other Drosophila mutants that had been characterized, develop into viable and fertile adults, because mutants were generally identified by their morphological or behavioral abnormalities as adults. This was a serious limitation to the scope of classical genetic analysis in Drosophila, because many developmentally important genes, including those controlling imaginal determination, are likely to generate mutants which are predominantly if not exclusively lethals. Therefore, a screen for lethal mutants affecting imaginal development was initiated in 1967 with ALLEN SHEARN, who had just completed his doctoral thesis on Neurospora genetics in NORMAN HOROWITZ's laboratory. Designing such a screen required assumptions about the mutant phenotype, which we anticipated would be a late larval lethal. The assumptions were that larval development involves a separate and independent pathway from imaginal development and therefore would not be affected by defects of imaginal development; also, that at least some of the genes controlling the imaginal pathway are specific for that pathway. Focusing first on zygotic-effect mutants which die as late third-instar larvae, we found that in about 50% of the mutants some or all of the imaginal discs were either missing or morphologically and developmentally defective, indicating that the assumptions were valid (SHEARN *et al.* 1971; SHEARN and GAREN 1974). It could be estimated that as many as 1000 zygotically active genes are specifically involved with the imaginal pathway, possibly including early steps of determination.

HADORN's studies with cultured imaginal cells had demonstrated that the cells were fully determined by the third-instar larval stage but did not provide information about earlier stages. To address that important point, HADORN and his students G. SCHUBIGER and M. SCHUBIGER-STAUB designed an elegant experiment which involved dissecting genetically marked 10-hr embryos to produce anterior and posterior halves, and then dissociating the embryonic cells to form cell suspensions. The dissociated cells from differently marked anterior and posterior halves were mixed together, cultured in adult hosts to allow the imaginal cells to reach maturity, and then tested for their developmental fates by transplantation into larval hosts. The results were clear and dramatic: anterior

head structures were formed only from cells of the anterior half and posterior genital structures were formed only from cells of the posterior half, showing that the imaginal cells are already autonomously determined as early as 10 hr after fertilization, although further processing is needed before the cells acquire the capacity to differentiate (SCHUBIGER, SCHUBIGER-STAUB and HADORN 1969). When HADORN's student WALTER GEHRING joined the laboratory as a postdoctoral fellow, we decided, together with graduate student LILLIAN LING-CHAN, to repeat HADORN's embryo culture experiment using younger embryos. The cellular blastoderm stage was chosen because it marks a major transition point in early development when the syncytial embryo becomes transformed into a multicellular embryo containing several thousand newly formed somatic cells arranged at fixed positions along the inner surface of the egg. During the syncytial blastoderm stage the nuclei are totipotent, because shifting their positions in the embryo results in a corresponding shift in their developmental fates. We expected the embryo culture experiment to provide equivalent information about the developmental potential of the blastoderm cells. The results obtained with cultured cellular blastoderm embryos were the same as those previously obtained with 10-hr embryos, showing that autonomous imaginal cell determination occurs concomitantly with blastoderm cell formation (CHAN and GEHRING 1971). Therefore, earlier stages of embryogenesis and oogenesis must have a key role in establishing the necessary positional information for determination.

Accordingly, we extended the genetic analysis of imaginal development to oogenesis, which traditionally had been neglected mainly for technical reasons because it would have involved an additional genetic cross using homozygous mutant females; the additional cross is not only labor-intensive but also requires homozygous mutant adults and therefore can only be performed with mutants that are not zygotic lethals. Nevertheless, encouraged by the possibility of identifying maternal-effect genes involved in providing positional information specifically for imaginal cell determination, THOMAS RICE, a graduate student, decided to focus his doctoral thesis on a large-scale screen for maternal-effect mutants involving such genes (RICE 1968). The screen was designed to detect a particular maternal-effect mutant phenotype which would exhibit apparently normal development until the cellular blastoderm stage, when imaginal determination occurs; defects of imaginal determination should result in late larval lethality or adult abnormalities as previously shown for zygotic-effect mutants. No mutant with that phenotype appeared in RICE's screen, nor in similar screens for maternal-effect mutants conducted by several other laboratories. It appears that the larval and imaginal pathways are initially interdependent, sharing maternally derived positional information, and that imaginal-specific functions are controlled entirely by zygotically active genes.

RICE's screen yielded 10 rare maternal-effect lethal mutants, representing eight complementation groups, which formed a morphologically normal syncytial blastoderm. In three of the groups blastoderm cell formation was either partially or totally blocked, probably because of a defect in cell membrane synthesis (RICE and GAREN 1975); the other five groups formed a morphologically normal cellular blastoderm but shortly afterward showed major abnormalities of gastrulation. Gastrulation-defective mutants have since been shown to involve genes controlling dorsal/ventral polarity in the embryo (ANDERSON and NÜSSLEIN-VOLHARD 1986). With the remarkable advances in elucidating the complex genetic control of early Drosophila development, it is becoming evident that maternal-effect genes have a key but limited role in providing positional information for imaginal development. Although the process of imaginal determination begins during oogenesis, it continues into the zygotic stage as zygotically active genes refine the rough maternal sketch for the imaginal homunculus. By the cellular blastoderm stage the individual imaginal cells have become autonomously determined entities, no longer dependent on positional cues in the embryo to pursue their developmental fates.

The phenotypes of RICE's mutants were sufficiently intriguing to attempt an identification of the products encoded by the maternal-effect genes. The strategy was to repair the mutant defect by injecting cytoplasm from normal eggs into the eggs produced by the homozygous mutant females, and then to apply this bioassay to fractions prepared from the normal cytoplasm in order to purify the active component. BRIGGS and CASSENS (1966) at the University of Indiana had already shown that the defect in a maternal-effect Axolotl mutant could be repaired in this way, although no purification experiments had been attempted. Since there was no precedent for an analogous experiment with Drosophila, I spent several months developing an injection technique suitable for the much smaller Drosophila egg. GEHRING and I tested the effectiveness of this technique with the maternal-effect lethal mutant *deep orange* (*dor*) which was chosen because, unlike RICE's mutants, the *dor* defect could be repaired by the zygotic activity of a paternal *dor*+ gene and therefore might respond similarly to injection of normal egg cytoplasm. The success of the *deep orange* tests (GAREN and GEHRING 1972) opened the way to similar tests with other mutants which were more relevant than *deep orange*

to the analysis of positional information in early development (ANDERSON and NÜSSLEIN-VOLHARD 1984).

The entire field of development would soon shift into high gear with the introduction of techniques for gene cloning and expression. Although we reported the cloning of the first Drosophila gene (LEPESANT, KEJZLAROVA-LEPESANT and GAREN 1978), our focus had changed by then and so the clone contained an ecdysone-inducible gene rather than a maternal-effect gene.

Early Drosophila development is now known to proceed via a highly complex network of coordinated interactions involving many maternally and zygotically expressed genes and their encoded products. A sophisticated understanding of the molecular bases of those interactions is rapidly emerging as a result of the brilliant contributions from several laboratories, notably those of NÜSSLEIN-VOLHARD, GEHRING, HOGNESS and their colleagues. The elusive homunculus is finally shaping up not as an object but rather as a dynamic process.

LITERATURE CITED

ANDERSON, K. V., and C. NÜSSLEIN-VOLHARD, 1984 Information for the dorsal-ventral pattern of the Drosophila embryo is stored as maternal mRNA. Nature **311:** 223–227.

ANDERSON, K. V., and C. NÜSSLEIN-VOLHARD, 1986 Dorsal-group genes of Drosophila, pp. 177–194 in *Gametogenesis and the Early Embryo*, edited by J. GALL. Alan R. Liss, New York.

BRIGGS, R., and G. CASSENS, 1966 Accumulation in the oocyte nucleus of a gene product essential for embryonic development beyond gastrulation. Proc. Natl. Acad. Sci. USA **55:** 1103–1109.

CHAN, L.-N., and W. GEHRING, 1971 Determination of blastoderm cells in *Drosophila melanogaster*. Proc. Natl. Acad. Sci. USA **68:** 2217–2221.

GAREN, A., and W. GEHRING, 1972 Repair of the lethal developmental defect in *deep orange* embryos of Drosophila by injection of normal egg cytoplasm. Proc. Natl. Acad. Sci. USA **69:** 2982–2985.

HADORN, E. , 1965 Problems of determination and transdetermination. Brookhaven Symp. Biol. **18:** 148–161.

LEPESANT, J-A., J. KEJZLAROVA-LEPESANT and A. GAREN, 1978 Ecdysone-inducible functions of larval fat bodies in Drosophila. Proc. Natl. Acad. Sci. USA **75:** 5570–5574.

RICE, T. B., 1973 Isolation and characterization of maternal-effect mutants: an approach to the study of early determination in *Drosophila melanogaster*. Ph.D. Thesis, Yale University.

RICE, T. B., and A. GAREN, 1975 Localized defects of blastoderm formation in maternal effect mutants of Drosophila. Dev. Biol. **43:** 277–286.

SCHUBIGER, G., M. SCHUBIGER-STAUB and E. HADORN, 1969 State of determination of imaginal blastemas in embryos of *Drosophila melanogaster* as revealed by mixing experiments. Wilhelm Roux' Arch. **163:** 33–39.

SHEARN, A., and A. GAREN, 1974 Genetic control of imaginal disc development in *Drosophila*. Proc. Natl. Acad. Sci. USA **71:** 1393–1397.

SHEARN, A., T. RICE, A. GAREN and W. GEHRING, 1971 Imaginal disc abnormalities in lethal mutants of *Drosophila*. Proc. Natl. Acad. Sci. USA **68:** 2594–2598.

June 1992

What Did Gregor Mendel Think He Discovered?

Daniel L. Hartl* and Vitezslav Orel†

*Department of Genetics, Washington University School of Medicine, St. Louis, Missouri 63110–1095;
and †Museum of the Mendelianum, Brno, Czechoslovakia

G REGOR MENDEL is accorded a special place in the history of genetics. His experiments, beautifully designed, were the first to focus on the numerical relationships among traits appearing in the progeny of hybrids; and his interpretation, clear and concise, was based on material hereditary elements that undergo segregation and independent assortment. Poignantly overshadowing the creative brilliance of MENDEL's work is the fact that it was virtually ignored for 34 years. Only after the dramatic rediscovery in 1900–16 years after MENDEL's death–was MENDEL rightfully recognized as the founder of genetics.

Mendelian mythmaking? This orthodox interpretation of MENDEL's contribution has recently been challenged as

. . . a myth created by the early geneticists to reinforce the belief that the laws of inheritance are obvious to anyone who looks closely enough at the problem (BOWLER 1989, p. 103).

This opinion reflects revisionist views of MENDEL and his intentions that have received considerable prominence in journals dealing with the history of science. The new perspectives come from several directions. One influential view is that MENDEL was not interested in heredity, as such, but in the role of hybrids in the generation of new species. This view of MENDEL's work

. . . strips it of inflated whiggish interpretations and places it squarely within the context of mid-nineteenth century biology (OLBY 1979, p. 53).

The iconoclastic conclusion is that if you define a Mendelian

. . . as one who subscribes explicitly to the existence of a finite number of hereditary elements which in the simplest case is two per hereditary trait, only one of which may enter a germ cell, then Mendel was clearly no Mendelian (OLBY 1979, p. 68).

A second view echoes the emphasis on MENDEL as hybridist

. . . concerned with the formation and development of hybrids . . . using empirical methods . . . [who did] not explain his results by employing invisible particulate determiners, paired or otherwise (MONAGHAN and CORCOS 1990, p. 268).

A third view imputes to MENDEL a dark motive in performing his experiments: that he had actually set out to prove that hybrids gave invariant progeny (essentially an antidarwinian rejection of descent with modification) and that his work with *Hieracium* was not undertaken to demonstrate agreement with his results with *Pisum* but rather to demonstrate the existence of constant (nonsegregating) hybrids (CALLENDER 1988). A fourth view goes well beyond the others in claiming that

[Mendel's monohybrid] experiments are fictitious in the sense that they have been carried out only on paper: the numerical data relative to them have been obtained by progressively disaggregating those from polyhybrid crosses. In other words, Mendel never carried out these experiments in the garden, but rather only on the pages of his notebooks (DI TROCCHIO 1991, p. 515).

We believe that it would be worthwhile to examine these claims in a forum accessible to geneticists. Most instructors in genetics, and most genetics textbooks, still put forth the orthodox interpretation of MENDEL's work. STERN and SHERWOOD (1966), in the foreword to their translation of MENDEL's *Versuche über Pflanzen-Hybriden*, point out that

. . . in the history of Mendelism the eternal is strongly confounded with the ephemeral. There is the neglect of Mendel's accomplishments during his lifetime and the futility of his years of writing to Nägeli. There is the uneven history of the rediscovery of his work 34 years after its publication and its striking reanalysis [by FISHER (1936)] another 36 years later.

Only time will tell whether the revisionist views of MENDEL's work are ephemeral, but if the orthodox interpretation of MENDEL's work is seriously flawed in any respect, then it ought to be adjusted.

Why the neglect? Although the main themes of this paper are paraphrases of FISHER's (1936) searching questions–What was MENDEL trying to discover? What did he discover? What did he think he discovered?–there are additional issues concerning MENDEL's work that warrant updating. First, why was the work neglected for so long? A comprehensive and thoughtful discussion of various categories of explanation is presented by SANDLER and SANDLER (1985). While granting a role to the relative inaccessibility of the *Verhandlungen des naturforschenden Vereines in Brünn (Brno)*, in which MENDEL's paper was published, to the overshadowing contemporary interest in organic evolution, and to the strangeness and novelty of MENDEL's experimental approach, SANDLER and SANDLER nevertheless conclude that MENDEL's paper was simply incomprehensible to his contemporaries since heredity and development were completely confounded conceptually in the latter half of the 19th century. The transmission of hereditary traits from parents to offspring was considered part of the same process as the development of traits in the offspring; heredity was but a moment in development with no need for a conceptual framework of its own. Hence, while

Mendel . . . defined his problem in purely genetic terms, and produced a correct and amazingly complete answer, [it was] to an as yet unformulated question! (SANDLER and SANDLER 1985, p. 69).

The all too goodness of fit: Another issue is the excessive goodness of fit of MENDEL's ratios (FISHER 1936; EDWARDS 1986). It is unfortunate that FISHER's

. . . painstaking analysis and his defense of Mendel's integrity have sometimes been incorrectly reported as having exposed a scientific fraud of major proportions . . . (EDWARDS 1986, p. 296).

The truth is that, while the data show a persistent lack of extreme segregations, as if there had been some trimming of highly deviant values (EDWARDS 1986), the bias toward expectation is slight (WRIGHT 1966). Considering the entirety of the evidence, EDWARDS (1986) agrees with DOBZHANSKY's conclusion:

Few experimenters are lucky enough to have no mistakes or accidents happen in any of their experiments, and it is only common sense to have such failures discarded. The evident danger is ascribing to mistakes and expunging from the record perfectly authentic experimental results which do not fit one's expectations. Not having been familiar with chi-squares and other statistical tests, Mendel may have, in perfect conscience, thrown out some crosses which he suspected to involve pollen contamination or other accident (DOBZHANSKY 1967, p. 1589).

More recently, MENDEL has also been accused of a more subtle kind of deception (DI TROCCHIO 1991). From his analysis of the *Versuche*, DI TROCCHIO supposes that MENDEL did not actually do the crosses he reported. What he actually did, according to this reconstruction, was to carry out no fewer than 484 crosses representing all pairwise reciprocal combinations of the 22 varieties of *Pisum* that MENDEL had available. Most of these crosses would have shown either no segregation or segregation for several traits. Among the latter, MENDEL pooled the marginal totals and reported them as monohybrid segregations. Even if MENDEL followed this procedure, the marginal totals were obtained in real crosses and could hardly be regarded as "fictitious." Furthermore, it is hard to believe that MENDEL actually followed this procedure without saying so, since he roundly criticized GÄRTNER for not describing his experiments in sufficient detail to allow MENDEL to repeat them:

The results which Gärtner obtained in his experiments are known to me; I have repeated his work and have reexamined it carefully to find, if possible, an agreement with those laws of development which I found to be true for my experimental plant. However, try as I would, I was unable to follow his experiments completely, not in a single case! It is very regrettable that this worthy man did not publish a detailed description of his individual experiments . . . However, in most cases, it can at least be recognized that the possibility of an agreement with *Pisum* is not excluded (letter to NÄGELI, December 31, 1866, p. 57). [In the present account, all citations to MENDEL's writings refer to the page numbers in STERN and SHERWOOD (1966).]

MENDEL as a hybridist: In considering MENDEL's contributions, the greatest weight must be placed on his own writing on hybridization, which is unfortunately limited to two papers (1866 and 1870) and 10 letters to CARL NÄGELI (1866–1873). The principal source of information is the *Versuche* (1966), which was the text of MENDEL's public lectures of February 8 and March 8, 1865, to fellow members of the Brno Natural History Society. In MENDEL's letter of April 18, 1867, to NÄGELI, he says,

I made every effort to verify, with other plants, the result obtained with *Pisum* . . . I attempted to inspire some control experiments, and for that reason discussed the *Pisum* experiments at the meeting of the local society of naturalists. I encountered, as was to be expected, divided opinion . . . When, last year [1866] I was asked to publish my lecture in the proceedings of the society, I agreed to do so, after having re-examined my records for the various years of experimentation, and not having been able to find a source of error. The paper which was submitted to you is the unchanged reprint of the draft of the lecture mentioned; thus the brevity of the exposition, as is essential for a public lecture (p. 60).

Therefore, while the *Versuche* is written in remarkably

clear German (STERN and SHERWOOD 1966), the account is abbreviated and addressed to a general audience. We have no way of knowing what revisions MENDEL might have made had he foreseen that every word and phrase in the paper would still be parsed and analyzed more than 125 years afterward. For example, DI TROCCHIO (1991, p. 516) readily admits that his allegation that MENDEL's monohybrid experiments were "fictitious" is based almost exclusively on the occurrence of two "unexpected" words: *eintheilung* ("breaking up into several parts"), which appears in the third subheading of the *Versuche* (p. 5); and *wesentlich* ("essential, substantial"), which appears in the statement that "plants were used which differed in only one essential trait" (p. 17).

Did MENDEL have an agenda to disprove descent with modification that led to his choice of Hieracium, with its constant hybrids, for his later experiments (CALLENDER 1988)? The Darwinian theory was well known by the time of MENDEL's presentation. The German translation of *On the Origin of Species* was published in 1863, and the monastery copy has marginal notes in MENDEL's handwriting. In January, 1965, at the monthly meeting of the Brno Natural History Society, A. MAKOWSKY, one of MENDEL's friends, lectured on the theory of natural selection. MENDEL gave the next two lectures, and thus he could easily have focused on the evolutionary angle had he wished. However, the *Versuche* mentions evolution on only three occasions: on page 2 in the phrase "the evolutionary history of organic forms," on page 41 in the phrase "the evolutionary history of plants," and on page 47 where MENDEL cites GÄRTNER's view that "a species has fixed limits beyond which it cannot change" and says that this statement cannot be accepted unconditionally. Furthermore, a number of plant species other than *Hieracium* were chosen in making "every effort to verify, with other plants, the result obtained with *Pisum*" (MENDEL's letter to NÄGELI, April 18, 1867, p. 60). The reason MENDEL chose *Hieracium* is given in his 1870 paper:

This genus possesses such an extraordinary profusion of distinct forms that no other genus of plants can compare with it (p. 51).

MENDEL's overriding interest was

. . . the question whether and to what extent hybridization plays a part in the production of this wealth of forms (p. 51)

knowing full well that

. . . we may be led into erroneous conclusions if we take rules deduced from observation of certain other hybrids to be laws of hybridization, and try to apply them to *Heiracium* without further consideration (p. 52).

At the beginning of his *Pisum* experiments MENDEL was certainly aware of the Linnean concept of constant hybrids and thought that they might be important exceptions to the laws deduced for *Pisum*. In the *Versuche* he remarked that there is

. . . an *essential difference* in those hybrids that remain constant in their progeny and propagate like pure strains (p. 41, emphasis his).

He also understood that

. . . this feature is of particular importance to the evolutionary history of plants, because constant hybrids attain the status of *new species* (p. 41, emphasis his).

On the other hand, he had

. . . proved experimentally that in *Pisum* hybrids form *different kinds* of germinal and pollen cells and that this is the reason for the variability of their offspring (p. 41, emphasis his).

Far from providing the constant hybrids that MENDEL was allegedly seeking, the experiments with *Hieracium*, as recounted in the letters to NÄGELI, were one long chronicle of failure and frustration.

On the other hand, there is no disputing that MENDEL was in the tradition of the plant hybridists, like KÖLREUTER and GÄRTNER, whose work, among that of others, he cites in the *Versuche*. The question is whether he was so engrossed in this tradition that the process of heredity itself was either unrecognized or of little interest (OLBY 1979; MONAGHAN and CORCOS 1990). OLBY (1979, p. 67) claims that

Mendel's overriding concern was with the role of hybrids in the genesis of new species . . . The laws of inheritance were only of concern to him in so far as they bore on his analysis of the evolutionary role of hybrids.

It is certainly true that MENDEL's main interest was in hybrids. The answer to the question "What was MENDEL trying to discover?" is clearly given in the introductory remarks in the *Versuche*, in which MENDEL describes the experimental program necessary to discover a

. . . generally applicable law of the formation and development of hybrids (p. 2)

which he considered as a law whose

. . . significance for the evolutionary history of organic forms must not be underestimated (p. 2).

On the other hand, in the very first sentence of the *Versuche*, MENDEL explains that the experiments were based on

. . . artificial fertilization undertaken on ornamental plants to obtain new color variants (p. 1),

which seems also to imply a significant interest in heredity for its role in practical breeding. MENDEL also had little concern for the systematic status of his pea plants. He remarks that, in the opinion of experts, most of the plants belong to the species *Pisum sativum*, but

> ... the rank assigned to them in a classification system is completely immaterial to the experiments in question (p. 5).

One will never know exactly what MENDEL was thinking, but one might reasonably have expected a less cavalier attitude toward species classification on the part of an author whose primary concern was the role of hybridization in the formation of new species. (MENDEL was not alone in regarding the distinction between species and varieties as purely arbitrary. The view was common among 19th century biologists, including DARWIN, and almost universal among the botanists. It was to cause MENDEL great trouble after 1866 when he began making hybrids between what would now be regarded as distinct species. We are indebted to ERNST MAYR for pointing this out in a letter of December 17, 1991, to DLH.)

The Moravian connection: If, as SANDLER and SANDLER (1985) point out, there was no clear conceptual distinction between heredity and development, then how could MENDEL have been interested in heredity for its own sake? Even before MENDEL's time, there had been great interest in Moravia in the practical breeding of sheep, fruit trees, and vines, partly through the leadership of the naturalist, C. C. ANDRÉ (1763–1831), who in 1806, through the patronage of COUNT SALM-REIFFERSCHEID (1776–1836), had organized in Brno the Royal and Imperial Moravian and Silesian Society for the Improvement of Agriculture, Natural Science and Knowledge of the Country (OREL and MATALOVÁ 1983). Many of the monks of the monastery of St. Thomas were active in this society, including MENDEL's predecessor as abbot, F. C. NAPP (1792–1867), and MENDEL himself. NAPP had organized the Brno Natural History Society as one of the sections in the larger organization until it become independent in 1861. If MENDEL had a mentor in Brno, it was NAPP: he had supported the teaching of agriculture in the context of natural science, and MENDEL attended these lectures in 1846; and he had MENDEL sent to the university in Vienna in 1851–1853 to study with, among others, the prominent plant physiologist F. UNGER and the physicist C. J. DOPPLER (of the DOPPLER effect). On the other hand, NAPP's role in shaping MENDEL's outlook and research agenda is uncertain. What is clear is that NAPP, motivated by issues in practical breeding, was interested in heredity as a problem in itself. In 1836 he attended a meeting of the Sheep Breeders Association and summarized the discussion of breeding methods by noting that the crucial questions were: What is inherited? How is it inherited? (OREL 1984). Later, in 1840, at a meeting of agriculturalists, NAPP defended hybridization as a method of obtaining new varieties of fruit trees and drew attention to the element of chance in

this process (OREL 1983). That MENDEL himself was interested in practical breeding can hardly be doubted, since he chose to memorialize these interests in ceiling paintings on the renovated monastery reception room as well as on his own tomb (MATALOVÁ 1983). MENDEL even ate the fruits of his pea breeding efforts:

> In 1859 I obtained a very fertile descendant with large, tasty, seeds from a first generation hybrid. Since, in the following year, its progeny retained the desirable characteristics and were uniform, the variety was cultivated in our vegetable garden, and many plants were raised every year up to 1865 (MENDEL letter of April 18, 1867 to NÄGELI, p. 61).

What did MENDEL discover? If MENDEL was trying to discover a "generally applicable law of the formation and development of hybrids," what did he actually discover? In the traditional view, MENDEL discovered that hereditary traits are determined by cellular elements, now called genes, that exist in pairs, undergo segregation and independent assortment, and persist unchanged through successive generations of hereditary transmission. A key passage in the *Versuche* that is relevant to this interpretation is as follows (p. 29ff):

> The difference of forms among the progeny of hybrids, as well as the ratios in which they are observed, find an adequate explanation in the principle [of segregation] just deduced. The simplest case is given by the series for *one pair of differing traits*. It is shown that this series is described by the expression: $A + Aa + a$, in which A and a signify the forms with constant differing traits, and Aa the form hybrid for both. The series contains four individuals in three different terms. In their production, pollen and germinal cells of form A and a participate, on the average, equally in fertilization; therefore each form manifests itself twice, since four individuals are produced. Participating in fertilization are thus:

> | Pollen cells | $A + A + a + a$ |
> | Germinal cells | $A + A + a + a$ |

> It is entirely a matter of chance which of the two kinds of pollen combines with each single germinal cell. However, according to the laws of probability, in an average of many cases it will always happen that every pollen form A and a will unite equally often with every germinal-cell form A and a; therefore, in fertilization, one of the two pollen cells A will meet a germinal cell A, the other a germinal cell a, and equally, one pollen cell a will become associated with a germinal cell A, and the other a.

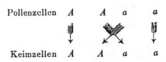

The result of fertilization can be visualized by writing the designations for associated germinal and pollen cells in the form of fractions, pollen cells above the line, germinal cells below. In the case under discussion one obtains

$$A/A + A/a + a/A + a/a$$

In the first and fourth terms germinal and pollen cells are alike; therefore the products of their association must be constant, namely A and a; in the second and third, however, a union of the two differing parental traits takes place again, therefore the forms arising from such fertilizations are absolutely identical with the hybrid from which they derive. *Thus, repeated hybridization takes place.* The striking phenomenon, that hybrids are able to produce, in addition to the two parental types, progeny that resemble themselves is thus explained. A/a and a/A both give the same association Aa, since, as mentioned earlier, it makes no difference to the consequence of fertilization which of the two traits belongs to the pollen and which to the germinal cell. Therefore

$$A/A + A/a + a/A + a/a = A + 2\,Aa + a$$

This represents the *average* course of self-fertilization of hybrids when two differing traits are associated in them. In individual flowers and individual plants, however, the ratio in which the members of the series are formed may be subject to not insignificant deviations.

In our opinion, this passage is strikingly perceptive and hardly betrays befuddlement or deep confusion as to whether the formative elements are paired in the plants and segregate in the reproductive cells. Although the passage does not use any of the words *gene, genotype, phenotype, homozygous, heterozygous,* or *segregation,* its meaning to modern geneticists is unmistakable. The only fault, which occurs on several occasions in the *Versuche,* is that the term *trait (Merkmal)* is used to mean either *phenotype* or *allele,* depending on the context, which indicates that the distinction may not always have been clear or entirely sharp in MENDEL's own mind.

Particulate inheritance: At this point it is necessary to discuss several issues bearing on the level of MENDEL's understanding of his own work (OLBY 1979; MEIJER 1983; MONAGHAN and CORCOS 1990; DI TROCCHIO 1991). One issue is whether MENDEL thought of his "potentially formative elements (*bildungsfähigen Elemente*)" (*Versuche,* p. 43) as particles rather than as fluids or emulsions (MEIJER 1983; MONAGHAN and CORCOS 1990). Nowhere in the *Versuche* is the physical nature of *die Elemente* discussed in enough detail to infer how MENDEL might have imagined them. On page 42, in the concluding remarks, MENDEL refers to "the material composition and arrangement of the elements . . . in the cell" ("*in der materiellen Beschaffenheit und Anordnung der Elemente . . . in der Zelle*"). This phrase would at least seem to imply that he was thinking in terms of some sort of material entities, but even this interpretation is disputed by KALMUS (1983), who dismisses it as "an afterthought" (p. 61) and argues instead that MENDEL must have been thinking of *die Elemente* in terms of nonmaterialistic scholastic metaphysics and invoking

the Aristotelian concept of the potential. But this opinion seems flatly contradicted by MENDEL's unselfconsciously materialistic statement that

. . . the distinguishing traits of two plants can, after all, be caused only by differences in the composition and grouping of the elements existing in dynamic interaction in their primordial cells (p. 43).

It does not matter whether MENDEL was thinking in terms or particles or fluids, since he emphasized repeatedly the key point that differing elements emerge unchanged from their association. For example, in the letter of April 18, 1867, to NÄGELI, MENDEL wrote,

The course of development consists simply in this; that in each generation the two parental traits appear, separated and unchanged, and there is nothing to indicate that one of them has either inherited or taken over anything from the other (p. 62).

(This passage also contains MENDEL's only known use of the term *inherited.*)

The use of *A* instead of *AA*: MENDEL routinely used the symbol A in genetic formulas in which a modern geneticist would use AA, and this notation has been interpreted as meaning that MENDEL did not believe that hereditary elements occur in pairs (OLBY 1979; MONAGHAN and CORCOS 1990). However, throughout most of the *Versuche,* MENDEL used the symbols A and a in a very different sense than used in modern genetics with reference to genes. In his usage, A refers to a plant that breeds true for the dominant trait, and similarly with a for the true-breeding recessive. Occasionally he used the same symbols to refer to the hereditary determinants, as in the quotation above from page 29ff, and in the context of this particular discussion it is quite clear that the expression

$$A/A + A/a + a/A + a/a = A + 2\,Aa + a$$

summarizes the expected genetic constitutions of the progeny on the left and gives their physical and breeding characteristics on the right. There are also other interpretations of MENDEL's symbolism, including that of MEIJER (1983), who argues that MENDEL's symbol A means "the potential for creating the dominant trait," and hence the use of AA for the homozygote would be redundant, since the two A's are logically equivalent. Lest we be too harsh in our anachronous criticism of MENDEL's somewhat inconsistent use of symbols, it is worthwhile to bear in mind that modern Drosophila geneticists routinely use unpaired symbols when referring to homozygous recessives; for example, in referring to Drosophila strains, the symbol al means the genotype al/al, and $cn\ bw$ means the genotype $cn\ bw/cn\ bw$.

Segregation in *AA* and *aa* genotypes: The segregation issue provides one of OLBY's (1979) principal arguments that Mendel was no Mendelian:

[Mendel] did not conceive of pairs of elements in the cell representing and determining the pairs of contrasted characters. If he had this conception he would have allowed a separation *between like members of such pairs as well as between unlike members* (OLBY 1979, p. 66, emphasis his).

The strongest evidence in the *Versuche* in support of OLBY's view is the following passage:

[The] differing elements [in hybrids] succeed in escaping from the enforced association only at the stage at which the reproductive cells develop. In the formation of these cells all elements present participate in completely free and uniform fashion, and only those that differ separate from each other (p. 43).

On the other hand, the context of this passage clearly refers to hybrids that produce variable progeny. MENDEL never specifically addresses the question whether segregation occurs in homozygous genotypes, and we have no way of knowing how he might have responded if queried directly about the matter. MENDEL's seeming indifference to segregation in homozygotes was entirely consistent with his primary interest in hybrids and the principle that the hereditary determinants emerge unchanged after their association together in hybrids. As ERNST MAYR has noted, "The homozygotes, not being hybrids, simply did not interest him" (personal communication to DLH, October 28, 1991). Also against OLBY's argument is MENDEL's formula

$$A/A + A/a + a/A + a/a = A + 2\,Aa + a$$

which clearly implies that the homozygous forms A and a each contain two hereditary determinants. In addition, MENDEL writes (p. 41),

. . . it seems permissible to assume that the germ cells of those [plants] that remain constant are identical, and also like the primordial cell of the hybrid.

The key question is whether the word *identical* (*gleichartig*) is intended to mean "identical in number" or "identical in type." We presume that MENDEL meant identical in both senses, otherwise some qualification would have been included, which would imply that the germ cells from homozygotes must contain only one of each of the paired determinants, since this is the case in "the primordial cell of the hybrid."

In a wider sense, whether or not segregation may be said to occur in homozygous genotypes is largely a matter of semantics. In the contemporary mind segregation is often confused with the process of chromosome separation during meiosis, but MENDEL knew nothing about chromosomes. Furthermore, in a precise technical sense, chromosomes undergo disjunction, not segregation. Segregation is a formal genetic phenomenon in which alleles are separated from one another and distributed into different germ cells (RIEGER, MICHAELIS and GREEN 1968; KING and STANS-

FIELD 1985). However, by definition, alleles must be different:

Allele . . . one of two or more alternate forms of a gene occupying the same locus on a particular chromosome . . . and differing from other alleles of that locus . . . . (RIEGER, MICHAELIS and GREEN 1968, p. 11);

Allele . . . one of a series of possible alternative forms of a given gene . . , differing in DNA sequence . . . . (KING and STANSFIELD 1985, p. 14).

Hence, MENDEL's view of segregation occurring only in the heterozygotes (*i.e.*, with different alleles) could easily be defended as being completely consistent even with the modern use of the term. Moreover, this usage provided MENDEL with the opportunity to summarize in the following way what he clearly regarded as his main result:

[Pea] hybrids form germinal and pollen cells that in their composition correspond in equal numbers to all the constant forms resulting from the traits united through fertilization (p. 29, emphasis his).

This summary is the subject of further discussion below.

The *Phaseolus* issue: In the *Versuche* MENDEL also commented on his results with flower color in *Phaseolus multiflorus*, in which the F_2 generation from an original cross of white × crimson consisted of a whole range of colors from purple to pale violet and white, in the ratio 30 colored to 1 white, instead of the expected 3:1. He then wrote,

But these puzzling phenomena, too, could probably be explained by the law valid for *Pisum* if one might assume that in *Ph. multiflorus* the color of flowers and seeds is composed of two or more totally independent colors that behave individually exactly like any other constant trait in the plant. With blossom color A composed of independent traits $A_1 + A_2 + . . .$, which produce the overall impression of crimson coloration, then, through fertilization with the differing trait of white color a, hybrid associations $A_1a + A_2a + . . .$ would have to be formed . . . (p. 35).

Hence, considering only A_1 and A_2, the

. . . terms of the [F_2 progeny] series can enter into 9 different combinations, each of which represents the designation for another color:

$1\ A_1\ A_2$	$2\ A_1a\ A_2$	$1\ A_2\ \ a$
$2\ A_1\ A_2a$	$4\ A_1a\ A_2a$	$2\ A_2a\ \ a$
$1\ A_1\ a$	$2\ A_1a\ \ a$	$1\ a\ \ a$

The numbers preceding the individual combinations indicate how many plants of corresponding coloration belong to the series (p 36).

OLBY (1979) discusses this example in some detail and wonders

. . . why [Mendel] made no apology for putting both A_1 and A_2 with the same contrasted character a . . . The chief reason for this obscurity was . . . that Mendel was thinking in terms of *the white colour* when he wrote down *a* . . . It may, of course, be objected that the way Mendel set out his *Phaseolus* series [the matrix above] shows that he was thinking of two gene loci for white, hence the genotype *a a* . . . [However, the layout of the table] makes clear the derivation of the classes of offspring from the multiplication of terms and no more (OLBY 1979, p. 60ff).

As is clear from OLBY's discussion, there is plenty of room for disagreement about MENDEL's intentions in summarizing the *Phaseolus* situation in this manner. Although MENDEL undoubtedly associated the symbol *a* with the color white, he also clearly stated that the two or more colors are "totally independent," that they "behave individually exactly like any other constant trait in the plant," and that "hybrid associations $A_1a + A_2a + \ldots$" would be formed by fertilization with germ cells from a white plant. These comments, and particularly the latter formula, clearly suggest that he had independent factors in mind, and that the *a* written as a partner for A_1 is different from the *a* written as a partner for A_2. MENDEL's matrix and the symbol *a a* makes perfect sense if he were using positional notation; otherwise, consistency would require the white plants to be symbolized simply as *a*.

At the risk of seeming whiggish, we will point out here that positional notation is commonly used in modern Drosophila genetics, although the wild-type alleles, rather than the mutant alleles, are designated with the single symbol, namely +. For example, to a modern Drosophila geneticist, the symbol $+ + +/y\,w\,f$ clearly means the triple heterozygote for *y*, *w*, and *f*, without any ambiguity, and $+ w +$ is the double recombinant chromosome with the wild-type alleles of *y* and *f*. We believe that it was this kind of positional notation that MENDEL had in mind when he wrote *a a* in his table of F_2 progeny in *Phaseolus*.

The Notizblatt argument: A good deal of discussion has centered on interpreting what appear to be genetic symbols in MENDEL's handwriting found on a document called the MENDEL Notizblatt (Figure 1), which bears the rough draft of a letter on the overleaf containing material that dates the letter (though possibly not the putative genetic symbols) to about 1875, or some seven years after MENDEL became abbot and two years after his last crossing experiments (RICHTER 1924). It is not at all clear what the symbols in the Notizblatt refer to: results from *Linaria*, *Phaseolus*, and *Pisum* have all been suggested (HEIMANS 1968). The *Pisum* suggestion comes from HEIMANS (1968) and is based on the observation that the number of individuals in the class *W* in the Notizblatt (166) agrees with the total for white seed coat color in the trifactorial cross in the *Versuche* (MENDEL, p. 21). The agreement could be coincidental, since the totals do not agree (601 progeny recorded in the Notizblatt *vs.* 639 in the trifactorial cross). Whatever the case, the

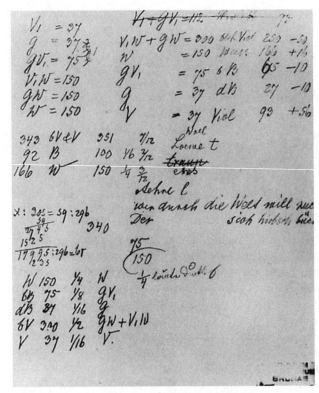

FIGURE 1.—The MENDEL Notizblatt, containing apparent genetic symbols in MENDEL's handwriting, dated to about 1875.

Notizblatt suggests that MENDEL was playing with the data, apparently trying various ways to group the phenotypes into classes, and he flirts briefly with a 7:3:2 ratio in the middle of the page (Figure 1). However, by the bottom of the page he has gotten to the ratio $1/4 : 1/8 : 1/16 : 1/2 : 1/16$, which is a perfectly respectable Mendelian ratio found among the 147 theoretically possible ratios in the F_2 progeny of a dihybrid cross (HARTL and MARUYAMA 1968).

It should also be noted that 7:2:3 is quite close to 9:3:4, which is one of the conventional examples of a modified 9:3:3:1. Nevertheless, much has been made of the 7:2:3 ratio, and OLBY (1979, p. 62) develops a model of what MENDEL might have been thinking when he wrote the markings and explains the model in a paragraph that OLBY imagines MENDEL might have written were this the model that MENDEL actually had in mind. However, MEIJER (1983) points out that OLBY's model does not really explain the 7:2:3 ratio anyway. These disagreements only serve to highlight the main problem with the Notizblatt: it is an unpublished page of markings pertaining to unknown traits in an unidentified organism written at an undetermined time and apparently of little importance to MENDEL himself since he used the page as scrap for drafting a letter about monastery business. Given these uncertainties, the Notizblatt is hardly the sort of thing to rely on in making inferences about MENDEL's understanding of his work in *Pisum*.

The issue of constant hybrids: In his argument

that MENDEL was an opponent of the fundamental principle of descent with modification, CALLENDER (1988) also puts great emphasis on MENDEL's discussion of "constant" hybrids as evidence that he did not regard his findings as generally applicable to other plant species. Indeed, in what CALLENDER (1988, p. 56) regards as MENDEL's "most important reference to constant hybrids," MENDEL wrote:

We encounter an *essential difference* in those hybrids that remain constant in their progeny and propagate like pure strains. According to Gärtner these include the *highly fertile* hybrids *Aquilegia atropurpurea-canadensis, Lavatera pseudolbia-thuringiaca, Geum urbano-rivale,* and some *Dianthus* hybrids . . . The correctness of these observations is vouched for by the eminent observers and cannot be doubted (p. 41).

However, later in the text of the *Versuche,* MENDEL also wrote:

Finally, the experiments performed by Kölreuter, Gärtner, and others on *transformation of one species into another by artificial fertilization* deserves special mention . . . Gärtner himself has carried out 30 experiments of this kind with plants from genera *Aquilegia, Dianthus, Geum, Lavatera, Lychnis, Malva, Nicotiana,* and *Oenothera* . . . If one may assume that the development of forms proceeded in these experiments in a manner similar to that for *Pisum,* then the entire process of transformation would have a rather simple explanation (p. 44).

It is important to emphasize that, in this passage, MENDEL pointedly and specifically includes all of the genera referred to earlier as containing constant hybrids as among those genera in which one may assume that the laws for *Pisum* hold.

While MENDEL may have been uncertain about the universal applicability of the laws for *Pisum,* particularly with regard to species with constant hybrids, he had already convinced himself that they were probably valid at least for all variable hybrids, since he asserted:

Whether variable hybrids of other plant species show complete agreement in behavior also remains to be decided experimentally; one might assume, however, that no basic difference could exist in important matters since *unity* in the plan of development of organic life is beyond doubt (p. 43, emphasis his).

What did MENDEL think he discovered? Whatever MENDEL thought he had discovered, he was certainly under the impression that it was important. In his letter of April 18, 1867, to NÄGELI he says,

I knew that the results I obtained were not easily compatible with our contemporary scientific knowledge, and that under the circumstances publication of one such isolated experiment was doubly dangerous; dangerous for the experimenter and for the cause he represented (p. 60).

In a paper containing as much data and interpretation as the *Versuche,* how should one decide what the author regarded as the main message? In our opinion, the key is found in the fact that the *Versuche* was written for oral presentation, and in an oral presentation the principal technique for emphasis is repetition. Thus, in order to discern what MENDEL regarded as the main message, one might examine the *Versuche* in order to identify any particular ideas or passages that are repeated. We have examined the document with this goal in mind, and have identified one idea that is expressed repeatedly in almost identical language. One version of the idea is as follows:

. . . *pea hybrids form germinal and pollen cells that in their composition correspond in equal numbers to all the constant forms resulting from the combination of traits united through fertilization* (p. 29, emphasis MENDEL's).

This statement, or close variants of it, is repeated no fewer than six times in the *Versuche,* on pages 24, 29, 32, twice on page 43, and 44. Furthermore, since MENDEL refers to this formulation as the "law of combination of differing traits according to which hybrid development proceeds" (p. 32), we may infer that he considered this statement as summarizing the "generally applicable law of the formation and development of hybrids" (p. 2), the elucidation of which he clearly regarded as his main goal of his experiments. That MENDEL regarded this law as widely applicable is supported by his statement that it

. . remains more than probable that a factor that so far has received little attention is involved in the variability of cultivated plants . . . [Our] cultivated plants, with few exceptions, are *members of different hybrid series* whose development along regular lines is altered and retarded by frequent intraspecific crosses (p. 37ff, emphasis his).

The context of this paragraph clearly points to segregation as "the factor that so far has received little attention."

MENDEL's own one-sentence summary of what he thought he discovered is remarkably general and concise. It contains both the laws of segregation and independent assortment in a form that is generally applicable to hybrids of any number of unlinked genes. Even a modern geneticist would be hard pressed to draft a sentence of comparable clarity without using terminology unavailable to MENDEL.

Conclusions: Our review of the issues and evidence regarding MENDEL as a Mendelian leads us to the following conclusions.

• MENDEL should certainly be regarded as a hybridist. He was in the hybridist tradition, and this is apparently how he regarded himself. However, his interest in hybridization did not blind him to the recognition of heredity as a process distinct from evolution. His outlook was conditioned by being in Brno, where there was a particular interest in the results of artificial fertilization for the improvement of sheep, fruit trees, and vines, in which colleagues of MENDEL, such as ABBOT NAPP, were leading participants, and conditioned also by MENDEL's own admitted interest in practical breeding as well as the coloration of ornamental flowers. On the other hand, MENDEL's hybridist tradition did result in his failure to emphasize the genetic composition of the constant (homozygous) forms, although the symbolism he used in the *Versuche*

$$A/A + A/a + a/A + a/a = A + 2\,Aa + a$$

implies to us that he was quite aware that the constant forms must contain paired hereditary determinants.

• Nowhere did MENDEL stipulate that the hereditary determinants are particulate, as opposed to fluid, vapor, colloid, gel, plasma, or whatever. He did, however, assume that they are material entities, rather than metaphysical "potentials," and asserted that the distinguishing traits of plants are caused only by differences in the composition and grouping of these hereditary elements.

• MENDEL clearly considered segregation as a phenomenon that characterizes the hybrids. On the other hand, the issue whether segregation of genes, as abstract entities, can be said to occur in homozygous genotypes is largely a matter of semantics and can be debated even today. For MENDEL, the clear cut segregation in heterozygotes carried the critical implication that the hereditary elements remain unchanged by their association together in heterozygous genotypes.

• The laws of inheritance for *Pisum* were regarded by MENDEL as quite generally applicable. He proposed explicitly that they would apply to all forms of variable (segregating) hybrids, and he also suggested that they might very well explain why genera that include constant (nonsegregating) hybrids can be transformed into new forms by means of artificial fertilization. According to MENDEL's own words, his studies of *Hieracium* and other species were undertaken in order to "verify, with other plants, the result obtained with *Pisum*" (MENDEL's letter to NÄGELI of April 18, 1867, p. 60).

• The key point of MENDEL's discovery is contained in a sentence that he repeated with minor variations no less than six times in the *Versuche:*

. . . pea hybrids form germinal and pollen cells that in their composition correspond in equal numbers to all the constant forms resulting from the combination of traits united through fertilization (p. 29, emphasis his).

This is the kind of "law of the formation and development of hybrids" (p. 2) that he had set out to discover, it is a remarkably concise statement of what he actually did discover, and it certainly represents the distillation of what he thought he discovered. We

conclude that MENDEL understood very clearly what his experiments meant for heredity. He deserves, not only the eponymic credit for Mendelism, but also the historical credit and a considerable measure of respect and admiration for his remarkable insights.

We are very grateful to ERNST MAYR for his advice, encouragement, and numerous helpful letters throughout the course of this study, and to MEL GREEN, ELENA LOZOVSKAYA, and DAN KRANE for their comments and suggestions.

LITERATURE CITED

BOWLER, P. J., 1989   *The Mendelian Revolution*. The Johns Hopkins University Press, Baltimore.

CALLENDER, L. A., 1988   Gregor Mendel: an opponent of descent with modification. Hist. Sci. **26:** 41–75.

DI TROCCHIO, F., 1991   Mendel's experiments: a reinterpretation. J. Hist. Biol. **24:** 485–519.

DOBZHANSKY, T., 1967   Looking back at Mendel's discovery. Science **156:** 1588–1589.

EDWARDS, A. W. F., 1986   Are Mendel's results really too close? Biol. Rev. **61:** 295–312.

FISHER, R. A., 1936   Has Mendel's work been rediscovered? Ann. Sci. **1:** 115–137.

HARTL, D. L., and T. MARUYAMA, 1968   Phenogram enumeration: the number of genotype-phenotype correspondences in genetic systems. J. Theor. Biol. **20:** 129–163.

HEIMANS, J., 1968   Ein Notizblatt aus dem Nachlass Gregor Mendel mit Analysen eines seiner Kreuzungsversuche. Folia Mendeliana **4:** 5–36.

KALMUS, H., 1983   The scholastic origins of Mendel's concepts. Hist. Sci. **21:** 61–83.

KING, R. C., and W. D. STANSFIELD, 1985   *A Dictionary of Genetics*. Oxford University Press, New York.

MATALOVÁ, A., 1983   Mendel's personality–still an enigma? pp. 299–308 in *Gregor Mendel and the Foundation of Genetics*, edited by V. OREL and A. MATALOVÁ. Mendelianum of the Moravian Museum, Brno, Czechoslovakia.

MEIJER, O. G., 1983   The essence of Mendel's discovery, pp. 123–172 in *Gregor Mendel and the Foundation of Genetics*, edited by V. OREL and A. MATALOVÁ. Mendelianum of the Moravian Museum, Brno, Czechoslovakia.

MONAGHAN, F. V., and A. F. CORCOS, 1990   The real objective of Mendel's paper. Biol. Philos. **5:** 267–292.

OLBY, R., 1979   Mendel, no Mendelian? Hist. Sci. **17:** 53–72.

OREL, V., 1983   Mendel's achievements in the context of the cultural pecularities of Moravia, pp. 23–46 in *Gregor Mendel and the Foundation of Genetics*, edited by V. OREL and A. MATALOVÁ. Mendelianum of the Moravian Museum, Brno, Czechoslovakia.

OREL, V., 1984   *Mendel*. Oxford University Press, Oxford.

OREL, V., and A. MATALOVÁ (Editors), 1983   *Gregor Mendel and the Foundation of Genetics*. Mendelianum of the Moravian Museum, Brno, Czechoslovakia

RICHTER, O., 1924   Ein kleiner Beitrag zur Biographie P. Gregor Mendel. Festschrift der Technischen Hochschule in Brünn **7:** 130–139.

RIEGER, R., A. MICHAELIS and M. M. GREEN, 1968   *A Glossary of Genetics and Cytogenetics*. Springer-Verlag, New York.

SANDLER, I., and L. SANDLER, 1985   A conceptual ambiguity that contributed to the neglect of Mendel's paper. Hist. Philos. Life Sci. **7:** 3–70.

STERN, C., and E. R. SHERWOOD, 1966   *The Origin of Genetics: A Mendel Source Book*. W. H. Freeman, San Francisco.

WRIGHT, S., 1966   Mendel's ratios, pp. 173–175 in *The Origin of Genetics: A Mendel Source Book*, edited by C. STERN and E. R. SHERWOOD. W. H. Freeman, San Francisco.

Molecular Genetics
○ # under an Embryologist's Microscope ○
Jean Brachet, 1909–1988

René Thomas

Laboratoire de Génétique, Université libre de Bruxelles, Brussels, Belgium

JEAN BRACHET, son of the well known Belgian embryologist ALBERT BRACHET, was himself fundamentally an embryologist by training. He remained so his entire life. But he was an unusual embryologist of the day; from the beginning he was convinced that development, and other biological phenomena, would eventually be understood in chemical terms.

BRACHET's entire career illustrated this conviction. His major books and monographs began with *Embryologie Chimique* (1944 and in English translation 1950), continued with *Le Rôle des Acides Nucléiques dans la Vie de la Cellule et de l'Embryon* (1952), *Biochemical Cytology* (1957), *The Biological Role of Ribonucleic Acids* (1960), *Introduction à l'Embryologie Moléculaire* (1974), and *Introduction to Molecular Embryology* (1974), and culminated with his monumental *Molecular Cytology* (1985). These are not the titles of a vitalist.

His fundamental biological interest was embryonic development. He focused this interest experimentally on the role of nucleic acids in protein synthesis, and the partitioning of morphogenetic determination between nucleus and cytoplasm. He thereby approached development "from the bottom up." From today's perspective, 30 years after the messenger-RNA hypothesis and 50 years after his germinal paper (BRACHET 1942), JEAN BRACHET was "the father of RNA."

Let us try to imagine the dark ages before the Golden Age of Molecular Biology. BRACHET (1987) tried to help us: ". . . I had of course read and reread the few pages that books on biochemistry dedicated to nucleic acids. They all stated that there exist two types (which was true), thymus nucleic acid in animals and zymonucleic acid in plants. The first one (DNA) has a mysterious sugar, deoxyribose, and the second one (RNA) a classical pentose, ribose . . . A rash and

false generalization had led to the conclusion that DNA was an 'animal' nucleic acid and RNA was 'vegetal' nucleic acid. Early observations had led me to a quite different view. But could a young student, 22 years old, be iconoclastic to the point of breaking the dogma, accepted by all, that plant and animal nucleic acids are distinct? Before doing so, I had the wisdom to consult Joseph Needham, the 'pope' of chemical embryology. My hypothesis appeared so daring to him that he turned to his 'boss,' the Nobel Laureate Sir F. G. Hopkins. The wise advice of 'Hoppy' was: 'Tell that young man that he should not believe everything he sees written in books; they are full of errors. Let him do the experiments to check his hypothesis.'

"Which I did, at the marine station in Roscoff in Brittany, my exams passed! I took with me an apparatus to measure pentoses . . . in straw . . . which prompted ironic remarks from my French friends, Ephrussi, Lwoff, and Monod. Experiments rapidly showed I was on the right track: sea urchin eggs did contain large amounts of pentoses, mostly in the form of RNA.

"Back in Brussels, I rushed into the office of my master, Albert Dalcq, to tell him my nice tale. He listened to me placidly and told me that he would believe the presence of plant nucleic acid in sea urchin eggs only when I could show it under the microscope."

Some of the initial confusion about the nucleic acids persists in BRACHET's early papers. But in 1942 the fog lifts. In a long paper in French, BRACHET provides us with: (1) a method that permits clear distinction between DNA and RNA on histological sections; (2) by application of this method to a wide variety of tissues and organisms, proof that both RNA and DNA are constituents of animal cells, yeasts, and protists; (3) a clear description of the localization of RNA and

DNA within the cell; and (4) two clear suggestions of the respective roles of the two nucleic acids, thymonucleic acid (DNA) as the genetic material and pentosenucleic acid (RNA) as an essential actor in protein synthesis.

How did BRACHET reach this clarification? In his words (1987), "After several not very encouraging attempts, I found in 1939 a simple cytochemical technique for detecting RNA in cells. To my great joy, I found RNA, like DNA, to be a universal constituent of cells–bacterial, vegetal, and animal. The intracellular localization of these two types of nucleic acid is, however, quite different: whereas DNA is found in chromatin and chromosomes, RNA accumulates in cytoplasm and nucleoli. In addition, whereas the amount of DNA per nucleus remains constant in a particular species (allowing for its doubling when cells prepare for division), the amount of RNA varies considerably from one tissue to another; I saw a completely unexpected correlation between the quantity of RNA in a cell and its capacity to synthesize proteins. This led me to another iconoclastic proposition: proteins are not synthesized by proteolytic enzymes operating backwards, as was generally thought, but by an unknown mechanism implicating RNA. The same conclusion was arrived at simultaneously (1941) by T. Caspersson in Stockholm, who was using a completely different technique for the cytochemical detection of nucleic acids."

What was that "simple cytochemical technique"? At the time, RNAse was one of the few enzymes that had been purified and crystallized, by KUNITZ. A fortunate property of RNAse was its heat stability, in contrast to most other enzymes. Thus, by heating to 100°, a crude "ferment" could be converted into an RNAse preparation presumed to be uncontaminated by other activities. "This specificity, together with the ease with which one isolates ferment in its active state thanks to its thermostability, suggested a simple way to detect pentosenucleic acid on slides: it would suffice to stain two cuts of the same organ with the UNNA mixture, one of them previously treated with the ferment" (BRACHET 1942).

The UNNA stain, a mixture of the red pigment pyronin and methyl green, was a happy choice: staining by pyronin is sensitive to RNAse, while that by methyl green coincides with that by the Feulgen reagent and is directed toward DNA. This permitted BRACHET to classify structures as containing RNA alone (red, sensitive to boiled ferment), DNA alone (green, insensitive to boiled ferment), or both (blue, converted to green by boiled ferment). The paper carefully validated the relationship between pyronin staining and chemically measured pentoses.

How did BRACHET convert his chemical determination into functional cellular information? Applying his simple method to a number of tissues and organisms, from yeasts to protists to vertebrates, he described the following pattern: the cytoplasm contains granules, then called "microsomes" (CLAUDE), whose basophilicity is due to RNA by the above criteria. Microsomes were later shown to be fragments of endoplasmic reticulum carrying ribosomes. The nuclear sap is not stained, but chromosomes are commonly stained blue, becoming pure green after RNAse treatment. These fundamental principles of the cellular deployment of the two nucleic acids were pursued in more cytological detail in this study. The RNA content of untreated chromosomes was quantitated as about 10% of the amount of DNA. In the giant chromosomes of Chironomus, BRACHET clearly distinguished euchromatin (bands staining green) from heterochromatin (which contains RNA in addition). The nucleoli were shown to contain RNA by BRACHET's criteria.

The central points distilled by BRACHET in his 1942 paper were that DNA is clearly localized in the chromosomes, and more specifically in the bands; and that the abundance of RNA in the cytoplasm is strongly correlated with the rate of protein synthesis. All the elements were in place for the so-called "central dogma" that DNA makes RNA which makes protein. What was lacking, 20 years before the messenger-RNA hypothesis, was a clear recognition of what is now known as genetic information, stored in one macromolecule and transferred to another. [The very word "information" had not moved from common parlance into the technical language of biologists. Indeed, a paper was sent to *Nature* as a joke pointing out that every biologist was using three combinatorial words–transformation, transduction, and induction–but nobody was using the fourth combination–information–which could neatly replace the other three (EPHRUSSI *et al.* 1953).]

It was clear to BRACHET that the relationship between DNA, RNA and protein was not a simple chemical transformation of one into another. Rather, his cytological analysis made it apparent that DNA played a role in the synthesis of RNA which, once transferred to the cytoplasm, would play a role in the synthesis of proteins.

Note that as late as 1960, the only strong argument for the existence of an informational intermediate between DNA and protein was the cytological separation between nucleus and the RNA-rich microsomes. In interpreting the classic experiments of PARDEE, JACOB and MONOD (1959) and RILEY *et al.* (1960) on expression from a conjugationally transferred *lacZ* gene, RILEY and her colleagues wrote: "The assumption that the z gene acts directly as a template in the synthesis of β-galactosidase would of course perfectly account for the observations. This assumption appears unlikely, however, in the face of a growing body of evidence suggesting that the seat of protein synthesis, in many types of cells including bacteria, is not the nucleus but rather certain cytoplasmic constituents (ribosomes). We are therefore left to consider the only other alternative, namely that the transfer of information involves functionally unstable intermediates, and to ask which cell constituents might be likely candidates for such a function." Soon afterward, as we know, this intermediate was identified as messenger RNA, and it was assumed always to be unstable.

Here again, BRACHET entered with an unorthodox observation. Continuing to focus on the dialog between nucleus and cytoplasm, a classic theme in embryology, he, a Professor of Animal Morphology, chose to work on *Amoeba proteus* and on the giant unicellular alga Acetabularia, because each could easily be cut into two parts, one with and one without a nucleus. When starved, the anucleate portion of *A. proteus* steadily decreased in RNA content, consistent with the notion that RNA is synthesized in the nucleus. However, protein synthesis continued for several days in the anucleate portion, indicating that at least some messenger RNAs are stable. With Acetabularia, a remarkable species-specific morphological marker is the "cap." HAMMERLING (1953) had shown previously that anucleates of Acetabularia could develop a cap and, by nuclear graft experiments, had shown that the morphology of the cap is determined by the nucleus. GOLDSTEIN and PLAUT (1955) and BRACHET (1955) resolved the apparent paradox by demonstrating that RNA is synthesized in the nucleus and chased into the cytoplasm. The messenger is not always unstable.

In persuing the issue of the life span of eukaryotic messenger RNAs, it was natural to focus on mammalian erythrocytes and their reticulocyte precursors as natural anucleates. BRACHET's disciple CHANTRENNE with his young colleagues BURNY and MARBAIX (1965) explicitly showed that a messenger RNA species could be purified from rabbit reticulocytes and injected into Xenopus oocytes to direct the synthesis of rabbit globin chains (in collaboration with GURDON). This tour de force, one of the crucial experiments in molecular biology, illustrated the breadth of biological material with which the school of BRACHET pursued the fundamental issue of the dialog between nucleus and cytoplasm.

As BRACHET remarks (1987), "It can be seen that as early as 1942 we already knew the fundamental principles of the 'central dogma of molecular biology.' However, during the war, my colleague R. Jeener and I tried to demonstrate biochemically the hypothesis of intervention of RNA in protein synthesis. The results of our experiments went the right way, but it was impossible for us to obtain definitive proof be-cause we did not have the necessary tool, radioactive amino acids. Just after 1950, several American laboratories demonstrated that the integrity of RNA was indispensable for radioactive amino acids to be incorporated into nascent proteins. Reading these papers made me as happy as if they had been mine. However, no one understood at the time how an RNA molecule could direct the synthesis of a specific protein. The astounding developments of molecular biology in the 1960s gave clues to this enigma."

From a local viewpoint, BRACHET and his colleague JEENER created the Belgian school of molecular biology. The small group, initially including their very first students WIAME, CHANTRENNE and ERRERA, gradually grew into a powerful institute of molecular biology on a new site of the Université libre de Bruxelles in Rhode-St-Genese. This group exerted a strong influence on the remarkable group in Ghent (FIERS, SCHELL and VAN MONTAGU). Till his death BRACHET remained *le patron* to all his students, including myself. An impressive personality, he clearly affirmed his scientific and political opinions. But, as in his science, he was able to free himself from dogma. Like many European scientists who had resisted the Nazi oppression, he was not only leftist, but for some time a member of the Communist party. Soon after his only visit to the USSR, he abruptly resigned the party because he was urged to support LYSENKO.

BRACHET was a very generous boss, never subjugating gifted young colleagues. He typically gave students complete freedom, seasoned with an occasional sharp but useful warning. He remained extremely careful to list himself as author only on papers to which he had contributed with his own hands. Those are the hands with which the embryologist JEAN BRACHET, *le patron* to me, developed his youthful iconoclasm and became the father of RNA.

LITERATURE CITED

BRACHET, J., 1942 La localisation des acides pentosennucléiques dans les tissus animaux et les oeufs d'Amphibiens en voie de développement. Arch. Biol. **53:** 207–257.

BRACHET, J., 1944 *Embryologie Chimique.* Masson, Paris, and Desoer, Liège.

BRACHET, J., 1950 *Chemical Embryology.* Interscience, New York.

BRACHET, J., 1952 *Le Rôle des Acides Nucléiques dans la Vie de la Cellule et de l'Embryon.* Desoer, Liege, and Masson, Paris.

BRACHET, J., 1955 Recherches sur les interactions biochimiques entre le noyau et le cytoplasme chez les organismes unicellulaires. I. *Amoeba proteus.* Biochim. Biophys. Acta **18:** 247–268.

BRACHET, J., 1957 *Biochemical Cytology.* Academic Press, New York.

BRACHET, J., 1960 *The Biological Role of Ribonucleic Acids,* Elsevier, Amsterdam.

BRACHET, J., 1974 *Introduction à l'Embryologie Moléculaire.* Masson, Paris.

BRACHET, J., 1974 *Introduction to Molecular Embryology.* The English Universities Press Ltd., London.

BRACHET, J., 1985 *Molecular Cytology, Vol. I, The Cell Cycle.* Vol.

II, Cell Interactions. Academic Press, New York.

BRACHET, J., 1987   Exposé: Souvenirs sur les origines de la biologie moléculaire. Bull. Cl. Sci. Acad. R. Belg. (5E Ser.) **73:** 441–449.

BURNY, A., and G. MARBAIX, 1965   Isolement du RNA messager des réticulocytes de lapin. Biochim. Biophys. Acta **103:** 409–417.

CASPERSSON, T., 1941   Studien über den Eiweissumsatz der Zelle. Naturwissenschaften **29:** 33–43.

EPHRUSSI, B., U. LEOPOLD, J. D. WATSON and J. J. WEIGLE, 1953   Terminology in bacterial genetics. Nature **171:** 701.

GOLDSTEIN, L., and W. PLAUT, 1955   Direct evidence for nuclear synthesis of cytoplasmic ribose nucleic acid. Proc. Natl. Acad. Sci. USA **41:** 874–879.

HAMMERLING, J., 1953   Nucleo-cytoplasmic relationships in the development of Acetabularia. Int. Rev. Cytol. **2:** 475–498.

PARDEE, A. B., F. JACOB and J. MONOD, 1959   The genetic control and cytoplasmic expression of "inducibility" in the synthesis of a β-galactosidase by *E. coli.* J. Mol. Biol. **1:** 165–178.

RILEY, M., A. B. PARDEE, F. JACOB and J. MONOD, 1960   On the expression of a structural gene. J. Mol. Biol. **2:** 216–225.

Sixty Years Ago
The 1932 International Congress of Genetics

James F. Crow

Genetics Department, University of Wisconsin–Madison, Madison, Wisconsin 53706

THE Sixth International Congress of Genetics, in Ithaca, New York in August, 1932 must have been an exciting experience in those dreary, depression, dust-bowl years. Five hundred and sixty-two people came to Cornell from 35 countries, often at considerable financial sacrifice, for in those days participants paid their own expenses.

The Congress (JONES 1932) featured demonstrations of living organisms, charts, photographs, and hundreds of microscopes for viewing specimens, especially cytological. Exhibits included 15 groups of invertebrates, including aphids, echinoderms, mollusks and tunicates, many with living specimens. There were 15 vertebrate species and 35 genera of plants. In addition there were an equal number of vegetable crops, flowers and fruits. The description of the exhibits took about 250 pages in the volume of abstracts available at the start of the Congress. The sheer magnitude and variety must have been overwhelming. The living plant exhibits, extending over about a hectare, attracted the most attention. These involved careful planning, with many of the types grown experimentally the year before to determine planting time so that demonstrations would peak in August. This was done under the supervision of MARCUS RHOADES, who did much of the field work himself, and that same year received his Ph.D. from Cornell. (RHOADES recently died and will be the subject of an obituary in a forthcoming issue.) The most popular exhibit was a "living chromosome map" in which mutant maize plants were arranged in positions corresponding to the locations of the mutations on the linkage map (Figure 1). The Congress set aside ample time for seeing the exhibits, including all day Sunday for those who didn't want to see Niagara Falls. Like the currently popular poster sessions, these offered the opportunity for individual discussions. According to the Congress description, "Even a most retiring person will easily find an opportunity to approach a person demonstrating his exhibits, in order to ask a question or to start a discussion."

My reason for featuring this particular Congress, however, is not the exhibits, but the number of outstanding addresses that have had a lasting influence. The year 1932 was near the end of the golden era of classical genetics, the period when the tools were breeding experiments and the microscope and when the riddles of genetic transmission were largely solved. The advances of the previous 32 years had created the new science of genetics.

Before discussing the Sixth Congress, I'll briefly mention some other early ones. The First antedated the rediscovery of MENDEL's laws. The "International Conference on Hybridisation and on the Cross-Breeding of Varieties" was held in London on July 11–12, 1899 at the instigation of the Royal Horticultural Society. The Congress featured a talk by WILLIAM BATESON, soon to become one of MENDEL's earliest and strongest supporters. The Second "International Conference on Plant Breeding and Hybridization" occurred in 1902, in New York City. Four years later the Royal Horticultural Society again convened an "International Conference on Hybridisation and Plant Breeding" in London in 1906, and again BATESON was featured, this time as President. In his talk he urged that his new verbal construct *genetics* be adopted. Accordingly, the printed volume was entitled *Report of the Third International Conference on Genetics*. For the first time, animal experiments were included. The Fourth Congress of Genetics took place in Paris in 1911. The Fifth was scheduled for 1916, five years later, but World War I intervened, and it was not held until 1927, in Berlin. By then genetics and geneticists had grown; 903 members from 35 countries attended, and the *Proceedings* include 148 papers.

The Sixth Congress, the subject of this essay, was held on schedule five years later. The Seventh was

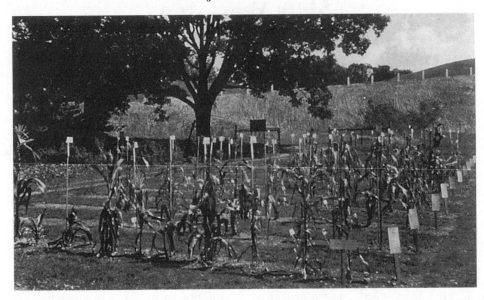

FIGURE 1.—A living chromosome map, with maize mutations planted in positions corresponding to their map locations. From COOK (1932).

planned for 1937 in Moscow, but was postponed a year by the National Academy of the USSR and was eventually held in Edinburgh in 1939. One month before the opening the Russian delegation withdrew and 50 papers were cancelled. On the second day of the Congress, British citizens living in Germany were advised to return home and several non-British delegations left. The Congress continued, however, with most of the members remaining. On September 1, the day after adjournment, fighting began on the Polish-German border. The *SS Athenia* with several geneticists aboard was torpedoed in the Atlantic. B. PRICE, C. W. COTTERMAN, W. LAWRENCE and W. R. SINGLETON survived but the F. W. TINNEYS of the University of Wisconsin perished.

To return to the 1932 Congress: the President was T. H. MORGAN (Figure 2). His attendance was greeted with great relief, for he had recently been in a severe automobile wreck and his friends feared that he would not recover in time. MORGAN's address dealt mainly with history, but he listed what he regarded as the five most important problems. They were: (1) "growth and duplication" of genes; (2) physical interpretation of synapsis and crossing over; (3) relation of genes to characters; (4) nature of the mutation process; (5) application to plant and animal breeding. This reflected the state of genetics at the time. Transmission genetics was essentially solved, and it was time to understand the gene and development in a more basic way. MORGAN had no way of knowing that the study of tiny organisms and enormous molecules would converge in the decades ahead.

One of the most exciting and influential addresses was delivered by H. J. MULLER. This was not long after his discovery of X-ray mutagenesis, and he exploited this tool to the fullest. He reviewed the induction of mutations and chromosome breakage by radiation, and among other things emphasized how the use of deletions enabled him to discern the difference between gain and loss of gene function. He introduced the now-standard vocabulary of amorphic, hypomorphic, hypermorphic, neomorphic and antimorphic mutations. MULLER also introduced the idea of dosage compensation and its elucidation by hypomorphic mutations. Although his preferred mechanism turned out to be wrong, the observation was remarkably astute and the generalizations from it to the meticulousness of evolution remarkably far-reaching. I have long enjoyed MULLER's reasoning from dosage compensation of *mutant* alleles to the conclusion, later abundantly confirmed, that *normal* alleles are not completely dominant. What a wealth of ingenuity of both concept and experimental trickery he displayed! Those who claim MULLER as *the* idea man of early genetics can find ample supporting evidence here.

A. H. STURTEVANT, with typical conciseness, discussed the possibility of using mosaics for elucidating developmental patterns. The newly discovered *claret* mutation in *Drosophila simulans*, which produced a high rate of nondisjunction in early cleavage, greatly facilitated this analysis. It was to be many years before the corresponding mutation was found in *Drosophila melanogaster*. The system was then exploited for fate mapping and neurogenetics, and SEYMOUR BENZER coined the eponymous unit *sturt*.

CURT STERN presented his famous experiment using translocations to demonstrate the physical reality of crossing over. His diagram from this Congress has been reproduced in one textbook after another. Essentially the same experiment had been done in maize by HARRIET CREIGHTON and BARBARA MC-

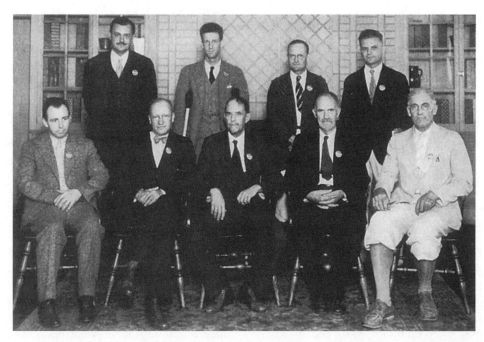

FIGURE 2.—The Executive Council. Front row: R. C. COOK, treasurer; E. M. EAST, program chairman; T. H. MORGAN, president; C. B. DAVENPORT, finances; R. A. EMERSON, local committee. Back row: C. C. LITTLE, secretary; L. C. DUNN, transportation; D. F. JONES, publications; M. DEMEREC, exhibits. From COOK (1932).

CLINTOCK, but was published elsewhere. At this Congress they went further and used doubly heteromorphic chromosomes to demonstrate four-strand crossing over. This was a subject of interest at the time because of BELLING's hypothesis of crossing over as a copying switch between newly replicated strands, which would not permit four-strand exchange. MC-CLINTOCK's name appears at many places in the proceedings. She gave a paper on nonhomologous chromosome associations. She also did the cytology for another important paper, that of L. J. STADLER. STADLER, deep and thoughtful as always, argued cogently that radiation produces mainly chromosome rearrangements and few, if any, "real" gene mutations.

In contrast, TIMOFÉEFF-RESSOVSKY discussed forward and backward mutations in great detail and believed that X-rays could indeed produce both. He ended his paper on a euphoric note: "We geneticists are in a very happy condition: our science is young, its 'development curve' is rising rapidly and the future will bring us the most interesting facts and views concerning the gene problem." Alas, this was one year before Hitler came to power and TIMOFÉEFF's life changed for the worse as he was caught up in both tragic dictatorships, Germany and USSR.

R. A. EMERSON gave a thorough review of maize genetics. All 10 linkage groups had by then been identified, some 100 mutations had been assigned to a group, and about 50 had been reasonably well mapped (Figure 1). The assignment of linkage groups to chromosomes was done mainly by MCCLINTOCK,

using trisomics. The trisomics, in turn, were obtained using GEORGE BEADLE's asynaptic gene, which produced abundant triploids from which all the primary trisomics were easily derived. EMERSON also described the variegated pericarp genes, now known to be the result of a transposable element. Later R. A. BRINK made this mutant the focus of his study, and variegated pericarp became a part of the MCCLINTOCK legend.

BEADLE was just deserting corn for Drosophila and was engaged in showing, through the use of attached-X chromosomes, that crossing over was a four-strand phenomenon and that chromatid interference was negligible. The genetical and cytological analysis of crossing over was an important subject at the time and several other papers were also devoted to it.

A. F. BLAKESLEE described a mountain of work on the jimsonweed, Datura. Cleverly starting with a doubled haploid, he systematically found all the primary trisomics and most of the possible secondaries (extra isochromosomes) and tertiaries (fusions of arms from different chromosomes). Each had a characteristic phenotype which, because the strain was isogenic to begin with, was caused solely by gene dosage effects. (I recall the euphoric but short-lasting belief shared with my late colleague KLAUS PÄTAU, after the discovery of the first human trisomic, that by analogy with Datura he would soon identify 22 more.) BLAKESLEE also used the trisomics to assign mutant genes to specific chromosome arms. All the Datura species had the same chromosome morphology and number, yet the hybrid meioses produced chromosome rings, showing that the chromosome arms had been extensively shuffled by translocations–a most convincing demonstration that translocations were an important part of the evolutionary process.

A high point of the 1932 Congress was the paper by N. I. VAVILOV, in which he reported extensive geographical studies of the wild relatives of cultivated plants. He described a series of polyploid potatoes in South America, wheat varieties in Abyssinia, and many others. In those premolecular days, he realized that one could compare noncrossable species by looking for homologous chromosome changes and genetic variants. He emphasized that the future of plant breeding must rely on wild varieties as sources of useful genetic variability and established foundation stocks in widely different latitudes in the USSR. Alas, VAVILOV's methods promised only hard work, more geographical expeditions, and slow (but certain) improvement of cultivated crops. In contrast LYSENKO's expansive promises based on his eccentric Lamarckian views caught Stalin's eye. It is ironic that, in his Congress paper, VAVILOV called attention to the "remarkable discovery" by LYSENKO of "simple physiological methods of shortening the period of growth, of transforming winter varieties into spring ones and late varieties into early ones by inducing processes of fermentation in the seeds before sowing them," thereby building up the man who would later be his ruination.[1] VAVILOV was the first of four speakers in a session on evolution. The other three were R. A. FISHER, J. B. S. HALDANE and SEWALL WRIGHT. This was one of the few times, if not the only one, that this triumvirate who founded the genetical theory of evolution appeared on the same platform. The session was organized by E. M. EAST, who asked each of the speakers to give a nonmathematical presentation. HALDANE asked, "Can evolution be explained in terms of known genetical facts?" He concluded that a great many facts can be explained qualitatively and quantitatively, and "while we cannot yet explain all evolutionary phenomena in terms of known genetical facts, the number of phenomena so explicable increases

every year, and there is no sign that the possibilities of explanation are reaching a limit." FISHER artfully noted that his title might well have been, in antiparallelism to HALDANE's, "Can genetical phenomena be explained in terms of known evolutionary causes?" and discussed the evolution of such genetic fundamentals as dominance and linkage. He accepted EAST's advice to suppress the mathematics and said, "As I am a mathematician by trade, perhaps I should explain that I shall use no mathematics, partly because I recognize that the first duty of a mathematician, rather like that of a lion tamer, is to keep his mathematics in their place." WRIGHT's paper has turned out to be the most influential of the three. This is partly because FISHER and HALDANE had both recently completed books that developed their ideas more completely, whereas WRIGHT had only written a paper that hardly anyone understood. His paper at the Congress was his first attempt to explain verbally the importance of population structure, random drift, and differential migration–what he later called the "shifting balance" theory of evolution, as controversial today as it was in 1932. WRIGHT spent much of the remainder of his long life restating the theory and arguing for it, but hardly changing it. My pleasure in writing this essay was enhanced by working with WRIGHT's well-worn copy of the *Proceedings* and inferring from his annotations on the abstracts which talks interested him most.

In addition to the plenary speakers, there were about 200 papers. T. S. PAINTER and MULLER reported a cytological map of Drosophila. This was made from metaphase chromosomes, salivary chromosomes having not yet been discovered, and showed a large variation in gene density in different chromosome regions. C. C. LITTLE, the founder of The Jackson Laboratory, argued against a highly publicized view that cancer in mice was a single recessive. DOBZHANSKY and STURTEVANT discussed variegated position effects produced by translocations. GEORGE SNELL, later to win a Nobel Prize for his work on histocompatibility, reported fertility reduction in irradiated mice, presumably the result of translocations. H. H. NEWMAN described 10 sets of identical twins who had been reared apart. D. F. JONES reported using two mutant genes to create a heterosexual strain of maize. (Some years later I explained the fundamentals of genetics to him, not knowing who he was. He was a quick study.) LILLIAN V. MORGAN described the properties of a ring chromosome, including the predicted absence of single exchanges. There were scores of papers using plants and animals other than Drosophila and maize. There was also a paper entitled "Genetical Engineering," meaning the application of genetic principles to animal and plant breeding. It is fascinating to see what kinds of problems were attracting attention in those days and what kinds of methods

---

[1] VAVILOV was named president of the 1939 Congress in Edinburgh. Shortly before the opening, he sent a letter noting that the Congress had been postponed for a year by the Academy of Sciences of the USSR so as to make better arrangements, and added, "The International Committee, however, postponed the Seventh International Congress of Genetics until 1939 and chose as its place of meeting not the USSR but another country. Under such circumstances Soviet geneticists and plant and animal breeders do not consider it possible to take part in the Congress." Nobody who knew VAVILOV thought this represented his true feelings. F. A. E. CREW was then chosen President and, with his usual grace, said, "I understand that in those places where films are made, every star has his shadow (technically known, I think, as a 'stand-in') who is required to look more or less like his principal and to take his place in the more arduous parts of his role. I would suggest to you that at the moment this is exactly what I am–a stand-in for a star. You invite me to play a part that VAVILOV would have so adorned. Around my unwilling shoulders you drape his robes, and if in them I seem to walk ungainly, you will not forget that this mantle was tailored for a bigger man" (PUNNETT 1939). Soon after, VAVILOV was arrested and died in prison.

were used. The variety of animal and plant species discussed was much greater than at a genetics meeting today.

What about the day-to-day aspects of this Congress? Remember that 1932 was the worst of the depression. Almost everybody was poor, and there were no grants to pay travel and living expenses. Nevertheless, 856 registered. The total expenses of the Congress were $17,583.58. For comparison, the 1988 Toronto Congress spent Can$1,396,701.16 (≈US$1,135,000) and 3702 attended.

The advance registration fee was $10 for full members and $6 for students. Those who couldn't afford the whole fee at one time could pay $5 down and the balance on arrival. Rooms in the residence halls at Cornell were $1.75 per day and rates in private rooming houses in the campus area ranged from $1.00 to $1.50. Those who traveled by car were told that "there are several very attractive camping places within thirty minutes' drive of Ithaca." Railroad fare from New York to Ithaca was $8.93 and attendees could get a round trip with various excursion privileges for 50% more. But the hard times took their toll; of 856 registered, only 562 were able to attend.

Despite great advances around the periphery, the central question of genetics–the nature of the gene, and how it replicates and mutates--was still elusive. In a review of the Congress, R. C. COOK (1932) said that "Oceans of words were spilled in formal and informal gatherings to discuss the vital question: 'What is the gene?' but that important entity is still elusive. Perhaps in 1937 the answer may be forthcoming." He was too optimistic; it would be two decades before WATSON and CRICK turned the trick.

Editors' Note: Regrettably the foldout group photograph and list of 389 of 562 registered participants of the Sixth International Congress of Genetics that appeared in the original essay could not be reproduced here. It can be found in GENETICS 131: 764–766.

LITERATURE CITED

COOK, R. C., 1932 The Genetics Congress. J. Hered. 23: 355–360.

JONES, D. F., ED., 1932 *Proceedings of the Sixth International Congress of Genetics. Vol. 1. Transactions and General Addresses. Vol 2. Condensed Articles and Descriptions of Exhibits.* Brooklyn Botanic Garden, Brooklyn, NY.

PUNNETT, R. C., ED. 1939 *Proceedings of the Seventh International Genetical Congress.* Cambridge University Press, Cambridge.

September 1992

On the Beginnings of Somatic Cell Hybridization
Boris Ephrussi and Chromosome Transplantation

Doris T. Zallen and Richard M. Burian

Center for the Study of Science in Society, Virginia Polytechnic Institute and State University, Blacksburg, Virginia 24061

TWO papers published in GENETICS in November, 1966 represent a key step in a decade of research in the laboratories of BORIS EPHRUSSI (1901–1979), research that helped transform mammalian genetics, especially human genetics. These papers, coauthored with MARY WEISS, then a graduate student in EPHRUSSI's laboratory at Western Reserve University in Cleveland (WEISS and EPHRUSSI 1966a,b), provided the first detailed reports of the formation of viable and self-perpetuating hybrids between somatic cells of two different species, mouse and rat (preliminary reports in EPHRUSSI and WEISS 1965; EPHRUSSI 1966). Such hybrids contributed crucially to the development of somatic cell genetics and soon provided an important tool for efforts to gain detailed information about the organization of genetic information in human chromosomes (WEISS and GREEN 1967).

Although the techniques described in these papers played an important role in the development of formal human genetics, this outcome was quite distant from EPHRUSSI's own scientific goals. His primary interest in constructing such "zoological oddities" as interspecific hybrids was to develop tools for analyzing the processes of determination, differentiation and regulation in development, including their bearing on oncogenesis. We will show that the work on interspecific hybrids was a natural culmination of investigations that occupied EPHRUSSI throughout his career and how the investigations described by WEISS and EPHRUSSI (1966a,b) grew out of the EPHRUSSI's lifelong effort to develop tools for understanding fundamental developmental processes (see BURIAN, GAYON and ZALLEN 1991; SAPP 1987, Chap. 5).

We will particularly emphasize EPHRUSSI's strategic use of methods involving variations on the theme of transplantation. Working with a great variety of organisms, he consistently found ways to explant, implant, or otherwise transfer organs, tissues, cells and nuclei into foreign organismal environments, combining these techniques with what he called "the genetical tool." He used the behavior of the transplant in the new context to test hypotheses about its regulation and control of its destiny, and about how it interacted with and was influenced by its host. In this respect, his work with somatic cell hybrids is best understood as a way of transplanting chromosomes, chromosome arms, or blocks of genes into a genetically and cytoplasmically foreign context. Although it fell short of the ideal of transplanting single genes, it was a natural extension of EPHRUSSI's approach and allowed him to gain insights (and develop tools for others to gain insights) into complexities of development that had eluded him ever since his early work with tissue culture and with sea urchin development as a young researcher in Paris in the 1920s.

Harnessing transplantation: From the start of his scientific training in France in 1920 as a Russian émigré, EPHRUSSI studied the initiation and regulation of embryological processes by intracellular and extracellular factors. A major strand of his early research concerned the effect of temperature on the development of fertilized sea urchin eggs (e.g., EPHRUSSI 1923, 1932). In this work he employed a relatively new apparatus, a micromanipulator. ROBERT CHAMBERS, an American biologist, had developed an accurate manipulator, enabling one to alter single cells by inserting (or extracting) small quantities of substances into (or from) them. In Paris in April, 1925, CHAMBERS personally instructed LOUIS RAPKINE, a fellow student and a close friend of EPHRUSSI's, in its use. RAPKINE, interested in chemical processes in the cell, employed the micromanipulator in a series of studies on cellular physiology during developmental change to probe the chemical state within individual cells. He and EPHRUSSI, working singly and together at the Collège de France and the Roscoff Marine Biological Station, studied chemical changes that occurred during the course of sea urchin development (e.g., EPHRUSSI and RAPKINE 1928). EPHRUSSI thus became familiar with the operation of the instrument and the opportunities it offered to track developmental changes by probing and altering internal and external cellular environments.

EPHRUSSI's second dissertation (two were then standard in France) was a project on tissue culture (EPHRUSSI 1933a; see also EPHRUSSI 1935a). Despite difficulties associated with the early unsatisfactory tissue culture techniques, EPHRUSSI concluded from this work and two explantation studies of brachyury in mice (EPHRUSSI 1933b, 1935b), that intrinsic factors (i.e., genes) play a key role in development.

Harnessing genetics: In the next phase of his career, EPHRUSSI coupled his embryological concerns to a firm conviction that one must understand the role of genes in order to decipher embryological processes. Supported by a Rockefeller Foundation fellowship, EPHRUSSI went to Caltech in 1934–1935 to learn genetics within the intellectual empire of T. H. MORGAN. While there, EPHRUSSI arranged a collaboration with GEORGE BEADLE, who joined him in Paris in the fall of 1935. They aimed at a genetic analysis of development, with BEADLE at first contributing genetic expertise and EPHRUSSI the insights and techniques of embryology. Their strategy was to subject *a single species* to both genetic and embryological attack. Since such traditional embryological organisms as sea urchins and frogs are ill-suited for standard genetic analysis, EPHRUSSI and BEADLE decided to apply experimental embryological techniques to a genetic organism *par excellence, Drosophila melanogaster* (HOROWITZ 1990, 1991). They were encouraged by STURTEVANT, who provided some leads from his work on flies mosaic for the *vermilion* mutation (STURTEVANT 1920, 1932). This work suggested that a diffusible substance, present in the wild type, could compensate for the absence of the wild-type product of the *vermilion* gene.

But could one do experimental embryology with Drosophila? Drosophila larvae seemed to be too small to permit use of the standard embryological technique of transplantation of parts of a developing embryo to learn about influences of location and of adjacent tissues on development. And difficulties in identifying imaginal disks added further complications. However, EPHRUSSI, aware of the implantation experiments of CASPARI, KÜHN, and PLAGGE on Ephestia (see CASPARI 1933; KÜHN, CASPARI and PLAGGE 1929, 1932) and thoroughly grounded in the use of the micromanipulator, was able to forge that instrument into a tool

that allowed implantation of imaginal disks into Drosophila larvae. As EPHRUSSI and BEADLE described the procedure they developed:

The essential part of the technique . . . is the actual operation of injection of the desired tissue by means of a micropipette. We have used the technique in implanting gonads and various imaginal disks . . . The assembly that we use is that of the standard Chambers micro-injection apparatus (EPHRUSSI and BEADLE 1936, pp. 218, 219, 221).

Striking results were obtained by implanting imaginal disks of various genotypes, fated to form eyes, into genetically foreign larvae. EPHRUSSI and BEADLE demonstrated that flies with wild-type alleles at the *vermilion* and *cinnabar* loci produced substances required in successive steps for the production of the brown eye pigment normally found in Drosophila. These and other results obtained by implanting various imaginal discs and organs, and injecting hemolymph, provided some insights into the pathways by which genes affect phenotypic characteristics by controlling the production of diffusible substances (see BURIAN, GAYON and ZALLEN 1988, pp. 389–400). Starting from this basis, BEADLE and TATUM, working with Neurospora and using more standard genetic approaches, were able to connect gene function with the production of specific enzymes as codified in their "one-gene:one-enzyme" hypothesis.

Yeast (and cytoplasmic) genetics: After World War II, EPHRUSSI, having spent most of the war as a refugee scientist at Johns Hopkins University, returned to France to reinstitute research aimed at disentangling the various influences, nuclear and cytoplasmic, on development. This time, EPHRUSSI eschewed the transplantation of cells and tissues between organisms, though he assigned his student PIOTR SLONIMSKI a thesis based on transplantation of sea urchin nuclei, an attempt that was unsuccessful (P. SLONIMSKI, personal communication). Given the failure of these efforts, he explained his choice of a new experimental organism as follows:

[W]hat is needed is direct genetic analysis of somatic cells, for the assumed functional equivalence of irreversibly differentiated somatic cells, however plausible, is only an hypothesis. Crosses between such cells being impossible, only nuclear transplantation from one somatic cell to another, or grafting of fragments of cytoplasm, could provide the required information; such experiments however will have to await the development of adequate technical devices. In the meantime, the closest approximation to the evidence we would like to have is provided by the study of lower forms which propagate by vegetative reproduction and possess no isolated germ line (EPHRUSSI 1953, p. 5; also in EPHRUSSI 1958, p. 37).

He selected the yeast *Saccharomyces cerevisiae* as a model system–that is, as a surrogate for his real concern with the development of distinct cell types with differing functions in higher organisms. He had the good fortune to stumble onto the ability of acriflavine to induce cytoplasmically inherited respiratory incompetence in yeast (EPHRUSSI 1949). The resultant "petite" mutation, so-called because of its small colony size, became a major object of study, playing a formative role in mitochondrial genetics (see BURIAN, GAYON and ZALLEN 1991; EPHRUSSI 1953 for an early review; SAPP 1987, Chap. 5). With this, EPHRUSSI managed to mimic the effects of transplantation, crossing wild-type with the respiration-deficient petite strains. This placed various nuclear genes in genetically distinct cytoplasms. Using such rearrangements of cellular parts with the full panoply of genetic and biochemical techniques, EPHRUSSI and his group at the Institut de Biologie Physicochimique (the Institut Rothschild in Paris), and later at the CNRS at Gif-sur-Yvette, studied the contribution of the cytoplasm to cell phenotype and pursued the interactions between nuclear and cytoplasmic genetic endowments needed to yield an intact, functioning (albeit single-celled) organism. Specifically, they were able to demonstrate the necessity of genetic information in cytoplasmic particles, ultimately identified as mitochondria, for the production of numerous enzymes in the respiratory chain.

The idea of transplantation was as fundamental to the yeast experiments as it was to the Drosophila program, though less obviously so. In yeast the effect of transplantation was accomplished not by surgically fusing different types of tissues, but by designing sexual crosses between yeasts whose cytoplasms exhibited genetic variation *independently* of the nucleus. Thus mating and budding, not micromanipulation, brought nuclei with defined constitutions into cytoplasmic environments with differing physiological and biochemical capabilities. And the micromanipulator still figured in some of the yeast experiments; it was used to isolate successively produced buds from individual yeast cells treated with acridine dyes to induce the petite phenotype. These bud analysis experiments demonstrated that the dyes act by increasing the rate of mutation to the petite phenotype rather than by altering selection (EPHRUSSI and HOTTINGUER 1950).

Somatic cell genetics[1]: EPHRUSSI's exploitation of the opportunities offered by the ability to "transplant" yeast nuclei between respiratory-competent and respiratory-incompetent cytoplasms did not permit him to get to the heart of his concerns about development. As he frequently pointed out (*e.g.*, EPHRUSSI 1970, pp. 19 *ff.*), there is an apparent conflict between the embryological concept of *the restriction of developmental potentiality in differentiation* and the genetic

concept of *the genotypic equivalence of virtually all cells of a metazoan.* He hoped to understand how differences in the determination of cells in various cell lineages (which he had long thought might be cytoplasmic in origin) are created, regulated, and perpetuated, and how overt differentiation is regulated and maintained. In 1971 he put the issue thusly:

> . . . if what Hershey (1970) calls the *unwritten* dogma is correct (*i.e.*, "the inference that *all* three-dimensional structure is encoded in nucleotide sequences"), the *establishment* of different epigenotypes [the restricted potentialities of determined cell lineages] in the course of development must be coded for [in] nuclear DNA . . . [But] whether the functional restriction of the total information, which results in different epigenotypes of different cell lineages, is due to a change in the chromosomes themselves . . . or is only a *reflection* of a change elsewhere in the cell (say in the cell membrane) is an entirely separate and largely unresolved question worthy of very serious consideration . . . In fact, this is *the* fundamental question to which I have no answer (EPHRUSSI 1972, p. 55).

So, during the 1950s, as the yeast work proceeded, EPHRUSSI sought a new system with which to study somatic cell differentiation. To this end he visited RENATO DULBECCO's laboratory in 1959–1960 to learn modern methods of handling cells in tissue culture. This choice was fortuitous since the new tool that fell into his hands for understanding somatic cell specialization depended on tissue culture.

The stimulus for this work came from a novel observation made by GEORGES BARSKI, SERGE SORIEUL and FRANCINE CORNEFERT at the Institut Gustave Roussy in Paris. BARSKI and his group were studying mouse cancer cell lines originally derived from a single mouse fibroblast cell (SANFORD, LIKELY and EARLE 1954). Two lines had evolved in tissue culture so as to display recognizably different phenotypes, chromosomal configurations, and tumor-producing abilities: the "high-cancer" line (N1) easily produced tumors, whereas the "low-cancer" line (N2) did so rather poorly. Hoping to find Pneumococcus-like transformation between the two lines, BARSKI, SORIEUL and CORNEFERT (1960, 1961) began a series of experiments on December 9, 1959, in which both cell types, N1 and N2, were grown together. After about 3 months of continuous cocultivation, they found an unexpected cell type, markedly different, growing vigorously in the mixed culture (BARSKI, SORIEUL and CORNEFERT 1960, 1961). The new cells appeared to be hybrids generated by a fusion between N1 and N2 cells, with the chromosomes contained in a single nucleus. The chromosome number was roughly the sum of those of N1 and N2 and the cells included chromosome types unique to each of the lines. With time in culture there was random loss of some chromosomes (about 10%), especially after pas-

---

[1] The work on somatic cell genetics during 1960–1970 in EPHRUSSI's laboratories has been usefully reviewed by EPHRUSSI (1970, 1972) and WEISS (1992).

sage into mice where the new cell type produced a high incidence of tumors.

Surprised by this result and unsure how to exploit it, BARSKI, who knew of EPHRUSSI's interests in tissue culture and somatic cell differentiation, turned to his colleague in Paris, explaining what he had found. EPHRUSSI was immediately fascinated with the opportunity presented by somatic cell hybridization. Should the phenomenon be reliably reproducible, it would provide a basis for genetic studies on differentiated cells that might shed light on the very questions that had driven his research for many years.

Many biologists, of course, had been hoping for just such a possibility. Among those who influenced EPHRUSSI were J. LEDERBERG and G. PONTECORVO. LEDERBERG, commenting partly on EPHRUSSI's views about determination and differentiation in a symposium on genetic approaches to somatic cell variation, explicitly argued that one should anticipate the mating of somatic cells followed by segregation of chromosomes since all of the "unit processes" required for such hybridization had been demonstrated separately on one system or another (LEDERBERG 1958, p. 384; see also LEDERBERG 1956, p. 663). PONTECORVO, partly in light of his experience with parasexuality in Aspergillus and other fungi, was a long-term advocate of the application of genetic analysis of mitotic recombination in somatic tissues of higher organisms (e.g., PONTECORVO and KÄFER 1958, p. 103; PONTECORVO 1961).

Working with SORIEUL in his own laboratory, EPHRUSSI started the search for somatic cell hybrids on January 3, 1961, only months after BARSKI's first report appeared. He set out to verify the original reports and, if possible, to convert the phenomenon into a genetic tool for probing the differentiated states of such cells. In a preliminary report, SORIEUL and EPHRUSSI (1961) wrote, "If this hope is justified hybridization may become a useful tool for the investigation of a number of problems of somatic cell genetics, of oncology and virology." In a number of subsequent publications, EPHRUSSI spelled out the characteristics which would allow these hybrids to meet his research needs. These included:

• Hybridization would have to occur often enough that cells of different genetic constitutions within a species–normal as well as neoplastic–could be readily "mated."

• It would have to be possible to detect and select the hybrid cells against the background of parental cell types.

• Hybrid cells would have to be stable and capable of persisting through many cycles of transfer in tissue culture.

• Genes contributed by both parental sets of chromosomes would have to be functional in the hybrid cells.

• Some form of "segregation," analogous to genetic exchange in microorganisms or recombination in sexual reproduction, would have to occur (perhaps via random chromosome loss or mitotic recombination) so that distinct gene combinations could be generated in different hybrid cells.

This last requirement is extremely important. It represents an extension of EPHRUSSI's transplantation methodology. By trapping different groups of chromosomes or chromosome segments in a single nucleus, somatic cell hybridization would mimic the transplantation of particular chromosomes or chromosome segments from one cell into another, allowing one to test the effects of their presence on cell functions and the regulatory controls altering the expression of their genes.

Over the next few years, while on prolonged leave at Western Reserve, EPHRUSSI developed his new research program. He and his group invested much effort to turn mouse somatic cell hybrids into a reliable system, running huge series of experiments on hybrid cells to establish control of the basic phenomena and the stability of appropriate markers. They proved that each of the desiderata listed above could be met, including, in particular, that segregation occurred through accidental loss of chromosomes during the cycles of mitoses that followed the original cell fusion events (EPHRUSSI and SORIEUL 1962a,b; EPHRUSSI et al. 1964).

But the system was still suboptimal. The selection of hybrids was a major problem. Unless hybrid cells enjoyed a significant growth advantage over the parental cells–which, in one frustrating case, was finally found to occur only at 28–29°, rather than the higher temperatures employed in tissue culture incubators (SCALETTA and EPHRUSSI 1965)–one could not find or isolate them. This problem limited the range of hybrid cells available for experiment. Also, the group had only karyological markers to work with, which made the protocols extremely laborious. Worse, since there were no distinctive chromosomes in most of the crosses they wanted to carry out, fusions between different parental cells were often indistinguishable from fusions between two similar cells.

The solution to this experimental dilemma came from another laboratory. JOHN LITTLEFIELD at Harvard developed the HAT system of the SZYBALSKIs (SZYBALSKI, SZYBALSKA and RAGNI 1962; SZYBALSKA and SZYBALSKI 1962) into a tool for selecting cell hybrids. When the de novo biosynthetic pathway for nucleotide precursors of DNA is blocked, the enzymes thymidine kinase (TK) and hypoxanthine-guanine phosphoribosyl transferase (HPRT) are required for production of pyrimidine and purine nucleotides, respectively, in the "salvage" pathway. LITTLEFIELD co-cultured two mutant lines of mouse cells in the SZY-BALSKIS' HAT medium, one TK⁻, the other HPRT⁻. This medium contains hypoxanthine (H, the substrate for HPRT), aminopterin (A, an inhibitor of *de novo* DNA synthesis) and thymidine (T, the substrate for TK). In these conditions, only cells simultaneously TK⁺ and HPRT⁺ (presumptive hybrids) are capable of utilizing thymidine *and* hypoxanthine to form DNA via the salvage pathway; all others die (LITTLEFIELD 1964). This system provided the means for selection, thus greatly expanding the search for mouse somatic cell hybrids. DAVIDSON and EPHRUSSI (1965) were able to adapt the LITTLEFIELD system to produce a "half-selective" system in which only one of the parent cells is HPRT⁻ or TK⁻. The other parent can come from any mouse cell line that displays contact inhibition in cell culture, including normal diploid cells. In this modification, the biochemical mutant cannot grow in the HAT medium and the normal cells will form a monolayer on the surface of the growth vessel. Hybrid cells can then be recognized by their ability to grow in clumps on top of the monolayer, from which they can be isolated and maintained in pure culture (DAV-IDSON and EPHRUSSI 1965).

EPHRUSSI and his co-workers applied the methods they had painstakingly developed during 4 years to address some larger questions about determination, differentiation, regulation of the cell cycle, and the onset and inheritance of neoplasticity. Some hints about regulatory phenomena began to emerge as they observed the gain and loss of particular antigens and enzyme bands in hybrids (*e.g.*, SPENCER *et al.* 1964; GREEN *et al.* 1966; DEFENDI *et al.* 1967) and other experiments were begun to test for dominance or recessiveness, or positive or negative regulation, of neoplasticity (*e.g.*, EPHRUSSI 1965; DEFENDI *et al.* 1967). The mouse hybrids with their "transplanted" chromosomes were beginning to yield interesting results, with the promise of more insights into the secrets of differentiation.

Interspecific cell hybrids: By his own account, EPHRUSSI was truly startled to learn from the *New York Times* (February 17, 1965) that HENRY HARRIS and J. F. WATKINS at Oxford had shown that inactivated Sendai virus could be used to facilitate the fusion of unlike cells, producing heterokaryons between human HeLa cells and mouse tumor cells (HARRIS and WAT-KINS 1965). The heterokaryons thus produced were not capable of division, although they manifested a few irregular mitoses and survived for up to 2 weeks. EPHRUSSI himself had earlier considered using viruses as agents to accomplish somatic cell fusion (see the speculations of EPHRUSSI and SORIEUL 1962a, p. 90), so the application of inactive virus to aid fusion was probably no surprise. But what galvanized him into

action was the use of fusion to cross species barriers. We have found no evidence that EPHRUSSI had considered creating interspecific hybrids in the four years he had devoted to somatic cell hybrids. The HARRIS and WATKINS report changed all that. As EPHRUSSI himself recollects: "[I]t was HARRIS and WATKINS' demonstration that cells of *different* species can be fused . . . that in 1965 led MARY WEISS and me to the isolation of the first viable interspecific hybrids" (EPHRUSSI 1972, p. 23, our emphasis). And the effect was immediate. According to WEISS:

[O]ne afternoon, rushing out to his airport-bound taxi, Ephrussi shouted to me, then a fledgling graduate student, "Order some rat fibroblasts from Microbiological Associates and set up a cross with (mouse) L cells." Within a few weeks we had the first viable proliferating interspecific hybrids (WEISS, 1992).

A brief report of this work (less than 600 words), which used the half-selection technique to detect hybrids between TK⁻ mouse L cells and explanted embryonic rat cells, was submitted on March 24, 1965 (EPHRUSSI and WEISS 1965). The interspecific hybrid cells, representing one cross, had been growing in culture for only about one month (about 25 cell divisions). The reports in GENETICS (WEISS and EPHRUSSI 1966a,b) were based on more substantial experience: seven different crosses between mouse and rat cells were studied and, in some cases, more than 200 division cycles had taken place. Careful karyotypic analysis confirmed beyond doubt that interspecific hybrids were formed. As with the intraspecific hybrids, there were some early chromosome losses (mainly rat chromosomes), with subsequent stabilization of the karyotype. Enzyme studies revealed that both rat and mouse enzymes–lactic dehydrogenase and β-glucuronidase–were produced in the hybrids, with mouse and rat subunits yielding hybrid molecules, providing a striking marker.

These papers dramatically changed the emerging field of somatic cell hybridization. As EPHRUSSI and many others quickly saw, the potential uses of the techniques of cell hybridization were enormously expanded. Somatic cell hybrids between different species vastly increased the markers that researchers could utilize because even the same enzyme would have somewhat different properties in different species, allowing the regulation and fate of the separate protein molecules in the hybrids to be accurately analyzed. Potentially, one could now study the regulation of many enzymes, not just those few with known mutant forms maintained in cell culture. Moreover, the robustness of interspecific hybrids, their coordination of gene expression, the ability to extinguish and restore their differentiated functions, and the coordinated mitotic division of hybrid cells all pointed to the existence of similar systems of cellular control even in distantly related organisms. These results suggested that general controls of cell division and gene expression, common across species barriers, could now be explored via cell hybridization; see the speculations on control of the cell cycle in EPHRUSSI and WEISS (1967). Similar hopes were expressed with regard to processes relating to determination, differentiation, and dedifferentiation of cells. In addition, there was considerable emphasis on the regulation of neoplastic transformation, with some bitter disagreements about whether the determinants of neoplasia acted in a dominant or recessive manner. Ironically, EPHRUSSI underestimated the importance of negative regulation for a few years, particularly in disagreement with H. HARRIS; this issue began to be clarified with the subsequent (and continuing) analysis of "tumor suppressor genes."

Conclusion: We have examined the first decade of somatic cell genetics from the perspective of one of its principal protagonists. After the field had developed to this point, limiting the focus to an individual's perspective is harder to justify. A new biological field had opened up, one that could no longer be dominated by the work of a small group of laboratories (WEISS 1992). As EPHRUSSI's research program moved on, so did that of others who were drawn to this area of study. The number of different interspecific combinations grew very rapidly, with mouse, Chinese hamster, Syrian hamster, rat and human cells all serving as "parents" of hybrids. In each of the resulting systems, there was a great variety of studies, formal and biochemical. A number of technical refinements, selective systems, enzyme systems, and approaches were introduced, placing experimental studies of the principal aspects of somatic cell genetics beyond the reach of any single laboratory.

Furthermore, the study of somatic cell hybrids was propelled into far greater prominence in genetics (with a corresponding increase in activity) by a new type of hybrid first produced by MARY WEISS and HOWARD GREEN, working at New York University School of Medicine (WEISS and GREEN 1967). They created a mouse/human hybrid using a TK⁻ mouse line and embryonic human lung fibroblasts. Such hybrid cells retained the mouse chromosome complement but exhibited a substantial loss of human chromosomes. As WEISS and GREEN pointed out, "Study of clones containing a small number of human chromosomes should permit the localization of other human genes" (WEISS and GREEN 1967, p. 1111). Indeed, that has been the case. Mouse/human hybrids, by effectively transplanting a few human chromosomes into a new cell type, have permitted detailed study of the organization of genes on human chromosomes and provided a substantial stimulus to research in human genetics–research that previously

had been stymied by the difficulty of conducting research on humans. The readers of this journal are certainly aware of the wide range of information that has been derived from such studies and from somatic cell genetics in general.

For his part, EPHRUSSI continued to work on the topics in which he was primarily interested into the late 1970s, using hybrids with teratomas to explore determination and differentiation (*e.g.*, FINCH and EPHRUSSI 1967; KAHAN and EPHRUSSI 1970), negative regulation of differentiated function (*e.g.*, DAVIDSON, EPHRUSSI and YAMAMOTO 1966; FOUGÉRE, RUIZ and EPHRUSSI 1972), and related topics. He continued to advocate cellular and genetic approaches over a direct attack at the molecular level (EPHRUSSI 1970, p. 12). Nonetheless, he lived long enough to recognize that his transformation of transplantation into a genetic tool would take on a new and more powerful aspect in the molecular era. Indeed, we suggest that it is useful to interpret recombinant DNA procedures as a form of transplantation that places individual genes or groups of genes into new cellular environments, thus facilitating detailed study of their structure, action, and regulation and the production of ·novel biological entities, processes, and products. EPHRUSSI could not have foreseen the new genetics emerging from recombinant DNA studies, but the many sorts of studies he set in motion played an important role in making such work possible.

D.T.Z.'s research was supported in part by a Creative Match Grant from Virginia Polytechnic Institute and State University, facilitating research in the Archives of the Institut Pasteur. These Archives and the Archives of the Rockefeller Foundation provided access to documents on which we have drawn. R.M.B.'s research was supported by a study/research leave from Virginia Polytechnic Institute and State University and a residential fellowship at the National Humanities Center, Research Triangle Park, North Carolina, funded by the National Endowment for the Humanities. We are grateful to all these institutions for their support. PIOTR SLONIMSKI, MARY WEISS and RENÉ WURMSER assisted us with interviews bearing directly on this paper. The former two also supplied us with useful documents. The text has been improved by the criticisms and suggestions of EDWARD BERNSTINE, JOSHUA LEDERBERG and HOWARD TEMIN.

LITERATURE CITED

BARSKI, G., S. SORIEUL and F. CORNEFERT, 1960 Production dans des cultures *in vitro* de deux souches cellulaires en association, de cellules de caractère "hybride." C. R. Acad. Sci. (Paris) **251:** 1825–1827.

BARSKI, G., S. SORIEUL and F. CORNEFERT, 1961 "Hybrid" type cells in combined cultures of two different mammalian cell strains. JNCI **26:** 1269–1277.

BURIAN, R. M., J. GAYON and D. T. ZALLEN, 1988 The singular fate of genetics in the history of French biology. J. Hist. Biol. **21:** 357–402.

BURIAN, R. M., J. GAYON and D. T. ZALLEN, 1991 Boris Ephrussi and the synthesis of genetics and embryology, pp. 207–227 in *A Conceptual History of Modern Embryology*, edited by S. GILBERT. Plenum Press, New York.

CASPARI, E., 1933 Über die Wirkung eines pleiotropen Gens bei der Mehlmotte *Ephestia kühniella* Z. Arch. Entwicklungsmech. Org. **130:** 353–381.

DAVIDSON, R. L., and B. EPHRUSSI, 1965 A selective system for the isolation of hybrids between L cells and normal cells. Nature **205:** 1170–1171.

DAVIDSON, R. L., B. EPHRUSSI and K. YAMAMOTO, 1966 Regulation of pigment synthesis in mammalian cells, as studied by somatic hybridization. Proc. Natl. Acad. Sci. USA **56:** 1437–1440.

DEFENDI, V., B. EPHRUSSI, H. KROPOWSKI and M. C. YOSHIDA, 1967 Properties of polyoma-transformed and normal mouse cells. Proc. Natl. Acad. Sci. USA **57:** 615–621.

EPHRUSSI, B., 1923 Action d'une température elevée sur la mitose de segmentation des oeufs d'oursin. C. R. Acad. Sci. (Paris) **177:** 152–154.

EPHRUSSI, B., 1932 Contribution à l'Analyse des Premiers Stades du Développement de l'Oeuf. Action de Température [Dissertation, University of Paris]. Imprimerie de l'Académie, Paris, and H. Vaillant-Carmanne, Liége.

EPHRUSSI, B., 1933a Croissance et régéneration dans les cultures des tissus. Arch. Anat. Microsc. **29:** 95–159.

EPHRUSSI, B., 1933b Sur le facteur léthal des souris brachyures. C. R. Acad. Sci. (Paris) **197:** 96–98.

EPHRUSSI, B., 1935a *Phénomènes d'Intégration dans le Cultures des Tissus.* Hermann, Paris.

EPHRUSSI, B., 1935b The behavior *in vitro* of tissues from lethal embryos. J. Exp. Zool. **70:** 197–204.

EPHRUSSI, B., 1949 Action de l'acriflavine sur les levures, pp. 165–180 in *Unités Biologiques Douées de Continuité Génétique.* Editions du CNRS, Paris.

EPHRUSSI, B., 1953 *Nucleo-Cytoplasmic Relations in Micro-Organisms: Their Bearing on Cell Differentiation.* Clarendon Press, Oxford.

EPHRUSSI, B., 1958 The cytoplasm and somatic cell variation. J. Cell. Comp. Physiol. **52** (Suppl. 1): 35–53.

EPHRUSSI, B., 1965 Hybridization of somatic cells and phenotypic expression, pp. 486–502 in *Developmental and Metabolic Control Mechanisms and Neoplasia,* University of Texas M. D. Anderson Hospital and Tumor Institute. Williams & Wilkins, Baltimore.

EPHRUSSI, B., 1966 Interspecific somatic hybrids. *In Vitro* **2:** 40–45.

EPHRUSSI, B., 1970 Somatic hybridization as a tool for the study of normal and abnormal growth and differentiation, pp. 9–28 in *Genetic Concepts and Neoplasia,* University of Texas M. D. Anderson Hospital and Tumor Institute. Williams & Wilkins, Baltimore.

EPHRUSSI, B., 1972 *Hybridization of Somatic Cells.* Princeton University Press, Princeton, N.J.

EPHRUSSI, B., and G. W. BEADLE, 1936 A technique of transplantation for Drosophila. Am. Nat. **70:** 218–225.

EPHRUSSI, B., and H. HOTTINGUER, 1950 A direct demonstration of the mutagenic action of euflavine on baker's yeast. Nature **166:** 956.

EPHRUSSI, B., and L. RAPKINE, 1928 Composition chimique de l'oeuf d'Oursin *Parvocentrotus lividus* Lk. et ses variations au cours du developpement. Ann. Physiol. Physicochim. Biol. **3:** 386–390.

EPHRUSSI, B., and S. SORIEUL, 1962a Mating of somatic cells *in vitro,* pp. 81–97 in *Approaches to the Genetic Analysis of Mammalian Cells,* edited by D. J. MERCHANT and J. V. NEEL. University of Michigan Press, Ann Arbor.

EPHRUSSI, B., and S. SORIEUL, 1962b Nouvelles observations sur l'hybridation *in vitro* de cellules de souris. C. R. Acad. Sci. (Paris) **254:** 181–182.

EPHRUSSI, B., and M. WEISS, 1965 Interspecific hybridization of somatic cells. Proc. Natl. Acad. Sci. USA **53:** 1040–1042.

EPHRUSSI, B., and M. WEISS, 1967 Regulation of the cell cycle in

mammalian cells: inferences and speculations based on observations of interspecific somatic hybrids. Symp. Soc. Dev. Biol. **26:** 136–169.

EPHRUSSI, B., L. J. SCALETTA, M. A. STENCHEVER and M. C. YOSHIDA, 1964 Hybridization of somatic cells *in vitro.* Symp. Int. Soc. Cell Biol. **3:** 13–25.

FINCH, B., and B. EPHRUSSI, 1967 Multiple developmental potentialities by cells of a mouse testicular teratocarcinoma during prolonged culture *in vitro* and their extinction upon hybridization with cells of permanent lines. Proc. Natl. Acad. Sci. USA **57:** 615–621.

FOUÉGERE, C., F. RUIZ and B. EPHRUSSI, 1972 Gene dosage dependence of pigment synthesis in melanoma × fibroblast hybrids. Proc. Natl. Acad. Sci. USA **69:** 330–334.

GREEN H., B. EPHRUSSI, M. YOSHIDA and D. HAMERMAN, 1966 Synthesis of collagen and hyaluronic acid by fibroblast hybrids. Proc. Natl. Acad. Sci. USA **55:** 41–44.

HARRIS, H., and J. F. WATKINS, 1965 Hybrid cells derived from mouse and man: artificial heterokaryons of mammalian cells from different species. Nature **205:** 640–646.

HOROWITZ, N. H., 1990 George Wells Beadle (1903–1989). Genetics **124:** 1–5.

HOROWITZ, N. H., 1991 Fifty years ago: the Neurospora revolution. Genetics **127:** 631–635.

KAHAN B. W., and B. EPHRUSSI, 1970 Developmental potentialities of clonal *in vitro* cultures of mouse testicular teratoma. JNCI **44:** 1015–1036

KÜHN, A., E. CASPARI and E. PLAGGE, 1929, 1932 Genetische Untersuchungen an der Mehlmotte *Ephestia kühniella* Zeller. I.-VII. Abh. Ges. Wiss. Göttingen **15:** 3–121, 127–219.

LEDERBERG, J., 1956 Prospects for a genetics of somatic and tumor cells. Ann. NY Acad. Sci. **63:** 662–665.

LEDERBERG, J., 1958 Genetic approaches to somatic cell variation: summary comment. J. Cell. Comp. Physiol. **52** (Suppl. 1): 383–402.

LITTLEFIELD, J. W., 1964 Selection of hybrids from matings of fibroblasts *in vitro* and their presumed recombinants. Science **145:** 709.

PONTECORVO, G., 1961 Genetic analysis via somatic cells, pp. 13–20 in *The Scientific Basis of Medicine.* Annual Reviews, Palo Alto, Calif.

PONTECORVO, G., and E. KÄFER, 1958 Genetic analysis by means of mitotic recombination. Adv. Genet. **9:** 71–104.

SANFORD, K. K., G. D. LIKELY and W. R. EARLE, 1954 The development of variations in transplantability and morphology within a clone of mouse fibroblasts transformed in sarcoma-producing cells *in vitro.* JNCI **15:** 215–237.

SAPP, J., 1987 *Beyond the Gene: Cytoplasmic Inheritance and the Struggle for Authority in Genetics.* Oxford University Press, New York.

SCALETTA, L. J., and B. EPHRUSSI, 1965 Hybridization of normal and neoplastic cells *in vitro.* Nature **205:** 1169.

SORIEUL, S., and B. EPHRUSSI, 1961 Karyological demonstration of hybridization of mammalian cells *in vitro.* Nature **190:** 653–654.

SPENCER, R. A., T. S. HAUSCHKA, D. B. AMOS and B. EPHRUSSI, 1964 Co-dominance of isoantigens in somatic hybrids of murine cells grown *in vitro.* JNCI **33:** 893–903.

STURTEVANT, A. H., 1920 The vermilion gene and gynandromorphism. Proc. Soc. Exp. Biol. Med. **17:** 70–71.

STURTEVANT, A. H., 1932 The uses of mosaics in the study of the developmental effects of genes. Proc. 6th Int. Congr. Genet. **1:** 304–307.

SZYBALSKA, E. H., and W. SZYBALSKI, 1962 Genetics of human cell lines. IV. DNA-mediated heritable transformation of a biochemical trait. Proc. Natl. Acad. Sci. USA **48:** 2026–2034.

SZYBALSKI, W., E. H. SZYBALSKA and G. RAGNI, 1962 Genetic studies with human cell lines, pp. 75–89 in *Analytical Cell*

Culture, edited by R. E. STEVENSON, National Cancer Institute Monograph No. 7. U.S. Public Health Service, Washington, D.C.

WEISS, M., 1992 Contributions of Boris Ephrussi to the development of somatic cell genetics. BioEssays **14:** 349–353.

WEISS, M., and B. EPHRUSSI, 1966a Studies of interspecific (rat × mouse) somatic hybrids. I. Isolation, growth and evolution of the karyotype. Genetics **54:** 1095–1109.

WEISS, M., and B. EPHRUSSI, 1966b Studies of interspecific (rat × mouse) somatic hybrids. II. Lactate dehydrogenase and β-glucuronidase. Genetics **54:** 1111–1122.

WEISS, M., and H. GREEN, 1967 Human-mouse hybrid cell lines containing partial complements of human chromosomes and functioning human genes. Proc. Natl. Acad. Sci. USA **58:** 1104–1111.

Forty Years Ago
The Discovery of Bacterial Transduction

Norton D. Zinder

The Rockefeller University, New York, New York 10021

FORTY years ago we published a paper describing bacterial transduction (ZINDER and LEDERBERG 1952). The work was done during the previous two years in JOSHUA LEDERBERG's laboratory at the University of Wisconsin where I was attempting to extend his discovery of bacterial conjugation. Since over many years one's memory can play tricks as well as be influenced by external circumstances, I've reconstructed the discovery from my notes. Although they are for the most part readable, we must remember that they were written at a time when concepts such as phage, lysogeny, and even the gene were obscure.

Getting started: With the discovery of the penicillin enrichment technique for isolating auxotrophic bacterial mutants (DAVIS 1948; LEDERBERG and ZINDER 1948), a number of strains of *Salmonella typhimurium* were marked so as to permit tests for bacterial conjugation. Marking the strains involved the isolation of two sets of nonoverlapping double mutants, most having amino acid requirements. Tests were done by mixing two cultures, plating on a minimal medium, and looking for prototrophic colonies. At that time, similarly marked mutant strains of *Escherichia coli* K-12 would give between 10^{-6} and 10^{-7} prototrophic recombinants. It is also important to note that the *E. coli* data strongly suggested that the bacteria were haploid (TATUM and LEDERBERG 1947).

This work really began when 22 phage-typed *S. typhimurium* strains arrived from LILLEENGEN in Sweden (LILLEENGEN 1948). From each of these strains large numbers of auxotrophic mutants were obtained by the penicillin enrichment procedure. Two mutagenesis protocols were used involving two UV dosages. Trying to reconstruct why I chose these dosages, my guess is that some of the strains carried UV-inducible phages and were readily killed but not readily mutagenized, necessitating a larger UV dose. There are no interpretable data in this part of my notes other than that the lower dose reduced the

viability of the test strain to 10^{-3} while the larger dose reduced it to 10^{-5}. This strain was probably noninducible, but at the time, of course, I knew nothing of phage induction. Over a period of months I accumulated a collection of mutant strain pairs and started intrastrain crosses.

Desperate moves: By June, 1950 I noted that all self-crosses had failed. That is, every cross within a strain for which I had a complementary pair of mutant markers failed to give prototrophs. I guess that out of desperation because there was little theory then, I started crossing different strains. Were I to get a cross to work between two different strains, it would already differ from the findings with *E. coli* K-12, because at that time none of the other laboratory strains would mate with K-12 while as far as tested, all K-12 strains were interfertile. There were many interstrain Salmonella crosses to try, a 20 × 20 set. They could only be done slowly and had to be analyzed in detail because there were always contaminants and partial revertants on the plates (false positives) that kept one busy. Crosses were done by washing overnight broth cultures and spreading 10^8 bacteria of each parental type on the surface of minimal agar Petri dishes. There were similar unmixed control plates. With double auxotrophs it was rare to find any real revertants, but during the four-day incubation contaminants would often appear. However, real signs soon appeared that some of the interstrain crosses were indeed producing prototrophs.

Discovery and confusion: We now come to the fall of 1950. On October 5 I did a cross between two of the LILLEENGEN strains, LT-2 and LT-22. It yielded recombinants at a frequency even higher than previously observed for *E. coli* crosses. Colonies appeared at a frequency of about 10^{-5}. This was exciting. We crossed all of our LT-2 and LT-22 derivatives with each other and with other mutant strains to try to understand the phenomenon. Slowly it became clear that the important element was that one of the parents be a particular mutant of LT-22, a double mutation in the pathway of aromatic amino acid synthesis. Next we compared the nature of the progeny with those from E. coli crosses. The E. coli recombinants not only had a prototrophic phenotype, that is, the four wild-type alleles of two pairs of markers being selected, but they also segregated a number of unselected markers such as for lactose fermentation and for phage resistance. In the Salmonella case I tested nine different markers. None of them segregated; all matched the LT-22 parent. What then seemed all the more remarkable was that one could always set up the cross in such a way as to select one of the previously unselected markers of the same LT-22 strain, and it would also give 10^{-5} recombinants while none of the other markers segregated, including previously selected ones. Again the markers recovered were always those of strain LT-22. It was an asymmetric recombination that involved only one marker at a time. It resembled pneumococcal transformation and this is why we decided to find out whether or not it required cell-to-cell contact for "mating" to occur. To decide this we did a U-tube experiment. This was first done by BERNARD DAVIS (1950) to ask the same question about E. coli K-12 conjugation. Two different cultures were grown in the separate arms of a glass U-tube. Between the arms was a sintered glass filter with pore size small enough to prevent bacterial passage. The medium was flushed back and forth between the arms as the bacteria grew, and those in each arm were sampled periodically for prototrophs. The LT-2 parent was an auxotroph requiring methionine and histidine while the LT-22 parent was a phenylalanine (tyrosine) and tryptophan auxotroph. Prototrophs were found among the LT-22 bacteria but not among the LT-2 bacteria.

Over the succeeding months the following observations were made. Supernatants from the separate cultures were without effect. When the two cultures were grown together, however, the filter-sterilized supernatant would convert, proportional to the amount used, about 10^{-6} of LT-22 mutants to prototrophy while being without effect on the LT-2 mutations. Some months later this could be understood. LT-22 carried a phage (PLT-22, now P22) that crossed the filter, grew on the LT-2 strain, and then returned through the filter, now carrying genes able to replace the fortuitously linked *arom* mutations in LT-22. At the time we floundered for an explanation. JOSH recalled the many stories in the bacterial literature about filterable L-forms (DIENES and WEINBERGER 1951; KLINEBERGER-NOBEL 1951), which looked like what we now call spheroplasts and which supposedly were induced when bacteria were stressed. Because they could regenerate, they must have had

genetic material and were somehow involved in what we were observing.

To confound matters, the effective lysates did indeed contain structures that looked like L-forms and that eventually turned out to be membranes from bacteria lysed by phage.

With the LT-22 strain as our assay, we found that when many of the Salmonella strains were stressed, for instance with chemicals such as crystal violet, by aging, or by the growth of certain Salmonella phages, varying amounts of an activity were produced which we called FA (filterable agent). The range of the effect was also extended. In fact, any single selectable marker from almost any Salmonella strain could be transduced (but this name was not proposed until the fall of 1951). We had clearly been using precisely the wrong procedure, a random collection of double markers, to find this phenomenon. Only two serendipitous occurrences allowed us to detect transduction at all. First, the original markers in LT-22 with which we found transduction were both in the pathway of aromatic amino acid biosynthesis and were probably linked so that they cotransduced. Second, the LT-22 strain carried a lysogenic transducing phage that could propagate on LT-2.

Cold Spring Harbor, 1951: The spring of 1951 brought little further insight into transduction as the notion of L-forms clouded our vision. Nevertheless we set off to the 1951 Cold Spring Harbor Symposium. I note, for those interested in the history of genetics, the most extraordinary volume documenting this symposium (Cold Spring Harbor 1951). If ever a science was in a prerevolutionary crisis (KUHN 1970) it was genetics in 1951. The symposium was opened by RICHARD GOLDSCHMIDT, who proclaimed that there was no such thing as a gene, rather that the chromosome was the unit of function and mutations were no more than analogs to stops on the string of a violin. This was in some ways supported by the mystifying studies of position effect pseudoallelism by LEWIS in Drosophila and STADLER in corn. This is also the Symposium that spawned the myth that Mc-CLINTOCK's description of transposition was not understood. There was in fact a separate meeting with BARBARA to discuss the details of her experiments. Moreover, R. A. BRINK, a corn geneticist, was there and had obtained similar results with what he then called *Mp*, but which later turned out to be homologous to MCCLINTOCK's *Ac*. As BRINK's colleagues from Wisconsin, we were certainly aware of transposition because we were all drafted to plant and pollinate his corn. For those who still believed in the gene, there were such as J. H. TAYLOR, who said, "I wish I could say something in behalf of the recently deceased, the gene, but . . . ." On the other hand some beautiful experiments by HOROWITZ and LEUPOLD provided substantial evidence for the one-gene, one-enzyme hypothesis. Still others accepted the one-gene, one-enzyme relationship but choked on the "one" in both phrases. EPHRUSSI presented a reasonable paper on cytoplasmic genes (mitochondria) in yeast while SPIE-GELMAN confused all with his discussion of long-term adaptation and plasmagenes in yeasts. LEDERBERG gave a paper from our laboratory which I believe has won all competition for incomprehensibility. He spoke for more than six hours. Only H. J. MULLER even began to follow it. There was also a lot on mutagenesis and particularly the new chemical mutagenesis, although most of the analysis was not directed toward the chemical nature of the gene but rather to chromosome damage and segregation effects. I've never found out why, but the Symposium closed with a defense of F. MOUWUS, the Chlamydomonas geneticist, by no less than T. SONNEBORN. MOEWUS's work was at best incompetent, at worst fraudulent.

For me personally, all of 22 years old, it was a revelation. I tried to believe everything I heard, which of course was impossible and left me confused. Still, when HARRIETT EPHRUSSI-TAYLOR said that transduction was due to a phage with some DNA stuck onto it, I knew what I had to do when I got back to the laboratory. From that moment on even a glance at my notes reveals that the experiments became highly focused.

Figuring it out: In addition to the idea that the FA was intimately related to the phage found in all my preparations, the many papers at Cold Spring Harbor on mutagenesis by a variety of mutagens raised the question whether FA was itself a mutagen rather than gene-like. We had so far done no experiment showing that the genetic events we detected were determined by the genotype of the donor bacteria. From August through October of 1951, experiments were done to clarify the nature of both the transduction event and the transducing particles. With the resolution of these questions we were able to give a cogent name to this phenomenon.

A search of phage stocks already in the laboratory revealed several with FA activity. Moreover, the transducing potential of any preparation reflected the genotype of the last host on which the phage had grown. For example, phage grown on a histidine-requiring mutant strain could transduce all genes except histidine. A further experiment showed that it was the genotype and not the phenotype that was determinant. A set of galactose-negative mutations was prepared and phage were grown on each one. Two groups of mutants were found which could mutually transduce each other to galactose fermentation, establishing that transduction reflected the underlying genotype and that there were at least two genes for galactose fermentation.

To this point, all of our transductions had been from mutant back to wild type. Using streptomycin resistance, a marker known to result from a recessive mutation in *E. coli*, we quickly showed that there was no mutant/wild-type directionality in the phenomenon. Additional clarification of the genetic nature of transduction came from studies of the Salmonella flagellar antigens. Different strains have characteristic antigens: *S. typhimurium* antigen i and *Salmonella paratyphi* A antigen a. With serum selection, *S. paratyphi* A could be transduced to carry flagellar antigen i, losing the a. Many other such antigens could be interchanged. The stability of the transductants, the recessive nature of streptomycin resistance and the interchangeability of flagellar antigens all pointed to gene replacement on a haploid background rather than gene addition as the genetic event of transduction.

While putting the genetics of transduction on a solid footing, we sought procedures to determine the nature of the particle involved. HOTCHKISS graciously provided us with purified DNase and we found it to be without effect against FA; however, our only control for DNase activity was its ability to decrease the visible viscosity of an *E. coli* DNA preparation. Antibody was prepared by injecting rabbits with an FA preparation. Neutralizing activity for plaque-forming ability and for transducing activity were both measured; they fell off at the same rate. Also at this time the lab had a large collection of different Salmonella strains. Those that adsorbed the phage also adsorbed FA and *vice versa*, and adsorption correlated with the presence of Salmonella somatic antigen XII.

Both FA and phage were retained by membrane filters with an average pore diameter of 0.1 μm, although both readily passed through bacteriological filter candles. Both were resistant to protease, nucleases, or chloroform treatment. Only UV irradiation inactivated plaque-forming activity at a much faster rate than transducing activity. In retrospect, we know that P22 requires many times as much genetic material to function as does the average bacterial gene, about 30 to 1. FA was obviously bacterial genetic material in a phage particle. Recall that this is all before the HERSHEY-CHASE experiment and the WATSON-CRICK model for DNA. Even LWOFF's critical experiments on the lysogenic state for some phages were just beginning to become known. Still, by the standards of 1951, we were convinced that we had a reasonable explanation for the Salmonella phenomenon and LEDERBERG suggested that we call it "transduction." Other words such as "entrainment" were considered and wisely rejected.

That fall BRUCE STOCKER joined the laboratory and we worked on the transduction of motility and flagellar antigens. The first clear example of a linked transduction then turned up. A nonmotile strain of *S.*

paratyphi B was transduced to motility. The flagella of some clones had the characteristic b antigen of para B while a third of the clones had the i antigen of the motile *S. typhimurium* donor. Evidently, some of the flagella mobility genes were linked to flagella antigen genes. Transduction progeny tests proved this point (STOCKER, ZINDER and LEDERBERG 1953).

Afterward: Shortly thereafter, I went to a meeting of the Society of American Bacteriologists (now the ASM) in Boston. Among those present were FRANCIS RYAN, ED TATUM, SOL SPIEGELMAN and others who were familiar with our findings. A place was created for me to talk at one of the symposia. I introduced a large and appreciative audience to phage PLT-22 and its works. What probably sold the group's true bacteriologists on the reality of what I said was the transduction of *Salmonella typhi* (agent of typhoid fever) from its classical IX, XII:d- (monophasic) to IX, XII:i (monophasic), something never seen in nature. To this day, however, I have never understood the quick acceptance of transduction as a phenomenon when the majority of the audience still believed in a Lamarckian mechanism for bacterial mutations, if they believed in bacterial genes at all, and only a few accepted the existence of conjugation in *E. coli*.

Within a few years of its discovery, transduction was used to study the linked genes specifying the enzymes of intermediate metabolism (operons) as well as the fine structure of a gene. "Transformations and transduction which deal directly with fragments of genetic material acting upon large populations might then provide the tools for genetic analysis at precisely the level wherein the analysis of higher forms become difficult" (ZINDER 1953). So in that strange way that science can absorb and quickly integrate that which it finds most useful, transduction became classical within a few years. Today it includes the cell-to-cell transfer of foreign genes by any virus, whether the laboratory constructs made by recombinant DNA technology or natural oncogenes in viral oncogenesis. "The ability of viruses to act in so many ways in the bacterial systems as bacterial genes resolves the intellectual difficulties of the mutation theory of the etiology of cancer and the viral theory, but in no way as yet ameliorates the medical problem" (ZINDER 1960).

LITERATURE CITED

Cold Spring Harbor, 1951 Genes and mutations. Cold Spring Harbor Symp. Quant. Biol. **16.**

DAVIS, B. D., 1948 Isolation of biochemically deficient mutants of bacteria by penicillin. J. Am. Chem. Soc. **70:** 4267.

DAVIS, B. D., 1950 Nonfilterability of the agents of recombination in *Escherichia coli*. J. Bacteriol. **60:** 507–508.

DIENES, L., and H. J. WEINBERGER, 1951 The L forms of bacteria. Bacteriol. Rev. **15:** 245–288.

KLINEBERGER-NOBEL, E., 1951 Filterable forms of bacteria. Bacteriol. Rev. **15:** 77–103.

KUHN, T., 1970 *The Structure of Scientific Revolutions.* University of Chicago Press, Chicago.

LEDERBERG, J., and N. D. ZINDER, 1948 Concentration of biochemical mutants of bacteria with penicillin. J. Am. Chem. Soc. **70:** 4267.

LILLEENGEN, K., 1948 Typing *Salmonella typhimurium* by means of bacteriophage. Acta Pathol. Microbiol. Scand. Suppl. **77.**

STOCKER, B. D., N. D. ZINDER and J. LEDERBERG, 1953 Transduction of flagellar characters in Salmonella. J. Gen. Microbiol. **9:** 410–433.

TATUM, E., and J. LEDERBERG, 1947 Gene recombination in the bacteria *E. coli*. J. Bacteriol. **53:** 673–684.

ZINDER, N. D., 1953 Infective heredity in bacteria. Cold Spring Harbor Symp. Quant. Biol. **18:** 261–269.

ZINDER, N. D., 1960 Virology, 1959. Am. Sci. **48:** 608–612.

ZINDER, N. D., and J. LEDERBERG, 1952 Genetic exchange in Salmonella. J. Bacteriol. **64:** 679–699.

November 1992

Forty Years Ago in *Genetics*
The Unorthodox Mating Behavior of Bacteria

L. Luca Cavalli-Sforza

Genetics Department, Stanford University, Stanford, California 94305

IN October, 1953 GENETICS published the first detailed report of a sex difference in *Escherichia coli*. This is a fitting time to look back at those years of simultaneous excitement and confusion when the genetics of bacteria was just beginning to be understood.

Looking at recent papers on bacterial genetics, I am surprised to still recognize the names of some of the markers and strains of *E. coli* K-12. So much has happened since that exciting time. *E. coli* is well on its way to becoming one of those few organisms for which we know the whole genome, incredible progress from what was understood around 1950 when we knew only a few linkages for less than a dozen markers.

Starting in 1941, bacteria had become my major interest and in 1948 I gave a paper at the International Congress of Genetics in Stockholm on cross resistance to radiation and nitrogen mustard in *E. coli* based on work done earlier in Milan with NICCOLO VISCONTI (CAVALLI and VISCONTI 1948). Italy was then, and for several decades, a scientific desert with a few oases. After much search I was lucky to have found one of these oases, with ADRIANO BUZZATI-TRAVERSO as my professor. In 1948 I received a scholarship from the Italian National Research Council to work with KENNETH MATHER at the John Innes Horticultural Institution, then at Merton and directed by C. D. DARLINGTON. This was the first time I was able to go abroad, a major success in post-war Italy, and I enjoyed enormously drinking directly at one of the original fountains of genetic and statistical knowledge.

It was in that eventful summer of 1948 that I had the surprise, immediately after introducing myself to R. A. FISHER at the Stockholm International Congress, of being offered a job in his laboratory. Very probably FISHER was one of the first readers of the GENETICS paper by JOSHUA LEDERBERG (1947) to be entirely convinced by it. The "Pope" of bacteriophage, MAX DELBRÜCK, who listened to the first communication by LEDERBERG at the famous 1946 Cold Spring Harbor Symposium, was initially skeptical of the *E. coli* K-12 crosses. SALVA LURIA, who was also present, tried to repeat LEDERBERG's experiments using *E. coli* B, but failed. Several years later ENRICO CALEF and I tested *E. coli* B and found it to be self-sterile but able to cross with *E. coli* K-12.

FISHER was immediately enthusiastic about K-12 genetics. He obviously was not scared by what JIM WATSON (1968) in The *Double Helix* called the "rabbinical complexity" of JOSHUA's papers. FISHER's main experimental interest was crossing over and gene mapping, which he studied mostly in mice. His laboratory was saturated with these smelly animals and his garden was full of various experimental plants, including MENDEL's peas. His hope was that *E. coli* would become an excellent organism for the study of crossing over.

I immediately accepted FISHER's offer and started working in Cambridge (at 44 Storey's Way, the address of the old Genetics Department) on October 1, 1948. My laboratory was carved out of the tea room and I must confess that I chose the equipment not so much on the basis of price or reliability as simply on early availability. In any case, there was very little difference in prices and reliability was hard to guess; moreover, a bacteriological laboratory at that time required only simple equipment. K-12 strains were sent by the LEDERBERGs and I began to make crosses in February, 1949.

It was perfectly easy to repeat the original experiments; people did not believe them because they did not try to duplicate them. But the skepticism around me was incredible. To classical bacteriologists, we (the very few bacterial geneticists could be counted on one or at most two hands) were lunatics. Bacteriologists had been taught that bacteria have no nucleus or chromosomes and besides, very few of them had clear ideas of Mendelism and, in particular, of recombination. Geneticists, such as D. G. CATCHESIDE and GUIDO

PONTECORVO, working with fungi were not so skeptical. GUIDO had developed a procedure for selecting recombinants in Ascomycetes very similar to the prototroph technique that permitted LEDERBERG to show bacterial recombination, mixing different mutant strains on a medium in which neither parent could grow but a recombinant would. On GUIDO's invitation, I went to Glasgow in 1950 and gave a demonstration of bacterial recombination to bacteriologists. At the time, it was customary to wash suspensions of the parent bacteria three times before plating them on minimal medium (without the nutritional supplements necessary for growth of the mutant strains), and the many bacteriologists who came to see had to stand for a long time during these simple but lengthy operations. I also kept them at some distance for fear of contaminations. They came back later to see the cultures after they had grown.

Recombination as observed at the beginning had a very low frequency. It stopped being rare when I found a mutant strain which I called Hfr for "high frequency of recombination." I found it accidentally in 1949 while I was selecting mutations resistant to nitrogen mustard and radiation. The first two resistant mutants, which had undergone a rather heavy treatment in the process of selecting for resistance to nitrogen mustard, proved to be exceptional in their mating behavior. One was Hfr and it showed immediately its remarkable mating ability, which was higher than that of normal crosses by a factor of 1000 or more. I repeated the experiment two more times before believing it. The other mutation, as I later proved, was an F$^-$ (self-sterile) mutation of an F$^+$ (fertile) strain.

Hfr was especially interesting but the biology of mating was difficult to understand. There was nothing to be seen microscopically on a plate or in mixed cultures; no distinguishable zygotes were formed. It was only in 1954 that LEDERBERG first proved by micromanipulation experiments that when mating took place there was something—an invisible thread—holding a male and a female together in a drop of saline, though at some distance from each other. Electron microscopy was for a long time negative or unclear. The genetics of the Hfr crosses were difficult to understand, not surprising in retrospect.

I wanted to publish only when I felt that I understood the phenomenon, and thus I published nothing about the finding of Hfr except for a short mention in an Italian journal (CAVALLI 1950). A year or so later, another independent Hfr turned up spontaneously in an old culture in Great Britain and was studied by W. HAYES. The two Hfrs are still around and are called by our two names or simply their initials, HfrC and HfrH. Much later, many more independent Hfrs were obtained, each with unique properties.

FISHER had planned to make bacterial genetics a major part of his research program, but despite his impassioned protestations the program was eliminated. It is ironic that FISHER, who pioneered both in blood groups (especially the Rh factor) and bacterial genetics, was unable to obtain support for sustained research in either area. It was not clear if I was going to keep my Cambridge position.

In this situation of uncertainty I was glad to accept an interesting offer to return to Milan in 1950, back to the laboratory of the Istituto Sieroterapico Milanese where I had started working in 1945 after the end of the war. Although this was a pharmaceutical firm, I was able to continue my genetic research on a part-time basis. I undertook the examination of other fertility mutations, which proved easier. The original K-12 strain is capable of mating with itself, but at a low frequency. I found several independent mutants that had lost this capacity to mate with themselves. To show this, I had to develop new biochemical mutants that would make it possible to test if a strain could or could not mate with itself. Self-sterile strains are called F$^-$. F$^+$ is the original K-12 strain, fertile at a low rate with all F$^-$ strains and at an even lower rate with itself. Hfr is a mutation of F$^+$ which has a high frequency of recombination. While the progeny of F$^+$ × F$^-$ crosses were consistently F$^+$ (except with some special F$^-$ strains, a phenomenon that I never got around to publishing), those of Hfr × F$^-$ were consistently F$^-$. But a very brief mixture of F$^+$ and F$^-$ cells, allowing contact between them, could pass the F$^+$ property to F$^-$ cells with high probability and without detectable recombination.

While I was doing these experiments I was in correspondence with JOSHUA LEDERBERG and wrote to him about these findings. He and ESTHER LEDERBERG had obtained very similar results, and we decided to publish them together. One joint paper was sent to GENETICS (LEDERBERG, CAVALLI and LEDERBERG 1952), the other to the *Journal of General Microbiology* (CAVALLI, LEDERBERG and LEDERBERG 1953). The LEDERBERGs and I had never met, and it was a strange but pleasant experience to write papers with people known only through air mail. We finally met when I was able to go to Madison, Wisconsin, in 1954, thanks to a Rockefeller Fellowship that allowed me to work with them for three months.

In England I had met BILL HAYES. I happened to give him the first *E. coli* K-12 strains and to show him the crossing and scoring techniques in the practicals of a course which was held at Cambridge. BILL and I also corresponded, though more rarely. He once wrote me the following on F$^+$ and F$^-$, about which I had written him: "I guess one can pass the F$^+$ property by infection to an F⁻." Both the LEDERBERGS and I had independently found this, and I hastened to write to him that he would find the experiment works quite well. He later told me that he was quite shocked when he received my answer because meanwhile he also had done the experiment. It was planned that the HAYES paper would appear in the same issue of the *Journal of General Microbiology* as ours, and it did (HAYES 1953).

In 1952 I had a student of KENNETH MATHER, JOHN L. JINKS, as a guest in my Milan laboratory. It was clear at the time that the Hfr × F⁻ cross yielded F⁻ progeny, as I said above. But we now found that the cross of HfrC with an F⁻ did generate some Hfr progeny, clearly linked to a galactose marker which only rarely segregated. The results could be summarized by saying that F is an infectious particle which could be easily transmitted by cell-to-cell contact and which showed no indication of linkage to other markers, but in some conditions would become irreversibly part of the bacterial chromosome at a specific site, losing the capacity to infect by cell-to-cell contact but acquiring the property of high-frequency recombination. We communicated this finding to the Bellagio 1953 International Congress of Genetics together with the first information on recombination and fitness (CAVALLI-SFORZA and JINKS 1954). The latter study was one of the original purposes of my work in FISHER's department. For example, all possible parental combinations of three markers were tried to test for effects of markers on viability. Until the mechanism of fertility became clear, research on *E. coli* recombination proved completely frustrating. JIM WATSON, who was then at Cambridge, spent a few days in Milan in 1952 to see my recombination data. He was convinced that a three-chromosome theory could explain the observations. He offered to write a paper together with HAYES and me on this theory, which he later published with HAYES (WATSON and HAYES 1953), but I was not persuaded by the theory and declined.

It became progressively more clear that there were some phenomena that could be interpreted on the basis of breaks and that a specific chromosome region was contributed only by female (F⁻) parents. This made the results of recombination difficult to understand. It took a long time for JINKS and me to agree on the formal interpretation of recombination data, and it was only in 1956 that we were able to publish a joint manuscript. The formal interpretation of detailed recombination results (CAVALLI-SFORZA and JINKS 1956) is, I think, correct to this day, and a *tour-*

de-force of recombination analysis. It showed how difficult it would have been to use the *E. coli* recombination system for the quantitative study of crossing over that FISHER was hoping to do. Nevertheless, FISHER followed with great interest and full open-mindedness the unexpected results that were coming out of bacterial crosses, and was more flexible than I in accepting the unorthodox behaviors of bacteria.

Up to this time bacterial genetics had been the province of a very small group. The stage was now set for a full-scale attack on *E. coli* and many joined in the fray. Phenomena that had seemed mysterious were soon understood, and *E. coli* became the best known species and the geneticist's favorite organism.

My position in the Istituto Sieroterapico Milanese was far from ideal for keeping up with the explosion of research on *E. coli* genetics. Beginning in 1952 I started flirting with human genetics while lecturing part time at the University of Parma, and I slowly left bacteria. The last Petri dish I touched must have been in 1960, working with JOSHUA and ESTHER LEDERBERG at Stanford on the effects of streptomycin on the phenotype of bacterial mutants, a very interesting phenomenon that we, as well as LUIGI GORINI, independently observed. Conversion to human genetics provided a completely different outlet for my scientific interests, replacing work at the laboratory bench with statistical and theoretical analysis, along with trips to such places as Africa to study human populations in their native habitats.

LITERATURE CITED

CAVALLI, L. L., 1950 La sessualità nei batteri. Boll. Ist. Sieroter. Milano **29:** 281–289.

CAVALLI, L. L., J. LEDERBERG and E. M. LEDERBERG, 1953 An infective factor controlling sex compatibility in *Bacterium coli.* J. Gen. Microbiol. **8:** 89–103.

CAVALLI, L. L., and N. VISCONTI, 1948 Variazioni di resistenza agli agenti mutageni in *Bacterium coli.* II. Azotoiprite. Ric. Sci. **18:** 1569–1574.

CAVALLI-SFORZA, L. L., and J. L. JINKS, 1954 Observations on the genetic and mating system of *E. coli* K-12. Atti IX Congr. Int. Genet. Caryol. Suppl. **1954:** 967–969.

CAVALLI-SFORZA, L. L., and J. L. JINKS, 1956 Studies on the genetic system of *E. coli* K-12. J. Genet. **54:** 87–112.

HAYES, W., 1953 Observations on a transmissible agent determining sexual differentiation in *Bacterium coli.* J. Gen. Microbiol. **8:** 72–88.

LEDERBERG, J., 1947 Gene recombination and linked segregation in *Escherichia coli.* Genetics **32:** 505–525.

LEDERBERG, J., L. L. CAVALLI and E. M. LEDERBERG, 1952 Sex compatibility in *Escherichia coli.* Genetics **37:** 720–730.

WATSON, J., 1968 *The Double Helix.* Atheneum, New York.

WATSON, J. D., and W. HAYES, 1953 Genetic exchange in *Escherichia coli* K-12; evidence for three linkage groups. Proc. Natl. Acad. Sci. USA **39:** 416–426.

Unicorns Revisited

Franklin W. Stahl

Institute of Molecular Biology and Department of Biology, University of Oregon, Eugene, Oregon 97403–1229

I N 1988, CAIRNS, OVERBAUGH and MILLER claimed to have evidence that some bacterial mutants arise as a specific, adaptive response to the selective environment of the moment, "adaptive" because the mutant has gained the ability to grow, and "specific" because other, irrelevant mutants do not accumulate during the selection. The environment appeared to "direct" the mutational process!

Whatever *you* may think, those who work on "directed" (or "adaptive") mutants seem to believe that the reality of their phenomenon has been securely established. In both hasty (HALL 1992) and responsible (STEELE and JINKS-ROBERTSON 1992) papers, even yeast has been claimed to show it. Thus, quite appropriately, FOSTER and CAIRNS (1992) have moved on to the next phase, testing the models that have been offered to explain "directed mutagenesis."

Since many otherwise intelligent people will doubt the phenomenon until its mechanism has been elucidated, FOSTER and CAIRNS are serving science well by directing their attention to the models. Not that they have identified the mechanism for the origin of directed mutants! That paper is yet to be written. However, FOSTER and CAIRNS have blown away several possibilities with further studies on the "directed" revertants of *lac* mutants.

The first model they go after is the one nobody liked anyway, because it would circumvent the Central Dogma. This model envisioned a feedback from "successful" protein to message that encoded it to gene that encoded the message. An undirected, propitious transcription error might thereby become immortalized as a DNA mutation. The experiment that disposes of this blasphemous model is tidy and convincing. It rests on the simple observation that among the directed revertants of a Lac⁻ amber are both true revertants, which could, in principle, be directed as described above, and tRNA suppressor mutants, which could not.

The second model challenged proposes that transcription is inherently mutagenic and that the lactose-induced Lac⁺ revertants are a consequence of the well known ability of lactose to induce transcription of the *lac* operon. Of course, the tRNA suppressors noted above already stand against this hypothesis. As further evidence, FOSTER and CAIRNS note that Lac⁻ mutants that are constitutive for transcription of the *lac* operon revert only in the presence of lactose. This experiment falls a bit short because there is no demonstration that the constitutive cells are, in fact, constitutive when they are starved. The argument that transcription plays no important role in the origin of these directed revertants is made more convincing by the demonstration that isopropyl thiogalactoside (IPTG), a gratuitous inducer of *lacZ*, does not by itself cause the accumulation of Lac⁺ cells. Furthermore, it cannot be argued that the starved (or semistarved) cells did not respond to the IPTG because the IPTG enhanced the ability of existing Lac⁺ cells to yield Lac⁺ colonies when the cells were exposed to lactose.

I was pleased to see those models crash. I was less pleased to see my model crash. That model (STAHL 1988) proposed that repair synthesis occurring here and there in stationary phase cells allows mutations. Postreplicational mismatch repair, proposed to act slowly in these cells, eventually repairs any irrelevant mutations. Mutations that allow the cell to escape its metabolic bind, however, lead to chromosome replication with the consequence that the mutation is fixed before it can be repaired. FOSTER and CAIRNS show, with minor caveats, that the postreplicational mismatch repair system as we know it (the Mut system) is not involved in the selective disappearance of irrelevant mutations (and see JAYARAMAN 1992). While they are at it, they demonstrate that selectivity does not depend on the alkylation repair pathway, either.

Where does that leave us? FOSTER and CAIRNS call our attention to the following two observations: (i)

Directed revertants of a Lac⁻ frameshift mutant arise at a reduced rate in a strain that carries a *recA* allele (CAIRNS and FOSTER 1991; and see JAYARAMAN 1992). (ii) The base change that results in reversion of one of the *lac* mutants studied almost certainly depends on DNA replication for its occurrence. Revertants of this *lac* mutant can be environmentally directed, telling us that DNA replication is required for the origin of some (maybe all) directed mutants. Because these revertants did not accumulate in the absence of lactose, the authors conclude that the replicated DNA is unstable if the cell cannot benefit from it.

These two observations suggest to the authors a model involving gene amplification:

. . . we can account for all the experimental evidence, at least in our system, with the following hypothesis. In stationary phase, cells may be amplifying limited regions of their genomes. We can imaging (sic) this as simple duplication, which is known to occur at frequencies of 10^{-3} to 10^{-4} per cell (ANDERSON and ROTH 1981), or as more extensive amplification. These extra DNA copies would be inherently unstable, but might have an increased chance of containing errors. The cell that achieves a useful mutation in one of these copies could exit stationary phase, begin to grow, and resolve the amplified region by a RecA-dependent process. This hypothesis predicts that anything that increases the error-rate of DNA synthesis will increase the rate of post-selection mutation, but the process will still be RecA-dependent. RecA could, in fact, be required for each step in this process (LARK and LARK 1979; TLSTY, ALBERTINI and MILLER 1984; DIMPFL and ECHOLS 1989).

Does this model really work? I have quoted the model in full so that you, Dear Reader, can judge whether I am being fair when I say, "Hardly, at least not if 'amplification' means the accumulation of tandem duplications as implied by the citation of ANDERSON and ROTH (1981)."

Although the paragraph quoted is unclear, I suppose that the tandem duplication model works like this: One element of the duplication mutates. If the mutation is irrelevant for cell growth under the selective conditions, there is an even chance that the mutation will be retained when the duplication is lost (as it will be) by some recombinational process ("looping out," unequal crossing over, etc.). On the other hand, if the mutation causes the cell to grow, it is virtually certain that at least one cell in the resulting clone will retain the beneficial, mutated allele when the duplication is lost. That cell will be the progenitor of a stable, "directed" mutant clone. The degree of "direction," however, is only twofold, which is a smaller factor than is observed.

In order for a beneficial mutant to enjoy a stimulation that is 20-fold (for instance) greater than that for a neutral mutant, the number of copies in the amplified array must be 20. There will then be a 1-in-20 chance of preserving an irrelevant mutation when the tandem array is reduced to single copy, while a beneficial mutation will again be preserved with near certainty. Thus, a tandem duplication model *could* work, but the authors have not told us how 20 (or more) tandem copies could accumulate when there is no apparent selective advantage to such a monstrous aberrancy.

The reason that the tandem duplication model does not work well is that there is no property of the moieties of a tandem duplication that allows one copy to be treated differently from any other. However, by introducing the concept of DNA amplification, the model offered does suggest a model that *could* work. (Who knows, maybe CAIRNS and FOSTER had models like this one in mind, too.) Let the required DNA synthesis be "stable DNA replication" (DEMASSY, FAYET and KOGOMA 1984). This DNA synthesis, which appears to be primed here and there by scraps of RNA, is RecA-dependent (WITKIN and KOGOMA 1984). In starving cells, this synthesis will not go far, I suggest, and a full replication fork will not arise from the D-loop. The new chain will be sooner-or-later expelled from the D-loop and degraded. However, if a life-saving mutation arises during the DNA synthesis, it will ensure the wherewithal for turning the D-loop into a full fork, the cell will replicate, and the beneficial mutation will be saved. Voila!

This model (call it "The Toe in the Water Model") can explain most of the data offered in the literature as evidence for the reality of directed mutants. It cannot account, however, for HALL's (1991) claim of strongly correlated reversion of the two mutant sites of a double *trp* mutant. In view of the great difficulty of explaining those revertants by *any* model, it is probably best to reject the observation. In fact, the failure of HALL (1991) to report the results of controls that measure growth of single revertants in colonies of the double *trp* mutant means we needn't take *that* sighting of the unicorn seriously.

How did unicorns get into the act (STAHL 1988, 1990)? In defense of *Nature*'s investigation of analytical procedures in BENVENISTE's laboratory (DAVENAS *et al.* 1988), THE AMAZING RANDI said ". . . what would you do if I said 'I keep a unicorn in my back yard'?" (MADDOX, RANDI and STEWART 1988). RANDI may have been alluding to JAMES THURBER's delightful short story. My allusion was to RANDI's rhetorical question, which invited the answer, "I would climb over the fence to have a look!" I was inviting the readers of *Nature* to have a look at CAIRNS, OVERBAUGH and MILLER (1988), whose claims were counter to conventional wisdom, although not to fundamental scientific laws. The allusion might have been more widely understood if I had retained the final line from the penultimate draft of *A Unicorn in the Garden* (STAHL 1988). That line wondered how far CAIRNS,

OVERBAUGH and MILLER (1988) could dilute the lactose and still see a lactose-directed mutation. By that musing I meant to imply that the authors could expect a reception rather like that received by DAVENAS *et al.* because of the unconventionality of their claims. I did not mean that the work of CAIRNS, OVERBAUGH and MILLER was intrinsically unbelievable.

Some critics (*e.g.*, SMITH 1992) appear to be blindly skeptical of the demonstrations offered in support of the view that cells can mutate in a directed way. By failing to provide a proven (or even attractive) hypothesis, the recent work of FOSTER and CAIRNS (1992) is unlikely to quiet such detractors.

Discussions with JOHN CAIRNS, PAT FOSTER and with members of my laboratory, especially ANDY KUZMINOV, LENA KUZMINOVA, JIM SAWITZKE and RIK MYERS, helped shape this review.

LITERATURE CITED

ANDERSON, R. P., and J. R. ROTH, 1981 Spontaneous tandem genetic duplications in *Salmonella typhimurium* arise by unequal recombination between rRNA (*rrn*) cistrons. Proc. Natl. Acad. Sci. USA **78:** 3113–3117.

CAIRNS, J., and P. L. FOSTER, 1991 Adaptive reversion of a frameshift mutation in *Escherichia coli*. Genetics **128:** 695–701.

CAIRNS, J., J. OVERBAUGH and S. MILLER, 1988 The origin of mutants. Nature **335:** 142–145.

DAVENAS, E., F. BEAUVAIS, J. AMARA, M. OBERBAUM, B. ROBINZON, A. MIADONNA, A. TEDESCHI, B. POMERANZ, P. FORTNER, P. BELON, J. SAINTE-LAUDY, B. POITEVIN and J. BENVENISTE, 1988 Human basophil degranulation triggered by very dilute antiserum against IgE. Nature **333:** 816–818.

DEMASSEY, B., O. FAYET and T. KOGOMA, 1984 Multiple origin usage for DNA replication in *sdr* (*rnh*) mutants of *Escherichia coli* K12: initiation in the absence of *oriC*. J. Mol. Biol. **128:** 227–236.

DIMPFL, J., and H. ECHOLS, 1989 Duplication mutation as an SOS response in *Escherichia coli*: enhanced duplication formation by a constitutively activated RecA. Genetics **123:** 255–260.

FOSTER, P. L., and J. CAIRNS, 1992 Mechanisms of directed mutation. Genetics **131:** 783–789.

HALL, B. G., 1991 Adaptive evolution that requires multiple spontaneous mutations: mutations involving base substitutions. Proc. Natl. Acad. Sci. USA **88:** 5882–5886.

HALL, B. G., 1992 Selection-induced mutations occur in yeast. Proc. Natl. Acad. Sci. USA **89:** 4300–4303.

JAYARAMAN, R., 1992 Cairnsian mutagenesis in *E. coli*: genetic evidence for two pathways regulated by *mutS* and *mutL* genes. J. Genet. **71:** 23–41.

LARK, K. G., and C. A. LARK, 1979 *recA*-dependent DNA replication in the absence of protein synthesis: characteristics of a dominant lethal replication mutation, *dnaT*, and requirement for *recA*+ function. Cold Spring Harbor Symp. Quant. Biol. **43:** 537–549.

MADDOX, J., J. RANDI and W. W. STEWART, 1988 "High dilution" experiments a delusion. Nature **334:** 287–290.

SMITH, K. C., 1992 Spontaneous mutagenesis: experimental, genetic and other factors. Mutat. Res. **277:** 139–162.

STAHL, F. W., 1988 A unicorn in the garden. Nature **335:** 112–113.

STAHL, F. W., 1990 If it smells like a unicorn . . . . Nature **346:** 791.

STEELE, D. F., and S. JINKS-ROBERTSON, 1992 An examination of adaptive reversion in *Saccharomyces cerevisiae*. Genetics **132:** 9–21.

TLSTY, D. T., A. M. ALBERTINI and J. H. MILLER, 1984 Gene amplification in the *lac* region of *E. coli*. Cell **37:** 217–224.

WITKIN, E., and T. KOGOMA, 1984 Involvement of the activated form of RecA protein in SOS mutagenesis and stable DNA replication in *Escherichia coli*. Proc. Natl. Acad. Sci. USA **81:** 7539–7543.

Felix Bernstein
and the First Human Marker Locus

James F. Crow

Genetics Department, University of Wisconsin–Madison, Madison, Wisconsin 53706

ACCUSTOMED as we now are to thousands of polymorphisms useful as human chromosome markers, it is hard to realize that in the first quarter century of Mendelism there was only one good marker. It is all the more remarkable that its simple mode of inheritance was not understood until the trait had been known for 25 years.

The human blood groups were discovered at the turn of the century (LANDSTEINER 1900), the year of the rediscovery of MENDEL's laws. Two others, MOSS and JANSKY, independently designated the four groups I, II, III and IV. This was fine except that MOSS's I was JANSKY's IV, and vice versa, leading to considerable transfusion confusion in the early days. LANDSTEINER was astute enough to invent a nomenclature that reflected the A and B antigens (and genes), or their absence, and this gradually prevailed–*very* gradually in at least some benighted quarters, for I remember learning about the four groups I, II, III and IV in the 1930s.

It was quickly recognized that the blood groups were inherited and the first plausible hypothesis was put forth by VON DUNGERN and HIRZFELD (1910). Studying 72 families with 102 children, they hypothesized that the A and B antigens were produced by two independent dominant alleles (Table 1). The correct hypothesis of multiple alleles at one locus was not demonstrated until BERNSTEIN did so in 1924 and 1925.

Let O, A, B and AB stand for the proportions of the four types. On the prevailing two-locus hypothesis with Hardy-Weinberg proportions and linkage equilibrium it is clear that the expected frequency of O × AB equals that of A × B, for both are equal to $p_a^2 p_b^2 (1 - p_a^2)(1 - p_b^2)$. BERNSTEIN used the equivalent relationship $(A + AB)(B + AB) = AB$. Applied to the observed proportions in Table 1, the left-hand quantity is $(0.500)(0.284) = 0.142$, about twice the observed proportion of AB, 0.078.

BERNSTEIN, noting the discrepancy and impressed by the frequency of multiple alleles in Drosophila, tried the single-locus, three-allele hypothesis shown in Table 1. He noted that on this assumption

$$[1 - \sqrt{A + O}] + [1 - \sqrt{B + O}] + \sqrt{O}$$
$$= p_B + p_A + p_O = 1.$$

As before, this expectation is easily verified by plugging in the expected proportions. Using the observed proportions in Table 1, the three quantities on the left side are 0.154, 0.293, and 0.542, which add up to 0.989.

The agreement with the multiple-allele hypothesis is clearly much closer than with the two-locus model, and BERNSTEIN went on to perform statistical tests. He also found a simple way of estimating the allele frequencies that gave values very close to the maximum likelihood estimates. Instead of following BERNSTEIN's procedures, however, I'll examine the two hypotheses by the methods now widely used for linkage analysis. Following EDWARDS (1992, pp. 39–42), the $\log_e$ likelihood on the two-locus model is -647.5 and on the multiple allele model is -627.5. The difference is 20.0. More familiar to human geneticists is the $\log_{10}$ of the odds (or lod score), which is $(20.0)(\log_{10} e) = 8.7$, so that the likelihood ratio is about 5×10^8, overwhelming support for the multiple-allele alternative.

BERNSTEIN's 1925 paper includes a summary of the already enormous literature of blood group frequencies throughout the world. One population after another showed close agreement with the frequencies expected with three alleles and Hardy-Weinberg proportions. The example in Table 1 is a very small part of the data, a population of Japanese living in Korea.

Why was the earlier incorrect hypothesis so widely accepted from 1910 to 1924? There is a clear difference in the predictions of the two hypotheses when

TABLE 1

Two hypotheses of blood group inheritance

| Group | VON DUNGERN and HIRZFELD | | BERNSTEIN | | Observed proportion |
	Genotype	Expected proportion	Genotype	Expected proportion	
O	$aa\,bb$	$p_a^2\,p_b^2$	OO	p_O^2	0.294
A	$A-\,bb$	$(1 - p_a^2)p_b^2$	$AA,\,OA$	$p_A^2 + 2p_O p_A$	0.422
B	$aa\,B-$	$p_a^2\,(1 - p_b^2)$	$BB,\,OB$	$p_B^2 + 2p_O p_B$	0.206
AB	$A-\,B-$	$(1 - p_a^2)(1 - p_b^2)$	AB	$2p_A p_B$	0.078
Total		1		1	1.000

The expected proportions assume Hardy-Weinberg ratios and linkage equilibrium. The observed proportions are from 502 Japanese (BERNSTEIN 1925).

one parent is AB. O children may be produced on the two-locus model (if the AB parent is doubly heterozygous), but not on the correct triallelic model. Such children actually were found. In WIENER's (1943) summary of the published data for the years 1924–1932 there were 10 such exceptions among 3205 children. These are now ascribed to errors in typing or misattributed paternity, but were once regarded as supporting the two-locus theory. (Earlier data, when methods were not well established, included a larger fraction of such exceptions.) The ease with which the correct answer was reached, using only population frequencies and simple assumptions, shows the power of BERNSTEIN's population genetic analysis. It is surprising that no one did this earlier, for the Hardy-Weinberg relationship and multiple alleles had been well known for a decade. I suspect that World War I was one cause.

FELIX BERNSTEIN, 1878–1956: FELIX BERNSTEIN was remarkable for his originality, his wide ranging interests, and his skills in both pure and applied mathematics. His grandfather, ARON BERNSTEIN (1812–1884), was a well known and multi-talented writer on, among other things, science and politics. When ALBERT EINSTEIN was a young man he was given one of BERNSTEIN's science books and became so fascinated that he gave up the idea of becoming a violinist in favor of science. If the stories about EINSTEIN's fiddle playing are correct, this was a salutary decision for both physics and music.

FELIX BERNSTEIN was born on February 24, 1878, in Halle, Germany, and spent his childhood and youth there. He was given the name FELIX because his mother, who composed music and was an accomplished pianist, hoped he would be a musician and named him after FELIX MENDELSSOHN. Music, however, was about the only field in which he did not become interested. His artistic love was painting and sculpture.

BERNSTEIN's becoming a mathematician is a fascinating story involving an improbable and fortunate coincidence. His father, JULIUS BERNSTEIN, was a

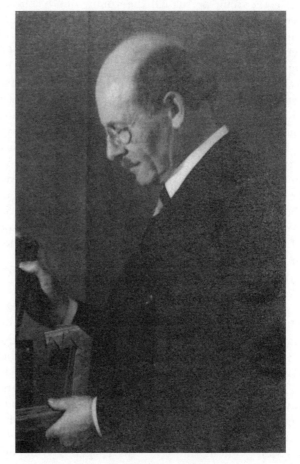

FELIX BERNSTEIN (1933)

friend of the mathematician GEORG CANTOR, and FELIX, while still in gymnasium in Halle, attended CANTOR's seminar. It was his good fortune to be introduced to set theory before the subject became popular.

In 1896 CANTOR took a holiday and left some proofs that young BERNSTEIN had volunteered to correct. As he was correcting the proofs, BERNSTEIN (while shaving, the story goes) thought of a proof of a theorem that CANTOR had been wrestling with and had been unable to prove to his satisfaction (NATHAN 1981). This "equivalence theorem of two sets" states that if each of two sets, A and B, is equivalent to a subset of the other, then A is equivalent to B. This has become a central theorem of set theory, first proved by this 18-year-old. For a contemporary discussion and proof, see STOLL (1963, p. 80*ff*). CANTOR was much impressed by the proof and communicated it to BOREL for the First International Mathematical Congress in Zurich. Meanwhile, BERNSTEIN, having finished his schooling in Halle, became a student of fine arts in Pisa, where he studied philosophy, archeology, and art history. His sister was an artist and studied with MATISSE. While he was at Pisa, two mathematicians there who had heard CANTOR discussing the equivalence theorem, persuaded the young BERNSTEIN to become a mathematician. He then went to Göttingen, where he was one of HILBERT's first doctorates and received his degree in 1901. He had a distinguished career in mathematics and showed his versatility by writing on a wide variety of mathematical topics. He retained his interest in art, though, spent many hours in museums and galleries, and entertained his family and friends by constructing statues of modeling clay.

He also had an interest in applied mathematics. After some years in Halle, he was appointed to Göttingen as Associate Professor of Mathematical Statistics in 1911. From 1921 to 1933 he was director of the Institute of Mathematical Statistics. After World War I he was head of the statistical branch of the office of rationing and in 1921 became Commissioner of Finance.

In 1928 BERNSTEIN came to the United States to work on epidemiology at Harvard, and during the next few years he had several visiting positions. In 1933 and 1934, having been dismissed from his position at Göttingen, he brought his family to this country. For a while he was guest professor at Columbia University. The anthropologist, FRANZ BOAS, had obtained a grant to support him for a year, with the understanding that Columbia would then hire him permanently. But Columbia never made good on this verbal commitment, and for the year 1945–1946 he was left without support. This elicited a comment from his friend, R. A. FISHER: "But Bernstein, why did you not come to England. In England, a handshake from a gentleman is as good as a signed contract." (Later, in 1954, FISHER happily wrote to inform BERNSTEIN of his election as an honorary fellow of the Royal Statistical Society.) From 1946 to 1949 he taught mathematics at Triple Cities College, now part of SUNY-Binghamton. On the hundredth anniversary of his birth, in 1978, the Department of Mathematical Sciences there announced the "Felix Bernstein Teaching Assistantship" in honor of this "pioneer in the development of mathematical set theory . . . and world renowned statistician and pioneer in the field of population genetics." He eventually returned to

Europe, spending time in Göttingen, Rome, and Freiburg, and died in Zurich on December 3, 1956.

The biography by FREWER (1981) lists 128 articles on an astonishing variety of subjects, including mathematics (set theory, convex functions, the Laplace transform, number theory, differential equations, Fermat's last theorem, the Fourier integral, mathematical statistics), economics, anthropology, tuberculosis therapy, human life span, assessing aging from eye lens refraction, polio, age and cancer, and, of course, genetics.

BERNSTEIN was a long-time close friend of EINSTEIN, starting in the 1910s in Germany and continuing throughout their lives (which ended at about the same time). Because of his involvement in pensions and insurance in Germany, he promoted attempts to establish unemployment insurance in the United States. He and Einstein also found positions for displaced European scholars in the 1930s.

Other contributions to genetics: BERNSTEIN's interest in genetics, if we can judge from his publications, began in the early 1920s. An early study (BERNSTEIN 1922a) involved the analysis of multiple factors in quantitative traits. In the same year (1922b) he published an amusing theory for inheritance of voice range, the first suggestion of inheritance of a sex-influenced character in man. He hypothesized a reverse sex-dependence such that bass and soprano represent one homozygous type, tenor and alto the other, and baritones and mezzo-soprano the heterozygotes. This idea has now been forgotten but I remember hearing it as a student.

BERNSTEIN's major contribution was blood group inheritance and he wrote extensively on this subject. Having found a marker, he naturally become interested in using it for linkage studies, and invented a way to get around the problem that in man the linkage phase is usually not known. For example, in a series of sibships from the mating $Aa\ Bb \times aa\ bb$, how do we measure recombination when the recombinant phenotypes under one linkage phase are the nonrecombinants with the other? BERNSTEIN (1931a) cleverly invented the statistic $y = (Aa\ Bb + aa\ bb)(Aa\ bb + aa\ Bb)$, the value of which depends on the degree of linkage but not on the linkage phase (nor does it require that the linkage phases be equally frequent). He prepared a series of tables of the expected value of y for different values of the recombination fraction and sibship size, with which the data could be compared. This method has been superseded by a series of advances starting with FISHER and leading to current computer-dependent likelihood ratio methods.

BERNSTEIN (1930) also considered the effects of consanguinity on Hardy-Weinberg expectations, particularly in the blood groups. His α is equivalent to WRIGHT's F. He discussed, as others did, the approach to linkage equilibrium under random mating.

He was the first to apply a mixture formula to determine the ancestry of racially mixed populations. If q_1, q_2 and q_m are the allele frequencies in the two parental populations and the mixed group, then the proportional contribution of the first population to the mixture is $M = (q_m - q_1)/(q_2 - q_1)$. This simple formula has been widely applied.

One of his major developments was a method of correcting for ascertainment bias in testing Mendelian ratios. When, for example, parents heterozygous for a recessive disease are ascertained through affected children, those heterozygous parents who happen to have no affected children are missed and the Mendelian ratio is distorted. BERNSTEIN worked out a procedure for correcting this error and testing the significance of the departure from Mendelian expectations when such a correction is made. This was presented as an alternative and compared to WEINBERG's sib method (BERNSTEIN 1931b). Better procedures were later developed by HALDANE, FISHER, MORTON, and others, so BERNSTEIN's work is now mainly of historical interest.

BERNSTEIN and WEINBERG were the two leaders in developing techniques for human genetic study, not only in Germany but throughout the world. The contrast in their backgrounds is striking. Both had other interests. While BERNSTEIN was a mathematician, WEINBERG was a busy obstetrician who somehow found time to think about human genetics. Yet each in his own way had a knack for finding ways to solve problems that are trivially easy in experimental plants and animals, but that called for a touch of genius in that genetically refractory species, *Homo sapiens*. This, of course, was long before molecular markers, computers, and CEPH families made things easier.

Final remark: I hope that someone will take advantage of BERNSTEIN's abundant published record to do a much more thorough study of this multifaceted man. His professional and personal relations with WEINBERG should be of great interest. Among other things, his correspondence with EINSTEIN, located at Boston University, is a gold mine.

FELIX BERNSTEIN, like so many German Jewish scientists, had his career disrupted by Nazi politics. Undoubtedly his life would have been quite different had history taken a different course and had he been able to spend his life in the cultural environment that

Göttingen supplied before the 1930s. As judged by number of published papers, his research productivity decreased greatly after his move to the United States. I suspect that this was caused, at least partially, by the necessity of moving from one temporary position to another. And, as I said, he spent a great deal of effort, often in collaboration with EINSTEIN, in social causes and in finding positions for other displaced European scientists. In one poignant note he asked that his name not be revealed in this context to protect his relatives still in Germany. Alas, they perished anyhow.

I am deeply indebted to MARIANNE BERNSTEIN-WIENER, who has generously supplied me with an abundance of personal information about her father.

LITERATURE CITED

BERNSTEIN, F., 1922a Die Theorie der gleichsinnigen Faktoren in der Mendelishen Erblichkeitslehre vom Standpunkt der mathematischen Statistik. Z. Indukt. Abstammungs. Vererbungsl. **28:** 295–323.

BERNSTEIN, F., 1922b Über die Tonlage der menschlichen Singstimme. Ein Betrag zur Statistik der sekundären Geschlechtsmerkmale beim Menschen. Sber. preuss. Akad. Wiss. Phys.-Math. Kl., pp. 30–37.

BERNSTEIN, F., 1924 Ergebnisse einer biostatistischen zusammenfassenden Betrachtung über die erblichen Blutstructuren des Menschen. Klin. Wochenschr. **3:** 1495–1567.

BERNSTEIN, F., 1925 Zusammenfassende Betrachtungen über die erblichen Blutstrukturen des Menschen. Z. Indukt. Abstammungs. Vererbungsl. **37:** 237–370.

BERNSTEIN, F., 1930 Fortgesetzte Untersuchungen aus der Theorie der Blutgruppen. Z. Indukt. Abstammungs. Vererbungsl. **56:** 233–273.

BERNSTEIN, F., 1931a Zur Grundlegung der Chromosomentheorie der Vererbung beim Menschen. Z. Indukt. Abstammungs. Vererbungsl. **57:** 113–138.

BERNSTEIN, F., 1931b Ist die Weinbersche Geschwistermethode neben der direkten Methode von Nutzen? Z. Indukt. Abstammungs. Vererbungsl. **58:** 434–437.

EDWARDS, A. W. F., 1992 *Likelihood*, Expanded Edition. Johns Hopkins Press, Baltimore.

FREWER, M., 1981 Felix Bernstein. Jahresber. Deut. Math. Verein. **83:** 84–95.

LANDSTEINER, K., 1900 Zur Kenntnis der antifermentative, lytischen und agglutinierenden Wirkungen des Blutserums der Lymphe. Zentralbl. Bakteriol. **27:** 357–362.

NATHAN, H., 1981 Felix Bernstein, pp. 58–59 in *Dictionary of Scientific Biography*. Charles Scribners Sons, New York.

STOLL, R. R., 1963 *Set Theory and Logic*. Dover, New York.

VON DUNGERN, E., and L. HIRZFELD, 1910 Über vererbung gruppenspezifischer Strukturen des Blutes. Zeits. Immunitätsforsch. **6:** 284–292.

WIENER, A. S., 1943 *Blood Groups and Transfusion*, Ed. 3. Charles C Thomas, Baltimore.

February 1993

Quantitative Genetics in Edinburgh
1947-1980

Douglas Falconer

Institute of Cell, Animal and Population Biology, University of Edinburgh, West Mains Road, Edinburgh, EH9 3JT, Scotland

FOOD rationing in the second world war brought home to everyone in Britain the need to improve agricultural output in order to reduce our dependence on imports. Seeing clearly the need for more government-funded research on animal breeding, the Agricultural Research Council (ARC) set up, in 1945, the Animal Breeding and Genetics Research Organization (ABGRO). The "Genetics" in the title signified the intention to pursue basic genetics with experimentation on laboratory animals, to be done by the Genetics Section of ABGRO. R. G. WHITE, then Professor of Agriculture in the University of North Wales at Bangor, was appointed Director, with C. H. WADDINGTON as Chief Geneticist in charge of the Genetics Section. WADDINGTON, then aged 42, was preeminent among the few geneticists in Britain at that time; his influential text, *An Introduction to Modern Genetics*, had been published in 1939. Soon after his appointment to ABGRO, WADDINGTON was offered the Buchanan Chair of Animal Genetics in the University of Edinburgh in succession to F. A. E. CREW. This was the reason it was decided to locate ABGRO in Edinburgh. WADDINGTON then held both positions, University Professor and Honorary Director of the Genetics Section of ABGRO.

The Genetics Section, which had been in temporary quarters in London, moved to Edinburgh in 1947. It was housed together with the University Department in a building named the Institute of Animal Genetics. The main part of ABGRO was accommodated in a large rented villa not far away until a new building on the University campus close to the Institute was opened in 1964.

The location of ABGRO in Edinburgh continued a distinguished tradition of animal breeding and genetics there. There were then (I think) only three university departments of genetics in the United Kingdom: London's University College (where J. B. S. HALDANE was Professor), Cambridge (with R. A.

FISHER), and Edinburgh (with F. A. E. CREW). Edinburgh's department was the first, established in 1919 as the Animal Breeding Research Department, with CREW as its Director but no other staff and no building. A forceful and persuasive speaker, CREW obtained money from various sources to expand the department, and he cajoled several wealthy industrialists into providing funds for a new building and to endow a chair. The Chair, founded in 1928 with CREW as its first occupant, was called the Buchanan Chair after Lord WOOLAVINGTON whose family name was Buchanan and whose business was whisky distilling; half the funds needed for the endowment were his gift. The title of the Chair was Animal Genetics, but it was changed to Genetics in WADDINGTON's time. The new building was formally opened in 1930 with 12 scientific staff and 13 visiting researchers.

CREW's enthusiasm attracted many visitors who came for short visits or for longer periods of research, among whom were some notable figures–LANCELOT HOGBEN, JULIAN HUXLEY, J. B. S. HALDANE, and H. J. MULLER (who was there from 1938 to 1940). On a handsome oak panel in the entrance hall of the Institute building in gilded carved letters are the names of those who obtained higher degrees from the Department. There are 66 up to 1947, and 5 more by 1950 when the inscriptions stopped. The first is CREW himself who is recorded as obtaining a D.Sc. in 1921 and a Ph.D. in 1923. Others who will be familiar to most geneticists are F. B. HUTT (Ph.D. 1929, D.Sc. 1939), CHARLOTTE AUERBACH (Ph.D. 1935, D.Sc. 1947), and H. J. MULLER (D.Sc. 1940).

Under CREW's leadership the Institute did pioneering work on sex determination, reproductive physiology, and many aspects of the husbandry and breeding of sheep, cattle, pigs, horses, and poultry. There was also work on cytology, on Drosophila genetics, and on the genetics of the color of budgerigars. (When I was a Ph.D. student in the Zoology Department in

Cambridge I found a set of CREW's budgerigar skins hidden away in a drawer. They made an impressive and beautiful illustration of all the main Mendelian principles, and were a major stimulus to my own interest in genetics.) CREW's era culminated in the holding of the Seventh International Congress of Genetics in Edinburgh in August, 1939. He was made President in default of N. VAVILOV who was unable to come (see the *Perspectives* of August, 1992). The outbreak of the second world war brought the Congress and most of the Institute's activities to an abrupt end. During the war CREW, who had a medical degree, worked in the War Office on medical statistics. He resigned his Chair in 1944 because, so he said, he felt himself to be too much out of date in genetics, but he returned to Edinburgh to take up the Chair of Public Health and Social Medicine.

When the ARC group came to Edinburgh after the war, CREW's Institute was much depleted in staff and funds. Soon after arrival in Edinburgh one of our technical staff, not renowned for his tact, found himself sitting next to an unknown person at coffee and, thinking that some conversation was called for, remarked, "I understand that this place has been pretty inactive recently." The unknown person was A. W. F. GREENWOOD who had been acting Director during CREW's absence. It is no wonder that those left of CREW's staff saw us newcomers as an arrogant lot intent on an aggressive take-over. I fear that at first we were a sore trial to them.

The ARC funded agricultural research in two main ways. There were large groups in their own buildings with a full-time director appointed by the ARC, and there were "units" which were small groups working in a university department under the direction of a senior member of the university staff, usually the professor. ABGRO was a large group, but the Genetics Section operated like a unit within it; its members were ABGRO staff but WADDINGTON, its director, was not. This anomalous situation was rectified in 1951 when H. P. DONALD, who had been in CREW's department, succeeded WHITE as Director of ABGRO. The Genetics Section was then formally separated; ABGRO lost its G and became ABRO. In 1957 the Genetics Section was designated the Unit of Animal Genetics.

In what follows I shall not discriminate between the Genetics Section and the Unit, and will refer to both as the Unit. It is about the Unit that I am writing here and I will not be able in this short article to say more about ABRO, though there was much fruitful collaboration between the members of the two groups, and the work of ABRO was a large component of quantitative genetics in Edinburgh.

To review adequately the work of the Unit would be impossible. Instead I shall summarize briefly the

earlier work done by its members. Those in the Unit at the beginning in 1947 who worked on quantitative genetics and related topics were the following:

C. H. WADDINGTON. His many diverse interests centered on developmental genetics. In quantitative genetics, he showed with Drosophila how what looked superficially like Lamarckian inheritance of an acquired character could result from straightforward selection.

ALAN ROBERTSON. With J. M. RENDEL he formulated improvement programs for dairy cattle, and the "contemporary comparison" by which bulls are selected for use in artificial insemination, which revolutionized dairy cattle breeding. His experiments with Drosophila tested the adequacy of current selection theory and located some of the genes responsible for the responses to selection, foreshadowing contemporary quantitative marker identification. Using KIMURA's stochastic theory, he developed a new theory of selection limits in a finite population.

J. M. RENDEL. After working with ROBERTSON on dairy cattle, he left in 1951 to join CSIRO in Australia and became head of its genetics section. He is well known for his work on developmental canalization in Drosophila.

D. S. FALCONER. I showed that selection for growth in mice was most effective when practiced in the environment in which the strain was expected to perform (as opposed to the frequently advocated practice of selecting in the most favorable environment), and that a character measured in two environments could be treated as two correlated characters. I introduced the use of realized heritability as a way of describing selection response.

R. A. BEATTY. In addition to studies of heteroploidy in mice and rabbits, he studied the genetics of spermatozoa, showing that metric characters of spermatozoa are determined by the genotype of the testis and not that of the spermatozoa.

F. W. ROBERTSON. In selecting for large and small body size in Drosophila he found strong asymmetry in the response to selection in the two directions, and showed that at the selection limit there was still considerable genetic variation. Chromosome assays of selected lines revealed strong epistatic interaction. Differences of body size were due to differences of cell number, not cell size. Later he worked on the ecological and physiological genetics of Drosophila growth. In 1970 he left for a chair in Aberdeen University.

E. C. R. REEVE. He worked with F. W. ROBERTSON on selection in Drosophila and showed that inbred lines were considerably more variable than F_1 hybrids. Later he worked on bacterial genetics.

J. H. SANG. He studied population growth of Drosophila in culture, and developed a synthetic culture medium which became an essential tool for physiological genetics. He left for a Chair in the University of Sussex in 1965.

Some later appointments in quantitative genetics were:

N. BATEMAN (1948). He selected for high and low milk production in mice and found very strong asymmetry of response. He transferred to ABRO in 1957.

I. L. MASON (1949). He studied dual-purpose cattle and advised on animal breeding programs in many countries. He cataloged the origins and characteristics of all livestock breeds. In 1972 he left to join FAO in Rome.

G. A. CLAYTON (1950). He worked with A. ROBERTSON on Drosophila selection and fitness experiments. They were, I think, the first to select with replicate lines and to test the observed responses against theoretical predictions. He also worked on turkey breeding. He transferred to the University staff in 1959.

A. L. MCLAREN (1958). She studied maternal effects, embryo transfer, early development, reproductive physiology, and chimeras in mice. In 1974 she left to be Director of the Medical Research Council's new Mammalian Development Unit in London.

R. C. ROBERTS (1959). He compared the life-time growth and reproduction of mouse lines selected for large and small body size and found that small mice had smaller litters, but more of them, than large mice, and produced nearly twice as many offspring in total. He characterized selected mouse lines using A. ROBERTSON's theory of selection limits.

W. G. HILL, who was appointed to the University staff in 1965, must be included here because he worked in close association with the Unit. His work covered many aspects of theoretical quantitative genetics, particularly in relation to selection and the estimation of parameters.

It was never the intention that the work of the Unit should be restricted to quantitative genetics. WADDINGTON believed, as CREW had, that any aspect of genetics might lead to advances in animal breeding. Accordingly there were other members of the Unit working on molecular genetics, cytology, development, and systematics, among whom were H. G. CALLAN who went to a chair at St. Andrews University in 1950 and J. L. SIRLIN from about 1962 to 1970.

We were generously provided with excellent technical assistance. A great advantage of working in the ARC. Unit was that funding was always assured; we did not have to spend time writing grant applications.

By the 1940s, partly because of the war, Britain had fallen far behind the United States in quantitative genetics and the theory underlying animal breeding. In the United States, J. L. LUSH's *Animal Breeding Plans* had been published in 1937, but the principles

it set forth were virtually unknown in the United Kingdom despite the presence of HALDANE and FISHER who had provided much of the mathematical background. There were few geneticists of any sort, and they tended to be regarded as eccentrics pursuing an incomprehensible subject. Consequently little or no genetics was taught in undergraduate courses. Most of us, therefore, joined the Unit with very little background in genetics. For example, the nearest thing to genetics in my zoology course at St. Andrews was the curious fact that Ascaris sheds most of its chromatin when it makes somatic cells. Some of us had not even a biological background; ALAN ROBERTSON started as a physical chemist, and REEVE as a mathematician. After joining the unit, however, ROBERTSON spent nine months with SEWALL WRIGHT and J. L. LUSH, the two who had done most to develop quantitative genetics in its application to animal breeding. Consequently, he was much better informed about quantitative genetics and animal breeding than the rest of us. In preparation for joining the Unit I spent 18 months with R. A. FISHER in Cambridge in order to learn about mouse genetics. FISHER was then mainly interested in linkage, and I did not learn much about quantitative genetics from him.

The original intention for the work on quantitative genetics was that there should be research on farm animals (but without farm facilities), on rabbits, on mice, and on Drosophila. The basic quantitative genetics would be done with Drosophila because it is cheap and quick. But the results from Drosophila could not be applied directly to farm animals because Drosophila is too different in physiology, in chromosome number, and in lacking crossing over in males. The rabbits and mice were to form a bridge, being similar in physiology, chromosome number, and male crossing over. Any breeding method that might be based on the Drosophila results would be tried with mice or rabbits and if it worked it could be applied with more confidence to farm animals. It soon became apparent, however, that there was no great difference in the quantitative genetics of Drosophila and mice. So the chromosome number, male crossing over, and indeed the physiology, were largely irrelevant.

No one "directed" our work. The ARC itself seemed to take no interest in what we did, or what we achieved. WADDINGTON, nominally our director, left us free to do what we each thought best. This was a wise policy, and it worked; I do not think that any of us wasted much time in doing the wrong things. And the freedom was greatly appreciated.

The first experiments done with Drosophila and mice were on selection. These take a long time, and when they finally produced results we were eager to publish them quickly. But in this we were frustrated. We sent the papers to the *Journal of Genetics*, the oldest of the two British journals publishing genetical work. It was owned and edited by J. B. S. HALDANE, who did the refereeing himself. But he was not well organized. It was said that when he was away for some time the cleaners, unwilling to disturb the piles of paper on his tables, covered them over with newspapers. When he returned he did not remove the papers, but started again on top. This was very useful to the geologists who, when HALDANE was away, took their students to his room to demonstrate stratification. It required several pleading letters of reminder before we eventually got our papers published. Continued difficulties with publication in British journals led WADDINGTON to found a new journal, *Genetical Research*, in 1960. Edited by E. C. R. REEVE, it has flourished and earned a high reputation.

In 1948 I. M. LERNER, a visitor from California, brought us new techniques from the United States. He unfolded the mystery of SEWALL WRIGHT's path coefficients, which were being used for deducing the necessary theoretical parameters for quantitative breeding. LERNER wrote most of his *Population Genetics and Animal Improvement*, published in 1950, while he was in Edinburgh. An important event in 1949 was a visit by SEWALL WRIGHT who also spent a sabbatical year in Edinburgh. I think, however, that his visit came too soon for some of us who did not have enough background to understand much of what he had to teach us, though it was a useful stimulus in showing us what a long way we had to go to catch up with current knowledge. He gave a long course of lectures and these formed the basis for part of his *Evolution and the Genetics of Populations*, the first volume of which was published in 1968.

In 1950, near the end of WRIGHT's visit, a symposium on quantitative inheritance was held in the Institute; it was published in 1952. WRIGHT gave a lengthy talk on the interactions between coat color genes in guinea pigs. But the manuscript was lost on his way home and a quite different paper appeared in the published symposium. It was a synopsis of the current state of quantitative genetics and was surely more generally useful than the guinea pig paper would have been. The symposium, however, had unforeseen and regrettable consequences of a political nature. KENNETH MATHER, then Professor of Genetics in Birmingham, was invited and talked about his chromosome-balance theory of quantitative inheritance. This asserted that + and − genes (those increasing and decreasing the trait) are arranged in repulsion linkages. The net effect of a chromosome is minimal but it holds a large amount of hidden variation that can be released by recombination. His theory was not well received by the audience and he was criticized in a forthright but injudicious manner. MATHER, as a guest speaker considerably senior to us, was understandably

affronted. I believe that the cool relationship between the Birmingham and Edinburgh schools that persisted for many years may have had its origin in this unfortunate episode.

The members of the ARC Unit, though ostensibly employed for research, contributed substantially to the Department's teaching. In respect of what we actually did in the Institute, there was little distinction between Unit and University staff, and those not familiar with the local arrangements often did not know to which group anyone belonged. The University authorities, however, were slow to recognize the existence of non-University staff and subjected us to petty restrictions. For example, we could not be official supervisors of Ph.D. students; there had to be a University supervisor, usually WADDINGTON who often knew little or nothing of what the student was doing. Eventually, however, the authorities were persuaded to be less narrow-minded. In 1949 a postgraduate Diploma in Genetics was started, allowing students with little previous training in genetics to embark on Ph.D. studies; it had a substantial component of quantitative genetics. Then, in 1975, an M.Sc. in animal breeding was started in collaboration with the Agriculture Department and was run by W. G. HILL, who had worked on animal breeding and had become a leading theorist in quantitative and population genetics. This was the only course of its kind in the United Kingdom. It attracted students (about six each year) from all over the world, many of whom went on to take Ph.D.s in Edinburgh and then went home to found nuclei of quantitative genetics or animal breeding in their own countries, notably in Australia and New Zealand. Not surprisingly, many of the staff of ABRO or its successor organization were recruited from among our students.

The Institute housed much more than just the ARC Unit. WADDINGTON rapidly increased the staff and the range of research, and there were several groups of workers with separate funding. The following is a very incomplete outline of the research staff of the Institute in the early 1960s, when the numbers were probably near their peak. The Unit then had nine staff members, and the University 13, among whom were the following. CHARLOTTE AUERBACH had been a research assistant to CREW; during the second world war she discovered the first chemical mutagen, mustard gas, and opened up a whole new field of research. G. H. BEALE worked on Paramecium, and later developed the new field of the genetics of the malarial parasite. H. KACSER studied the genetics and enzymology of metabolic pathways. B. WOOLF helped many people with his statistical advice, and was the originator of the idea of realized heritability. W. G. HILL's work has already been outlined. A later addition was D. J. BOND, who worked on fungal development.

From 1947 till 1955 there was a group of four, funded by the Medical Research Council (MRC), working on the mutagenic effects of radiation on mice. This was an outpost of the MRC's Radiobiology Research Unit at Harwell in Oxfordshire. Among its members were T. C. CARTER, who later became director of the ARC's Poultry Research Center, and M. F. LYON, known for her work on X inactivation and the *t* locus in mice. Then, in 1958, the MRC set up another group, the Mutagenesis Research Unit, of which AUERBACH was director. It had five members among whom were B. M. CATTANACH and B. J. KILBY. And finally, in 1963, the MRC founded the Epigenetics Research Group under WADDINGTON's direction with M. BIRNSTIEL as his deputy. There were initially four MRC staff in the group, but others with different funding worked in the group, among whom were K. W. JONES and, from the University staff, J. O. BISHOP, R. M. CLAYTON, J. JACOB, A. JURAND and G. G. SELMAN. The group worked on development and molecular genetics.

WADDINGTON was an inveterate traveler and was widely known throughout the world. His interests were wide-ranging, and not only in science. Among his 17 books was a lavishly illustrated one showing how modern art had been influenced by the ideas of science (WADDINGTON 1969). WADDINGTON's breadth of interests, and the reputation of the Institute, attracted many visiting research workers and Ph.D. students, so that there were usually more visitors than indigenous staff. New people seemed to be arriving almost every day and it was hard to keep track of who was who and doing what. An idea of the numbers can be got from a list of people present in June, 1962. There were 22 permanent staff and 36 temporary research workers. The visitors came from 13 different counties in addition to the United Kingdom. Their fields of work are recorded as: development (12), quantitative genetics and animal breeding (10), mutation (7), Paramecium (4) Neurospora (2), and gametes (1). With so many people of such diverse interests the Institute was a lively and stimulating place. It was a great privilege to work there during that time. Naturally, lots of papers were published. In the period 1961–1965 there were an average of 85 papers and 8 Ph.D. theses per year.

Meeting for coffee in the canteen was an important activity which kept staff and visitors in touch with each other. Some might say that this was a waste of research time, but it was not; often we got valuable ideas and advice. At first nearly everyone came, but later, as we got to know each other, the meetings broke up into specialist groups. Of these, ALAN ROBERTSON's coffee sessions became world famous and continued until his final illness. He died in 1989; his personality and wisdom are greatly missed.

Did WADDINGTON keep in touch with all the many staff and visitors? With the permanent staff he did, to some degree. We in the Unit seldom had any conversation with him, yet he often surprised us by knowing what we were doing and what we had found. He did this mainly, he said, by reading our papers. Of most of the visitors, however, he knew very little. It was not unknown for a visitor to have spent three years in the Institute and never to have spoken to him. Many of the Ph.D. students came expecting to work under WADDINGTON's supervision. But often he was away on his travels, and then the rest of us had to come to the rescue, hastily think up suitable projects, and find space and facilities for them.

Although WADDINGTON seemed to take little day-to-day interest in what we did, he took great pride in the achievements of his staff. He was immensely proud of the fact that in 1975 there were five Fellows of the Royal Society among the Institute staff (WADDINGTON, AUERBACH, BEALE, A. ROBERTSON, FALCONER) with a sixth (MCLAREN) being elected shortly after leaving. HILL was elected after WADDINGTON had died. This was out of a total of about 19 in the whole University and it elicited an article by a columnist in a newspaper (TAYLOR 1975) in praise of the Institute.

Most organizations go through a cycle of growth and decline. The Institute was no exception. There were three reasons why it grew the way it did: first, and most important, WADDINGTON's drive to expand; second, the ready availability of funds at the time; and third, good fortune in the selection of staff. It reached the peak of its activities in the late 1960s and then started a gradual decline, for which I can see several reasons. Possibly the prime reason was that WADDINGTON's interests moved from genetics and the Institute to futurology. In 1970 he went for two years to the Center for Theoretical Biology at Buffalo, and when he returned he set up a new "School of the Man-Made Future" in the University. In consequence he was seldom seen in the Institute from then till his death in 1975. Fewer visitors came. Interest in most areas of research was shifting to the more molecular. Embryo transfer and, later, the prospect of transgenic animals made classical quantitative genetics of less interest to animal breeding. Working in Edinburgh had been so attractive that few staff members had moved elsewhere. Consequently most of us were of an age when change becomes difficult. Funds were increasingly hard to get and, in the absence of new posts, very few young people could be recruited to rejuvenate the Institute.

To complete the history: before he went to Buffalo WADDINGTON wanted to shed his responsibilities in the Institute and in 1968 he resigned as Director of the Unit. I was made Director in his place and at the same time was transferred to the University Department in a personal chair; a year later I was made head of the Department and held this position until J. R. S. FINCHAM came to the Buchanan Chair in 1977. T. F. C. MACKAY joined the Department in 1980 when I retired. ARC Units are normally terminated when their directors retire. That our unit survived a change of director may have been due partly to its beginning as part of ABGRO and partly to the ARC's difficulty in finding new posts for its members. It did not, however, survive my retirement. By then most of its members had left or retired, and the Unit was finally terminated in 1980. Very fortunately W. G. HILL was on the University staff and was not directly affected by the closure of the Unit. A new cycle of quantitative genetics has started under his leadership, with a new and strong group.

I am very grateful indeed to R. C. ROBERTS and W. G. HILL for reading the drafts and offering many helpful suggestions, and to B. JAMIESON of the AFRC (formerly the ARC) for supplying some dates. I ask forgiveness of any of my colleagues who find errors, omissions, or misunderstandings.

LITERATURE CITED

LUSH, J. L., 1937 *Animal Breeding Plans*, Ed. 3. Iowa State College Press, Ames, Ia.

TAYLOR, W., 1975 More jolly good fellows; a Scotsman's log. *The Scotsman*, Edinburgh, 17 April.

WADDINGTON, C. H., 1939 An *Introduction to Modern Genetics*. Allen & Unwin, London.

WADDINGTON, C. H., 1969 *Behind Appearance*. Edinburgh University Press, Edinburgh.

SOURCES

Anonymous, 1950 Research in animal breeding and quantitative genetics. A review of work in progress at the Institute of Animal Genetics, Edinburgh. Anim. Breed. Abstr. **18:** 347–357.

CREW, F. A. E., 1971 The genealogy of the Poultry Research Centre, Edinburgh. Br. Poult. Sci. **12:** 289–295.

FALCONER, D. S., 1977 Conrad Hal Waddington. Yearb. R. Soc. Edinb., pp. 58–60.

HILL, W. G., 1990 Alan Robertson. Biogr. Mem. Fellows R. Soc. **36:** 465–488.

HOGBEN, L., 1974 Francis Albert Eley Crew. Biogr. Mem. Fellows R. Soc. **20:** 135–153.

PUNNETT, R. C. (Editor), 1939 *Procedings of the VII International Congress of Genetetics*. Cambridge University Press, Cambridge.

ROBERTSON, A., 1977 Conrad Hal Waddington. Bibliogr. Mem. Fellows R. Soc. **23:** 575–622.

ROBERTSON, F. W., 1983 Genetics (in *Two Hundred Years of the Biological Sciences in Scotland*). Proc. R. Soc. Edinb. **84B:** 211–229.

WADDINGTON, C. H., 1973 Professor F. A. E. Crew. *The Times*, London, 2 June.

WADDINGTON, C. H., and T. L. MASON, 1951 Institute of Animal Genetics Edinburgh. Research **4:** 315–319.

UNPUBLISHED

DEACON, MARGARET (undated) The Institute of Animal Genetics at Edinburgh–The First Twenty Years.

Institute of Animal Genetics, University of Edinburgh, Research Reports. Five quinquennial reports for the years 1947 to 1965.

MASON, I. L., 1950 The History and Work of the Institute of Animal Genetics, Edinburgh.

March 1993

Thirty Years Ago in *Genetics*
Prophage Insertion into Bacterial Chromosomes

Allan M. Campbell

Department of Biological Sciences, Stanford University, Stanford, California 94305

OVER 30 years ago, a model for insertion of λ prophage into the host chromosome during lysogenization was first proposed (CAMPBELL 1961a). The model was developed during the writing of a review on episomes, major inputs being experimental work on prophage gene order by CALEF and LICCIARDELLO (1960), studies on the genetic content of λ*gal* phages (culminating in a March, 1963 paper in GENETICS) and some provocative ideas of FRANK STAHL's about chromosome circularity in prokaryotes. Retrospectively, the event can be viewed as one incident in the understanding of chromosome structure, and as one argument for a position that has now been accepted so completely that it may seem surprising there was ever dissent.

The issue was whether the chromosome is unidimensional (linear or circular) and, if so, whether added elements such as proviruses are integral parts of it. The two questions are closely intertwined. Had it transpired (as was frequently supposed prior to 1962, *e.g.*, JACOB and WOLLMAN 1961) that a prophage could establish a permanent association with a chromosomal site by some means other than intercalation, it would have been illogical to deny that chromosomal genes might employ the same mode of association. Whereas classical linkage analysis and cytogenetics provided definitive evidence that genes were linearly disposed along the length of the chromosome, and fine structure genetics was equally convincing as to the linearity of very small, gene-sized segments, the physical studies of the time did not exclude models of chromosome structure where DNA genes were attached laterally to a protein backbone or joined end to end by protein connectors (FREESE 1958) or where chromosomes were composed of parallel DNA double helices held in register by lateral protein bonds (CAVALIERI and ROSENBERG 1961). The latter model needed only minor extensions to accommodate side-by-side synapsis of a prophage to a segment of homeologous chromosomal DNA (JACOB and WOLLMAN 1961). Autoradiography of bacterial chromosomes, although indicating a circular DNA-containing structure, lacked the necessary resolution to settle the issue; and traditional biochemistry left open the possibility that lateral elements attached noncovalently might be lost during purification.

Although various physical studies in the 1970s encouraged the current view that each chromosome (prokaryotic or eukaryotic) contains a single DNA molecule, joined throughout by phosphodiester bonds, the proof awaited restriction mapping, chromosome walking, and sequencing.

Current techniques of course also demonstrate that added elements (proviruses, transposons, integrating plasmids) are part of the continuity of the chromosome. However, it was already possible 30 years ago to provide convincing genetic arguments on this score, and bacteriophage λ was the first element to which such arguments were applied. The goal of the genetic experiments was to construct an integrated map of a chromosome containing an added element. The prerequisites were an element marked with several mutations and a chromosome that was genetically marked in the flanking DNA.

It was shown early on that λ prophage could be mapped close to the *gal* and *bio* operons of *Escherichia coli* K-12, in which mutations were available. In λ, plaque morphology mutations could be used; or more conveniently, conditionally lethal mutations. Hfr × F⁻ bacterial crosses consistent with intercalation of λ between *gal* and the fairly distant *trp* locus (CALEF and LICCIARDELLO 1960) were followed by P1 transductions with the closely flanking loci *gal* and *bio* (ROTHMAN 1965). Selection for mutations inactivating nearby chromosomal genes provided nested sets of deletions that penetrate into and through the prophage, first in a λ-related phage (FRANKLIN, DOVE and YANOFSKY 1965), then in λ itself (ADHYA, CLEARY and CAMPBELL 1968).

Most of the above experiments came some time after the initial proposal for λ insertion. The earlier evidence (besides the work of CALEF and LICCIARDELLO) came from examination of λgal specialized transducing phages, which had been discovered a few years earlier by MORSE, LEDERBERG and LEDERBERG (1956), and from segregation patterns of double lysogens containing one normal λ and one λgal in tandem (CAMPBELL 1963a). The interpretation of the λgal results was logically equivalent to the "topological" mapping used with deletions (BENZER 1959), the basic assumption being that each λgal isolate represented a connected segment of the lysogenic chromosome. The enzymology behind the rare excisions that produce λgal's is still unknown. It was clear 30 years ago that λgal's have a large number of different endpoints, both at the phage and the bacterial end, and that specific λgal types are probably generated at the time of excision, rather than earlier in the development of the bacterial clone (CAMPBELL 1963b).

The detailed analysis of λgal phages required the availability of a large collection of mutations distributed over the phage genome; and to be practical, it required that prophage genotypes be easy to score. This approach was greatly facilitated by the use of conditional-lethal mutants, which allowed scoring by spot tests rather than by making lysates and checking plaque morphology.

A digression on the discovery of conditional lethals in λ: they were first observed in 1958, quite by accident. For the studies on λgal gene content, I wanted mutations at many sites of the λ genome, and decided it might help to induce small-plaque mutations by SOS mutagenesis (WEIGLE 1953). The standard strain for plating λ was C600, a K-12 derivative. I isolated two small-plaque mutants and made lysates of them. When I assayed these lysates, I had run out of C600 and used instead a second λ-sensitive K-12 strain, W3350. No plaques were visible. Checking, I found that the mutants formed plaques only on C600, not on W3350. I had no idea why the host specificity, but it made the mutants very useful for the kind of mapping studies I contemplated; and it proved simple to collect more of them. From the first 15 mutations, it was clear that they mapped to many parts of the λ genome, and that most mutant pairs complemented in mixed infection.

I sent some of the mutants to JEAN WEIGLE at CalTech, where my own work on λ transduction had started. In 1959, BOB EDGAR told me about some results of DICK EPSTEIN's on T4. At CalTech, EPSTEIN had looked for T4 mutations that allowed plaque formation on K-12 but not on the standard T4 plating host, E. coli B, and had later found that such "amber"

mutants plated only on some K-12 strains, the same ones on which my λ mutants plated. BOB thought this might be a general method for finding mutations whose products were essential for phage development. This encouraged me to isolate many more mutations, arrange them into complementation groups, test the effect of E. coli suppressors on mutant phage growth, and isolate thermosensitive mutants for comparison (CAMPBELL 1961b). When I sent my manuscript to BOB, he wrote back, "Great minds run in the same tracks," and explained that he had been isolating ts mutants of T4 for several months.

Later, in a semihistorical note (EDGAR 1966), BOB raised the question of why there was such a long time lag between the isolation of ts mutations in Neurospora crassa (HOROWITZ and LEUPOLD 1951) and rediscovery of the principle with T4. In my case, rediscovery was not necessary. The Neurospora experiments came to mind in my initial conversation with BOB, and I suspect that he may have had a subliminal recollection as well. At any rate, as noted elsewhere (BERG 1990), my own explanation for the time lag is that neither BOB nor I would have proceeded in these studies without the example of BENZER's work on fine structure genetics, which raised our consciousness of the manner in which conditional lethals could be most constructively classified and analyzed. The T4 group, led by EPSTEIN and EDGAR, proceeded to a comprehensive analysis of mutant function, whereas I employed the mutations primarily as genetic markers. In the late 1960s, many members of the λ group carried the physiological analysis of my mutants to a similar level of sophistication, apparently stimulated less by my original paper or the T4 work than by the thesis work of one of my students (BROOKS 1965), which initiated analysis of λ replication genes. BROOKS' paper, coming at a time when λ regulation seemed ripe for investigation, found an audience prepared to respond.

Returning to λ insertion, the model postulated that the ends of the linear phage genome became joined prior to insertion, thereby allowing a single crossover to insert the prophage with the observed cyclic permutation of gene order. Direct evidence for endjoining, by ligation of sticky ends, soon became available (KAISER and WU 1968).

A few years later, specialized transducing phages provided direct molecular evidence of DNA insertion. When the DNA from a λgal of known gene content formed a heteroduplex with λ DNA, the physical extent of the gal substitution could be used to locate genes on a DNA map. More fundamentally, the results argued strongly that phage DNA and bacterial DNA are covalently joined, and that no non-DNA linkers separate prophage from host DNA (DAVIDSON and SZYBALSKI 1971). Eventually, λgal and λbio specialized transducing phages provided junction fragments

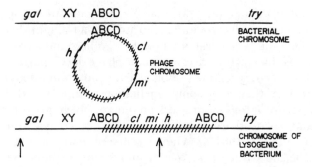

FIGURE 1.—Prophage insertion as proposed in CAMPBELL (1961a). The original legend reads "Possible mechanisms of lysogenization by reciprocal crossing over between a circular phage chromosome and a linear bacterial chromosome. Arrows indicate rare points of breaking and joining in the formation of transducing lambda. The genes ABCD are hypothetical and indicate a small region of homology between host and phage. X and Y are unspecified bacterial genes." Thirty years later, ABCD is identified as the 15-mer "GCTTTTTTATACTAA" and X and Y could be *chlD* and *pgl*.

whose sequences define the insertion event with precision (LANDY and ROSS 1977).

Genetic control: As originally formulated, the insertion model postulated crossing over between a unique sequence of the circular phage genome and a homolog on the bacterial chromosome (Figure 1). Thus it used the known process of homologous recombination to explain the unknown mechanism of prophage insertion. The reasonable assumption that such a crossover should require the RecA protein was soon tested and proven incorrect. The work led instead to the discovery that RecA is needed for repressor destruction following SOS induction (BROOKS and CLARK 1967). Another prediction was that increasing the extent of homology should increase the rate of insertion; instead, even extensive homology had little effect if repressor was present, indicating that a phage-coded protein might be required. A search for mutations affecting insertion identified a single phage gene (*int*); later a second gene (*xis*) was identified whose product was needed (in addition to Int) for excision from the chromosome. Two host-coded proteins (the heterodimeric integration host factor IHF and the Fis protein) were later shown to play a role in the integrase reaction, both by *in vivo* genetics and *in vitro* biochemistry (reviewed in CRAIG 1988).

Enzymology: This genetic work set the stage for the identification of the *int* gene product, which proved to be a site-specific recombinase (NASH 1981). A number of elegant biochemical experiments defined the reaction mechanism. Integrase causes a two-strand exchange at a precise nucleotide position by way of a transient DNA-protein bond on a tyrosine residue of the integrase, to generate a Holliday cross-bridge. Branch migration across a 7-bp segment that is identical in both partners occurs next, then the Holliday structure is resolved by exchange between the other two strands. The result is a precise crossover.

The whole reaction proceeds in a concerted manner, requiring neither an external energy source nor repair synthesis.

The substrate requirements for the reaction are a 21-bp segment from the bacterial site (*attB*) and a 235-bp segment from the phage (*attP*). The *in vitro* reaction works best when *attP* is supercoiled. The initial step in integration is binding of Int to *attP*, followed by association of the complex with *attB*. The reaction is then catalyzed by the C-terminal domains of integrase molecules associated with DNA sequences (core sites) symmetrically around the 7-bp overlap segment. Binding of integrase to core sites is enhanced by high affinity binding of the N-terminal integrase domain to arm sites in the flanking DNA of *attP* 60–140 bp from the crossover point, as well as by protein-protein interactions.

Proper positioning of integrase molecules is facilitated by binding of IHF, a DNA-bending protein, at specific sequences between the core and arm sites. Xis and Fis are also DNA-bending proteins, which promote formation of the complex in the excision reaction. The system provides an instructive model for DNA looping (KIM and LANDY 1992).

Soon after the discovery of excisionase, a physical chemical question was raised (DOVE 1970): if the insertion reaction comes about simply through catalysis of DNA recombination by an enzyme (integrase), then the second law of thermodynamics requires that the catalyst work equally well in both directions, approaching an equilibrium position depending solely on the energy contents of reactants and products. If Xis were a second catalytic component, it could not change the equilibrium position. The thermodynamic driving force has still not been identified with certainty. However, the question is circumscribed by the demonstration that branch migration proceeds in the same direction in excision as in insertion (NUNES-DUBY, MATSUMOTO and LANDY 1987). Therefore, excision is not the true reversal of insertion; but the failure of integrase to promote the direct reversal efficiently remains unexplained.

Regulation: Both insertion and excision are efficient. Insertion takes place in almost every cell surviving infection; and even transient derepression can induce excision in most cells of a lysogenic culture (WEISBERG and GALLANT 1967). Nevertheless, only some years after the discovery of integrase and excisionase was it discovered that their expression is differentially regulated.

It was known early on that the two genes could be transcribed from the major leftward promoter (pL), which was turned on following either infection of a sensitive host or derepression of a lysogen. Obligatory coexpression of these two genes seemed ill suited to the dissimilar enzyme requirements for insertion *vs.* excision. An indication that integrase might have a second promoter came from characterization of rare lysogens with λ inserted into the *trpC* gene rather than at its normal location (SHIMADA and CAMPBELL 1974). SHIMADA found that such lysogens transcribe the adjacent *trpB* gene at a low constitutive rate, and that this transcription is eliminated by internal prophage deletions penetrating *int*. Selection for a high rate of *trpB* expression produces phage mutants (*int-c*) that transcribe *int* even as prophages. Later sequencing showed that the *int-c* mutation improves the −10 region of the normal *int* promoter (pI).

The importance of pI became apparent only after the discovery that it is strongly stimulated by the the λ CII protein (reviewed in ECHOLS and GUARNEROS 1983). (SHIMADA's *int-c* mutant is not stimulated by CII, for reasons that remain obscure.) It was known that CII is the principal macromolecular effector driving an infected cell toward lysogeny rather than lysis, by turning on transcription of the repressor gene *cI*. Stimulation of pI by the same effector ensures a high rate of integrase production in cells surviving infection but not in those that lyse. Deletion analysis located the CII-responsive element very close to pI (HEFFERNAN, BENEDIK and CAMPBELL 1979); we now know it is the −35 region of pI.

On the other hand, when a lysogen is derepressed, transcription from pL results in coordinate expression of *int* and *xis*, directing the reaction toward excision. The system turned out to have an additional refinement. Coordinate expression of *int* and *xis* is desirable following derepression of a lysogen but not in an infected cell before commitment to lysis or lysogeny. It turns out that very little integrase is formed from pL transcription of infecting DNA, because pL mRNA degradation is initiated by host RNAse III-mediated cleavage at a site (sib) downstream from *int*. In the inserted prophage, sib is separated from *int* because it lies on the opposite side of *attP*; thus the pL transcript from a derepressed lysogen is more stable (ECHOLS and GUARNEROS 1983).

λ insertion thus became the first well characterized example of a programmed DNA rearrangement.

Impact on other research areas: As a demonstrated specific DNA rearrangement, λ insertion provided encouragement for the belief that such re-arrangements might be used elsewhere. For example, DREYER and BENNETT (1965) invoked λ insertion as a precedent for their novel proposal (later proven correct in principle) that gene rearrangement underlies the determination of immunoglobulin specificity.

λ insertion also influenced work on the insertion of transposable elements, including phage Mu and retroviruses. As the mechanism turned out to be different, some of the parallels proved misleading. Transposons insert from linear rather than circular substrates, and no homology is needed at the target site. Retrovirologists retained an affection for a circular

integration substrate like λ's until quite recently, and I have enjoyed an intermittent dialog with them over the years. In an early edition of *The Molecular Biology of the Gene*, JIM WATSON (1965) bravely diagrammed the insertion of another cancer virus (polyoma) as a λ-like event. In retroviral infection, a minor fraction of the viral DNA prior to insertion is in circular form, resulting either from ligation of the terminal repeats or from recombination between them. Some retroviruses can use the genetic sequence of the ligated ends as an integration substrate (PANGANIBAN and TEMIN 1984); however, the major pathway, strongly supported by *in vitro* data, is through insertion of the linear molecule into the target site (BROWN *et al.* 1987).

Evolution and natural variation: λ has many natural relatives (collectively known as lambdoid phages), which have a common genetic map and presumed common ancestry but exhibit extensive variation in specific traits. Some lambdoid phages (such as λ and 434) insert at a common chromosomal site and encode interchangeable integrase and excisionase proteins. Others insert at various sites and encode proteins with corresponding specificities. As all their integrase genes are related, this raises the question of how specificities have changed and why natural selection might have favored variants with altered specificities.

The simplest answer to the "why" question is frequency-dependent selection (which has often been invoked for other host-parasite interactions). When two phages have the same specificity, each can sometimes expel the other when it inserts. A rare variant with a new specificity is never expelled by other phages—an advantage that lasts only until it becomes as common as other types. The "how" question has been approached by studying the properties of natural phages with overlapping specificities. The best examples are λ *vs.* HKO22, which share the same specificity for excisionase and arm binding but differ in core binding; and phage 21 *vs.* defective element e14, which insert at the same site but differ in recognition specificity, so that neither one can expel the other from the chromosome. Current research is defining the molecular determinants of specific recognition in the two cases (CAMPBELL 1992; NAGARAJA and WEISBERG 1990).

While λ inserts into intergenic DNA, some lambdoid phages insert within structural genes for proteins or tRNAs. In those cases, the phage DNA includes on one side of the crossover point a duplicate (either precise or imprecise) of the 3′ end of the target gene. Thus, the lysogen expresses a functional gene whose 3′ end is phage-derived. The simplest historical scenario is that the ancestral phage arose in a strain with a preexisting duplication of the gene in question; and that the phage later picked up a short segment of flanking host DNA by the same mechanism used in λgal formation, thus enabling it to lysogenize other strains where the gene was unique (CAMPBELL 1992).

In a wider context, λ integrase can be placed by DNA and protein homology into a large family of site-specific recombinases, the integrase family, which is represented in both prokaryotes and eukaryotes. (A second family, responsible for DNA inversions and transposon resolution, is not detectably related to the integrase family.) All of the prokaryotic elements that insert by site-specific recombination use enzymes that belong to the integrase family; and the existing data indicate that, despite extensive sequence divergence, they all have similar attributes, such as a 7-bp overlap segment. A currently popular notion is that all these elements are derived from an ancestral phage that inserted into the anticodon loop of a tRNA gene (where a unique 7-bp sequence is flanked by short inverted repeats). This fits with the widespread use of tRNA insertion sites by elements with diverse hosts. Work currently underway in many laboratories should fill some of the gaps in the evolutionary picture.

I am grateful for continuous support since 1959 from the National Institute of Allergy and Infectious Diseases, grant AI08573.

LITERATURE CITED

ADHYA, S., P. CLEARY and A. CAMPBELL, 1968 A deletion analysis of prophage lambda and adjacent genetic regions. Proc. Natl. Acad. Sci. USA **61:** 956–962.

BENZER, S., 1959 On the topology of the genetic fine structure. Proc. Natl. Acad. Sci. USA **45:** 1607–1620.

BERG, D. E., 1990 Conditional mutations in procaryotes, pp. 15–26 in *The Bacterial Chromosome*, edited by K. DRLICA and M. RILEY. American Society for Microbiology, Washington, D.C.

BROOKS, K., 1965 Studies in the physiological genetics of some suppressor-sensitive mutants of bacteriophage λ. Virology **26:** 489–499.

BROOKS, K., and A. CLARK, 1967. Behavior of λ bacteriophage in a recombination deficient strain of *Escherichia coli.* J. Virol. **1:** 283–293.

BROWN, P. O., B. BOWERMAN, H. E. VARMUS and J. M. BISHOP, 1987 Correct integration of retroviral DNA *in vitro.* Cell **49:** 347–356.

CALEF, E., and G. LICCIARDELLO, 1960 Recombination experiments on prophage host relationships. Virology **12:** 81–103.

CAMPBELL, A. M., 1961a Episomes. Adv. Genet. **11:** 101–145.

CAMPBELL, A., 1961b Sensitive mutants of bacteriophage λ. Virology **14:** 22–32.

CAMPBELL, A., 1963a Segregants from lysogenic heterogenotes carrying recombinant lambda prophages. Virology **20:** 344–356.

CAMPBELL, A., 1963b Distribution of genetic types of transducing lambda phages. Genetics **48:** 409–421.

CAMPBELL, A., 1992 Chromosomal insertion sites for phages and plasmids. J. Bacteriol. **174:** 7495–7499.

CAVALIERI, L. F., and B. H. ROSENBERG, 1961 The replication of DNA. III. Changes in the number of strands in *E.coli* DNA during its replication cycle. Biophys. J. **1:** 337–351.

CRAIG, N. L., 1988 The mechanism of conservative site-specific recombination. Annu. Rev. Genet. **22:** 77–105.

DAVIDSON, N., and W. SZYBALSKI, 1971 Physical and chemical characteristics of lambda DNA, pp. 45–82 in *The Bacteriophage* λ, edited by A. D. HERSHEY. Cold Spring Harbor Laboratory, Cold Spring Harbor, N.Y.

DOVE, W., 1970 An energy level hypothesis for λ prophage insertion and excision. J. Mol. Biol. **47:** 585–589.

DREYER, W. J., and J. C. BENNETT, 1965 The molecular basis of antibody formation: a paradox. Proc. Natl. Acad. Sci. USA **54:** 864–869.

ECHOLS, H., and G. GUARNEROS, 1983 Control of integration and excision, pp. 75–92 in *Lambda II*, edited by R. W. HENDRIX, J. W. ROBERTS, F. W. STAHL and R. A. WEISBERG. Cold Spring Harbor Laboratory, Cold Spring Harbor, N.Y.

EDGAR, R. S., 1966 Conditional lethals, pp. 167–172, in *Phage and the Origins of Molecular Biology*, edited by J. CAIRNS, G. S. STENT and J. D. WATSON. Cold Spring Harbor Laboratory, Cold Spring Harbor, N.Y.

FRANKLIN, N. C., W. F. DOVE and C. YANOFSKY, 1965 The linear insertion of a prophage into the chromosome of *E. coli* shown by deletion mapping. Biochem. Biophys. Res. Commun. **18:** 910–923.

FREESE, E., 1958 The arrangement of DNA in the chromosome. Cold Spring Harbor Symp. Quant. Biol. **23:** 13–18.

HEFFERNAN, L., M. BENEDIK and A. CAMPBELL, 1979 Regulatory structure of the insertion region of bacteriophage λ. Cold Spring Harbor Symp. Quant. Biol. **43:** 1127–1134.

HOROWITZ, N. H., and O. LEUPOLD, 1951 Some recent studies bearing on the one gene-one enzyme hypothesis. Cold Spring Harbor Symp. Quant. Biol. **33:** 677–687.

JACOB, F., and E. WOLLMAN, 1961 *Sexuality and the Genetics of Bacteria*. Academic Press, New York.

KAISER, A. D., and R. WU, 1968 Structure and function of DNA cohesive ends. Cold Spring Harbor Symp. Quant. Biol. **33:** 729–734.

KIM, S., and A. LANDY, 1992 Lambda Int protein bridges between higher order complexes at two distinct chromosomal loci *attL* and *attR*. Science **256:** 198–203.

LANDY, A., and W. ROSS, 1977 Viral integration and excision. Structures of the lambda *att* sites. Science **197:** 1147–1160.

MORSE, M., E. LEDERBERG and J. LEDERBERG, 1956 Transduction in *Escherichia coli* K-12. Genetics **41:** 121–156.

NAGARAJA, R., and R. A. WEISBERG, 1990 Specificity determinants in the attachment sites of bacteriophages HK022 and λ. J. Bacteriol. **172:** 6540–6550.

NASH, H. A., 1981 Integration and excision of bacteriophage lambda: the mechanism of conservative site-specific recombination. Annu. Rev. Genet. **15:** 143–167.

NUNES-DUBY, S. E., L. MATSUMOTO and A. LANDY, 1987 Site-specific recombination intermediates trapped with suicide substrates. Cell **50:** 779–788.

PANGANIBAN, A. T., and H. M. TEMIN, 1984 Circles with two tandem LTRs are precursors to integrated retrovirus DNA. Cell **36:** 673–679.

ROTHMAN, J. L., 1965 Transduction studies on the relation between prophage and host chromosome. J. Mol. Biol. **12:** 892–912.

SHIMADA, K., and A. CAMPBELL, 1974. Int-constitutive mutants of bacteriophage lambda. Proc. Natl. Acad. Sci. USA **71:** 237–241.

WATSON, J. D., 1965 *The Molecular Biology of the Gene*. W. A. Benjamin, New York.

WEIGLE, J., 1953 Induction of mutations in a bacterial virus. Proc. Natl. Acad. Sci. USA **39:** 628–636.

WEISBERG, R., and J. GALLANT, 1967 Dual function of the λ prophage repressor. J. Mol. Biol. **25:** 537–544.

William Ernest Castle
Pioneer Mammalian Geneticist

George D. Snell* and Sheldon Reed†

*21 Atlantic Avenue, Bar Harbor, Maine 04609; and †1588 Vincent Street, St. Paul, Minnesota 55108

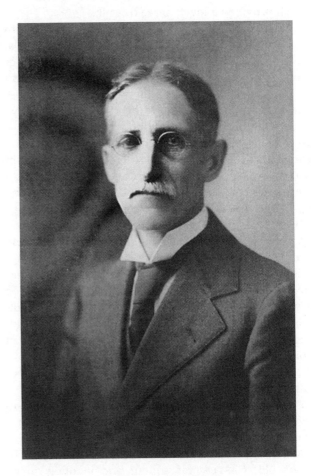

WILLIAM ERNEST CASTLE, Professor of Genetics at Harvard and Director of Harvard's Bussey Institution, was born on a farm in Ohio on October 25, 1867. He was one of six children, two of whom, in addition to William, followed academic careers. As a boy he collected flowers, and learned to graft trees and to identify the bones of animals which he came across. He graduated in 1889 from Denison University in nearby Granville, Ohio, a Baptist college that emphasized the classics and ancient languages, and went on to teach Latin at another Baptist college, Ottawa University in Ottawa, Kansas.

Through all of his early years he kept up his interest in botany. Using his personal copy of Gray's manual he recorded in his first scientific paper several hundred flowering plants he had identified in the prairies surrounding Ottawa. After three years of teaching Latin in the morning and botanizing in the afternoons his hobby finally won out. Aided by a scholarship, he entered the senior class of Harvard in 1892 and in 1893 took a second A.B. degree with honors. This was followed by an appointment as laboratory assistant in Zoology, an A.M. degree in 1894, and a Ph.D. in 1895. After a year teaching zoology at the University of Wisconsin and another at Knox College in Galesburg, Illinois, he was called back to Harvard in 1897.

CASTLE's early work at Harvard was concerned with vertebrate embryology, but with the rediscovery of Mendel's laws in 1900, his interest soon shifted to mammalian genetics. Interestingly, CASTLE was the first to use Drosophila for genetic experiments. With some colleagues, he did an extensive study of inbreeding and selection, which was published in 1906. It was through CASTLE's influence that Drosophila became known to geneticists, most notably T. H. MORGAN, and this species became the basis of MORGAN's 1933 Nobel Prize. CASTLE soon decided to concentrate his own genetic studies on mammals, and chose mice,

rats, rabbits and guinea pigs as appropriate for this work.

CASTLE's early work on mammalian genetics was carried out in the basement of Harvard's Museum of Comparative Zoology in Cambridge. In 1908, however, he moved his animals to the Bussey Institution for Applied Biology in Jamaica Plains, about ten miles from Cambridge. The Bussey, a gray stone building built originally as a private mansion, had served as an undergraduate school of husbandry and gardening from 1871 to 1908. Besides Professor CASTLE, the staff included I. W. BAILEY, a plant anatomist, E. M. EAST, a plant geneticist, and W. M. WHEELER, an entomologist. CASTLE's rat colony was housed in a room on the ground floor, his rabbits and guinea pigs in the basement, and his mice in what had been a greenhouse attached to the building.

There was a house on the Bussey grounds that served as a dormitory for students. An elderly couple lived on the ground floor; the second story provided quarters for eight students, plus a kitchen where they could get their meals. The Bussey grounds adjoined The Arnold Arboretum, another adjunct of Harvard, which provided a lovely place to walk.

Efforts to accommodate all of these renowned individuals and their students were fraught with political hazards and left some wounds and hard feelings among some of the prima donnas. There was an attempt, in 1929, to bring the world famous biometrician, RAYMOND PEARL, to be the Director. However, scientific and political opposition prevented this from being achieved. PEARL was strongly opposed by the mathematician E. B. WILSON, who had been critical of a claim by PEARL that cancer and tuberculosis were negatively associated. PEARL had also made some egregious mistakes in his early papers on inbreeding.

CASTLE became the Director because of his soft-spoken, kindly but firm, even-handed diplomacy. He was a prudent spender of the large funds at his disposal, but very generous to his students and the underlings who did the chores around the Bussey. He never forgot his old biology mentor, Professor MARK, who was still tottering around the new Biology Building in Cambridge at age 100! Professor MARK had trained CASTLE in embryology at Harvard.

After the completion of the new Biological Laboratories in Cambridge, Harvard shut down the Bussey in 1936 and moved research in genetics and entomology, though not CASTLE's mice, rats, rabbits and guinea pigs, to the new building. CASTLE's retirement was timed to coincide with the move. Although 70 years old, CASTLE was still fit and mentally alert. Happily for all concerned, the University of California offered him a position as Research Associate in mammalian genetics. He accepted the offer and moved to California. He died June 3, 1962, at the age of 95.

In 1896, CASTLE married CLARA SEARS BOSWORTH, whom he had met while teaching at Ottawa. They had three sons. One of them died as a teen-ager. The oldest, WILLIAM B. CASTLE, was a professor at Harvard Medical School and received great recognition for his work in the isolation of vitamin B_{12}. The third

son EDWARD was a professor of plant physiology at Harvard.

As early as 1903, CASTLE published a paper on "The Heredity of Albinism" and another on "The Heredity of Angora Coat in Mammals." As he put it in 1951, the theoretical question of concern to him at this time "was whether Mendelian characters are, as generally assumed, incapable of modification by selection, whether or not attended by outcrossing. My own early observation indicated that they were modifiable and to this view I stubbornly adhered, like Morgan in his early opposition to Mendelism, until the contrary view was established by crucial experiment." The "crucial experiment" was one suggested by his student SEWALL WRIGHT, who disagreed with his professor's view. WRIGHT often commented on CASTLE's friendly tolerance of a student who argued persistently for a position contrary to his own.

As the number of identified loci in mammals increased, the problem of linkage and chromosome mapping assumed increasing importance. In 1914, CASTLE published in the *American Naturalist* a paper, "The Theoretical Distinction Between Allelomorphs and Close Linkage," and in 1915 with SEWALL WRIGHT, "Two Color Mutants of Rats Which Show Partial Coupling." From then on, although only one of the many areas in which CASTLE was involved, linkage became an area of growing concern. For a while he constructed three-dimensional chromosome maps, much to the annoyance of the Drosophila school.

CASTLE's contributions to genetics centered in two areas: the students he trained, especially those who ended with a Harvard Sc.D. or Ph.D., and his published works. He published 242 papers, three books, and a genetics laboratory manual. Most of his papers dealt with the genetics of mice, rats, rabbits and guinea pigs, but he also wrote on the genetics of horses, sheep and humans, and on race crossing and hybrid vigor. His textbook on *Genetics and Eugenics* went through four editions. Late in life he became interested in the genetics of the Palomino horse. His last two papers, both on horses, were published in 1961 when he was 94 years old. His first paper, on the plants he had collected while teaching in Ottawa, had been published in 1893, 68 years earlier.

Altogether, 21 students received their doctoral degrees under Professor CASTLE:

1912 JOHN A. DETLEFSEN
       E. CARLETON MACDOWELL
1914 CLARENCE C. LITTLE
1915 SEWALL WRIGHT
1920 L. C. DUNN
1923 TAGE U. H. ELLINGER
1925 HORACE W. FELDMAN
1926 W. H. GATES

CLYDE E. KEELER
LAURENCE H. SNYDER
1927 GREGORY PINCUS
1928 P. W. GREGORY
ROBERT C. ROBB
E. A. LIVESAY
1930 GEORGE D. SNELL
1931 PAUL B. SAWIN
NELSON F. WATERS
1934 FRANK H. CLARK
1935 SHELDON C. REED
1937 SUMNER A. BURHOE
LLOYD W. LAW

CASTLE's work lives on, not only in his contributions to our knowledge but in his students and students' students. The Jackson Laboratory, founded in 1929 by CLARENCE COOK LITTLE, one of his students, is the recognized world center for mammalian (especially mouse) genetics and the natural heir to the Bussey.

It is of interest to readers of GENETICS that CASTLE was one of the ten original founders of the journal in 1916, and the last survivor.

SOURCES

DUNN, L. C., 1965 William Ernest Castle. Biographical Memoirs of the National Academy of Sciences 38: 34–80. This includes a chronology and a complete list of publications.

WRIGHT, S., 1963 WILLIAM ERNEST CASTLE, 1867–1962. Genetics 48: 1–5.

N. I. Vavilov, Martyr to Genetic Truth

James F. Crow

Genetics Department, University of Wisconsin–Madison, Madison, Wisconsin 53706

FIFTY years ago, on January 26, 1943, NIKOLAI IVANOVITCH VAVILOV, near starvation, died in a Soviet prison hospital. He was 55, at what should have been the peak of his career. On this 50th anniversary of his death, the most short-sighted of the many genetics tragedies in the STALIN-LYSENKO era, it is fitting that he be memorialized in this journal. This comes at a time of dissolution of the USSR, with its enormous problems which we hope are temporary, and its augury of a better political and scientific tomorrow.

Genetics was fated to be caught up in the two most devastating European dictatorships of the century. HITLER's notorious racist policies deprived Germany and the world of some of our greatest minds and clouded human genetics for decades. STALIN, by supporting LYSENKO's bizarre Lamarckism, set Soviet genetics a generation behind.

I first heard the VAVILOV story from H. J. MULLER while visiting him at Amherst College during World War II. He had spent four years in Russia, from 1933 to 1937, at VAVILOV's invitation. He had gone there with high hopes for an expanded, well supported genetic research program and had come back thoroughly discouraged. Geneticists had been disappearing–18 of VAVILOV's staff members were arrested between 1934 and 1940–and the program was devastated. At the time of our conversations MULLER knew of VAVILOV's arrest, but not whether he was still alive. In those years Russia was our ally and MULLER was unwilling to say things that would undermine the US-USSR cooperation. Furthermore, he was reluctant to speak out against the state of genetics in the USSR for fear of further jeopardizing his friends and students there; but he was happy to talk privately. Later, after the war, when he decided that his silence was not helping, he became an outspoken opponent of the LYSENKO fiasco.

VAVILOV was a man of prodigious energy, personal charm, contagious enthusiasm, retentive memory, encyclopedic knowledge and linguistic talent. He spoke all the major European languages, and on his trips he managed to learn enough words to get along in one country after another as he traveled in search of wild relatives of cultivars. MULLER spoke of VAVILOV's great physical energy, his sleeping only 4–5 hours per night and his writing articles while traveling. An early favorite of LENIN, he headed the All-Union Institute of Plant Breeding. He had written more than 350 articles and books. He had won awards throughout the world. He was Vice-President of the Sixth International Congress of Genetics and had been elected President of the Seventh. How could such a man be challenged?

His downfall came from the ambitious TROFIM LYSENKO, who managed to win favor with STALIN. LYSENKO had attracted attention with the technique of vernalization, by which cold treatment of seeds altered development in a way said to hasten maturity and increase yields. VAVILOV actually promoted LYSENKO by praising these results at the Sixth International Genetics Congress in 1932. By this time VAVILOV was being criticized for failing to produce the hoped-for increases in agricultural productivity. His method of collecting wild relatives of cultivars from around the world would yield only slow (but certain) improvement. LYSENKO, with his naive Lamarckian views, promised quick results. The debates were vigorous and even MULLER got into the act. I have always liked something he said in one of the debates. He asked what hope there could be for a proletarian revolution when the poor had suffered generations of bad environments, which on a Lamarckian interpretation would have ruined their genetic potential. The answer is not recorded.

LYSENKO came from a peasant background, which gave him prestige. (In contrast, VAVILOV came from a wealthy family.) LYSENKO's Lamarckian ideas fitted

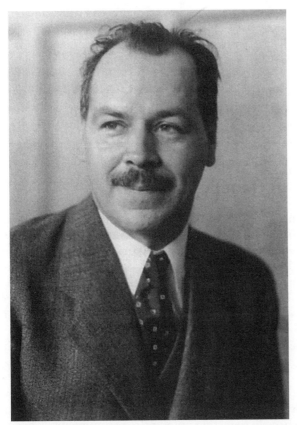

FIGURE 1.—A photograph of N. I. VAVILOV from the 1932 International Genetics Congress. Reprinted from MANGELSDORF (1953).

the political climate. Most important, he had STALIN's support. A major reason for LYSENKO's ascent was his promise of quick crop improvement compared to VAVILOV's slow process of systematic collection of wild varieties, hybridization, testing, and selection. The public criticisms brought against VAVILOV also included such things as giving too much attention to "fascistic" foreign science, wasting government money on useless collecting trips, and holding idealist Mendelian theories. VAVILOV was removed from his high post in the Central Executive Committee in 1935. His successor was A. I. MURALOV, who was arrested in July, 1937; his successor was G. K. MEISTER, who was arrested in February, 1938. Not a very safe line of work. Then LYSENKO took over. I have mentioned earlier (CROW 1992) that VAVILOV was prevented from attending the Seventh International Congress, held in Edinburgh in 1939, despite being its President. VAVILOV never heard the words of high praise given by F. A. E. CREW and others at the Congress.

VAVILOV refused to follow the politically expedient path of supporting LYSENKO's theories. He clearly knew that trouble lay ahead, but he did not retreat from his scientific views. He advised MULLER to leave, which MULLER did by working in a blood bank in Spain. He thought that supporting the Spanish loyalists would be the best way not to be branded a bourgeois reactionary deserter; it didn't help. MULLER said that the last conversation between the two of them, in 1937, was held outside VAVILOV's apartment, lest they be overheard. MULLER also carried a secret message from VAVILOV to N. TIMOFEEFF-RESSOVSKY warning him to stay away from Russia. TIMOFEEFF-RESSOVSKY was a Russian geneticist, then working in Germany and wanting to leave for his homeland; but return would have meant certain imprisonment.

VAVILOV was arrested on August 6, 1940, while on a collecting trip in the Ukraine. He was tried and sentenced to be shot for, among other things, belonging to a rightist organization, spying for England, sabotaging agriculture and maintaining links with émigrés. After a short time in a Moscow prison he was moved 450 miles southeast to Saratov, where 20 years earlier he had been Professor at Saratov University and first attained prominence. The British Royal Society elected him to membership in the hope that this might save his life. His supporters, especially his mentor PRYANISHNIKOV, made a strong plea for clemency and VAVILOV also had help from his physicist brother SERGEI, later to be president of the Soviet Academy of Sciences. The death sentence was rescinded in June, 1942, but VAVILOV remained imprisoned until his death in 1943. His name was removed from the list of members of the Soviet Academy of Sciences in 1945.

Many other geneticists were also victims at about the time of VAVILOV's arrest, including his famous associate G. D. KARPECHENKO. KARPECHENKO had hybridized radish and cabbage to produce the enormously luxuriant allopolyploid Raphanobrassica, a textbook example of extreme heterosis. An earlier "liquidation" was SOLOMON LEVIT, the leading Soviet human geneticist.

According to POPOVSKY (1984, p. 181), VAVILOV, while confined to a crowded prison cell, "brought a measure of discipline into things. He tried to cheer up his companions. To take their minds off grim reality he arranged a series of lectures on history, biology and the timber industry. Each of them delivered a lecture in turn. They had to speak in a very low voice because if the guard heard them he would order them to talk only in a whisper." It is reminiscent of TIMOFEEFF-RESSOVSKY's lectures to fellow prisoners a few years later after he had returned to Russia and had been arrested as VAVILOV warned. It is vividly described by SOLZHENITSYN in The Gulag Archipelago.

VAVILOV was born in Moscow on November 25, 1887, and graduated from high school in 1906. He then became a student at the Moscow Agricultural Institute and graduated in 1911, winning a prize for his thesis on garden slugs. The greatest scientific influence on his career, he said, came from his study with WILLIAM BATESON in England. His first work, on his return to Russia, was on disease resistance in plants. He was particularly interested in identifying resistant varieties, in some cases finding that a single gene was responsible. One of his discoveries was *Triticum timopheevii,* a wheat variety resistant to several diseases, which has been widely used as a source of resistant germ plasm. He also had the idea that if a parasitic fungus has a wide range of hosts, it is less likely that resistant varieties will be found in any of the host varieties than if it were host-specific.

VAVILOV's interest in wild relatives of cultivated species led to ambitious expeditions throughout the world. By 1940 more than 250,000 plants had been collected. These were not just museum specimens, but seeds and live plants. They were studied taxonomically, cytologically and genetically in more than 400 experiment stations throughout the Soviet Union. The idea was to provide breeders with the full genetic potential of the species and the means for creating new and better varieties. He had a program of testing each variety in many habitats to find those best suited to each particular environment. He was especially interested in finding strains that would mature and produce high yields in the short growing season that plagues much of the Soviet Union. In short, he carried out on an unprecedented scale the kind of plant breeding program that has since been practiced in agricultural experiment stations throughout the world. The All-Union Institute of Plant Breeding, of which he was the head, at one time had some 20,000 workers.

VAVILOV noted that closely related species had similar variations. In those pre-molecular days, similarity of variants was one of the best indicators of genetic relationship. His law of "homologous variation" held that the more similar species are, the more similar are their patterns of variation. This way of classification became very popular, and he was sometimes able to predict that a particular variant would be found. This predictive idea was even compared to MENDELEEV's periodic table. The theory was naturally controversial, and some took it as evidence against Darwinism. L. S. BERG, for example, regarded similar variations in related species as evidence for a predetermined evolution, "nomogenesis" as he called it. Later, VAVILOV relied on additional techniques, such as cytogenetics; but he always regarded homologous variation as an important measure of genetic relationship.

The work of greatest lasting influence was his search for the origins of domestic plants. He formulated the hypothesis that locales in which there is the largest amount of genetic variability are the ones from which new varieties, the future cultivars, arose. VAVILOV found some parts of the world to be particularly rich in varieties, and he regarded these as the centers from which the crop plants were descended. These areas also were often the sites of origin of civilizations.

In retrospect, the hypothesis has not stood up very well. Cultivated varieties have not regularly come from the areas of greatest diversity. But, such centers have turned out to be of great utility in the search for sources of new germ plasm for plant improvement. VAVILOV's foresight shines through in these times of concern for preservation of genetic diversity. Ironically, the work that was tarred as idealistic has turned out to be of great practicality, far more so than LYSENKO's fanciful schemes.

LYSENKO was an unmitigated disaster, not only for Soviet genetics but for agriculture as well. He fostered one hare-brained scheme after another, each being put into practice on a wide scale. Controlled experiments and the efficient experimental designs introduced by R. A. FISHER were no part of his program. His lack of controlled pollination led to varieties losing their identity. Hybrid corn, derived from puny inbred parents, was derided as fatuous Morgan-Mendelism. VAVILOV's efforts to introduce American corn-breeding methods were totally rejected. The wonder is that agricultural production did not fall still lower.

VAVILOV was a strong believer in the importance of selection, both for evolution and as a tool for the plant breeder. Finding diverse types, hybridizing them, and especially selecting among the recombinants, gave the best hope for producing better plants. And, of course, he was right. But the slow and certain program he was advocating could not compete in the political arena with those who promised instant gratification. Here lies a lesson for all science.

VAVILOV's foresight is preserved in the Vavilov Institute in St. Petersburg, now one of the world's largest and most varied repositories of plant germ plasm. It is located in one of the central squares and VAVILOV now holds a position of high respect, one more example of the custom–not confined to the Soviet Union–of killing people before honoring them.

Throughout his tragically truncated life, VAVILOV had both scientific and utilitarian goals. He thought of his wide-ranging geographical studies–more than 40 trips outside the Soviet Union and many more within–as adding to our understanding of evolution by natural selection. But it was also a way of improving plants and adapting them to new areas. He had the resources to carry out such a program, and in time would surely have produced the results he foresaw. He believed that the Soviet Union gave scientists a better opportunity to advance knowledge and serve mankind than any other country, and for this reason overlooked the crudities and cruelties of the regime. Alas, the crudities and cruelties soon predominated. VAVILOV's favorite saying, particularly poignant as it turned out, was: "Life is short; hurry."

Several perceptive and useful suggestions from DIANE PAUL,

ALEXEY KONDRASHOV and ALEXANDER KOLKER have been incorporated in this article and it is much improved thereby. I thank JOHANNES SIEMENS for calling the attention of geneticists to this being the 50th anniversary of VAVILOV's death. Finally, I register here my indebtedness to H. J. MULLER, who half a century ago broadened my genetic horizons and opened my eyes to the tragic state of genetics in the Soviet Union.

REFERENCES

Information not identified as to source has come mainly from the book by POPOVSKY and the articles by ADAMS and MANGELSDORF.

ADAMS, M. B., 1978 Vavilov, Nikolay Ivanovich. *Dictionary of Scientific Biography* **15:** 505–513. Charles Scribner's Sons, New York.

CROW, J. F., 1992 Sixty years ago: the 1932 International Congress of Genetics. Genetics **131:** 761–768.

MANGELSDORF, P. C., 1953 Nikolai Ivanovich Vavilov, 1887–1942. Genetics **38:** 1–4.

POPOVSKY, M. A., 1984 *The Vavilov Affair*. Archon Books, Hamden, Conn.

The Discovery of Mustard Gas Mutagenesis by Auerbach and Robson in 1941

Geoffrey Beale

Institute of Cell, Animal and Population Biology, University of Edinburgh, West Mains Road, Edinburgh, EH9 3JT, Scotland

GENETICS in 1940: The notion of the gene as a unit of heredity was well established by 1940, but its material basis was far from clear at that time. Proof of the chromosome theory made it reasonable to believe that genes were components of the chromosomes, presumably proteins, nucleic acids or nucleoproteins. The work of GRIFFITH and AVERY *et al.* showing the special importance of nucleic acids had not yet been assimilated into genetic theory, and the naive concept of chromosomes as "strings of beads" was the best that geneticists of those times could suggest. One of the properties of genes was that of mutation, the change of one form (allele) into another, and it had been shown by MULLER and STADLER that such gene mutation, in addition to occurring spontaneously, could be induced by ionizing radiation (*e.g.*, X-rays) or ultraviolet light. It was thought that such mutation experiments might throw light on the nature of the gene, and in this connection the target theory of TIMOFEEFF-RESSOVSKY, ZIMMER and DELBRÜCK (1935) had been proposed. It was thought possible that the size of the gene might be determined on the basis of this theory. X-ray-induced mutation, however, was found to be mainly the result of inactivation or deletion of genes. The hope had been expressed by MULLER (see below) that some kind of directional mutagenesis might be obtained in the future, perhaps by treating germ cells with chemical substances, and if successful would yield more definite information about the nature of the gene. However, in spite of many attempts, only negative or at best marginally significant results had been obtained from experiments on chemical mutagenesis prior to 1940. The success of AUERBACH and ROBSON in 1941, described in this paper, in obtaining mutations in Drosophila by treatment with mustard gas, was therefore an outstanding event in the history of genetics, even though publication had to be delayed till 1946, after World War II had ended.

The aim of this article is to describe–as far as is possible 50 years after the event–how the discovery was made and to analyze the circumstances leading up to it. As will be shown, these circumstances involved the concurrence of a number of unusual factors, such as political events, war and the chance proximity of key individuals–factors which are not often thought to be responsible for scientific discoveries. It is therefore an excellent example of the unpredictability of some major scientific advances.

AUERBACH: CHARLOTTE (LOTTE) AUERBACH was born in 1899 to a Jewish family in Krefeld on the Rhine in Germany. She went to school in Berlin and, following the custom in Germany at that time, attended lectures in a number of different universities– in Berlin, Würzburg and Freiburg. She remembers receiving instruction from KNIEP in Würzburg and Berlin (in botany), from SPEMANN in Freiburg (Entwicklungsmechanik), and from HEIDER and MAX HARTMANN in Berlin. She took her "Staatsexamen" in 1924 in Berlin and then spent a short time working in developmental physiology under O. MANGOLD at the Kaiser-Wilhelm-Institut in Berlin-Dahlem. However, she found this uncongenial, MANGOLD being a Nazi. On one occasion when she suggested to him that her project might be changed, MANGOLD reacted, according to LOTTE, in a "typical German-Nazi way," saying "Sie sind meine Doktorantin; Sie müssen machen was *ich* sage. Was Sie denken hat nichts damit zu tun." When recounting this incident to me, LOTTE suddenly burst into German, with some feeling. Even after 65 years, MANGOLD's words remained in her mind. As a Jewish woman without private means, she felt she had no chance of making a career in a German university at that time, though with the aid of a small legacy she had been able to start with MANGOLD.

The only geneticist in Berlin that she remembers is CURT STERN, from whom she received a few lectures, but apparently soon abandoned them to go off singing in a choir. When H. J. MULLER came to Berlin in 1932 and delivered a lecture on the *ClB* technique, LOTTE knew nothing about it.

Her main interest at that time was school-teaching, and after passing the qualifying examination, she spent some years teaching in various schools in Berlin. In 1933, however, HITLER became Chancellor and a law was passed prohibiting the employment of Jews in all state schools in Germany. LOTTE learned about this through the newspapers, and was not allowed to return to her school to collect her belongings. After that she had the opportunity of teaching in a school for Jews only, but was advised against this by her mother–fortunately for, as she later learned, those who did this were afterward killed by the Nazis.

In view of the threatening situation in Germany, especially for Jews, LOTTE decided to leave the country. Through a close Anglo-German family friend (H. FREUNDLICH, Professor of Chemistry in London) she arranged to come to Britain in 1933. Initially she wanted to go to Cambridge and study embryology under C. H. WADDINGTON, but this was not possible as it could have involved too many years of study for a Ph.D. degree. Through FREUNDLICH and G. BARGER (Professor of Chemistry in Relation to Medicine at Edinburgh), she was introduced to F. A. E. CREW, head of the Institute of Animal Genetics at Edinburgh. This Institute was the subject of an earlier essay (FALCONER 1993). CREW offered LOTTE a very modest position at his Institute. On arrival, he gave her some reprints of papers on Drosophila and casually invited her to choose a project. She decided to study the development of the legs of Drosophila. After two years, in 1935, she wrote a thesis entitled "Development of the legs, wings and halteres in wild type and certain mutant strains of *D. melanogaster*" and was awarded a Ph.D. by the University of Edinburgh.

After this, CREW tried to persuade LOTTE to move elsewhere but, thanks again to the intercession of BARGER, was persuaded to keep her on to look after the mice and especially the budgerigars in which CREW was particularly interested (see FALCONER 1993). LOTTE was also able to get a little more money by acting as an assistant to H. P. DONALD, working on pig records, and giving evening classes in biology.

It happened that the Institute was one of the few places in Britain at that time where genetics research was going on. Plant genetics was being actively pursued at the John Innes Horticultural Institution at Merton, S. London. At Cambridge, it was alleged by the irreverent that the Professor of Genetics, R. C. PUNNETT, was more interested in social activities and tennis than genetics. But in Edinburgh, CREW had collected a group of what LOTTE called "waifs and strays" on minimal salaries, from various continental European countries–notably P. C. KOLLER from Hungary, G. PONTECORVO from Italy, R. LAMY from Trinidad, and later B. M. SLYZINSKI and H. SLYZINSKA from Poland. Most important of all was H. J. MULLER who arrived in Edinburgh from the USSR and Spain in 1938. The intellectual atmosphere was very lively, and CREW liked everyone to stay in the laboratory late at night discussing their work (and other things), drinking tea or coffee, and even playing ping pong. With the help of her colleagues, especially LAMY and KOLLER, LOTTE taught herself some genetics and did some experiments with Drosophila and mice.

At the outbreak of World War II in 1939, with CREW's help LOTTE was able to acquire British nationality and was therefore spared the fate of many distinguished German and Italian scientists of being incarcerated in an internment camp on the Isle of Man. However, on one occasion she did receive a visit from the police, who had been informed that mysterious tapping noises had been heard late at night coming from a room occupied by a lady with a strong German accent. At that time–especially after the fall of France to HITLER's troops–there was a paranoid spy fever in Britain, and it was expected that German parachutists (possibly disguised as nuns) would be descending from the skies. Fortunately, LOTTE was able to persuade the police that her tapping was quite innocent and came from her typewriter. The professor of astronomy, a personal friend, was able to certify that she was not an enemy agent.

Some time in 1938, CREW brought MULLER to LOTTE's room and peremptorily announced that she was to work with him. Later, however, MULLER returned and said it was up to LOTTE to do what she thought interesting. He sat down and discussed her work. He thought that future developments in genetics, particularly with regard to the nature of the gene, would be more likely to follow from studies on mutation than from the developmental studies which had previously been LOTTE's main interest (see AUERBACH 1978). MULLER advised her to try to obtain mutations in Drosophila by chemical treatments, and suggested that a number of carcinogens should be tested. LOTTE carried out such experiments with three known carcinogens, 1:2:5:6-dibenzanthracene, 9:10-dimethyl-1:2-benzanthracene, and methyl-cholanthrene, but obtained only negative results (AUERBACH 1940). Following these attempts, LOTTE began experiments with mustard gas, as will be discussed in the next section.

LOTTE received the prestigious D.Sc. from the University of Edinburgh in 1947, largely for her published work on chemical mutagenesis, and continued research in this area for the remainder of her career, publishing many papers and several books. She was elected a Fellow of the Royal Society of Edinburgh in 1949 and of London in 1957, and in 1970 she became a Foreign Associate of the U.S. National Academy of Sciences. After acquiring a worldwide reputation, she received invitations to return to Germany to take up a senior position there. She declined these offers, however, and informed me that she would "rather work as a lab girl in Scotland than as a professor in Germany."

In 1969 LOTTE became an Emeritus Professor of the University of Edinburgh, but continued to supervise research on mutagenesis even then. Now aged 93, she still lives in Edinburgh and maintains a lively interest in science though she is much handicapped by poor eyesight. She is much loved and respected by us all.

ROBSON: J. M. ROBSON (see ADAM 1984) (hereafter denoted "RAB") was born in Belgium in 1900 to a Russian family named RABINOVICH. He came to England before World War I and attended school and university in Leeds, where he studied medicine. In 1929 he moved to Edinburgh, changing his name to ROBSON on the advice of CREW, and was appointed an assistant to B. P. WIESNER who was working on gonadotrophic hormones at the Institute of Animal Genetics. For a time RAB was in charge of a unit on pregnancy diagnosis, which CREW had set up. In 1934, however, the grant for work on sex hormones was withdrawn and RAB then moved to the Pharmacology Department in Edinburgh (headed by A. J. CLARK). RAB was a man with many interests, and worked on toxicology and chemotherapy as well as sex hormones. Some of his work led ultimately to the development of the contraceptive pill.

In one experiment, which was apparently never published (see ADAM 1984), RAB applied hormonal stimulation to the vaginal epithelium of rats, some of which were exposed to minute doses of mustard gas. The hormonal treatment alone produced a burst of mitoses, but this was inhibited by mustard gas. Thus, RAB showed that mustard gas, like X-rays, inhibited mitosis. The question was whether mustard gas did this by causing lesions in the chromosomes.

In 1940 RAB began a collaboration with LOTTE on the mutagenic effect of mustard gas, as will be described in detail below. In 1946 he moved to the Pharmacology Department at Guy's Hospital Medical School in London, and continued to work on sex hormones and other things, but did nothing further in genetics. He died in 1982.

The experiments of AUERBACH and ROBSON on mutagenesis with mustard gas: The first experiments on the effect of mustard gas on Drosophila were done under conditions that now seem extraordinarily prim-

itive. The initial exposures were done on the roof of the Pharmacology Department in Edinburgh. Liquid mustard gas was heated over a bunsen burner in an open vessel, and the flies were exposed to the gas in a large chamber. As a result, all of the people doing this work developed serious burns on their hands, which were then treated with gentian violet. After a short time LOTTE was warned by a dermatologist not to expose her hands to mustard gas any more or she would develop serious injuries. RAB took to wearing gloves. On one occasion LOTTE recalls how she went into a room where RAB and his wife SARAH were eating lunch and said, "There must be mustard gas here. I can smell it." "Nonsense," was RAB's answer. Then LOTTE went round the room and found a beaker of mustard gas bubbling away over a gas burner, filling the room with what she described as a "garlic-like" smell. This did not seem to worry RAB at all. Later, LOTTE left all the exposure work to RAB or his assistants. One of the latter, M. GINSBURG, who was then a Ph.D. student (later becoming Professor of Pharmacology at King's College, London) told me that he was "ordered" by RAB to expose flies to mustard gas.

Eventually a somewhat safer system was devised (AUERBACH and ROBSON 1947a). Nevertheless, it was never possible to control precisely the amount of mustard gas to which the flies were exposed. Sometimes all were killed. After treatment, the survivors, if any, were taken by LOTTE from the Pharmacology Department to the Institute of Animal Genetics, about two miles away in another part of the University, and analyzed by MULLER's *ClB* method, which detects *X*-linked visible and lethal mutations.

The experiments were begun in November, 1940. On February 1, 1941, LOTTE wrote to MULLER, who had moved to Amherst College from Edinburgh in 1940 and was aware of the work planned by LOTTE and RAB. It was therefore unnecessary to use the words "mustard gas" in letters (which would have contravened the secrecy rule imposed by government regulation).

Dear Dr. Muller and Thea,

In November I started the experiments suggested by CLARK. Unfortunately I had not been warned sufficiently of the danger . . . I was punished with an allergic rash on both hands . . . which lasted many weeks. The substance appears to have many similarities to X-rays . . . It seems worth while trying its possible effect on mutation rates. ROBSON has promised to do the exposures for me . . . and if I treat mature sperm and use the *ClB* method I think I may manage to keep the labour involved within the limits at my disposal. Ponte [G. PONTECORVO, who was no longer in Edinburgh; he was interned from June, 1940 till January, 1941] would have been a person with whom one can discuss Drosophila work and plans. There is nobody else in the Institute with whom this can be done satisfactorily. Peo [P.

C. KOLLER] is, of course, absolutely unfitted for his role of director of Drosophila research . . . .

Yours, as always,

Lotte A.

In April, 1941 the first tests were carried out, as mentioned in another letter to MULLER dated June 7, 1941:

Dear Dr. Muller,

ROBSON was right after all with his hunch about his substance . . . I got heaps of lethals and am quite excited . . . Doses which are not lethal for imagines prevent eggs exposed in the body of the mother from hatching and sperm exposed in the body of the father from fertilizing eggs . . . but the sperm is not killed as the spermathecae of [untreated] ♀♀ mated to treated ♂♂ contain plenty of motile sperm . . . The observations on ♂♂ and ♀♀ taken together suggest that treatment interferes with the orderly process of cell division. This gives one courage to undertake a large-scale mutation experiment using the *ClB* method and a dose which does not interfere too much with fertility of ♂♂ (reduced to something like 1/2 of normal). The following mutation rate was obtained (the figures are not quite final yet).

	Nbr. of chromosomes tested	Nbr. of lethals
Controls	1216	3
Treated	1213	93

In addition there were 10 semilethals among the offspring from treated fathers, none among the controls, most having visible abnormalities.

Robson has been doing all the exposures for me, as I have become hypersensitive. He is very triumphant that his idea came right. They [*i.e.*, RAB and SARAH] often talk of you and Thea [Mrs. MULLER] . . . .

With kind regards, as always,

Lotte Auerbach

MULLER responded by sending a congratulatory telegram in June, 1941. This cannot be traced now but LOTTE thinks it stated, "Congratulations on your major discovery," and says this telegram was "her greatest reward" as MULLER was her hero.

After this first result, LOTTE had a lot of trouble repeating the experiment. RAB insisted this should be done before sending an official report to the Ministry of Supply. On March 27, 1942, LOTTE again wrote to MULLER:

Dear Dr. Muller,

I am afraid you will be disappointed how little further I have progressed with my work since I last wrote. It was not however my fault through laziness, but terrible difficulties with the dosage. From May to December I have done one experiment after the other without being able to reproduce the right dosage again . . . Robson insisted on a repetition of the original experiment for sex-linked lethals. As I expected, the result when it at last came off was completely confirmatory: 68 lethals and four semi-lethals in 790 tested

chromosomes. In addition there were some visible mutations among the semi-lethals . . . .

Yours very sincerely,

Lotte Auerbach

Apparently MULLER did not reply to LOTTE's letter of March 27, 1942 (or perhaps his reply was sunk crossing the Atlantic), for on January 29, 1943 LOTTE wrote again:

Dear Dr. Muller,

. . . I hope you won't think me ungrateful if I admit that in spite of my pleasure I was disappointed that there was no word from you or Thea . . . It is such a long time since we last heard from you, and I often wonder how life is treating you two just now. I hope, very kindly. In any case, here are my sincerest wishes that it will do so in 1943.

I also was hoping for a word from you on my work. I am getting rather discouraged by the lack of interest I encounter everywhere. And the fact that you don't write about it makes me suspect that I have disappointed you very much by my various reports . . .

All the same–hearty thanks once more, and the kindest regards for Thea and you.

Yours,

Lotte A.

Of course, it was unreasonable to expect much interest in the work from others since nothing could be published, and even when talking in the laboratory the words "mustard gas" could not be mentioned. Instead, the expression "substance H" was used.

On March 14, 1942, the results of the first experiment were sent to the Ministry of Supply in London (headed by LORD BEAVERBROOK). In the first report, LOTTE and RAB stated, as mentioned above, that sex-linked lethal mutations had been produced by treatment with substance H, as well as breaks and rearrangements of chromosomes as shown by the occurrence of inversions and translocations. The ratio of translocations to sex-linked lethals was considerably smaller than would have been obtained by equivalent doses of X-rays.

In the second report (June 4, 1942), some differences in susceptibility to mustard gas of different Drosophila strains were mentioned. It was shown that the basis of these differences was not the chromosomal constitution of the sperm, but genetically determined differences presumed to act "by way of anatomy, metabolism, and behavior." In the third report, sent the same day, it was shown that mustard gas acted directly on the chromosomes rather than by some indirect effect on treated cytoplasm. In the fourth report, again sent on June 4, 1942, the induction of visible mutations was described. This report also contained a preliminary general discussion of the genetic action of mustard gas, thus: "The main genetical effects produced by X-rays, namely lethals, visible mutations, gross and minute chromosomal re-arrangements, are obtained after mustard gas treatment. So far only three differences from X-ray effects have been observed, namely: (1) a relative shortage of translocations, (2) a high percentage of fractionals, and (3) the absence of certain visible mutations, which however is based on too small a sample to be taken as more than suggestive."

A fifth report (December 23, 1942) dealt with the action of certain other vesicant substances. Negative results were obtained with Lewisite and osmic acid, while ammonia had a slight effect which was not, however, proved to be significant.

Nothing seems to be known about the reaction of the Ministry of Supply to these reports. Presumably their significance for the war effort was considered to be negligible.

Publication: After the war, permission was at last given to LOTTE and RAB to publish their work. Even before this, however, a hint was dropped in a letter to *Nature* (AUERBACH and ROBSON 1944) where it was mentioned that "in the course of the last few years we have examined a number of chemical substances for their ability to produce mutations. Some substances were found to be highly effective, producing mutation rates of the same order as those with X-rays, 6–24 percent sex-linked lethals developing in treated X-chromosomes. These data will be published later." They went on to report that they had obtained mutations by treatment with a substance, allyl isothiocyanate, a naturally occurring mustard oil found in Brassica and other plants. The inference from this was that some "spontaneous" mutations might be caused by chemical mutagens occurring naturally in plants and also that mustard gas itself was mutagenic.

On January 4, 1944, LOTTE attended a meeting of the (British) Genetical Society in London, and presented a paper entitled "The effects of chemicals on the chromosomes of Drosophila." How much was revealed at that meeting is not known, but she may have mentioned mustard gas, because J. B. S. HALDANE complained that she should not have done so in public.

When permission to publish was given in 1946, LOTTE and RAB sent another letter to *Nature* (AUERBACH and ROBSON 1946) stating, "in a previous letter, chemical substances were mentioned which were as effective as X-rays in inducing mutations and chromosome re-arrangements. The chemical nature of the main substance used can now be stated. It is dichloro-diethyl-sulphide or mustard gas." This was followed by more detailed accounts in the *Proceedings of the Royal Society of Edinburgh* (AUERBACH and ROBSON 1947a,b). LOTTE also wrote a paper by herself (AUERBACH 1947), which she now considers the most important one, dealing with the induction of chromosomal

instabilities in Drosophila. Finally, at the 8th International Congress of Genetics in Stockholm in 1948. LOTTE delivered a comprehensive review paper entitled "Chemical induction of mutations" (AUERBACH 1949). At the same meeting the President, MULLER, stated: "We shall perhaps mention first the dramatic opening up by Auerbach and Robson of the great field of chemical mutagenesis." This gave LOTTE enormous satisfaction.

Priorities in formulating proposals for work on chemical mutagenesis with mustard gas: It is interesting to consider, in retrospect, how it came about that so unlikely and hazardous a substance as mustard gas came to be used as a chemical mutagen. According to LOTTE's statement to me, the originator of the idea was the pharmacologist A. J. CLARK, who had earlier been interested in the biological effects of radiation. At the outbreak of World War II he had a research contract with the Chemical Defense Establishment of the British War Office to study the effects of mustard gas, especially in regard to eye injuries. At that time it was generally expected that gas warfare would be resorted to in the coming war, as it had been in the war of 1914–18. Those of us who were around in 1939, at the beginning of World War II, remember how we were compelled to carry around gas masks in square cardboard boxes, wherever we went at that time. Actually, gas was never used in that war and the boxes were later used for other, more innocent purposes.

According to LOTTE, CLARK was impressed by the long-lasting effects of mustard gas. It produced wounds that were slow to heal and liable to break out again later. In 1939, ophthalmologists were still treating ulcers of the cornea that had been produced by mustard gas in World War I. These long-lasting effects seemed to resemble the somatic effects of X-rays. Thus CLARK got the idea that mustard gas, like X-rays, whose mutagenic action had been shown by MULLER and others, might act on the genetic material in the cell nuclei.

Sometime in 1940, CLARK summoned LOTTE and P. C. KOLLER from the Institute of Animal Genetics to the Pharmacology Department to discuss the possibility of analyzing the effect of mustard gas by genetic tests. According to LOTTE, RAB was not present at this first meeting. Following this and later discussions among CLARK, LOTTE, RAB and KOLLER, it was decided that genetic tests on Drosophila exposed to mustard gas should be done by LOTTE in collaboration with RAB, while KOLLER should carry out cytological studies on the chromosomes of Tradescantia pollen in flowers treated with mustard gas. KOLLER was initially rather half-hearted about the work on Tradescantia when he announced, with his very characteristic Hungarian accent, "All the chromosomes are broken."

Later, however, this part of the work was done at the John Innes Horticultural Institution, then at Merton, South London, in collaboration with C. D. DARLINGTON (DARLINGTON and KOLLER 1947).

The situation in Edinburgh was uniquely favorable for this work. CLARK, who died in 1942, had supplies of mustard gas, and the Institute of Animal Genetics was one of the few places in the U.K. where research in genetics was going on. The presence of MULLER, even for a short time, was outstandingly important. He, however, was unwilling to embark on work with chemical mutagens at that time. Although (as previously mentioned) LOTTE's position was very poor and she had to spend most of her time looking after mice and other experimental animals, her experiments with RAB were successful in spite of many difficulties.

In the genetics literature, the credit for the work on the mutagenic effect of mustard gas is mostly given to LOTTE. A recent Russian visitor to Edinburgh dramatically exclaimed to LOTTE, "You are the mother of mutagenesis" (the "father" being the Soviet scientist I. A. RAPOPORT). For her work, LOTTE was awarded the Keith Prize of the Royal Society of Edinburgh in 1948. In making the award, the President, SIR WILLIAM WRIGHT SMITH, stated:

Miss Auerbach has contributed extensively to our knowledge of mutation processes. Many of the results of her investigations have been published in the Proceedings of the Society . . . she is distinguished for her researches into the genetical effect of the mustard gases, and in these experiments was associated closely with Dr. Robson . . . Her publications in the Society have attracted world-wide notice. It might be of some interest to state that Dr. Auerbach received her training for this special field of research from Professor Muller, Nobel Laureate . . . .

This award caused great offense to RAB and even more to his wife SARAH, who wrote a furious letter to LOTTE complaining that the prize should have been awarded jointly to LOTTE and RAB. LOTTE informed me that she wrote back apologetically, "I completely agree with you, but I had to accept the prize because I needed the money" (actually only £50). LOTTE later stated that "They never forgave me," and she did not succeed in having any further contact with the ROBSONs, who had left for London in 1946. RAB's pique is fully understandable. In an interview in 1971, he stated (rather bombastically, perhaps),

I discovered the mutagenic action of mustard gas. I had the idea that mustard gas would be mutagenic. I suggested to Muller he should do it. He suggested I should approach Lotte Auerbach . . . I knew Joe Muller very well. My wife and I were the only people at the wedding [of MULLER and THEA] . . . . (Taped unpublished interview with MARGARET DEACON in 1974, quoted by permission.)

LOTTE herself on numerous occasions has stated that she does not wish to be remembered principally for the discovery of mustard gas mutagenesis, modestly pointing out that, had she not done it, someone else would have, and in any case this was only one chemical among many others which were shown to be mutagenic then or later. She prefers to be remembered for her subsequent work on the study of mutagenesis in depth, especially on the production of "replicating instabilities."

No doubt many factors contributed to the proposal (and successful prosecution) of the work. Among these we may mention: (1) the imminence of World War II, leading to the support for CLARK's work on mustard gas in Edinburgh; (2) the presence in Edinburgh at the same time of CLARK, RAB, LOTTE, and above all MULLER, who met frequently for discussion of research; and (3) the existence of CREW's Institute of Animal Genetics, at which there was a lively group creating an atmosphere favorable for scientific work. LOTTE herself informed me that, speaking ironically, even HITLER could be held to some degree responsible, as he had forced her to leave Germany and abandon school teaching for scientific research. But there seems no doubt that it was the expertise in Drosophila research methods and perseverance of LOTTE along with the intrepid, perhaps foolhardy handling of the chemical that were mainly responsible for the success of the work.

Discussion: After World War II was over and communications were reestablished between scientists in different European countries, it became apparent that several other chemical substances, in addition to mustard gas, had been shown to be capable of breaking chromosomes and/or causing gene mutations. Among these substances, the most significant was probably urethane, which was studied extensively by OEHLKERS (1943, 1949) in Germany and found to cause chromosome breaks in Oenothera, and was also found by VOGT (1948) to cause recessive lethal and visible mutations in Drosophila. According to LOTTE, OEHLKERS felt very hurt that she was always given the credit for the discovery of chemical mutagenesis, and not he.

Formaldehyde (in the food) was shown by RAPOPORT (1946) in the USSR to produce mutations in Drosophila larvae, though this work was much hindered by the rise to power of T. D. LYSENKO, who attained total domination over biology in the USSR during and for some years after World War II. RAPOPORT was strongly opposed to LYSENKO's crazy ideas and consequently was prevented from carrying on research on mutagenesis. Another mutagenic substance was phenol, discovered in Switzerland during the war by HADORN (1949) to produce mutations in Drosophila ovaries treated in the third instar larval stage. These results, however, were uncontrollably variable; numerous visible mutations were produced in some experiments, but none were found following treatment of males subsequently tested by the *ClB* method. LOTTE says that HADORN was at first suspicious that she wanted to "hog" the field of mutagenesis.

Subsequently, of course, many other substances have been shown to be mutagenic (see AUERBACH 1976). It is beyond the scope of this article to discuss them. Expansion of the work on mutagenesis was particularly great after the discovery of the structure of DNA by WATSON and CRICK in 1953, which made possible a more rational approach than previously. In this connection, however, LOTTE expressed herself trenchantly. She wrote (AUERBACH 1978),

... mutation is a process that takes place inside living cells, and as such cannot be described fully by a purely physical or chemical model, however ingenious, and the advent of the double helix has meant a tremendous break-through in our understanding of mutation, but it has neither been the beginning nor the end of mutation research. One gets the impression that molecular geneticists labour under two misapprehensions: (1) that no meaningful questions about mutation could be asked, even less answered, before 1953, and (2) that all questions were answered by the Watson-Crick model . . . .

Probably one reason for this outburst was the failure of LOTTE or anyone else to explain some aspects of chemical mutagenesis in terms of base substitutions or other changes in DNA structure. This applies particularly to the tendency of mustard gas and other chemicals to produce the so-called "replicating instabilities," that is, unstable genes that not only continue over many cell cycles to throw off the same mutation, but also can replicate the unstable state. This phenomenon continued to be studied by LOTTE and her research group at Edinburgh right up to the time of her retirement, but was never satisfactorily explained. Thus, it is to some extent understandable that she was hostile to the idea that mutagenesis could be interpreted solely in physical or chemical terms, though such an attitude in this matter is quite unfashionable at the present time. The mechanism of replicating instabilities remains unknown.

In conclusion, it should be pointed out that the main significance of the work of AUERBACH and ROBSON is the clear demonstration that gene mutations can be induced by treatment of Drosophila with a chemical agent, mustard gas. Although the discovery did not increase our knowledge of the chemical nature of the gene, as had earlier been thought possible, it led to the later discovery of many other chemical mutagens which became vitally important tools for genetic research. It also had an important impact on the use of some chemicals, such as nitrogen mustard and other alkylating agents, in the treatment of cancer. Most remarkable, perhaps, were the unusual circumstances leading to the planning of the work and the long period during which the results remained classified as "secret."

The author acknowledges the enormous help he has received from CHARLOTTE AUERBACH in preparing this paper and allowing him to quote excerpts from her letters to H. J. MULLER. Grateful thanks are also extended to HENRY ADAM (Edinburgh) and MICHAEL GINSBURG (London) for their recollections of ROBSON, and to MARGARET DEACON (Mrs. SEWARD) and the Science Studies Unit of Edinburgh University, for permission to use some information in her unpublished report and taped interviews on the history of the Institute of Animal Genetics, Edinburgh. The excerpts from correspondence between AUERBACH and MULLER are quoted from the MULLER Mss. by kind permission of the Lilly Library, Indiana University.

LITERATURE CITED

ADAM, H., 1984 John Michael Robson. Obit. Not. R. Soc. Edinb., pp. 209–212.

AUERBACH, C., 1940 Tests of carcinogenic substances in relation to the production of mutations in *Drosophila melanogaster*. Proc. R. Soc. Edinb. B **60:** 164–173.

AUERBACH, C., 1947 The induction by mustard gas of chromosomal instabilities in *Drosophila melanogaster*. Proc. R. Soc. Edinb. B **62:** 307–320.

AUERBACH, C., 1949 Chemical induction of mutations. Proc. 8th Intern. Congr. Genet. Hereditas (Suppl. Vol.), pp. 128–147.

AUERBACH, C., 1976 *Mutation Research.* Chapman & Hall, London.

AUERBACH, C., 1978 Forty years of mutation research. A pilgrim's progress. Heredity **40:** 177–187.

AUERBACH, C., and J. M. ROBSON, 1944 Production of mutations by allyl isothiocyanate. Nature **154:** 81.

AUERBACH, C., and J. M. ROBSON, 1946 Chemical production of mutations. Nature **157:** 302.

AUERBACH, C., and J. M. ROBSON, 1947a The production of mutations by chemical substances. Proc. R. Soc. Edinb. B **62:** 27.

AUERBACH, C., and J. M. ROBSON, 1947b Tests for chemical substances for mutagenic action. Proc. R. Soc. Edinb. B **62:** 284–291.

DARLINGTON, C. D., and P. C. KOLLER, 1947 The chemical breakage of chromosomes. Heredity **1:** 187–221.

FALCONER, D., 1993 Quantitative genetics in Edinburgh: 1947–1980. Genetics **133:** 137–142.

HADORN, E., G. BERTANI and S. ROSIN, 1949 Ergebnisse der Mutationsversuche mit chemischer Behandlung von *Drosophila* ovarien *in vitro*. Proc. 8th Intern. Congr. Genet. Hereditas (Suppl. Vol.), pp. 256–266.

OEHLKERS, F., 1943 Die Auslösung von Chromosomenmutationen in der Meiosis durch Einwirkung von Chemikalien. Z. Indukt. Abstammungs. Vererbungsl. **81:** 313–341.

OEHLKERS, F., 1949 Mutationsauslösung durch Chemikalien und die Bedeutung des Plasmas. Proc. 8th Intern. Congr. Genet. Hereditas (Suppl. Vol.), pp. 635–637.

RAPOPORT, I. A., 1946 Carbonyl compounds and the chemical mechanism of mutations. Dok. Acad. Nauk. SSSR, Ser. Biol. **54:** 65–67.

TIMOFEEFF-RESSOVSKY, N. W., K. G. ZIMMER and M. DELBRÜCK, 1935 Über die Natur der Genmutation und der Genstruktur. Nachr. Ges. Wiss. Göttingen (Math. Physik. Klass, Fachgruppen VI Biol.) **1:** 234–241.

VOGT, M., 1948 Mutationsauslösung bei Drosophila durch Äthylurethan. Experientia **4:** 68–69.

July 1993

Morgan's Hypothesis
of the Genetic Control of Development

Raphael Falk[*,†] **and Sara Schwartz**[†]

*Department of Genetics and †Program for the History and Philosophy of Science, The Hebrew University of Jerusalem, Jerusalem, Israel

A NY student of genetics who has read STURTE-
VANT's classical paper of 1913, "The linear arrangement of six sex-linked factors in Drosophila, as
shown by their mode of association," must have been
puzzled by the odd terminology that he used for the
wing mutants miniature and rudimentary: "The normal wing is RM. The rM wing is known as miniature,
the Rm as rudimentary, and the rm as rudimentary-
miniature" (STURTEVANT 1913). Why did he confuse
the notation, assigning to the miniature phenotype
the mutant gene r and to the rudimentary phenotype
the mutant gene m, rather than the other way around,
as is customary nowadays?

The terminology was also used by MORGAN, as in
the paper in which he examined the results of crosses
between the two sex-linked traits miniature and rudimentary (MORGAN 1912). A careful reading of the
paper reveals that this oddity actually expressed a
sophisticated hypothesis of gene action in the embryological development of Drosophila.

MORGAN was very conscious of the epistomological
importance of the notation that he used to describe
his experimental results. Thus, in his first Mendelian
paper, where he reported his breeding results with
the white-eyed mutant of Drosophila, he initially suggested the assumption "that all of the spermatozoa of
the white-eyed male carried the single 'factor' for
white eyes 'W' [and] all of the eggs of the red-eyed
females carry the red-eyed 'factor,' R" (MORGAN
1910, p. 120), rather than the more common convention that had been introduced by MENDEL, R for red
eyes and r for white eyes. That this was not a frivolous
act, but rather indicated MORGAN's awareness that
white eye-color was not the only genetically determined alternative to red eye-color, is obvious from his
other papers at that time (*e.g.*, MORGAN 1912, 1913a),
in which he noted that the problem had not existed
for MENDEL "for none of his paired characters involved two changes in kind in the same organ" (MOR-

GAN 1913a, p. 7).[1] In fact, toward the end of the 1910
paper he went one step further in assigning developmental meaning to his symbolic representation of the
white-eyed factor when he denoted it by O rather
than by W. The reason for this change was MORGAN's
acceptance of BATESON's popular notion that the appearance of a trait, such as color, was due to the
presence of a gene, and white, *i.e.*, no color, to its
absence. The substitution of O for W indicated to
MORGAN the likelihood that the white-eye condition
resulted from the absence (loss) of the red factor, R
(ALLEN 1978).

MORGAN introduced his wing-shape mutants as follows: "If M stand for Miniature, the miniature wing
will occur when M is present, and R is absent (r), *i.e.*,
rM. If R is the symbol for Rudimentary, the rudimentary wing will be Rm" (MORGAN 1912, pp. 324–325).
Obviously, R is needed to convert the miniature phenotype to normal, and similarly M is needed to convert
another phenotype, rudimentary, into normal. MOR-
GAN signifies here his embryological notion that it was
not a single gene but rather the whole genome of an
organism that was involved in the development of any
trait. He attempted to incorporate this notion by
adopting a terminology that diverted the attention
from the missing (or defective) genetic determinant
to the remaining ones. The mutant wing phenotypes
were then the result of changes in the gene array of
the long-wing trait as a whole. Once one of the genes
mutated (was absent) it could no longer affect the
trait, and the phenotype was determined by those
genes that remained intact (the *residuum*).

MORGAN's developmental concept was that the min-

---

[1] We suspect that, although MORGAN adopted the Mendelian methodology
in 1910, he had not studied MENDEL's original paper or its translation as late
as 1913. If he had been familiar with the paper, it is hard to believe that he
would have symbolized the wild-type red eye-color by R and the white-eye
color mutant by W in the first place, nor would he have written, "According
to the scheme that Mendel followed, red, R, and vermilion, V, are symbolized
as complete and contrasting characters carried by the germ-plasm of the
hybrid" (MORGAN 1913a, p. 6).

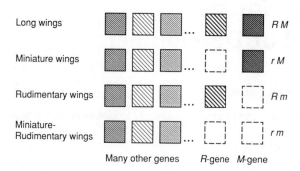

Long wings

Miniature wings

Rudimentary wings

Miniature-
Rudimentary wings

Many other genes   *R*-gene   *M*-gene

FIGURE 1.—MORGAN's concept of the genes affecting wing size and shape.

iature phenotype is a genetically determined intermediate step in the development of the perfect long-wing wild phenotype, while rudimentary is another such intermediate step. Thus, when *M* mutated to *m* (*M* becoming inactive, or more probably, absent, according to the prevailing "presence and absence" hypothesis of BATESON), only the developmental steps going as far as the rudimentary phenotype could be carried out, and the phenotype remained that of rudimentary. Similarly, when *R* mutated to *r*, the rudimentary developmental step could not be completed, and the phenotype remained that of the intact complementary pathway, namely that of miniature. It takes the action of *R* to convert the miniature wing to normal wing. Likewise, the action of the gene responsible for the developmental step of converting the rudimentary phenotype to normal is *M*. Note that he treated each gene as controlling a specific developmental step, each such developmental step being complementary to, but independent of others. The notation for the mutants clearly reveals MORGAN's developmental hypothesis of gene action in normal wing differentiation (Figure 1).

Morgan explicated his developmental hypothesis as follows (Morgan 1912, p. 331):

It may seem, on first thought, that no wings at all should appear with M and R absent; but such an interpretation would rest on a false conception, as I take it, of Mendelian factors; for, the absence of R and M does not mean that all factors for wings are lost–there may be hundreds of factors that enter into the production of wings–but only that when a certain factor, R, is lost from the complex, a miniature wing is produced by the remainder; and when the factor M is lost from the complex of wing-factors, a rudimentary wing is produced by the remainder. When both R and M are absent the remaining factors are still capable of forming much of the wing as is shown by the rudimentary-miniature wing. In fact, this last type of wing bears the same relation to miniature wing that ordinary rudimentary bears to long wing.

It did not take long, however, for MORGAN to realize that this nomenclature was not only too cumbersome but, more seriously, was inadequate. This notational crisis arose when more than two mutations affecting the same organ were discovered. Consider, for example, a third mutation affecting the same trait as

miniature and *rudimentary*, that in combination with the other two would give a compound mutant wing phenotype (*i.e.*, is *not* epistatic or hypostatic to those mutations), like that of the gene *vestigial* (*Vg*). This would have uncovered a third developmental step leading to normal wing form. Accordingly the three single-mutant phenotypes should be described as miniature-rudimentary for the *M R vg* genotype, rudimentary-vestigial for the *m R Vg* genotype, and miniature-vestigial for the *M r Vg* genotype (along with the corresponding genotypic notations for the phenotypes of the double mutants and the additional phenotype for the *m r vg* genotype). MORGAN (1913a) presented these difficulties through his attempt to accommodate a third eye-color mutant, *eosin*, into a similar scheme suggested for the two eye-color mutants *vermilion* (symbolized by *V*) and *pink* (originally symbolized by *R* and subsequently by *P*).

When CASTLE (1913) complained that the meaning of "residuum" was not clearly explicated in MORGAN's paper, MORGAN could not understand "why I failed to make clear what I meant by 'residuum' "(MORGAN 1913b, p. 374). Indeed, in his 1912 paper MORGAN had made quite clear what he meant by "residuum": the phenotype that appeared when one developmental step was aborted by the mutation and only the effects of the putative numerous remaining steps were carried out ("there may be hundreds of factors that enter into the production of wing"). That is to say, the phenotype was that of the wild-type minus the step aborted by the mutation. By using such a nomenclature MORGAN hoped to counter the reductionist Weismannian factorial concept that "identified each character of the organism as the product of a special determinant." Moreover, when MORGAN (1913a, p. 9) wrote, "A change in a factor may have far-reaching consequences. Every part of the organization capable of reacting to the new change is affected," he goes even further than indicated in his nomenclature: not only do many genes affect each trait, but also many traits are affected by each gene. In other words, a change in a genetic factor may affect many more traits than the one picked out as its marker.

Obviously MORGAN already had a profound comprehension of the many-many relationship between phenotype and genotype. On the other hand, the notion of epistatic interactions, such as those caused by sequential developmental pathways, is missing from MORGAN's nomenclature-model. He noted, however, that extending his notation based on multiple developmental steps beyond the simple cases of two factors acting independently on a character led into a paradoxical position in regard to the use of factors: "a double meaning was attached to *P*, for it stood both for the *P*-factor . . . and also for the residuum [that gave pink] as a whole" (MORGAN 1913a, p. 9).

As MORGAN noted, the nomenclature oriented toward multiple developmental steps was "not sufficiently elastic to allow the introduction of a new term in the series" because a complete revision of the method was necessary each time a new mutation in kind was added (MORGAN 1913a, p. 12). By 1913 MORGAN had good reasons to doubt the generality of the "presence and absence" hypothesis that provided one of the aspects of his hypothesis of the genetic control of development. Thus, he admits that

It is with much reluctance that I suggest this change in our present nomenclature. It has become necessary, however, in the case of the *Drosophila* to find some way to represent consistently those cases in which three or more factors are involved in the same organ. The change is not one of any theoretical importance, but a practical necessity for all cases of this kind (MORGAN 1913a, p. 14).

The simplified method that he recommended was that "[t]he first letter . . . of the name of the new character stands as heretofore, as its symbol; thus *P* stands for the pink factor and small *p* stands for the correlative factor of the pink-eyed fly. Whether small *p* represents the loss of the *P* factor, or a change in that factor when the pink eye appears, is immaterial" (MORGAN 1913a, p. 13). MORGAN reluctantly gave up most of the attempt to indicate in his nomenclature the functional role of the Mendelian transmission factors.

WILLIAM E. CASTLE, however, strongly disapproved of assigning developmental or functional meaning to the genetic factors via the nomenclature: "It is most unfortunate . . . that the small letters, having lost their original significance, were not discarded altogether, for under the presence and absence hypothesis they have done nothing but cause mischief" (CASTLE 1913, p. 171). He found great support in MORGAN's revision of the genetic nomenclature, but claimed that MORGAN did not go far enough. CASTLE suggested a further simplification of MORGAN's terminology, so that it would have the advantage that "it commits us to no physiological theory, but simply states the facts" (CASTLE 1913, p. 181). CASTLE asserted that

That terminology evidently is most desirable which states demonstrated facts most clearly and simply, and makes fewest assumptions as to their explanation. Otherwise the investigator may be led to conclusions based on his terminology rather than his facts, and this can lead only to disaster (CASTLE 1913, p. 182).

Yet, as MORGAN (1913b) noted, such a Baconian ideal was a price that we could hardly afford, because it jeopardized basic information about the *genetic* hypothesis that we wish to transmit by the nomenclature adopted. As a matter of fact, geneticists have continued ever since, for better or worse, to include in their nomenclature facts, if not hypotheses, about the action of the genetic factors (the genes) in the development of traits (the phenotype). Even CASTLE did not give up the advantage of denoting dominant mutations with capital letters and recessives with small letters.

Strictly seen, recessivity and dominance relate to the phenotypic expressions of the genes rather than to their hereditary properties.

It is significant that the original multi-developmental-steps hypothesis of MORGAN and his students, reflected in their nomenclature, was resurrected some 15 years later when BEADLE and EPHRUSSI (1936) interpreted their experimental results from the study of the genetic control of pigments in Drosophila eyes. The wild-type eye color is the end product of two developmental pathways, one producing the red pteridines, the other the brown ommochrome. Bright-red-eyed mutants, like those in the genes *v*, *cn* and *st*, do not produce the brown ommochrome, while brown-eyed mutants, like *bw*, do not produce the red pteridines. In other words, red-eyed flies have no brown pigment and brown-eyed flies have no red pigment, just like miniature flies that lack the rudimentary product and rudimentary flies that lack the miniature product. However, in contradistinction to MORGAN's early conception of the genes' control of development, BEADLE and EPHRUSSI introduced into their hypothesis not only complementary effects of different genes but also the concept of developmental (and metabolic) sequential pathways. And, of course, BEADLE and EPHRUSSI did not use the original MORGAN notation. Thus *v*, *cn* and *st* were considered to affect three steps in the same sequence, and *w* and its alleles were considered to affect an early step common to both the pteridine and the ommochrome pathways.

MORGAN had always seen a close relationship between problems of development, heredity, and evolution, and in his writings in the period between 1900 and 1910 he was highly critical of the then-prevailing theories of heredity and evolution. As an embryologist MORGAN claimed that "any theory which referred adult traits to hereditary particles was nothing more than an up-dated version of preformism" (ALLEN 1984, pp. 723–724). ALLEN suggested that behind all of MORGAN's objection to Mendelism as "preformationist" lies one fundamental problem, namely his confusion of the phenotype and genotype of an individual. As a consequence, he confused the inherited factor with the actual adult character (ALLEN 1966, p. 53; 1978, pp. 306–307).

By 1910 the experiments with the white-eye Drosophila mutant forced Mendelism on MORGAN the embryologist. JOHANSSEN's book *Elemente der exakten Erblichkeitslehre* was published in 1909. MORGAN heard JOHANSSEN's talk and met him when JOHANSSEN spent the winter term of 1911 at Columbia University. As STURTEVANT recalled in his autobiographical notes, prepared for the National Academy of Sciences (quoted by BEADLE 1970), "One event that did much to stimulate [current rethinking in the fly room] was a series of lectures given at Columbia by W. Johanssen in the winter of 1911–12. Johanssen had a critical mind, a broad knowledge of the field, and a stimulating manner of presentation." The insight contributed by JOHANSSEN's distinction between genotype and phenotype played a crucial role in MORGAN's efforts to adapt the Mendelian conceptual framework to his embryological thinking, and to incorporate in his concept of the genetic factors–and accordingly in his nomenclature–his earlier developmental notions, so that these factors could be related to embryological development. Until 1913 MORGAN hoped to reconcile embryological and Mendelian research. By then, however, his difficulties with the nomenclature forced him to realize that it was not only nomenclature, but also empirical considerations that required him to abandon efforts to deal simultaneously with genetics as transmission and genetics as development. It took him some time to realize that he could not eat the cake and still have it. From that moment on he reluctantly adopted the heuristic of carefully segregating discussions of the possible functions of genes from their role in transmission.[2]

---

[2] It is noteworthy that T. H. MORGAN never published a scientific paper in GENETICS, which was founded in 1916, although his name appeared on the cover of all issues as one of the persons who cooperated in founding and supporting it, and in spite of the fact that his students, BRIDGES, STURTEVANT and MULLER, as well as his wife L. V. MORGAN, contributed extensively to the journal from the day of its foundation. MORGAN's only contribution was an obituary of C. B. BRIDGES (MORGAN 1940).

LITERATURE CITED

ALLEN, G. E., 1966 Thomas Hunt Morgan and the problem of sex determination. Proc. Am. Philos. Soc. 110: 48–57.

ALLEN, G. E., 1978 *Thomas Hunt Morgan: The Man and His Science.* Princeton University Press, Princeton, N.J.

ALLEN, G. E., 1984 Thomas Hunt Morgan: materialism and experimentalism in the development of modern genetics. Soc. Res. 51: 709–738.

BEADLE, G. W., 1970 Alfred Henry Sturtevant. Yearb. Am. Philos. Soc., pp. 166–171.

BEADLE, G. W., and B. EPHRUSSI, 1936 The differentiation of eye pigments in *Drosophila* as studied by transplantation. Genetics 21: 225–247.

CASTLE, W. E., 1913 Simplification of Mendelian formulae. Am. Nat. 47: 170–182.

MORGAN, T. H., 1910 Sex limited inheritance in *Drosophila*. Science 32: 120–122.

MORGAN, T. H., 1912 A modification of the sex ratio, and of other ratios, in *Drosophila* through linkage. Z. Indukt. Abstammungs. Vererbungsl. 7: 323–345.

MORGAN, T. H., 1913a Factors and unit characters in Mendelian heredity. Am. Nat. 47: 5–16.

MORGAN, T. H., 1913b Simplicity versus adequacy in Mendelian formulae. Am. Nat. 47: 372–374.

MORGAN, T. H., 1940 CALVIN BLACKMAN BRIDGES. Genetics 25: i-v.

STURTEVANT, A. H., 1913 The linear arrangement of six sex-linked factors in *Drosophila* as shown by their mode of association. J. Exp. Zool. 14: 43–59.

August 1993

The Gene, the Polygene, and the Genome

William F. Dove

McArdle Laboratory for Cancer Research, University of Wisconsin–Madison, Madison, Wisconsin, 53706–1599

THIS month, geneticists will assemble in Great Britain for the XVIIth International Congress of Genetics. The last British Congress, in Edinburgh in 1939, was abruptly terminated by the outbreak of World War II. From the perspective of 1993, we can see a series of triumphs in Britain that have shaped our science over this century. In the distant background, the physician GARROD (1904) enunciated inborn errors of human metabolism, presaging the one gene/one enzyme formalism (see BEARN 1993). The tradition of monitoring mammalian phenotypes by urinalysis led to the identification of phenylketonuria as a recessive metabolic disorder by PENROSE and QUASTEL (1937); this continues in this issue of GENETICS (SHEDLOVSKY et al. 1993). The major postwar British scientific campaigns that have matured our science are broadly known to all: the elucidation of the linear and three-dimensional structures of proteins (SANGER 1955; KENDREW et al. 1958; PERUTZ et al. 1960) and DNA (WATSON and CRICK 1953), the triplet code (CRICK et al. 1961), mRNA (BRENNER, JACOB and MESELSON 1961), X chromosome inactivation (LYON 1961), and gametic imprinting (SEARLE and BEECHEY 1978; CATTANACH and KIRK 1985). Readers of this column will be familiar with some of the field generals in these British campaigns: HALDANE (CROW 1992), FISHER (CROW 1990), HARRIS (ZALLEN and BURIAN 1992), AUERBACH (BEALE 1993), WADDINGTON, ROBERTSON, CREW, HILL, and their Edinburgh colleagues in quantitative genetics (FALCONER 1993), PONTECORVO (WAELSCH 1989), and BRENNER (HODGKIN 1989; HORVITZ and SULSTON 1990). More will come.

One guerrilla campaign continues unabated, claiming neither victors nor victims. If the genes are the "atoms" of the genome, what are the "compounds"? The issue of subgenomic ensembles comes up in many guises:

• How important are the effects of genetic background in understanding genes controlling development?

• To what extent do genes exist in quasi-redundant sets, obscuring their individual detection by qualitatively distinct mutant phenotype (see BRENNER et al. 1990)?

• Are quantitative trait loci distinct in nature from those controlling qualitative variation?

At the midpoint of this century–indeed, in the midst of World War II–a heated debate arose between two distinguished British geneticists, K. MATHER and C. H. WADDINGTON. MATHER (1943) proposed, "Major or switch genes may determine which of the paths will be followed, but systems of other genes, the buffering action of which can be adapted by natural selection, will delimit the possible paths with greater or less precision. The familiar genes of genetical experiment fall into the category of what we have called switch genes . . . [We] distinguish them from the minor genes controlling quantitative characters. These two classes have also been called oligogenes and polygenes respectively from the oligogenic and polygenic nature of the variation which they determine." WADDINGTON (1943) responded, "There is a true distinction between polygenic variation (determined by numerous genes) and oligogenic variation (determined by few genes); but this is certainly not a distinction between the kinds of genes involved, and need not correspond to a distinction between the modes of action of these genes during development."

In the extreme, the notion of interacting genes becomes a truism: "When we try to pick out anything by itself, we find it hitched to everything else in the universe" (MUIR 1911). Thus, WILKINS (1990) summarizes the current view: "Today, [background effects on the expressivity and/or penetrance of mutations] are usually treated as either an irrelevance or a nuisance." Clearly, one must distinguish between strong and weak interactions. In contemporary research, the issue of gene ensembles is stated in any of the following forms:

- What genes control the major alternatives of development, including disease states?
- What genes can generate continuous changes in phenotype?
- Are null alleles of genes in each set equally likely to be homozygous lethal?
- When genes interact strongly, does it involve contact between gene products, or joint participation in a pathway (*trans* effects), or clustering in the genome (*cis* effects), or both?

WADDINGTON's (1957) notions of canalization in development have an active contemporary reincarnation. On one side, detailed analysis of the regulatory interactions among developmental genes has identified situations of positive feedback stimulation (loosely termed autoregulation) wherein gene activities self-reinforce (BERGSON and MCGINNIS 1990). On the other side, negative feedback regulation in development–colloquially called checkpoint regulation–serves to organize sets of independent activities into a coherent developmental series (WEINERT and HARTWELL 1993; CUTTING *et al.* 1990). It is too soon to estimate the proportion of lethal null phenotypes among switch genes with positive feedback function and among the genes with a checkpoint function in development. The dramatic finding from contemporary saturation genomic analyses in yeast is that a large proportion of the expressed genome has no strong null phenotype in the laboratory (GOEBL and PETES 1986).

MATHER's notion of the clustered polygene has resurfaced in surprising ways. The operons of enteric bacteria exhibit clustering of functions belonging to common metabolic pathways, offering the opportunity for coordinate regulation. The individual genes involved in these operons, however, are just as major in their phenotypic effects as are solo metabolic genes. The clusters of related functions in bacteriophage genomes can be explained by notions closer to that of the polygene: the component genes are polymorphic in the species, and recombinant genomes lose fitness (STAHL *et al.* 1966; THOMAS 1964). In metazoans, related metabolic functions are not commonly clustered. However, the homeobox clusters that are conserved from Drosophila to mammals (SCOTT 1992), the β-globin cluster (GROSVELD *et al.* 1987), and the major histocompatibility complex in mammals may contain elements of regional coordination. Again, the issue is whether an interaction is strong (affecting function as assayed in the laboratory or the clinic), or weak (affecting function over evolutionary time).

It is interesting that evidence is emerging for one of the properties proposed by MATHER for members of polygene clusters: null alleles of certain *Hox* genes in the mouse show a less severe laboratory phenotype than their expression patterns would naively predict (CHISAKA and CAPECCHI 1991). A contemporary interpretation of this situation is that *Hox* genes and other putative mammalian regulatory genes are partially redundant in function (KESSEL and GRUSS 1990; RUDNICKI *et al.* 1992). Is this interpretation different in principle from the developmental buffering proposed by MATHER?

The notion of integrated multigenic domains is substantiated by numerous contemporary studies of long-range position effects in mammalian genomes. The "spreading effect" of X inactivation can apparently extend over centiMorgans (megabase pairs) (CATTANACH 1974; RUSSELL 1983). The physical structure and rules for replication in the gray zone between the nucleosome and the chromosome call for attention!

WADDINGTON found complete agreement with MATHER in using the adjective *polygenic* even if they disagreed fundamentally on the noun *polygene*. Not surprisingly, we find considerable contemporary activity in analyzing polygenic determination in lower metazoans by modifier genetics (see KENNISON and TAMKUN 1988) and foresee equivalent excitement for mammals with the advent of facile genome-wide mapping methods (WEBER and MAY 1989; DIETRICH *et al.* 1992). Some cases of polygenic determination of development in the mouse are being discovered inadvertently when mixed genetic backgrounds are used in screening gene-knockout mutations (LE MOUELLIC, LALLEMAND and BRÛLET 1992; RUDNICKI *et al.* 1992) or ENU-induced mutations (MOSER *et al.* 1992). For lower metazoans, the molecular identities of the products of modifier loci are becoming identified, as well as the null phenotypes, which are often lethal. For the mouse, neither gene product nor null phenotype is known as yet for a modifier locus, even for the classical modifiers of the *short-ear* mutation in the bone morphogenetic protein 5 gene (KINGSLEY *et al.* 1992; GREEN 1957). The maps–genetic and physical–will change this.

Our circuit through British genetics can be interestingly closed by returning to issues in human medical genetics. Recall GARROD (1904), the practitioner whose interpretation of families with aberrant urines was enhanced by the popularization of Mendelism in Britain at the turn of the century. In his synoptic Huxley Lecture, GARROD (1927) focused on the side of human genetics that complements the search for "disease genes" as follows: "Again, I have said little of the converse of diathesis, the benign mutations which favor the individual in the struggle for existence. Difficult as it is to detect an error of the body chemistry by its evil effects, which may be long postponed, it must needs be more difficult to detect those which are harmless or have only good effects."

In experimental mammalian genetics with the laboratory mouse, we find from today's perspective an investigator of great interest, HANS GRÜNEBERG. His synoptic volume on *The Pathology of Development* (1963) gathers together an impressive combination of concrete and abstract analyses of the development of the vertebrate skeleton. Major changes in phenotype can be created by alteration of the genetic background. GRÜNEBERG was trained on the continent as a physician and was brought to Britain as a World War II exile, fostered by Sir HENRY DALE and J. B. S. HALDANE. He commented (GRÜNEBERG 1947) on the intellectual gulf between geneticists and physicians: "The majority of inherited diseases in animals have been discovered by geneticists without a medical background. Much of the material has thus not yet been utilized to its full advantage and now lies dormant in genetical journals which are rarely consulted by the medical profession."

Surely the genetics of the laboratory mouse will synergize with that of the human, not only in the identification of "disease genes" but also of their modifiers. The molecular identification by KINGSLEY *et al.* (1992) of *short ear* signals the beginning of stronger ties between clinical and experimental genetics. Soon, one may be able systematically to identify the beneficial genes of which GARROD spoke. SCRIVER (1988) suggested that ". . . to dissect out the genetic determinants of multifactorial disease is an essential first step toward understanding pathogenesis, dealing with manifestations, and designing treatments."

The major efforts being made to establish high resolution genetic and physical maps of the human and mouse genomes promise to change this situation. Whether or not complete genomic nucleotide sequence information comes into our computers, maps with a resolution of a centiMorgan (see DARVASI *et al.* 1993) and large insert DNA clones approaching a megabase pair (JAKOBOVITZ *et al.* 1993; SCHEDL *et al.* 1993; STRAUSS *et al.* 1993) will give us the necessary tools to study at the molecular level the polygenic biological processes in mammals in which we are interested.

The 1993 International Congress of Genetics in Birmingham brings the science of genetics back to the intellectually fertile British ground, at a somewhat more hopeful time in history than was 1939. The words *polygene* and *oligogene* have not served to clarify the science. In contrast, other effective neologisms have been contributed by British geneticists: allele, heterozygote, homozygote, F_1, F_2, *cis-* and *trans-*, genetics, epistasis, variance, Chi-square, Hardy-Weinberg equilibrium, inborn errors, and incomplete penetrance (see STURTEVANT 1965). And the dramatic advances that British molecular genetics have brought to the science create new life for classic issues in genetics.

LITERATURE CITED

BEALE, G., 1993 The discovery of mustard gas mutagenesis by AUERBACH and ROBSON in 1941. Genetics **134:** 393–399.

BEARN, A. G., 1993 *Archibald Garrod and the Individuality of Man.* Clarendon Press, Oxford.

BERGSON, C., and W. MCGINNIS, 1990 An autoregulatory enhancer element of the Drosophila homeotic gene *Deformed.* EMBO J. **9:** 4287–4297.

BRENNER, S., F. JACOB and M. MESELSON, 1961 An unstable intermediate carrying information from genes to ribosomes for protein synthesis. Nature **190:** 576–581.

BRENNER, S., W. DOVE, I. HERSKOWITZ and R. THOMAS, 1990 Genes and development: molecular and logical themes. Genetics **126:** 479–486.

CATTANACH, B. M., 1974 Position effect variegation in the mouse. Genet. Res. **23:** 291–306.

CATTANACH, B. M., and M. KIRK, 1985 Differential activity of maternally and paternally derived chromosome regions in mice. Nature **315:** 496–498.

CHISAKA, O., and M. R. CAPECCHI, 1991 Regionally restricted developmental defects resulting from targeted disruption of the mouse homeobox gene *hox-1.5.* Nature **350:** 473–479.

CRICK, F. H. C., L. BARNETT, S. BRENNER and R. J. WATTS-TOBIN, 1961 General nature of the genetic code for proteins. Nature **192:** 1227–1232.

CROW, J. F., 1990 R. A. FISHER, a centennial view. Genetics **124:** 207–211.

CROW, J. F., 1992 Centennial: J. B. S. HALDANE, 1892–1964. Genetics **130:** 1–6.

CUTTING, S., V. OKE, A. DRIKS, R. LOSICK, S. LU and L. KROOS, 1990 A forespore checkpoint for mother cell gene expression during development in *B. subtilis.* Cell **62:** 239–250.

DARVASI, A., A. WEINREB, V. MINKE, J. I. WELLER and M. SOLLER, 1993 Detecting marker-QTL linkage and estimating QTL gene effect and map location using a saturated genetic map. Genetics **134:** 943–951.

DIETRICH, W., H. KATZ, S. E. LINCOLN, H. S. SHIN, J. FRIEDMAN, N. C. DRACOPOLI and E. S. LANDER, 1992 A genetic map of the mouse suitable for typing intraspecific crosses. Genetics **131:** 423–447.

FALCONER, D., 1993 Quantitative genetics in Edinburgh: 1947–1980. Genetics **133:** 137–142.

GARROD, A. E., 1904 On black urine. Practitioner **72:** 383–396.

GARROD, A. E., 1927 The Huxley lecture on diathesis. Br. Med. J. **ii:** 967–971.

GOEBL, M. G., and T. D. PETES, 1986 Most of the yeast genomic sequences are not essential for cell growth and division. Cell **46:** 983–992.

GREEN, M. C., 1957 Modifiers of the pleiotropic effects of the short ear gene in the mouse. J. Hered. **48:** 205–212.

GROSVELD, F., G. B. VAN ASSENDELFT, D. R. GREAVES and G. KOLLIAS, 1987 Position-independent, high-level expression of the human β-globin gene in transgenic mice. Cell **51:** 975–985.

GRÜNEBERG, H., 1947 *Animal Genetics and Medicine.* Paul B. Hoeber, New York.

GRÜNEBERG, H., 1963 *The Pathology of Development.* Blackwell, Oxford.

HODGKIN, J., 1989 Early worms. Genetics **121:** 1–3.

HORVITZ, H. R., and J. E. SULSTON, 1990 "Joy of the worm." Genetics **126:** 287–292.

JAKOBOVITZ, A., A. L. MOORE, L. L. GREEN, G. J. VERGARA, C. E.

MAYNARD-CURRIE, H. A. AUSTIN and S. KLAPHOLZ, 1993 Germ-line transmission and expression of a human-derived yeast artificial chromosome. Nature 362: 255–258.

KENDREW, J. C., G. BODO, H. M. DINTZIS, R. G. PARRISH, H. WYCKOFF and D. C. PHILLIPS, 1958 A three-dimensional model of the myoglobin molecule obtained by X-ray analysis. Nature 181: 662–666.

KENNISON, J. A., and J. W. TAMKUN, 1988 Dosage-dependent modifiers of Polycomb and Antennapedia mutations in Drosophila. Proc. Natl. Acad. Sci. USA 85: 8136–8140.

KESSEL, M., and P. GRUSS, 1990 Murine developmental control genes. Science 249: 374–379.

KINGSLEY, D. M., A. E. BLAND, J. M. GRUBBER, P. C. MARKER, L. B RUSSELL, N. G. COPELAND and N. A. JENKINS, 1992 The mouse short ear skeletal morphogenesis locus is associated with defects in a bone morphogenetic member of the TGFβ super-family. Cell 71: 399–410.

LE MOUELLIC, H., Y. LALLEMAND and P. BRLET, 1992 Homeosis in the mouse induced by a null mutation in the Hox-3.1 gene. Cell 69: 251–264.

LYON, M. F., 1961 Gene action in the X-chromosome of the mouse (Mus musculus L.). Nature 190: 372–373.

MATHER, K., 1943 Polygenic balance in the canalization of development. Nature 151: 68–71.

MOSER, A. R., W. F. DOVE, K. A. ROTH and J. I. GORDON, 1992 The Min (multiple intestinal neoplasia) mutation: its effect on gut epithelial cell differentiation and interaction with a modifier system. J. Cell Biol. 116: 1517–1526.

MUIR, J., 1911 My First Summer in the Sierras. Houghton Mifflin, Boston.

PENROSE, L., and J. H. QUASTEL, 1937 Metabolic studies in phenylketonuria. Biochem. J. 31: 266–274.

PERUTZ, M. F., M. G. ROSSMANN, A. F. CULLIS, H. MUIRHEAD, G. WILL and A. C. T. NORTH, 1960 Structure of haemoglobin: a three-dimensional Fourier synthesis at 5.5 Å resolution, obtained by X-ray analysis. Nature 185: 416–422.

RUDNICKI, M. A., T. BRAUN, S. HINUMA and R. JAENISCH, 1992 Inactivation of MyoD in mice leads to up-regulation of the myogenic HLH gene Myf-5 and results in apparently normal muscle development. Cell 71: 383–390.

RUSSELL, L. B., 1983 X-autosome translocations in the mouse: their characterization and use as tools to investigate gene inactivation and gene action, pp. 205–250 in Cytogenetics of the Mammalian X Chromosome. Part A. Basic Mechanisms of X Chromosome Behavior, edited by A. A. SANDBERG. Alan R. Liss, New York.

SANGER, F., 1955 The chemistry of simple proteins. Symp. Soc. Exp. Biol. 9: 10–31.

SCHEDL, A., L. MONTOLIU, G. KELSEY and G. SCHÜTZ, 1993 A yeast artificial chromosome covering the tyrosinase gene confers copy number-dependent expression in transgenic mice. Nature 362: 258–261.

SCOTT, M. P., 1992 Vertebrate homeobox gene nomenclature. Cell 71: 551–553.

SCRIVER, C. R., 1988 Nutrient-gene interactions: the gene is not the disease and vice versa. Am. J. Clin. Nutr. 48: 1505–1509.

SEARLE, A. G., and C. V. BEECHEY, 1978 Complementation studies with mouse translocations. Cytogenet. Cell Genet. 20: 282–303.

SHEDLOVSKY, A., J. D. MCDONALD, D. SYMULA and W. F. DOVE, 1993 Mouse models of human phenylketonuria. Genetics 134: 1205–1210

STAHL, F. W., N. E. MURRAY, S. NAKATA and J. M. CRASEMANN, 1966 Intergenic cis-trans position effects in bacteriophage T4. Genetics 54: 223–232.

STRAUSS, W. M., J. DAUSMAN, C. BEARD, C. JOHNSON, J. B. LAWRENCE and R. JAENISCH, 1993 Germ line transmission of a yeast artificial chromosome spanning the murine alpha-1 (I) collagen locus. Science 259: 1904–1907.

STURTEVANT, A. H., 1965 A History of Genetics. Harper & Row, New York.

THOMAS, R., 1964 On the structure of the genetic segment controlling immunity in temperate bacteriophages. J. Mol. Biol. 8: 247–253.

WADDINGTON, C. H., 1943 Polygenes and oligogenes. Nature 151: 394.

WADDINGTON, C. H., 1957 The Strategy of the Genes. Macmillan, New York.

WAELSCH, S. G., 1989 In praise of complexity. Genetics 122: 721–725.

WATSON, J. D., and F. H. C. CRICK, 1953 Molecular structure of nucleic acids. A structure for deoxyribose nucleic acids. Nature 171: 737–738.

WEBER, J. L., and P. E. MAY, 1989 Abundant class of human DNA polymorphisms which can be typed using the polymerase chain reaction. Am. J. Hum. Genet. 44: 388–396.

WEINERT, T. A., and L. H. HARTWELL, 1993 Cell cycle arrest of cdc mutants and specificity of the RAD9 checkpoint. Genetics 134: 63–80.

WILKINS, A. S., 1990 Position effects, methylation and inherited epigenetic states. BioEssays 12: 385–386.

ZALLEN, D. T., and R. M. BURIAN, 1992 On the beginnings of somatic cell hybridization: BORIS EPHRUSSI and chromosome transplantation. Genetics 132: 1–8.

Francis Galton
Count and Measure, Measure and Count

James F. Crow

Genetics Department, University of Wisconsin–Madison, Madison, Wisconsin 53706

WOULD DARWIN have understood and appreciated MENDEL's work had he known of it? The question is often asked. But DARWIN was so convinced of the continuous nature of inheritance that he might not have been receptive. There is a better candidate, FRANCIS GALTON. In 1965 A. H. STURTEVANT wrote:

The question has often been raised: Would any biologist have appreciated Mendel's work if he had seen the paper before 1900? My own candidate for the most likely person to have understood it is Galton, because of his interest in discontinuous variation, his mathematical turn of mind, and his acceptance of Weismann's view that the hereditary potentialities of an individual must be halved in each germ cell.

GALTON lived long enough to learn about the rediscovery of MENDEL's laws, but by this time his genetic work was largely finished.

GALTON was the founder of biometry. Regression and correlation were his ideas and he used them to study inheritance and the similarity of relatives. He pioneered in the use of the Gaussian distribution, and realized that the methods developed to study measurement errors were just what was needed to study biological variability. He showed that one measured trait after another was normally distributed, or close to it. He did monumental studies of stature, eye color, and hereditary disease in humans. From the extensive records of coat color in basset hounds he formulated his law of ancestral heredity, a nice idea but superseded by Mendelism. He was the first to use twins to separate genetic from environmental effects. Along the way, he developed techniques for classifying fingerprints, interesting to him as a neutral trait. GALTON's high place in the history of genetics is shown by a biographical memoir and portrait (Figure 1) in the second volume of GENETICS, following MENDEL who was honored in the first.

GALTON's great work on heredity and biometry came late in his life. He published his *Hereditary Genius* when he was nearly 50 and *Natural Inheritance* when

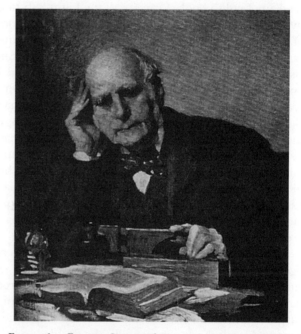

FIGURE 1.—FRANCIS GALTON, from a painting by C. W. FURSE. Reproduced from the frontispiece of GENETICS, Volume 2, 1917.

he was well into his 60s. The last third of his long life was spent almost entirely on heredity, biometry, and eugenics, and it is these for which he is known. Yet his earlier life and accomplishments are also remarkable, although less well known to geneticists, and I will mention some of them. Much of this comes from his fascinating autobiography, *Memories of My Life*, published in his 88th year.

I have also been dipping into a four-volume, 15-pound biography comprising 1345 pages, plus foldouts and page after page of photographs. It was written by KARL PEARSON (1914, 1924, 1930a,b). In the preface PEARSON says, "The indolent reader will find much in this work which he does not want and which is of little interest to him . . . this work is not written to gain a public." And in Volume III he says further,

"I will paint my portrait of a size and colouring to please myself, and disregard at each stage circulation, sale or profit." As the publishers later rued, "This quaint notion of the author's, which some would call integrity, resulted in a rather small sale." The overstocked vender finally offered the entire set for $17.50. A set now sells for several hundred dollars.

GALTON (1822–1911) was born the same year as MENDEL (1822–1884). DARWIN (1809–1882) and GALTON were half-cousins, grandsons of ERASMUS DARWIN. GALTON was the youngest of nine children and was carefully attended by a sister. She had a spinal deformity and was confined to her bed, from which she directed his early studies. He was a precocious child. On his fifth birthday, uninhibited by false modesty, he wrote, "I am four years old (sic) and I can read any English book. I can say all the Latin Substantives and Adjectives and active verbs besides 52 lines of Latin poetry. I can cast up any sum in addition and can multiply by 2, 3, 4, 5, 6, 7, 8, [9], 10, [11]. I can also say the pence table. I read French a little and I know the Clock." The numbers in brackets were erased from the letter; in his exuberance he had claimed too much. In school he led his class, although there were comments, then and later, that he had neglected his classics in favor of natural history and science. His intense curiosity about *everything* and his determination to experiment were apparent at an early age and continued throughout his life. His conviction that counting and measurement were the secret of success grew with the years.

At his parents' urging he began medical studies at age 16. He wrote feelingly about the brutalities of surgery–this was before anesthetics–and wondered why more patients were not made dead drunk before surgery, which in one instance seemed to provide succor. Always the experimentalist, he decided to find out for himself the effects of all the medicines by taking very small doses. Going through the list alphabetically, he reached the letter C; but even a minute dose of croton oil was too much for him. He also flirted with hypnotizing people and discovered, contrary to the conventional wisdom of the time, that intense concentration on his part was unnecessary; he was just as effective when he deliberately let his mind wander.

GALTON was admitted to Trinity College, Cambridge, and started to concentrate on mathematics. A high point was a study-vacation tour with mathematics taught by ARTHUR CAYLEY, inventor of matrix algebra. Unfortunately, GALTON's plans for further study were halted by illness. Later when he returned to his studies, he gave up his mathematical ambitions and settled for a medical degree. At about this time his father died, leaving him with a fortune sufficient to make medical practice unnecessary, and immediately he abandoned it.

The next few years were spent traveling, mostly in Africa. He rode on horses, oxen and camels, and on a barge up the Nile. His trips included areas not previously traveled by Europeans. Everywhere he went he made notes and measurements. Latitude and longitude were determined by astronomy and altitude by the temperature of boiling water. He wrote several books about traveling, and for many years was active in the Royal Geographical Society.

Always, even on trips, he read widely. He wrote frequent articles, often for *Nature*, on all manner of subjects. He also was an inventor. He invented a new type of heliostat, for sending signals by sun reflection. He made a trip to Spain to study a total eclipse of the sun with a newly invented instrument for measuring temperature changes; it failed, but this, he said, gave him time to revel in the beauty of the eclipse. He developed stereoscopic maps, better to show relief. He experimented with trying to make breathing entirely voluntary, and almost succeeded, to his terror.

He became interested in the ability of animals to hear frequencies too high for human ears and designed supersonic whistles to measure this. In order to measure the hearing of zoo animals without being noticed by human visitors, he contrived a whistle in his cane that he could unobtrusively activate from the handle. The results, however, were "disappointing." He wondered why, with all the selection in dogs for special traits and bizarre shapes, no one had ever selected for intelligence; but he did not have the resources for a study and could not elicit interest from anyone else. He studied a calculating prodigy and learned about the geometrical pattern in which this person arrayed numbers in his mind.

GALTON's curiosity and efforts to satisfy it exceeded all bounds. He once decided to study the efficacy of prayer. To do this he studied mortality rates of royalty, whose subjects prayed for their health, and compared insurance charges for vessels with and without (presumably praying) missionaries.

Another of GALTON's inventions was to combine photographs of different individuals into a single print. In this way he could wash out the noise of special features and reinforce the general ones. This enabled him more readily to perceive familial and ethnic resemblances. As usual, he invented a machine to make the composites. This foreshadowed modern computer programs for removing noise from images.

This superficial summary may give the impression that these various experiments were done casually, which is not true. Almost always they involved careful, repeated measurements, and were usually published. GALTON's hard-working habits paid off in a list of 183 articles and memoirs, including 12 books.

GALTON's most famous experiment is his test of DARWIN's pangenesis hypothesis. In the later editions of his book DARWIN postulated that minute "gemmules" pass from body cells to the germ cells, thus providing a mechanism for the Lamarckian inheritance that he was increasingly drawn to. GALTON tested this by massive transfusions in rabbits. The experiments involved cross connections of the blood vessels, leading to a thorough mixing. He praised the skill of his friends who did the tricky surgery; his own part "was confined to inserting cannulae and the like." (GALTON always seemed to have friends willing to help him.) The results were unequivocal: there were no inherited effects of the transfusions. DARWIN was not convinced. He said that gemmules need not travel by way of the blood stream and that his theory was supposed to apply as well to organisms without blood. GALTON was himself largely convinced of the nonexistence, or at least the non-importance, of Lamarckian inheritance, although, perhaps out of respect for his cousin, he kept an open mind. He did, however, retain part of the pangenesis theory, but confined the particles to the germ line. If only he had understood Mendelian segregation and recombination!

Another of GALTON's lasting contributions was the development of fingerprints. At this time BERTILLON was using body measurements as a way of identifying people. GALTON pointed out a fundamental error, that the various measurements were not independent and the simple multiplication of probabilities could give an erroneous impression of accuracy of identification, the same issue that sometimes arises today in DNA forensics. Looking for something better, GALTON had the idea of trying fingerprints, which had been used by, among others, the ancient Chinese. GALTON's great contribution was developing a systematic way of cataloging fingerprints to permit ready comparison. His methods and derivatives therefrom are now standard. He was fascinated by this trait because of its apparent selective neutrality. How, he wondered, could such seemingly useless patterns be so precisely determined, as evidenced by the regeneration of the same pattern when the finger tip had been mutilated? GALTON had originally thought of fingerprints as a way to aid racial classification. They turned out to be useless for this purpose, but far more important as a means of individual identification.

Although GALTON did all of these things, and much more, his deep interest in the last part of his life was heredity. Increasingly he emphasized counting and measurement. His greatest accomplishments were the discovery of regression and correlation, the foundations of biometry. Filial regression is now so familiar that it is hard to imagine that its significance was so slow to be appreciated. GALTON noted that the progeny or other relatives of individuals who deviated from the population mean in either direction also deviated in the same direction *but to a lesser extent.* If the parental measurement deviated by an amount x, say, the progeny deviated by an amount kx ($0 < k < 1$). The fraction k is the regression coefficient, remarkably constant for all values of x. This discovery solved the dilemma that had been bothering GALTON: if the progeny means were the same as the parental, the population should become more variable each generation as extreme parents produced some progeny that were still more extreme. Regression, he delightedly realized, prevented this. Thus the population distribution remained stable.

GALTON believed that regression always tended toward an unchanging population mean, and this would swamp out any effects of selection. He therefore concluded that evolution depended on discontinuous saltations, or "sports," and that DARWIN's continuous variation was not the basis of evolution.

In the 1890s the biological community was divided between advocates of Darwinian gradualism and those supporting Galtonian "evolution by jerks." The conflict became more bitter after the rediscovery of Mendelism in 1900. GALTON was in the honored, but at the same time delicate, position of being quoted and courted by both sides. The Mendelists called attention to his emphasis on discrete differences. The biometricians lauded him for the invention of biometry. He somehow managed to retain friendships on both sides.

In 1905, *Nature* refused to accept any more polemics on this subject. Yet the controversy continued, much longer than it should have, especially in England (PROVINE 1971). The definitive answer came with FISHER's famous 1918 paper, which demonstrated the consistency of the data with Mendelian inheritance when dominance, epistasis, and assortative mating were taken into account. But by this time Mendelism had won and the argument had stopped.

The two great innovations, regression and correlation, both involved mathematical methods that were beyond GALTON's skills. Yet, he understood the problems clearly and was able to call on mathematicians for the necessary help. GALTON was the first student of heredity to use the normal Gaussian distribution creatively. He expressed deviations from the population mean in units of half the interquartile range (he objected to the use of the "uncouth" term, probable error). For each multiple of this unit he could calculate the proportion of the population exceeding this value from the normal integral. Here is one example, showing GALTON's cleverness but lack of rigor. From the number of outstanding persons in various populations, by his rather elaborate scheme of classification, he calculated that British ability exceeded that of some races. At least he was not a chauvinist, for he classified the people of Scotland as higher than those of his own

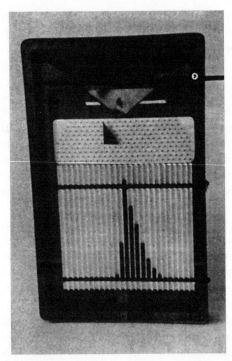

FIGURE 2.—A quincunx. In this example a triangular block has been introduced to produce a skewed distribution. (Reprinted by permission of the Quantum Company.)

England. From the large number of outstanding people (*e.g.*, Plato, Socrates, Sophocles, Arisophanes) in a small population he calculated that the average aptitude in ancient Greece was about 2 units (1.35 standard deviations) above that of contemporary Britain. Viewed by 1993 standards this seems loose and naive. But it illustrates beautifully GALTON's obsession with measuring everything and using whatever trick he could think of.

One of GALTON's most appealing inventions was a device for dropping pellets through a hole, where they bounced off strategically located pins (Figure 2). At the bottom they accumulated in slots and generated a binomial distribution, which became Gaussian as the number of pellets and slots increased. He called this a quincunx after the geometrical pattern of the pins. By suitable modifications he could demonstrate selection, regression, and various statistical principles. The most ingenious was his use of a two-stage quincunx to demonstrate that the sum of a number of normal distributions is itself normal.

GALTON's delightful account of how he came to invent the concept of correlation was published in 1890 and has been reprinted with an introduction by STIGLER (1989). For a discerning discussion of GALTON's central role in the history of statistics see STIGLER (1986).

GALTON believed firmly in the importance of heredity, and reacted strongly against the prevailing view that mental traits were not inherited. "I have no patience with the hypothesis occasionally expressed, and often implied, especially in tales written to teach children to be good, that babies are born pretty much alike, and that the sole agencies in creating differences . . . are steady application and moral effort. It is in the most unqualified manner that I object to pretensions of natural equality." His books are full of statements that are today regarded as excessively hereditarian or racist. There is a cottage industry of books and articles critical of this. But I say it is unfair to judge a Victorian Britisher, a creature of his time, by political and social standards of the 1990s. I prefer to admire him for his achievements. The subject of biometry is a lasting monument, unaffected by the changing winds of political correctness.

My greatest debt is to STEVE STIGLER who has made a detailed study of GALTON. I also thank CARTER DENNISTON and BILL ENGELS for helpful comments on the manuscript and BRIAN JOINER for helping me find a quincunx.

LITERATURE CITED

FISHER, R. A., 1918 The correlation between relatives on the supposition of Mendelian inheritance. Trans. R. Soc. Edinb. **52:** 399–433.

GALTON, F., 1869 *Hereditary Genius*, Ed. 2, 1892. Mamillan, London.

GALTON, F., 1889 *Natural Inheritance.* Macmillan, London.

GALTON, F., 1909 *Memories of My Life*. Menthuen, London. (This includes a nearly complete list of GALTON's publications, but even GALTON himself could not keep track of all that he wrote.)

PEARSON, K., 1914, 1924, 1930a, 1930b *Life, Letters, and Labours of Francis Galton.* The University Press, Cambridge.

PROVINE, W. B., 1971 *The Origins of Theoretical Population Genetics.* University of Chicago Press, Chicago.

STIGLER, S. M., 1986 *The History of Statistics.* Harvard University Press, Cambridge.

STIGLER, S. M., 1989 Francis Galton's account of the invention of correlation. Statist. Sci. **4:** 73–86.

STURTEVANT, A. H., 1965 *A History of Genetics.* Harper & Row, New York.

YULE, G. U., 1902 Mendel's laws and their probable relations to intra-racial heredity. New Phytol. **1:** 193–207, 222–238.

Roland Thaxter's Legacy and the Origins of Multicellular Development

Dale Kaiser

Departments of Biochemistry and of Developmental Biology, Stanford University, Stanford, California 94305

ROLAND THAXTER published a bombshell in December, 1892. He reported that *Chondromyces crocatus*, before then considered an imperfect fungus because of its complex fruiting body, was actually a bacterium (Figure 1). THAXTER had discovered the unicellular vegetative stage of *C. crocatus*; the cells he found were relatively short and they divided by binary fission. *C. crocatus* was, he concluded, a "communal bacterium." THAXTER described the locomotion, swarming, aggregation and process of fruiting body formation of *C. crocatus* and its relatives, which are collectively called myxobacteria, with an accuracy that has survived 100 years of scrutiny. He recognized the behavioral similarity to the myxomycetes and the cellular slime molds, drawing attention in all three to the transition from single cells to an integrated multicellular state. He described the behavior of myxobacteria in fructification in terms of a "course of development" because it was "a definitely recurring aggregation of individuals capable of concerted action toward a definite end" (THAXTER 1892). This essay will emphasize some implications of THAXTER's demonstrations, often apparently unrecognized.

The striking similarities to cellular slime mold development probably led JOHN TYLER BONNER and KENNETH B. RAPER, 50 years after THAXTER's discovery, to take independent forays into myxobacterial development. RAPER, an eminent mycologist, had in fact discovered *Dictyostelium discoidium*, recognizing it as a superb subject for the study of morphogenesis, cellular differentiation and intercellular communication. BONNER was fascinated by morphogenesis and sought unifying principles behind the bewildering diversity (BONNER 1952, 1974). Both RAPER and BONNER seemed to be intrigued by the unusual example of morphogenetic movements exhibited by the myxobacteria as they formed fruiting bodies. RAPER saw "examples of interdependent cellular behavior that involve purposeful orientation, morphogenetic move-

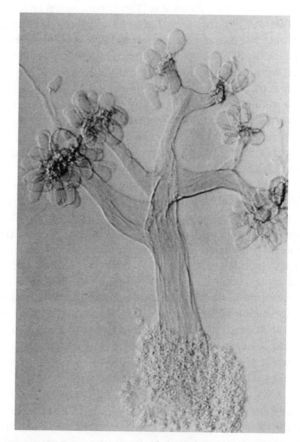

FIGURE 1.—*Chondromyces crocatus* fruiting body. Photograph by HANS REICHENBACH, GBF, Braunschweig.

ments, intercellular integration and finally coordinated differentiation that are in some ways comparable to higher forms" (QUINLAN and RAPER 1965). Both BONNER and RAPER sought the factors in *C. crocatus* that coordinated and guided the morphogenetic cell movements, noting that individual myxobacterial swarm cells retained their physical individuality throughout the process of cooperative morphogenesis, and in that respect differed from the myxomycetes but resembled the cellular slime molds.

Their search was extended by HANS KUHLWEIN and his students, particularly REICHENBACH, who prepared a series of time-lapse films of the behavior of different types of myxobacteria (REICHENBACH, HEUNERT and KUCZKA 1965a,b,c,d; REICHENBACH, GALLE and HEUNERT 1976). Using time-lapse photography to condense the roughly day-long process of fruiting body development into a few minutes of running time, as BONNER had done for *D. discoideum*, brought the morphogenesis into a time scale more suggestive and intriguing to the human psyche. The myxobacterial movies showed the simplest fruiting bodies to be mounds of myxospores covered by slime, while the more complex fruiting body structures enclosed myxospores within acellular skins of slime that either rested directly on the substratum or were raised on slime stalks. REICHENBACH (1962) concluded that the formation of fruiting bodies generally passed through several stages: vegetative growth of a multicellular swarm, induction by starvation to begin development, cell accumulation, rearrangement of cells within the originally undifferentiated mass (including production of slime stalks or sporangiole walls) and, finally, myxospore formation. REICHENBACH (1965) also discovered that the ripples noted in myxobacterial swarms were traveling waves generated by many myxobacteria during the aggregation phase.

Work with dispersed (*i.e.*, non-clumping) strains of *Myxococcus xanthus* enabled DWORKIN, ROSENBERG and their students to study this bacterium's nutrition and metabolism, prerequisites for understanding the role of starvation in the induction phase of fruiting body development (summarized by DWORKIN 1984). Genetic studies of mutants defective in fruiting body development became possible through the isolation of transducing myxophages (CAMPOS and ZUSMAN 1975; MARTIN *et al.* 1978), the introduction of transposons from *Escherichia coli* into *M. xanthus* (KUNER and KAISER 1981) and the infusion of gene cloning techniques (GILL and SHIMKETS 1993).

THAXTER's discovery called attention to the transition from single cells to an integrated multicellular unit. There is general agreement that this step has been taken many times in the course of organic evolution. For example, the sponges probably arose from solitary cells separately from all other animals, and the seed plants, the fungi, and the algae all gained their multicellular condition independently (WHITTAKER 1969). Comparing these independent experiments of nature should provide insight into the general attributes of multicellular life.

Myxobacteria, which belong to the δ subgroup of purple bacteria, are a well defined and unique experiment in multicellularity. All myxobacteria construct multicellular fruiting bodies (LUDWIG *et al.* 1983), which is to say that no aerobic gliding bacterial species are known which form spores, have a high G·C content in their DNA, but do not build fruiting bodies, even though gliding bacteria have been systematically examined (REICHENBACH *et al.* 1988). That all the myxobacteria arose from the same ancestor within the δ subgroup of purple bacteria is supported by an extensive set of characters they hold in common: swarming behavior, closely related 16S ribosomal RNA sequences (LUDWIG *et al.* 1983; WOESE 1987; SHIMKETS 1993), high (66–72) mole % G·C content in their DNA (MANDEL and LEADBETTER 1965; MCCURDY and WOLF 1967; BEHRENS, FLOSSDORF and REICHENBACH 1976) and a set of notable chemosystematic markers (REICHENBACH and DWORKIN 1981). None of the other members of the δ subgroup of purple bacteria form fruiting bodies or spores; in addition to the myxobacteria, this phylogenetic subgroup includes the bdellovibrios and the mesophilic sulfate-reducing bacteria (WOESE 1987; STACKEBRANDT 1992; WIDDEL and BAK 1992).

In contrast to the monophyletic origin of myxobacteria, cell aggregation of eukaryotes leading to fruiting bodies appears, on cytostructural grounds, to have evolved several times among the cellular slime molds (OLIVE 1975). BONNER (1982) has argued that there is likely to have been an independent origin from single-celled amoebae for each group because of unique aggregation attractants; he distinguishes at least eight different attractants.

No matter how many independent events there were among the cellular slime molds, it is clear that the changes from single to multicellular organism were taken independently from the myxobacteria. To date there has been no report of lateral gene transfer between myxobacteria and the slime molds. The cell biology of the slime molds and the myxobacteria are very different, as THAXTER first discovered. The former are eukaryotic amoebae with a flexible cell membrane and a well defined cytoskeleton. We now recognize that the latter are rigid-walled, rod-shaped, Gram-negative procaryotic cells that lack the structural anatomic features of a cytoskeleton. Molecular studies of small ribosomal rRNA sequences as well as physiological and morphological studies show that the myxobacteria arose among the purple sulfur eubacteria, while the cellular slime molds arose among the protists. The two groups are thus separated by a wide evolutionary gap (Figure 2) (WOESE 1987). Features common to these two types of microorganisms promise insight into basic biological attributes of multicellular development. The width of the phylogenetic gap decreases the effects of chance evolutionary "tinkering" (JACOB 1982), the accidents of mutational history. The point is that features shared by different organisms will be the more robust and functionally informative the less the organisms share a common descent.

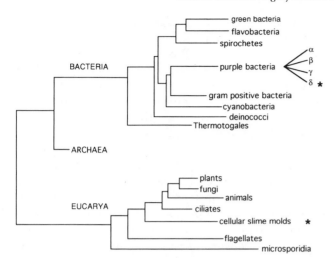

FIGURE 2.—Phylogeny of myxobacteria (∗ in δ purple bacteria) and the cellular slime molds (∗ in Eucarya). Adapted from Woese (1992) and Stackebrandt (1992).

Common qualities: As understood today, cellular slime molds (exemplified by *D. discoideum*) and myxobacteria have these similarities:

• Fruiting body development is asexual. The growing cells are haploid and the fruiting bodies are filled with haploid spores. As expected, the genome sizes are different. The sizes of several myxobacterial genomes have been determined by pulsed-field gel electrophoresis and include the closed circular genome of *M. xanthus* at 9.4 Mb (Chen *et al.* 1991), *Stigmatella aurantiaca* at 9.2–9.9 Mb and *Stigmatella erecta* at 9.7–10 Mb (Neuman, Pospiech and Schairer 1992). The genome of *D. discoideum* consists of six (possibly seven) (Darcy *et al.* 1993) linkage groups that total 40 Mb of DNA (Kuspa *et al.* 1992).

• Both move on surfaces, neither can swim. Slime mold cells translocate by amoeboid movement that involves dynamic changes in their cytoskeleton. Myxobacteria move by gliding on surfaces without apparent rotation or change in cell shape; they lack flagella or any other obvious organelles of movement. The mechanism of gliding is currently unexplained even though many bacteria can do so (McBride, Hartzell and Zusman 1993).

• Cell division is separate from development. Cells grow and divide when food is abundant. Starvation stops growth and induces development. Amino acid starvation appears to be a prime factor in the induction of development. Addition of a complete set of the amino acids required for *D. discoideum* growth delays the initiation of development (Marin 1976). In *M. xanthus*, limitation for any of the amino acids induces fruiting body development (Manoil and Kaiser 1980).

• The program of morphological change and development begins with recognition of starvation, aggregation of preexisting cells, arrangement of cells within the aggregate in a species-specific pattern, then differentiation of individual cells into spores.

• Both pass several chemical signals between their cells. In *D. discoideum*, the signals include cAMP and DIF (Williams and Jermyn 1991). cAMP seems not to be significant in myxobacteria in the way it is in *D. discoideum*. Instead, in *M. xanthus* a mixture of eight amino acids (called A-factor) is a signal early in development, and a 17-kDa surface protein known as C-factor is a signal later during the aggregation and sporulation phases (Kim, Kaiser and Kuspa 1992; Kaiser and Kroos 1993).

• The cells respond to signal reception by expressing new batteries of genes. In *D. discoideum* there are cAMP-dependent and DIF-dependent genes (Devreotes 1989; Williams and Jermyn 1991). In *M. xanthus* there are A-factor-dependent and C-factor-dependent genes (reviewed in Kroos, Kuspa and Kaiser 1986; Kaiser and Kroos 1993).

• During aggregation, cells are swept into a fruiting body from neighboring regions. The mechanisms of sweeping are similar in several ways, including the generation of traveling waves. In *D. discoideum*, the traveling waves are generated by pulses of cAMP that emanate from an aggregation center (Tomchik and Devreotes 1981), while in *M. xanthus* the traveling waves are local accumulations of cells, which depend for their formation on C-factor (Shimkets and Kaiser 1982).

• Stalk formation differs. In *C. crocatus*, cells migrate upward inside a tube of "slime" (apparently mostly polysaccharide), depositing more slime at the top and elongating the stalk as they pass into the cell mass resting on the top (Quinlan and Raper 1965; Reichenbach, Heunert and Kuczka 1965b; Thaxter 1892). In *D. discoideum*, prestalk cells move up the outside of the preexisting cellulose tube (Raper and Fennell 1952). As these cells migrate over the lip of the tube, they deposit more cellulose, elongating the tube (Williams and Jermyn 1991). Though Dictyostelium stalks contain specialized, differentiated stalk cells, the stalk of another dictyostelid, Acytostelium, is acellular like those of the myxobacteria (Raper 1984).

• The fruiting bodies of the cellular slime molds and the myxobacteria cover the same morphological range of spheres and cylinders ordered and combined in various ways (Reichenbach and Dworkin 1981; Bonner 1982; Raper 1984). The fruiting bodies of *D. discoideum* and *M. xanthus* each contain up to 100,000 cells.

Selective forces: Slime molds and myxobacteria are found in the same habitats, and are often isolated from the same soil samples by enrichment culture (Singh 1947). Both feed on bacteria in the soil. However, the slime molds ingest bacteria by endocytosis while the myxobacteria secrete their digestive enzymes, then take up the products of extracellular digestion (SUDO and DWORKIN 1972; LOOMIS 1975). The observed evolutionary convergence of these two disparate groups is presumably a consequence of natural selection in a common habitat. Both organisms are less insulated from their environment than flowering plants or higher animals and are haploid, so that natural selection can constantly play a role in shaping their development. What might the selective forces have been? Several have been suggested:

Social feeding: The selective advantage for the evolution of multicellularity in myxobacteria is likely to have been cooperative feeding. Myxobacteria feed on particulate organic matter in the soil by means of extracellular bacteriolytic, proteolytic, cellulolytic and other digestive enzymes (REICHENBACH 1984). Based on their secretion of lytic enzymes, DWORKIN (1973) proposed that myxobacteria feed like "packs of microbial wolves." ROSENBERG, KELLER and DWORKIN (1977) measured the growth rate when the only source of carbon and nitrogen for *M. xanthus* cells in liquid culture was the polymeric substrate casein, so that proteolysis was required for growth. The growth rate increased twofold as the cell density was raised above 10^4 cells/ml. When intact casein was replaced with enzymatically hydrolyzed casein, the cells grew at the more rapid rate independently of cell density. Evidently, extracellular digestion of protein is enhanced by cooperation between cells.

A swarm may be the unit of efficient cooperative feeding. REICHENBACH has shown that a single germinating sporangiole of a *Chondromyces apiculatus* fruiting body forms an active swarm that behaves much like a swarm of bees (BONNER 1952; QUINLAN and RAPER 1965; KUHLWEIN and REICHENBACH 1968). Forming a multicellular fruiting body ensures that, when conditions favorable for growth are restored, the myxospores can germinate and the new phase of growth can start as a preformed community of efficiently feeding cells. The success of the myxobacterial design is evident in their distribution; they are common inhabitants of soils drawn from all over the world regardless of climate (REICHENBACH 1984).

Dispersal: BONNER (1982) has suggested that the cellular slime molds evolved from solitary soil amoebae to multicellular forms under selection for an efficient means of dispersal. He argues that " . . . selection pressure for fruiting bodies in small organisms, be they amoebae, hyphae, plasmodia, swarms of bacteria, or even ciliate protozoa (Olive, 1978), must be enormous, and the scale of convergent evolution vast" (BONNER 1982). Rain water, wind, or movement of small soil invertebrates could disperse fruiting bodies. Stalks, multiple sorogens and sporangioles might be explained this way. Mites have been observed to carry

myxobacterial fruiting bodies (REICHENBACH 1984).

Survival under marginal conditions in a fluctuating environment: STEPHEN BARCLAY (University of Wisconsin) has pointed out to me that soil amoebae often find themselves in nutritional conditions that are marginal, neither rich enough for rapid growth nor poor enough to trigger efficiently the encystment of individual cells. Marginal conditions may encourage slow growth that would leave cells incapable of completing a final mitotic cycle, with death as the consequence. One strategy to cope with marginal conditions may be to aggregate and construct a fruiting body, withdrawing cells from the ambiguous environment and allowing them to continue starvation-induced development.

Increased reliability of perceiving starvation: The A-factor of *M. xanthus*, which is a mixture of eight amino acids, is a cell-density signal (KUSPA, PLAMANN and KAISER 1992b). The amount of A-factor released is proportional to the number of cells per unit volume, and a certain minimum quantity of A-factor is required to continue development. Thus, the A-signal ensures a cell density sufficient to complete a proper fruiting body (KUSPA, PLAMANN and KAISER 1992a). A-factor, which is released about 2 hr after the beginning of starvation, is also a way for cells to vote their individual assessment of nutritional conditions. Because new proteins must be made during aggregation and sporulation, some protein synthetic capacity must be retained, and the cells must begin to aggregate before they have exhausted all their sources of amino acids and energy. To initiate development or to grow slowly is an important choice on which long-term survival depends. An optimal choice is one that anticipates the future. When this decision is jointly made by a population of cells, it is likely to be more reliable than that made by one cell. A protein, CMF, secreted by starved Dictyostelium cells plays a similar role (JAIN et al. 1992).

These forces, and others, can be discriminated by experiment because myxobacteria and cellular slime molds are microbes that can be conveniently handled in large numbers. Moreover, the set of molecular genetic tools currently available in both organisms includes physical/genetic maps, tools for random insertional mutagenesis to identify genes and to provide genetic markers, methods for homologous gene replacements including construction of null alleles, and the capacity to clone genes in *E. coli* or *Saccharomyces cerevisiae* for manipulation before returning them to their proper host for expression; see GILL and SHIMKETS (1993) for myxobacteria and KUSPA and LOOMIS (1992) for Dictyostelium.

The selective forces, whichever may have been effective, will have acted within a set of biological and physical constraints. Unexpected convergence on related body plans and systems for control of multicellular development by cellular slime molds and myxobacteria suggests that the structural differences between eukaryotic and procaryotic cells may in fact be secondary to deeper similarities. We are aware of many metabolic similarities. We are becoming aware that there are also rules for the folding, structuring and assembly of proteins. Perhaps there are also rules about the way development and morphogenesis are regulated for reliability in relatively harsh or changing environments. Use of cellular oscillators revealed by traveling waves and the expression of genes in batteries, triggered by different extracellular signals, are cases in point. Part of ROLAND THAXTER's legacy is the notion that comparisons of eukaryotes and prokaryotes may give insights that would come from neither examined alone.

LITERATURE CITED

BEHRENS, H., J. FLOSSDORF and H. REICHENBACH, 1976 Base composition of deoxyribonucleic acid from *Nannocystis exedens* (Myxobacterales). Int. J. Syst. Bacteriol. **26:** 561–562.

BONNER, J. T., 1952 *Morphogenesis. An Essay on Development.* Princeton University Press, Princeton, N.J.

BONNER, J. T., 1974 *On Development. The Biology of Form.* Harvard University Press, Cambridge, Mass.

BONNER, J. T., 1982 Evolutionary strategies and developmental constraints in the cellular slime molds. Am. Nat. **119:** 530–552.

CAMPOS, J., and D. ZUSMAN, 1975 Regulation of development in *Myxococcus xanthus*: effect of cAMP, AMP, ADP, and nutrition. Proc. Natl. Acad. Sci. USA **72:** 518–522.

CHEN, H., A. KUSPA, I. M. KESELER and L. J. SHIMKETS, 1991 Physical map of the *Myxococcus xanthus* chromosome. J. Bacteriol. **173:** 2109–2115.

DARCY, P. K., Z. WILCZYNSKA and P. R. FISHER, 1993 Phototaxis genes on linkage group V in *Dictyostelium discoideum*. FEMS Lett., in press.

DEVREOTES, P., 1989 *Dictyostelium discoideum*: a model system for cell-cell interactions in development. Science. **245:** 1054–1058.

DWORKIN, M., 1973 Cell-cell interactions in the *Myxobacteria*. Symp. Soc. Gen. Microbiol. **23:** 125–147.

DWORKIN, M., 1984 Research on the *Myxobacteria*, pp. 221–245 in *Myxobacteria*, edited by E. ROSENBERG. Springer-Verlag, New York.

GILL, R. E., and L. J. SHIMKETS, 1993 Genetic approaches for analysis of myxobacterial behavior, pp. 129–155 in *Myxobacteria II*, edited by M. DWORKIN and D. KAISER. American Society for Microbiology, Washington, D.C.

JACOB, F., 1982 *The Possible and the Actual.* Random House, New York.

JAIN, R., I. YUEN, C. TAPHOUSE and R. GOMER, 1992 A density-sensing factor controls development in *Dictyostelium*. Genes Dev. **6:** 390–400.

KAISER, D., and L. KROOS, 1993 Intercellular signaling, pp. 257–283 in *Myxobacteria II*, edited by M. DWORKIN and D. KAISER. American Society for Microbiology, Washington, D.C.

KIM, S. K., D. KAISER and A. KUSPA, 1992 Control of cell density and pattern by intercellular signalling in Myxococcus development. Annu. Rev. Microbiol. **46:** 117–139.

KROOS, L., A. KUSPA and D. KAISER, 1986 A global analysis of developmentally regulated genes in *Myxococcus xanthus*. Dev. Biol. **117:** 252–266.

KUHLWEIN, H., and H. REICHENBACH, 1968 Swarming and mor-

phogenesis in *Myxobacteria*. Film C893/1965. Institut Wissenschaftliche Film, Göttingen.

KUNER, J., and D. KAISER, 1981 Introduction of transposon Tn5 into Myxococcus for analysis of developmental and other nonselectable mutants. Proc. Natl. Acad. Sci. USA **78:** 425–429.

KUSPA, A., and W. F. LOOMIS, 1992 Tagging developmental genes in Dictyostelium by restriction enzyme mediated integration of plasmid DNA. Proc. Natl. Acad. Sci. USA **89:** 8803–8807.

KUSPA, A., L. PLAMANN and D. KAISER, 1992a A-signalling and the cell density requirement for *Myxococcus xanthus* development. J. Bacteriol. **174:** 7360–7369.

KUSPA, A., L. PLAMANN and D. KAISER, 1992b Identification of heat-stable A-factor from *Myxococcus xanthus*. J. Bacteriol. **174:** 3319–3326.

KUSPA, A., D. MAGHAKAIN, P. BERGESCH and W. F. LOOMIS, 1992 Physical mapping of genes to specific chromosomes in *Dictyostelium discoideum*. Genomics **13:** 49–61.

LOOMIS, W. F., 1975 *Dictyostelium Discoideum. A Developmental System.* Academic Press, New York.

LUDWIG, W., K. SCHLEIFER, H. REICHENBACH and E. STACKEBRANDT, 1983 A phylogenetic analysis of the myxobacteria *Myxococcus fulvus, Stigmatella aurantiaca, Cystobacter fuscus, Sorangium cellulosum* and *Nannocystis exedens*. Arch. Microbiol. **135:** 58–62.

MANDEL, M., and E. R. LEADBETTER, 1965 Deoxyribonucleic acid base composition of Myxobacteria. J. Bacteriol. **90:** 1795–1796.

MANOIL, C., and D. KAISER, 1980 Guanosine pentaphosphate and guanosine tetraphosphate accumulation and induction of *Myxococcus xanthus* fruiting body development. J. Bacteriol. **141:** 305–315.

MARIN, F. T., 1976 Regulation of development in *Dictyostelium discoideum*. 1. Initiation of the growth to development transition by amino acid starvation. Dev. Biol. **48:** 110–117.

MARTIN, S., E. SODERGREN, T. MASUDA and D. KAISER, 1978 Systematic isolation of transducing phages for *Myxococcus xanthus*. Virology **88:** 44–53.

McBRIDE, M. J., P. HARTZELL and D. R. ZUSMAN, 1993 Motility and tactic behavior of *Myxococcus xanthus*, pp. 285–305 in *Myxobacteria II*, edited by M. DWORKIN and D. KAISER. American Society for Microbiology, Washington, D.C.

McCURDY, H. D., and S. WOLF, 1967 Deoxyribonucleic acid base compositions of fruiting Myxobacteria. Can. J. Microbiol. **13:** 1707–1708.

NEUMAN, B., A. POSPIECH and H. U. SCHAIRER, 1992 Size and stability of the genomes of the myxobacteria *Stigmatella aurantiaca* and *Stigmatella erecta*. J. Bacteriol. **174:** 6307–6310.

OLIVE, L. S., 1975 *The Mycetozoans.* Academic Press, New York.

OLIVE, L. S., 1978 Sorocarp development by a newly discovered ciliate. Science **202:** 530–532.

QUINLAN, M. S., and K. B. RAPER, 1965 Development of the myxobacteria. Handb. Pflanzenphysiol. **15:** 596–611.

RAPER, K. B., 1984 *The Dictyostelids.* Princeton University Press, Princeton, N.J.

RAPER, K. B., and D. I. FENNELL, 1952 Stalk formation in *Dictyostelium*. Bull. Torrey Bot. Club **79:** 25–51.

REICHENBACH, H., 1962 Problems of the developmental physiology of the myxobacteria. Ber. Dtsch. Bot. Ges. **75:** 90–95.

REICHENBACH, H., 1965 Rhythmic motion in swarms of Myxobacteria. Ber. Dtsch. Bot. Ges. **78:** 102–105.

REICHENBACH, H., 1984 *Myxobacteria*: a most peculiar group of social prokaryotes, pp. 1–50 in *Myxobacteria*, edited by E. ROSENBERG. Springer-Verlag, Berlin.

REICHENBACH, H., and M. DWORKIN, 1981 The order Myxobacterales, pp. 328–355 in *The Prokaryotes*, edited by M. STARR, H. STOLP, H. TRUPER, A. BALOWS and H. SCHLEGEL. Springer-Verlag, New York.

REICHENBACH, H., H. K. GALLE and H. H. HEUNERT,

1976 *Stigmatella aurantiaca* (Myxobacterales). Schwarmentwicklung und Morphogenese. Film E2421. Institut Wissenschaftliche Film, Göttingen.

REICHENBACH, H., H. H. HEUNERT and H. KUCZKA, 1965a *Archangium violaceum* (Myxobacterales)–Schwarmentwicklung und Bildung von Protocysten. Film E777. Institut Wissenschaftliche Film, Göttingen.

REICHENBACH, H., H. H. HEUNERT and H. KUCZKA, 1965b *Chondromyces apiculatus* (Myxobacterales)–Schwarmentwicklung und Morphogenese. Film E779. Institut Wissenschaftliche Film, Göttingen.

REICHENBACH, H., H. H. HEUNERT and H. KUCZKA, 1965c *Myxococcus spp.* (Myxobacteriales)–Schwarmentwicklung und Bildung von Protocysten. Film E778. Institut Wissenschaftliche Film, Göttingen.

REICHENBACH, H., H. H. HEUNERT and H. KUCZKA, 1965d Schwarmentwicklung und Morphogenese bei Myxobacterien–*Archangium, Myxococcus, Chondrococcus, Chondromyces.* Film C893. Institut Wissenschaftliche Film, Göttingen.

REICHENBACH, H., K. GERTH, H. IRSCHIK, B. KUNZE and G. HOFLE, 1988 Myxobacteria: a source of new antibiotics. Trends Biotechnol. **6:** 115–121.

ROSENBERG, E., K. KELLER and M. DWORKIN, 1977 Cell-density dependent growth of *Myxococcus xanthus* on casein. J. Bacteriol. **129:** 770–777.

SHIMKETS, L. J., 1993 The myxobacterial genome, pp. 85–108 in *Myxobacteria II*, edited by M. DWORKIN and D. KAISER. American Society for Microbiology, Washington, D.C.

SHIMKETS, L., and D. KAISER, 1982 Induction of coordinated movement of *Myxococcus xanthus* cells. J. Bacteriol. **152:** 451–461.

SINGH, B. N., 1947 Myxobacteria in soils and composts; their distribution, number and lytic action on bacteria. J. Gen. Microbiol. **1:** 1–9.

STACKEBRANDT, E., 1992 Unifying phylogeny and phenotypic diversity, pp. 19–47 in *The Prokaryotes*, edited by A. BALOWS, H. G. TRUPER, M. DWORKIN, W. HARDER and K.-H. SCHLEIFER, Springer-Verlag, New York.

SUDO, S., and M. DWORKIN, 1972 Bacteriolytic enzymes produced by *Myxococcus xanthus*. J. Bacteriol. **110:** 236–245.

THAXTER, R., 1892 On the Myxobacteriaceae, a new order of Schizomycetes. Bot. Gaz. **17:** 389–406.

TOMCHIK, K. J., and P. N. DEVREOTES, 1981 Adenosine 3′,5′-monophosphate waves in *Dictyostelium discoideum*: a demonstration by isotope dilution-fluorography. Science **212:** 443–446.

WHITTAKER, R. H., 1969 New concepts of kingdoms of organisms. Science **163:** 150–160.

WIDDEL, F., and F. BAK, 1992 Gram-negative mesophilic sulfate-reducing bacteria, pp. 3352–3378 in *The Prokaryotes*, edited by A. BALOWS, H. G. TRUPER, M. DWORKIN, W. HARDER and K.-H. SCHLEIFER. Springer-Verlag, New York.

WILLIAMS, J. G., and K. A. JERMYN, 1991 Cell sorting and positional differentiation during *Dictyostelium* morphogenesis. Symp. Soc. Dev. Biol. **49:** 261–272.

WOESE, C. R., 1987 Bacterial evolution. Microbiol. Rev. **51:** 221–271.

WOESE, C. R., 1992 Prokaryotic systematics, pp. 3–18 in *The Prokaryotes*, edited by A. BALOWS, H. TRUPER, M. DWORKIN, W. HARDER and K.-H. SCHLEIFER. Springer-Verlag, New York.

See also page 704 in Addenda et Corrigenda.

November 1993

Meiosis as an "M" Thing
Twenty-five Years of Meiotic Mutants in Drosophila

R. Scott Hawley

Department of Genetics, University of California, Davis, California 95616

FIVE years ago, at the Annual Drosophila Conference in New Orleans, talks on Drosophila meiosis were squeezed into a session entitled *Muscles, Meiosis and Morphogenesis* (in other words, meiosis as an "M" thing; hence, the title of this piece). Although that session represented perhaps the nadir of interest in meiotic phenomena by Drosophila workers (there were simply too many more interesting slides of zebra-striped embryos to watch), the field has significantly regained its momentum in the ensuing years. Papers on meiosis in flies are now common in major journals and the number of labs working on meiosis seems to increase each year. Perhaps now, as the field matures, it is worth looking back at the publication that continues to guide work on the genetic analysis of meiosis in Drosophila.

This month marks the 25th anniversary of the publication of SANDLER, LINDSLEY, NICOLETTI and TRIPPA (1968), the paper that has served as a cornerstone of the genetic analysis of meiosis in *Drosophila melanogaster*. What follows is an appreciation of that paper and also of its intellectual companion, BAKER and CARPENTER (1972). It is not intended to be a review of the genetic study of meiosis in Drosophila (I have done that elsewhere: HAWLEY and THEURKAUF 1993 and HAWLEY, MCKIM and ARBEL 1993), but rather an attempt to put SANDLER *et al.* (1968) and BAKER and CARPENTER (1972) into perspective as truly fundamental works. My comments are based on the works themselves, a series of oral histories of varying reliability, and a yellowed copy of DAN LINDSLEY's application for the sabbatical funding that supported this study.

SANDLER *et al.* (1968) as a classic paper: In a parochial sense, SANDLER *et al.* (1968) remains the standard for the mutational analysis of meiosis in Drosophila; it served as the first report of a direct screen for meiotic mutations in flies and it established the standards by which future mutations would be characterized. In a more general sense, the paper represents one of the first heralds of modern genetic analysis in higher eukaryotes; it reframed the process by which genetics in Drosophila was done.

As noted by B. S. BAKER, SANDLER *et al.* (1968) is one of the earliest examples of a *systematic* search for, and study of, mutations affecting a complex regulatory process in higher eukaryotes. To the best of my knowledge, the only precedents for this systematic mutational approach in higher eukaryotes were the screens for early embryonic lethals at the *t* locus performed by SALOME WAELSCH and her colleagues in the mouse and the studies of mutations at the *bithorax* complex by ED LEWIS.

Those notable exceptions aside, much of the prior work in this century had focused on the analysis of mutations encountered by chance. Moreover, in many cases the focus was centered more on the nature of the mutants and the mutational processes themselves than on the biological function of the wild-type gene and the role of genes in regulatory hierarchies.

This was certainly true of the genetic analysis of meiosis. Although STURTEVANT, DOBZHANSKY, NOVITSKI, GRELL, SANDLER and LINDSLEY had certainly conducted detailed studies of the meiotic behavior of existing chromosome aberrations, there were very few data on mutations that affected meiosis in Drosophila. Indeed, there were only three recessive mutations known to affect the meiotic process (*c(3)G*, *ca^{nd}* and *eq*). Although each of these mutations had been studied in detail, all of those studies were based on the analysis of single alleles. Moreover, there is no published evidence of an attempt to determine whether or not these mutations were true null alleles.

Certainly there had been no systematic approach to

identify other, perhaps equally important genes in the meiotic process. To quote from the grant proposal that funded this work, "The existence of these three autosomal recessive mutations that profoundly affect meiosis, which were encountered purely by chance, encourages one to suspect that a systematic search for meiotic genes might prove fruitful."

How the screen for new meiotic mutants was done: The mutations were recovered from wild populations collected in and around Rome at such locales as a winery in Salaria and the city's wholesale fruit market. LARRY SANDLER claimed for years that the collections were made entirely by DAN LINDSLEY while LARRY conversed with the vintners or the fruit merchants. (Having been LARRY's student, I have no reason to doubt this description of the division of labor). In a story that, until recently, I had always viewed as too apocryphal to be repeated in print, LARRY also claimed that while the fruit sellers were initially suspicious of DAN and his butterfly net, they were reassured by LARRY's claims, in the vernacular, that this was the only therapy that DAN's physicians at the asylum found effective. DAN did not speak Italian and was thus fortunately unaware of these conversations.

The decision to search for meiotic mutations in natural populations was based on the assumption that recessive mutations would be found as heterozygotes in natural populations at a frequency equal to the square root of their mutation rate, a frequency high enough to be detected in screens. To quote from LINDSLEY's grant application, "In ordinary ranges of mutation rates this should lead to an incidence of such mutations in nature in excess of that obtainable with most mutagens." Given that EMS would not be introduced to Drosophila geneticists until 1968, this frequency of mutations seemed greatly in excess of what could be obtained with existing mutagens such as γ- or X-rays. Moreover, a screen of wild populations seemed desirable because in addition to providing the desired mutations, it would also provide information on the types and prevalence of such mutations in natural populations.

The basic scheme was straightforward. Using a *2-3* translocation and crossover-suppressing marker chromosomes, lethal-free second and third chromosome complements would be extracted from several natural populations in Italy, and homozygotes for these *2-3* complements would be tested for their effects on segregation in both males and females and on recombination in females. Indeed, a significant number of meiotic mutants were recovered; of the 118 *2-3* complements tested in females, 11 significantly increased the rate of nondisjunction. Some 123 such *2-3* complements were tested in males, along with 177 half-complements (either *2* or *3*), and of these, four had strong effects on segregation. In addition a new *Segregation Distorter* chromosome was found.

As successful as these screens were, it is reasonable to ask why SANDLER and LINDSLEY felt the need to do them in Rome (as opposed to their home institutions in Seattle and San Diego). LINDSLEY's grant application presents two justifications for this decision. First, "If the incidence of autosomal recessive lethals in North America can be considered general, then southern populations might be expected to have more mutations than northern ones." Given that Rome is well north of San Diego, this rationale only makes sense if one is already committed to a European sabbatical. I find more truth in his second justification, "As an investigator demonstrates competence in his chosen field, the demands for him to devote his efforts to nonresearch efforts become incessant. This is especially true as long as he is at his home institution." (It might help us to consider the significance of this statement during the next 10 or so committee meetings.)

The recovered mutations: As stated above, SANDLER *et al.* (1968) recovered 15 mutations that affected disjunction in one or both sexes. Of these, only one, *mei-S332*, affected disjunction in both sexes; the remainder affected only females (11) or males (3). Two of these mutations, both of which specifically affect the disjunction of chromosome *4*, proved to be allelic and to define the *mei-S8* locus. Of the mutations affecting female meiosis, the most notable are *mei-S282* and *mei-S51*, both of which are described below.

As important as these mutations have subsequently proven to be, an equal or perhaps even greater yield was produced by the screen of EMS-treated *X* chromosomes performed by B. S. BAKER and A. T. C. CARPENTER who were, at that time, graduate students in LARRY SANDLER's laboratory (BAKER and CARPENTER 1972). This screen of 209 EMS-treated *X* chromosomes yielded a set of meiotic mutations whose study has supported much of the last 20 years of work on meiosis in Drosophila. These include *mei-9*, *mei-41*, *mei-218*, *mei-352* and *nod*.

There also appear to have been at least two small screens of EMS-treated autosomes in the SANDLER lab, one of which is reported in SANDLER (1971). Although these screens examined a very limited number of chromosomes, 35 in the first instance and 24 in the second, they yielded a number of very important mutations, namely *c(3)G68*, *pal*, *mei-W68* and *ord*. These mutations, as well those produced in the two screens described above, were to provide research materials for generations of students in LARRY's laboratory (cf. BAKER 1975; HALL 1972; PARRY 1973).

What did these mutations tell us? There was more at issue in this search than simply finding the mutations. At the time this work was initiated, the existing cytogenetic work had begun to lead to some rather specific models of meiotic processes in Drosophila.

For example, it was widely accepted at that time that there were two systems for ensuring segregation in Drosophila females: a chiasmate system, and the so-called distributive system (GRELL 1976) that guaranteed the segregation of homologous or heterologous achiasmate chromosomes. According to GRELL, the choice of partners in the distributive system was determined not by homology, but rather in a manner that was determined by the availability, size and shape of these chromosomes. Buried in LINDSLEY's grant proposal, and thus presumably in the intent of the authors, is a direct test of that hypothesis. To quote again from the proposal, "If indeed there are two distinct pairing processes that obey different rules, then there should be different though probably overlapping, constellations of genes that control these phenomena."

Indeed, two mutations serving exactly this function, nod and mei-S51, were found in the course of these initial screens. The mei-S51 mutation was found in the screen of natural populations reported in the SANDLER et al. (1968) paper. The nod mutation was found in the parallel screen of EMS-treated chromosomes by BAKER and CARPENTER (1972). Studies of nod would indeed confirm that the process of achiasmate disjunction was truly separate from that which ensured chiasmate segregation (CARPENTER 1973). Moreover, in a manner not appreciated for almost two decades, the study of mei-S51 by L. G. ROBBINS would provide the first evidence that there was not one but rather two separate processes of achiasmate segregation in females (ROBBINS 1971; HAWLEY et al. 1993).

The work reported in SANDLER et al. (1968) also revealed that, although the control of meiosis I appears to be quite different between males and females, the processes that ensure sister chromatid adhesion and segregation at meiosis II appear to be under common control in the two sexes. This is exemplified by the mei-S332 mutation, first reported in this paper, which affects the control of sister chromatid separation in both sexes. A second mutation, ord, which also affects sister chromatid cohesion in both sexes, was recovered in a separate screen of 24 EMS-treated second chromosomes performed by JIM MASON (1976) as a graduate student in LARRY SANDLER's laboratory. Work on both mei-S332 and ord was continued by L. S. B. GOLDSTEIN (1980) and the loci are now under intensive study in the lab of T. ORR-WEAVER (KERREBROCK et al. 1992; MIYAZAKI and ORR-WEAVER 1992).

Finally, the phenotypes of several of the male meiotic mutations suggested the existence of at least some chromosome-specific functions acting during male meiosis. Most notably, the two alleles of mei-S8 recovered by SANDLER et al. (1968) affect only the disjunction of chromosome 4 in males. Similarly, BAKER and CARPENTER (1972) recovered a large number of mutations that affect only the disjunction of the sex chromosomes. This may define a crucial difference between the two meiotic processes in that, with the quite possibly spurious exception of mei-1, there are no chromosome-specific meiotic mutations in females.

Most crucially, the analysis of the original set of mutants recovered in the screen of natural populations allowed SANDLER et al. (1968) to produce a pair of flow charts, or pathways, describing the deduced pathway of wild-type functions (see their Figures 3 and 4). The descriptions of these pathways are couched in terms, such as landmarks and control points, which seem to presage more modern discussions of the cell cycle. The term landmark was used to describe major events in the meiotic cycle, while the term control points was defined by SANDLER et al. (1968) as "points at which a genetic effect is necessary for the normal process of meiosis to continue." The analysis of the mutants recovered by BAKER and CARPENTER (1972) allowed these diagrams to be refined to the point where they became invaluable road maps of the meiotic processes in Drosophila, for example Figure 6 of BAKER and HALL (1976).

I might, however, point out that Figure 3 was more a source of anxiety than pride to LARRY SANDLER. He opened his issue of GENETICS only to find that this figure was upside down. Apparently, LARRY was concerned that someone had played an elaborate practical joke on him, and checked with his colleague DAVID STADLER, whose issue also contained the inverted Figure 3. I am told that LARRY was eventually calmed and reassured by the conviction that the defective copies had only been sent to those individuals whose last name started with S. I am happy if LARRY was indeed reassured by that conviction. However, honesty requires me to note that the copy on the desk next to me, which belongs to and was sent to M. M. GREEN, also contains an inverted Figure 3, as does the copy in our library.

Where are the mutants now? In the decade or so after their recovery, these mutations provided investigators with an incalculable wealth of information. This is perhaps best understood in terms of the use of these mutations to elucidate both the genetic control of recombination and the mechanism of the process itself.

CARPENTER used the existing array of recombination-defective mutants in genetic studies of both the recombination process itself and the mechanisms that control the number and distribution of recombinants. She also exploited these mutations in the course of detailed ultrastructural studies on the formation of the synaptonemal complex and analyses of recombination nodule structure (CARPENTER 1988, 1989). Finally, her detailed analysis of the effects of several recombination-defective mutations on various parameters of gene conversion provided crucial insights into the underlying mechanism (CARPENTER 1982). Taken together, and in light of data arising from the study of meiosis in yeast, these studies of recombination-deficient meiotic mutations in Drosophila served as linchpins in the modern synthesis of the relationship between chromosome pairing and the initiation of recombination (CARPENTER 1987; HAWLEY and ARBEL 1993).

In addition, the detailed analysis of the relationships between exchange and segregation in females homozygous for recombination-defective mutations provided crucial details for the now commonly accepted notion that normal levels of exchange are both necessary and sufficient to ensure regular segregation (BAKER and HALL 1976; HAWLEY 1988). They also provided data on the mechanisms that control the number and distribution of exchanges, which would have been impossible to glean in the absence of the mutations. More crucially, they also generated important insights into the functional significance of those controls: the extraordinary control of chiasma position probably reflects a compromise between the difficulties inherent in resolving proximal chiasmata and the low ability of very distal chiasmata to ensure disjunction.

These studies of the phenotypes of recombination-defective mutations were augmented by the finding that the set of recombination-defective mutations in Drosophila overlapped significantly with the set of mutagen-sensitive or repair-defective mutations (BAKER et al. 1976). Initially this finding generated enormous enthusiasm, both because it linked together two emerging new areas in Drosophila genetics and because it seemed to predict that the ongoing biochemical studies of repair would provide rapid insights into the nature of the recombinational defects, and thus into the nature of the recombination process itself. Although much has been learned, that later promise remains to be fulfilled. Recent progress on the cloning of such genes (mei-41 and mei-9) by BOYD and his collaborators seems likely to provide truly significant insights into the mechanisms of both recombination and repair.

Finally, in a series of collaborative papers, BRUCE BAKER and MAURIZIO GATTI elegantly demonstrated that many of the recombination-defective or repair-defective strains also exhibit severe defects in mitotic chromosome behavior (BAKER, CARPENTER and RIPOLL 1978; GATTI and BAKER 1980). This work again served to interlock two emerging fields and to provide significant new insights into the roles the wild-type alleles of these genes play in the proper development of the fly.

With all of this work in the literature, why did only four or five labs present at the 1988 meeting in New Orleans? What happened? Perhaps the loss of apparent interest reflected refocusing of major workers in the field toward new problems. Perhaps the field was simply eclipsed by exploding developments in the study of various aspects of gene function during embryogenesis. Regardless of the cause of that decline, the last five years have witnessed a renaissance in the analysis of meiosis.

This rebirth has been characterized by three types of efforts. The first has been the detailed characterization of many of these loci at the genetic level: large searches for additional alleles have been reported for nod (ZHANG and HAWLEY 1990), mei-S332 (KERREBROCK et al. 1992), ord (MIYAZAKI and ORR-WEAVER 1992) and mei-218 (K. S. MCKIM and R. S. HAWLEY, unpublished data). Second, the development of confocal microscopy has allowed detailed analysis of the normal meiotic process in females, which had previously been impossible (THEURKAUF and HAWLEY 1992).

Perhaps the most instructive case of the power of combining the new microscopy with the analysis of a well characterized meiotic mutation is the analysis of the nod mutation. In this case the cytological description of the nod phenotype, together with the finding that the nod locus encodes a kinesin-like protein (ZHANG et al. 1990), provided truly important insights into the role that the wild-type nod protein plays in the process of achiasmate segregation.

But perhaps the most important addition to the field has been the application of the now traditional methods of molecular genetics to the genes defined by meiotic mutations. As noted above, this process has been accomplished for the nod mutation (ZHANG et al. 1990) and for the ncd mutation (MCDONALD and GOLDSTEIN 1990; ENDOW, HENIKOFF and NIEDZIELLA 1990). To the best of my knowledge, none of the genes defined by the mutants recovered by SANDLER et al. (1968) have so far been characterized at the molecular level. However, mei-S332 has been characterized extensively at the cytological level by GOLDSTEIN (1980) and by KERREBROCK et al. (1992). In addition, multiple alleles of this mutation have now been obtained and the molecular analysis should be considered as imminent, if indeed it has not been completed at the time of this writing. A similar set of assertions can be made about the ord mutation which, like mei-S332, defines a crucial component of sister chromatid separation (MIYAZAKI and ORR-WEAVER 1992).

This molecular assault on the mutations provided by the original screen even extends to reviving the dead. Sadly, both alleles of *mei-S8* were lost shortly after the paper was published. I'm aware of at least two laboratories seriously looking for new alleles of this locus. Similarly, my own laboratory has become deeply interested in recovering new alleles of *mei-T3*, a semi-sterile line recovered in the original SANDLER *et al.* (1968) screen.

Reflections from a cloudy crystal ball: One hopes that the enormous progress in the study of meiosis observed during the last five years is predictive of the next 25. Curiously, though, my strongest perception of the present is an uneasy feeling that we are running out of the past. The legacy of meiotic mutants left to us by SANDLER *et al.* (1968) and by BAKER and CARPENTER (1972) is nearly exhausted. It is clear that to take the next few steps in this process, we will once again need to perform large screens for meiotic mutations in both sexes. My own laboratory, and I suspect those of others as well, has now begun exactly this task.

Perhaps the most significant praise I can place on SANDLER *et al.* (1968) and on BAKER and CARPENTER (1972) is to note that they still serve as the most useful guide-posts as we embark in this effort. These more modern searches will use higher-tech mutagens (enhancer-traps and the like) and they will be combined with a more molecularly oriented and technically sophisticated analysis. Unlike SANDLER *et al.* (1968) and BAKER and CARPENTER (1972), our most immediate goals will be molecular descriptions of the genes in question.

Nonetheless, both the general schemes and the rationales remain unchanged. We still seek to dissect the meiotic process through the systematic collection and analysis of a large number of meiotic mutants. I suspect that those of us involved in these mutant hunts secretly hope that the mutants recovered in our screens will prove as valuable in the next 25 years as did those of our predecessors in the last 25 years.

I wish to thank BRUCE BAKER, ADELAIDE CARPENTER, JIM MASON and especially DAN LINDSLEY for sharing their memories and insights. I also thank DEAN PARKER, from whose reprint collection I unearthed the sabbatical grant application written by DAN LINDSLEY. Finally, I want to thank ADELAIDE CARPENTER, BRUCE BAKER, KENNETH BURTIS, BARRY GANETZKY, JENNIFER FRAZIER and KIM MCKIM for their valuable comments on the manuscript. Due to space limitations I have had to omit references to many of the studies done by various students in the SANDLER laboratory and by other workers. I deeply regret this limitation. This paper is dedicated to the memory of LARRY SANDLER, whose presence remains undiminished.

LITERATURE CITED

BAKER, B. S., 1975 Paternal loss (*pal*): a meiotic mutant in *Drosophila melanogaster* causing loss of paternal chromosomes. Genetics **80:** 267–296.

BAKER, B. S., and A. T. C. CARPENTER, 1972 Genetic analysis of sex chromosome meiotic mutants in *Drosophila melanogaster*. Genetics **71:** 255–286.

BAKER, B. S., A. T. C. CARPENTER and P. RIPOLL, 1978 The utilization during mitotic cell cycle of loci controlling meiotic recombination and disjunction in *Drosophila melanogaster*. Genetics **90:** 531–578.

BAKER, B. S., and J. C. HALL, 1976 Meiotic mutants: genic control of meiotic recombination and chromosome segregation, pp. 351–434 in *Genetics and Biology of Drosophila Ia*, edited by E. NOVITSKI and M. ASHBURNER. Academic Press, New York.

BAKER, B. S., J. B. BOYD, A. T. C. CARPENTER, M. M. GREEN, T. D. NGUYEN, *et al.*, 1976 Genetic controls of meiotic recombination and somatic DNA metabolism in *Drosophila melanogaster*. Proc. Natl. Acad. Sci. USA **73:** 4140–4143.

CARPENTER, A. T. C., 1973 A mutant defective in distributive disjunction in *Drosophila melanogaster*. Genetics **73:** 393–428.

CARPENTER, A. T. C., 1982 Mismatch repair, gene conversion and crossing-over in two recombination-defective mutants in *Drosophila melanogaster*. Proc. Natl. Acad. Sci. USA **79:** 5961–5965.

CARPENTER, A. T. C., 1987 Gene conversion, recombination, and the initiation of meiotic synapsis. BioEssays **6:** 232–236.

CARPENTER, A. T. C., 1988 Thoughts on recombination nodules, meiotic recombination and chiasmata, pp. 526–548 in *Genetic Recombination*, edited by R. KUCHERLAPATI and G. SMITH. American Society for Microbiology, Washington, D.C.

CARPENTER, A. T. C., 1989 Are there abnormal recombination nodules in the *Drosophila melanogaster* meiotic mutant *mei-218*? Genome **31:** 74–80.

ENDOW, S. A., S. HENIKOFF and L. S. NIEDZIELLA, 1990 Mediation of meiotic and early mitotic chromosome segregation in *Drosophila* by a protein related to kinesin. Nature **345:** 81–83.

GATTI, M., S. PIMPINELLI and B. S. BAKER, 1980 Relationships between chromatid interchanges, sister chromatid exchanges, and meiotic recombination in *Drosophila melanogaster*. Proc. Natl. Acad. Sci. USA **77:** 1575–1579.

GOLDSTEIN, L. S. B., 1980 Mechanisms of chromosome orientation revealed by two meiotic mutants in *Drosophila melanogaster*. Chromosoma (Berl.) **78:** 79–111.

GRELL, R. F., 1976 Distributive pairing, pp. 435–486 in *Genetics and Biology of Drosophila Ia*, edited by E. NOVITSKI and M. ASHBURNER. Academic Press, New York.

HALL, J. C., 1972 Chromosome segregation influenced by two alleles of the meiotic mutation *c(3)G* in *Drosophila melanogaster*. Genetics **71:** 367–400.

HAWLEY, R. S., 1988 Exchange and chromosome segregation in eukaryotes, pp. 497–525 in *Genetic Recombination*, edited by R. KUCHERLAPATI and G. SMITH. American Society for Microbiology, Washington, D.C.

HAWLEY, R. S., and T. ARBEL, 1993 Yeast genetics and the fall of the classical view of meiosis. Cell **72:** 301–303.

HAWLEY, R. S., K. S. MCKIM and T. ARBEL, 1993 Meiotic segregation in *Drosophila melanogaster* females: molecules, mechanisms, and myths. Annu. Rev. Genet. **27:** 281–317.

HAWLEY, R. S., and W. E. THEURKAUF, 1993 Requiem for the distributive system: achiasmate segregation in Drosophila females. Trends Genet. **9:** 310–316.

HAWLEY, R. S., H. IRICK, A. E. ZITRON, D. A. HADDOX, A. LOHE, *et al.*, 1993 There are two mechanisms of achiasmate segregation in *Drosophila*, one of which requires heterochromatic homology. Dev. Genet. **13:** 440–467.

KERREBROCK, A. W., W. Y. MIYAZAKI, D. BIRNBY and T. L. ORR-WEAVER, 1992 The Drosophila *mei-S332* gene promotes sister-chromatid adhesion in meiosis following kinetochore differentiation. Genetics **130:** 827–841.

MASON, J. M., 1976 *Orientation disrupter (ord)*: a recombination-defective and disjunction-defective meiotic mutant in *Drosophila melanogaster*. Genetics **84:** 545–572.

MCDONALD, H. B., and L. S. B. GOLDSTEIN, 1990 Identification and characterization of a gene encoding a kinesin-like protein in Drosophila. Cell **61:** 991–1000.

MIYAZAKI, W. Y., and T. L. ORR-WEAVER, 1992 Sister chromatid misbehavior in Drosophila *ord* mutants. Genetics **132:** 1047–1061.

PARRY, D. M., 1973 A meiotic mutant affecting recombination in female *Drosophila melanogaster*. Genetics **73:** 465–486.

ROBBINS, L. G., 1971 Nonexchange alignment: a meiotic process revealed by a synthetic meiotic mutant of *Drosophila melanogaster*. Mol. Gen. Genet. **110:** 144–166.

SANDLER, L. M., 1971 Induction of autosomal meiotic mutants by EMS in *Drosophila melanogaster*. Genetics **39:** 365–377.

SANDLER, L. M., D. L. LINDSLEY, B. NICOLETTI and G. TRIPPA, 1968 Mutants affecting meiosis in natural populations of *Drosophila melanogaster*. Genetics **60:** 525–558.

THEURKAUF, W. E., and R. S. HAWLEY, 1992 Meiotic spindle assembly in *Drosophila* females: behavior of nonexchange chromosomes and the effects of mutations in the *nod* kinesin-like protein. J. Cell Biol. **116:** 1167–1180.

ZHANG, P., and R. S. HAWLEY, 1990 The genetic analysis of distributive segregation in *Drosophila melanogaster*. II. Further genetic analysis of the *nod* locus. Genetics **125:** 115–127.

ZHANG, P., B. A. KNOWLES, L. S. B. GOLDSTEIN and R. S. HAWLEY, 1990 A kinesin-like protein required for distributive chromosome segregation in *Drosophila*. Cell **62:** 1053–1062.

December 1993

A Notable Triumvirate of Maize Geneticists

Oliver E. Nelson

Laboratory of Genetics, University of Wisconsin–Madison, Madison, Wisconsin 53706

WITH the current explosive rate of progress in genetics, we are less likely than ever before to devote much thought to those whose research established the firm foundation on which our science has been built. In this essay, I pay tribute to a distinguished figure in the development of plant genetics, EDWARD M. EAST, and to two of his first graduate students, ROLLINS A. EMERSON and DONALD F. JONES. All three figured prominently in research that made maize a model system for plant genetics and transformed the methods used by plant breeders to improve the yield and agronomic qualities of the maize species. Each was from the Midwest–East from Illinois, EMERSON from Nebraska, and JONES from Kansas–so it is ironic that virtually all the research on a quintessentially Midwestern crop for which they are known was carried out in the Northeast. All were much honored by their contemporaries, including their election to the National Academy of Sciences, and each served as president of the Genetics Society of America.

EDWARD EAST had been educated in another discipline, like all of the first generation of geneticists. EAST was trained as a chemist at the University of Illinois. He became interested in maize breeding in his position at Illinois as an assistant to C. G. HOPKINS, who was engaged in experiments to change the oil and protein content of maize through selection. This effort is continuing to the present time and is still making progress in the lines selected for higher contents. EAST's task was to conduct the chemical analyses of the various samples, a task he apparently regarded as thoroughly routine. He was rescued by the offer of a position by the director of the Connecticut Agricultural Experimental Station in New Haven, E. H. JENKINS. JENKINS, also a chemist, had been impressed by the Illinois selection experiments. Desiring to initiate such research at Connecticut, he hired EAST on HOPKINS's recommendation.

EAST joined the staff of the Connecticut Station in 1905, a year after receiving his M.S. degree at Illinois on a study of how streams purify themselves. It was still two years before he was to receive his Ph.D. degree from Illinois! His thesis involved a study of variation in an asexually propagated plant, the potato; he initiated this study in New Haven together with research on Nicotiana species and on inbreeding and outbreeding in maize. His tenure at New Haven was brief; he accepted an invitation in 1909 to join the staff of the Bussey Institute, Harvard's version of an agricultural experiment station. But his New Haven work was remarkably productive: a number of reports on potato improvement and inbreeding in maize were published during his stay at the Connecticut Station or shortly thereafter. He had grown some crosses between his lines of inbred maize in 1908 and thus had his own observations of the phenomenon of hybrid vigor. His explanation, as outlined in his 1909 paper in the *American Naturalist*, was the "stimulus of heterozygosis." EAST had followed closely the research of G. H. SHULL at the Cold Spring Harbor Laboratory and agreed with SHULL's interpretation (1908) that the loss of vigor in inbred maize was owing to the isolation of homozygous biotypes. He also believed that SHULL's proposed method of hybrid corn seed production by crossing inbred lines (1909), though theoretically correct, was impractical. He recommended that the farmer who was to grow the hybrid should produce the seed himself by crossing two elite open-pollinated varieties.

Another notable contribution was EAST's explanation in 1910 of quantitative inheritance in Mendelian terms, on the basis of results from inheritance studies of endosperm color and row number in corn. This report appeared the year after NILSSON-EHLE's 1909 paper on the same subject, a report that EAST cites although noting that his interpretation antedated the appearance of NILSSON-EHLE's work. The studies ini-

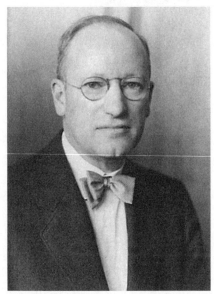
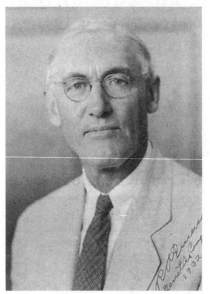
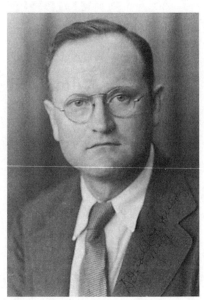

EDWARD M. EAST (left), ROLLINS A. EMERSON (center) and DONALD F. JONES (right) in portraits taken at the 1932 International Congress of Genetics.

tiated at Connecticut, particularly those on maize and tobacco, formed the interests that EAST was to pursue for the remainder of his career, together with numerous studies of self-sterility in plants.

EAST's studies of the effects of inbreeding in corn and subsequent crosses between the inbred lines culminated in the publication of the monograph *Inbreeding and Outbreeding* in 1919 with his student, DONALD JONES. He had been impressed with JONES's argument (1917) that, contrary to EAST's previously stated views, the basis of heterosis was the dominance of favorable alleles from each parent, which compensated for the deleterious recessive alleles present in the other parent. JONES pointed out that relatively few loci at which such deleterious alleles were present would be required to make it very difficult to select for favorable alleles at all the loci, especially in light of linkage, then recently discovered. This led to EAST's invitation to Jones to join in writing the above volume. In the chapter in which they discuss the basis of hybrid vigor, they accepted the complementary action of dominant factors as the cause while noting that the stimulation hypothesis must be held in abeyance. For maize, most subsequent research has tended to validate the dominant-factor hypothesis.

In his biographical memoir of EAST, DONALD JONES (1944) suggested that, while EAST's research at Harvard was productive, it was to a certain extent overshadowed by his influence as a mentor of graduate students. The students who received advanced degrees at Harvard under his guidance include a number whose names are known to most geneticists owing to their manifold contributions to plant genetics. R. A. EMERSON, O. E. WHITE, D. F. JONES, H. K. HAYES, EDGAR ANDERSON, KARL SAX, R. A. BRINK, PAUL

MANGELSDORF, RALPH SINGLETON, ERNEST SEARS and HAROLD SMITH constitute a distinguished group who not only received an education in genetics, but also imbibed their mentor's critical attitude and insistence on accuracy.

ROLLINS A. EMERSON was the first of EAST's students to receive a doctorate (1913). He was an unusual graduate student in that he was older than his major professor; as a member of the University of Nebraska faculty (professor of horticulture), he had considerable prior research experience in genetics, utilizing beans as the experimental organism. MARCUS RHOADES (1949) in his biographical memoir of EMERSON relates that an unexpected turn of events sparked EMERSON's interest in the genetics of corn. As an exercise, he had prepared for a class in genetics at Nebraska the F_2 generation of a cross between Rice popcorn and sweet corn (*su1/su1*), expecting this material to serve as an example of monogenic segregation. To his chagrin, the counts of the students showed a significant deficiency of sugary kernels from the expected 25%. His desire to learn the basis of this anomalous result led him to maize as an experimental organism for genetic research. However, his explanation of the deficiency of sugary kernels did not appear until 1934, some years after JONES and MANGELSDORF (1926) had arrived at a similar conclusion. The effect is due to the linkage of *su1* with *ga1*, a gametophyte allele that makes *ga1* microspores ineffective when competing against *Ga1* microspores on the silks of plants that are *ga1/Ga1* or *Ga1/Ga1*.

EMERSON's first publication (1910) dealing with maize genetics concerned a latent color factor, *pr*, present in a strain with colorless aleurone. The introduction to this report notes that other topics were under investigation. These were the nature of inheritance of the red and white variegation of "calico" corn, the modifiers of aleurone color intensity, and the appearance of mottled aleurone seeds in some crosses between purple and nonpurple stocks. EMERSON was also interested at the time in quantitative inheritance in maize, mentioned also as a concern of EAST's, and the two collaborated on a large and notable study published in 1913. They used the data from F_2 and F_3 generations of crosses of two vastly dissimilar varieties of corn (usually Tom Thumb popcorn and Missouri Dent) to demonstrate that the almost continuous range observed in the F_2 generation for such characters as height and days to flowering was explicable as the segregation of multiple Mendelian factors.

EMERSON had taken a leave from the University of Nebraska in 1910–1911 to pursue graduate studies at Harvard. It was obviously a period in which residence requirements were not as rigid as at present. Following his year at Harvard, he returned to Lincoln, but in 1914 he accepted an invitation to become head of the Department of Plant Breeding at Cornell University, where he was to remain for the rest of his career and where his most important research was carried out. Much of his research centered on the genetic control of plant and seed colors in maize and on the P-vv allele, where he demonstrated that the variegation was conditioned by a mutable gene. The variegated pericarp allele, P-vv, was a problem that engaged the attention of several maize geneticists, until the demonstration by BRINK and NILAN (1952) of the insertion into the P locus of what is now called a transposable element.

One of EMERSON's major contributions to genetics also resides in the students who received their graduate training under his tutelage. His group at Cornell became a major center for genetics research. When he moved to Cornell, two of his students, E. G. ANDERSON and E. W. LINDSTROM, went with him. Others whose names are familiar to geneticists were to join the group over the next few years: MILISLAV DEMEREC, GEORGE BEADLE, GEORGE SPRAGUE and MARCUS RHOADES, as well as a number of competent but less well known scientists, many of whom were to concentrate their efforts in plant breeding projects. By all accounts, EMERSON insisted that students select their own problems, trusting that good students would select significant areas in which to pursue their thesis research. Other Cornell scientists, who were students or postdoctoral fellows in other laboratories but working in maize genetics or cytogenetics, such as HARRIET CREIGHTON, BARBARA MCCLINTOCK, and CHARLES BURNHAM, interacted closely with the EMERSON group in the late 1920s and early 1930s, adding to the sense of excitement prevailing in that period. A widely

circulated photograph from 1929 shows EMERSON, BEADLE, BURNHAM, MCCLINTOCK and RHOADES at the edge of their corn plot. Note that it was Cornell University that hosted the notable 1932 International Congress of Genetics (CROW 1992).

Cornell University, by EMERSON's efforts, became a focal point for maize genetics research. In addition to the ongoing research in his group, he initiated two services that have benefited maize genetics greatly and continue to do so to the present day. He started the *Maize Newsletter*, which has been published annually since 1932 and includes progress reports, notes and unpublished data from researchers. No doubt this has been a major factor in the sense of community and openness that characterizes maize genetics. EMERSON also was responsible for the Maize Genetics Cooperation, which maintains and distributes the existing maize mutants and cytological aberrations. EMERSON directed these enterprises until his death. Several years later, MARCUS RHOADES took responsibility for both services and moved them to the University of Illinois, where he was then on the faculty. The Maize Genetics Cooperation remains at the University of Illinois, but when RHOADES moved to Indiana University, the *Maize Newsletter* moved with him. In 1975, when E. H. COE assumed the editorial responsibility, the *Newsletter* moved to the University of Missouri. Another service of considerable importance to maize genetics was the 1935 compendium, *A Summary of Linkage Studies in Maize* by EMERSON, BEADLE and FRASER, which brought together all the mapping information available at that time.

DONALD JONES received his Sc.D. degree at Harvard in 1918, five years after EMERSON. He was working as an alfalfa breeder at the Arizona Experiment Station when he read the 1912 bulletin by EAST and HAYES entitled *Heterozygosis in Evolution and Plant Breeding*. Intrigued, JONES wrote to EAST inquiring about the possibility of doing graduate work under his direction. Because the opportunity was not available immediately, he spent 1913–1914 at Syracuse University working toward a master's degree and teaching before enrolling at Harvard in the fall of 1914. In the fall of 1915, he moved to the Connecticut Experiment Station to succeed H. K. HAYES, who had moved to the University of Minnesota, and to carry on the plant breeding program under EAST's direction. He remained at the Experiment Station for the remainder of his career. His position at an agricultural experiment station undoubtedly accounted for the fact that his interests were divided almost equally between basic research and the application of genetic principles to plant improvement.

One of JONES's important contributions to genetic theory came while he was still a graduate student. His 1917 paper in GENETICS on the genetic basis of heterosis in maize and the apparent impression it had on EAST has been mentioned, but his findings are worth discussing in greater detail. Both EAST and SHULL in their reports of heterosis in crosses between inbred lines proposed that heterosis was generated by interaction between unlike alleles. In explaining the increase in height of the F_1 cross between two varieties of peas, KEEBLE and PELLEW (1910) suggested that it was because each variety had the dominant allele at one of two loci at which the other variety had the recessive allele, and that this was a model for hybrid vigor. EAST and HAYES (1912) had argued against this hypothesis on the grounds that selection should then make it possible to combine the favorable alleles at all pertinent loci into one line. EMERSON and EAST (1913) also noted that, if dominance of favorable alleles played a major role, one should observe an asymmetrical distribution in the F_2 generation for the character being measured. JONES pointed out that these arguments were negated by the recent discovery of linkage. If the pertinent loci were distributed randomly on all the chromosomes and if it were possible that a locus might contain either a favorable dominant or an unfavorable recessive allele, then neither objection was valid. The hypothesis of complementary dominant factors then offered a plausible basis for heterosis, while it was difficult to envision a mechanism for stimulus by heterozygosis.

In 1922, JONES suggested the procedure that was to stimulate serious interest in hybrid corn as a means of enhancing production. G. H. SHULL in his 1909 paper "A pure line method of corn breeding" had outlined essentially the method used today by corn breeders except for the methods of inbred improvement. The first inbreds, few in number, were notably weak and derived from one or several varieties. While the first F_1s illustrated the possibility of a large increase in yield over the parental inbreds compared with a lesser increase over the variety from which the inbreds were extracted, hybrid seed production seemed to be impractical as a method of corn improvement because of the limited seed production of the inbreds. JONES used examples from his research to point out that the solution was to produce the seed that the farmer was to plant by crossing an F_1 made by crossing two inbreds from one variety with an F_1 made from two inbreds derived from another variety to make double cross hybrids. It was this demonstration that interested corn breeders in hybrid production. Virtually all the hybrids were double crosses through the decade of the 1940s, by which time hybrids were grown on nearly 100% of the acreage in the principal corn-growing areas of the United States. It was only later that improved inbreds with greater vigor made feasible the production initially of three-way crosses (an F_1

female times an inbred male) and later of single crosses.

Two other contributions to hybrid corn seed production show JONES's interest in extending genetic principles into practice. Hybrid corn seed was first produced by emasculating (detasseling) the plants of the female parent in three or four rows planted between two rows of the male parent. JONES and MANGELSDORF (1951) suggested that part of the hybrid seed could be produced with a female parent that had Texas cytoplasmic male sterility, making detasseling unnecessary. Then seed of the sterile hybrid could be mixed with one-half or one-third as much seed of the same hybrid that was fertile, and the fertile plants would produce sufficient pollen to result in full seed sets on all plants. In another report in the same year, JONES showed that it was possible to use a male parent that had nuclear fertility-restoring factors for the Texas male-sterile cytoplasm so that the F_1 progeny were fertile. This procedure soon became the preferred method for producing hybrid corn seed and was used for some years until 1970, when a new strain of the Southern corn leaf blight fungus, *Helminthosporium maydis* a.k.a. *Cochiobolus heterostrophus*, attacked hybrids with the Texas sterile cytoplasm, causing serious losses in fields in which the fungus became established early in the season. This epiphytotic forced an end to seed production by this system.

It should not be thought, however, that JONES's interest in the application of genetic principles to plant improvement diverted him from research on basic aspects of genetics. He was intensely interested in somatic segregation in relation to atypical growth, in genetic control of the male gametophyte, and in the control of sexual differentiation in plants. He showed (1934) that by manipulation of the allelic state at two loci it was possible to convert maize, which is monoecious, into a dioecious plant. This suggested to him that monoecism was an intermediate step between plants with perfect flowers and the dioecious state. He also served the genetics community well as the second editor of GENETICS, holding the post from 1926 until 1935, and as the editor of the *Proceedings of the Sixth International Congress of Genetics* in 1932.

DONALD JONES was the only one of this notable trio with whom I was acquainted. I was one of the relatively few students whose graduate training was under his tutelage, because he did not have a formal affiliation with a university. All of his students were supported by fellowships at the Connecticut Agricultural Experiment Station while studying at Yale. So my major professor of record was E. W. SINNOTT. Several others, including WARREN GABELMAN and HERBERT EVERETT who also were to go into academia, followed the same path. JONES believed, as did EMERSON, that students should not be assigned topics for research but should find their own way to a thesis problem. This made for some uncomfortable moments in the early stages of graduate study but was salutary in preparing one for a career in research. He also imbued his students with the sense that one could and should contribute to both applied and theoretical research.

JONES was a modest man without a trace of ostentation. He was described by one author as "a Yankee from Kansas," and he did have the independence of thought and disregard for public acclaim that prompted that description. On one occasion when I commented on an effusive magazine article on his research, his response was, "Flattery is like poison; it can't hurt you if you don't swallow it." My colleague, JIM CROW, has recounted his first meeting with DONALD JONES, and the story nicely illustrates JONES's modesty. CROW's first faculty position was at Dartmouth, where JONES's son, LORING, was then a student. On one occasion when DONALD JONES visited Dartmouth, he was introduced by another faculty member simply as "MR. JONES, who is interested in genetics." JIM, as was his custom with visitors who evinced an interest in the subject, proceeded in explain what the science of genetics was about and what geneticists did, without any word or show of impatience from JONES to indicated that he was well acquainted with the subject. It was only later that JIM learned to whom he had been talking.

Plant genetics in general and maize genetics in particular owe a considerable debt to these geneticists, who left us a solid legacy of basic knowledge and critical standards that fostered progress by their successors. It has been illuminating to reread their most important papers, and my respect for their scientific acumen is reinforced as it would be for any geneticist delving into this early literature.

I am indebted to the *Biographical Memoirs* of the National Academy of Sciences for much of the information concerning these geneticists. E. M. EAST's memoir was written by D. F. JONES (1944), R. A. EMERSON's by MARCUS RHOADES (1949), and D. F. JONES's by PAUL MANGELSDORF (1975).

LITERATURE CITED

BRINK, R. A., and R. A. NILAN, 1952 The relation between light variegated and medium variegated pericarp in maize. Genetics 37: 519–544.

CROW, J. F., 1992 Sixty years ago: the 1932 International Congress of Genetics. Genetics 131: 761–768.

EAST, E. M., 1909 The distinction between development and heredity in inbreeding in maize. Am. Nat. 43: 173–181.

EAST, E. M., 1910 A Mendelian interpretation of variation that is apparently continuous. Am. Nat. 44: 65–82.

EAST, E. M., and H. K. HAYES, 1912 Heterozygosis in evolution and plant breeding. U. S. Dept. Agric. Bur. Plant Indust. Bull. 243: 1–58.

EAST, E. M., and D. F. JONES, 1919 *Inbreeding and Outbreeding.* J. B. Lippincott, Philadelphia.

EMERSON, R. A., 1910 Latent colors in corn. Am. Breeders Assoc. Rep. 6: 233–237.

EMERSON, R. A., 1934 Relation of the differential fertilization genes, *Ga, ga,* to certain other genes of the *Su-Tu* linkage group in maize. Genetics 19: 137–156.

EMERSON, R. A., G. W. BEADLE and A. C. FRASER, 1935 A summary of linkage studies in maize. Cornell Univ. Agric. Exp. Sta. Memoir 180.

EMERSON, R. A., and E. M. EAST, 1913 The inheritance of quantitative characters in maize. Bull. Nebraska Agric. Exp. Sta. 2.

JONES, D. F., 1917 Dominance of linked factors as a means of accounting for heterosis. Genetics 2: 466–479.

JONES, D. F., 1922 The productiveness of single and double first generation corn hybrids. J. Am. Soc. Agron. 14: 242–252.

JONES, D. F., 1934 Unisexual maize plants and their relation to dioecism in other plants. Proc. Natl. Acad. Sci. USA 20: 39–41.

JONES, D. F., 1944 Edward Murray East (1879–1938). National Academy of Sciences, *Biographical Memoirs* 23: 217–242.

JONES, D. F., 1951 The induction of cytoplasmic pollen sterility and restoration of fertility in maize. Genetics 36: 557.

JONES, D. F., and P. C. MANGELSDORF, 1926 The expression of Mendelian factors in the gametophyte of maize. Genetics 11: 423–455.

JONES, D. F., and P. C. MANGELSDORF, 1951 The production of hybrid corn without detasseling. Conn. Agric. Exp. Sta. Bull. 550.

KEEBLE, F., and C. PELLEW, 1910 The mode of inheritance of stature and of time of flowering in peas (*Pisum sativum*). J. Genet. 1: 47–56.

MANGELSDORF, P. C., 1975 Donald Forsha Jones (1890–1963). National Academy of Sciences, *Biographical Memoirs* 46: 135–156.

NILSSON-EHLE, H., 1909 Kreuzungsuntersuchungen an Hafer und Weizen. Lunds Univ. Aarskr. N. F. 5 (2): 1–122.

RHOADES, M. M., 1949 ROLLINS ADAMS EMERSON (1873–1947). National Academy of Sciences, *Biographical Memoirs* 25: 313–325.

SHULL, G. H., 1908 The composition of a field of maize. Am. Breeders Assoc. Rep. 4: 296–301.

SHULL, G. H., 1909 A pure line method of corn breeding. Am. Breeders Assoc. Rep. 5: 51–59.

Allozymes in Evolutionary Genetics
Self-Imposed Burden or Extraordinary Tool?

Ward B. Watt[1]

Department of Biological Sciences, Stanford University, Stanford, California 94305–5020,
and Rocky Mountain Biological Laboratory, Crested Butte, Colorado 81224

THE controversial history of allozyme studies: Alternative heritable forms of enzymes, differing in charge or shape, have been known since the 1940s; these may be alleles of one gene (allozymes) or products of distinct but related genes (isozymes). LEWONTIN and HUBBY (1966), finding an unexpected bonanza of allozyme variation in Drosophila, re-cast the existing debate about the evolutionary meaning of genetic variation in terms of allozymes. A torrent of like data followed; its interpretation was dominated at first by the notorious "neutralist-selectionist" debate. Population-genetic theory alone proved unable to resolve this debate; pure genetic-statistical analyses lacked power to test deviations from neutrality (EWENS and FELDMAN 1976), and neutralist and selectionist models predicted convergent distributions of allelic/genotypic frequencies (GILLESPIE 1991). Too little *biology* was present in the debate, and studying the impacts of allozymes on biological mechanisms in the wild promised to help. Mechanistic study of allozymes has indeed ensued, and its practitioners are mostly optimistic. LEWONTIN (1991), in contrast, stigmatized allozyme study since 1966 as a "fardel" or frustrating burden. Some others share his skepticism. Such clashing views bespeak varying awareness of what has been found, or else paradigm differences or other communication barriers. Here, I summarize progress in mechanistic allozyme study, critique reservations about it and explore its promise for new research.

What has been learned from mechanistic study of allozymes? A thorough review is impossible here. I illustrate points with a subset of well analyzed cases, apologizing to those whose important work is omitted or discussed cursorily. I often cite recent summaries rather than original references.

Function of allozymes in metabolic context: Consider a 1-substrate-1-product enzyme-catalyzed reaction described by

$$v = \frac{(V_{\max_f}/K_{m_f})[A] - (V_{\max_r}/K_{m_r})[B]}{1 + [A]/K_{m_f} + [B]/K_{m_r}}$$

where v is net reaction rate, f and r mark parameters of forward and reverse reactions, $[A]$ and $[B]$ are substrates/products, K_ms are composite constants which index substrate affinity (but are not strict dissociation constants), and $V_{\max}$, the maximum velocity, is the product of enzyme concentration $[E]$ and catalytic rate constant k_{cat}. The ratio $V_{\max}/K_m$ is the limiting pseudo-first-order rate constant as $[A]$ (or $[B]$) decreases. Enzyme stability differences may change $[E]$. Variants in transcriptional or translational regulation, changing $[E]$, may co-occur with allozymes' peptide-specific differences (*e.g.*, LAURIE and STAM 1988); this can mimic variation in k_{cat}, but not variation in K_m.

How do metabolic effects arise from changes in these allozyme parameters? Metabolic network theory (KACSER and BURNS 1973; EASTERBY 1973; SAVAGEAU and SORRIBAS 1989) is central to a clear answer. Metabolism may be in steady state (all rates in the pathway equal to the system flux rate, metabolite pool sizes unchanging) or transient state (rates and metabolite pools changing). In either case, most ("intervening") steps must evolve high (*not* "excess") catalytic power (= high $V_{\max}/K_m$) if control of steady state flux, or of speed of transient response, is to be focused on a few steps which thus are "rate-limiters" and whose properties may then be refined *coadaptively*. No allozymes have been studied at rate-limiting steps (except for Hb), so high $V_{\max}/K_m$ has been a performance criterion for allozyme studies. $V_{\max}/K_m$ can increase *via* tighter binding, *i.e.*, low K_m (too low K_m may be harmful, HOCHACHKA and SOMERO 1973), or by increased $V_{\max}$, through higher $[E]$ or k_{cat} ($V_{\max} = k_{cat}[E]$).

---

[1] Use Stanford address for correspondence.

Thermal stability changes [E] *via* effects on enzyme half-life. Location of an enzyme in a "branch point" among pathways may intensify the impact of change in its metabolic parameters. Connection to fitness measures (WATT 1986), mutation-selection balance models (CLARK 1991), etc., promises more evolutionary utility of this theory.

Mechanistic study of allozymes' evolutionary impact: Case studies may be thought of in terms of FEDER and WATT's (1992) view of evolution as a recursion of four stages, from the starting genetic makeup of one generation to the same point of the next: a) genotypes → phenotypes, how genetic variants change organisms' "design" (*e.g.*, protein structure, body form, etc.); b) phenotypes → performance, how organismal design supports important activity such as feeding, locomotion, or regulation; c) performance → fitness, how organisms' performance translates through demography into survivorship or fecundity, thence into net fitness; d) fitness → genotypes, how fitnesses set (or fail to set, if genetic drift or inbreeding forestall them) the next generation's genetic makeup. The whole recursion has been traced in the case of human Hb. Some newer case studies are nearly complete, and others are close behind:

• Ten genotypes of the glycolytic enzyme phosphoglucose isomerase (PGI) in lowland Colias butterflies differ strikingly in kinetics and thermal stability, often trading off between these qualities as anticipated by HOCHACHKA and SOMERO (1973). Some but not all heterozygotes are superior in kinetics; PGI genotypes *4/4* and *4/5* are equally kinetically poor and thermally stable compared to "sister" genotypes, thus being neutral with respect to one another even while they differ sharply from others at the same gene. The major V_{max}/K_m advantage of *3/4* over *4/4* genotypes of Colias PGI is reflected, as predicted, in a severalfold advantage of *3/4* over *4/4* in flux response (detected with radioisotope tracers) through Colias' flight muscle glycolysis during flight. Differences among the PGI genotypes in daily flight capacity, predicted from the biochemical differences, were found in extensively replicated field experiments. The flight differences in turn were predicted to translate into genotypic differences in survival, male mating success, and female fecundity; predictions have been tested and confirmed in replicate among seasons, years, populations, and two semi-species. Genotype frequencies, reflecting the fitness component results in genotype-specific fashion, have shown closely similar values across western North America for 36–100[+] generations, depending on local demography. More fitness component trials in extreme habitats, then quantitative synthesis of the components into net fitness, will complete analysis of this selection regime [WATT (1992) and references therein].

• LABATE and EANES (1992) have recently found major effects of Drosophila glucose-6-phosphate dehydrogenase (G6PD) allozymes *in vivo*: a 32% difference in pentose shunt flux among genotypes arises from 40% difference in their kinetics.

• In a clinal lactate dehydrogenase (LDH) polymorphism of the fish Fundulus, the heterozygote enzyme's kinetics are more like the cold-specialist homozygote at low temperature (10°) and more like the warm-specialist homozygote at high temperature (40°). At 10°, the kinetic differences between genotypes successfully predict their carriers' erythrocyte ATP/hemoglobin (Hb) ratios, hence Hb O₂ loading (ATP being used by fish to modify Hb function), and predicted differences among the genotypes in egg hatch and in swimming speed are experimentally confirmed. At 25°, allozymes' similarity leads to a *lack* of difference in ATP/Hb values. These functional differences have been used successfully to predict survivorship differences among the LDH-B genotypes. A cline of Fundulus' LDH frequencies along the Atlantic coast of North America, from northern near-fixation of the cold-specialist allele to southern fixation of the warm-specialist allele, follows directly from the lower-level analysis [POWERS *et al.* (1991) and references therein].

• Other such cases include Drosophila alcohol dehydrogenase (ADH) (VAN DELDEN 1982; FRERIKSEN *et al.* 1991; LAURIE and STAM 1988), Metridium sea anemones' PGI (ZAMER and HOFFMANN 1989), α-Hb in Peromyscus mice (CHAPPELL and SNYDER 1984), Tigriopus copepods' glutamate-pyruvate transaminase (GPT) (BURTON and FELDMAN 1983), and leucine aminopeptidase (LAP) of Mytilus mussels (KOEHN 1987) [see WATT (1985, 1991) and POWERS *et al.* (1991) for yet others and more detail].

• Major allozyme differences are not universal. There is little kinetic difference at 37° among PGI allozymes of *Escherichia coli*; in turn, these alleles are the same in fitness at 37° in chemostat competition to within *s* (selection coefficient) ≈ 0.002 (DYKHUISEN and HARTL 1983). This result is sometimes said to "oppose" other case studies, but does no such thing: obviously, lack of difference in allozymes' function should yield lack of difference in allozymes' fitness (WATT 1985)!

These results undermine extreme neutralist and selectionist views alike: allozymes' biochemical function differs often *but not always*; non-additive heterozygote intermediacy is most usual, but overdominance also occurs. These functional differences have *specifically predictable* impacts on metabolic and physiological performance, and in turn on diverse fitness components.

Challenges faced by mechanistic evolutionary study of allozymes: If the above is so, why is the approach still controversial? Some workers still harbor reservations, whether or not stated in print. Concerns should be addressed, and naiveté requires correction, but also, mistaken concerns should be identified.

Null alleles: LANGLEY *et al.* (1981) studied these in two wild Drosophila samples. Nulls at 25 allozyme loci had frequencies of 0.0–1.2% among 357–912 alleles. Assuming mutation/selection frequency balance, phenotypic effects of the null heterozygotes were estimated, on average, as minimal. How, some ask, can recessiveness of nulls be consistent with findings of strong phenotypic effects of allozyme variants?

As the authors' statistics show, these null frequencies are heterogeneous within, and similarly so between, samples. Of 58 nulls, 41 were at 5 of the 25 loci, while 10 loci had 0 or 1 null. These data provide no meaningful average for heterozygous effect of nulls, yet the question about strong effects of allozymes relies on just such an average. (Also, for the rarer nulls, a frequency estimated from, *e.g.*, one sample of 1/716 and one of 0/436 is likely to be an *over*estimate, *under*estimating heterozygous phenotypic effect.) Next, it is a *non sequitur* to say that if null mutants are recessive at some loci in one taxon, variants at other loci or in other taxa must also be recessive. This study of null variants needs follow-up in terms of differing protein structures or functional roles of loci *vs.* null frequency, but its results do not conflict with evidence of other variants' phenotypic and/or fitness-related effects.

Metabolic aspects of dominance: KACSER and BURNS (1981) restated WRIGHT's (1934) argument for a metabolic cause of dominance: an intervening metabolic step working in steady state may have enough catalytic power to be "haplo-sufficient" (two copies of an impaired allele needed to produce major phenotypic damage). Going beyond WRIGHT, they claimed that allozymes should therefore have little phenotypic effect, but this does not follow because:

• Many pathways are not selected to focus control on a few rate-limiting steps, so no one step has enough catalytic power that its mutants are recessive.

• Enzymes' kinetics, stability, and [*E*] will change in pathway evolution only so far as selection dictates (WATT 1986; CLARK and KOEHN 1992). This will often entail functional compromise between mean and extreme conditions. Thus, haplo-sufficiency may often be narrowly limited, such as within a thermal optimum (*cf.* WATT 1991).

• Pathways often operate in transient-state conditions, which are much more demanding and much less likely to allow haplo-sufficiency.

Thus, when dominance occurs, the WRIGHTian mechanism often explains it, but embedding allozymes in metabolic networks does not, *per se*, render their phenotypic effects recessive, nor does it imply that allozymes usually are without metabolic effect.

Genetic load: LEWONTIN and HUBBY (1966) posed the problem thus: if balancing selection acted on allozymes at thousands of loci in a population, the cumulative disadvantage of homozygotes might wipe out the population. Besides reduction of this problem by diverse assumptions or selection regimes (*e.g.*, GILLESPIE 1991), the argument does not undermine allozyme studies because we do not find, in one species, thousands of varying allozymes *or* uniform selection on them. Most studied allozymes work in energy processing or biosynthesis; while centrally important, there are only 300–500 such loci in a species. Usually ≤25% of these are polymorphic at once, and the nature and strength of selection varies widely among loci (above). Thus, genetic load arguments do not clash with specific findings of major allozymic effect.

Linkage disequilibrium: Effects attributed to allozymes might instead be caused associatively by tightly linked variants of unknown genes. Linkage disequilibrium is unstable to recombination, but special conditions can produce it, so it merits consideration in each study of natural genetic variation. In purely structural-genetic terms, only DNA-sequence-level finding of linkage equilibrium between a selected site and its neighbors can fully test associative alternatives. However, associative alternatives can also be tested with great power on other grounds.

One major associative effect is "hitchhiking" wherein a directionally selected allele is followed in its frequency rise by a neutral allele at a closely linked gene (THOMSON 1977). This might confound apparent differences among allozymes, especially those lacking clear functional cause, but again, recombination opposes it. Neutral variants hitchhike with old, selected variants in a narrow range, *e.g.*, Drosophila ADH accumulates plausibly neutral "silent" variants (which do not change amino acids) only within ≈200 base pairs of the selected site, well within the ADH gene (HUDSON, KREITMAN and AGUADÉ 1987; AQUADRO 1992). Strong selection may extend this range, but asymmetric selection narrows it (ASMUSSEN and CLEGG 1981).

Moreover, any view of allozymes as neutral associates of other genes strongly predicts the *absence* of connections between allozymes' properties and organism-level or fitness differences. Given the diversity of genes and the general eukaryotic absence of linkage among genes controlling a process (save for some multi-gene families), there is minimal chance of correlation between genotypic patterns of even one enzyme property (*e.g.*, V_{max}/K_m) at a truly neutral gene and patterns of selection on a linked gene. So, when allozymes' functional differences can predict performance and fitness-related effects in a genotype-specific way, associative hypotheses (*e.g.*, hitchhiking) require additional postulates: (a) tightly linked genotypes, which actually cause observed effects and realistic mechanisms for their action, and (b) mechanistic reasons why the allozymes' differences do not cause the effects predicted from them. Without evidence for these postulates, associative views of functionally and fitness-distinct allozymes are negated by Ockham's razor: "Do not multiply entities needlessly."

Complications of pleiotropy or epistasis: "Fitnesses at one gene vary with fitnesses at others." This does not, as some claim, preclude meaningful study of allozymes. If pleiotropy or epistasis were impenetrable, genetics would be impossible. Allozymes are powerful tools just because they are specific probes of metabolic hierarchies in Darwinian context. Background effects and genetic or phenotypic correlations do occur, and mean effects of allozymes may be complicated by interaction with other variation, but these issues may be analyzed empirically (*e.g.*, CARTER and WATT 1988; WATT 1992).

Are allozyme studies "adaptationist"? Naive adaptationism, seeking separate explanation for each "atomized" trait of an organism, deserves critique. But this pitfall can be avoided, *e.g.*, if allozymes alter a trait without altering fitness, then to the extent of the change, the trait's state is not adaptive. *E. coli*'s PGI K_m is not differently adaptive among its allozymes at 37° (DYKHUISEN and HARTL 1983), while Colias' PGI V_{max}/K_m is adaptive with precision down to the 20–30% difference between *3/4* and *3/3* genotypes, which leads to, *e.g.*, major genotypic fecundity effects (WATT 1992). Using allozymes to probe adaptation need not entail adaptationist bias.

Are allozymes peripheral to modern evolutionary study? LEWONTIN (*e.g.*, 1980) and others say that adaptation is peripheral to the logic of evolution, which would lessen the utility of allozyme studies. They claim that three propositions are necessary and sufficient for natural selection: (1) phenotypic variation, (2) heritability of the variants and (3) differential reproduction of the variants. But, as is clear from DARWIN (1859; *cf.* BRANDON 1990), *this claim is wrong*: these three propositions, while *necessary* for natural selection, are *sufficient* only for *arbitrary* selection, wherein we do not know the cause of differential reproduction. DARWIN held that natural selection resides in the demographic *results* of differences among heritable variants in suitedness to their environment, *i.e.*, *differences in adaptation*.

KRIMBAS (1984) claimed that this makes evolution "circular" or "tautological." This charge may fit the confused aphorism "survival of the fittest" but it fails against DARWIN's basic concept. The evolutionary recursion is not circular unless causative adaptive and resulting fitness differences have been mistakenly conflated. As for tautology, do not confuse the tautological nature of well defined, logically (or algebraically) true statements, such as DARWIN's argument, with the empirical issue: do these statements, or this argument, rightly describe the world? DARWIN was neither circular nor tautological in posing adaptation as a central *empirical* problem for evolutionary study.

Some question whether allozymes typify traits of most evolutionary interest: complex morphologies or performances, which many expect to be under polygenic control. But allozymes have large fitness-related effects through such complex performances as, *e.g.*, locomotion (Fundulus LDH, Colias PGI), cold stress tolerance (Peromyscus Hb), or osmoregulation (Mytilus LAP, Tigriopus GPT). This also suggests that major fractions of the genetic variance in complex traits may be neither additive nor polygenic, and hence ill described by usual quantitative genetic models.

Others argue that study of adaptation, hence of allozymes, is particularist. If so, it is better to know about specific cases than to know nothing about adaptation; but beyond that, generality is seldom found unless sought. If few generalities about allozymes have yet been made, that does not imply futility of future attempts.

Is evolution too complex to measure? One anonymous skeptic, perhaps speaking for others, remarked of mechanistic evolutionary genetics that it " . . . is heuristic, but ignores the true complexity of evolution . . . . " But is this really so? What difficulties could lead to this claim, and are they real or illusory?

Demographic or genetic-transmission subtleties can be accounted for. Subpopulation mixing effects may mimic genotypic survivorship differences, but can be ruled out when population structure is known and allelic covariances can be calculated (WATT 1983). Segregation distortion or assortative mating can be studied during the progeny analysis of mating success testing, as for Colias PGI, where neither effect was found (WATT, CARTER and BLOWER 1985). Genetic drift and inbreeding cause irreproducibility of genotypic differences, or characteristic distortion of genotypic frequency patterns.

Catastrophism is said to preclude evolutionary prediction, but it is not at issue here. A population's extinction by a stochastic hundred-year weather event (*e.g.*, EHRLICH *et al.* 1972) erases its evolutionary history, but our task is to explore what *is* predictable about evolution, not to despair in the face of stochastic complications.

Habitat diversity concerns some workers in relation to possible variation or antagonism of selection pressures, but one may replicate performance or fitness studies across microhabitats; proper field work accounts for this in its designs. Allozymes' effects may indeed be antagonistic, as in red deer whose IDH allozymes reciprocally change female survival and fertility, but this may maintain the variation (PEMBERTON *et al.* 1991). One must evaluate all major, ecologically relevant performances and fitness components before making final conclusions about maintenance of genetic variation, but this may be easier than has been feared. Where organisms' niche structure is well understood, rigorous experiments can be done with statistical testing against explicit null hypotheses (above; FEDER and WATT 1992).

The mechanistic study of evolution, using allozymes as tools or probes, in no way ignores complexity either of allozymes' phenotypic expressions or of their translation into large, small, or zero fitness differences. Rather, like all other science, it moves by successive refinement toward full understanding of relevant complexity. A quasi-vitalistic reluctance to believe that this is possible will help no one.

Where can we go from here? WATT (1985, 1986) and CLARK and KOEHN (1992) stress a bioenergetic focus on allozymes' impacts. More work in this line will be fruitful, *e.g.*, can bioenergetic cost-benefit theory of metabolic evolution evaluate which alternatives of change in $[E]$, k_{cat}, and K_m should be favored by selection in specific cases? Of course, this is not the only possible context for allozyme evaluation. Overall adaptation might well be a supervenient (ROSENBERG 1978) "umbrella" under which bioenergetic, mating-system, or other contexts for allozyme evaluation might be co-important.

Nucleic-acid analysis may complement allozyme work and *vice versa* (KREITMAN, SHORROCKS and DYTHAM 1992). DNA-sequence analysis of allozymes, together with coalescence theory, allows inference of selection or its absence, though alone it gives no clue to biological causes (AQUADRO 1992). The combination of these approaches has much to offer, *e.g.*, DNA sequencing easily reveals the amino acid variation underlying allozymes' properties. Conversely, mechanistic study of allozymes gives the biological sources of selection (or its absence) whose statistical correlates may be found by sequencing. Also, sequencing is basic to studying the extent of linkage disequilibrium, D, around selected sites in allozymes (above). Complementary functional study of the allozymes can then probe how D varies with the nature or strength of selection.

Further exploration of habitat variation will greatly aid allozyme work, *e.g.*, food supply variation selects on allozymes in Apodemus mice (LEIGH BROWN 1977), and Colias' esterase-D allozymes covary with food plant use, suggesting a role in detoxifying plants' chemical defenses (BURNS 1975). The opportunity for new insight is immense if physiological and behavioral ecology are more used in evolutionary genetics.

Allozymes' mechanisms have not yet been much studied in phylogenetic context, yet they could be. For example, the "adaptation to neutral limits" concept of metabolic evolution (HARTL, DYKHUISEN and DEAN 1985) may apply widely to *E. coli* allozymes, yet it does not hold for eukaryotes studied so far (WATT 1991). What phyletically consistent aspects of these taxa, or of their proteins' evolutionary history, might explain this?

Final remarks: Many, but not all, allozymes differ in function. These differences translate *predictably* through metabolic and physiological performance into fitness component differences, eventually leading to net fitness differences. In this work, neutrality is the null model. Where allozymes do not differ, this null model is the mechanistic prediction and has been sustained; where allozymes differ significantly, the null model has been falsified as the mechanistic prediction has been sustained. Thus, these studies are not correlational, but follow the alternative-hypotheses decision strategy of PLATT (1964). Among empirical or *a priori* reservations about such studies, some are mistaken, while others must always be considered but can be tested empirically. None pose general barriers to the probing of evolution with allozymes.

The mechanistic study of allozymes (or other natural variants) offers great power for asking and answering both integrative and specific questions that other approaches have not recognized or resolved. Far from being a self-imposed burden, allozymes' functional and fitness-related diversity affords a extraordinary intellectual tool for experimental, genetically informed study of evolution.

I thank CAROL BOGGS, ANDREW CLARK, JOHN ENDLER, JOHN GILLESPIE, DEBORAH GORDON, MARC JACOBS, EGBERT LEIGH, MARK NIELSEN, SARAH OTTO, PETER PARSONS, DAVID POLLOCK and LOREN RIESEBERG for stimulating discussions, and the U.S. National Science Foundation for research support (DEB 91-19411).

LITERATURE CITED

AQUADRO, C. F., 1992 Why is the genome variable? Insights from *Drosophila*. Trends Genet. **8:** 355–362.

ASMUSSEN, M. A., and M. T. CLEGG, 1981 Dynamics of the linkage disequilibrium function under models of gene-frequency hitchhiking. Genetics **99:** 337–356.

BRANDON, R. N., 1990 *Adaptation and Environment.* Princeton University Press, Princeton, N.J.

BURNS, J. M., 1975 Isozymes in evolutionary systematics, pp. 49–62 in *Isozymes IV: Genetics and Evolution*, edited by C. L. MARKERT. Academic Press, New York.

BURTON, R. S., and M. W. FELDMAN, 1983 Physiological effects of an allozyme polymorphism: glutamate-pyruvate transaminase and response to hyperosmotic stress in the copepod *Tigriopus californicus*. Biochem. Genet. **21:** 239–251.

CARTER, P. A., and W. B. WATT, 1988 Adaptation at specific loci. V. Metabolically adjacent enzyme loci may have very distinct experiences of selective pressures. Genetics **119:** 913–924.

CHAPPELL, M. A., and L. R. G. SNYDER, 1984 Biochemical and physiological correlates of α-chain hemoglobin polymorphisms. Proc. Natl. Acad. Sci. USA **81:** 5484–5488.

CLARK, A. G., 1991 Mutation-selection balance and metabolic control theory. Genetics **129:** 909–923.

CLARK, A. G., and R. K. KOEHN, 1992 Enzymes and adaptation, pp. 193–228 in *Genes in Ecology*, edited by R. J. BERRY, T. J. CRAWFORD and G. M. HEWITT. Blackwell Scientific Publications, Oxford.

DARWIN, C. R., 1859 *The Origin of Species.* Modern Library, Random House, New York.

DYKHUISEN, D. E., and D. L. HARTL, 1983 Functional effects of PGI allozymes in *E. coli*. Genetics **105:** 1–18.

EASTERBY, J. S., 1973 Coupled enzyme assays: a general expression for the transient. Biochim. Biophys. Acta **293**: 552–558.

EHRLICH, P. R., D. E. BREEDLOVE, P. F. BRUSSARD and M. A. SHARP, 1972 Weather and the "regulation" of subalpine populations. Ecology **53**: 243–247.

EWENS, W. J., and M. W. FELDMAN, 1976 The theoretical assessment of selective neutrality, pp. 303–337 in *Population Genetics and Ecology*, edited by S. KARLIN and E. NEVO. Academic Press, New York.

FEDER, M. E., and W. B. WATT, 1992 Functional biology of adaptation, pp. 365–392 in *Genes in Ecology*, edited by R. J. BERRY, T. J. CRAWFORD and G. M. HEWITT. Blackwell Scientific Publications, Oxford.

FRERIKSEN, A., D. SEYKENS, W. SCHARLOO and P. W. H. HEINSTRA, 1991 Alcohol dehydrogenase controls the flux from ethanol into lipids in *Drosophila* larvae: a ^{13}C NMR study. J. Biol. Chem. **266**: 21399–21403.

GILLESPIE, J. H., 1991 *The Causes of Molecular Evolution*. Oxford University Press, New York.

HARTL, D. L., D. E. DYKHUISEN and A. M. DEAN, 1985 Limits of adaptation: the evolution of selective neutrality. Genetics **111**: 655–674.

HOCHACHKA, P. W., and G. N. SOMERO, 1973 *Strategies of Biochemical Adaptation*. W. B. Saunders, New York.

HUDSON, R. R., M. KREITMAN and M. AGUADÉ, 1987 A test for neutral molecular evolution based on nucleotide data. Genetics **116**: 153–159.

KACSER, H., and J. M. BURNS, 1973 The control of flux. Symp. Soc. Exp. Biol. **27**: 65–104.

KACSER, H., and J. M. BURNS, 1981 The molecular basis of dominance. Genetics **97**: 639–666.

KOEHN, R. K., 1987 The importance of genetics to physiological ecology, pp. 170–185 in *New Directions in Ecological Physiology*, edited by M. E. FEDER, A. F. BENNETT, W. W. BURGGREN and R. B. HUEY. Cambridge University Press, Cambridge.

KREITMAN, M., B. SHORROCKS and C. DYTHAM, 1992 Genes and ecology: two alternative perspectives using *Drosophila*, pp. 281–312 in *Genes in Ecology*, edited by R. J. BERRY, T. J. CRAWFORD and G. M. HEWITT. Blackwell Scientific Publications, Oxford.

KRIMBAS, C. B., 1984 On adaptation, neo-Darwinian tautology, and population fitness. Evol. Biol. **17**: 1–57.

LABATE, J., and W. F. EANES, 1992 Direct measurement of *in vivo* flux differences between electrophoretic variants of G6PD from *Drosophila melanogaster*. Genetics **132**: 783–787.

LANGLEY, C. H., R. A. VOELKER, A. J. LEIGH BROWN, S. OHNISHI, B. DICKSON and E. MONTGOMERY, 1981 Null allele frequencies at allozyme loci in natural populations of *Drosophila melanogaster*. Genetics **99**: 151–156.

LAURIE, C. C., and L. STAM, 1988 Quantitative analysis of RNA produced by Slow and Fast alleles of *Adh* in *Drosophila melanogaster*. Proc. Natl. Acad. Sci. USA **85**: 5161–5165.

LEIGH BROWN, A. J., 1977 Physiological correlates of an enzyme polymorphism. Nature **269**: 803–804.

LEWONTIN, R. C., 1980 Adaptation, pp. 236–251 in *Conceptual Issues in Evolutionary Biology*, edited by E. SOBER. M.I.T. Press, Cambridge, Mass.

LEWONTIN, R. C., 1991 Electrophoresis in the development of evolutionary genetics: milestone or millstone? Genetics **128**: 657–662.

LEWONTIN, R. C., and J. L. HUBBY, 1966 A molecular approach to the study of genetic heterozygosity in natural populations. II. Amount of variation and degree of heterozygosity in natural populations of *Drosophila pseudoobscura*. Genetics **54**: 595–609.

PEMBERTON, J. M., S. D. ALBON, F. E. GUINNESS and T. H. CLUTTON-BROCK, 1991 Countervailing selection in different fitness components in female red deer. Evolution **45**: 93–103.

PLATT, J. R., 1964 Strong inference. Science **146**: 347–353.

POWERS, D. A., T. LAUERMAN, D. CRAWFORD and L. DIMICHELE, 1991 Genetic mechanisms for adapting to a changing environment. Annu. Rev. Genet. **25**: 629–659.

ROSENBERG, A., 1978 The supervenience of biological concepts. Phil. Sci. **45**: 368–386.

SAVAGEAU, M. A., and A. SORRIBAS, 1989 Constraints among molecular and systemic properties-implications for physiological genetics. J. Theor. Biol. **141**: 93–115.

THOMSON, G., 1977 The effect of a selected locus on linked neutral loci. Genetics **85**: 753–788.

VAN DELDEN, W., 1982 The alcohol dehydrogenase polymorphism in *Drosophila melanogaster*. Selection at an enzyme locus. Evol. Biol. **15**: 187–222.

WATT, W. B., 1983 Adaptation at specific loci. II. Demographic and biochemical elements in the maintenance of the Colias PGI polymorphism. Genetics **103**: 691–724.

WATT, W. B., 1985 Bioenergetics and evolutionary genetics: opportunities for new synthesis. Am. Nat. **125**: 188–143.

WATT, W. B., 1986 Power and efficiency as indexes of fitness in metabolic organization. Am. Nat. **127**: 629–653.

WATT, W. B., 1991 Biochemistry, physiological ecology, and population genetics–the mechanistic tools of evolutionary biology. Funct. Ecol. **5**: 145–154.

WATT, W. B., 1992 Eggs, enzymes, and evolution–natural genetic variants change insect fecundity. Proc. Natl. Acad. Sci. USA **89**: 10608–10612.

WATT, W. B., P. A. CARTER and S. M. BLOWER, 1985 Adaptation at specific loci. IV. Differential mating success among glycolytic allozyme genotypes of Colias butterflies. Genetics **109**: 157–175.

WRIGHT, S., 1934 Physiological and evolutionary theories of dominance. Am. Nat. **34**: 24–53.

ZAMER, W. E., and R. J. HOFFMANN, 1989 Allozymes of glucose-6-phosphate isomerase differentially modulate pentose-shunt metabolism in the sea anemone *Metridium senile*. Proc. Natl. Acad. Sci. USA **86**: 2737–2741.

February 1994

The Transformation of Genetics by DNA
An Anniversary Celebration
of Avery, MacLeod, and McCarty (1944)

Joshua Lederberg[1]

The Rockefeller University, New York, New York 10021–6399

THE publication of AVERY, MACLEOD and MC-CARTY (1944) just 50 years ago marked the opening of the contemporary era of genetics, its molecular phase. The reverberations continue, now dominating large sectors of biomedical science and biotechnology, and have established the centrality of genetics in biological thought (LEDERBERG 1959, 1993a).

AVERY *et al.* (1944) can be dissected into the following observations, claims and tacit extrapolations, which may be paraphrased as:

a) Certain bacteria (pneumococci) have clonally inherited attributes, notably serospecific polysaccharide capsules. These are associated with virulence and can be selected accordingly, by inoculation into mice or by serological reagents.

b) The genetic Anlage of these attributes can be transferred from clone to clone by cell-free extracts: the phenomenon of transformation. The transformed cells faithfully transmit their new phenotype to succeeding clonal generations, as had been established by GRIFFITH (1928) with crude, heat-killed cell suspensions.

c) The chemical structure of that transforming principle is DNA, to the exclusion of protein or other macromolecules.

Founded on these claims, the following radical ideas emerged:

d) Bacteria have discrete, autonomous genes analogous to those of higher life forms (*viz.* Drosophila).

e) The gene is DNA, and the transformation phenomenon affords the first bioassay for genes extractable *in vitro*.

f) Accordingly, bacteria might be favored subjects for genetic investigation and eventually for technological application of molecular genetic science.

I recite these principles with some nostalgia: they are precisely how they came across to me as an undergraduate already working on Neurospora in FRANCIS RYAN's laboratory at the Columbia University Zoology Department in Morningside Heights, New York's upper West Side. Elsewhere, I have noted how they vectored my own career aspirations into the pioneering of bacterial genetics (LEDERBERG 1987).

Studying in the academic archipelago called New York, I was uniquely well situated to observe and sometimes participate in the debate. The Rockefeller Institute was across town, overlooking the East River near the 59th Street bridge. ALFRED MIRSKY, likewise a senior member there, was a frequent visitor to Columbia to collaborate with ARTHUR POLLISTER. From 1942 on I heard a good deal of the progress in AVERY's laboratory. Reprints of the AVERY *et al.* (1944) article were circulated in the department. I borrowed one from HARRIETT TAYLOR (later EPHRUSSI), a graduate student working on yeast budding kinetics, who would shortly join AVERY's laboratory for her postdoctoral research. My personal exclamatory notes were ". . . unlimited in its implications, . . . Direct demonstration of the multiplication of transforming factor . . . Viruses are gene-type compounds [sic]. . . ."

While MIRSKY was the principal herald, he was also a dogged critic of the claim that DNA, alone, had been proven to be the exclusive chemical substance of transforming activity (MIRSKY and POLLISTER 1946). That was indeed a difficult proposition: AVOGADRO's number is a formidable protagonist in that contest. My stance was sympathetic to MIRSKY's: I felt that so crucial a claim should not be impulsively engrafted into the corpus of science as if by first intention. More important than doctrinal conversion was that the issue was squarely on the table and could be settled by

[1] Raymond and Beverly Sackler Foundation Scholar.

overwhelming experimental analysis. Previous fiascoes had darkened the history of biopolymers: WILLS-TATTER's claim of enzymatic activity of protein-free preparations and WENDELL STANLEY's initial claim in 1935 that crystallized tobacco mosaic virus was a pure protein. AVERY himself was an epitome of caution, having had to weather similar skepticism of his conclusion that pneumococcal polysaccharide, devoid of protein, was a type-specific antigen. The main fruit of the debate was to stimulate a range of further enquiries: CHARGAFF on the base composition of DNA and my own on other modes of gene recombination in *E. coli*. And MACLYN McCARTY, later joined by ROLLIN HOTCHKISS, added much to the repertoire of enzymatic and analytical refinements for the exclusion of protein from the DNA preparations (McCARTY 1946; HOTCHKISS 1979). WATSON and CRICK perhaps owe some debt to MIRSKY's obstinacy. PAULING, who had collaborated with MIRSKY on protein denaturation, was led to delay entering the marathon for solving the DNA structure (WATSON 1968).

Conceptually, DNA in the 1940s was an unlikely candidate for biological specificity. The root problem was the unavailability of any homogeneous sample of DNA appropriate for detailed chemical analysis. This would have to await studies with tiny DNA viruses, and much help from precisely targeting restriction enzymes. DNA was then believed to be a monotonous structure, perhaps even merely a tetranucleotide, harkening back to PHOEBUS LEVENE's analyses. The protein-enthusiasm evoked by the successful crystallization of enzymes in the 1930s then dominated most biochemists' attention.

In fact, DNA was more popular at the turn of the century: "A tempting hypothesis, suggested by Mathews on the basis of Kossel's work, is that nuclein, or one of its constituent molecular groups, may in a chemical sense be regarded as the formative centre of the cell which is directly involved in the process by which food-matters are built up into the cell-substance" (WILSON 1906, p. 340).

By 1925, WILSON was discouraged and misled by the apparent loss of chromatin (basophilia) in the nucleus of the growing oocyte:

These facts afford conclusive proof that the individuality and genetic continuity of chromosomes does not depend upon a persistence of 'chromatin' in the older sense (*i.e.*, basichromatin). It is the expression of a morphological organization that is not destroyed by those chemical and physical transformations that lead to a netlike structure and a change from the basophilic to the oxyphilic condition (WILSON 1925, p. 351).

Just as these words were being written, ROBERT FEULGEN developed the fuchsin-bisulfite cytochemical reaction that offered the first authentic cytochemical indicator for DNA and restored confidence in the continuity of the DNA content of the chromosome. (CLARK and KASTEN 1983).

The biological interpretation of the pneumococcus transformation was also fraught with uncertainty. DOBZHANSKY, and later BOIVIN, persisted in describing the phenomenon as a "directed mutation," and it was given overtones of "cytoplasmic inheritance" by SONNEBORN–these were all rhetorical devices intended to seal off a vaguely understood phenomenon from the sureties of chromosomal inheritance. Nothing was known of chromosomes or genes in bacteria at that time: a certain leap of faith was required to relate the transformation (and therefore, in turn, DNA) to mendelizing genes. For many years, the only marker studied was the capsular polysaccharide. In that setting, even HARRIETT TAYLOR (1951), reporting from the Rockefeller Institute, remarked, "No bridge can be seen leading over into classical genetics," and in private correspondence criticized my own efforts to do precisely that. Among early comments from geneticists, MULLER's (1947) was the closest to the mark:

. . . the most probable interpretation of these . . . pneumococcus results then becomes that of [a] type of crossing over, though on a more minute scale . . . [involving] viable bacterial 'chromosomes' or parts of chromosomes [penetrating] the capsuleless bacteria and in part at least taken root there . . . However, unlike what has so far been possible in higher organisms, viable chromosome threads could also be obtained from these lower forms for *in vitro* observation, chemical analysis, and determination of the genetic effects of treatment.

In a retrospection over prior hypothetical interpretations of the transforming principle, seven alternatives could be listed (LEDERBERG 1956):

1. It was a specific mutagen with a special ability to direct a particular gene to mutate in a definite direction.

2. It was a polysaccharide autocatalyst (perhaps as a complex with DNA) that primed an enzymatic reaction for polysaccharide synthesis.

3. It was a bacterial virus, which on infecting the bacteria provoked capsular synthesis as a host reaction.

4. It was an autonomous cytoplasmic gene or a morphogenetic inducer.

5. It acted at a distance without penetrating the bacterium.

6. It was a fragment of the genetic makeup of the bacterium, the only one to have been tested to that time.

7. It was an element *sui generis* for which no general conception should be adduced.

Some of these were not logically distinguishable, but were no less strongly held semantic strongholds. The notion that the transformation was indeed a gene transfer by DNA was eventually solidified by new work with markers other than the capsule, and especially by the linkage of mannitol fermentation and streptomycin resistance (HOTCHKISS and MARMUR 1954). It was also bolstered by other phenomena of gene transfer, such as conjugal exchange in *E. coli* (LEDERBERG 1947) and virus-mediated transduction in Salmonella (ZINDER and LEDERBERG 1953). Finally, the monopoly of the pneumococcus on transformation—and this was a notoriously difficult experimental system—was broken by ALEXANDER and LEIDY's (1951) report on Hemophilus, so that a stream of other workers could provide mutual confirmation and reinforcement about the biological interpretations.

The debate about DNA chemistry petered out by sheer exhaustion of the critics and by the conceptual plausibility of DNA as gene, introduced by WATSON and CRICK's double helix model (1953). HERSHEY and CHASE's (1952) study of the injection of phage DNA into *E. coli* lent further support to the "DNA only" view; however, this was quantitatively less rigorous than MCCARTY and HOTCHKISS' prior work on the pneumococcus. Even after 1953, HERSHEY himself was still referring to something more than DNA as a possibility. It might be said that rigorous proof was concluded only with the enzymatic and chemical synthesis *in vitro* of biologically active DNA (KORNBERG 1960; KHORANA 1969).

AVERY *et al.* (1944) was originally published in a medical journal of The Rockefeller Institute that was not habitually read by geneticists of that time. This has led some commentators to compare the launching and reception of AVERY *et al.*'s claims to the so-called prematurity of MENDEL's ideas in the last third of the 19th century (STENT 1972; WYATT 1975). Mendel was little known and for the most part ignored by his contemporaries. But I would argue that the critical reception initially given to AVERY *et al.* (1944) exemplifies the critical scientific method at its most functional (MERTON 1973). Far from being ignored, the paper enjoyed almost 300 citations between 1945 and 1954 (Science Citation Index 1945–1954), not to mention many more earned by MCCARTY's elaborations (1946). The first in GENETICS was LEDERBERG (1947). The *Annual Review of Genetics* did not exist at that time, but SEWALL WRIGHT (1945) reviewed the work in the *Annual Review of Physiology* and it was also noted by no less than three reviewers (GULLAND, MUELLER and KALCKAR) in the *Annual Review of Biochemistry* that same year. It was so well known during that decade that, as I can tell from my own experience, it was often cited by indirection, without specific reference (*e.g.*, LEDERBERG and TATUM 1946; LEDERBERG 1959).

To return, then, to attributions of "prematurity," this might mean either that the data do not exist to explain all of the paradoxes and challenges of a new discovery, and the claims then meet critical resistance, or that the audience is incapable of understanding the challenge. The touchstone is plainly the operational reaction. For AVERY *et al.* (1944), and MCCLINTOCK (1953) as well, this comprised open controversy and active inquiry. For MENDEL, this was oblivion and a long delay before rediscovery. Happily, such examples are few and far between. In the long run of scientific advance, for a work to be ignored is perhaps only slightly worse than to be swallowed whole. A lot of revision looms ahead even for our well established dogmas (LEDERBERG 1993b).

That AVERY and his colleagues failed to win the Nobel Prize has repeatedly been a subject of critical remark. WENDELL STANLEY (1970) openly apologized for not having been more attentive to that lack of recognition, after he had won his own prize in 1946. In 1958, it came to me to plan my own Nobel lecture, the first in the field of genetics since MULLER in 1946. Rather than recite my own work on bacterial recombination, I thought it more important to acknowledge how genetics had been totally transformed by these discoveries: this was embodied in the lecture entitled "A view of genetics" (LEDERBERG 1959). AVERY had consummated this research at the very end of his career and died in 1955 before a full round of recognition could be fulfilled. The survivor of that team, MACLYN MCCARTY, has written a vibrant memoir (1985) that is a model for expert and methodical tackling of very difficult technical problems. It displays the highest ideals of the scientific personality and leaves no doubt of the importance of his role, together with that of his colleagues, in the pivotal discovery of Twentieth Century biology.

Spanning more than a decade of often frustrating effort, that discovery is an outstanding example of the feedback of clinically motivated inquiry to the most basic issues of fundamental biomedical science (BEECHER 1960). Genetics, especially as we explore the human genome, will be fraught with many more like opportunities, and precisely because of their pervasive applications with commensurate dilemmas. Many institutional arrangements today nurture such transdisciplinary and vertically integrated research, which is often the arena of the most revolutionary advances. Before the federalization of biomedical research financing since World War II, The Rockefeller Institute was very nearly the only site where this could have taken root.

BIBLIOGRAPHICAL NOTE

A vast effort of scholarship and erudition on the history of DNA offers easily accessible guides to the primary sources; see: OLBY (1974, 1990), JUDSON (1979), PORTUGAL and COHEN (1977), CLARK and KASTEN (1983), MOORE (1985), SAPP (1990), WOLFF and LEDERBERG (1944) and WATSON and TOOZE (1981). In addition, memoirs by DUBOS (1976), HOTCHKISS (1979), MCCARTY (1985), CHARGAFF (1978), KORNBERG (1989), WATSON (1968) and CRICK (1988) add indispensable personal perspectives. I have referred to primary sources primarily to document or accent particular items under debate.

LITERATURE CITED

ALEXANDER, H. E., and G. LEIDY, 1951 Determination of inherited traits of *H. influenzae* by desoxyribonucleic acid fractions isolated from type-specific cells. J. Exp. Med. **93**: 345–359.

AVERY, O. T., C. M. MacLEOD and M. McCARTY, 1944 Studies on the chemical nature of the substance inducing transformation of pneumococcal types. J. Exp. Med. **79**: 137–158.

BEECHER, H. K., 1960 *Disease and the Advancement of Basic Science.* Harvard University Press, Cambridge, Mass.

CHARGAFF, E., 1978 *Heraclitean Fire. Sketches from a Life before Nature.* The Rockefeller University Press, New York.

CLARK, G., and F. H. KASTEN, 1983 *History of Staining.* Williams & Wilkins, Baltimore.

CRICK, F., 1988 *What Mad Pursuit. A Personal View of Scientific Discovery.* Basic Books, New York.

DUBOS, R. J., 1976 *The Professor, The Institute, and DNA.* The Rockefeller University Press, New York.

GRIFFITH, F., 1928 The significance of pneumococcal types. J. Hyg. **27**: 113–159.

HERSHEY, A., and M. CHASE, 1952 Independent functions of viral proteins and nucleic acid in growth of bacteriophage. J. Gen. Physiol. **36**: 39–56.

HOTCHKISS, R. D., 1979 The identification of nucleic acids as genetic determinants. Ann. N. Y. Acad. Sci. **325**: 321–342.

HOTCHKISS, R. D., and J. MARMUR, 1954 Double marker transformations as evidence of linked factors in desoxyribonucleate transforming agents. Proc. Natl. Acad. Sci. USA **40**: 55–60.

JUDSON, H. F., 1979 *The Eighth Day of Creation.* Simon & Schuster, New York.

KHORANA, H. G., 1969 Nucleic acid synthesis in the study of the genetic code, pp. 196–220 in *Les Prix Nobel en 1968.* Imprimerie Royale P. A. Norstedt & Soner, Stockholm.

KORNBERG, A., 1960 The biologic synthesis of deoxyribonucleic acid, pp. 165–179 in *Les Prix Nobel en 1959.* Imprimerie Royale P. A. Norstedt & Soner, Stockholm.

KORNBERG, A., 1989 *For Love of an Enzyme.* Harvard University Press, Cambridge, Mass.

LEDERBERG, J., 1947 Gene recombination and linked segregations in *Escherichia coli.* Genetics **32**: 505–525.

LEDERBERG J., 1956 Genetic transduction. Am. Sci. **44**: 264–280.

LEDERBERG, J., 1959 A view of genetics, pp. 170–189 in *Les Prix Nobel en 1958.* Imprimerie Royale P. A. Norstedt & Soner, Stockholm.

LEDERBERG, J., 1987 Genetic recombination in bacteria: a discovery account. Annu. Rev. Genet. **21**: 23–46.

LEDERBERG, J., 1993a What the double helix (1953) has meant for basic biomedical science. A personal commentary. J. Am. Med. Assoc. **269**: 1981–1985.

LEDERBERG, J., 1993b The anti-expert system: hypotheses an AI program should have seen through, in *Artificial Intelligence and Molecular Biology,* edited by L. HUNTER. AAAI Press, Menlo Park, Calif. (in press).

LEDERBERG, J., and E. L. TATUM, 1946 Gene recombination in *Escherichia coli.* Nature **158**: 558.

McCARTY, M., 1946 Chemical nature and biological specificity of the substance inducing transformation of pneumococcal types. Bacteriol. Rev. **10**: 63–71.

McCARTY, M., 1985 *The Transforming Principle.* W. W. Norton, New York.

McCLINTOCK, B., 1953 Induction of instability at selected loci in maize. Genetics **38**: 579–599.

MERTON, R. K., 1973 *The Sociology of Science. Theoretical and Empirical Investigations.* University of Chicago Press, Chicago.

MIRSKY, A. E., and A. W. POLLISTER, 1946 Chromosin, a desoxyribose nucleoprotein complex of the cell nucleus. J. Gen. Physiol. **30**: 117–148.

MOORE, J. A., 1985 Science as a way of knowing–genetics. Am. Zool. **25**: 1–165.

MULLER, H. J., 1947 The gene. Proc. R. Soc. Lond. Biol. **134**: 1–37.

OLBY, R. C., 1974 *The Path to the Double Helix.* University of Washington Press, Seattle.

OLBY, R. C., 1990 The molecular revolution in biology, pp. 503–520 in *Companion to the History of Modern Science,* edited by R. C. OLBY *et al.* Routledge, London.

PORTUGAL, F. H., and J. S. COHEN, 1977 *A Century of DNA.* MIT Press, Cambridge, Mass.

SAPP, J., 1990 *Where the Truth Lies. Franz Moewus and the Origins of Molecular Biology.* Cambridge University Press, Cambridge.

SCIENCE CITATION INDEX, 1945–1954 *Ten Year Cumulation.* Institute for Scientific Information, Philadelphia.

STANLEY, W. M., 1970 The "undiscovered" discovery. Arch. Environ. Health **21**: 256–262.

STENT, G. S., 1972 Prematurity and uniqueness in scientific discovery. Sci. Am. **227**: 84–93.

TAYLOR, H., 1951 Genetic aspects of transformations of pneumococci. Cold Spring Harbor Symp. Quant. Biol. **16**: 445–456.

WATSON, J. D., and F. H. C. CRICK, 1953 Molecular structure of nucleic acid. A structure for deoxyribose nucleic acid. Nature **171**: 737–738.

WATSON, J. D., and J. TOOZE, 1981 *The DNA Story.* W. H. Freeman, San Francisco.

WATSON, J. D., 1968 *The Double Helix.* Atheneum Publishers, New York.

WILSON, E. B., 1906 *The Cell in Development and Inheritance,* Ed. 2. Macmillan, New York.

WILSON, E. B., 1925 *The Cell in Development and Heredity,* Ed. 3. Macmillan, New York.

WOLFF, J. A., and J. LEDERBERG, 1994 A history of gene transfer and therapy, in *Gene Therapeutics,* edited by J. A. WOLFF. Birkhauser, Boston (in press).

WRIGHT, S., 1945 Physiological aspects of genetics. Annu. Rev. Physiol. **7**: 75–106.

WYATT, H. V., 1975 Knowledge and prematurity: the journey from transformation to DNA. Perspect. Biol. Med. **18**: 149–156.

ZINDER, N. D., and J. LEDERBERG, 1953 Genetic exchange in Salmonella. J. Bacteriol. **64**: 679–699.

See also page 705 in Addenda et Corrigenda.

Sturtevant's Mantle and the (Lost?) Art of Chromosome Mechanics

John C. Lucchesi

Department of Biology, Rollins Research Center, Emory University, Atlanta, Georgia 30322

. . . not even the most skeptical of readers can go through the Drosophila work unmoved by a sense of admiration for the zeal and penetration with which it has been conducted, and for the great extension of genetic knowledge to which it has led–greater far than has been made in any one line of work since Mendel's own experiments (BATESON 1916).

Drosophila is the organism of choice for this research because of the wealth of genetic information available and because of the ease with which its genome can be manipulated (generic sentence included in countless grant proposals).

IT all started, of course, in the "Fly Room" around 1910. That year, two remarkable undergraduates joined THOMAS HUNT MORGAN's laboratory at Columbia University. One of them, CALVIN BRIDGES, was beginning a brilliant if sadly brief career, the most singular highlight of which was the proof of the chromosome theory of inheritance. The other undergraduate, ALFRED STURTEVANT, would be fortunate enough to remain actively engaged in research for over half a century. BRIDGES was the first to discover autosomal linkage. He was the first to identify correctly the X and Y chromosomes in the *Drosophila melanogaster* genome and to propose that sex in this species is determined by the number of X chromosomes relative to the number of autosomes. He was the first to translate the discovery of the giant larval salivary gland chromosomes into a set of cytological maps. His untimely death, in 1938, prevented him from exploiting this new finding in a hoped-for collaboration with HERMAN J. MULLER, whom he had met in the early days of the Fly Room (CROW 1991).

STURTEVANT's contributions covered an amazing range of biological subjects, from the demonstration of maternal inheritance to the use of mosaicism for the study of development, from the discovery of position effect variegation to the analysis of sexual transformation. His abiding interest in evolutionary biology led to investigations of hybrid sterility, the genetic control of mutation rates, the frequency of lethal alleles in populations and, in collaboration with TH. DOBZHANSKY, the use of inversions to retrace phylogeny. Although necessarily performed in formal genetic and occasionally in classical cytological terms, STURTEVANT's experiments laid the cornerstones in many areas of modern quantitative and developmental biology;

the reader is referred to a collection of STURTEVANT's papers selected and edited by LEWIS (1961).

STURTEVANT's contribution to transmission genetics began with nothing less than the realization that differences in the strength of the linkage between genes could be used to determine their linear arrangement along a chromosome. Having invented genetic mapping, he proceeded to demonstrate that inversions are "crossover reducers"; in collaboration with GEORGE BEADLE, he suggested a simple mechanism for this effect. These discoveries led to the development of one of the most useful tools in genetic research, the balancer chromosomes. Soon, other classes of chromosomal aberrations were characterized, and each of them enabled the establishment of a fundamental concept or the development of another important tool. Translocations, for example, were used by CURT STERN (1931) and, independently, by HARRIET CREIGHTON and BARBARA McCLINTOCK (1931) for the cytological demonstration of crossing over; deletions were used to map the physical location of genes on the polytene chromosomes of larval salivary glands (SLIZYNSKA 1938), leading to the creation of cytological maps. The field of genetics was ready to enter the golden era of chromosome mechanics, an era that would produce an experimental corpus accurately characterized by one of STURTEVANT's students, EDWARD NOVITSKI, as "the epitome of sophistication in a rather esoteric field."

The period in question spans approximately 25 years, from the early 1940s to the late 1960s. Some of the work that was performed during this period on chromosome movement, gene function, mutagenesis, and the genetic characteristics of populations, to name a few areas, provided the framework for the subsequent or current redefinition of these phenomena in molecular, mechanistic terms. Center stage, though, was certainly occupied by genetics' first generation of engineers. Some of the special chromosomes that they discovered or constructed were useful for a variety of purposes. The discovery of the first attached-X chromosome by L. V. MORGAN (1922) was most propitious in that it could be used to study the relation of crossing over to meiosis, and as a tool with which one could force the transmission of normal X chromosomes from fathers to sons. Attached-XY chromosomes (STERN 1927;

NEUHAUS 1935; LINDSLEY and NOVITSKI 1959) were used to map and characterize the Y-linked fertility factors and to generate XO males. An unstable ring-X chromosome (HINTON 1955) allowed the creation of sexual mosaics or gynandromorphs. And yet, enormous amounts of creative energy, time, and effort were also spent on problems whose solution, today, could be considered an intellectual exercise carried out for its own sake.

It soon became apparent that five additional compound-X chromosomes could exist, differing from one another in the orientation of their two X chromosomes in relation to the single centromere. (MORGAN's attached-X is a reversed metacentric; the other possible combinations are the tandem metacentric, the reversed or tandem acrocentric, and the reversed or tandem compound ring.) Ingenious schemes were devised for the synthesis of all of these compound chromosomes, and laborious experiments were carried out for the purpose of studying their segregation properties and their recombination products.

Unsurpassed in skill and imagination were ED NOVITSKI, who was the original motivating force and guiding genius in this field, and his former student, LARRY SANDLER. Their laboratories and those of others, notably DAN LINDSLEY, vied with one another for the prize of being the first to synthesize a new compound combination (see NOVITSKI 1963a, b; LINDSLEY and SANDLER 1963; and references therein). Although compound-XY chromosomes, ring-X chromosomes, and ring-Y chromosomes (MULLER 1948) had been induced by exposure to ionizing radiation, no ring compound-XY chromosome existed, and the race to synthesize it was on. (As a postdoctoral fellow in NOVITSKI's laboratory from 1963 to 1965, I joined the long list of those who had an unsuccessful crack at it.) This chromosome was finally generated by a procedure involving two induced and three spontaneous consecutive recombinational events (NOVITSKI and CHILDRESS 1976). Although compound chromosomes were generated consisting of two left or two right arms of the major autosomes (RASMUSSEN 1960), the real challenge was the creation of compound autosomes with the two entire homologous elements attached to a single centromere. Better yet, why not attempt to attach both pairs of the major autosomes to each other and to a single centromere? All of these combinations were eventually synthesized by NOVITSKI, who provided an account of the wizardry needed to perform these particular feats (NOVITSKI 1963a, b; NOVITSKI et al. 1981).

The problems that gave birth to chromosome mechanics and were its *raison d'être*–pairing, crossing over, segregation–are no longer studied to any extent (with one or two notable exceptions) in Drosophila. A few of the intellectual descendants of the scions of the great dynasties of chromosome mechanics (in addition to the STURTEVANT line, those established by MULLER and DOBZHANSKY come to mind) have continued to practice the traditional craft in order to create new genetic tools. Even so, their use of chromosome mechanics is sporadic, at best, and their scientific interests are focused on gene function, cellular dif-

ferentiation, organismal development, genome organization, or the genetic basis of adaptation. The predominant techniques that they use are those of recombinant DNA, molecular cloning, and immunology. It is natural, therefore, that in looking back over that particular period in the history of genetics that is best referred to as "the age of Drosophila chromosome mechanics," one cannot help wondering whether it was a crucial passage without which our current understanding of genetic mechanisms could not have been reached or whether it represents a dead end that contributed little if anything to the evolution of our field. I tend to favor the former possibility; given the relative brevity of one's professional life, the latter possibility, representing a significant waste of time, is perhaps too difficult to accept.

I had the good fortune of running into JIM PEACOCK and DAVID SUZUKI at the recent International Congress of Genetics. This encounter led to an evening of reminiscing and of recounting of the "good(?) old days"; it also provided the opportunity for JIM PEACOCK to read a draft of this *Perspectives* and to make useful suggestions for which I am grateful.

LITERATURE CITED

BATESON, W., 1916 The mechanism of Mendelian heredity (a review). Science 44: 536–543.

CREIGHTON, H. B., and B. MCCLINTOCK, 1931 A correlation of cytological and genetical crossing over in *Zea mays*. Proc. Natl. Acad. Sci. USA 17: 492–497.

CROW, J. F., 1991 Our diamond birthday anniversary. Genetics 127: 1–3.

HINTON, C. W., 1955 The behavior of an unstable ring chromosome of *Drosophila melanogaster*. Genetics 40: 951–961.

LEWIS, E. B. (Editor), 1961 *Genetics and Evolution: Selected Papers of A. H. Sturtevant*. W. H. Freeman, San Francisco.

LINDSLEY, D. L., and E. NOVITSKI, 1959 Compound chromosomes involving the X and Y chromosomes of *Drosophila melanogaster*. Genetics 44: 187–196.

LINDSLEY, D. L., and L. SANDLER, 1963 Construction of compound-X chromosomes in *Drosophila melanogaster* by means of the *Bar-Stone* duplication, pp. 390–403 in *Methodology in Basic Genetics*, edited by W. J. BURDETTE. Holden-Day, San Francisco.

MORGAN, L. V., 1922 Non-criss-cross inheritance in *Drosophila melanogaster*. Biol. Bull. 42: 267–274.

MULLER, H. J., 1948 The construction of several new types of Y chromosomes. Drosophila Inform. Serv. 22: 73–74.

NEUHAUS, M. J., 1935 Data concerning crossing over between the X and Y chromosomes in females of *melanogaster Drosophila* [sic]. C. R. Acad. Sci. USRSS 3: 41–44.

NOVITSKI, E., 1963a The construction of new chromosomal types in *Drosophila melanogaster*, pp. 381–389 in *Methodology in Basic Genetics*, edited by W. J. BURDETTE. Holden-Day, San Francisco.

NOVITSKI, E., 1963b The construction of an entire compound two chromosome, pp. 562–568 in *The Genetics and Biology of Drosophila*, Vol. 1b, edited by M. ASHBURNER and E. NOVITSKI. Academic Press, London.

NOVITSKI, E., and D. CHILDRESS, 1976 Compound chromosomes involving the X and the Y chromosomes, pp. 487–503 in *The Genetics and Biology of Drosophila*, Vol. 1b, edited by M. ASHBURNER and E. NOVITSKI. Academic Press, London.

NOVITSKI, E., D. GRACE and C. STROMMEN, 1981 The entire compound autosomes of *Drosophila melanogaster*. Genetics 98: 257–273.

RASMUSSEN, I. E., 1960 Report on new mutants. Drosophila Inform. Serv. 34: 53.

SLIZYNSKA, H., 1938 Salivary gland chromosome analysis of the white-facet region of Drosophila. Genetics 23: 291–299.

STERN, C., 1927 Ein genetischer und zytologischer Beweis für Vererbung im Y-Chromosom von *Drosophila melanogaster*. Z. Indukt. Abstammungs. Vererbungsl. 44: 187–231.

STERN, C., 1931 Zytologisch-genetische Untersuchungen als Beweise für die Morgansche Theorie des Faktorenaustauschs. Biol. Zentralbl. 51: 547–587.

Harvard, Agriculture, and the Bussey Institution

J. A. Weir

Division of Biology, University of Kansas, Lawrence, Kansas 66045

The genes are units useful in concise descriptions of the phenomena of heredity. Their place of residence is the chromosomes. Their behavior brings about the observed facts of genetics. For the rest, what we know about them is merely an interpretation of crossover frequency. In terms of geometry, chemistry, physics, or mechanics we can give them no description whatever. E. M. EAST (1926)

GENETICS had its first influence in agriculture and first achieved independent status in agricultural colleges. The main training ground was the Bussey Institution of Harvard University.

By his will of 1835, BENJAMIN BUSSEY left his extensive farm (now the Arnold Arboretum) to Harvard to be held forever as a Seminary for "instruction in practical agriculture, in useful and ornamental gardening, in botany, and in such other branches of natural science, as may tend to promote a knowledge of practical agriculture, and the various arts subservient thereto and connected therewith." The government of the University is also "to cause courses of lectures to be delivered there . . . and also to furnish gratuitous aid . . . to such meritorious persons as may resort there for instruction."

The bequest did not become available until 1861, and the school did not open until 1871, following the construction of a suitable building. The initial appointments included, as instructor of farming, BUSSEY's grandson-in-law, THOMAS MOTLEY, who came with the farm; FRANCIS STORER, brother-in-law of Harvard's President ELIOT, as professor of agricultural chemistry and dean; and FRANCIS PARKMAN, the famous historian, as professor of horticulture.

The resources for the school were seriously depleted when a number of Bussey estate rental properties were destroyed in the Great Boston Fire of November 9–10, 1872. The meager income was augmented by growing vegetables, cutting firewood, and boarding horses. The school never did come up to Harvard undergraduate standards, which were not all that high, at best.

From a movement led by the physicist WALLACE SABINE, a Graduate School of Applied Science was organized in 1906 to replace the undergraduate Lawrence Scientific School. As part of the reorganization in 1908, "Bussey" became a graduate school for advanced instruction and research in scientific problems that relate and contribute to practical agriculture and horticulture–this just at the time when the claims of genetics could no longer be ignored. In recommending to President ELIOT that W. E. CASTLE's work be transferred from Cambridge to the Bussey Institution, Dean SABINE wrote, "The University has Professor Castle to start with; to lose him will be to lose the best man in the country in genetics." So instead of going to Wisconsin or Yale, CASTLE moved his animals to Forest Hills, soon to be joined by the noted plant geneticist EDWARD MURRAY EAST from the Connecticut Agricultural Experiment Station. CASTLE and EAST have been the subjects of recent *Perspectives* (SNELL and REED 1993; NELSON 1993); see also the biographies by WRIGHT (1963) and JONES (1944).

WILLIAM MORTON WHEELER, an erudite scholar who rated artistry in taxonomy above all his other powers, left Texas in 1908 to join the Bussey as Professor of Economic Entomology. He was appointed dean in 1915 when the Bussey was separated from the other schools of applied sciences, but in 1929 he resigned in favor of the more congenial atmosphere of the Museum of Comparative Zoology. IRVING W. BAILEY, who came to the Bussey from the defunct School of Forestry, acted as secretary. Between 1912 and 1939, 44 doctorates in genetics were awarded.

Animal genetics had its roots in liberal arts, not agriculture, with Johns Hopkins University as the early leader. E. B. WILSON, the cytologist (Ph.D. 1881), T. H. MORGAN (Ph.D. 1890), E. G. CONKLIN (Ph.D. 1891), and R. G. HARRISON (Ph.D. 1894), ostensibly students of the morphologist W. K. BROOKS, came under the influence of the physiologist H. NEWELL MARTIN and, except for CONKLIN, furthered their studies in Europe. (MORGAN, who retained his interest in embryology, was the only one to become a member of the Genetics Society of America.)

At Harvard, C. B. DAVENPORT (Ph.D. 1892) and W. E. CASTLE (Ph.D. 1895) were students of EDWARD L. MARK, whose doctorate in 1876 from the University of Leipzig was under RUDOLPH LEUCKART, an early proponent of the need to combine morphology and physiology. Their theses, based on morphological studies, were published in the *Bulletin of the Museum of Comparative Zoology*. Both DAVENPORT and CASTLE had farm backgrounds and later worked with laboratory and farm animals. DAVENPORT, with a B.S. degree in civil engineering, brought quantitative methods to biology but turned his attention to eugenics and administration. CASTLE, who assisted DAVENPORT as a student and succeeded him at Harvard when DAVENPORT departed in 1899, had little interest in eugenics and none in administration, but they remained close friends, and DAVENPORT, through control of Carnegie funds, provided assistance to CASTLE at the Bussey. Both men were interested in heredity even before 1900, so their grasp of Mendelism, after its rediscovery in 1900, was not immediate because they carried a considerable baggage of seemingly conflicting evidence.

After the rediscovery of MENDEL's laws, there ensued lively debate about the extent to which the laws applied to animals, including man. Naturally it was the conspicuous characters that attracted attention at first, but, as the inheritance of more and more characters was shown to behave according to simple Mendelism or one of its easily understood modifications, attention shifted to the materials in their own right–on one hand, as sources for new problems; on the other, as a new approach to the solution of old problems, such as the limits of selection or the consequences of inbreeding.

From 1901 to 1905, CASTLE, with the cooperation of four students in successive years, followed the effects of inbreeding in *Drosophila melanogaster* through 59 generations of brother-sister mating. After the move to the Bussey, no one used Drosophila for thesis research, but it became the favorite material for Harvard undergraduate teaching in Cambridge, so the graduate students were familiar with its usefulness. They kept abreast of developments and some, notably E. C. MACDOWELL, L. C. DUNN, and S. C. REED, later used Drosophila for research.

Although he emphasized the importance of laboratory animals in the study of inheritance, CASTLE retained an interest in farm animals. Between 1940 and 1961 (after retiring to Berkeley) he published 17 papers on coat colors in horses, and while at the Bussey he published on inheritance in sheep and dairy cattle and on various aspects of animal breeding.

After graduation, a number of CASTLE's students and two of EAST's worked with economic animals. JOHN DETLEFSEN worked with rats, mice, and cattle at Illinois. SEWALL WRIGHT went to the Bureau of Animal Industry, while L. C. DUNN went to the Connecticut Agricultural Experiment Station at Storrs, where he worked with poultry. TAGE ELLINGER from Denmark became a plant breeder, whereas H. C. MCPHEE (EAST's student) became Chief of the Animal Husbandry Division of the U.S. Bureau of Animal Industry. P. W. GREGORY went to Davis, where he investigated the genetics of cattle, including size inheritance, and also worked with rats. EDWARD LIVESAY became professor of animal husbandry at West Virginia. NELSON WATERS went on to a career in poultry research. Four of CASTLE's 23 doctoral candidates spent their entire careers after graduation working with economic species; four others were so engaged over a period of years. EAST's student, W. R. SINGLETON, studied coat color inheritance in horses in collaboration with CASTLE. The first generation of geneticists were able to pursue problems in pure and/or applied research.

CASTLE's own favorite species was the rat. He had come to distrust the concept of gametic purity on finding that the Mendelizing guinea pig characters, polydactylism, long hair, and rough coat were not exactly the same when extracted from crosses. To test his hypothesis, he undertook a selection experiment with hooded rats and by 1914 had reared and studied the color pattern of over 25,000 rats. With great persistence he defended his hypothesis in the face of mounting criticism–some rather heated. EMERSON and EAST's classic paper on maize, showing that quantitative characters are inherited in Mendelian fashion, appeared in 1913, a year before the completion of CASTLE and PHILLIPS' monograph (1914). The concept was debated in Bussey seminars, with CASTLE and EAST holding opposing views. CASTLE was not convinced until he performed the critical experiments suggested by WRIGHT. His retraction appeared in the *American Naturalist* in 1919 (CASTLE 1919). In L. C. DUNN's words, "Castle cured himself of disbelief in the integrity of the gene the hard way–by 15 years of arduous experimentation."

It is noteworthy that both CASTLE and EAST considered it the function of the professor to provide space, materials, encouragement, and little else, with course work in diverse areas only sufficient to broaden the students' perspective. CASTLE's first graduate students, JOHN A. DETLEFSEN, who arrived in 1908 and worked with guinea pigs, and EDWIN CARLETON MACDOWELL, who arrived a year later and worked with rabbits, received their doctorates in 1912. They did not share CASTLE's skepticism concerning the multiple-factor theory, and MACDOWELL's thesis, published as a monograph (1914), carried a prefatory note by CASTLE: "While not entirely sharing his views, I have tried not to bias his judgment either for or against the multiple-factor hypothesis which he adopts in this paper. But to avoid misunderstanding, I wish to say that in my own opinion the theory of the purity of the gametes has not been established." CASTLE was aware that the top signer of the thesis is not the only or even the chief source of guidance. He himself had been influenced more by C. B. DAVENPORT than by his professor, E. L. MARK.

The only students to use rats exclusively for doctoral thesis research were H. W. FELDMAN on sterility and fertility, GREGORY PINCUS on cytological studies, and LIVESAY on hybrid vigor, while DUNN and W. L. WACHTER worked on linkage in rats and mice. CLYDE KEELER's thesis was on rodless retina in mice, but he published 18 papers between 1940 and 1949 on rats. LAURENCE SNYDER published on the effects of X-rays on rats while at the Bussey, but his doctoral thesis was on blood groups in man, and he remained a human geneticist. With great persistence himself and tolerance on the part of others, CASTLE continued to collect and study mutants in the rat, even after moving to California in 1936.

Rabbits and guinea pigs were natural choices at the turn of the century because both species thrive under ordinary laboratory conditions. CASTLE assembled and studied a number of traits before the Bussey was reorganized, but about the only ones to stick mainly to one species were SEWALL WRIGHT with guinea pigs and PAUL SAWIN with rabbits. C. C. LITTLE, founder of The Jackson Laboratory, was the first graduate student to work with mice, but eventually most of CASTLE's students adopted the mouse, as did WRIGHT's. W. H. GATES' thesis was on the Japanese waltzing mouse, later shown by T. S. PAINTER to involve a chromosome deletion. In the 1930s, SHELDON REED worked on harelip, FRANK CLARK on hydrocephalics, siderocyte anemia and brachyury, SUMNER BURHOE on waved coat, and LLOYD LAW on size inheritance. It became increasingly evident that the mouse would serve as a model for human diseases. At Columbia University DUNN picked up work on the mouse where he had left off as a student (having published on black-and-tan in 1916, on yellow in 1919, and on sable and white spotting in 1920). He brought the much debated role of modifying genes to a satisfactory state by his thorough analysis of "sub-threshold alleles" that modify spotting. He early perceived that the t-complex was uniquely fitted for intensive study of gene action, while the discovery of t mutants in feral populations led to studies in population genetics and distorted segregation ratios.

Even though their attendance at the Bussey Institution was separated by 10 years, the careers of DUNN (S.D. 1920) and GEORGE D. SNELL (S.D. 1930) were strikingly similar. Both became interested in genetics under the influence of JOHN H. GEROULD at Dartmouth College; both had experience with mice before attending the Bussey, and their dissertations involved linkage in rodents; both later came to concentrate on a very small segment of a mouse chromosome, and in the process each developed stocks that are highly prized. In 1980, GEORGE SNELL, age 77, shared the Nobel Prize in Physiology or Medicine for his work on histocompatibility genes. Similarities between the HLA system in humans and the major histocompatibility complex in mice have reinforced the fundamental nature of SNELL's painstaking efforts over many years.

E. M. EAST was trained as a chemist, but as assistant to C. G. HOPKINS at Illinois he became interested in plant breeding with emphasis on maize. (His doctoral research was on the potato.) In 1905 EAST joined the Connecticut Agricultural Experiment Station where he remained until the call to Harvard in 1909.

Relations between EAST and his student, R. A. EMERSON (S.D. 1913), were unusual in that EMERSON, 6 years older than EAST, was already an established investigator at the University of Nebraska. The two remained close friends and collaborators.

Although EMERSON was the first to earn the doctorate degree in plant genetics at the Bussey, he was not EAST's first graduate student. That distinction goes to H. K. HAYES, who joined the Connecticut Station as assistant to EAST on July 1, 1909. EAST had already accepted the offer from Harvard but remained at the Connecticut Station until the fall. With the Harvard master's degree in 1911, HAYES did not submit his doctoral thesis until 1921, using data on wheat and corn from the University of Minnesota, the institution he joined in 1915.

As successor to HAYES, DONALD JONES (S.D. 1918) was the sole geneticist at the Connecticut Station from 1915 until 1921, when PAUL MANGLESDORF came as his assistant. With materials left behind by EAST and HAYES, prior experience in practical horticulture, and friendly relations with EAST and E. H. JENKINS, JONES was in a particularly favorable position. With an undiminished passion for gardening and plant breeding, JONES became involved in theoretical genetics–the theory of heterosis, cytoplasmic male sterility, fertility-restoring genes, somatic segregation, and sex differentiation–but he is best known as the inventor of the double-cross method of corn breeding and as co-author with EAST of *Inbreeding and Outbreeding* (EAST and JONES 1919). For further information on EAST, EMERSON, and JONES, see NELSON (1993).

Before mechanization, the horse was the unit of power, animal husbandry was in the driver's seat, and vocational subjects prevailed. Consequently, even though he majored in chemistry and physics, R. A. BRINK's degree from the Ontario Agricultural College was not accepted by Cornell University. So he went to Illinois, where he became a botanist, obtained a master's degree, and was recommended to the Bussey by DETLEFSEN.

At the time, EAST's experimental work was confined almost exclusively to studies on self sterility in tobacco. J. B. PARK (S.D. 1916), and EDGAR ANDERSON (S.D. 1922) before BRINK and E. R. SEARS (S.D. 1936) after, worked on different aspects of the problem. BRINK's assignment was the physiology of pollen. That the matching of problem and student was not a perfunctory matter is evident from EAST to SEARS (June 14, 1937): "I am sorry that, with the amount of work you have gone through, there are so many negative results . . . You begin to see how difficult it is to set out problems for graduate students where the problem is worth while and results can be more or less guaranteed inside of three years." The thesis problem was by no means an end in itself, and most

Bussey students pursued quite different lines of research in later life. BRINK's distinguished career at Wisconsin, with contributions to plant breeding and theoretical genetics, is described by OWEN and NELSON (1986).

KARL SAX (S.D. 1922) and PAUL MANGLESDORF (S.D. 1925) channeled their research to conform to Harvard directions. On appointment in 1928 as Associate Professor of Plant Cytology at the Arnold Arboretum, SAX abandoned work with wheat, dividing his efforts between horticulture and comparative chromosomal studies. Later he turned his attention to radiation cytology, a line followed by a number of his graduate students. In 1940, when MANGLESDORF returned to Harvard, he made the transition from practical breeding to study of the ancestry of corn, an interest he acquired at Texas A and M.

RALPH SINGLETON (S.D. 1936), like SAX, received his B.Sc. and M.Sc. from Washington State College and was steered to the Bussey by E. F. GAINES. His doctoral thesis was on tetraploid hybrids in tobacco. As senior geneticist (1948–1955) at the Brookhaven National Laboratory, he studied induced mutations in growing plants laid out in concentric circles around a central cobalt-60 source.

E. R. SEARS and HAROLD SMITH (Ph.D. 1936) were among the last of the Bussey students. (J. D. BEASLEY's Ph.D. was awarded in 1939.) SMITH ended up as Professor of Plant Genetics at Cornell, while SEARS spent his entire career after graduation at the University of Missouri. Picking up where SAX left off, SEARS launched a research program in wheat cytogenetics that remained at the cutting edge throughout his lifetime. He developed the complete series of wheat aneuploids, nullisomic through tetrasomic, for all 21 chromosomes. Also, combining a number of techniques, including X-irradiation, he was able to transfer disease resistance to wheat from a wild relative.

EDGAR ANDERSON's career was unlike that of any other Bussey graduate student. Shy, precocious, introspective, independent, disliked by Bussey classmates, but a favorite of EAST's–whom he admired but with reservations– ANDERSON was fitted to break new ground in a field eschewed by other students from agricultural colleges. Since the secrets of inheritance had come from artificially cultivated forms, it is not surprising that geneticists were unsympathetic to the methodologies of taxonomy. ANDERSON used genetics as a tool rather than an end in itself and was primarily a naturalist. Of graduate school he said, "My thesis [the genetic behavior of cross sterility in Nicotiana] was not particularly interesting: the topic was largely a question of what was available. I don't think it did me any harm and it did give me an insight into a certain field" (ROE 1952, p. 98). After graduation, ANDERSON spent his entire professional career attached to the Missouri Botanical Garden in St. Louis (1922–1931 and 1935 on) and the Arnold Arboretum (1931–1935).

Staking out for himself the much neglected classification of weeds and cultivated plants, ANDERSON made contributions to methodology, theory, and teaching methods. Impressed by the rarity of hybrids under natural conditions in contrast to the survival of hybrid swarms in "hybridized habitats," he emphasized the role of introgressive hybridization in plant evolution. His closest friend, G. L. STEBBINS, with similar interests, was never connected directly with the Bussey, although KARL SAX was on his thesis committee.

At the Sixth International Congress of Genetics held in Ithaca, New York, in 1932, there were 399 participants from the United States, including CASTLE, EAST, and 32 of their students (Figure 1). T. H. MORGAN, from Cal Tech, was president of the Congress, but former Bussey student C. C. LITTLE was chairman and general secretary, L. C. DUNN was secretary of the council, E. M. EAST was chairman of the program committee, and D. F. JONES was chairman of the publications committee. Because the conference was held at Cornell, with R. A. EMERSON as chairman of the local committee, the selection of Bussey men is not surprising, but it is significant that this carried over to the organization of the Genetics Society of America later in the same year.

Up through 1931 genetics was affiliated with the American Society of Zoologists and the Botanical Society of America. Because a number of geneticists were members of neither Society, it was decided in 1931 to reorganize the Joint Genetics Sections as an independent society. A cordial invitation was tendered to "geneticists interested in agriculture" to apply for membership. R. A. BRINK was chosen to organize symposia of interest to agriculturists, but "Geneticists Interested in Agriculture" was discontinued as a separate group. The first seven presidents of the Society had Bussey connections:

Year	President	Location
1932	L. C. DUNN	Columbia University
1933	R. A. EMERSON	Cornell University
1934	SEWALL WRIGHT	University of Chicago
1935	D. F. JONES	Connecticut Agricultural Experiment Station
1936	P. W. WHITING	University of Pennsylvania
1937	E. M. EAST	Harvard University
1938	L. J. STADLER	University of Missouri

(WHITING was a research worker at the Bussey in 1927, STADLER in 1925–1926.)

At the Seventh International Congress held in London, Cambridge, and Edinburgh in 1939, the Bussey was again well represented. In addition to nine holders of the Bussey doctorate, the program included presentations by 12 Bussey visiting scientists, most of whom had spent 1 or 2 years there.

To declare financial exigency as the reason for closing an institution is like saying the candidate lost because he didn't get enough votes. The tide in the affairs of men began in earnest in 1924, the year that Harvard failed to

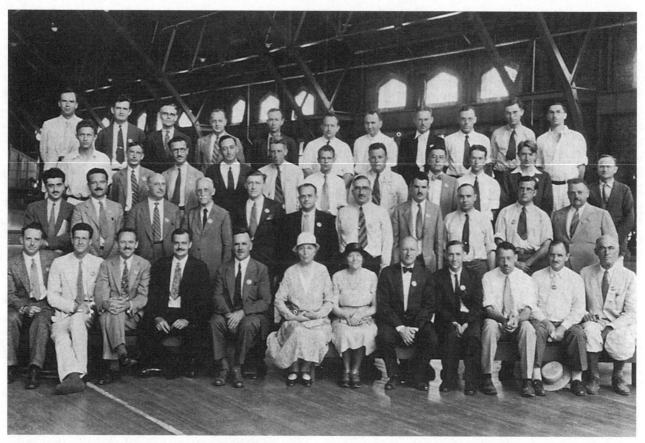

FIGURE 1.—A group picture of attendees at the 1932 International Congress of Genetics at Cornell University who had been associated with the Bussey Institute. Its influence is apparent. *Front row:* KARL SAX, L. C. DUNN, P. W. WHITING, C. C. LITTLE, O. E. WHITE, Mrs. W. E. CASTLE, Mrs. KARL SAX, E. M. EAST, N. F. WATERS, F. H. CLARK, D. W. DAVIS, R. A. EMERSON. *Second row:* G. G. PINCUS, E. C. MacDOWELL, R. B. GOLDSCHMIDT, W. E. CASTLE, H. W. FELDMAN, L. H. SNYDER, H. C. McPHEE, G. L. SLATE, E. F. GAINES, R. A. BRINK, E. N. WENTWORTH. *Third row:* A. MARSHAK, J. BEN HILL, HAIG DERMEN, L. J. STADLER, P. C. MANGELSDORF, S. C. REED, EDGAR ANDERSON, J. B. PARK, G. D. SNELL, J. I. KENDALL, D. F. JONES. *Back row:* M. R. IRWIN, W. R. SINGLETON, S. H. YARNELL, H. P. RILEY, T. W. WHITAKER, L. C. STRONG, WILLIAM GATES, P. W. GREGORY, C. R. BURNHAM, P. B. SAWIN, R. C. ROBB.

respond to the Rockefeller Foundation's willingness to invest up to $20,000,000 as an endowment for a broadly conceived program of fundamental biological research. Although the Bussey lingered on until 1936, the final paroxysm occurred in September 1929 when, by a vote of 10 to 9, the Board of Overseers turned down the Harvard Corporation's decision to appoint RAYMOND PEARL as dean of the Bussey Institution.

Joining the University of California in 1936 as research associate in mammalian genetics, CASTLE became the first recipient of the Kimber Genetics Award of the National Academy of Sciences in 1955 and continued to work almost up to his death in 1962.

On April 20, 1937, WILLIAM MORTON WHEELER collapsed on the Harvard Square subway and died within a few minutes. On November 8, 1938, RALPH W. WETMORE spent the evening with EAST in the hospital where EAST's operation was scheduled for the following morning. Recalling events of his career in genetics and grasping WETMORE's hand in both of his, EAST said, "Tomorrow it will be all over." It was.

LITERATURE CITED

CASTLE, W. E, 1919   Piebald rats and selection, a correction. Am. Nat. **53:** 370–375.

CASTLE, W. E., and J. C. PHILLIPS, 1914   Piebald rats and selection. Publication No. 195, Paper No. 21. Carnegie Institution of Washington, Washington, D.C.

EAST, E. M., 1926   The concept of the gene. Proc. Int. Congr. Plant Sci. **1:** 889–895.

EAST, E. M., and D. F. JONES, 1919   *Inbreeding and Outbreeding.* J. B. Lippincott, Philadelphia.

EMERSON, R. A., and E. M. EAST, 1913   The inheritance of quantitative characters in maize. Bull. Nebraska Agric. Exp. Sta. **2:** 1–120.

JONES, D. F., 1944   Edward Murray East (1879–1938). Biogr. Mem. Natl. Acad. Sci. **23:** 217–242.

MACDOWELL, E. C., 1914   Size inheritance in rabbits. Publication No. 195, Paper No. 22. Carnegie Institution of Washington, Washington, D.C.

NELSON, O. E., 1993   A notable triumvirate of maize geneticists. Genetics **135:** 937–941.

OWEN, R. D., and O. E. NELSON, 1986   ROYAL ALEXANDER BRINK, 1897–1984. Genetics **112:** 1–10.

ROE, A., 1952   *The Making of a Scientist.* Dodd, Mead & Co., New York.

SNELL, G. D., and S. REED, 1993   WILLIAM ERNEST CASTLE, pioneer mammalian geneticist. Genetics **133:** 751–753.

WRIGHT, S., 1963   WILLIAM ERNEST CASTLE, 1867–1962. Genetics **48:** 1–5.

Archibald Edward Garrod
The Reluctant Geneticist

Alexander G. Bearn

The Rockefeller University, New York, New York 10021-6399

THE name ARCHIBALD EDWARD GARROD (1857–1936) is familiar to most geneticists, particularly those interested in the historical roots of biochemical and human genetics. The seminal work by which GARROD is identified, *Inborn Errors of Metabolism*, was delivered as the Croonian Lectures in June, 1908 to the Royal College of Physicians in London and was published the following year [GARROD (1909), reprinted in HARRIS (1963)].

The substance of these lectures is now a genetic commonplace: errors in metabolism are often inherited in a recessive fashion and are due to the absence of a critical enzyme in a metabolic pathway. The lectures failed to arouse any enthusiasm from his audience and were received only perfunctorily by the medical press.

The extension of these ideas to the important concept of biochemical individuality may have originated when GARROD read CARL HUPPERT's (1834–1904) impressive rectorial address at the Carl Ferdinand University in Prague in 1895, entitled "On the Maintenance of the Characteristics of Species" (HUPPERT 1896). HUPPERT, a physiological chemist who had been trained by CARL LEHMANN (1812–1863), advanced the view that chemical differences between species must exist and that these differences express themselves as unique chemical structures. In the course of his lectures, HUPPERT suggested that interspecies differences in susceptibility to infective agents resided in the species' possessing different chemical structures that were probably protein in nature. Resistance to infection in certain species could be laid at the door of unique chemical structures that were inhospitable to the invading infectious agent. HUPPERT's evolutionary interest led him to assert with foresight, "The nucleins and nucleoalbumins which derive from the cell nucleus ... play the primordial role in life itself ... an uninterrupted chain of specific chemical characteristics linking antecedents and descendants."

When HUPPERT made these far-sighted remarks, ARCHIBALD GARROD, whose father was a Harley Street physician who discovered that uric acid played a prominent role in the causation of gout, had launched his consulting practice in London and was intent on honing his medical skills. In addition to pursuing the purely clinical work necessary to support a growing family, GARROD was energetically applying spectroscopic methods, which he had originally learned while an undergraduate at Oxford, as an aid to medical diagnosis. His immediate goal was to explore the nature of the chemical substances that conferred the distinctive coloration to the urine in normal individuals as well as in patients with a variety of diseases. Working collaboratively with GOWLAND HOPKINS, a future Nobel Laureate in medicine or physiology, GARROD noticed that patients who had been treated with sulfonal, a sedative drug, excreted a reddish-colored urine whose color he and HOPKINS went on to identify as hematoporphyrin. In 1900, while GARROD was continuing his spectroscopic studies on colored urine, the celebrated trio of DE VRIES, CORRENS and TSCHERMAK rediscovered the works of GREGOR MENDEL and, almost immediately, the naturalist WILLIAM BATESON became GARROD's most articulate and spirited disciple.

A year earlier, pursuing his interest in colored urine, GARROD had presented a paper to the Royal Medical and Chirurgical Society in London that would mark the beginning of a life-long career devoted to the study of human metabolic disease and led, a decade later, to his Croonian Lectures. GARROD's paper was on alkaptonuria, a rare condition then colloquially known as "black urine disease." Those with the disease were usually free of symptoms, but they "advertised their condition," to use GARROD's phrase, by passing urine that turned black on standing because of the presence of homogentisic acid. Without explanatory comment, GARROD (1900) recorded that the condition was usually congenital and frequently occurred in brothers and sisters. While continuing his clinical practice, GARROD became increasingly fascinated by the disease. On November 30, 1901, GARROD, in an article in *The Lancet* entitled "About Alkaptonuria," made the trenchant observation, "I am able to bring forward evidence which seems to point, in no uncertain manner, to a very special liability of alkaptonuria to occur in the children of first cousins"

(GARROD 1901). This association, he wrote, "can hardly be ascribed to chance and further evidence bearing upon this point would be of great general interest." Further evidence was soon to come. The following month, BATESON referred directly to GARROD's work on alkaptonuria. In a footnote to his Report to the Evolution Committee of the Royal Society, he pointed out that one-quarter of the cases of alkaptonuria reported by GARROD were the offspring of cousin marriages (BATESON and SAUNDERS 1901). This fact could be simply and easily accounted for if the condition was inherited in a recessive fashion, according to the recently discovered laws of MENDEL.

GARROD immediately recognized the evident truth of BATESON's suggestion. The familial aggregation of patients with alkaptonuria, the rare transmission of the trait from parent to offspring, and the consanguinity could all be explained on the basis of recessive inheritance. He understood clearly the implications of recessive inheritance, and in a playful moment he wrote slyly to BATESON, "I do not see any way of introducing any marriageable alkaptonurics to each other with a view to matrimony."

Extending the concept of Mendelian inheritance, GARROD proposed that inherited variations could lead either to a relatively simple "metabolic sport" such as alkaptonuria or, more complicatedly, to structural abnormalities including congenital malformations, such as Down's syndrome. As he adroitly put it, "Bodily form and chemical structure go hand in hand." GARROD, particularly in his later years, is so often portrayed as a genial, white-haired, unassuming, patriarchal physician of extreme modesty, that it is wonderfully refreshing to read in one of his early letters to BATESON, "I would ask that you kindly not speak of [my ideas] to others, insofar as they may contain anything new."

With enthusiasm and dogged determination, and by writing to physicians throughout the world, GARROD collected, in addition to patients with alkaptonuria, families with albinism, cystinuria and pentosuria, conditions he also regarded as recessively inherited. It was these four metabolic diseases that formed the core of his Croonian lectures. In addition to summarizing his extensive experience with these diseases, GARROD made a bold and novel intellectual leap. These thoughts were summarized in a landmark paper in *The Lancet*, published in 1902. He proposed that the concept of inherited deficiencies of an enzyme as a cause of recessively inherited diseases could be made biologically generalizable. Individual biochemical variation was not only the biological norm, but also the sovereign hallmark of human nature.

Only occasionally would the hereditary biochemical individuality be so extreme that it would result in overt disease. With these thoughts GARROD's medical fascination with inborn errors of metabolism continued but, as

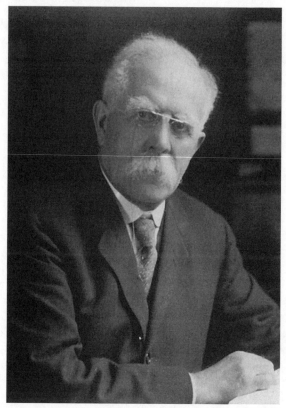

FIGURE 1.—ARCHIBALD EDWARD GARROD

the years passed, he became increasingly absorbed by the broad spectrum of individuality, its chemical and biological as well as its medical significance, and what it might mean from an evolutionary point of view.

Although GARROD was a pillar of the medical establishment who had received the highest honors and had become Regius Professor of Medicine at Oxford, the profession never appreciated the broad biological significance of his work. A well respected, competent physician, he never enjoyed the routine, often monotonous, aspects of the profession. He frequently wondered why he had chosen to pursue a career in clinical medicine and consultant practice. He was, as he freely admitted, "a wanderer down the by-paths of medicine," and that is exactly the way his contemporaries regarded him.

GARROD gradually became more and more convinced that biochemical variation was an essential clue to an understanding of evolution and that even human disease must be considered and taught in an evolutionary perspective. In the final analysis, it was biological individuality that determined susceptibility or resistance to human disease.

After GARROD retired in 1927 as Regius Professor of Medicine, released from the daily responsibilities of a busy professional life, he had more time to assemble the ideas that had been steadily forming during his 40 years as a practicing physician. He now wrote what was his crowning intellectual achievement.

GARROD (1931) could not bring himself to dignify *The Inborn Factors in Disease* as a book, preferring instead to call it "an essay." There is no evidence that this elegant and perceptive essay was appreciated any more than *Inborn Errors of Metabolism*. When GARROD first proposed to the Oxford University Press that they publish *The Inborn Factors in Disease*, they "assented palely" and agreed to do so only because GARROD was a Delegate to the Press and they had already published *Inborn Errors of Metabolism*. The Secretary continued, "He will not pay for it. I don't see how we can very well avoid doing this. It ought not to cost more than £100, and might even sell a few copies." In the event, they printed 1250 copies. Even GOWLAND HOPKINS, to whom he had dedicated the second edition of *Inborn Errors of Metabolism* (1923) and who a year later linked GARROD's name with JUSTUS LIEBIG as one of two Fathers of Biochemistry, did not refer to *Inborn Factors in Disease* in his otherwise sensitive and appreciative obituary of GARROD for the Royal Society. The recent facsimile publication of this "essay," edited and thoughtfully annotated by CHARLES SCRIVER and BARTON CHILDS (1989), should do much to rekindle interest in this wise and insightful book.

After GARROD's death in 1936, physicians continued to remember him as the author of *Inborn Errors*, but it was the biochemists who were the first to recognize the biological importance of GARROD's work. Alkaptonuria made its way into MEYER BODANSKY's *Introduction to Physiological Chemistry* in 1927, although he did not refer specifically to GARROD. ROGER J. WILLIAMS, also a biochemist, devoted a paragraph to alkaptonuria in his *Introduction to Biochemistry* in 1931, but did not develop the concept of biochemical individuality until he wrote his influential text, *Biochemical Individuality*, in 1956, 20 years after GARROD's death.

Despite GARROD's profound impact on the field of genetics, he remained a busy practitioner of medicine who preferred to stand on the sidelines while BATESON battled furiously with the biometricians. When the Genetical Society was founded in 1919, GARROD did not become a member, nor did he attend meetings of the Society, even as a guest. Although he, with his friend GOWLAND HOPKINS, was one of the Founding Committee Members of the Biochemical Club that met in March, 1911, he soon resigned from the Committee and, surprisingly, does not seem to have played an active role in the Society thereafter. Less surprisingly, GARROD had similarly shown no interest in joining the Eugenics Education Society inspired by GALTON and founded in 1907. That Society was largely devoted to popularizing the eugenic doctrine, and GARROD wanted no part in it. When the horticultural geneticist, CHARLES C. HURST, created a Council to further research in human genetics in 1931, he urged GARROD to become a founding member. GARROD was supportive and encouraging, but he was now 74 years old, and his age and deteriorating health deterred him from getting actively involved.

GARROD, ever careful to avoid giving the impression that he understood the mathematical consequences of Mendelian inheritance, wrote in a letter to LIONEL PENROSE in 1934, "Hogben in his paper on alkaptonuria in the *Edin.* (sic) *Royal Society Proceedings* and in his 'Nature and Nurture' has, I think, given me more credit than I am entitled to, seeing that it was Bateson who saw daylight." A year earlier, in a letter to E. A. COCKAYNE, a friend and dermatologist, he wrote, "I find myself quite out of my depth in the new Mendelism of Hogben and Haldane . . . He [HOGBEN] refers too kindly to a thirty year old paper of mine [GARROD's 1902 paper]. It is curious to look back to the old Bateson-Weldon controversies and the position of Mendelism today."

Although reference by geneticists to GARROD's work on inherited metabolic diseases was initially sparse, there was an early and notable exception. SEWALL WRIGHT, who had begun his work on the coat color of guinea pigs in WILLIAM E. CASTLE's department at Harvard and who was to become one of the world's leading population geneticists, became aware of GARROD's work through reading BATESON's *Mendel's Principles of Heredity*, published in 1909, although he did not refer to GARROD when he wrote his Ph.D. thesis at Harvard in 1916. However, by the time WRIGHT took up his position in the Department of Zoology at the University of Chicago in 1929, he promptly introduced his students to a course on "physiological genetics." This consisted of 30 lectures, three of which were devoted to ARCHIBALD GARROD and inborn errors of metabolism (PROVINE 1986, p. 172).

T. H. MORGAN was rather less interested than WRIGHT in biochemical aspects of gene action and, as late as 1934, in delivering his Nobel lecture on "The Relation of Genetics to Physiology and Medicine" (MORGAN 1934) to a largely medical audience, did not refer to GARROD's work. MORGAN was preoccupied more with genetic linkage than with the physiology of gene action, and he clearly perceived the relevance of linkage analysis to human disease: "Even the phenomenon of linkage may some day be helpful in [medical] diagnosis . . . There can be little doubt that there will, in time, be discovered hundreds of linkages and some of these, we may anticipate, will tie together visible and invisible hereditary characteristics."

It was probably GEORGE W. BEADLE who brought GARROD to the attention of geneticists with his generous references to GARROD in his 1958 Nobel lecture (BEADLE 1959): "In this long round about first in Drosophila and then in Neurospora we had rediscovered what Garrod had seen so clearly so many years before." He even suggested that it was GARROD who first proposed a direct relation between genes and enzymes. This was not quite true. The enunciation of the one gene-one enzyme hypothesis by BEADLE and TATUM followed from their experiments on nutritional mutants in Neurospora. Despite some legitimate skepticism on the part of DELBRÜCK and also LEDERBERG (1956), this concept proved to be of enduring importance and ushered in a new field, biochemical genetics. In his Nobel lecture BEADLE expressed regret that he had been tardy in recognizing the importance of GARROD's work, although BEADLE had first referred to GARROD in 1939 in a lecture at the Seventh International Congress of Genetics, and again in 1941, when he gave a paper on Drosophila at a meeting of the American Association for the Advancement of Science (BEADLE and TATUM 1941).

HALDANE, who had long pondered the nature of gene action, certainly since 1920 when he gave a paper to the Oxford University Junior Science Club entitled "Some Recent Work on Heredity," made no evident recorded reference to GARROD until 1937 when, in a commemorative volume of essays in honor of the 75th birthday of GOWLAND HOPKINS, he accorded GARROD his rightful place as one of the pioneers of biochemical genetics (HALDANE 1937). It was another five years before HALDANE would refer to him again, at least in print.

HALDANE was appointed geneticist to the John Innes Horticultural Research Station in 1927 and became a champion of the work of MURIEL WHELDALE and ROSE SCOTT-MONCRIEF on the biosynthetic pathways of the anthocyanin pigments of plants. Whether they discussed GARROD's highly relevant work on metabolic pathways is not known, but these authors never referred to GARROD and his work; neither did BEADLE remember talking about GARROD when he visited HALDANE at the Institute in 1936, six years before the publication of *New Paths in Genetics* (HALDANE 1942).

In 1909 GARROD had postulated that the metabolic abnormality in alkaptonuria was an inherited deficiency of an enzyme that in normal individuals split the benzene ring of homogentisic acid. This hypothesis was finally proved in 1958, 22 years after GARROD's death, when BERT LA DU and his colleagues (1958) demonstrated the absence of an enzyme, homogentisic acid oxidase, in the liver of a patient with the disease.

ARCHIBALD GARROD will not be forgotten; the biological truths that he uncovered will endure. His role in the development of the field of biochemical genetics is secure. For those in medicine, his life represents the best of clinical investigation, a subject desperately in need of resuscitation and modern interpretation. The extension of his ideas, based on emerging genetic knowledge, to the diagnosis and prevention of human disease is already apparent and will take on even more importance as the map of the human genome unfolds. The twenty-first century, soon to be upon us, will continue to build

on GARROD's pioneering thoughts; patients and medical education will be the beneficiaries of the remarkable insights of this physician-scientist who was also a reluctant geneticist (BEARN 1993).

LITERATURE CITED

BATESON, W., 1909   *Mendel's Principles of Heredity.* Cambridge University Press, Cambridge.

BATESON, W., and E. R. SAUNDERS, 1901   *Report to the Evolution Committee of the Royal Society,* Footnote, Vol. 1, pp. 133–134.

BEADLE, G. W., 1959   Genes and chemical reactions in Neurospora, pp. 587–597 in *Nobel Lectures Including Presentation Speches and Laureates' Biographies,* Physiology or Medicine, 1942–1962. Elsevier, Amsterdam (also in Science **129:** 1715–1719)

BEADLE, G. W., and E. L. TATUM, 1941   Experimental control of development and differentiation: genetic control of developmental reactions. Am. Nat. **75:** 107–116.

BEARN, A. G., 1993   *Archibald Garrod and the Individuality of Man.* Oxford University Press, New York.

BODANSKY, M., 1927   *Introduction to Physiological Chemistry.* Wiley, New York.

GARROD, A. E., 1900   A contribution to the study of alkaptonuria. Proc. R. Med. Chirurg. Soc. (NS) **11:** 130–135.

GARROD, A. E., 1901   About alkaptonuria. Lancet **2:** 1484–1486.

GARROD, A. E., 1902   The incidence of alkaptonuria: a study in chemical individuality. Lancet **2:** 1616–1620.

GARROD, A. E., 1909   *Inborn Errors of Metabolism: The Croonian Lectures Delivered Before the Royal College of Physicians of London in June 1908,* Ed. 2, 1923. Frowde, Hodder & Stoughton, London.

GARROD, A. E., 1931   *The Inborn Factors in Disease: An Essay.* Clarendon Press, Oxford.

HALDANE, J. B. S., 1937   The biochemistry of the individual, pp. 1–10 in *Perspectives in Biology: Thirty-one Essays Presented to Sir Gowland Hopkins by Past and Present Members of His Laboratory,* edited by J. NEEDHAM and D. E. GREEN. Cambridge University Press, Cambridge.

HALDANE, J. B. S., 1942   *New Paths in Genetics.* Harper, New York.

HARRIS, H., 1963   *Garrod's Inborn Errors of Metabolism,* reprinted with a supplement. Oxford University Press, London.

HUPPERT, C. H., 1896   Rectorial address delivered 16 November 1895, in *Die Erhaltung der Arteigenschaften.* Carl Ferdinand University Press, Prague.

LA DU, B. N., V. G. ZANNONI, L. LASTER and J. E. SEEGMILLER, 1958   The nature of the defect in tyrosine metabolism in alcaptonuria. J. Biol. Chem. **230:** 251–260.

LEDERBERG, J., 1956   Comments on gene-enzyme relationships, pp. 161–174 in *Enzymatic Units of Biological Structure and Function,* Henry Ford Hospital International Symposia, edited by O. H. GAEBLER. Academic Press, New York.

MORGAN, T. H., 1934   The relation of genetics to physiology and medicine, pp. 313–328 in *Nobel Lectures Including Presentation Speeches and Laureates' Biographies,* Physiology or Medicine, 1922–1941. Elsevier, Amsterdam.

PROVINE, W. B., 1986   *Sewall Wright and Evolutionary Biology.* University of Chicago Press, Chicago.

SCRIVER, C. R., and B. CHILDS, 1989   *Garrod's Inborn Factors in Disease.* Oxford University Press, London.

WILLIAMS, R. J., 1931   *An Introduction to Biochemistry.* Van Nostrand, New York.

WILLIAMS, R. J., 1956   *Biochemical Individuality: The Basis for the Genetotrophic Concept.* Wiley, New York.

Transparent Vertebrates and Their Genetic Images

William F. Dove

McArdle Laboratory for Cancer Research and Laboratory of Genetics, University of Wisconsin–Madison, Madison, WI 53706

NO organism is phenotypically screened more intensively and extensively than the human. From continual self-screening to the modern teaching hospital, over a billion of the world's human population participate in this screen. Objective methods emerge to deal with hypochondria in the patient and with the subjective judgment of the consulting physician. For example, in a recent report on an ocular phenotype associated with certain alleles of the *Adenomatous polyposis coli* (*APC*) gene, it is reassuring to read that "at the time of the examination, the ophthalmologist was not informed of the conclusions of the genetic analysis" (OLSCHWANG *et al.* 1993). With continual progress in establishing the map of the human genome (COHEN *et al.* 1993), the possibility is being created for extensive correlation between phenotype and genotype. If these correlations are made "blind," with appropriate statistical analysis, confidence increases.

Despite the surge of medical genetics, many a human phenotype remains invisible. Mutations leading to embryonic lethality are not generally discovered even in pediatric clinics. Post-embryonic phenotypes that respond quantitatively to multiple polymorphic loci seldom lend themselves to a strict phenotype/genotype correlation within the available human kindreds (see DIETRICH *et al.* 1993). Improvements in the objective phenotyping of subtle human traits are in great demand, as we shall see later in this essay. But first we shall note a surge in the phenotyping and genetics of embryonic and post-embryonic development in the genetically facile vertebrates of the laboratory–the mouse and the zebrafish.

Under the microscope, the developing embryos of Drosophila and the nematode have each gained a measure of optical transparency. For Drosophila, a major simplification in descriptive molecular embryology was created by the ability to perform *in situ* hybridization analysis with nucleic acid probes on whole-mount embryos (HAFEN *et al.* 1983; AKAM 1983). For the nematode, the direct observation of embryonic and post-embryonic patterns of cell division and differentiation was made possible through Nomarski optics, courtesy of ROGER FREEDMAN and SIMON PICKVANCE (HORVITZ and SULSTON 1990). But description is not enough, even if transparent.

Geneticists reading this journal are each well aware of the power of mutational analysis, as well as the barriers to its full implementation. With mutational analysis, the temporal and spatial descriptive molecular embryology is transformed into a network of cause and effect: the "genetic image" of the developing organism. Whether the networks in extant organisms have deep structures with the elegant simplicity of the genetic code is a matter of active biological and mathematical investigation (see KAUFFMAN 1973, 1993; THOMAS and D'ARI 1989). For the experimental vertebrates, how transparent are the current genetic images?

In mouse genetics, the invention of gene targeting has created opportunities to observe the phenotype of recessive mutant alleles in which a particular gene product of interest has lost function either partially (HASTY *et al.* 1991) or fully (WILLIAMSON *et al.* 1992). Rather often, individual mutant loci have little if any phenotypic manifestation, owing to compensation (RUDNICKI *et al.* 1993) or to other forms of genetic redundancy (see THOMAS 1993). Along the other route to connect phenotypes with causative molecules, steady progress continues in creating new mutant lines defined by their interesting phenotypes. These involve undirected mutagenesis with insertion elements (see MEISLER 1992), enhancer and promoter traps (see BEDDINGTON 1992), or the point mutagen ethylnitrosourea (ENU) (see RINCHIK 1991). The former mode of mutagenesis permits ready identification of the salient gene product involved in the phenotype. By contrast, ENU mutagenesis achieves very high mutant frequencies–of crucial logistical importance–but requires positional cloning with its unpredictable relationship between map distance and physical distance [see DOVE (1987); *cf.* KING *et al.* (1991) and MALO *et al.* (1993)]. One wonders to how many non-human mammals these methods of molecular genetics will be extended in the upcoming few decades; note that an initial genetic map of the sheep is reported in this issue of GENETICS (CRAWFORD *et al.*, 1994). The major improvements in the creation of the genetic image of the mouse are joined by important technical improvements in the molecular description of the embryo by whole-mount hybridization *in situ* (see WILKINSON 1992). However, the molecular description of the mouse embryo confronts major barriers to exploiting the transparency of the developing mammal. The mother obscures the embryo, particularly around the stage of implantation when the embryo is difficult even to dissect away from maternal tissue.

The zebrafish, externally fertilized, presents a fully transparent embryo. As with the nematode under Nomarski optics, the living zebrafish embryo can be visualized under the dissecting microscope. Thus, both spatial and temporal descriptions can be made at a resolution of individual cells. In the present year, two major mutational analyses of the developing zebrafish embryo have been launched (MULLINS *et al.* 1994; SOLNICA-KREZEL *et al.* 1994). Optimizing ENU mutagenesis of the zebrafish germline to forward mutation rates similar to those of the mouse germline, *ca.* 1.5×10^{-3} per locus, MULLINS and her colleagues provide evidence that ENU is a point mutagen in this organism as it is in others. Although the zebrafish permits homozygosis of mutations either during oogenesis or at the first cleavage division of a haploid egg, many of the current mutant screens formally resemble classical $F_2 \times F_2$ sibling crosses (see DRIEVER *et al.* 1994). The majority of the developmental mutants found in the initial screens displayed general abnormalities; about 30% of the mutants, by contrast, showed abnormalities in the development of particular structures or tissues. Neither MULLINS nor SOLNICA-KREZEL and their respective colleagues have yet reported zygotically controlled recessive lethal mutations that affect the establishment of the embryonic axes or the formation of the germ layers of the early embryo (see DRIEVER *et al.* 1994). Are these processes in vertebrates determined by redundant gene sets? Or by maternally expressed genes? Interestingly, these two zebrafish mutagenesis efforts are being directed by CHRISTIANE NÜSSLEIN-VOLHARD and WOLFGANG DRIEVER, the two protagonists in elucidating the properties of the maternally acting pattern-formation gene of Drosophila, *bicoid*. A new layer of interest in this gene can be seen in this issue of GENETICS (LUK *et al.* 1994).

The incidence of embryonic lethal mutations in the zebrafish, compared with the range of mutant frequencies for specific visible loci, can be interpreted on the basis of *ca.* 1500 genes that can mutate to an embryonic lethal phenotype (SOLNICA-KREZEL *et al.* 1994). This number is small compared with the total genome size of the zebrafish, 1.6 $\times 10^9$ base pairs (see DRIEVER *et al.* 1994). As with the mouse genome (see DOVE 1987), it seems that the vast majority of expressed genes do not readily display their mutant phenotype. The genetic image is being observed through a peephole! Again, genetic redundancy may obscure the genetic image until the phenotypic characterizations become more penetrating.

Genetics began with careful phenotyping, and there it continues. Despite the opacity of the mammalian embryo *in utero*, developmental steps of great interest are being discovered by careful postnatal phenotyping. The *shortear* gene of the mouse controls not only the proportionation of the ear, but also the formation of particular vertebral ramifications (KINGSLEY *et al.* 1992). The *brachypodism* gene of the mouse controls the lengths of the limbs but not of the axial skeleton (STORM *et al.* 1994). Interestingly, the classical morphological observations of the action of the *shortear* and the *brachypodism* genes have involved rendering the mouse transparent and staining the skeleton with alizarin (see STORM *et al.* 1994). Positional cloning has identified the product of the *shortear* gene as the bone morphogenetic protein BMP5 and that of the *brachypodism* gene as growth-differentiating factor GDF7 (STORM *et al.* 1994). Note that in these two cases the diagnostic phenotype is postnatal, not prenatal.

Much of behavior is developed postnatally. However, phenotypic screens for behavioral mutants must confront major sources of environmental variation. One striking response to this challenge has recently been reported from the Laboratory of Biological Timing at Northwestern University, headed by JOSEPH TAKAHASHI (VITATERNA *et al.* 1994). The circadian locomotor activity pattern of the mouse can be determined to high precision by monitoring activity for many days under controlled light/dark conditions and performing a Fourier analysis of the temporal cycles. Given a highly precise diurnal periodicity, an ENU-induced, semi-dominant mutation *Clock* was identified, mapped, and made homozygous. *Clock/Clock* mice can be synchronized by an external light/dark regimen, but rapidly lose memory of it when caged in total darkness. The map position of the *Clock* mutation, on mouse chromosome 5 near the well studied dominant spotting locus *W* or c-*kit*, bodes well for the positional cloning of a molecule essential for the circadian activity system of mammals. Any success in this venture must pay an essential debt to the thoroughness of the initial phenotypic screen. Humans who *know* their mice will create such screens.

Can the emergent genetics of the mouse and the zebrafish contribute to a deeper understanding of human biology? Here, too, there is no substitute for careful phenotypic observation. In the end, this observation must be robust enough to be carried out blind to the genotype. The zebrafish and the mouse will efficiently offer candidate genes for analyzing particular vertebrate traits. Those candidates can then be effectively tested individually within human kindreds that segregate for traits of interest. Altogether, the fruits of knowledge of individual human genotypes are being anticipated with varied attitudes. Will the inescapable surge of this knowledge be matched by a gentle but thorough self-scrutiny of individual human phenotypes (see GOETHE 1808)? We must not avert our eyes.

I thank DAVID KINGSLEY for sharing his morphogenetic analysis of the mouse skeleton, and LILIANNA SOLNICA-KREZEL for cheerfully informing me what she sees under her microscope, from *Physarum polycephalum* to *Brachydanio rerio*.

LITERATURE CITED

AKAM, M. E., 1983 The location of *Ultrabithorax* transcripts in *Drosophila*. EMBO J. **2**: 2075–2084.

BEDDINGTON, R., 1992 Transgenic mutagenesis in the mouse. Trends Genet. **8**: 345–347.

COHEN, D., I. CHUMAKOV and J. WEISSENBACH, 1993 A first-generation physical map of the human genome. Nature **366**: 698–701.

CRAWFORD, A. M., G. W. MONTGOMERY, C. A. PIERSON, T. BROWN, K. G. DODDS *et al.*, 1994 Sheep linkage mapping: nineteen linkage groups derived from the analysis of paternal half-sib families. Genetics **137**: 571–577.

DIETRICH, W. F., E. S. LANDER, J. S. SMITH, A. R. MOSER, K. A. GOULD *et al.*, 1993 Genetic identification of *Mom-1*, a major modifier locus affecting *Min*-induced intestinal neoplasia in the mouse. Cell **75**: 631–639.

DOVE, W. F., 1987 Molecular genetics of *Mus musculus*: point mutagenesis and millimorgans. Genetics **116**: 5–8.

DRIEVER, W., D. STEMPLE, A. SCHIER and L. SOLNICA-KREZEL, 1994 Zebrafish: genetic tools for studying vertebrate development. Trends Genet. **10**: (in press).

GOETHE, J. W. v., 1808 *Faust*, translated by W. KAUFMANN, 1961. Doubleday, New York.

HAFEN, E., M. LEVINE, R. L. GARBER and W. J. GEHRING, 1983 An improved *in situ* hybridization method for the detection of cellular RNAs in *Drosophila* tissue sections and its application for localizing transcripts of the homeotic *Antennapedia* gene complex. EMBO J. **2**: 617–623.

HASTY, P., R. RAMÍREZ-SOLIS, R. KRUMLAUF and A. BRADLEY, 1991 Introduction of a subtle mutation into the *Hox-2.6* locus in embryonic stem cells. Nature **350**: 243–246.

HORVITZ, H. R., and J. E. SULSTON, 1990 Joy of the worm. Genetics **126**: 287–292.

KAUFFMAN, S. A., 1973 Control circuits for determination and transdetermination. Science **181**: 310.

KAUFFMAN, S. A., 1993 *The Origins of Order: Self-Organization and Selection in Evolution*. Oxford University Press, Oxford.

KING, T. R., W. F. DOVE, J.-L. GUÉNET, B. G. HERRMANN and A.

SHEDLOVSKY, 1991 Meiotic mapping of murine chromosome **17**: the string of loci around *l(17)-2Pas*. Mamm. Genome **1**: 37–46.

KINGSLEY, D. M., A. E. BLAND, J. M. GRUBBER, P. C. MARKER, L. B. RUSSELL *et al.*, 1992 The mouse *short ear* skeletal morphogenesis locus is associated with defects in a bone morphogenetic member of the TGF superfamily. Cell **71**: 399–410.

LUK, S. K.-S., M. KILPATRICK, K. KERR and P. M. MACDONALD, 1994 Components acting in localization of *bicoid* mRNA are conserved among *Drosophila* species. Genetics **137**: 521–530.

MALO, D., S. VIDAL, J. H. LIEMAN, D. C. WARD and P. GROS, 1993 Physical delineation of the minimal chromosomal segment encompassing the murine host resistance locus *Bcg*. Genomics **17**: 667–675.

MEISLER, M. H., 1992 Insertional mutation of 'classical' and novel genes in transgenic mice. Trends Genet. **8**: 341–344.

MULLINS, M. C., M. HAMMERSCHMIDT, P. HAFFTER and C. NÜSSLEIN-VOLHARD, 1994 Large-scale mutagenesis in the zebrafish: in search of genes controlling development in a vertebrate. Curr. Biol. **4**: 189–202.

OLSCHWANG, S., A. TIRET, P. LAURENT-PUIG, M. MULERIS, R. PARC *et al.*, 1993 Restriction of ocular fundus lesions to a specific subgroup of *APC* mutations in adenomatous polyposis coli patients. Cell **75**: 959–968.

RINCHIK, E. M., 1991 Chemical mutagenesis and fine-structure functional analysis of the mouse genome. Trends Genet. **7**: 15–21.

RUDNICKI, M. A., P. N. J. SCHNEGELSBERG, R. H. STEAD, T. BRAUN, H.-H. ARNOLD *et al.*, 1993 MyoD or Myf-5 is required for the formation of skeletal muscle. Cell **75**: 1351–1359.

SOLNICA-KREZEL, L., A. F. SCHIER and W. DRIEVER, 1994 Efficient recovery of ENU-induced mutations from the zebrafish germline. Genetics **136**: 1401–1420.

STORM, E. E., T. V. HUYNH, N. G. COPELAND, N. A. JENKINS, D. M. KINGSLEY *et al.*, 1994 Limb alterations in *brachypodism* mice are due to mutations in a new BMP-related member of the TGF superfamily. Nature **368**: 639–643.

THOMAS, J. H., 1993 Thinking about genetic redundancy. Trends Genet. **9**: 395–399.

THOMAS, R., and R. D'ARI, 1989 *Biological Feedback*. CRC Press, Boca Raton, Fla.

VITATERNA, M. H., D. P. KING, A.-M. CHANG, J. M. KORNHAUSER, P. L. LOWREY *et al.*, 1994 Mutagenesis and mapping of a mouse gene, *Clock*, essential for circadian behavior. Science **264**: 719–725.

WILKINSON, D. G., 1992 *In Situ Hybridization: A Practical Approach*. IRL Press, New York.

WILLIAMSON, D. J., M. L. HOOPER and D. W. MELTON, 1992 Mouse models of hypoxanthine phosphoribosyltransferase deficiency. J. Inherit. Metab. Dis. **15**: 665–673.

A Century of Homeosis
A Decade of Homeoboxes

William McGinnis

Department of Molecular Biophysics and Biochemistry, Yale University, New Haven, Connecticut 06520–8114

ONE hundred years ago, while the science of genetics still existed only in the yellowing reprints of a recently deceased Moravian abbot, WILLIAM BATESON (1894) coined the term homeosis to define a class of biological variations in which one element of a segmentally repeated array of organismal structures is transformed toward the identity of another. After the rediscovery of MENDEL's genetic principles, BATESON and others (reviewed in BATESON 1909) realized that some examples of homeosis in floral organs and animal skeletons could be attributed to variation in genes. Soon thereafter, as the discipline of Drosophila genetics was born and was evolving into a formidable intellectual force enriching many biological subjects, it gradually became clear that fruit flies contained multiple "homeotic" genes (*e.g.*, *bithorax*, *aristapedia* and *proboscipedia*) (BRIDGES and MORGAN 1923; BALKASCHINA 1929; BRIDGES and DOBZHANSKY 1933), some of which appeared to be loosely clustered on the third chromosome. These genetic studies culminated in the systematic analyses of LEWIS (1978) and KAUFMAN *et al.* (1980), which provided preliminary definitions of the many homeotic genes of the Bithorax and Antennapedia complexes, and also showed that the mutant phenotypes for most of these genes could be traced back to patterning defects in the embryonic body plan.

Ten years ago, a sudden stream of papers (McGINNIS *et al.*, 1984a,b,c; SCOTT and WEINER 1984; LAUGHON and SCOTT 1984; SHEPHERD *et al.* 1984; CARRASCO *et al.* 1984; LEVINE *et al.* 1984) introduced the homeobox to developmental genetics and sketched its basic outlines. In retrospect, each of these studies contained relatively few data for the impact they had. Putting the best face on it, one could claim they are reports of exemplary brevity. These reports defined homeoboxes as members of a highly conserved family of DNA sequences that appeared to be preferentially associated with homeotic and segmentation genes of Drosophila. Homeobox sequences were highly conserved in other animals, including mammals, and were proposed to encode DNA-binding homeodomains because of a faint resemblance to mating-type transcriptional regulatory proteins of budding yeast and an even fainter resemblance to bacterial helix-turn-helix transcriptional regulators.

The initial stream of papers was a prelude to a flood concerning homeobox genes and homeodomain proteins, a flood that has channeled into a steady river of homeo-publications, fed by many tributaries. A major reason for the continuing flow of studies is that many groups, working on disparate lines of research, have found themselves swept up in the currents when they found that their favorite protein contained one of the many subtypes of homeodomain. This was in part because the definition of what proteins belonged to the homeodomain family expanded to include proteins that had only marginal amounts of sequence similarity to the founder members in the Drosophila Antennapedia and Bithorax gene complexes. Many of the proteins that have homeodomains have nothing to do with BATESON's version of homeosis, although there is a loosely defined structural subgroup of homeodomains that is closely linked to homeotic genetic functions in animals.

The initial stream of reports immediately explained (or purported to explain) some of the burning questions concerning homeotic genes. They seemed to be a fairly closely conserved gene family, and the sequence that validated their family membership, the homeobox, provided a plausible biochemical function for their action. They were likely to be DNA-binding transcriptional regulators that would modulate the expression of many downstream genes. The conservation of very similar homeobox sequences in other animals suggested that homeotic-like genetic functions might exist in structurally homologous genes other than in Drosophila. That is, perhaps a conservation of developmental genetic circuitry could be detected at the molecular level that was invisible at the level of comparative embryological morphology. All of these things had been suggested before in either explicit or vague terms by those with insight, prescience, and/or theoretical leanings (WOLPERT 1969; GARCIA-BELLIDO 1977; GARCIA-BELLIDO et al. 1979; LEWIS 1978; RAFF and KAUFMAN 1983), but a bit of molecular evidence goes a long way toward swaying opinion (especially the opinion of molecular biologists), so that much was made of the homeobox discovery.

In the original set of reports, the evidence for any of the conclusions was incomplete at best, which did not prevent the original authors from discussing them as quite likely to be true. There was even more hope expressed (and a bit of metaphorical hyperbole, at least in the titles) in a variety of review articles that suggested variously that the homeobox might be a biological equivalent of the Rosetta stone, the universal genetic key to body plan, and so on (e.g., STRUHL 1984; SLACK 1984). There were even articles in newspapers and popular magazines announcing that something important had happened in developmental biology that might be relevant even to those sophisticated mammals that perform a daily perusal of The New York Times. All of this attention jump-started homeobox gene research in Drosophila, where it would be defined and enriched beyond anyone's wildest dreams by the rich genetics of that animal. But perhaps the most hope, and the most rapid and concerted jump out of the homeobox research starting gate, occurred in laboratories studying development in those vertebrates that had a rich history of descriptive and experimental embryology, but rudimentary genetic tool kits compared with Drosophila. Here the homeobox seemed to provide a toehold halfway up what had seemed to be a slippery and impassable barrier of developmental genetics.

Not all concurred with the blinkered enthusiasm over the meaning and utility of the homeobox homology. Some fancifully suggested that many developmental biologists were in the grip of "homeobox madness" or "homeobox fever" (RAFF and RAFF 1985; ROBERTSON 1985; WILKINS 1986), apparently a horizontally transmitted disease that caused a loss of one's critical faculties. Some geneticists and evolutionary biologists were thought to be immune to this syndrome. Many of those with cool heads who read the original homeobox papers carefully, and interpreted them critically, found some of the arguments specious. And some were, if the results within a particular paper are considered in isolation. In those days, however, the results were coming along so fast that by the time one paper was written, the results for the next, or the next two or three, were already in one's notebook. So the temptation was to "speculate" rather boldly on behalf of some of the early general conclusions described above, this being much safer than it looked since additional evidence to support them was already in hand.

Many people working on a variety of developing animals quickly realized that the homeobox, whatever its ultimate meaning, should be exploited as a useful tool to clone genes. This was especially true in Drosophila, which already had a mother lode of genetic and cytogenetic studies as a biological treasure. And this rich lode of genetics was indeed mined for all it was worth by anyone with a homeobox probe and a hypothesis (e.g., FJOSE et al. 1985; LEVINE et al. 1985; REGULSKI et al. 1985; MACDONALD et al. 1986). For those of us who were doing something with homeoboxes as students or postdocs with WALTER GEHRING in Basel, Switzerland (which included MICHAEL LEVINE, ATSUSHI KUROIWA, ERNST HAFEN, ANDERS FJOSE, MAREK MLODZIK, and me), it will be difficult to forget the feeling of guilty pleasure when we realized how incredibly easy it might be to clone and identify the coding regions of the Drosophila homeotic genes and many of the segmentation genes. That this suspicion wasn't entirely a Swiss chocolate-inspired delusion was fortified by a chance conversation with GINES MORATA at a Swiss-USGEB meeting. Some of us, in collaboration with FRANCOIS KARCH and WELCOME BENDER, had found only three homeoboxes in Bithorax complex DNA (REGULSKI et al., 1985). At the time, the number of protein-coding transcription units in the Bithorax complex was thought to be eight or more, but MORATA, ERNESTO SANCHEZ-HERRERO, and their co-workers had just discovered that the Bithorax complex contained only three lethal complementation groups (SANCHEZ-HERRERO et al. 1985), suggesting correctly that the three bithorax homeoboxes corresponded to those three lethal genes, now known as Ubx, abd-A and Abd-B.

One of the most exciting outcomes of the early homeobox research in Drosophila was the general way it confirmed some of E. B. LEWIS's speculations about the evolution of the Bithorax complex. In an article that is oft cited but rarely read in its complex entirety, LEWIS (1978) proposed that the Bithorax complex genes were members of a gene family, having duplicated and diverged from a common ancestor and in the process having acquired divergent functions that accounted for some of the morphological differences that distinguish the Drosophila body plan from that of more primitive arthropods. Luckily for some of us, LEWIS put that speculation in the first paragraph instead of in the middle of the article among the terse and tortuous genetics. T. C. KAUFMAN (RAFF and KAUFMAN 1983) had also proposed an extension of this to embrace the homeotic genes of the Antennapedia complex controlling head and thoracic development. It is still unclear how much the variation in homeotic protein function or expression pattern can account for evolutionary changes in arthropods, but it was eventually shown that the eight homeotic genes of the Antennapedia and Bithorax complexes (now conceptually grouped as the Homeotic Complex, or HOM-C genes; AKAM 1989) contained eight structurally similar homeobox sequences, sometimes designated as the Antp-class of homeoboxes (GEHRING et al. 1990; McGINNIS and KRUMLAUF 1992).

Conservation of anterior-posterior axial patterning:
One important thread in homeobox gene research has
been the studies on the *Antp*-class *Hox* genes in other
animals, particularly in the mouse. It was found early on
that *Hox* genes were expressed in discrete anterior-
posterior regions of embryos (*e.g.*, AWGULEWITSCH *et al.*
1986; GAUNT *et al.* 1986), that some of the *Hox* genes
mapped in clusters (LEVINE *et al.* 1985; HART *et al.* 1985),
and that some Drosophila genes were much more
closely related in structure to certain mammalian *Hox*
genes than to other Drosophila homeobox genes
(REGULSKI *et al.* 1987). But it took the comprehensive
and insightful studies of BONCINELLI *et al.* (1988),
GRAHAM *et al.* (1989), and DUBOULE and DOLLÉ (1989)
to put it all together. All three groups provided convincing evidence that individual *Hox* genes mapped in the
same relative positions in one of the four *Hox* complexes
as did (some of) their homologs in Drosophila. In addition, the latter two groups showed that the embryonic expression boundaries of many of the mouse *Hox* complex
genes mimicked their map order within the complexes,
again strikingly similar in a general sense to the properties
of the *HOM*-type homeobox genes of Drosophila.

Though many found all this to be compelling evidence that the *Hox* genes must be doing something similar to the Drosophila *HOM-C* genes, it was still correlative molecular evidence. The first strong biological
evidence as to the role of the *Hox* genes came from
inducing their expression anterior to their normal limits, or artificially reducing their levels of expression, both
of which caused some interpretable and some uninterpretable defects in the development of more anterior
regions of the frog or mouse (WRIGHT *et al.* 1989;
RUIZ I ALTABA and MELTON 1989; KESSEL *et al.* 1990). By
expressing Hox proteins in developing Drosophila, one
could also get mouse and human Hox proteins to phe-
nocopy specific Drosophila HOM gain-of-function mutations (MALICKI *et al.* 1990; MCGINNIS *et al.* 1990), which
indicated that the Hox proteins certainly had homeotic
genetic functions in the context of Drosophila cells,
though still saying little or nothing about their role in
mouse or human cells. However, in many recent studies
performed over the past few years (*e.g.*, CHISAKA and
CAPECCHI 1991; LUFKIN *et al.* 1991; LEMOUELLIC *et al.*
1992; RAMIREZ-SOLIS *et al.* 1993), mouse *Hox* genes have
been mutated by gene targeting, and many of these loss-
of-function mutations result in either loss of axial structures or subtle to obvious homeotic transformations of
skeletal elements and/or rhombomere elements of the
hindbrain. These studies have represented one of the
principal success stories for the practice of "reverse genetics," a discipline that has resulted in a "reversal of
fortune" for more than one long-suffering graduate student or postdoc who has not been so fortunate as to have
the mouse *Hox* genes as the focus of his or her mutant
screen.

Also adding to the same intellectual picture are the
highly influential studies indicating that both beetles
and nematodes encode an important part of the genetic
circuitry that controls their anterior-posterior axial patterning in clusters of *HOM/Hox*-type homeobox genes
(BEEMAN *et al.* 1989; WANG *et al.* 1993). With the finding
that some of the most primitive animals like hydra have
Antp-class homeobox genes that are expressed in localized body regions (SHENK *et al.* 1993), it seems possible
that many or all animals use *Antp*-class genes in *HOM/
Hox* clusters to assign positional identities on the
anterior-posterior axis (or oral-aboral axis where head is
more difficult to define). Thus, only one hundred years
after BATESON finished analyzing some bizarre variations
in skeletons, and insightfully grouped a class of them as
homeotic variations, we now have plausible molecular
explanations for the homeotic defects, and a near certainty
that many of the variations that he originally noticed in a
variety of invertebrates and vertebrates are due to variations in the same basic underlying genetic circuitry.

Homeodomain proteins as transcription factors:
Much of the current research that concerns homeobox
gene function has been substantially enriched by the
work on homeodomain proteins as transcription factors.
The Antp-type homeodomain proteins are a relatively
small subset of the total spectrum of proteins grouped
in the homeodomain family. The only criterion for admission to this family is the conservation of a few crucial
amino acid residues that tend to reside in the same positions in the 60-amino-acid primary sequence of known
homeodomains. Structural studies of highly divergent
homeodomains suggest that most of the family members
defined by these criteria will have extremely similar
three-dimensional structures and similar interactions
with DNA binding sites (GEHRING *et al.* 1990; KISSINGER
et al. 1990; WOLBERGER *et al.* 1991). There are many
hundreds of homeodomain proteins, in many separate
subclasses (SCOTT *et al.* 1989). It seems likely that hundreds exist even within a single genome–the current
count in Drosophila is >60 and climbing (KALIONIS and
O'FARRELL 1993; DESSAIN and MCGINNIS 1993)–and these
proteins are surely involved in a myriad of biological
control circuits. Many of these are understood quite
poorly at the genetic level.

Evidence was not long in coming that homeodomain
proteins actually did have the ability to bind specific
DNA sites and that proteins with different homeodomain sequences had different preferred binding sites
(DESPLAN *et al.* 1985, 1988; HOEY and LEVINE 1988). How
much these different DNA binding preferences have to
do with their functional specificity is still rather mysterious. The most widely accepted model (or class of models) explaining homeodomain protein functional specificities is largely derived from the biochemical studies on
yeast Matα2, mammalian Oct1 and Oct2 and other POU
proteins (*e.g.*, TREACY *et al.* 1992; POMERANTZ *et al.* 1992;

VERSHON and JOHNSON 1993; CLEARY *et al.* 1993), with much support from genetic studies on chimeric HOM proteins in Drosophila embryos (*e.g.*, LIN and MCGINNIS 1992; FUROKUBO-TOKUNAGA *et al.* 1993; CHAN and MANN 1993). This model has the homeodomain presenting one face to DNA and acquiring a bit of its specificity from that interaction. The other face, a sociable but discriminating face, is free to interact with one or many other proteins either on or off DNA. Only when the right set of interactions takes place on both faces is a given homeodomain protein interpreted as part of an active or inactive transcriptional regulatory complex that is capable of flipping a developmental switch.

Some questions that might have been answered in 10 years, but might take another 10 (or 100, until BATESON's second centennial anniversary): Though the amount of research that has been done on HOM/Hox-type homeodomain proteins is enormous, it is still unknown how many genetic or cofactor inputs are *required* for a homeotic switch to be thrown that changes cells (or even a single gene for that matter) from being assigned to a head, thoracic, or abdominal fate. Another way to look at this is that the genetic and molecular interactions between the homeotic proteins and the proteins that control other equally (or more) important developmental decisions such as sex determination, muscle or nerve cell identity, the timing of developmental events, or conserved signal transduction pathways are largely unexplored and mysterious.

We still don't really understand why the *HOM/Hox* genes tend to be arranged in a colinear array that (usually) correlates with the order of their domains of expression and function in embryos. There are some appealing ideas about how these clusters might have arisen and the forces that might tend to keep them together, involving shared regulatory regions (*e.g.*, CELNIKER *et al.* 1990), but there is not enough evidence as yet to provide a convincing explanation for the persistent colinear arrangements.

We have only a primitive understanding of how HOM/Hox proteins, or any other homeodomain proteins for that matter, might have the wholesale but coordinated effects that they exert on morphogenesis. In Drosophila, the HOM proteins are known to regulate the expression of other genes that encode other transcription factors, growth factors, homophilic membrane proteins, and proteins of unknown function (reviewed in BOTAS 1993), but how is this all coordinated to result in an antenna instead of a leg, or even a gut constriction?

One interesting curiosity is that despite the importance that the human *Hox* genes must have during development, there is surprisingly little direct or indirect evidence that their proper function is relevant to known human heritable developmental defects or human teratology (*e.g.*, WOLGEMUTH *et al.* 1989). In addition, to my knowledge there are as yet no naturally occurring mouse developmental defects that map to the *Hox* clusters, de-spite the obvious involvement of some other homeodomain protein subgroups in mouse (and human) heritable morphological abnormalities.

Disclaimer: This essay is definitely not intended to be a scholarly review of homeobox gene research over the past 10 years, just an admittedly biased look back at what happened 10 years ago, and to look at how a few of the questions that were interesting then have either been answered (or not) in the ensuing period. I've benefited enormously from talking to all of the people working on *HOM* and *Hox* genes and proteins and to many of those working on other classes of homeobox genes, and I have been influenced by nearly everyone. Thus, they all bear a highly diffuse responsibility for the opinions expressed here, though certainly no blame for the manner in which they are expressed.

LITERATURE CITED

AKAM, M., 1989 *Hox* and HOM: homologous gene clusters in insects and vertebrates. Cell **57:** 347–349.

AWGULEWITSCH, A., M. F. UTSET, C. P. HART and F. H. RUDDLE, 1986 Spatial restriction in expression of a mouse homeo box locus within the central nervous system. Nature **320:** 328–335.

BALKASCHINA, E. I., 1929 Ein Fall der Erbhomeosis (die Genovarition "aristopedia") bei *Drosophila melanogaster.* Wilhelm Roux' Arch. Entwicklungsmech. Org. **115:** 448–463.

BATESON, W., 1894 *Materials for the Study of Variation Treated with Especial Regard to Discontinuity in the Origin of Species.* Macmillan, London.

BATESON, W., 1909 *Mendel's Principles of Heredity.* University Press, Cambridge, England.

BEEMAN, R. W., J. J. STUART, M. S. HAAS and R. E. DENELL, 1989 Genetic analysis of the homeotic gene complex (HOM-C) in the beetle *Tribolium castaneum.* Dev. Biol. **133:** 196–209.

BONCINELLI, E., R. SOMMA, D. ACAMPORA, M. PANNESE, M. F. A. D'ESPOSITO *et al.*, 1988 Organization of human homeobox genes. Hum. Reprod. **3:** 880–886.

BOTAS, J., 1993 Control of morphogenesis and differentiation by HOM/Hox genes. Curr. Opin. Cell Biol. **5:** 1015–1022.

BRIDGES, C. B., and T. DOBZHANSKY, 1933 The mutant "proboscipedia" in *Drosophila melanogaster*–a case of hereditary homeosis. Wilhelm Roux' Arch. Entwicklungsmech. Org. **127:** 575–590.

BRIDGES, C. B., and T. H. MORGAN, 1923 The third-chromosome group of mutant characters of *Drosophila melanogaster.* Carnegie Inst. Washington Publ. **327:** 93.

CARRASCO, A. E., W. MCGINNIS, W. J. GEHRING and E. M. DEROBERTIS, 1984 Cloning of a *Xenopus laevis* gene expressed during early embryogenesis coding for a peptide region homologous to Drosophila homeotic genes. Cell **37:** 409–414.

CELNIKER, S. E., S. SHARMA, D. J. KEELAN and E. B. LEWIS, 1990 The molecular genetics of the bithorax complex of *Drosophila*: *cis*-regulation of the *Abdominal-B* domain. EMBO J. **9:** 4277–4286.

CHAN, S., and R. S. MANN, 1993 The segment identity functions of Ultrabithorax are contained within its homeo domain and carboxy-terminal sequences. Genes Dev. **7:** 796–811.

CHISAKA, O., and M. R. CAPECCHI, 1991 Regionally restricted developmental defects resulting from targeted disruption of the mouse homeobox gene *hox-1.5.* Nature **350:** 473–479.

CLEARY, M. A., S. STERN, M. TANAKA and W. HERR, 1993 Differential positive control by Oct-1 and Oct-2: activation of a transcriptionally silent motif through Oct-1 and VP16 co-recruitment. Genes Dev. **7:** 72–83.

DESPLAN, C., J. THEIS and P. H. O'FARRELL, 1985 The Drosophila developmental gene, engrailed, encodes a sequence-specific DNA binding activity. Nature **318:** 630–635.

DESPLAN, C., J. THEIS and P. H. O'FARRELL, 1988 The sequence specificity of homeodomain-DNA interaction. Cell **54:** 1081–1090.

DESSAIN, S., and W. MCGINNIS, 1993 Drosophila homeobox genes. Adv. Dev. Biochem. **2:** 1–55.

DUBOULE, D., and P. DOLLÉ, 1989   The structural and functional organization of the murine *HOX* gene family resembles that of Drosophila homeotic genes. EMBO J. **8:** 1497–1505.

FJOSE, A., W. McGINNIS and W. J. GEHRING, 1985   Isolation of a homeobox-containing gene from the engrailed region of Drosophila and the spatial distribution of its transcripts. Nature **313:** 284–289.

FUROKUBO-TOKUNAGA, K., S. FLISTER and W. J. GEHRING, 1993   Functional specificity of the Antennapedia homeodomain. Proc. Natl. Acad. Sci. USA **90:** 6360–6364.

GARCIA-BELLIDO, A., 1977   Homeotic and atavic mutations in insects. Am. Zool. **17:** 613–629.

GARCIA-BELLIDO, A., P. A. LAWRENCE and G. MORATA, 1979   Compartments in animal development. Sci. Am. (July): 102–110.

GAUNT, S. J., J. R. MILLER, D. J. POWELL and D. DUBOULE, 1986   Homeo box gene expression in mouse embryos varies with position by the primitive streak stage. Nature **324:** 662–664.

GEHRING, W. J., M. MULLER, M. AFFOLTER, A. PERCIVAL-SMITH, M. BILLETER *et al.*, 1990   The structure of the homeodomain and its functional implications. Trends Genet. **6:** 323–329.

GRAHAM, A., N. PAPALOPULU and R. KRUMLAUF, 1989   The murine and Drosophila homeobox gene complexes have common features of organization and expression. Cell **57:** 367–378.

HART, C. P., A. AWGULEWITSCH, A. FAINSOD, W. McGINNIS and F. H. RUDDLE, 1985   Homeo box gene complex on mouse chromosome 11: molecular cloning, expression in embryogenesis, and homology to a human homeo box locus. Cell **43:** 9–18.

HOEY, T., and M. LEVINE, 1988   Divergent homeo box proteins recognize similar DNA sequences in Drosophila. Nature **332:** 858–861.

KALIONIS, B., and P. H. O'FARRELL, 1993   A universal target sequence is bound *in vitro* by diverse homeodomains. Mech. Dev. **43:** 57–70.

KAUFMAN, T. C., R. LEWIS and B. WAKIMOTO, 1980   Cytogenetic analysis of chromosome *3* in *Drosophila melanogaster*: the homeotic gene complex in polytene chromosome interval 84A-B. Genetics **94:** 115–133.

KESSEL, M., R. BALLING and P. GRUSS, 1990   Variations of cervical vertebrae after expression of a *Hox-1.1* transgene in mice. Cell **61:** 301–308.

KISSINGER, C. R., B. LIU, E. MARTIN-BLANCO, T. B. KORNBERG and C. O. PABO, 1990   Crystal structure of an engrailed homeodomain-DNA complex at 2.8 Å resolution: a framework for understanding homeodomain-DNA interactions. Cell **63:** 579–590.

LAUGHON, A., and M. P. SCOTT, 1984   Sequence of a Drosophila segmentation gene: protein structure homology with DNA-binding proteins. Nature **310:** 25–31.

LE MOUELLIC, H., Y. LALLEMAND and P. BRULET, 1992   Homeosis in the mouse induced by a null mutation in the *Hox-3.1* gene. Cell **69:** 251–264.

LEVINE, M., G. RUBIN and R. TIJAN, 1984   Human DNA sequences homologous to a protein coding region conserved between homeotic genes of Drosophila. Cell **38:** 667–673.

LEVINE, M., K. HARDING, C. WEDEEN, H. DOYLE, T. HOEY *et al.*, 1985   Expression of the homeo box gene family in Drosophila. Cold Spring Harbor Symp. Quant. Biol. **50:** 209–222.

LEWIS, E. B., 1978   A gene complex controlling segmentation in Drosophila. Nature **276:** 565–570.

LIN, L., and W. McGINNIS, 1992   Mapping functional specificity in the Dfd and Ubx homeodomains. Genes Dev. **6:** 1071–1081.

LUFKIN, T., A. DIERICH, M. LEMEUR, M. MARK and P. CHAMBON, 1991   Disruption of the *Hox-1.6* homeobox gene results in defects in a region corresponding to its rostral domain of expression. Cell **66:** 1105–1119.

MACDONALD, P. M., P. INGHAM and G. STRUHL, 1986   Isolation, structure and expression of *even-skipped*: a second pair-rule gene of Drosophila containing a homeo box. Cell **47:** 721–734.

MALICKI, J., K. SCHUGHART and W. McGINNIS, 1990   Mouse *Hox 2.2* specifies thoracic segmental identity in Drosophila embryos and larvae. Cell **63:** 961–967.

McGINNIS, N., M. A. KUZIORA, M. REGULSKI and W. McGINNIS, 1990   Human *Hox-4.2* and Drosophila *Deformed* encode similar regulatory specificities in Drosophila embryos and larvae. Cell **63:** 969–976.

McGINNIS, W., and R. KRUMLAUF, 1992   Homeobox genes and axial patterning. Cell **68:** 283–302.

McGINNIS, W., M. LEVINE, E. HAFEN, A. KUROIWA and W. J. GEHRING, 1984a   A conserved DNA sequence found in homeotic genes of the Drosophila Antennapedia and Bithorax complexes. Nature **308:** 428–433.

McGINNIS, W., R. L. GARBER, J. WIRZ, A. KUROIWA and W. J. GEHRING, 1984b   A homologous protein-coding sequence in Drosophila homeotic genes and its conservation in other metazoans. Cell **37:** 403–408.

McGINNIS, W., C. P. HART, W. J. GEHRING and F. H. RUDDLE, 1984c   Molecular cloning and chromosome mapping of a mouse DNA sequence homologous to homeotic genes of Drosophila. Cell **38:** 675–680.

POMERANTZ, J. L., T. M. KRISTIE and P. A. SHARP, 1992   Recognition of the surface of a homeo domain protein. Genes Dev. **6:** 2047–2057.

RAFF, E. C., and R. A. RAFF, 1985   Possible functions of the homeobox. Nature **313:** 185.

RAFF, R. A., and T. C. KAUFMAN, 1983   *Embryos, Genes, and Evolution*. Macmillan, New York.

RAMIREZ-SOLIS, R., H. ZHENG, J. WHITING, R. KRUMLAUF and A. BRADLEY, 1993   *Hoxb-4* (*Hox-2.6*) mutant mice show homeotic transformation of a cervical vertebra and defects in closure of the sternal rudiments. Cell **73:** 279–294.

REGULSKI, M., K. HARDING, R. KOSTRIKEN, F. KARCH, M. LEVINE *et al.*, 1985   Homeo box genes of the antennapedia and bithorax complexes of Drosophila. Cell **43:** 71–80.

REGULSKI, M., N. McGINNIS, R. CHADWICK and W. McGINNIS, 1987   Developmental and molecular analysis of *Deformed*: a homeotic gene controlling Drosophila head development. EMBO J. **6:** 767–777.

ROBERTSON, M., 1985   Mice, mating types and molecular mechanisms of morphogenesis. Nature **318:** 12–13.

RUIZ I ALTABA, A., and D. A. MELTON, 1989   Involvement of the Xenopus homeobox gene Xhox3 in pattern formation along the anterior-posterior axis. Cell **57:** 317–326.

SANCHEZ-HERRERO, E., I. VERNOS, R. MARCO and G. MORATA, 1985   Genetic organization of Drosophila bithorax complex. Nature **313:** 108–113.

SCOTT, M. P., and A. WEINER, 1984   Structural relationships among genes that control development: sequence homology between the Antennapedia, Ultrabithorax, and fushi tarazu loci of *Drosophila*. Proc. Natl. Acad. Sci. USA **81:** 4115–4119.

SCOTT, M. P., J. W. TAMKUN and I. G. W. HARTZELL, 1989   The structure and function of the homeodomain. Biochim. Biophys. Acta **989:** 25–48.

SHENK, M. A., H. R. BODE and R. E. STEELE, 1993   Expression of *Cnox-2*: a HOM/HOX homeobox gene in hydra, is correlated with axial pattern formation. Development **117:** 657–667.

SHEPHERD, J. C. W., W. McGINNIS, A. E. CARRASCO, E. M. DEROBERTIS and W. J. GEHRING, 1984   Fly and frog homeo domains show homologies with yeast mating type regulatory proteins. Nature **310:** 70–71.

SLACK, J., 1984   A Rosetta stone for pattern formation in animals? Nature **310:** 364–365.

STRUHL, G., 1984   A universal genetic key to body plan? Nature **310:** 10–11.

TREACY, M. N., L. I. NEILSON, E. E. TURNER, X. HE and M. G. ROSENFELD, 1992   Twin of I-POU: a two amino acid difference in the I-POU homeodomain distinguishes an activator from an inhibitor of transcription. Cell **68:** 491–505.

VERSHON, D., and A. D. JOHNSON, 1993   A short, disordered protein region mediates interactions between the homeodomain of the yeast α2 protein and the MCM1 protein. Cell **72:** 105–112.

WANG, B. B., M. M. MULLER-IMMERGLUCK, J. AUSTIN, N. T. ROBINSON, A. CHISHOLM *et al.*, 1993   A homeotic gene cluster patterns the anteroposterior body axis of C. elegans. Cell **74:** 29–42.

WILKINS, A. S., 1986   Homeobox fever, extrapolation and developmental biology. Bioessays **4:** 147–148

WOLBERGER, C., A. K. VERSHON, B. LIU, A. D. JOHNSON and C. O. PABO, 1991   Crystal structure of a MATα2 homeodomain-operator complex suggests a general model for homeodomain-DNA interactions. Cell **67:** 517–528.

WOLGEMUTH, D. J., R. R. BEHRINGER, M. P. MOSTOLLER, R. L. BRINSTER and R. D. PALMITER, 1989   Transgenic mice overexpressing the mouse homoeobox-containing gene *Hox-1.4* exhibit abnormal gut development. Nature **337:** 464–467.

WOLPERT, L., 1969   Positional information and the spatial pattern of cellular differentiation. J. Theor. Biol. **25:** 1–47.

WRIGHT, C. V. E., K. W. Y. CHO, J. HARDWICKE, R. H. COLLINS and E. M. DE ROBERTIS, 1989   Interference with function of a homeobox gene in Xenopus embryos produces malformations of the anterior spinal cord. Cell **59:** 81–93.

See also page 705 in Addenda et Corrigenda.

Hitoshi Kihara, Japan's Pioneer Geneticist

James F. Crow

Genetics Department, University of Wisconsin–Madison, Madison, Wisconsin 53706

The history of the earth is recorded in the layers of its crust; the history of all organisms is inscribed in the chromosomes.

THIS striking aphorism, engraved in a bronze relief at the Kihara Institute in Yokohama, was coined by KIHARA in 1946. It has a remarkably modern ring; replace chromosomes by DNA and it could have been written today.

HITOSHI KIHARA was born in Tokyo on October 21, 1893 and died on July 27, 1986 at the age of 92. Were he alive today he would be starting his second century. During his long research career–some 65 years– his main interest was the genetics of wheat, but his versatility and wide-ranging curiosity led him along many paths.

KIHARA went through grade school and high school in Tokyo. Then, because he didn't conform to the highly competitive custom of aiming for high grades and essaying difficult entrance examinations, he did not enter the prestigious Imperial Universities of Tokyo or Kyoto. Instead, he went to far-off Sapporo on Japan's Northern Island to enroll at Hokkaido University. In a biographical note he mentions a brilliant but late-blooming physicist and then says of himself that "I did not so much mature late but rather matured hardly at all." In a sense this is true, for throughout his life he retained a small boy's curiosity about everything.

In 1918 the pioneer Hokkaido wheat geneticist, TETSU SAKAMURA, had just cleaned up a cytogenetic morass by determining the correct chromosome numbers for different wheat varieties. He identified diploid, tetraploid, and hexaploid varieties with zygotic chromosome numbers 14, 28, and 42, and made crosses among them. KIHARA's entry into wheat genetics was through the cultivation of a pentaploid hybrid. Interrupted by a year in the army, he resumed his work in Hokkaido

and in 1921 transferred to Kyoto University. This was the beginning of 35 highly productive years there. Ultimately, he was to author more than 400 papers and 20 books.

It was KIHARA's good fortune to receive SAKAMURA's entire collection of wheat stocks. In 1918 SAKAMURA was promoted to the Chair of Plant Physiology, entailing two years of study in Europe. He never returned to his wheat work, one more example of being promoted out of a promising scientific career. KIHARA never failed to acknowledge his indebtedness to SAKAMURA and dedicated his major book (KIHARA 1982) to him. It is this chance circumstance that led to KIHARA's paradoxical emphasis on wheat in a rice-growing country. He did, however, do several studies on rice and its ancestry, and on other grains, but these were minor relative to his monumental studies of wheat.

At the time of KIHARA's appointment in Kyoto, a potential faculty member was required to spend two years abroad in order to qualify for a position at an Imperial University. A personable, adventurous, ambitious, and intellectually curious young man, KIHARA made the most of his opportunities abroad. The bulk of his time was spent at the Kaiser Wilhelm Institut in Berlin-Dahlem, working with C. CORRENS, one of the three who rediscovered MENDEL's laws. KIHARA also met the other two, VON TSCHERMAK in Austria and DE VRIES in Holland. In Russia he visited KOLTZOV and KARPECHENKO, but missed his counterpart VAVILOV, who was away. Later, the two men met in Japan. They shared a deep interest in the wild relatives of cultivated plants, and both organized extensive expeditions to discover them. On the way back to Japan, KIHARA visited Columbia University in New York, meeting T. H. MORGAN and E. B. WILSON. While in Germany, he sharpened his cytological skills in chromosome studies of *Rumex acetosa* and several other species of sorrel. Among other things, he determined chromosome numbers and described X and Y chromosomes

This essay is dedicated to MOTOO KIMURA in honor of his 70th birthday. He was responsible for my getting acquainted with KIHARA.

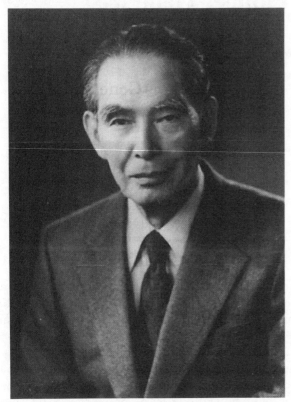

FIGURE 1.—HITOSHI KIHARA.

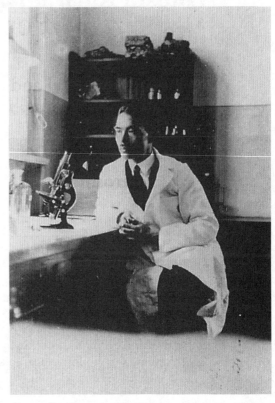

FIGURE 2.—KIHARA while he was studying in Germany.

in sorrels. He was thus one of first to find sex chromosomes in angiosperms.

Returning to the University of Kyoto, he remained there until 1955. During this time Kyoto became a world genetics center, and KIHARA was soon the best known geneticist in Japan. Although there were severe hardships during World War II and work was greatly inhibited, his research did not stop. Reaching retirement age in 1955, he became director of the National Institute of Genetics in Mishima, retiring a second time in 1969. He continued research for the rest of his long life in Yokohama in his own Institute for Biological Research.

From hybridization of polyploid wheat varieties, KIHARA discovered that only those with a multiple of seven chromosomes were normally viable, and only those with 14 or a multiple of 14 were fully fertile. He adopted WINKLER's newly coined word, "genome," designating the basic monoploid chromosome set, but he gave it a functional meaning as the minimum set containing all the essential genes. By studying the cytology of meiosis, he confirmed the irregular assortment of univalents in hybrids with an odd ploidy level, in contrast to orthodox segregation in those with an even number of genomes.

KIHARA soon realized that the degree of meiotic synapsis could be used as an index of similarity and relationship, and designated the three main wheat genomes as A, B, and D. Thus, diploid einkorn wheat (*Triticum monococcum*) is AA, tetraploid emmer (*Triticum dicoc-*

cum) is AABB, and hexaploid bread wheat (*Triticum aestivum*) is AABBDD. A fourth genome, the G group from *Triticum timopheevi*, was added later. One of KIHARA's outstanding discoveries was the ancestry of bread wheat. Having identified the D group from genome analysis, he suspected that the key to wheat ancestry lay in the Middle East. Going there, he found diploid DD goat grass (*Aegilops squarrosa*) growing as a weed in tetraploid emmer AABB wheat fields. In his words, "This observation opened our eyes to the possibility that if *Aegilops squarrosa* (2x) grew as a weed in an emmer (4x) wheat field, the two different grains might very well produce a hybrid (3x) and in the next generation join to generate the bread wheat 6x." He proceeded then to construct such a hexaploid and found that it was completely fertile with cultivated bread wheat and the chromosomes paired perfectly. Thus the whole story–sympatric growth of parental species, hybrid formation, production of unreduced gametes, and union of these gametes to produce a hexaploid–was confirmed (TSUNEWAKI 1989). During the 20-year period starting in 1930, KIHARA determined the genome composition of all known wheat and goat grass species.

While KIHARA was determining the ancestry of wheat in Asia, ERNEST SEARS was making the same discovery at the University of Missouri. Sears had admired KIHARA's work since his student days in the 1930s. He recalled that during World War II he dreamed of being shot down over Kyoto, being forced to parachute, and hoping he could find KIHARA and be welcomed as a fellow cytogeneticist. The two never met until KIHARA's trip to the United States in 1951, the first postwar visit by a Japanese geneticist (SEARS 1987).

KIHARA's trip to Pakistan, Afghanistan, and Iran was widely publicized in Japan, and a documentary film, *Karakoram*, was shown throughout the country. His name was well known to the Japanese populace. An important spin-off from these trips was a large collection of wild relatives of various cultivated plants, material that has been of use to many plant breeders. Along with VAVILOV, he played a major role in popularizing this now-common practice.

In 1951 KIHARA found cytoplasmic male sterility in several varietal and species crosses. He was able to identify both the cytoplasmic sterility factors and the specific nuclear restoring genes. Needless to say, this work, reported at the International Congress of Genetics in Montreal in 1958, attracted a great deal of attention from companies interested in developing hybrid wheat. As the preeminent wheat geneticist, KIHARA was the founder and first chairman of the International Wheat Symposium in 1958. He attended the regular meetings at five-year intervals, his last being in 1983. At age 90 he addressed the group and discussed the origin of "Daruma," a variety that has provided genetic material for many of the semi-dwarfs that have been so important in the green revolution. Daruma is a folk figure to which foreign visitors are often introduced in the form of a roly-poly seated doll. The custom is for Daruma to have only one eye at the beginning of a conference; if the meeting is successful, the second eye is painted at the conclusion. Using this name for the wheat is especially appropriate, for the Daruma doll recovers its upright posture when tipped; a striking feature of semi-dwarf wheats is that they remain standing after strong winds and heavy rains.

Although wheat was KIHARA's main interest throughout his working life, it was by no means his only one. As mentioned earlier, he was one of the first to identify sex chromosomes in flowering plants. He developed several methods for producing haploids. He had interest in rare plants and living fossils. Another interest was variegation, including that found in historical writings. And, as expected of Japan's leading geneticist, he also studied rice and its origins. His early work in 1918 provided the technique and incentive for studying polyploidy in other crop genera, and he himself discovered a polyploid series in oats.

KIHARA was an early advocate of polyploidization as a tool in plant breeding. Noting that many domestic varieties (such as oats, wheat, and strawberry) are polyploid, he argued that this should become a regular part of plant breeding technology. This was a far-sighted suggestion, later becoming routine after the discovery of colchicine and other chromosome-doubling treatments.

He also recognized the desirability of seedless varieties of edible plants, such as bananas, grapes, and pineapples. The explanations are diverse. Pineapples, for example, are self-incompatible, so that clones of vegetatively propagated and therefore identical plants are seedless. KIHARA was especially interested that vegetatively propagated, cultivated bananas are triploid while their wild relatives with seeds are diploid. So he decided to construct a seedless triploid watermelon. He started in 1939, first obtaining a tetraploid from a normal diploid by colchicine treatment. Then, using pollen from a diploid on a tetraploid stigma (the reciprocal mating didn't work), he got triploid progeny. As expected, these did not produce seeds; but without pollination they didn't produce melons either, and triploid plants did not produce appreciable amounts of functional euploid pollen. So he grew diploid plants in the same field to supply the needed pollen. But the only way to distinguish seeded from seedless melons was to cut them open. Simple Mendelism came to the rescue. KIHARA used a color-pattern gene to distinguish diploids from triploids. Seedless watermelons attracted a great deal of attention in Japan, and KIHARA became almost as well known for this as for his collecting expeditions. The melons also attracted attention elsewhere, and in 1952 the American Society of Horticulture gave KIHARA its annual award for this work.

Another of KIHARA's interests was the direction of spiraling in such places as flowers, spikelets, and climbing vines (KIHARA 1982). He collected data from the literature and from the field, and performed various experimental and genetic tests. For example, in alfalfa the direction was a simple Mendelian trait. KIHARA forced some vines to coil in the wrong direction, producing bizarre shapes that clearly showed the frustrated plant's attempt to do what its genes told it to do. Typically, his curiosity went beyond biology and he made historical studies such as examining the direction of coiling of ropes in Japanese history. Because of his interest in spiraling he noted things that most of us overlook. I remember the delight with which he showed me a painting by a European master in which a rope changed its twist from right-handed to left-handed as it went through a pulley. He was also surprised to find wrongly coiled DNA diagrams in about a fourth of the genetics textbooks he examined, including–much to his amusement–a diagram in JIM WATSON's book.

KIHARA had a life-long interest in athletics. As a student he was active in many sports. His book of photographs (KIHARA 1985) shows him involved in baseball, archery, racing, and javelin throwing. He was a skilled skier and traveled with the Kyoto University Alpine club to the snowy heights of Japanese mountains. The group planned to climb K2, but World War II intervened. Later, KIHARA led the Japanese ski team at the Winter Olympics in 1960 and 1964.

His interest in archery led to a fascinating paper (reprinted in KIHARA 1982) on the traditional contest in an ancient Kyoto temple, Sanjusan-gendo. The archer sat on a small box at one end of a 120-meter veranda, and the object was to shoot as many arrows as possible to the other end in a 24-hour period. Only those arrows that traveled the entire distance in the air counted. An assistant handed bamboo arrows as fast as they were shot. The record was 8,133 out of 13,053 attempts, or an arrow every 6.6 seconds. Shooting an arrow every 6.6 seconds for 24 hours seems an almost unbelievable feat of endurance. The training was long and arduous. This record, set in 1686, was never equaled, and the games finally stopped with the Meiji restoration nearly 200 years later. A visitor to the Sanjusan-gendo can still see marks on the rafters made by misdirected arrows. KIHARA also studied the physiology of these super-athletes. From studies of contemporary archers he calculated the amount of energy expended in 24 hours as about 8000 calories. He also computed the necessary initial velocity for the arrows to traverse the long veranda, which was only 5.2 meters high.

KIHARA was an active, public spirited, and influential citizen, strongly committed to conservation. In his later years he devoted a great deal of time to preservation of the landscape, a much-needed activity in that crowded and environmentally fragile country. He was especially active in preserving the native vegetation in the Hakone area not far from Mount Fuji. A particular concern was the increasing number of golf courses, which were interfering with the normal pattern of water runoff. As a botanist he was largely responsible for the Hakone Arboretum and edited a book of trees and other plants in this area (KIHARA 1971). He had a deep interest in a "living fossil" sequoia (*Metasequoia glyptoboides*) found in China and transplanted some trees to Japan. His favorite plant in the Hakone area was the dogwood (*Cornus kousa*), and he also transplanted American dogwood (*Cornus florida*) to the grounds of the National Institute of Genetics in Mishima.

KIHARA was far and away the best known Japanese geneticist in pre-molecular days. He was an honorary member of no less than 20 societies outside of Japan, including those in Russia, Britain, Sweden, Germany, and India. In the United States he was a foreign member of the National Academy of Sciences, the American Academy of Arts and Sciences, and the American Philosophical Society. I believe his nearest counterpart was N. I. VAVILOV. Both had great self-confidence, tremendous enthusiasm, and boundless energy. Their work was characterized, not so much by its brilliance and depth of insight as by its thoroughness and breadth, and by a willingness to try big things–large-scale experiments and long expeditions. And, most important, both had the ability to lead and inspire followers. Fortunately, in contrast to VAVILOV'S tragically truncated career (CROW 1993), KIHARA lived a long life. He was intellectually vigorous until the end.

KIHARA liked to characterize himself figuratively as "a grain of wheat" and his photographic biography bears this title (KIHARA 1985). He had remembered the biblical parable of the sower whose seeds flourished and multiplied only when they fell on good ground.

Although I had met KIHARA on his trip to the United States in 1951, I first became well acquainted with him in 1957, when I had the good fortune to spend the summer at the National Institute of Genetics in Mishima working with MOTOO KIMURA. KIHARA was director at the time. I have vivid memories of his generous hospitality, his enthusiasm and physical energy on trips to see interesting plants and geological formations, his pleasure in leading foreign geneticists on a tour through a Sapporo brewery, and his delight in serving seedless watermelons to his guests. Wherever we went he seemed to know everybody and to be instantly recognized. He was Mishima's leading citizen, a role that I think he enjoyed. One anecdote will serve. Impelled by curiosity as to how the Japanese did such things, I went to a large public gathering at which Miss Mishima was to be chosen. And who turned out to be the judge to select the most personable and comely young woman? KIHARA, of course.

I am happy to acknowledge the help of YURIKO KIHARA. She not only furnished pictures of her father but also made many helpful comments on the manuscript. I also thank NAOYUKI TAKAHATA and KOICHIRO TSUNEWAKI, who provided materials and, along with OLIVER NELSON and BOB FORSBERG, commented on earlier drafts. I should also like to offer belated thanks to WARREN WEAVER and the Rockefeller Foundation for supporting a summer's work with KIMURA at the National Institute of Genetics, headed by KIHARA, in 1957.

LITERATURE CITED

CROW, J. F., 1993   N. I. VAVILOV, martyr to genetic truth. Genetics **184:** 1–4.

KIHARA, H., 1971   *Trees in Hakone*. Hakone Arboretum. (In Japanese with color illustrations and an English summary.)

KIHARA, H., 1982   *Wheat Studies–Retrospect and Prospects*. Elsevier, New York. (This includes as appendices reprints of papers on handedness in plants, Japanese archery, seedless fruits, the history of biology in Japan, and a biographical note.)

KIHARA, H., 1985   *A Grain of Rice, an Album of Photographs*. Kihara Institute, Yokohama. (In Japanese.)

SEARS, E. R., 1987   Professor Hitoshi Kihara. Jpn. J. Genet. **62:** 3–4.

TSUNEWAKI, K., 1989   Hitoshi Kihara, pp. 209–224 in *American Philosophical Society Yearbook*. American Philosophical Society, Philadelphia.

September 1994

A Reconsideration of the Mechanism of Position Effect

Steven Henikoff

Howard Hughes Medical Institute, Fred Hutchinson Cancer Research Center, Seattle, Washington 98104

THE title of this article was chosen for two reasons. First, it is the title of a remarkable article published 50 years ago by BORIS EPHRUSSI and EILEEN SUTTON aimed at explaining a widely studied but enigmatic phenomenon (EPHRUSSI and SUTTON 1944). But in addition, by highlighting ideas presented in that article, I will be reconsidering the mechanism of position effect in light of recent work suggesting that EPHRUSSI and SUTTON's explanations were largely correct. Reconsideration includes resuscitation: while their article received attention in an early review on position effect (LEWIS 1950), it is barely mentioned in most reviews written since (BAKER 1968; SPOFFORD 1976; EISSENBERG 1989; TARTOF et al. 1989; SPRADLING and KARPEN 1990; GRIGLIATTI 1991; REUTER and SPIERER 1992).

Position effects on gene expression fall into two classes. Somatically stable position effects were originally seen as rare spontaneous occurrences, such as the *Bar* locus duplication (STURTEVANT 1925). With the advent of germline transformation, stable position effects on transgenes were found to be very common (WILSON et al. 1990). These examples of position effect have proven to be extremely valuable, both for generating "enhancer trap" lines where these position effects are used to detect genes of developmental interest (O'KANE and GEHRING 1987) and for identifying boundary elements that insulate against position effects (KELLUM and SCHEDL 1991). Stable position effects on transgenes can be understood in terms of the interaction between tissue-specific regulatory elements and promoters of position-affected genes.

In contrast to stable position effects, somatically unstable, or variegated, position effects associated with chromosomal rearrangements (MULLER 1930) have resisted explanation. Position-effect variegation (PEV) is observed as a random mixture of mutant and wild-type tissue that occurs for genes close to a newly created euchromatin-heterochromatin junction. In squashes of salivary gland polytene chromosomes, a position-affected gene typically appears to lie immediately adjacent to or within heterochromatin, the unbanded chromatin that comprises the chromocenter. PEV is a very common phenomenon, accounting for a large fraction of mutations in X-ray screens. In 1944, PEV was so familiar to geneticists that EPHRUSSI and SUTTON did not find it necessary to describe the phenomenon to readers.

EPHRUSSI and SUTTON were by no means the first to speculate on the basis for position effects. They discussed "kinetic" diffusion hypotheses for PEV put forward by others, which would encompass the more modern heterochromatin "spreading" model. By this spreading model, gene silencing occurs because the chromosomal proteins responsible for the condensed state of heterochromatin spread from the junction with euchromatin, leading to condensation and silencing of euchromatic genes. Kinetic diffusion hypotheses represent attempts to account for the polarity of silencing, which is seen as a stronger effect for genes closer to the junction than for genes farther away. Currently popular versions of this model suppose that there are elements in heterochromatin that promote spreading and elements in euchromatin that can terminate spreading (TARTOF et al. 1984; EISSENBERG 1989; GRIGLIATTI 1991). Because no such elements have been identified, this model remains speculative.

Another type of model supposes that the gene is absent from tissue in which no activity is seen (SCHULTZ 1936; PROCUNIER and TARTOF 1978; SPRADLING and KARPEN 1990). However, gene sequences are indeed present in affected tissues in several cases (HENIKOFF 1981; RUSHLOW et al. 1984; HAYASHI et al. 1990; UMBETOVA et al. 1991).

The Ephrussi-Sutton model was one they described as "structural." In a structural model, position effects are thought to result from altered gene conformation, not from altered movement of a substance along the chromosome as in kinetic models. EPHRUSSI and SUTTON supposed that conformational changes occur in PEV because normal somatic pairing is disrupted by rearrangement breakpoints (MULLER 1941). Somatic pairing is easily visualized in salivary gland polytene chromosomes: bands are present and homologs are paired because the individual chromatids are precisely aligned. Although nothing was known about DNA sequences in 1944, it was nevertheless possible to infer that there are forces that cause identical genes on polytene chromatids to come together precisely. A chromosomal rearrangement that causes a position effect on a gene would do so because the gene and its homolog are no longer correctly paired with each other, and this mispairing causes an alteration in the gene that interferes with its normal activity. This model assumes that somatic pairing forces also operate in interphase diploid cells, and recent cytological studies with molecular probes support this assumption (KOPCZYNSKI and MUSKAVITCH 1992; HIRAOKA *et al.* 1993).

EPHRUSSI and SUTTON first applied their structural model to account for position effects involving the *cubitus interruptus* (*ci*) gene. The *ci* mutation causes a gap to appear in the cubital vein of the wing. The length of the gap is a measure of the strength of the *ci* phenotype. Although the *ci* allele is recessive to ci^+, and so was thought to be a loss-of-function mutation, translocations that move either *ci* or ci^+ show the *ci* phenotype to a greater or lesser degree in heterozygotes (DUBININ and SIDOROV 1934; KHVOSTOVA 1939; STERN and HEIDENTHAL 1944). Heterozygosity is needed, because homozygous or hemizygous translocations involving ci^+ are wild type. This requirement for heterozygosity distinguishes *ci* position effect from PEV. According to the Ephrussi-Sutton model, separating the alleles, and not simply moving one allele to a new position, is responsible for the apparent reduction in dominance of ci^+ over *ci*. Thus, pairing disruptions can interfere with either the allele on the translocated chromosome or the allele on the normal homolog, or both.

Ten years after this model was published, LEWIS (1954) described a phenomenon he termed "trans-vection" (not always hyphenated) involving the *bithorax* locus. Trans-vection resembles *ci* position effect in that chromosomal rearrangements increase the mutant effect in heterozygotes. In trans-vection, however, the mutant effect is seen in particular heteroallelic mutant combinations, rather than between a wild-type and mutant allele. Although LEWIS has preferred a kinetic hypothesis (LEWIS 1985), more recent molecular studies favor a structural explanation for trans-vection similar to what EPHRUSSI and SUTTON proposed for *ci* position effect. Modern structural models for trans-vection are based on shared features of allele-specific *trans* interactions at different loci (ZACHAR *et al.* 1985; JUDD 1988; WU and GOLDBERG 1989). It is thought that in these cases, DNA-binding proteins can act across paired but not unpaired homologs.

The clearest example of heteroallelic complementation mediated by a DNA-binding protein comes from studies of mutations at the *yellow* (*y*) locus (GEYER *et al.* 1990). The y^2 mutation is associated with a *gypsy* transposon that blocks tissue-specific enhancers upstream of the transposon from interacting with the promoter downstream. When y^2 is paired with a deletion that removes the *y* promoter and coding region but not the enhancers, y^+ transcription is restored. This heteroallelic complementation appears to be mediated by a DNA-binding protein encoded by the *suppressor-of-Hairy-wing* [*su(Hw)*] locus, which binds to multiple sites in the *gypsy* transposon. This protein is thought to have special properties (yet unknown) that cause it to respond to the presence of enhancer elements on a paired homolog. Thus, in the paired heterozygote, su(Hw) protein would mediate activation of the intact structural gene in *cis* via the action of enhancer elements in *trans*. Unpairing would disturb the communication between su(Hw) protein and the enhancers in *trans*, causing an increased mutant effect. It seems likely that a similar interaction occurs at the *bithorax* locus because, like y^2, a *gypsy* element is present in the regulatory region of the affected allele with an intact structural gene (BENDER *et al.* 1983).

It is impressive that the Ephrussi-Sutton structural model successfully accounts for phenomena discovered years later. How successful was it in explaining *ci* position effect? An answer comes from a very recent molecular study of *ci* itself. An initial clue that *ci* might not be a simple loss-of-function allele was drawn from the observation that it is suppressed by mutations in the *su(Hw)* locus and therefore might be caused by insertion of a *gypsy* transposon (MODOLLEL *et al.* 1983). Molecular analysis of *ci* confirmed the presence of a *gypsy* transposon upstream of the ci^+ transcription unit, and, together with examination of other alleles at the locus, a structural model was proposed for *ci* position effect (LOCKE and TARTOF 1994). Earlier work had suggested that ci^+ expression is confined to the anterior compartment of embryonic segments and imaginal discs (ORENIC *et al.* 1990; EATON and KORNBERG 1990). Because the cubital vein is in the posterior compartment of the wing, the phenotype could be caused by misexpression of the *ci* gene in that compartment (LOCKE and TARTOF 1994). The *ci* phenotype would thus result from *gypsy*-mediated gene expression in the posterior compartment of the wing, not from loss of gene function. To explain why *ci* is recessive to ci^+, these authors postulated that posterior-specific silencer elements present at ci^+ repress transcription of the *ci* allele across paired homologs. One might suppose that the special properties of su(Hw) protein bound to the *gypsy* transposon present at *ci* mediate this interaction. In this way, *ci* position effect would be similar to y^2 complementation, except that the interaction is between su(Hw) protein and compartment-specific silencers rather than tissue-specific enhancers.

Pairing-dependent effects associated with *gypsy* elements belong to a growing class of phenomena thought to depend on direct interactions between homologs, termed "*trans*-sensing" effects (TARTOF and HENIKOFF 1991). Recent insight into some of these phenomena comes from the discovery that certain gene regulatory elements can mediate silencing of a reporter gene across homologs. When an enhancerless "mini-*white*" eye pigment gene was placed downstream of an *engrailed* gene regulatory element, paired, but not unpaired, copies of the chimeric transgene were repressed (KASSIS *et al.* 1991). A similar observation has been made for a regulatory element of the *polyhomeotic* gene (FAUVARQUE and DURA 1993). The basis for pairing-dependent repression is not clear, although as yet unknown features of regulatory proteins that bind to these elements are probably involved. The zeste protein, which mediates other *trans*-sensing effects (GANS 1953; GELBART and WU 1982), might serve as a paradigm. Zeste is a transcription factor that can form aggregates, a feature that correlates with pairing sensitivity of target *white* genes (BICKEL and PIRROTTA 1990).

While *trans*-sensing effects require the pairing of homologs, PEV can occur in the absence of a homolog, which is the case for genes on the male *X* chromosome. The Ephrussi-Sutton structural model was specifically intended to explain PEV, but its apparent failure to do so probably contributed to its subsequent obscurity. An example of this apparent failure is EPHRUSSI and SUTTON's explanation for the exceptional dominance of *brown* gene PEV alleles over wild-type *brown* (GLASS 1933). EPHRUSSI and SUTTON imagined that heterochromatic rearrangements leading to pairing disruptions should identically affect the homologous copies of *brown*, so that a position effect in *trans* should be just as strong as in *cis*. However, a test of this prediction revealed that the position effect on *brown* is typically stronger in *cis* than in *trans* (SLATIS 1955). This asymmetry can now be understood in light of recent work that leads to a modified structural model based on somatic pairing (DREESEN *et al.* 1991). Whereas the *cis* copy is inactivated by heterochromatin formation, the *trans* copy is thought to be affected via a transcription factor that is sensitive to contact with heterochromatin in the paired state. Thus, the exceptional dominance of *brown* gene PEV is now thought to be a pairing-dependent phenomenon mediated by a (hypothetical) DNA-binding protein with special properties, analogous to the situation for *trans*-sensing effects involving *gypsy* elements.

In addition to providing a basis for understanding *trans*-sensing effects, EPHRUSSI and SUTTON proposed a tentative explanation for the nature of heterochromatin. The precise banding and pairing seen for polytene chromosome euchromatin do not extend into the peri-centric heterochromatin. Rather, all of the heterochromatin from different chromosomes is coalesced into a single diffuse chromocenter, an example of heterologous pairing. Noting this, EPHRUSSI and SUTTON pointed out that "if the forces responsible for this pairing are operative between any two heterochromatic regions, they must act not only between regions in non-homologous chromosomes, but also between heterochromatic bands in the same chromosome." Thus, heterochromatin might differ from euchromatin by showing promiscuous pairing of non-homologous regions both within and between chromosomes. In modern terms, somatic pairing, which we now know occurs between identical sequences, would also occur between sequence repeats in tandem along the chromosome and shared between non-homologous chromosomes. By observing polytene chromosomes, EPHRUSSI and SUTTON inferred features of heterochromatin without knowing about DNA sequences, sequence repeat families, and their abundance in heterochromatin.

The possibility that somatic pairing underlies heterochromatin formation is supported by recent studies of PEV. Genes normally located in heterochromatin show PEV when moved to euchromatin. It has been proposed that some feature of repetitive sequences in heterochromatin provides a suitable nuclear environment for expression of heterochromatic genes (DEVLIN *et al.* 1990), and this environment is disrupted in rearrangements that move blocks of heterochromatin to distal locations (BAKER 1953; HESSLER 1958; WAKIMOTO and HEARN 1990; EBERL *et al.* 1993; TALBERT *et al.* 1994). Creation of a heterochromatic environment might involve pairing associations as envisioned by EPHRUSSI and SUTTON. Direct evidence is now available that repetitive sequences induce heterochromatin formation, possibly because these sequences can pair with one another (DORER and HENIKOFF 1994). Inverted duplications of a mini-*white*-bearing transgene induced by *P*-transposase were found to cause repression of the transgenes very similar to that observed for *engrailed*-mini-*white* homozygotes. This similarity in phenotype suggested that the adjacent copies were forming paired (hairpin) structures in *cis* similar to the *trans* paired structures hypothesized to be mediated by the *engrailed* and *polyhomeotic* regulatory elements. For paired copies in *cis*, association might be tighter than in *trans*, so that repression can occur without the involvement of special regulatory elements. More extreme silencing was found for transgene arrays of up to seven copies, an effect that strengthened with increasing transgene copy number. These multicopy arrays showed PEV phenotypes, confirmed by demonstration of sensitivity to PEV genetic modifiers. So it appears that heterochromatin capable of causing PEV can be synthesized *in vivo* simply by generating direct or inverted repeat arrays of a transposon entirely lacking sequences derived from natural heterochromatin. Similar observations have been made for the *brown* gene, in that repeat arrays show stronger PEV with increases in copy number (J. SABL, unpublished results). In both cases, more copies of the locally duplicated transposon caused a stronger mutant effect. Because the transposon copies appear to be interacting with one another, pairing of closely linked homologous sequences provides an attractive model. It thus appears that somatic pairing forces underlie heterochromatin formation and PEV as hypothesized by EPHRUSSI and SUTTON 50 years ago.

Repetitive DNA is by no means limited to the pericentric heterochromatin of Drosophila; rather, this is a general feature of higher eukaryotic chromosomes. Does somatic pairing of repeats drive heterochromatin formation in general? Somatic pairing can be difficult to observe cytologically outside of Dipterans (METZ 1916). For example, in humans, somatic pairing between homologs is not ordinarily seen (LEITCH *et al.* 1994). However, under special conditions (SCHMID *et al.* 1983) or in a particular cell type (ARNOLDUS *et al.* 1989), homologous associations are seen that involve pericentric heterochromatic regions of certain chromosomes. These loose associations between homologs might be a byproduct of the tight associations that cause heterochromatin to condense along the length of repeated segments. Hopefully, it will not require another 50 years to elucidate the molecular basis of somatic pairing and determine whether the Ephrussi-Sutton model accounts for a central feature of higher eukaryotic chromosomes.

LITERATURE CITED

ARNOLDUS, E. P. J., A. C. B. PERTERS, G. T. A. M. BOTS, A. K. RAAP and M. VAN DER PLOEG, 1989   Somatic pairing of chromosome 1 centromeres in interphase nuclei of human cerebellum. Hum. Genet. **83:** 231–234.

BAKER, W. K., 1953   V-type position effects of a gene in *Drosophila virilis* normally located in heterochromatin. Genetics **38:** 328–344.

BAKER, W. K., 1968   Position-effect variegation. Adv. Genet. **14:** 133–169.

BENDER, W., M. AKAM, F. KARCH, P. A. BEACHY, M. PEIFER *et al.*, 1983   Molecular genetics of the bithorax complex in *Drosophila melanogaster*. Science **221:** 23–29.

BICKEL, S., and V. PIRROTTA, 1990   Self-association of the *Drosophila zeste* protein is responsible for transvection effects. EMBO J. **9:** 2959–2967.

DEVLIN, R. H., B. BINGHAM and B. WAKIMOTO, 1990   The organization and expression of the *light* gene, a heterochromatic gene of *Drosophila melanogaster*. Genetics **125:** 129–140.

DORER, D. R., and S. HENIKOFF, 1994   Expansions of transgene repeats cause heterochromatin formation and gene silencing in Drosophila. Cell **77:** 993–1002.

DREESEN, T. D., S. HENIKOFF and K. LOUGHNEY, 1991   A pairing-sensitive element that mediates *trans*-inactivation is associated with the *Drosophila brown* gene. Genes Dev. **5:** 331–340.

DUBININ, N. P., and B. N. SIDOROV, 1934   Relation between a gene and its position in the system. Am. Nat. **68:** 377–381.

EATON, S., and T. B. KORNBERG, 1990   Repression of *ci-D* in posterior compartments of *Drosophila* by *engrailed*. Genes Dev. **4:** 1068–1077.

EBERL, D. F., B. J. DUYF and A. J. HILLIKER, 1993   The role of heterochromatin in the expression of a heterochromatic gene, the *rolled* locus of *Drosophila melanogaster*. Genetics **134:** 277–292.

EISSENBERG, J. C., 1989   Position effect variegation in *Drosophila*: towards a genetics of chromatin assembly. Bioessays **11:** 14–17.

EPHRUSSI, B., and E. SUTTON, 1944   A reconsideration of the mechanism of position effect. Proc. Natl. Acad. Sci. USA **30:** 183–197.

FAUVARQUE, M.-O., and J.-M. DURA, 1993   *polyhomeotic* regulatory sequences induce developmental regulator-dependent variegation and targeted *P*-element insertions in *Drosophila*. Genes Dev. **7:** 1508–1520.

GANS, M., 1953   Étude génétique et physiologique du mutant z de *Drosophila melanogaster*. Bull. Biol. Fr. Belg. Suppl. **38:** 1–90.

GELBART, W. M., and C.-T. WU, 1982   Interactions of zeste mutations with loci exhibiting transvection effects in *Drosophila melanogaster*. Genetics **102:** 179–189.

GEYER, P. K., M. M. GREEN and V. G. CORCES, 1990   Tissue-specific transcriptional enhancers may act in *trans* on the gene located in the homologous chromosome: the molecular basis of transvection in *Drosophila*. EMBO J. **9:** 2247–2256.

GLASS, H. B., 1933   A study of dominant mosaic eye color mutants in *Drosophila melanogaster*. II. Tests involving crossing-over and non-disjunction. J. Genet. **28:** 69–112.

GRIGLIATTI, T., 1991   Position-effect variegation. An assay for nonhistone chromosomal proteins and chromatin assembly and modifying factors, pp. 587–627 in *Functional Organization of the Nucleus: A Laboratory Guide*, edited by B. A. HAMKALO and S. C. R. ELGIN. Academic Press, San Diego.

HAYASHI, S., A. RUDDELL, D. SINCLAIR and T. GRIGLIATTI, 1990   Chromosomal structure is altered by mutations that suppress or enhance position effect variegation. Chromosoma **99:** 391–400.

HENIKOFF, S., 1981   Position-effect variegation and chromosome structure of a heat shock puff in *Drosophila*. Chromosoma **83:** 381–393.

HESSLER, A., 1958   V-type position effects at the light locus in *Drosophila melanogaster*. Genetics **43:** 395–403.

HIRAOKA, Y., A. S. DERNBURG, S. J. PARMELEE, M. C. RYKOWSKI, D. A. AGARD *et al.*, 1993   The onset of homologous chromosome pairing during *Drosophila melanogaster* embryogenesis. J. Cell Biol. **120:** 591–600.

JUDD, B. H., 1988   Transvection: allelic cross talk. Cell **53:** 841–843.

KASSIS, J. A., E. P. VANSICKLE and S. M. SENSABAUGH, 1991   A fragment of *engrailed* regulatory DNA can mediate transvection of the *white* gene in Drosophila. Genetics **128:** 751–761.

KELLUM, R., and P. SCHEDL, 1991   A position-effect assay for boundaries of higher order chromosomal domains. Cell **64:** 941–950.

KHVOSTOVA, V. V., 1939   The role played by the inert chromosome regions in the position effect of the cubitus interruptus gene in *Drosophila melanogaster*. Izv. Akad. Nauk SSSR Otd. Ser. Biol. **4:** 541–574.

KOPCZYNSKI, C. C., and M. A. T. MUSKAVITCH, 1992   Introns excised from the *Delta* primary transcript are localized near sites of *Delta* transcription. J. Cell Biol. **119:** 503–512.

LEITCH, A. R., J. K. M. BROWN, W. MOSGOLLER, T. SCHWARZACHER and J. S. HESLOP-HARRISON, 1994   The spatial localization of homologous chromosomes in human fibroblasts at mitosis. Hum. Genet. **93:** 275–280.

LEWIS, E. B., 1950   The phenomenon of position effect. Adv. Genet. **3:** 73–115.

LEWIS, E. B., 1954   The theory and application of a new method of detecting chromosomal rearrangements in *Drosophila melanogaster*. Am. Nat. **88:** 225–239.

LEWIS, E. B., 1985   Regulation of genes of the bithorax complex in *Drosophila*. Cold Spring Harbor Symp. Quant. Biol. **50:** 155–164.

LOCKE, J., and K. D. TARTOF, 1994   Molecular analysis of *cubitus interruptus* (*ci*) mutations suggests an explanation for the unusual *ci* position effects. Mol. Gen. Genet. **243:** 234–243.

METZ, C. W., 1916   Chromosome studies on the Diptera. II. The paired association of chromosomes in the diptera, and its significance. J. Exp. Zool. **21:** 213–280.

MODOLLEL, J., W. BENDER and M. MESELSON, 1983   *Drosophila melanogaster* mutations suppressible by the suppressor of Hairy-wing are insertions of a 7.3-kilobase mobile element. Proc. Natl. Acad. Sci. USA **80:** 1678–1682.

MULLER, H. J., 1930   Types of visible variations induced by X-rays in *Drosophila*. J. Genet. **22:** 299–334.

MULLER, H. J., 1941   Induced mutations in Drosophila. Cold Spring Harbor Symp. Quant. Biol. **9:** 151–165.

O'KANE, C., and W. J. GEHRING, 1987   Detection *in situ* of genomic regulatory elements in *Drosophila*. Proc. Natl. Acad. Sci. USA **84:** 9123–9127.

ORENIC, T. V., D. C. SLUSARKSI, K. L. KROLL and R. A. HOLMGREN, 1990 Cloning and characterization of the segment polarity gene *cubitus interruptus Dominant* of Drosophila. Genes Dev. **4:** 1053–1067.

PROCUNIER, J. D., and K. D. TARTOF, 1978 A genetic locus having *trans* and *contiguous cis* functions that control the disproportional replication of ribosomal RNA genes in *Drosophila melanogaster.* Genetics **88:** 67–79.

REUTER, G., and P. SPIERER, 1992 Position effect variegation and chromatin proteins. Bioessays **14:** 605–612.

RUSHLOW, C. A., W. BENDER and A. CHOVNICK, 1984 Studies on the mechanism of heterochromatic position effect at the *rosy* locus of *Drosophila melanogaster.* Genetics **108:** 603–615.

SCHMID, M., D. GRUNERT, T. HAAF and W. ENGEL, 1983 A direct demonstration of somatically paired heterochromatin of human chromosomes. Cytogenet. Cell Genet. **36:** 554–561.

SCHULTZ, J., 1936 Variegation in Drosophila and the inert heterochromatic regions. Proc. Natl. Acad. Sci. USA **22:** 27–33.

SLATIS, H. M., 1955 Position effects at the brown locus in *Drosophila melanogaster.* Genetics **40:** 5–23.

SPOFFORD, J. B., 1976 Position-effect variegation in *Drosophila,* pp. 955–1019 in *Genetics and Biology of Drosophila,* edited by M. ASHBURNER and E. NOVITSKI. Academic Press, London.

SPRADLING, A. C., and G. H. KARPEN, 1990 Sixty years of mystery. Genetics **126:** 779–784.

STERN, C., and G. HEIDENTHAL, 1944 Materials for the study of the position effect of normal and mutant genes. Proc. Natl. Acad. Sci. USA **30:** 197–205.

STURTEVANT, A. H., 1925 The effects of unequal crossing over at the Bar locus in Drosophila. Genetics **10:** 117–147.

TALBERT, P. B., C. D. S. LECIEL and S. HENIKOFF, 1994 Modification of the Drosophila heterochromatic mutation *brown^{Dominant}* by linkage alterations. Genetics **136:** 559–571.

TARTOF, K. D., and S. HENIKOFF, 1991 Trans-sensing effects from Drosophila to humans. Cell **65:** 201–203.

TARTOF, K. D., C. HOBBS and M. JONES, 1984 A structural basis for variegating position effects. Cell **37:** 869–878.

TARTOF, K. D., C. BISHOP, M. JONES, C. A. HOBBS and J. LOCKE, 1989 Towards an understanding of position effect variegation. Dev. Genet. **10:** 162–176.

UMBETOVA, G. H., E. S. BELYAEVA, E. M. BARICHEVA and I. F. ZHIMULEV, 1991 Cytogenetic and molecular aspects of position effect variegation in *Drosophila melanogaster.* IV. Underreplication of chromosomal material as a result of gene inactivation. Chromosoma **101:** 55–61.

WAKIMOTO, B., and M. HEARN, 1990 The effects of chromosome rearrangements on the expression of heterochromatic genes in chromosome *2L* of *Drosophila melanogaster.* Genetics **125:** 141–151.

WILSON, C., H. G. BELLEN and W. J. GEHRING, 1990 Position effects on eukaryotic gene expression. Annu. Rev. Cell Biol. **6:** 679–714.

WU, C.-T., and M. L. GOLDBERG, 1989 The *Drosophila zeste* gene and transvection. Trends Genet. **5:** 189–194.

ZACHAR, Z., C. H. CHAPMAN and P. M. BINGHAM, 1985 On the molecular basis of transvection effects and the regulation of transcription. Cold Spring Harbor Symp. Quant. Biol. **50:** 337–346.

See also page 703 in Addenda et Corrigenda.

October 1994

The Holliday Junction on Its Thirtieth Anniversary

Franklin W. Stahl

Institute of Molecular Biology, University of Oregon, Eugene, Oregon 97403–1229

IN the 1940s and 50s, the apparent lack of reciprocality in the production of bacteriophage recombinants led to the ascendancy of copy-choice schemes for recombination in those little creatures (STURTEVANT, cited in HERSHEY and ROTMAN 1949). The subsequent description of gene conversion (non-4:4 meiotic segregation) in Neurospora (MITCHELL 1955a,b) was viewed by some as an illustration of the applicability of such schemes to meiotic exchange (*e.g.*, FREESE 1957).

However, to ROBIN HOLLIDAY, copy-choice was not a decent explanation for meiotic conversion. He found the potential for a different explanation in the embryonic field of DNA repair. The trick was to make recombination involve a heteroduplex, in which a marked segment of one chain carries information from one chromosome while the corresponding segment of the other chain carries information from its homolog. [The word "strand" is used by classical geneticists to denote a chromosome or a chromatid. It is used by those lacking a classical education to refer to a polynucleotide chain as defined by WATSON and CRICK (1953). We'll avoid confusion by not using it at all.] Such locally heteroduplex products of recombination had been hypothesized to account for heterozygous particles of phage T4 (LEVINTHAL 1954). Then, enzymes analogous to enzymes proposed to repair UV damage could recognize violations of Watson-Crick pairing at the marked site and operate on the heteroduplex, removing a bit from one chain or the other. Deviations from 4:4 segregation would (or, at least, could) result. Failure of the hypothetical mismatch correction enzymes to operate on a given heteroduplex site would result in meiotic products that would segregate alleles in the first post-meiotic mitosis. The demonstrated occurrence in some fungi of such post-meiotic segregations (PMS) fully justified the assumption of heteroduplexes in meiotic recombination.

In fungi, about half of the tetrads manifesting either deviations from a 4:4 ratio (conversion) or 4:4 tetrads with PMS at a given site in two of the four haploid products are reciprocally recombined for markers flanking that site (they are usually tetratype for those markers). The crossover typically involves the chromatid that is converted or the two chromatids that are enjoying PMS. The remaining tetrads are parental type (*i.e.*, nonrecombinant ditype). The apparent equality of these two types (the precision of which was later shown to be bogus) provoked the notion of a structurally symmetric four-chained intermediate that could be resolved to give crossover or noncrossover chromatids with equal probability. The structure proposed by HOLLIDAY (1964) fit the bill in all essential respects. It was, as HOTCHKISS (1974) exclaimed, "... the only sophisticated way in which two homologous DNAs can become covalently joined."

Wed to the classical notion that crossing over is a reciprocal process, HOLLIDAY envisioned processes for forming and for resolving the Holliday junction intermediate that were symmetric at each step. Thus, he proposed that chains of the same polarity were simultaneously cut on homologous chromatids at the same site (Figure 1). Each cut chain was then unwound on one side of the cut and rewound on the complementary chain vacated by the other. The four-chained structure (the Holliday junction), which could be modeled in a tidy way (SIGAL and ALBERTS 1972), was resolved either by cutting the pair of chains that were swapped (to give chromatids that were parental for flanking DNA) or by cutting the other two chains (giving chromatids that were recombinant for flanking DNA). The structural symmetry that could underlie equality for these two modes of resolution was specified by SOBELL (1974), who noted that the swapped and unswapped chains could exchange positions by isomerization of the structure through the open, four-way junction intermediate visualized in phage T4 by BROKER and LEHMAN (1971).

HOLLIDAY's model had attractive features beyond those specifically identified by him. (i) The two-step feature of the model was nice. First, the Watson chains (say) could be cut. They could then engage their partners' Crick chains to verify that the cut sites on the two participants were truly homologous. If they were, permanent partner swapping could be effected. If they were not, each could retreat to its old partner with no harm

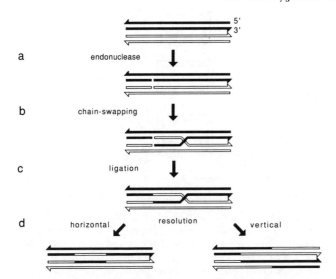

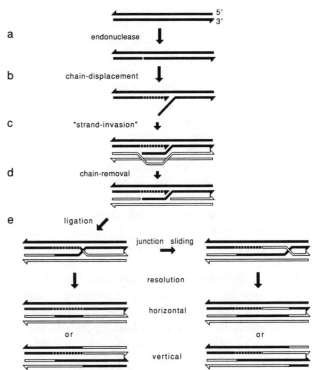

FIGURE 1.—The Holliday model. (a) Paired homologs are cut at the same level on corresponding chains. (b) The cut chains swap pairing partners. (c) Nicks are ligated, completing the formation of a Holliday junction. (d) The four-chained intermediate is resolved either by cutting the two swapped chains ("horizontal") or by cutting the two originally unswapped chains ("vertical"). Products are ligated. Horizontal resolution produces a pair of duplexes that are parental except for the short region in which they have swapped single chains (patches). The patches will be heteroduplex if the two parents differed in the patched region. Vertical resolution produces a pair of crossover duplexes that are spliced together. The splice will be heteroduplex if the two parents differed in the spliced region. Conversion can result from mismatch correction operating on heteroduplex patches or splices.

FIGURE 2.—The Meselson-Radding model. (a) A duplex is cut on one chain. (b) DNA polymerase operates in the chain-displacement mode. (c) The resulting single chain invades the homolog, displacing its counterpart. (d) This displaced chain is enzymatically digested. (e) Ligation completes the formation of a Holliday junction, which is genetically asymmetric in that only one of the two duplexes has a region of potentially heteroduplex DNA. If the junction slides, heteroduplex DNA can arise on both duplexes. (f) Resolution of the junction occurs as in the Holliday model.

done. (This feature of the model might not have struck ROBIN as very relevant. He had apparently envisioned a prerecombinational pairing of homologs that was sufficient to avoid such embarrassments.) (ii) The requirement that the initiating cuts be precisely isolocal could be relaxed. Once chain swapping had been effected, appropriate enzymes could trim or fill as necessary. (However, such trimming and filling could be a source of gene conversion, and ROBIN was conspicuously reluctant to allow for any conversion mechanisms other than mismatch correction. In fact, his adherence to that perspective often led him to equate the words "correction" and "conversion.")

Like any truly fine model, ROBIN's was testable. The structural symmetry in each of the steps and in the intermediate predicted symmetric consequences. In his model, heteroduplex DNA on one chromatid is invariably accompanied by heteroduplex on the other. Evidence of this symmetry might be lost through mismatch correction, but shadows of the initial symmetry would be likely to remain in the resulting types of tetrads. Data from some fungi supported the model. However, as data on yeast tetrads were released (mostly from the laboratories of SY FOGEL, BOB MORTIMER and PHIL HASTINGS), it became apparent that HOLLIDAY's model was too symmetric to deal with data of *Saccharomyces cerevisiae*, in

which little or no evidence of reciprocal heteroduplex could be found (but see ALANI *et al.* 1994).

Rather than abandoning the possibility of a universal recombination mechanism, MATT MESELSON and CHARLEY RADDING (1975) altered ROBIN's model to give it the flexibility required to handle data both from yeast and from fungi that did show appreciable reciprocality in heteroduplex formation (Figure 2). In their model, a recombinogenic single chain was displaced from a chromatid by the action of polymerase operating in the chain-displacement mode. This chain invaded the homolog (exploiting the supercoiled nature of the latter and/or using the as yet to be discovered "strand-invasion" activity of RecA protein), displacing the resident chain of like polarity. Nuclease activity was postulated to remove this displaced chain, and a genetically asymmetric but structurally symmetric Holliday junction resulted. A marker in this region would show half conversion (segregate 5:3) if it were not mismatch-corrected. Diffusion-driven or enzyme-driven sliding of the junction away from the point of initiation would result in segments of reciprocal (symmetric) heteroduplex DNA. (In 1974, HOLLIDAY grafted sliding junctions onto his own model.) By appropriate adjustment of the relative durations of the initial asymmetric phase and the subsequent symmetric phase, a wide range of fungal data could be embraced by the model. For yeast, the paucity of evidence for symmetric heteroduplex DNA was simply accounted for by supposing that the symmetric phase was vanishingly short relative to the asymmetric one. The relative shortage of 5:3 tetrads in yeast was accounted for by supposing that correction enzymes in yeast were more active than they are in other fungi.

Just as ROBIN's model had dominated the recombination field for a decade, CHARLEY and MATT's model ruled for the next decade. It is, of course, a mark of the importance of the Holliday model that it was replaced by evolution rather than by revolution, and both of HOLLIDAY's innovations, the junction and mismatch correction of heteroduplex DNA, retained central roles in the new model.

However, the Meselson-Radding model, in its turn, ran into troubles. Some of these troubles are easy to appreciate and will serve to introduce the next generation of models. In the Meselson-Radding model, in contrast to that of HOLLIDAY, one participating chromatid is identifiable as the aggressor and the other as the responder. [Asymmetry in the early steps of recombination had been postulated earlier by HOTCHKISS (1973), among others.] The mechanism proposed for recombination initiation, DNA synthesis in the chain displacement mode, results in a net gain of one (simplex) copy of information from the initiating chromatid with the loss of one simplex copy from the responder. This results in an incipient 5:3 tetrad, which can be mismatch-corrected to give a full conversion tetrad (6:2) or to restore the Mendelian ratio of 4:4.

In the Meselson-Radding model, the aggressor chromosome blows information into the responding chromosome. Studies on recombination-promoting sites in *Schizosaccharomyces pombe* (GUTZ 1971) and Neurospora (CATCHESIDE and ANGEL 1974) correctly foretold the behavior of all subsequently discovered "recombinator" sites by showing that, rather than blowing, these genetic elements suck information from the responding chromosome. This troubles the Meselson-Radding model. [RADDING (1982) later modified the model to fit this new fact.] A second finding troubling the Meselson-Radding model was the evidence from yeast that, when incipient 5:3 tetrads were acted upon by presumptive mismatch-correction enzymes, they were (almost) always converted to 6:2 tetrads. Somehow, within the framework of the model, the correction enzymes could identify the invading chain and effect correction in its favor (giving 6:2) rather than in favor of the invaded chromatid (restoring 4:4). That made some of us wonder whether correction really played a role in yeast conversion. If the symmetric phase is vanishingly short, and if correction is hyperactive, evidence for correction of a heteroduplex intermediate vanishes. Might not one

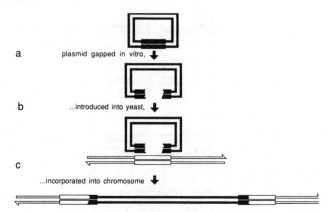

FIGURE 3.—Repair of a gapped plasmid (ORR-WEAVER *et al.* 1981). (a) A plasmid carrying a segment of yeast DNA was gapped within the yeast DNA by a restriction enzyme cut at the site of a deletion. (b) The gapped (linearized) plasmid was introduced into yeast cells, which were then plated under conditions that select for a different gene carried by the plasmid. (c) Since the plasmid could not replicate in yeast, all the selected transformants were a result of incorporation of the plasmid into the chromosome by homologous recombination between the gapped segment of yeast DNA and its undeleted wild-type homolog in the yeast chromosome. Plasmid incorporation was accompanied by repair of the gap, so that the plasmid was found flanked by two full, wild-type copies of the DNA segment.

chromatid simply donate two chains' worth of information directly to the other? One class of models based on this concept (STAHL 1969, 1979) was given little respect. Another, however, started a revolution.

In 1981, ORR-WEAVER *et al.* confirmed the observation of HICKS *et al.* (1979) that a double-chained break in a fragment of yeast DNA carried by a plasmid stimulated crossing over that incorporated the plasmid into the chromosome. The incorporated plasmid was flanked by a duplication of the region corresponding to the yeast fragment carried by the plasmid. These demonstrations of the recombinogenicity of a double-chained break confirmed, in an especially dramatic way, a conclusion reached earlier by RESNICK and MARTIN (1976) on the basis of X-ray stimulation of recombination in yeast. Especially significant in the revolution was the demonstration (ORR-WEAVER *et al.* 1981) that a sizable double-chained gap engineered into the region of homology stimulated incorporation of the plasmid into the chromosome and that both copies of the duplicated region were complete in the final product (Figure 3). This repair of a double-chained gap is equivalent to full conversion without mismatch correction—the information for repairing each of the chains is derived directly from the intact homolog. Furthermore, the aggressor element (the gapped plasmid) sucks information from the responding element (the intact host chromosome). This demonstration was just what seemed to be needed for meiotic recombination in yeast: full conversion without correction and aggressor chromosomes that sucked. The double-chain-break/gap-repair model for yeast

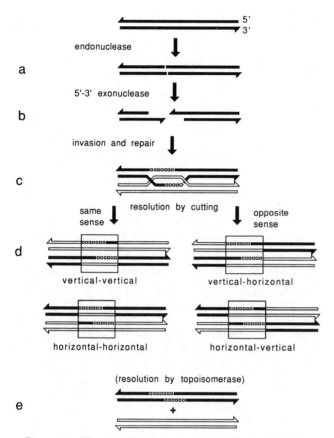

FIGURE 4.—The double-chain-break repair model. (a) A chromatid (or duplex) is cut on both chains, at an enzyme-accessible recombinator site. (b) Exonucleolytic digestion in the 5' to 3' direction exposes 3' overhangs. These overhangs may sometimes be digested, too. (c) The 3' ends invade the intact homolog. In yeast, sequence differences between the two participants may provoke further digestion of the 3' overhangs. The 3' ends prime DNA synthesis that replaces the DNA lost from the aggressor duplex. Ligation completes a four-chained intermediate in which duplexes are held together by a pair of Holliday junctions. (d) The junctions can be resolved either vertically or horizontally. When each is resolved in the same sense, no crossover results, but markers near the recombinator site will manifest either half or full conversion. When the junctions are resolved in the opposite sense, crossing over results, and the tetrad will again manifest conversion for markers near the recombinator site. The squares indicate the region between the two resolved junctions. In contrast to intermediates with one Holliday junction, the double Holliday junction structure of this model may be resolved without crossing over by the action of topoisomerase (THALER *et al.* 1987). This route is attractive for its unique ability to yield one pristine product.

soon followed and was published (SZOSTAK *et al.* 1983) after ORR-WEAVER and SZOSTAK (1983) confirmed an important prediction of the model, that about half the instances of plasmid repair occurred without incorporation of the plasmid into the chromosome. Thus, conversion by double-chain-gap repair modeled meiotic conversion in yeast in every important respect.

The double-chain-break/gap-repair model, too, made use of Holliday junctions (Figure 4). In this respect, it differed from the double-chain-break model offered earlier by RESNICK (1976). (Models without Holliday junctions have rarely made it to first base.)

Thus, HOLLIDAY's junction survived the revolution, embodied in a model that rejected most of the features of his model for recombination. (i) Initiation was no longer symmetric. (ii) Both chains of a duplex, rather than one chain, were cut to initiate recombination. (iii) Heteroduplex DNA was relegated to a minor role, and conversion occurred without a requirement for mismatch correction. This perspective put Saccharomyces outside the fungal pale, within which the Meselson-Radding model was doing very well (*e.g.*, HAMZA *et al.* 1981). Subsequent developments, described below, drew yeast and other fungi onto common ground.

The importance of double-chain breaks in the initiation of meiotic recombination in yeast was confirmed by the demonstration that meiotic initiators of recombination, whose presence was inferred by the gradients of gene conversion emanating from them, were sites for spontaneous meiosis-specific double-chain breaks (SUN *et al.* 1989; NICOLAS *et al.* 1989). Deletion of these break sites eliminated both the breaks and the high rates of recombination in their vicinity. Double-chain breaks were shown to be effective stimulators of recombination in *Escherichia coli* and phage, as well. However, the double-chain-gap repair version of the model was soon challenged. WILLIAMSON *et al.* (1985) isolated mutant yeasts in which aberrant 5:3's, normally rare for most markers in yeast, were as common as 6:2 tetrads. BISHOP *et al.* (1987) showed that these strains were deficient in mismatch-correction activity. The implication was clear—many of the 6:2 tetrads seen in wild-type yeast are the result of mismatch rectification of incipient 5:3 tetrads. Thus, in many instances, the initiating double-chain break (Figure 4) is not appreciably enlarged to a gap, so that much conversion is the result of heteroduplex DNA formation followed by correction. However, even the repair-deficient strains give appreciable numbers of 6:2 tetrads, and some of these may represent tetrads in which double-chain breaks were enlarged to double-chain gaps prior to interaction with the homolog.

If, as argued above, much conversion in yeast is the result of mismatch correction, how can we account for the apparent shortage of restorations, tetrads in which the heteroduplex is rectified so as to restore the 4:4 ratio of alleles? The very structure of the intermediate postulated in Figure 4 suggests the answer, which experiments by HABER *et al.* (1993) support. In the intermediate, the invading chains from the cut duplex are discontinuous for a time. Like the new, discontinuous chains at a replication fork, they could be recognized as targets for correction not by enzymes that replace a bit of mispaired chain but by the post-replicational repair system, which removes hundreds of bases from a growing chain. Thus, if the correction enzymes acted concurrently with intermediate formation, the invading chain might be removed from its tip to beyond the mismatch. The break would thus be enlarged to a gap, and the genetic consequences of conversion by such mismatch correction would be difficult to distinguish from the predictions of the original double-chain-gap repair model of SZOSTAK et al. (1983).

Work by SCHWACHA and KLECKNER (1994) supports the notion of the four-chained intermediate flanked by Holliday junctions that was proposed by SZOSTAK et al. (1983). The former investigators isolated and examined a four-chained structure that arises at a prominent double-chain-break hot spot in yeast. The four single chains in each intermediate are parental for markers flanking the hot spot at some remove (SCHWACHA and KLECKNER 1994). Some of these same chains, however, are recombinant with respect to each of these flanking markers and to a marker located close to the break site, consistent with conversion accompanying repair of the double-chain break. Furthermore, exposure of the four-chained structures in vitro to a Holliday junction resolvase from E. coli converts them to an essentially equal mixture of duplexes (presumably nicked) that are parental and recombinant respectively for the flanking markers (A. SCHWACHA and N. KLECKNER, personal communication).

Note that the double-chain-break repair model (Figure 4) retains not only the Holliday structure but central features of the Meselson-Radding model, as well. (i) Thanks to the 3′ overhangs created at the break site (SUN et al. 1989, 1991), there is a region of asymmetric heteroduplex DNA (on each side of the break). (ii) Once a Holliday junction is formed, it may slide outwards, forming a region of symmetric heteroduplex DNA.

HOLLIDAY's junction has been a cornerstone of recombination models since its introduction. Consequently, it has been a focus for biochemical investigations, as well. The ability of junctions to slide, postulated by MESELSON (1972) and assumed in the Meselson-Radding model, was confirmed by in vitro studies on isolated structures (THOMPSON et al. 1976). Subsequent studies revealed enzymes in bacteria that promote such sliding (IWASAKI et al. 1992; WHITBY et al. 1993).

Enzymes capable of resolving Holliday junctions in vitro were sought and found in phage T4 (MIZUUCHI et al. 1982), in E. coli (DUNDERDALE et al. 1991; IWASAKI et al. 1991), and elsewhere. Mutants lacking these enzymes are frequently recombination deficient.

MAX DELBRÜCK presented HOLLIDAY's recombination model at a meeting at Lake Arrowhead. MAX liked much of the model but objected that mismatch correction, if it operated by removing a mispaired bit of chain, would prevent the construction of intragenic linkage maps. MAX scorned a suggestion that the relevant correction enzymes might remove stretches of DNA of appreciable and variable length, preserving intragenic mapability. [HOLLIDAY (1964) dealt with mapability by proposing

marker-dependent pairing problems.] MAX dictated against the invention of an enzyme just because genetic phenomenology called for it. He was wrong again–a major mismatch-correction system does remove long, variable stretches of DNA. My goodness, even the oocyte of the African clawed toad has such a system (LEHMAN et al. 1994). Furthermore, the history of recombination studies is replete with the discovery of enzymes that were previously posited just to make the models work.

So, just which ideas from HOLLIDAY's (1964) model are retained in the reigning double-chain-break/gap model? (i) The junction is there (except now there are two of them). (ii) Mismatch correction of heteroduplex DNA contributes to conversion (except that now there is an additional contribution to the conversion process in terms of mismatch-independent generation of 3′ overhangs and the subsequent replacement of the DNA lost in that reaction, and, perhaps, DNA from both chains may sometimes be lost independently of any mismatches, so that the entire conversion occurs without mismatch correction). That's an impressive record, really. ROBIN's model was the lightning rod for 30 years of research, and its central assumptions, though modified, have survived every strike. Congratulations, ROBIN!

CHARLES RADDING and members of my laboratory graciously offered suggestions for improvement of this essay.

LITERATURE CITED

ALANI, E., R. A. G. REENAN and R. D. KOLODNER, 1994 Interactions between mismatch repair and genetic recombination in Saccharomyces cerevisiae. Genetics 137: 19–39.

BISHOP, D. K., M. S. WILLIAMSON, S. FOGEL and R. D. KOLODNER, 1987 The role of heteroduplex correction in gene conversion in Saccharomyces cerevisiae. Nature 328: 362–364.

BROKER, T. R., and I. R. LEHMAN, 1971 Branched DNA molecules: intermediates in T4 recombination. J. Mol. Biol. 60: 131–149.

CATCHESIDE, D. G., and T. ANGEL, 1974 A histidine-3 mutant, in Neurospora crassa, due to an interchange. Aust. J. Biol. Sci. 27: 219–229.

DUNDERDALE, H. J., F. E. BENSON, C. A. PARSONS, G. J. SHARPLES, R. G. LLOYD et al., 1991 Formation and resolution of recombination intermediates by E. coli RecA and RuvC proteins. Nature 354: 506–510.

FREESE, E., 1957 The correlation effect for the histidine locus of Neurospora crassa. Genetics 42: 671–684.

GUTZ, M., 1971 Site specific induction of recombination in Schizosaccharomyces pombe. Genetics 69: 317–337.

HABER, J. E., B. L. RAY, J. M. KOLB and C. I. WHITE, 1993 Rapid kinetics of mismatch repair of heteroduplex DNA that is formed during recombination in yeast. Proc. Natl. Acad. Sci. USA 90: 3363–3367.

HAMZA, H., J. HAEDENS, A. MEKKI-BERRANDA and J.-L. ROSSIGNOL, 1981 Hybrid DNA formation during meiotic recombination. Proc. Natl. Acad. Sci. USA 78: 7648–7651.

HERSHEY, A. D., and R. ROTMAN, 1949 Genetic recombination between host-range and plaque-type mutants of bacteriophage in single bacterial cells. Genetics 34: 44–71.

HICKS, J. B., A. HINNEN and G. R. FINK, 1979 Properties of yeast transformation. Cold Spring Harbor Symp. Quant. Biol. 43: 1305–1313.

HOLLIDAY, R., 1964 A mechanism for gene conversion in fungi. Genet. Res. 5: 282–304.

HOLLIDAY, R., 1974 Molecular aspects of genetic exchange and gene conversion. Genetics 78: 273–287.

HOTCHKISS, R. D., 1973 Genetic unity and biochemical diversity in genetic recombination mechanisms. Stadler Genet. Symp. **5:** 145–160.

HOTCHKISS, R. D., 1974 The evolution of recombination models, pp. 439–443 in *Mechanisms in Recombination*, edited by R. F. GRELL. Plenum, New York.

IWASAKI, H., M. TAKAHAGI, T. SHIBA, A. NAKATA and H. SHINAGAWA, 1991 *Escherichia coli* RuvC protein is an endonuclease that resolves the Holliday structure. EMBO J. **10:** 4381–4389.

IWASAKI, H., M. TAKAHAGI, A. NAKATA and H. SHINAGAWA, 1992 *Escherichia coli* RuvA and RuvB proteins specifically interact with Holliday junctions and promote branch migration. Genes Dev. **6:** 2214–2220.

LEHMAN, C. W., S. JEONG-YU, J. K. TRAUTMAN and D. CARROLL, 1994 Repair of heteroduplex DNA in *Xenopus laevis* oocytes. Genetics **138:** 459–470.

LEVINTHAL, C., 1954 Recombination in phage T2: its relationship to heterozygosis and growth. Genetics **39:** 169–184.

MESELSON, M., 1972 Formation of hybrid DNA by rotary diffusion during genetic recombination. J. Mol. Biol. **71:** 795–798.

MESELSON, M. S., and C. M. RADDING, 1975 A general model for genetic recombination. Proc. Natl. Acad. Sci. USA **72:** 358–361.

MITCHELL, M. B., 1955a Aberrant recombination of pyridoxine mutants of Neurospora. Proc. Natl. Acad. Sci. USA **41:** 215–220.

MITCHELL, M. B., 1955b Further evidence of aberrant recombination in Neurospora. Proc. Natl. Acad. Sci. USA **41:** 935–937.

MIZUUCHI, K., B. KEMPER, J. HAYS and R. A. WEISBERG, 1982 T4 endonuclease VII cleaves Holliday structures. Cell **29:** 357–365.

NICOLAS, A., D. TRECO, N. P. SCHULTES and J. W. SZOSTAK, 1989 An initiation site for meiotic gene conversion in the yeast *Saccharomyces cerevisiae*. Nature **338:** 35–39.

ORR-WEAVER T. L., and J. W. SZOSTAK, 1983 Yeast recombination: the association between double strand gap repair and crossing over. Proc. Natl. Acad. Sci. USA **80:** 4417–4421.

ORR-WEAVER, T. L., J. W. SZOSTAK and R. J. ROTHSTEIN, 1981 Yeast transformation: a model system for the study of recombination. Proc. Natl. Acad. Sci. USA **78:** 6354–6358.

RADDING, C. M., 1982 Homologous pairing and strand exchange in genetic recombination. Annu. Rev. Genet. **16:** 405–437.

RESNICK, M. A., 1976 The repair of double-strand breaks in DNA: a model involving recombination. J. Theor. Biol. **59:** 97–106.

RESNICK, M. A., and P. MARTIN, 1976 The repair of double strand

breaks in the nuclear DNA of *Saccharomyces cerevisiae* and its genetic control. Mol. Gen. Genet. **143:** 119–129.

SCHWACHA, A., and N. KLECKNER, 1994 Identification of joint molecules that form frequently between homologs but rarely between sister chromatids during yeast meiosis. Cell **76:** 51–63.

SIGAL N. and B. ALBERTS, 1972 Genetic recombination: the nature of the crossed strand exchange between two homologous DNA molecules. J. Mol. Biol. **71:** 789–793.

SOBELL, H. M., 1974 Concerning the stereochemistry of strand equivalence in genetic recombination, pp. 433–438 in *Mechanisms in Recombination*, edited by R. F. GRELL. Plenum, New York.

STAHL, F. W. 1969 *Mechanics of Inheritance*, Ed. 2, pp. 173–179. Prentice-Hall, Englewood Cliffs, N.J.

STAHL, F. W. 1979 *Genetic Recombination: Thinking About It in Phage and Fungi*, pp. 229–233. W. H. Freeman, San Francisco.

SUN, H., D. TRECO, N. P. SCHULTES and J. W. SZOSTAK, 1989 Double strand breaks at an initiation site for meiotic gene conversion. Nature **338:** 87–90.

SUN, H., D. TRECO and J. W. SZOSTAK, 1991 Extensive 3′-overhanging, single-stranded DNA associated with the meiosis-specific double-strand breaks at the *ARG4* recombination initiation site. Cell **64:** 1155–1161.

SZOSTAK, J. W., T. L. ORR-WEAVER, R. J. ROTHSTEIN and F. W. STAHL, 1983 The double-strand-break repair model for recombination. Cell **33:** 25–35.

THALER, D. S., M. M. STAHL and F. W. STAHL, 1987 Tests of the double-strand-break model for Red-mediated recombination of phage and plasmid dv. Genetics **116:** 501–511.

THOMPSON, B. J., M. N. CAMIEN and R. C. WARNER, 1976 Kinetics of branch migration in double-stranded DNA. Proc. Natl. Acad. Sci. USA **73:** 2299–2303.

WATSON, J. D., and F. H. C. CRICK, 1953 Molecular structure of nucleic acids: a structure for deoxyribose nucleic acid. Nature **171:** 737–738.

WHITBY, M. C., L. RYDER and R. G. LLOYD, 1993 Reverse branch migration of Holliday junctions by RecG protein: a new mechanism for resolution of intermediates in recombination and DNA repair. Cell **75:** 341–350.

WILLIAMSON, M. S., J. C. GAME and S. FOGEL, 1985 Meiotic gene conversion mutants in *Saccharomyces cerevisiae*. I. Isolation and characterization of *pms1-1* and *pms1-2*. Genetics **110:** 609–646.

November 1994

Discovery and Genetic Definition
of the Drosophila Antennapedia Complex

Rob Denell

Division of Biology, Kansas State University, Manhattan, Kansas 66506–4901

ONE day in 1976 THOM KAUFMAN called me in great excitement. KAUFMAN and I shared an interest in Drosophila homeotic genes located near the third chromosome centromere. He had recently arrived at Indiana University, and the results of his first set of crosses convinced him that these genes were part of a complex important to anterior developmental commitments (KAUFMAN *et al.* 1980), just as ED LEWIS's bithorax complex controlled fate in more posterior regions. He invited me to Bloomington the next summer to join him in a genetic study of this Antennapedia complex (ANT-C).

In the late 1960s, KAUFMAN and I had been graduate students together in BURKE JUDD's lab at the University of Texas. Although my interest in segregation distortion was far from the focus of the lab, KAUFMAN worked at its very center: a mutational analysis of the *zeste-white* region. JUDD was and remains interested in genome organization, and in this pre-molecular era he wished to ascertain all zygotically active functions in this *X* chromosome interval necessary for normal morphology and/or viability and to examine the distribution of these loci along the polytene chromosome map (JUDD *et al.* 1972). In addition to the genetic aspects of this "saturation mutagenesis" effort, KAUFMAN joined MARY SHANNON in a study of the developmental consequences of the recessive-lethal variants isolated (SHANNON *et al.* 1972).

I left Austin in 1970 for postdoctoral studies with DAN LINDSLEY at UCSD and arrived there at a particularly exciting time. LINDSLEY and long-time collaborator LARRY SANDLER were also interested in functional aspects of genetic organization, and I joined their massive effort to systematically generate and study small deficiencies and duplications distributed throughout the genome (LINDSLEY *et al.* 1972). LINDSLEY has served as a repository and chronicler of Drosophila genetic knowledge and takes seriously his responsibility to impart this lore to his students. He pointed out to me an apparent enrichment of homeotic and sex-transforming genes near the third chromosome centromere. These genes were fascinating from a developmental standpoint, and it had been ar-

gued for decades that they must play key regulatory roles in assigning developmental commitments realized through the action of downstream genes. Moreover, the apparent clustering of genes of similar function in a higher eukaryote was potentially very interesting. However, uncertainties as to allelic relationships and mapping difficulties due to centromeric inhibition of recombination in this region (HANNAH-ALAVA 1969) left the number of homeotic genes and their spatial relationships in considerable doubt.

All known homeotic loci in that region had been recognized by adult transformations, and included *Extra sex combs* (*Scx*), *proboscipedia* (*pb*), *Antennapedia* (*Antp*), *Polycomb* (*Pc*), *Multiple sex combs* (*Msc*), and *Nasobemia* (*Ns*) (Figure 1A). [That *Deformed* (*Dfd*) and *Humeral* (*Hu*) were homeotic mutations was not then recognized.] Many *Antennapedia* mutant alleles shared a common dominant antenna → leg transformation phenotype, rearrangement breakpoint, and recessive lethality. WALTER GEHRING (1966) had discovered a mutation associated with a similar (albeit more extreme) transformation that was free of recessive lethality and gross chromosomal rearrangement. He believed this variant to identify a locus separate from *Antennapedia* and named it *Nasobemia* after MORGENSTERN's mythological creature that walked on its nose. ELIEZER LIFSCHYTZ, then also in LINDSLEY's lab, had recently shown that the dominant phenotype of a gain-of-function allele could be "reverted" by loss-of-function mutations isolated at rates characteristic of forward mutation (LIFSCHYTZ and FALK 1969). LINDSLEY suggested that I use LIFSCHYTZ's approach for the sex-transforming mutation then known as *transformer-dominant* (which proved to be *doublesex-dominant* instead), and I also applied it to *Nasobemia*. Most revertants were associated with recessive lethality that failed to complement the lethality of *Antennapedia* mutations, showing that *Nasobemia* was an *Antennapedia* allele and that the phenotype that was its namesake was neomorphic (DENELL 1973). *Extra sex combs* appeared to be an *Antennapedia* allele as well. A very similar reversion analysis was done independently by KAUFMAN and IAN DUNCAN, then an undergraduate at the University of British Columbia (DUNCAN and KAUFMAN 1975). [In this issue, TALBERT and GARBER (1994) discuss the molecular nature of *Nasobemia* revertants.] These results clarified the picture a little, but the question of relationships in the genome and their potential significance remained unsolved.

At this time ED LEWIS was performing his well known and elegant work at Caltech on other homeotic mutations. In this case, a large number of recessive and dominant variants causing homeotic transformations of the adult thorax and abdomen were unambiguously very tightly clustered within the bithorax complex (BX-C), which mapped more distally on the right arm of chromosome 3. LEWIS (1978) argued that loss-of-function variants caused anteriorly directed transformations, whereas those associated with gain-of-function variants were posteriorly directed. Moreover, the mutations mapped along the chromosome in an order colinear with their mutant effects along the anterior-posterior body axis. This distribution led Lewis to the hypothesis that the number of genes corresponded to the number of thoracic and abdominal segments. He suggested a model in which the middle thoracic segment was a "ground state" characteristic of no BX-C activity in the context of an otherwise normal genotype, and the expression of a progressively greater number of BX-C genes defined successively more posterior segments. He interpreted gain-of-function mutations as being due to the expression of a gene in an inappropriate domain. For me at least, this idea provided one satisfying explanation for the difficult question of how neomorphic mutations could acquire "a new function" (MULLER 1932). Noting that Japanese geneticists studying the silk moth equivalent of the BX-C had placed emphasis on larval mutant phenotypes (TAZIMA 1964), LEWIS also stressed the importance of examining the terminal lethal syndromes of genotypes dying at preadult stages.

KAUFMAN's first crosses at Indiana used a small deficiency isolated as a revertant of *Nasobemia* (*Df(3R)Ns+R17*), and an overlapping deletion isolated at the University of British Columbia by DON SINCLAIR called *Df(3R)Scr*. The latter was associated with a reduction in the size of the sex combs of the male proleg shared by *Multiple sex combs*, and KAUFMAN postulated that deletion of a haplo-insufficient *Sex combs reduced* gene caused a partial transformation of first to second leg. Complementation analysis using the deficiencies indicated that polytene chromosome region 84A-B included all of the homeotic loci known in the proximal third chromosome region except *Polycomb*, which by then had been shown to reside on the other side of the centromere (PURO and NYGREN 1975). This exciting definitive evidence of clustering led Kaufman to propose that these genes were part of a complex controlling anterior determinative decisions, and to predict similarities to the

BX-C. He envisaged the middle thoracic segment as a ground state, such that the loss-of-function phenotype of *Sex combs reduced* caused posteriorly directed changes of the first thoracic leg, and dominant gain-of-function variants *Multiple sex combs* and *Extra sex combs* caused opposing changes (KAUFMAN *et al.* 1980).

How could the structure and function of this complex be elucidated? KAUFMAN recognized that the available collection of variants, isolated on the basis of adult homeotic phenotypes, probably had been strongly influenced by ascertainment bias. Except for some *proboscipedia* alleles, all available visible mutations were neomorphs, and null alleles were needed to assess their normal developmental significance. Moreover, he anticipated that additional functionally related genes existed within the complex that could be recognized by the embryonic or larval phenotypes of recessive lethal alleles. Thus, he proposed that we apply JUDD's concept of saturation mutagenesis to identify and characterize all loci in this region that mutate to yield recessive lethal or visible adult phenotypes. When I arrived in Bloomington in the summer of 1976, KAUFMAN and graduate student RICKI LEWIS had set up an experiment to isolate X-ray- and EMS-induced mutations that failed to complement *Df(3R)Ns+R17*. Later, graduate student BARBARA WAKIMOTO screened for additional mutations using *Df(3R)Scr*. Both sets of variants were subjected to complementation and recombinational analysis, and the map shown in Figure 1B was generated (LEWIS *et al.*, 1980a,b). As predicted, point mutations associated with a dominant adult T1 → T2 transformation were isolated at the *Sex combs reduced* locus. The results also suggested that the *EbR11* complementation group included the *Deformed* mutation, and preliminary observations showed that the lethal syndromes associated with the *EbR11* and *EfW36* complementation groups included larval head abnormalities.

The description of complementation groups with arbitrary names generated little widespread excitement. The real payoff began when WAKIMOTO and KAUFMAN (1981) and WAKIMOTO *et al.* (1984) described the phenotypes of lethal larvae and adult clones homozygous for recessive lethal alleles (see KAUFMAN *et al.* 1990). KAUFMAN (1978) had earlier made the unexpected observation that *proboscipedia* function is dispensable for normal embryonic development, so it was satisfying that the null phenotypes of *Antennapedia* and *Sex combs reduced* were associated with larval homeotic transformations. The *EfR14* complementation group was associated with aberrant embryos missing half of the normal number of segments. Wishing to give this gene a descriptive Japanese name, WAKIMOTO and KAUFMAN consulted colleague BOB TOGASAKI as well as WAKIMOTO's father and settled on *fushi tarazu* (*ftz*), a term that roughly translates to describe a shortening of bamboo by loss of segments. This segmentation gene has been among the most intensively studied in Drosophila. They also found that the *EfW36* complementation group caused abnormalities in

A. Recombinational map positions, from LINDSLEY and GRELL (1967)

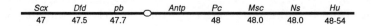

B. Complementation groups, after LEWIS *et al.* (1980a)

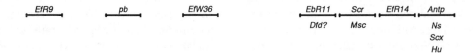

C. Post-molecular organization, after KAUFMAN *et al.* (1990)

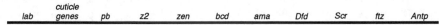

FIGURE 1.—Conceptual evolution of the Drosophila Antennapedia complex. (A) Map positions of the homeotic mutations (as well as *Deformed* and *Humeral*) recognized in 1967 in the proximal region of chromosome *3*, with the centromere position indicated by a circle. Because of centromeric inhibition of recombination, the region from *Scx* to *Ns* potentially spanned salivary chromosome map region 77–84. All recognized *Antp* alleles were associated with rearrangements sharing breakpoints in proximal 84, and its relative position was assigned on that basis. Likewise, *Humeral* is associated with an inversion of salivary chromosome map region 84–86 and was placed at recombinational map position 48–54. Later studies would show that *Pc* is in the left arm and all others in the right arm at salivary map position 84B1,2. (B) Complementation groups recognized by LEWIS *et al.* (1980a). They have been aligned with the current version of the map (based on molecular as well as genetic studies) shown in (C), although LEWIS *et al.* showed them in a slightly different order.

morphogenetic rearrangements associated with gastrulation, and renamed the locus *zerknüllt* (*zen*) (German for crumpled). Later work has defined the importance of this gene in dorsal-ventral patterning. Studies of the *EbR11* complementation group (later to be *Deformed*) detected anterior abnormalities that were not obviously homeotic in nature, and later work on the *EfR9* or *labial* (*lab*) group also demonstrated similar nonhomeotic head defects.

Which of these loci associated with diverse mutant phenotypes potentially belonged to a complex of functionally related genes? KAUFMAN argued that all of the genes necessary for early embryonic development (as well as *proboscipedia*) were members of the ANT-C. He believed that the lack of overt embryonic homeotic phenotypes of *labial* and *Deformed* was a consequence of the highly derived nature of the maggot head; *labial* and *Deformed* mutations were later shown to cause head transformation in homozygous adult clones. He further argued that the interspersion of *fushi tarazu* and *zerknüllt* among the homeotic genes could not be merely fortuitous.

Off the record, membership of the complex (or indeed the idea that there was more than a chance proximity of developmentally significant genes) was sometimes questioned, but additional work proved KAUFMAN correct. Molecular analysis showed that the homeotic genes (and indeed all other interspersed nonhomeotic genes except the cuticle cluster mentioned below) shared homeoboxes encoding sequence-specific DNA-binding domains important to the function of their proteins as transcription factors. Further, it was realized that a cluster of homeobox genes regulating developmental commitments in an

integrated manner is an ancient feature of the Metazoa. In 1987 my colleague DICK BEEMAN mapped the homeotic mutations then extant in the red flour beetle, *Tribolium castaneum*. He found that apparent homologs of both ANT-C and BX-C genes were tightly linked, suggesting that a single homeotic complex (HOM-C) was the ancestral organization among insects. As recently related by McGINNIS (1994), the homeobox facilitated comparative molecular studies that showed that this complex arose very early in animal evolution and that (with the single recognized exception of Drosophila) its integrity had been maintained over hundreds of millions of years. Until recently, homologs of the nonhomeotic members of the complex had not been detected outside of the Diptera, suggesting that these genes originated as a concomitant of evolutionarily advanced aspects of early development in higher flies. However, a homolog of *fushi tarazu* has now been recognized in Tribolium (BROWN *et al.* 1994), and probable homologs have been described in the brine shrimp and grasshopper (AVEROF and AKAM 1993; DAWES *et al.* 1994), leading to the hypothesis that this and other nonhomeotic members of the complex show a rate of sequence divergence much higher than do homeotic genes. Thus, the question of their origin remains unresolved.

The kind of saturation mutagenesis effort devoted to the Antennapedia complex could not detect all of the functions included (Figure 1C). Screening for zygotic effects failed to identify the maternal effect gene *bicoid* (*bcd*) (FROHNHÖFER and NÜSSLEIN-VOLHARD 1987), which plays a critical role in the establishment of embryonic anterior/posterior polarity. The gene *amalgam* (*ama*) and the *zerknüllt* paralog *z2* were discovered molecularly, but mutant effects have not yet been described. Perhaps most enigmatic is a molecularly ascertained cluster of genes putatively affecting cuticle synthesis and structurally unrelated to any other members of the complex.

Saturation mutagenesis also proved very important to our understanding of the BX-C. Independent work by three groups detected only three lethal complementation groups (SÁNCHEZ-HERRERO *et al.* 1985; TIONG *et al.* 1985; KARCH *et al.* 1985). Molecular studies showed that they correspond to the only protein-coding transcription units in the complex and that many mutations giving adult transformations affect complex *cis*-regulatory regions. Earlier views that the BX-C (and some ANT-C) genes function within segmental domains were also modified by the discovery that mutant phenotypes correspond to metameric units offset from segments (HAYES *et al.* 1984; STRUHL 1984) and later called parasegments (MARTINEZ-ARIAS and LAWRENCE 1985).

The facility with which homeo genes can be molecularly cloned and studied (see MCGINNIS 1994) has allowed an investigation of the roles of these developmentally significant genes in phylogenetically diverse animals, as well as insights into the evolution of transcriptional regulatory mechanisms. In the past, some of my colleagues have questioned how the arcane results from Drosophila studies could possibly be relevant to more important matters such as mammalian development. Thus, it is especially satisfying to contemplate how the genetic and molecular characterization of these bizarre mutations has led to the discovery of a gene complex that is providing ever increasing insight into mammalian regulatory mechanisms and incidentally has been proposed as the criterion that defines members of the animal kingdom (SLACK *et al.* 1993).

Many thanks to THOM KAUFMAN, BARBARA WAKIMOTO and RICKI LEWIS for helpful suggestions, as well as to MONICA JUSTICE and MARNETTE DENELL for comments on the manuscript.

LITERATURE CITED

AVEROF, M., and M. AKAM, 1993 *HOM/Hox* genes of *Artemia*: implications for the origin of insect and crustacean body plans. Curr. Biol. **3**: 73–78.

BEEMAN, R. W., 1987 A homoeotic gene cluster in the red flour beetle. Nature **327**: 247–249.

BROWN, S. J., R. B. HILGENFELD and R. E. DENELL, 1994 The beetle, *Tribolium castaneum*, has a *fushi tarazu* homolog expressed in stripes during segmentation. Proc. Natl. Acad. Sci. USA **91**: (in press).

DAWES, R., I. DAWSON, F. FALCIANI, G. TEAR and M. AKAM, 1994 *Dax*, a locust Hox gene related to *fushi-tarazu* but showing no pair-rule expression. Development **120**: 1561–1572.

DENELL, R. E., 1973 Homeosis in Drosophila. I. Complementation studies with revertants of *Nasobemia*. Genetics **75**: 279–297.

DUNCAN, I. W., and T. C. KAUFMAN, 1975 Cytogenetic analysis of chromosome *3* in *Drosophila melanogaster*: mapping of the proximal portion of the right arm. Genetics **80**: 733–752.

FROHNHÖFER, H. G., and C. NÜSSLEIN-VOLHARD, 1987 Maternal genes required for the anterior localization of *bicoid* activity in the embryo of *Drosophila*. Genes Dev. **1**: 880–890.

GEHRING, W., 1966 Bildung eines vollständigen Mittelbeines mit Sternopleura in der Antennenregion bei der Mutante *Nasobemia*

(Ns) von *Drosophila melanogaster*. Arch. Julius Klaus-Stift. Vererbungsforsch. Sozialanthropol. Rassenhyg. **41**: 44–54.

HANNAH-ALAVA, A., 1969 Localization of Pc and Scx. Drosophila Inf. Ser. **44**: 75–76.

HAYES, P. H., T. SATO and R. E. DENELL, 1984 Homoeosis in *Drosophila*: the Ultrabithorax larval syndrome. Proc. Natl. Acad. Sci. USA **81**: 545–549.

JUDD, B. H., M. W. SHEN and T. C. KAUFMAN, 1972 The anatomy and function of a segment of the *X* chromosome of *Drosophila melanogaster*. Genetics **71**: 139–156.

KARCH, F., B. WEIFFENBACH, M. PEIFER, W. BENDER, I. DUNCAN *et al.*, 1985 The abdominal region of the bithorax complex. Cell **43**: 81–96.

KAUFMAN, T. C., 1978 Cytogenetic analysis of chromosome *3* in *Drosophila melanogaster*: isolation and characterization of four new alleles of the *proboscipedia* (*pb*) locus. Genetics **90**: 579–596.

KAUFMAN, T. C., R. LEWIS and B. WAKIMOTO, 1980 Cytogenetic analysis of chromosome *3* in *Drosophila melanogaster*. The homeotic gene complex in polytene interval 84A-B. Genetics **94**: 115–133.

KAUFMAN, T. C., M. A. SEEGER and G. OLSON, 1990 Molecular and genetic organization of the Antennapedia gene complex of *Drosophila melanogaster*. Adv. Genet. **27**: 309–362.

LEWIS, E., 1978 A gene complex controlling segmentation in Drosophila. Nature **276**: 141–152.

LEWIS, R. A., T. C. KAUFMAN, R. E. DENELL and P. TALLERICO, 1980a Genetic analysis of the Antennapedia gene complex (ANT-C) and adjacent chromosomal regions of *Drosophila melanogaster*. I. Polytene chromosome segments 84B-D. Genetics **95**: 367–381.

LEWIS, R. A., B. T. WAKIMOTO, R. E. DENELL and T. C. KAUFMAN, 1980b Genetic analysis of the Antennapedia gene complex (ANT-C) and adjacent chromosomal regions of *Drosophila melanogaster*. II. Polytene chromosome segments 84A-84B1,2. Genetics **95**: 383–397.

LIFSCHYTZ, E., and R. FALK, 1969 A system for screening of rare events in genes of *Drosophila melanogaster*. Genetics **63**: 343–352.

LINDSLEY, D. L., and E. H. GRELL, 1968 *Genetic Variations of Drosophila melanogaster*. Carnegie Inst. Wash. Publ. 627.

LINDSLEY, D. L., L. SANDLER, B. S. BAKER, A. T. C. CARPENTER, R. E. DENELL *et al.*, 1972 Segmental aneuploidy and the genetic gross structure of the Drosophila genome. Genetics **71**: 157–184.

MARTINEZ-ARIAS, A., and P. A. LAWRENCE, 1985 Parasegments and compartments in the *Drosophila* embryo. Nature **313**: 639–642.

MCGINNIS, W., 1994 A century of homeosis, a decade of homeoboxes. Genetics **137**: 607–611.

MULLER, H. J., 1932 Further studies on the nature and causes of gene mutations, pp. 213–255 in *Proceedings of the Sixth International Congress of Genetics*, edited by D. F. JONES. Brooklin Botanic Gardins, Menasha, Wisc.

PURO, J., and T. NYGREN, 1975 Mode of action of a homoeotic gene in *Drosophila melanogaster*. Localization and dosage effect of *Polycomb*. Hereditas **81**: 237–248.

SÁNCHEZ-HERRERO, E., I. VERNÓS, R. MARCO and G. MORATA, 1985 Genetic organization of the *Drosophila* bithorax complex. Nature **313**: 108–113.

SHANNON, M. P., T. C. KAUFMAN, M. W. SHEN and B. H. JUDD, 1972 Lethality patterns and morphology of selected lethal and semi-lethal mutations in the zeste-white region of *Drosophila melanogaster*. Genetics **72**: 615–638.

SLACK, J. M. W., P. W. H. HOLLAND and C. F. GRAHAM, 1993 The zootype and the phylogenetic stage. Nature **361**: 490–493.

STRUHL, G., 1984 Splitting the bithorax complex of *Drosophila*. Nature **308**: 454–457.

TALBERT, P. B., and R. L. GARBER, 1994 The Drosophila homeotic mutation *nasobemia* (*Antp^{Ns}*) and its revertants: an analysis of mutational reversion. Genetics **138**: 000–000.

TAZIMA, Y., 1964 E-group as a tool of developmental genetics, pp. 6075 in *The Genetics of the Silkworm*, edited by Y. TAZIMA. Logo Press, London.

TIONG, S., L. M. BONE and J. R. S. WHITTLE, 1985 Recessive lethal mutations within the *bithorax* complex in *Drosophila melanogaster*. Mol. Gen. Genet. **200**: 335–342.

WAKIMOTO, B. T., and T. C. KAUFMAN, 1981 Analysis of larval segmentation in lethal genotypes associated with the Antennapedia gene complex in *Drosophila melanogaster*. Dev. Biol. **81**: 51–64.

WAKIMOTO, B. T., F. R. TURNER and T. C. KAUFMAN, 1984 Defects in embryogenesis in mutants associated with the Antennapedia gene complex of *Drosophila melanogaster*. Dev. Biol. **102**: 147–172.

December 1994

The Evolution of Somatic Selection
The Antibody Tale

Gerald M. Edelman

Department of Neurobiology, The Scripps Research Institute, La Jolla, California 92037

IT is a piece of good luck if one is working in a branch of science at a time of crisis or when a far-reaching technique has been introduced. It is even better luck when ideas and data lock together to reveal a new horizon. By the late 1950s such a time had arrived in immunology. Up to that time, this field was largely a subdiscipline of microbiology with a strong emphasis on serology and vaccines. Its basic underpinnings came from the work of KARL LANDSTEINER, whose demonstration that organic chemical groupings could serve as hapten antigens revealed the remarkable range of immune specificity [see LANDSTEINER (1945) for a review]. Proteins, peptides, carbohydrates, and even new molecules that almost certainly never existed during evolution could be distinguished by immune sera. The prevailing theories to account for this were instructionist–by one means or another, the antigen or hapten served as a template for the folding of the antibody-combining site. An outstanding example was the proposal of PAULING (1940).

Within the 10-year period from 1959 to 1969, the whole picture changed. Immunology was thrust into prominence as a source of ideas [see EDELMAN (1973)], of techniques for molecular biology and pathology, and as a major source of insight into a vast set of diseases.

During that period, instructionist theories were abandoned in favor of selectional theories that took their inspiration from the Darwinian two-step, variation and selection, leading to alterations in population structure. Two developments played a key role in the change: the clonal selection theory of immunity (BURNET 1959) and the analysis of antibody structure. The coupling of these efforts gave rise to new insights not only into the immune system [see ADA (1966)], but also into a series of problems of great interest to geneticists.

In this article, I want to review briefly how this coupling came about, emphasizing first the chemical and structural challenges facing those who wished to understand the nature of antibodies. Then I want to comment on certain consequences of this work for thinking about the evolution and genetics of gene families. My purpose is not to give an exhaustive historical account, but rather to highlight some intellectual and methodological turning points. The exercise will, I hope, show how specific insights in one subject can open up a general horizon in another. Viewing such a horizon is one of the sudden glories afforded by a scientific career.

Two short reports that appeared in *Biochemistry* and the *Journal of the American Chemical Society* in 1959 were to have a strong impact on the direction of immunological thinking. The first was by the late RODNEY PORTER, who used the enzyme papain to cleave the antibody molecule into what are now called the Fab (antigen-binding) and F_C (crystallizable) fragments (PORTER 1959). The other paper was by me and showed that reduction of the disulfide bonds of antibodies in the presence of denaturing agents led to dissociation of the molecule into smaller pieces, now known to be the light (L) and heavy (H) chains (EDELMAN 1959). These two papers were short but seminal–after their appearance, an explosion of effort spread its effects in many directions. But it was not yet clear what they had to do with each other. PORTER still believed that the antibody molecule was one long polypeptide chain, and despite the differences in our interpretations, I had not then succeeded in separating L and H chains. Nevertheless, the possibility of linking immunoglobulin structure to immune function unquestionably pointed to a grand horizon. Within a short time, glimpses of that horizon were to reveal connections between immunology and a series of other areas in a series of linkages that had previously not been suspected.

It is, I believe, particularly revealing to consider the methodological problems confronting us at the time. Their eventual solution was to involve unusual biological

Address for correspondence: Department of Neurobiology, The Scripps Research Institute, 10666 North Torrey Pines Road, La Jolla, CA 92037.

insight as well as chemical ingenuity. Three such problems were blocking progress in determining the structure of antibodies. I shall call these the heterogeneity problem, the size problem, and the specificity problem. Their solutions were linked eventually in a most beautiful way that required tying many fields together–chemistry, medicine, and biological theory as it pertained to genetics and evolution.

The heterogeneity problem had been noted several times in one form or another by serologists and immunologists. It was posed most clearly by TISELIUS and his co-workers, using free boundary electrophoresis to analyze serum (TISELIUS 1937). γ-Globulin, as the main fraction of immunoglobulin was then called, showed a broad spread of net charge at various pH values; this was unlike other serum proteins such as albumin, whose spreading during electrophoresis could be attributed to diffusion. Successive subfractions of γ-globulin ran "true" to their original modal position but also displayed charge heterogeneity. It was not clear whether this was the result of folding differences in the same antibody chain–consistent with PAULING's version (1940) of the instructive theory of immunity–or whether it was the result of sequence differences in different antibodies. If it was the latter, no structural work was possible unless individual antibodies could be successfully fractionated. An additional kind of heterogeneity in size was also recognized as new kinds of immunoglobulins of high molecular weight (e.g., the so-called 19 S antibody) were found. Members of each of these families also revealed the microheterogeneity seen for γ-globulin. γ-Globulin certainly was large enough (150,000 Da) to strike terror in the hearts of the structurally inclined protein chemist, but these new molecules had molecular weights close to a million!

The size problem is simple to state in terms of comparatives. The only protein molecule to have been successfully sequenced at the time was insulin (molecular weight 6,000 Da), a triumph achieved by FRED SANGER and his colleagues (SANGER 1964). γ-Globulin, with its molecular weight of 150,000, had a size that made it seem like Everest to local hill climbers. As if that were not daunting enough, the shape of the mountain–its specificity–seemed almost beyond grasp.

The specificity problem was the one about which there was the most theoretical dispute. If one believed with the instructionists that each antibody was a single long chain which folded differently around antigens as a template, then specificity was acquired by information transfer. If, on the other hand, one believed in selectionist theories, different antibodies were already synthesized *before* encounter with the antigen. If one accepted this view, the specificity problem then became: How?

As things turned out, all three problems were solved relatively rapidly by applying medical knowledge, protein chemical techniques, and, finally, molecular biology. The solutions came as each of these fields exploded into progress, and each solution in turn contributed to that progress in a recursive fashion.

My own efforts in these arenas began in naiveté. After reading an immunology text that emphasized antigens but left antibodies as shadowy abstractions, I came to the conclusion that, in unraveling the puzzle of specificity in the immune response, antibodies, not antigens, were the central elements. I set to work to see what I could learn about the molecular structure of antibodies, starting with γ-globulin fractions. My first efforts were aimed at measuring the number of disulfide bonds in each molecule. While examining the effects of disruption of these bonds in the ultracentrifuge, I found that there was a sharp drop in the apparent sedimentation coefficient, indicating either a radical unfolding or a drop in molecular weight. In the ultracentrifuge, the apparent molecular weight dropped to one-third that of the untreated γ-globulin, a value difficult to reconcile with unfolding (EDELMAN 1959). Unfortunately, the 6 M urea necessary to keep the protein soluble made for a nonideal solution, and there was no completely worked out theory for sedimentation in such three-component solvents. After resorting to many empirical comparisons, measuring other proteins' molecular weights in and out of urea, I concluded that the molecule was indeed dissociated into its component polypeptide chains. This conclusion, that there were multiple chains, went against the prevailing dogma. But I was convinced that they existed and that a key problem was to fractionate and characterize them.

With starch gel electrophoresis in 6 M urea, a technique pioneered by OLIVER SMITHIES (1995), a clear fractionation pattern was obtained. It consisted of a broad band of what are now known as heavy chains preceded by a long diffuse smear of light chains (EDELMAN and POULIK 1961). These experiments and some knowledge of medicine provided the bases for a simultaneous solution of the heterogeneity and size problems. It was known that patients with a cancer of plasma cells known as multiple myeloma produced large amounts usually of a single γ-globulin, called myeloma protein, that appeared to lack the heterogeneity of the molecules from normal individuals. Moreover, some of these patients excreted a smaller protein in their urine that had unusual solubility properties during heat denaturation. When heated, it precipitated like albumin but then went back into solution at higher temperature. This so-called Bence Jones protein was named after HENRY BENCE JONES, a London practitioner who had studied with LIEBIG, the discoverer of albumin. JONES received a note from two Scottish physicians who were treating a rich grocer who had multiple myeloma. His urine showed the peculiar solubility properties of the protein. The note ended with a question: "What is it?" JONES performed some elemental analysis and answered that the urinary protein was the "hydrated deutoxide of albumin." Bence Jones protein was, in fact, the second protein to be characterized after LIEBIG's albumin. The name has a fine ring to it, but it is not as alliteratively grand as that of JONES' uncle, BENCE BENCE, Bishop of Beccles.

From my medical experience, I knew about Bence Jones proteinuria and also about the sometimes huge amounts of myeloma protein in the serum of myeloma patients. I decided to study these proteins. After I compared reduced myeloma proteins from a number of different patients on urea gels, it became clear that each had a sharp, light-chain band at a different position within the range of the normal light-chain smear (EDELMAN and POULIK 1961). I surmised that each myeloma protein had a unique light chain and that each sample from normal individuals consisted of a vast mixture of different molecules, each with a different light chain. This conclusion fit MACFARLANE BURNET's recently announced clonal selection theory (BURNET 1959), which assumed that one cell made one kind of antibody *before* seeing any antigen and that a particular antigen selected those cells bearing antibodies that happened to fit and somehow induced clonal proliferation.

These experimental findings and thoughts hinted at a solution to the heterogeneity problem and a possible resolution of the dilemmas of the specificity problem: one might be able to study a single myeloma protein as a pure example of an antibody. But the myeloma protein was huge: 150,000 Da compared with insulin's 6000 Da. The size problem had to be resolved, and it turned out that the experiments I had carried out on the breakage into chains provided a possible way of doing so. The picture was nevertheless confusing. RODNEY PORTER had shown that the molecule could be cleaved by papain into pieces of about 50,000 Da (PORTER 1959). These could not be the natural units (the L and H chains), which I knew were produced without peptide bond breakage. PORTER, a superb protein chemist, later turned his attention to these units and found a simple way of fractionating L and H chains (FLEISHMAN *et al.* 1963). With the puzzle constantly in mind, it occurred to me that Bence Jones proteins were simply excreted light chains, not PORTER's pieces. I heated a sample of light chains obtained from normal human serum γ-globulin, and they had the behavior of Bence Jones proteins: they became insoluble and then resolubilized with continued heating (EDELMAN and GALLY 1962). *A fortiori*, the same had to be true of the light chains of myeloma proteins, and it was: Bence Jones proteins from each patient had mobilities in starch gels identical to the light chain of that patient's serum myeloma protein. Moreover, peptide maps of such pairs were identical, although maps of different patients' proteins were different (SCHWARTZ and EDELMAN 1963). Bence Jones proteins (each now

identified as a pure light chain) had molecular weights of around 20,000 Da. The size problem was still daunting but not hopelessly irresolvable. It was conceivable that one could analyze the amino acid sequence of pure light chains and learn about their structure.

At around this time (1962), I received a visit from BURNET. I told him that I was delighted with his theory, that I too was a selectionist, and I briefly described my findings. He said, "Why are you doing this? Chemistry only makes things more complicated." I replied, "But, if we are to believe in selection, we have to know how many different antibodies are present in a person's repertoire and exactly how they differ. There not only has to be diversity, there has to be a lot of it." He replied, "Mathematics is even worse than chemistry. Don't worry, you don't need it, my theory is right." It was right, although it was only with longer acquaintance that I could persuade him that my work not only made sense but provided some of his theory's key underpinnings.

The resolution of the heterogeneity problem brought with it another insight: antibodies of higher molecular weight showed heavy-chain bands of different mobility, each characteristic of a given immunoglobulin class. This picture, along with the work by PORTER's group showing how papain cleaved the heavy chain (FLEISHMAN *et al.* 1962, 1963), provided a basis for attacking the specificity problem. It was likely that different antibodies had chains of different amino acid composition, as did Bence Jones proteins from different patients. (Gels of the chains of specifically purified antibodies looked like those of different mixtures of myeloma proteins–not a diffuse smear as seen for normal serum γ-globulin.) That different Bence Jones proteins were actually different in their peptide sequences was shown by FRANK PUTNAM [see PUTNAM *et al.* (1967)]. A satisfying clue to the nature of their heterogeneity from protein to protein came when HILSCHMANN and CRAIG did partial amino acid sequences of two Bence Jones proteins and showed that the NH₂-terminal regions differed, whereas the COOH termini were identical (HILSCHMANN and CRAIG 1965).

The suggestion that there were variable (V) and constant (C) regions in immunoglobulin chains married heterogeneity to specificity under the auspices of clonal selection. It remained to be shown that heavy chains were also variable; this was accomplished later both in our laboratory (CUNNINGHAM *et al.* 1969) and in PORTER's (PRESS and HOGG 1969). One experiment had been done earlier in my group to suggest a combinatorial possibility: one could dissociate antibodies of a given specificity and then reconstitute them with the same or different light or heavy chains (OLINS and EDELMAN 1964). This "p × q experiment" suggested that the combined contributions of each chain type to the binding site for antigens might multiplicatively increase the heterogeneity of the antibody repertoire.

With these developments, the stage was set to try to analyze the complete primary structure of an antibody. Our group picked one IgG myeloma protein that we had obtained in over 200-g amounts from a patient who had been exchange-transfused because his myeloma protein was causing viscosity problems, impeding his blood flow. PORTER's group attacked the heavy chain of another patient. By 1969, my colleagues and I had completed the sequence of the whole molecule (EDELMAN et al. 1969), and PORTER's group had most of their heavy chain (PRESS and HOGG 1969). Comparison of the data from both laboratories with those on other heavy chains confirmed the idea that there were V and C regions for these chains. Our work on the entire structure provided a basis for a detailed model of the IgG molecule that was to prove useful in relating the various functions of antibodies to their structures (EDELMAN 1970).

As a result of the combined insights obtained from the union of the protein structural data with the clonal selection theory, the specificity problem was transformed into one of molecular genetics (see GALLY and EDELMAN 1972). This transformation, in turn, prompted new insights into the co-evolution of gene families. A veritable ecstasy of theory making was prompted by this union between fields. Limitations of space do not permit even a reduced account of that state of affairs. But in retrospect one may say that theories of antibody diversity came in two main types: somatic and germ line. The somatic theories, in turn, came in two flavors: mutational and recombinational. Key examples of mutational theories were the proposals of SYDNEY BRENNER and CÉSAR MILSTEIN (1966) and also of MELVIN COHN (1971). These theories stated that, in each lymphocyte, somatic mutations occurred in DNA specifying V regions. The alternative recombinational theories were provided by JOSEPH GALLY and me (EDELMAN and GALLY 1967), who suggested somatic recombination of a small number of germ line genes (as many as eight or so for each subclass of chains), and by SMITHIES (1967) [championed by CRICK (CRICK et al. 1967)], who suggested one and a half genes: one for a V region gene recombining somatically with one VC gene having a different V region.

Genetic analysis [see GALLY and EDELMAN (1972)] indicated that there had to be multiple germ line genes for each light and each heavy chain, effectively ruling out SMITHIES' version of recombination. Nevertheless, there was no indication that the germ line would contain hundreds or thousands of V region genes, as suggested by the germ line theory of DREYER and HOOD (HOOD et al. 1967). Furthermore, their proposal posed a profound problem in genetics. How could multiple copies of germ line genes for antibodies be kept alike *within* a species and still be more or less alike when compared *among* evolutionarily related species? In the absence of selection by each particular antigen for specific V regions during evolution (a selection prohibited by the clonal selection theory), variants would accumulate and deviate greatly in their structure. This highlighted the problem of accounting for the co-evolution of duplicated genes, a problem that at the time presented an enormous challenge not just for antibodies, but for other proteins as well.

Before discussing how this challenge was met, it may be useful to mention that, once the primary structure of antibodies was in hand, solutions to some less thorny evolutionary problems fell nicely into line. Not only could one see that there were V and C regions for L and H chains, but computer comparisons revealed regions of homology within V and C regions about 100 amino acids in length. On the basis of the similarities among many such regions in immunoglobulin polypeptide chains, I proposed the domain hypothesis, which put forth three key tenets related to the structure, function, and evolution of antibodies (EDELMAN 1970; CUNNINGHAM et al. 1969). This hypothesis predicted that the amino acid sequence in each region would fold into a compact domain with a single disulfide bond in its interior. This was later confirmed in 1973 by X-ray crystallography. The hypothesis also proposed that each pair of domains across a symmetry axis (L-H or H-H) would carry out a distinct function. (One pair of C domains might carry out complement binding, the paired unlike V_L V_H domains carried out antigen binding, etc.) Subsequent work also validated this functional proposal. Finally, domains were presumed to have arisen by gene duplication of an ancestral gene coding for a single domain. Duplication and divergence would then have led to all the Ig chains and families, each of which had a set of characteristic heavy chain C regions. The evidence available to this date remains consistent with this evolutionary mechanism.

By the late 1960s it was clear that this work and that of many other laboratories had allied immunology to molecular genetics as closely as the work of LANDSTEINER had previously allied immunology to organic chemistry (see GALLY and EDELMAN 1972). It is revealing to consider some of the key questions raised by these developments. Answers to these questions revealed that, while certain remarkable mechanisms were unique to Igs, in other instances Igs were harbingers of key details of protein structure and synthesis, and observations made on them could rapidly be generalized to other proteins.

What was not unique was the pattern of amino acid substitutions in V regions: it resembled the mutation patterns of homologous non-immunoglobulin proteins as they were compared across different species. No completely novel mechanism to generate antibody diversity therefore seemed necessary. Nevertheless, the usual mechanism of gene duplication and unequal crossing over that had been proposed (HILL et al. 1966) to generate all of the different immunoglobulin genes in the genome during evolution was open to doubt and required revision. Indeed, the gene arrangement that emerged from the evolutionary emergence that I mentioned above posed profound questions concerning the origin of multigene families.

One of the major paradoxes came from the fact that there could be no selection of each chain by each possible antigen. As the number of different immunoglobulin genes grew, the selective pressure maintaining the sequence of any given gene would decrease, and the probability of unequal crossing over events would increase. The problem of how such reiterated gene families could nevertheless be maintained thus came to the fore. Close examination of Ig sequences showed that repeated DNA sequences within a family in one species were more similar than they were to the homologous gene families in other species. Moreover, although the members of an Ig family did not diverge greatly from one another in a given species, they could diverge from ancestors at about the same rate as the products of non-repeated genes. Furthermore, although examination of Ig chain sequences showed that they deviated one from the other, the chains bore enough family resemblance to be recognized as human, as distinguished from rabbit, for example. The results of such comparisons posed a great difficulty for any purely germ line theories of antibody diversity. It was difficult to see how a very large number of Ig genes could have *co-evolved* as a set with family resemblances while each member kept its structural uniqueness.

These and other observations directed attention to those somatic theories for the origin of diversity that started from the assumption of a relatively small number of Ig genes (*i.e.*, of the order of 100 or so). While this number was considerably less than that required by germ line theories of diversity, it still faced the problem of how family members could co-evolve. In 1968, JOSEPH GALLY and I (EDELMAN and GALLY 1968, 1970) suggested a mechanism consistent with our somatic recombination theory. We proposed that the mechanisms of *cis* recombination that we previously suggested would operate somatically in lymphoid cells to generate diversity also operated in the germ line during evolution. Such gene conversion or recombination between similar but not identical family members would tend to maintain family resemblances while evolutionary changes in a family would still be able to occur. Although gene conversion would keep particular subgroups of family members alike, selection pressure could still act to maintain differences among germ line Ig genes, *i.e.*, they could still favor an increase in sequences providing a basis for the different types of antigen-binding specificities–via electrostatic interactions of charged groups, hydrophobic interactions, etc. Such germ line genes could then be further diversified by somatic recombination and variation in each animal.

At the time that this hypothesis was advanced and elaborated (1968–1970), gene conversion had already been discovered by scientists working on fungi, but no evidence was available for such a process in animal cells. Nevertheless, it seemed to us that such a process not only could account for the antibody data, but could even explain the co-evolution of gene families other than those of Ig genes. Because we felt that such systems of tandem genes could act as "mutation nets" in which favorable mutations could rapidly be spread into family members during evolution, we generalized our proposal to the evolution of all multiprotein gene families and to repetitious RNA families. A dozen years later, two articles with the same ideas were published (EGEL 1981; BALTIMORE 1981) in apparent ignorance of our original proposals.

Since the time of our proposals, strong evidence has appeared that gene conversion events actually do play an important role in the evolution of multigene families. SLIGHTOM et al. (1980) provided the earliest sequence data for gene conversion among two linked human γ-globulin genes. In short order, similar examples were elaborated for a variety of proteins: cytochromes, rhodopsin, haptoglobins, neurophysins, keratins, histones, γ-crystallin, actin, and members of the major histocompatibility complex. Actual demonstration of gene conversion was achieved by transfecting cultured mammalian cells with cloned DNA segments that would generate selectable markers following conversion (LISKAY and STACHELEK 1983; RUBNITZ and SUBRAMANI 1986).

This period of intense theorizing about the generation of diversity (or G.O.D.) was followed by a particularly fruitful set of molecular biological investigations of antibody genes. The earliest stimulus came from TONEGAWA, who isolated the gene for a light chain in 1976. His studies [for review, see TONEGAWA (1983)] and those of others made it clear that the genes for V regions were on the same chromosome as those for C regions, but at different locations. This confirmed DREYER and BENNETT's previous proposal for separate V and C genes (DREYER and BENNETT 1965) and contradicted the prevalent dogma of "one gene-one polypeptide chain." TONEGAWA's ongoing studies in lymphoid cells also showed that a DNA rearrangement actually must have occurred to join V and C regions, since the genes in lymphoid cells showed V-C proximity, but those in the germ line gene did not.

An extensive set of studies was then carried out in many laboratories, revealing in detail how Ig diversity is achieved. The results, when taken together with the Clonal Selection Theory and ongoing work on the biology of lymphoid cells, resolved the specificity problem. It was shown that, in immune cells that are not yet committed to antibody production, a functional gene for an Ig chain contains a series of exons (one for each homologous domain). DNA encoding the V domains consists of three separate segments: V (about 95% of the domain), J (coding for about 10 amino acids), and D (coding for a short stretch between V and J that was known to be part of the antigen-binding site).

Commitment of a cell may be illustrated for heavy chains. In one of the two chromosomes of an uncommitted lymphoid cell, one D (diversity) segment is joined at random to a J (junctional segment). Intervening DNA is cleaved out and discarded. By this recombinant process, a large number of different DJ sequences can be generated. At the same time, this joining reaction can create further diversity by adding, subtracting, or substituting nucleotides. The result of this junctional diversity is that a large number of amino acid sequences are possible in this part of the V region. After formation of a DJ sequence, a splicing out reaction occurs to join one of the adjacent V genes to that sequence, creating additional diversity. Moreover, somewhere in this set of events, multiple somatic mutations can also occur in another part of the V region.

Formation of the VDJ gene segment is followed by heavy chain synthesis, cessation of rearrangement, and the elaboration of a signal to create light chains. By a process similar to that of heavy chain, a complete light chain is formed and the Ig molecule is assembled. Since, by the p × q hypothesis, light chains and heavy chains can associate in many combinations, additional diversity is created across different cells. In any one cell, further splicing is inhibited by the synthesis of a single Ig which can be displayed on the cell surface or secreted.

The enormous diversity required by the Clonal Selection Theory (one cell-one antibody with lots of different cells, each presenting a different antibody) is thus provided by a variety of mechanisms including somatic recombination, somatic mutation, and p × q assembly of L and H chains. These somatic mechanisms act on a set of Ig germ line genes that are kept alike within each family by gene conversion during evolution. Interestingly, gene conversion has actually been shown to occur somatically for light chains in chickens and thus can provide an additional source of antibody diversity (MAIZELS 1987). It is notable that conversion events also seem to be able to generate diversity in another system of the Ig superfamily, the class I histocompatibility genes encoded by the MHC locus (GELIEBTER and NATHENSON 1988).

I began this short account by mentioning the good fortune of being in a scientific field at the "right time." But, in this essay, I also wanted to illustrate how one particular well chosen biological example in a biological field can open up many horizons in other fields. In one sense, antibodies are to immunology what DNA is to genetics. Analysis of antibody structure and genetics not only unified the picture of immunology in a very satisfying way, but also provided a large number of views of key problems in disparate areas. The clarifying nomenclature of much of the field came directly from the structural work, and it remains useful to this day. Immunoglobulins were among the first large multichain proteins to be dissected, and they also provided the first clear-cut picture of the nature of protein domains. Structural

analysis of antibodies and the ensuing domain hypothesis accounted for many of their previously unexplained functional properties, including their attachment to the cell surface. They were also examples for study of other proteins: Igs were among the first proteins shown to have signal sequences and genes with intron and exon arrangements.

Above all, the structural and molecular genetic analyses of antibodies gave a satisfying basis for the clonal selection theory while also accounting for the evolution of multigene families. One is lucky indeed to have participated in these developments and also to witness the extraordinary convergent accomplishments of so many different laboratories, each with its own style of work.

Finally, a description of a recent piece of luck may serve as a coda to this antibody tale, which could be entitled, "Thought is good but you can never be smart enough." In formulating the domain hypothesis, I was aware of the fact that antibodies were seen only in vertebrate species. But what was their origin in earlier ancestor species? We did not know. After 1974, I left immunology to work in developmental biology and had decided, for various reasons, to study cell adhesion. In 1977, my colleagues and I isolated N-CAM, the neural cell adhesion molecule, the first of its kind to be characterized [see EDELMAN (1983) for a review]. N-CAM was present in many locations in the embryo, but in particular it was an important molecule serving to link cells of the central nervous system. Other CAMs were soon characterized in our laboratories and those of many others. When, together with B. A. CUNNINGHAM (a key colleague in the elucidation of Ig structure), we analyzed the cDNA of N-CAM (CUNNINGHAM et al. 1987), we were astounded and delighted to note a 27% homology with Ig domains! I promptly suggested that the whole Ig superfamily arose in evolution from a precursor gene leading to a cell adhesion molecule of the N-CAM type (EDELMAN 1987a). Recent findings of N-CAM-like molecules in species of invertebrates that lack Ig-based adaptive immunity, such as Drosophila and Aplysia, provide strong support for this hypothesis (GRENNINGLOH et al. 1990; MAYFORD et al. 1992). When we viewed these results, we experienced an epiphany second only to the day we viewed our first gels of Bence Jones and myeloma proteins.

Population thinking in the Darwinian mode was crucial to understanding the role of somatic selection in the immune system. As I have discussed elsewhere (EDELMAN 1987b, 1992), population thinking has much to contribute to our understanding of the nervous system. Mechanisms of somatic selection other than those of the immune system appear to have evolved to assure neural development and may even be crucial to thought itself (EDELMAN 1993).

I conclude this antibody tale with a truism, obvious but worth repeating. Thinking is central to science but can never be exhaustive. It helps to have luck. For luck, make observations, do experiments, and, above all, associate with the right colleagues at the right time. And then, think again.

LITERATURE CITED

ADA, G. L., 1966 Relationship of antigen to the formation of antibodies. Australas. Ann. Med. **15:** 17–23.

BALTIMORE, D., 1981 Gene conversion: some implications for immunoglobulin genes. Cell **24:** 592–594.

BRENNER, S., and C. MILSTEIN, 1966 Origin of antibody variation. Nature **211:** 242–243.

BURNET, F. M., 1959 *The Clonal Selection Theory of Acquired Immunity.* Vanderbilt University Press, Nashville.

COHN, M., 1971 The take home lesson. Ann. N.Y. Acad. Sci. **190:** 529–584.

CRICK, F. H. C., L. HOOD, O. SMITHIES, W. J. DREYER, C. MILSTEIN *et al.,* 1967 General discussion on theories of antibody variability. Cold Spring Harbor Symp. Quant. Biol. **32:** 169–172.

CUNNINGHAM, B. A., M. N. PFLUMM, U. RUTISHAUSER and G. M. EDELMAN, 1969 Subgroups of amino acid sequences in the variable regions of immunoglobulin heavy chains. Proc. Natl. Acad. Sci. USA **64:** 997–1003.

CUNNINGHAM, B. A., J. J. HEMPERLY, B. A. MURRAY, E. A. PREDIGER, R. BRACKENBURY *et al.,* 1987 Neural cell adhesion molecule: structure, immunoglobulin-like domains, cell surface modulation and alternative RNA splicing. Science **236:** 799–806.

DREYER, W. J., and J. C. BENNETT, 1965 The molecular basis of antibody formation: a paradox. Proc. Natl. Acad. Sci. USA **54:** 864–869.

EDELMAN, G. M., 1959 Dissociation of γ-globulin. J. Am. Chem. Soc. **81:** 3155.

EDELMAN, G. M., 1970 The covalent structure of a human γG-immunoglobulin. XI. Functional implications. Biochemistry **9:** 3197–3204.

EDELMAN, G. M., 1973 Antibody structure and molecular immunology, pp. 145–170 in *Les Prix Nobel en 1972.* Nobel Foundation, Stockholm.

EDELMAN, G. M., 1983 Cell adhesion molecules. Science **219:** 450–457.

EDELMAN, G. M., 1987a CAMs and Igs: cell adhesion and the evolutionary origins of immunity. Immunol. Rev. **100:** 11–45.

EDELMAN, G. M., 1987b *Neural Darwinism: The Theory of Neuronal Group Selection.* Basic Books, New York.

EDELMAN, G. M., 1992 *Bright Air, Brilliant Fire: On the Matter of the Mind.* Basic Books, New York.

EDELMAN, G. M., 1993 Neural Darwinism: selection and reentrant signaling in higher brain function. Neuron **10:** 115–125.

EDELMAN, G. M., and J. A. GALLY, 1962 The nature of Bence-Jones proteins. J. Exp. Med. **116:** 207–227.

EDELMAN, G. M., and J. A. GALLY, 1967 Somatic recombination of duplicated genes: a hypothesis on the origin of antibody diversity. Proc. Natl. Acad. Sci. USA **57:** 353–358.

EDELMAN, G. M., and J. A. GALLY, 1968 Antibody structure, diversity, and specificity. Brookhaven Symp. Biol. **21:** 328–344.

EDELMAN, G. M., and GALLY, J. A., 1970 Arrangement and evolution of eukaryotic genes, pp. 962–972 in *Neuroscience: Second Study Program,* edited by F. O. SCHMITT. Rockefeller University Press, New York.

EDELMAN, G. M., and M. D. POULIK, 1961 Studies on structural units of the globulins. J. Exp. Med. **113:** 861–884.

EDELMAN, G. M., B. A. CUNNINGHAM, W. E. GALL, P. D. GOTTLIEB, U. RUTISHAUSER *et al.,* 1969 The covalent structure of an entire γG-immunoglobulin molecule. Proc. Natl. Acad. Sci. USA **63:** 78–85.

EGEL, R., 1981 Intergenic conversion and reiterated genes. Nature **290:** 191–192.

FLEISHMAN, J. B., R. H. PAIN and R. R. PORTER, 1962 Reductions of γ-globulins. Arch. Biochem. Biophys. Suppl. **1:** 174–180.

FLEISHMAN, J. B., R. R. PORTER and E. M. PRESS, 1963 The arrangement of the peptide chains in gamma-globulin. Biochem. J. **88:** 220–228.

GALLY, J. A., and G. M. EDELMAN, 1972 The genetic control of immunoglobulin synthesis. Annu. Rev. Genet. **6:** 1–46.

GELIEBTER, J., and S. G. NATHENSON, 1988 Microrecombinations generate sequence diversity in the murine major histocompatibility complex: analysis of the K^{bm3}, K^{bm4}, K^{bm10}, and K^{bm11} mutants. Mol. Cell. Biol. **8:** 4342–4352.

GRENNINGLOH, G., A. BIEBER, J. REHM, P. SNOW, Z. TRAQUINA *et al.,* 1990 Molecular genetics of neuronal recognition in Drosophila: evolution and function of immunoglobulin superfamily cell adhesion molecules. Cold Spring Harbor Symp. Quant. Biol. **55:** 327–340.

HILL, R. L., R. DELANEY, R. R. FELLOWS, JR., and H. E. LEBOVITZ, 1966 The evolutionary origins of immunoglobulins. Proc. Natl. Acad. Sci. USA **56:** 1762–1769.

HILSCHMANN, N., and L. C. CRAIG, 1965 Amino acid sequence studies with Bence-Jones proteins. Proc. Natl. Acad. Sci. USA **53:** 1403–1409.

HOOD, L., W. R. GRAY, B. G. SANDERS and W. J. DREYER, 1967 Light chain evolution. Cold Spring Harbor Symp. Quant. Biol. **32:** 133–146.

LANDSTEINER, K., 1945 *The Specificity of Serological Reactions,* Ed. 2. Harvard University Press, Cambridge, Mass.

LISKAY, R. M., and J. L. STACHELEK, 1983 Evidence for intrachromosomal gene conversion in cultured mouse cells. Cell **35:** 157–165.

MAIZELS, N., 1987 Diversity achieved by diverse mechanisms: gene conversion in developing B cells of the chicken. Cell **48:** 359–360.

MAYFORD, M., A. BARZILAI, F. KELLER, S. SCHACHER and E. R. KANDEL, 1992 Modulation of an NCAM-related adhesion molecule with long-term synaptic plasticity in *Aplysia.* Science **256:** 638–644.

OLINS, D. E., and G. M. EDELMAN, 1964 Reconstitution of 7S molecules from L and H polypeptide chains of antibodies and γ-globulins. J. Exp. Med. **119:** 799–815.

PAULING, L., 1940 Theory of structure and process of formation of antibodies. J. Am. Chem. Soc. **62:** 2643–2657.

PORTER, R. R., 1959 The hydrolysis of rabbit γ-globulin and antibodies with crystalline papain. Biochem. J. **73:** 119–126.

PRESS, E. M., and N. M. HOGG, 1969 Comparative study of two immunoglobulin G-Fd-fragments. Nature **223:** 808–810.

PUTNAM, F. W., K. TITANI, M. WIKLER and T. SHINODA, 1967 Structure and evolution of kappa and lambda light chains. Cold Spring Harbor Symp. Quant. Biol. **32:** 9–30.

RUBNITZ, J., and S. SUBRAMANI, 1986 Extrachromosomal and chromosomal gene conversion in mammalian cells. Mol. Cell. Biol. **6:** 1608–1614.

SANGER, F., 1964 The chemistry of insulin, pp. 544–556 in *Nobel Lectures.* Elsevier Press, New York.

SCHWARTZ, J., and G. M. EDELMAN, 1963 Comparisons of Bence-Jones proteins and L polypeptide chains of myeloma globulins after hydrolysis with trypsin. J. Exp. Med. **118:** 41–54.

SLIGHTOM, J. L., A. E. BLECHL and O. SMITHIES, 1980 Human fetal G-gamma and A-gamma globin genes: complete nucleotide sequences suggest that DNA can be exchanged between these duplicated genes. Cell **21:** 627–638.

SMITHIES, O., 1967 The genetic basis of antibody variability. Cold Spring Harbor Symp. Quant. Biol. **32:** 161–168.

SMITHIES, O., 1995 Early days of gel electrophoresis. Genetics **139:** 1–3.

TISELIUS, A., 1937 Electrophoresis of serum globulin. Biochem. J. **31:** 313–317.

TONEGAWA, S., 1983 Somatic generation of antibody diversity. Nature **302:** 575–581.

Early Days of Gel Electrophoresis

O. Smithies

Department of Pathology, University of North Carolina, Chapel Hill, North Carolina 27599–7525

I suppose that few experimental scientists refuse an invitation to remember and to write about an exciting time in their life in front of the bench. I certainly did not when JIM CROW suggested that the fortieth anniversary of starch-gel electrophoresis was an appropriate occasion on which to reminisce.

At the present time, about 0.2 microgram of protein is quite sufficient for performing a high-resolution gel electrophoresis experiment, when the gel is silver stained. In the early 1950s, when I was a postdoctoral fellow in JACK WILLIAMS' laboratory in the Department of Physical Chemistry at the University of Wisconsin, we needed about 1,000,000 times more protein (0.2 gram) for electrophoresis in the department's (only) Tiselius moving boundary electrophoresis apparatus—itself a complex and elegant piece of equipment over five meters in length. Nor were the results particularly convincing when it came to assessing protein purity; anomalies in moving boundary electrophoresis caused large quantitative changes in the analysis to the extent that "it would ... be impractical to use the method to follow further purification" (SMITHIES 1954).

When I moved to the Connaught Laboratories at the University of Toronto shortly thereafter, my immediate superior and later friend, DAVID A. SCOTT, allowed me to choose any project I wished, provided that it was related to insulin, which was of course discovered in Toronto. I decided to look for a precursor to insulin (I never found it!). My Wisconsin experiences had shown me that the quantity of material required for moving boundary electrophoresis, together with its potential anomalies, precluded my using it as an assay, so I turned to the literature and found that the newly invented procedure of zone electrophoresis had many advantages over the moving boundary method. The chief distinction between the two methods lies in the fact that, starting with a complex mixture of proteins, the boundary method gives *overlapping* boundary separations of the type

$$[A + B + C] \rightarrow [A + B + C] \cdots B + C] \cdots C]$$

whereas zone electrophoresis gives *discrete* zone separations,

$$[A + B + C] \rightarrow [A] + [B] + [C].$$

Furthermore, zone electrophoresis on filter paper required 100 times less material. Thus, one could hope to take a complex mixture of proteins, separate them by filter paper electrophoresis, stain a strip of the paper, and test the biological activity of the separated proteins on the remaining portion of the paper. But insulin was recalcitrant: it absorbed to filter paper under all the conditions that I could devise, giving results rather like a carpet unrolling—the length of the resulting smear was proportional to the amount of protein, not to its electrophoretic mobility.

Then on Saturday, January 23rd, 1954, I visited the laboratory of ANDREW SASS-KORTSAK at the Hospital for Sick Children, Toronto, to see a new method of zone electrophoresis that he was using (KUNKEL and SLATER 1952). The method used starch *grains* as a support for the electrophoresis. It was rather like carrying out electrophoresis in a wet bed of sand, with migration occurring through the buffer in the spaces *between* the grains. I noted with envy that the starch grains were gloriously free from absorption problems, and I thought that for this reason starch might solve my problems with insulin. Unfortunately, in order to detect the protein zones after starch grain electrophoresis, it was necessary to carry out Folin chemical assays for protein on about 40 transverse slices of the moist starch bed. This I could not manage to do, for I had no technical help of any type, not even a dishwasher. Fortunately, however, my childhood memories are strong, and I recalled one day when I was about 12 years old helping my mother with the laundry and observing that the starch she used for my father's shirts was liquid when hot but turned to a jelly when cold. Remembering this, I thought that if I cooked the starch and allowed it to cool, then the proteins could migrate *through* the resulting jelly, and could subsequently be detected by

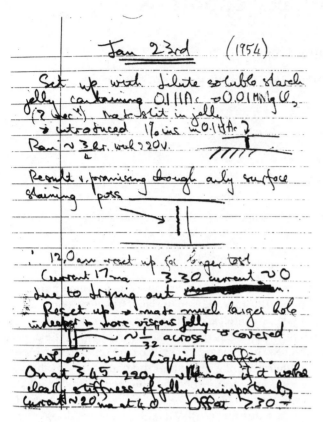

FIGURE 1.—A page from laboratory notebook I, January 23, 1954.

staining, in the way that worked with filter paper electrophoresis.

Previous nightly forays had made me cognizant of the whereabouts of all the chemical storerooms in Connaught Labs, and in one of them I found a bottle of "Starch according to Lintner." I tried cooking this Lintner starch with my electrophoretic medium (0.1 M acetic acid and 0.01 M $MgCl_2$) and found that at a concentration of about 15 g per 100 ml it gave a gooey liquid that set into a nice gel when cold. The first starch gel electrophoresis experiment was promptly performed in the afternoon of that same Saturday with purified insulin, using 220 V across the electrodes for $^3/_4$ hour. (In 1954, the University of Toronto still had 220-V *direct* current in some electric outlets, so that power supplies were not needed.) Figure 1 shows my lab notebook page of that day with a sketch of the resulting gel (no Polaroids!) and the happy comment, "Result v. promising."

About two months later, on Tuesday, March 23rd at 10:30 p.m. (with a bachelor's disregard for the time of day and night), out of curiosity I tried a short run with serum, "just for rough test." It looked good, and at midnight I had set up my first real test of starch gel electrophoresis of serum. On the following day my notebook contains the comment "Total ~11 components!" (Figure 2). Since at that time we always talked about five serum proteins (albumin and α_1, α_2, β, and γ globulins), it was with neither qualms nor regrets that I forever left my search for the precursor of insulin and concentrated on serum. (DAVID SCOTT was a tolerant boss, and we weren't dependent on grants.)

Then followed a busy seven months tuning up the method. In doing this I used serum from myself and from my two graduate-student friends, GORDON H. DIXON, now a distinguished professor at the University of Calgary, and GEORGE E. CONNELL, now a highly regarded past president of the University of Toronto. The results were very similar with these various sera (Figure 3) and I was about ready to publish when, on October 26th, I ran a gel on the serum of BETH WADE, CHARLIE HANES' technician. Figure 4 shows the result. "Most odd—many extra components."

At first, I thought the difference was sex determined, to the surprise of all and sundry. But after a week or so of running daily tests on serum from a male and from a female, my M and F patterns reversed, with a notebook comment, "must have muddled sera." But I had not, and I began to suspect the existence of genetic differences (later shown to be in the plasma protein haptoglobin), as indicated by the brief comment, "Hereditary factors may determine the serum groups" in my paper describing the starch gel procedure and the results obtained with it (SMITHIES 1955).

To investigate this possibility, I joined forces with NORMA FORD WALKER, who was Head of the Department of Genetics at the Hospital for Sick Children. She was to a large degree my first real, albeit informal teacher of genetics. In truth, we just learned together about what eventually became the new field of protein polymorphisms (SMITHIES and WALKER 1955). We also learned the hard way that the haptoglobin levels of infants are usually very low, and that nonpaternity in a family will challenge (but eventually confirm) a good genetic hypothesis. Serum haptoglobin types are still used as a common polymorphic trait in forensic situations, and their molecular biology has proved almost inexhaustibly interesting (MAEDA and SMITHIES 1986).

For quite some time after the starch gel technique was working, we did not know the correct identity of the protein bands that were resolved. Only when my friend and collaborator M. DAVID POULIK set out to compare the results of filter paper electrophoresis and starch gel electrophoresis were the true properties of the starch gels recognized (POULIK and SMITHIES 1958). We found that many proteins migrated through starch gels in an order different from their migration through the strictly aqueous buffer surrounding filter paper fibers. We realized that "the high degree of resolution obtained [in the starch gels] . . . appears to be

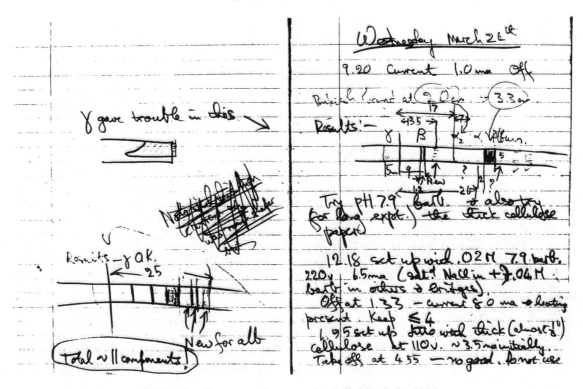

FIGURE 2.—Two pages from notebook II, March 24, 1954.

due to the use of a supporting medium the pore size of which approaches the molecular dimensions of some of the proteins." Two-dimensional electrophoresis was conceived and born as a result of this realization, with filter paper in one dimension and starch gel in the other (SMITHIES and POULIK 1956). With it we proudly resolved about 20 protein spots in serum. A measure of progress since those halcyon days is that two-dimensional electrophoresis of serum can now resolve more than 750 protein spots (ANDERSON and ANDERSON 1991).

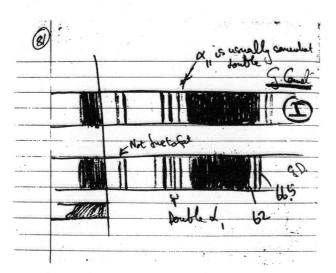

FIGURE 3.—A page from notebook IV, October 15, 1954.

It took GEORGE CONNELL, GORDON DIXON and me about another three years to work out the molecular genetics of the serum haptoglobins at the protein level, by which time I was back in Wisconsin, now a molecular geneticist rather than a physical chemist. There are still many stories to tell about those days, but they must wait for another time—although I cannot close without recalling the day (after returning to Madison from a consultation in Toronto with GEORGE and GORDON) on which I asked JIM CROW, "Is it possible for two allelic genes on homologous chromosomes to join together and give a double-sized gene?" His response was to introduce me to the *Bar* locus in Drosophila, with its long and fascinating history of homologous and nonhomologous recombination and gene duplication (STURTEVANT 1925; BRIDGES 1936). This introduction served me well. With it as a clue, we solved the intricacies of the "many extra components" of haptoglobin (SMITHIES *et al.* 1962). Extensions of the ideas of homologous and nonhomologous recombination continue to be enthralling in these days of gene targeting. My most recent paper, as it happens, talks about using homologous recombination (gene targeting) to duplicate genes in order to analyze quantitative genetic traits in mice (SMITHIES and KIM 1994). We find that simply duplicating a gene at its normal chromosomal locus is sufficient to cause a modest increase in the amount of gene product without any obvious changes in gene regulation. I imagine that JIM CROW will enjoy this continuity of

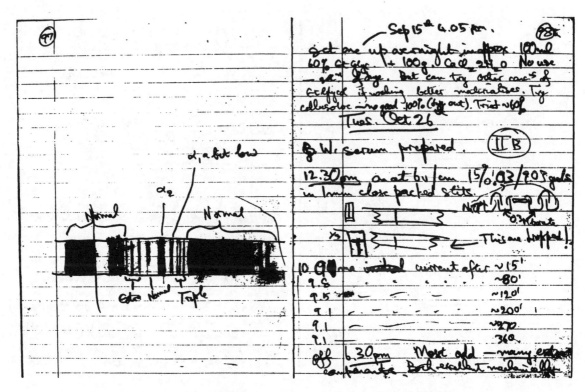

FIGURE 4.—Three days later, the first evidence of genetic differences.

thought, as I do, and as the mother of the 12-year-old boy would have done if she were still alive.

LITERATURE CITED

ANDERSON, N. L., and N. G. ANDERSON, 1991 A two-dimensional gel database of human plasma proteins. Electrophoresis **12:** 883–906.

BRIDGES, C. B., 1936 The "bar" gene, a duplication. Science **83:** 210–211.

KUNKEL, H. G., and R. J. SLATER, 1952 Zone electrophoresis in a starch supporting medium. Proc. Soc. Exp. Biol. Med. **80:** 42–44.

MAEDA, N., and O. SMITHIES, 1986 The evolution of multigene families: human haptoglobin genes. Annu. Rev. Genet. **20:** 81–108.

POULIK, M. D., and O. SMITHIES, 1958 Comparison and combination of the starch-gel and filter-paper electrophoretic methods applied to human sera: two-dimensional electrophoresis. Biochem. J. **68:** 636–643.

SMITHIES, O., 1954 The application of four methods for assessing protein homogeneity to crystalline β-lactoglobulin: an anomaly in phase rule solubility tests. Biochem. J. **58:** 31–38.

SMITHIES, O., 1955 Zone electrophoresis in starch gels: group variations in the serum proteins of normal human adults. Biochem. J. **61:** 629–641.

SMITHIES, O., and KIM, H.-S., 1994 Targeted gene duplication and disruption for analyzing quantitative genetic traits in mice. Proc. Natl. Acad. Sci. USA **91:** 3612–3615.

SMITHIES, O., and M. D. POULIK, 1956 Two-dimensional electrophoresis of serum proteins. Nature **177:** 1033.

SMITHIES, O., and N. F. WALKER, 1955 Genetic control of some serum proteins in normal humans. Nature **176:** 1265–1266.

SMITHIES, O., G. E. CONNELL and G. H. DIXON, 1962 Chromosomal rearrangements and the evolution of haptoglobin genes. Nature **196:** 232–236.

STURTEVANT, A. H., 1925 The effects of unequal crossing over at the bar locus in Drosophila. Genetics **10:** 117–147.

February 1995

The Fifties and the Renaissance
in Human and Mammalian Cytogenetics

Orlando J. Miller

Center for Molecular Medicine and Genetics and Department of Obstetrics and Gynecology,
Wayne State University School of Medicine, Detroit, Michigan 48201

THE period from 1956 to 1962 was seminal for human and mammalian cytogenetics. The human chromosome number and normal human karyotype were established, along with those of many other mammals. The high incidence and severe effects of human aneuploidy were discovered, along with the critical importance of the Y chromosome in mammalian sex determination, the nature of the sex-chromatin (Barr) body, the mechanism of dosage compensation for genes on the X chromosome, and the late replication of constitutive and facultative heterochromatin. The involvement of chromosome changes in malignancy began to be clarified, setting the stage for understanding their role in activating cellular oncogenes and the discovery of tumor suppressor genes. The single active X hypothesis (LYON 1961) remains the most powerful theoretical statement in mammalian cytogenetics.

The watershed publication by JOE HIN TJIO and AL-BERT LEVAN (1956) established the correct human chromosome number as $2n = 46$, not 48 as stated in all the textbooks at that time. This discovery was made possible by advances in cell culture technique and by the use of colchicine as a spindle poison and hypotonic treatment prior to fixation as a way to improve the spreading of metaphase chromosomes (the serendipitous discovery of T. C. HSU in 1952). It also took courage to deny a universally accepted ''fact.'' The renaissance of mammalian cytogenetics was marked by several bold rejections of accepted observations or hypotheses, and this was the first. TJIO and LEVAN pointed out that their finding might not be completely general, because it was based on the study of somatic cells in culture. It was, therefore, important that CHARLES FORD and JOHN HAMERTON (1956) found $2n = 46$ in human spermatogonia and $n = 23$ in testicular first meiotic divisions, thus ruling out the presence of germline-limited chromosomes and confirming $2n = 46$. Their chiasma counts (mean of 56 per cell) provided a still-useful minimum estimate of 28 morgans as the genetic length of human chromosomes in older males.

The human chromosome number, $2n = 46$, was confirmed in at least 74 individuals by 1958. Mitotic chromosomes showed clear morphologic features, such as length and arm ratio, that enabled workers to distinguish three to five chromosome pairs individually and to place all the chromosomes into seven groups: *1–3, 4–5, 6–12 + X, 13–15, 16–18, 19–20,* and *21–22 + Y*. A standard nomenclature for the karyotype was proposed in Denver by the seven groups who had published papers on the normal karyotype by early 1960. This was almost universally accepted and used with minimal modification for ten years. A number of methodological improvements, such as the air-drying technique for flattening chromosomes that K. H. ROTHFELS and L. SIMINOVICH introduced in 1958, made chromosome studies easier. Most important was the discovery by MOORHEAD *et al.* (1960) that phytohemagglutinin is a potent mitogen for human peripheral blood lymphocytes; this made it possible to do a chromosome study on virtually anyone, using only a few drops of blood instead of a tissue or bone marrow biopsy. The demonstration by STEELE and BREG (1966) that amniotic fluid cells could be grown in culture and karyotyped opened the floodgates still wider, permitting prenatal screening of pregnancies at high risk for chromosomally unbalanced complements.

There was great excitement when JEROME LEJEUNE and associates announced in late 1958 that individuals with Down syndrome, then called mongolism, have 47 chromosomes, as first suggested by WAARDENBURG in 1932, and are trisomic for a G-group chromosome, which they called number *21*. They confirmed this in a total of nine patients with Down syndrome and published the results in January, 1959. The race was on to find other disease states due to a chromosome imbalance, and some journals pushed the pace by publishing particularly timely reports in as little as two weeks from receipt of the manuscript. That's how long my first chromosome paper (FORD *et al.* 1959a) took, in April of that year.

The presence of multiple malformations involving almost every organ system in *21*-trisomic individuals led to the idea that trisomy for other chromosomes might cause malformation syndromes as distinctive as Down syndrome. Sure enough, two such syndromes were reported in 1960 in back-to-back papers, the one by EDWARDS *et al.* dealing with trisomy for an E-group chromosome and the one by PATAU *et al.* with trisomy for a D-group chromosome. Despite vigorous efforts, no further autosomal trisomies (nor any monosomies) were found in people until 1966, when THORBURN and JOHNSON reported a case of G-group monosomy. Because there was no reason to expect nondisjunction to be limited to only three of the 22 autosomes, an alternative explanation for the failure to observe most trisomies or monosomies gained favor: that most of these severe chromosome imbalances have lethal effects during embryonic or fetal development. Indeed, PENROSE and DELHANTY (1961) had found a macerated fetus to be triploid. DAVID CARR (1963 and later) carried out an intensive study of aborted embryos and fetuses and found that about 40% of these were chromosomally abnormal, with trisomy being most common, and involving chromosomes of every group. Because 15% of recognized pregnancies are spontaneously aborted, these results indicated that about 3% of pregnancies are trisomic, 1% triploid, and 1% *XO*, almost all being embryonic lethals. The meiotic process was errorprone!

LEJEUNE's original observations on Down syndrome were quickly confirmed by other groups, who then turned their attention to the exceptional cases: those born to young mothers (the incidence rising exponentially with increasing maternal age), and familial cases. In 1960, three groups reported Down syndrome in patients with 46 chromosomes, including what they interpreted as a D/G or a G/G Robertsonian-type translocation. The report by PENROSE *et al.* (1960) included examples of both types, and one parent had not only the same G/G translocation as the affected child, but also a tiny fragment thought to represent the reciprocal translocation product, an extremely rare finding. The slightly earlier report by MARCO FRACCARO, K. KAIJSER and JAN LINDSTEN illustrates some of the limitations of nonbanded karyotype analysis. The affected child had 46 chromosomes, but the father had 47: both had an extra F-group (*19–20*) chromosome, probably a G/G translocation, but that would have meant the father had two extra G-group (*21–22 + Y*) chromosomes. Was he also *XYYY*? The authors did not suggest that, but concluded he might be *19*-trisomic, even though that left his normal phenotype and the translocation trisomic child unexplained. Most of us experienced similar difficulties in interpretation because of the limited ability to identify extra or rearranged chromosomes. Fortunately, interphase sex chromatin bodies provided an

independent means to evaluate the *X* chromosome complement.

Sex chromosome abnormalities were quickly found to be quite common in humans and responsible for relatively mild phenotypic abnormalities. PATRICIA JACOBS and J. A. STRONG's report of an *XXY* complement in a chromatin-positive male with Klinefelter syndrome appeared in January 1959, and three months later CHARLES FORD *et al.* (1959a,b) reported an *XXY, 21*-trisomic complement in a man with both Klinefelter and Down syndromes, and an *XO* complement in a female with Turner syndrome. The choice of these patients for karyotype analysis was based on the earlier observations that females with Turner syndrome, like normal males, lack a sex chromatin body (are chromatin negative), and males with Klinefelter syndrome, like normal females, are chromatin positive. Each was considered a type of sex reversal by some investigators, although in 1956 PAUL POLANI and associates suggested that chromatin-negative Turner females were *XO*, and E. R. PLUNKET and M. L. BARR suggested that chromatin-positive Klinefelter males were *XXY*. In 1957, MATILDA DANON and LEO SACHS observed patches of skin that were chromatin-positive mixed with patches that were chromatin-negative in two females with Turner syndrome and suggested that these patients were *XO/XX* or *XY/XX* mosaics. Chromosome studies in 1959 led CHARLES FORD and associates to the direct demonstration of *XO* and *XO/XX* mosaic karyotypes in Turner females.

My involvement in human cytogenetics began in 1958 when, after an obstetrics and gynecology residency at Yale, I went to the Galton Laboratory in London to work with LIONEL PENROSE to delineate genetic causes of infertility and sexual abnormality. The slight degree of mental subnormality of some men with Klinefelter syndrome led us, and others, to screen institutions for the mentally retarded, PENROSE's favorite place for research. In this way, we identified a large number of males with Klinefelter syndrome and variants and were thus well positioned to apply the new chromosome techniques in collaborative studies with CHARLES FORD and DAVID HARNDEN. This led to the identification of the first *XXY, 21*-trisomic male (FORD *et al.* 1959a) and the first *XXYY* male (ELLIS *et al.* 1961). (I also screened a prison, with comparable results, probably reflecting a comparable concentration of mildly retarded individuals in both types of institution.) I continued this approach after moving to Columbia University and, with ROY BREG (Yale), analyzed other sex chromosome abnormalities. In 1961, we reported a chromatin three-positive *XXXXY* male who was phenotypically similar to the one MARCO FRACCARO and JAN LINDSTEN had first reported in 1960 as an *XXY, 8*-trisomic, *11*-trisomic Klinefelter male but later reinterpreted after finding three Barr bodies in some cells. This case serves to re-emphasize the limitations of the techniques and the lack of information on the phenotypic effects of most autosomal trisomies in 1960.

The discovery of individuals with unusual sex chromosome complements provided the key to understanding mammalian sex determination. XO individuals were female and XXY individuals male, indicating that the Y chromosome is male-determining. This is quite different from the situation in Drosophila, where sex is determined by the balance between the number of X chromosomes and the number of autosome sets. Thus, in Drosophila, diploid XO flies are male and XXY flies female, just the reverse of the human situation. Even the presence of three or four X chromosomes in the human complement did not overcome the male-determining effect of a single Y chromosome. However, intersexual development could occur when only a fraction of the cells had a Y chromosome, as in an XO/XY mosaic (KURT HIRSCHHORN et al. 1960) and an XX/XY chimera produced by double fertilization (STAN GARTLER et al. 1962).

Individuals with three or four X chromosomes in their diploid complement provided a critical insight into the nature of the sex chromatin (Barr) body discovered by MURRAY BARR and M. A. BERTRAM in 1949. This was present as a nucleolus-associated chromatin mass in the neurons of female, but not male, cats and other mammals, and as a nuclear membrane-associated chromatin mass in epithelial cells of female mammals. Barr suggested that this frequently bipartite body arose from paired heterochromatic segments of the two X chromosomes. This hypothesis became so well established it initially led SUSUMU OHNO and his associates in 1958 to interpret the single heteropycnotic X chromosome of mouse mitotic prophase cells in the following way: "At prophase the two X chromosomes, in positively heteropycnotic state, were found, without exception, to be in end-to-end association." Hypothesis influences (and sometimes misguides) observation! However, a year later, OHNO et al. (1959) offered a different interpretation of identical findings in the rat, reporting that these showed a single heteropycnotic prophase chromosome, and proposing that the sex chromatin body arises from a single X chromosome. What led to this critical reinterpretation? The authors never said. However, at about the same time, JACOBS et al. (1959) reported an XXX female who had two sex chromatin bodies in many cells, and in the same year Murray Barr's group reported the presence of two sex chromatin bodies in three males with Klinefelter syndrome (later shown to be XXXY). Seven more XXX females were reported in 1960; they, as well as the two XXXY males reported by FERGUSON-SMITH et al. (1960), had two chromatin masses, while the XXXXY males referred to above had three. OHNO's hypothesis offered a simple explanation of these results and was an important precursor of the LYON hypothesis.

The most profound theoretical insight to come out of the renaissance in mammalian cytogenetics was the single-active-X hypothesis formulated by MARY LYON (1961). This short paper in Nature is a model of terse, critical argument: (1) XO mice have a normal female phenotype (reported by WILLIAM WELSHONS and LIANE B. RUSSELL in 1959); (2) all sex-linked mutants affecting coat color in the mouse have a mottled or dappled phenotype, with patches of normal color and patches of mutant color; (3) a similar phenotype, described as "variegated," is seen in female mice heterozygous for coat color mutants translocated on to the X chromosome (reported by RUSSELL and BANGHAM in 1959 and 1960).

MARY LYON's hypothesis followed: "It is here suggested that this mosaic phenotype is due to the inactivation of one or the other X-chromosome early in embryonic development. If this is true, pigment cells descended from cells in which the chromosome carrying the mutant gene was inactivated will give rise to a normal-coloured patch and those in which the chromosome carrying the normal gene was inactivated will give rise to a mutant-coloured patch." The utter simplicity of this formulation allowed no misinterpretation. Furthermore, the two final arguments she presented indicate her awareness that the single-active-X hypothesis applied to all mammals: (4) in embryos of the cat, monkey, and human, sex chromatin is first found in nuclei of the late blastocyst stage (with reference to two 1957 papers); (5) the sex chromatin is thought to be formed from one X chromosome in the rat and opossum (referring to 1959 and 1960 papers of OHNO et al.).

In 1962, LYON gave a fuller discussion of the various components of her powerful hypothesis, with particular reference to human disease phenotypes. In this paper, she tried to share some credit, pointing out that, simultaneously with the original publication of her own hypothesis, L. B. RUSSELL (1961) put forward a very similar but more limited one concerning variegation due to sex-linked translocations in the mouse. Russell considered that the variegation was "presumably a heterochromatic effect" and, from the fact that two X chromosomes were essential for its expression, together with cytological evidence, postulated that "in animals, genic balance requires the action of one X in a manner which precludes realization of its heterochromatic potentialities, so that only additional X's present assume the properties characteristic of heterochromatin." In this paper and another published the same year in GENETICS, RUSSELL called this phenomenon "some kind of V-type position effect," a well known but poorly understood phenomenon in Drosophila. In fact, transcriptional inactivation of the variegating gene was first demonstrated by STEVEN HENIKOFF in Drosophila only in 1979.

Although her formulations lacked the clarity and generality that has made the LYON hypothesis so useful, L. B. RUSSELL was closer, in 1961, to understanding X inactivation than anyone else. More limited attempts had been made to account for the sexual dimorphism in sex chromatin. In a short letter to *Lancet* in 1960, J. S. S. STEWART stated, "There is a very simple explanation for the presence of the sex chromatin body: In the intermitotic metabolic nucleus the heterochromatin of one X chromosome is apparently necessary for and engaged in the metabolic business of the cell and therefore not stainable. The heterochromatin of any other X chromosome is, however, superfluous to metabolic requirements, functionally inert at this time, and therefore stainable." Little attention was paid to this hypothesis because no supporting evidence was presented, and heterochromatin was generally regarded as having no metabolic functions; "facultative heterochromatin" was not yet an established concept in mammals.

MARY LYON's 1961 paper in *Nature* was like a bolt out of the blue, providing the insight that allowed the rest of us to make sense out of a diverse array of findings. For example, J. HERBERT TAYLOR (1960) had observed asynchronous replication of one arm of the two X chromosomes of the Chinese hamster, which GEORGE YERGANIAN said bolstered his own hypothesis, based on morphologic differences, of an $X_1 X_2 / X_1 Y$ sex-determining mechanism in this species. The LYON hypothesis favored a different explanation: that the arm of the X chromosome which replicates early in XY cells but late in XX cells is active and euchromatic in XY cells but inactive and heterochromatic in XX cells. This fit well with the finding by LIMA-DE-FARIA (1959) that heterochromatin is late-replicating in the insect Melanoplus and the plant Secale, and was supported by later studies, such as that of GRUMBACH in 1963, showing that the number of late-replicating X chromosomes in humans is the same as the number of Barr bodies and one less than the number of X chromosomes.

Tests of the LYON hypothesis were not long in coming. MEL GRUMBACH and associates showed in 1962 that the level of X-linked G6PD enzyme activity was the same in individuals with one, two, three, or four X chromosomes. ERNEST BEUTLER and his associates demonstrated in the same year that two populations of red blood cells are present in G6PD heterozygotes, and the following year RON DAVIDSON and associates showed the clonal nature of G6PD-A and G6PD-B fibroblasts in such heterozygotes, using a method that has been used many times since then to determine whether an X-linked gene shows "Lyonization" or escapes X inactivation. BARID MUKHERJEE and ANIL SINHA showed in 1964 that X inactivation was random in XX cells, taking advantage of the dimorphic X chromosomes in a horse–ass hybrid, the mule. Exceptions to one or another aspect of the LYON hypothesis have been discovered,

such as non-random inactivation in X-autosome translocation heterozygotes and reactivation of the second X in oocytes, but despite such exceptions this hypothesis continues to spark novel experiments and lead to new insights. One of these was the clonal origin of many neoplasms, such as chronic myeloid leukemia, and the common origin of erythroid and granulocyte lineages (FIALKOW *et al.* 1967). One of the most interesting was OHNO's recognition that the presence of a single active X in mammalian somatic cells would greatly restrict the transfer of genes between X and autosomes because of dosage effects, and his resultant hypothesis that the X chromosome of all placental mammals should carry the same genes and have the same amount of euchromatin. Measurements in a diverse series of mammals supported this hypothesis (OHNO *et al.* 1964), as have more recent mapping studies.

Throughout the 1950s, SAJIRO MAKINO, ALBERT LEVAN, GEORGE KLEIN, and others had demonstrated that ascites and some other cancer cell lines tend to be mitotically unstable and show highly variable chromosome numbers. Aneuploid cells with a specific number were usually most common within a line and tended to persist, leading to a "stem cell" concept, the precursor of today's much better established "clonal" origin of most cancer cell lineages. The first definitive evidence of an association between a specific chromosome change and a particular malignancy was the discovery of a partially deleted G-group chromosome in human chronic myeloid leukemia (CML) cells by PETER NOWELL and DAVID HUNGERFORD (1960). They initially interpreted this as a deletion involving the Y (both patients being male), but soon discovered the same Ph1 (Philadelphia) chromosome in CML in females. The occcurrence of a constitutional deletion involving a D-group chromosome in one of six patients with a retinoblastoma was described by LELE *et al.* (1963), who pointed out that the deletion might be causal and indicate the location of the retinoblastoma gene. In fact, although only a small number of such deletions have been studied, their cytogenetic analysis guided the mapping of the autosomal dominant retinoblastoma gene to the 13q14 region, its positional cloning, and its recognition as a tumor suppressor gene.

Despite much effort, additional insights into chromosomal causes of cancer were slow in coming in the pre-banding era. Increased chromosome breakage and rearrangement was observed in 1964 in two autosomal recessive disorders associated with an increased risk of cancer: Fanconi anemia by TRAUTE SCHROEDER and Bloom syndrome by JAMES GERMAN. Perhaps the first evidence for tumor suppressor genes was derived by chromosome segregation analysis in somatic cell hybrids between malignant and nonmalignant murine cells (HARRIS *et al.* 1969). HENRY HARRIS showed that these hybrids were initially nonmalignant but tended to regain their ability to grow as tumors when injected into histocompatible mice. While on sabbatical leave with HARRIS, I showed that the return of the malignant phenotype was associated with loss of chromosomes from the nonmalignant parent, suggesting that loss of a specific tumor suppressor gene on one chromosome was responsible. Unfortunately, the methods then available did not permit identification of individual mouse chromosomes.

Improvement in methods for chromosome identification was very limited throughout the sixties. Symbolic of this were the minimal modifications adopted at the Conference on Standardization in Human Cytogenetics in 1966 at the International Congress of Human Genetics in Chicago: (1) "chromosome short arms are designated p and long arms q" (p for petite, at JEROME LEJEUNE's suggestion, and q because all geneticists know that p + q = 1!); and (2) "autoradiographic DNA replication patterns may help identify chromosomes *4, 5, 13, 14, 15, 17* and *18.*" Thus, GERMAN et al. (1964) showed that the deleted (*5p*) chromosome in the cri du chat syndrome discovered the year before by JEROME LEJEUNE had a characteristic replication pattern, and WOLF et al. (1965) emphasized that the deleted (*4p*) chromosome in their patient with a clinically different syndrome had the other replication pattern found in the B group. We and others identified abnormal chromosomes in B, D, and E groups in this way, but were unwilling to accept unusual conclusions by another group on the basis of this rather limited technique! The excitement of the early years was gradually replaced by increasing frustration at the severe limitations imposed by the inability to identify individual chromosomes or chromosome segments in the mammals of most interest, the human and the mouse. Clearly, most inversions and translocations were being missed, and those detected were often difficult to interpret. The location of most deleted segments could not be determined, nor could the identity of extra or missing chromosomes in highly aneuploid cancer cells. Thus, by the mid to late sixties, it seemed that little more could be learned by cytogenetic analysis with the existing methods.

This rather gloomy state of mind was quickly abolished by TORBORN CASPERSSON's discovery of chromosome banding, which permitted accurate identification of every normal human chromosome and of an impressive array of structural abnormalities. His original findings, in 1968, were made in plants and enabled a distinction to be made only between euchromatin and heterochromatin. Application of his quinacrine mustard fluorescent staining technique to human chromosomes (CASPERSSON et al. 1970) revealed the power of the method to delineate a hitherto unknown level of diploid mitotic and meiotic chromosome organization, the band. Each band contains 1 to 50 or more megabase

pairs of DNA, roughly 10 to 100 or more genes, and is thus totally different from a band in polytene chromosomes. JOHN EVANS, MARINA SEABRIGHT, JEROME LEJEUNE, and others quickly discovered methods to produce a very similar banding pattern (G banding) or the reverse pattern (R banding) using Giemsa stain, and my group showed that almost every banding pattern could be produced by selective denaturation of chromosomal DNA and binding of labeled single-strand-specific antinucleoside antibodies. Most exciting was the discovery by SAM LATT and BERNARD DUTRILLAUX of a nonradioactive method for analyzing replication timing. This produced either a G-band or an R-band pattern, depending on whether BrdU is incorporated early or late in the S phase, and demonstrated that G bands replicate late and R bands replicate early.

The introduction of chromosome banding made individual identification of every chromosome routine and led to an explosive growth in knowledge. Trisomies of every chromosome were identified in abortuses. Translocations, deletions and inversions were identified in great abundance in malformation syndromes or cancer. The specific chromosome change in chronic myelogenous leukemia was shown by JANET ROWLEY to be a specific translocation. The role of this translocation in activating the *c-abl* proto-oncogene by placing it 3′ to the strong promoter of the *bcr* gene was demonstrated in the present molecular era. Dozens of additional translocations have since been shown to be specifically associated with other cancers, some activating other proto-oncogenes. Banding analysis made it possible to identify any human chromosome remaining in mouse-human hybrid cells and thus to map a specific gene quickly (MILLER et al. 1971b). This technique has been widely used to maps hundreds of genetic markers to specific chromosomes in the human and a few other mammals, and it set the stage for the Human Genome Initiative. We showed that even the 20 pairs of similarly sized telocentric chromosomes of the mouse could be individually identified by their banding patterns, and we were able to assign mouse linkage groups to specific chromosomes by identifying the chromosomes involved in a series of translocations involving known linkage groups (MILLER et al. 1971a). JONASSON, HARRIS, KLEIN and their colleagues showed in 1974 that specific loss of mouse chromosome *4* contributed by the nonmalignant parent of hybrid cells led to malignancy, *i.e.*, mouse chromosome *4* carries a tumor suppressor gene.

Chromosome banding made possible a second renaissance in human and mammalian cytogenetics, but in retrospect we can only marvel at how much was accomplished with the simple tools available in the prebanding days of the fifties and early sixties, a time that truly deserves to be called the first renaissance in this field.

LITERATURE CITED

BEUTLER, E., M. YEH and V. F. FAIRBANKS, 1962 The normal human female as a mosaic of X-chromosome activity: studies using the gene for G-6-PD deficiency as a marker. Proc. Natl. Acad. Sci. USA 48: 9–16.

CARR, D. H., 1963 Chromosome studies in abortuses and stillborn infants. Lancet ii: 603–606.

CASPERSSON, T., L. ZECH and C. JOHANSSON, 1970 Analysis of human metaphase chromosome set by aid of DNA-binding fluorescent agents. Exp. Cell Res. 62: 490–492.

DAVIDSON, R. G., H. M. NITOWSKY and B. CHILDS, 1963 Demonstration of two populations of cells in the human female heterozygous for glucose-6-phosphate dehydrogenase variants. Proc. Natl. Acad. Sci. USA 50: 481–485.

EDWARDS, J. H., D. G. HARNDEN, A. H. CAMERON, V. M. CROSSE and O. H. WOLFE, 1960 A new trisomic syndrome. Lancet ii: 787–790.

ELLIS, J. R., O. J. MILLER, L. S. PENROSE and G. E. B. SCOTT, 1961 A male with XXYY chromosomes. Ann. Hum. Genet. 25: 145–151.

FERGUSON-SMITH, M. A., A. W. JOHNSTON and S. D. HANDMAKER, 1960 Primary amentia and micro-orchidism associated with an XXXY sex-chromosome constitution. Lancet ii: 184–187.

FIALKOW, P. J., S. M. GARTLER and A. YOSHIDA, 1967 Clonal origin of chronic myelocytic leukemia in man. Proc. Natl. Acad. Sci. USA 58: 1468–1471.

FORD, C. E., and J. L. HAMERTON, 1956 The chromosomes of man. Nature 178: 1020–1023.

FORD, C. E., K. W. JONES, O. J. MILLER, U. MITTWOCH, L. S. PENROSE et al., 1959a The chromosomes in a patient showing both mongolism and the Klinefelter syndrome. Lancet i: 709–710.

FORD, C. E., K. W. JONES, P. E. POLANI, J. C. DE ALMEIDA and J. H. BRIGGS, 1959b A sex-chromosome anomaly in a case of gonadal dysgenesis (Turner's syndrome). Lancet i: 711–713.

FRACCARO, M., K. KAIJSER and J. LINDSTEN, 1960 Chromosomal abnormalities in father and mongol child. Lancet i: 724–727.

GARTLER, S. M., S. H. WAXMAN and E. GIBLETT, 1962 An XX/XY human hermaphrodite resulting from double fertilization. Proc. Natl. Acad. Sci. USA 48: 332–335.

GERMAN, J., 1964 Cytological evidence for crossing-over in vitro in human lymphoid cells. Science 144: 298–301.

GERMAN, J. L., J. LEJEUNE, M. N. MACINTYRE and J. DEGROUCHY, 1964 Chromosomal autoradiography in the cri du chat syndrome. Cytogenetics 3: 347–352.

GRUMBACH, M. M., P. A. MARKS and A. MORISHIMA, 1962 Erythrocyte glucose-6-phosphate dehydrogenase activity and X-chromosome polysomy. Lancet i: 1330–1332.

HARRIS, H., O. J. MILLER, G. KLEIN, P. WORST and T. TACHIBANA, 1969 Suppression of malignancy by cell fusion. Nature 223: 363–368.

HIRSCHHORN, K., W. H. DECKER and H. L. COOPER, 1960 Human intersex with chromosome mosaicism of type XY/XO. N. Engl. J. Med. 263: 1044–1048.

JACOBS, P. A., and J. A. STRONG, 1959 A case of human intersexuality having a possible XXY sex-determining mechanism. Nature 183: 302–303.

JACOBS, P. A., A. G. BAIKIE, W. M. COURT BROWN, T. N. MACGREGOR, N. MACLEAN et al., 1959 Evidence for the existence of the human "super female." Lancet ii: 423–425.

LEJEUNE, J., M. GAUTIER and R. TURPIN, 1959 Etude des chromosomes somatique de neuf enfantes mongoliens. Compt. rend. acad. sci. 248: 1721–1722.

LELE, K. P., L. S. PENROSE and H. B. STALLARD, 1963 Chromosome deletion in a case of retinoblastoma. Ann. Hum. Genet. 27: 171–174.

LIMA-DE-FARIA, A., 1959 Differential uptake of tritiated thymidine into hetero- and euchromatin in Melanoplus and Secale. J. Biophys. Biochem. Cytol. 6: 457–466.

LYON, M. F., 1961 Gene action in the X-chromosome of the mouse (Mus musculus L.). Nature 190: 372–373.

LYON, M. F., 1962 Sex chromatin and gene action in the mammalian X-chromosome. Am. J. Hum. Genet. 14: 135–148.

MILLER, O. J., W. R. BREG, R. D. SCHMICKEL and W. TRETTER, 1961 A family with an XXXXY male, a leukemic male, and two 21-trisomic mongoloid females. Lancet ii: 78–79.

MILLER, O. J., P. W. ALLDERDICE, D. A. MILLER, W. R. BREG and B. R. MIGEON, 1971a Human thymidine kinase gene locus: assignment to chromosome 17 in a hybrid of man and mouse cells. Science 173: 244–245.

MILLER, O. J., D. A. MILLER, R. E. KOURI, P. W. ALLDERDICE, V. G. DEV et al., 1971b Identification of the mouse karyotype and tentative assignment of seven linkage groups. Proc. Natl. Acad. Sci. USA 68: 1530–1533.

MOORHEAD, P. S., P. C. NOWELL, W. J. MELLMAN, D. M. BATTIPS and D. A. HUNGERFORD, 1960 Chromosome preparations of leukocytes cultured from human peripheral blood. Exp. Cell Res. 20: 613–616.

MUKHERJEE, B. B., and A. K. SINHA, 1964 Single-active-X hypothesis: cytological evidence for random inactivation of X-chromosomes in a female mule complement. Proc. Natl. Acad. Sci. USA 51: 252–259.

NOWELL, P. C., and D. A. HUNGERFORD, 1960 Chromosome studies on normal and leukemic leukocytes. J. Natl. Cancer Inst. 25: 85–109.

OHNO, S., W. D. KAPLAN and R. KINOSITA, 1958 Somatic association of the positively heteropycnotic X-chromosomes in female mice (Mus musculus). Exp. Cell Res. 15: 616–618.

OHNO, S., W. D. KAPLAN and R. KINOSITA, 1959 Formation of the sex chromatin by a single X-chromosome in liver cells of Rattus norvegicus. Exp. Cell Res. 18: 415–418.

OHNO, S., W. BEÇAK and M. L. BEÇAK, 1964 X-autosome ratio and the behavior pattern of individual X-chromosomes in placental mammals. Chromosoma 15: 14–30.

PĀTAU, K., D. W. SMITH, E. THERMAN, S. L. INHORN and H. P. WAGNER, 1960 Multiple congenital anomaly caused by an extra autosome. Lancet i: 790–793.

PENROSE, L. S., and J. D. A. DELHANTY, 1961 Triploid cell cultures from a macerated foetus. Lancet i: 1261–1262.

PENROSE, L. S., J. R. ELLIS and J. D. A. DELHANTY, 1960 Chromosomal translocations in mongolism and in normal relatives. Lancet ii: 409–410.

RUSSELL, L. B., 1961 Genetics of mammalian sex chromosomes. Science 113: 1795–1803.

SCHROEDER, T. M., F. ANSCHÜTZ and A. KNOPP, 1964 Spontane Chromosomenaberrationen bei familiarer Panmyelopathie. Humangenetik 1: 194–196.

STEELE, M. W., and W. R. BREG, 1966 Chromosome analysis of human amniotic fluid cells. Lancet i: 383–385.

STEWART, J. S. S., 1960 Genetic mechanisms in human intersexes. Lancet i: 825.

TAYLOR, J. H., 1960 Asynchronous duplication of chromosomes in cultured cells of Chinese hamster. J. Biophys. Biochem. Cytol. 7: 455–463.

TJIO, J. H., and A. LEVAN, 1956 The chromosome number of man. Hereditas 42: 1–6.

WOLF, U., H. REINWEIN, R. PORSCH, R. SCHRÖTER and H. BAITSCH, 1965 Defizienz an den kurzen Armen eines Chromosoms Nr. 4. Humangenetik 1: 397–413.

The Cold Spring Harbor
○ Phage Course (1945–1970) ○
A Fiftieth Anniversary Remembrance

Millard Susman

Laboratory of Genetics, Medical School and College of Agricultural and Life Sciences,
University of Wisconsin–Madison, Madison, Wisconsin 53706

THIS year marks the 50th anniversary of the birth of the Cold Spring Harbor Phage Course and the 25th anniversary of its demise. The course was first taught in 1945 by MAX DELBRÜCK (with the assistance of A. H. DOERMANN and J. REYNOLDS) and last taught in 1970 by WILLIAM F. DOVE and RENÉ THOMAS. In its 25-year lifespan, the Phage Course was remarkably productive. Graduates included MARK ADAMS, MARTHA BAYLOR, SEYMOUR BENZER, ROBERT EDGAR, HERMAN KALCKAR, AARON NOVICK, FRANK STAHL, GUNTHER STENT, LEO SZILARD, NORTON ZINDER, and dozens of others whose names evoke pleasant and reverent memories of the infancy of molecular biology. The lifetime of the Phage Course coincided with a time when new ideas emerged almost as abundantly as new details, when students could be more or less familiar with the entire literature, and when field representatives from NIH frequently visited university campuses looking for ways to invest federal research funds.

The Phage Course was started by DELBRÜCK, whose missionary devotion to bacteriophage biology led to an explosion in the population of phage workers between 1940 and 1965 (LURIA 1966). The course was essential training for more than a generation of phage biologists. For some of us, it was truly an introductory course in which we learned the arts of sterile technique, serial dilution, soft agar plating, and plaque counting. For others, already skilled in basic microbiological methods, the Phage Course was a rite of passage through which ordinary microbiologists could become members of the Phage Group, a rather exclusive circle with DELBRÜCK at its center.

For DELBRÜCK, the only biology was "quantitative biology." It was not surprising, therefore, that his course for new phage workers was founded at the Cold Spring Harbor Laboratory of Quantitative Biology. Nor was it surprising that DELBRÜCK, who was trained as a physicist, looked to physics as a source of prospective quantitative biologists. He believed that the complexities of biological systems might conceal new principles of physics and that the researchers most likely to discover these new principles were physicists. He actively sought converts, and among the most distinguished students of the Phage Course were a number of physicists, coaxed by DELBRÜCK to take a little taste of biology and discover how delicious it could be.

I took the Phage Course in 1957 at Caltech, which is about as far from the Long Island home of the Course as you can get in the contiguous United States. The precedent for teaching the Cold Spring Harbor Phage Course at remote sites was established early in its history. In 1949, for example, DELBRÜCK himself offered a cloned Phage Course at Caltech for a very small class, consisting of JEAN WEIGLE and OLE MAALØE (MAALØE 1966). When I took the course, it was taught by RENÉ COHEN, a French nuclear physicist recently turned phage geneticist, and FRANK STAHL, a postdoc in the phage group. COHEN was a teacher in the DELBRÜCK tradition, bringing to the course a convert's devotion and a physicist's rigor. I retain just two vivid recollections of discussions with COHEN: in one, he explained his aversion to the "sandveetch," which was a barbarism because it had to be eaten with the fingers; in the other, he explained why it would be impossible to manufacture an optical device that could scan a petri dish and count phage plaques. The other instructor, FRANK STAHL, was working with MESELSON on ways to test the idea that DNA synthesis was semi-conservative. My clearest memory of STAHL's teaching is a chalk-talk he gave on "mating theory," a mathematical analysis of recombination in phage. The theory had appeared first in a very difficult paper by VISCONTI and DELBRÜCK (1953)—a paper Stahl considered "one of the worst ever written"—and, together with CHARLEY STEINBERG, STAHL had reworked the old problem and produced a comparatively clear and lucid theory (STEINBERG and STAHL 1958). Standing at the blackboard and explaining the mathematics, STAHL did an imitation of

DELBRÜCK. I do not know if the imitation was calculated or unconscious, but the likeness was certainly evident to anyone who had seen DELBRÜCK lecture. The exposition moved slowly, interrupted by long pauses (eyes shut tight to show intense concentration), mumbled soliloquies, and sighs of satisfaction when the pieces finally fell into place. I have always loved the STEINBERG-STAHL solution to "mating theory," partly because STAHL gave it to us that day in 1957 as if it were a gift he had received directly from the gods. DELBRÜCK himself took little part in the course—he had turned his attention by that time to phototaxis in Phycomyces—but his office was just across the hall from the teaching lab, and he dropped in from time to time to offer encouragement.

The students in this class were, I believe, DENNIS BARRETT, JOHN CAIRNS, LEA SEKELY, ILGA LIELAUSIS, ANN ROLLER, EDWARD SIMON, BARBARA SUSMAN, and me. There is some dispute about ED SIMON's exact role in the course. LEA SEKELY says he was her lab partner at the beginning of the course, but that he dropped out soon after the course began. DENNIS BARRETT, BARBARA, and I also believe that SIMON was a member of the class, but SIMON himself says he did not take the course and suggests that he was simply a "groupie." We worked in pairs. My lab partner was ILGA LIELAUSIS, who at the time was the lead worker in the phage kitchen. She was a gifted lab worker who eventually became ROBERT EDGAR's co-author on a series of papers describing temperature-sensitive mutants of phage T4. Our experiments in the Phage Course always worked because ILGA did all the pipetting. My wife, BARBARA, who at the time was MATTHEW MESELSON's technician, was paired with DENNIS BARRETT, a biochemistry graduate student who is now an Associate Professor of Biology at the University of Denver. DENNIS loved folk songs and group dancing and instigated much of the social life of Caltech graduate students. I feel that I must record here an act of heroism for which DENNIS deserves to be remembered. A large group of us graduate students organized a picnic one summer on the beach at Playa del Rey, and DENNIS volunteered to shop for the food. Everyone but DENNIS showed up on time. We spent a long, hungry afternoon watching the planes from LAX take off over our heads and wondering why DENNIS and the hot dogs had not arrived. DENNIS finally appeared, laden with grocery bags and wrapped in bandages. He had purchased our provisions and then, bags in hand, had walked through a plate glass window of the grocery store. After visiting the Emergency Room and enduring over 100 stitches, conscientious DENNIS retrieved the bags of food from the grocery store and joined the picnic.

EDWARD SIMON is now a Professor of Biology at Purdue. He was one of several students in our class who decided to confirm the MESELSON-STAHL experiment in organisms other than bacteria; ED showed with BrdU labeling that DNA synthesis was semi-conservative in HeLa cells. LEA SEKELY is now Program Director in the Chemical and Physical Carcinogenesis Program at NCI; her specific area of interest is hormonal carcinogenesis. ILGA LIELAUSIS retired from Caltech a few years ago. Unfortunately, I have not been able to trace ANN ROLLER.

Certainly the most sophisticated member of the class was JOHN CAIRNS. CAIRNS was already a well-known animal virologist. He had come to Caltech from Canberra for a four-month visit to learn from RENATO DULBECCO how to grow animal viruses in tissue culture. On discovering that the famous Cold Spring Harbor Phage Course was to be offered during that four months, CAIRNS decided to become a member of the class. He was good-looking, self-assured, spoke with an accent that was British rather than Australian, and had an innovative flair. He was admirably modest, generous and collegial, but he certainly stood out in our class. It was rather as if SIR LANCELOT had decided to attend the senior prom. JOHN and his partner, ANN ROLLER, did all the experiments with such ease that they could always manage to do something extra. It was ANN who shared the news with the class. "JOHN and I tried two higher multiplicities of infection to see if that affected the latent period." "JOHN and I think we found a few new plaque morphology mutants." Even within the confines of a scripted laboratory course, CAIRNS found ways to be original.

Graduation parties were part of the tradition of the Phage Course, probably because DELBRÜCK liked parties and looked for opportunities to arrange them (Figure 1). BARBARA and I missed the party celebrating our graduation from the Phage Course because she was pregnant and felt queasy that night. The party was at the Prufrock House—so called because it was discreetly listed in the Pasadena telephone directory under "J. A. PRUFROCK." The house was occupied by MATT MESELSON, HOWARD TEMIN, JAN DRAKE, CHARLEY STEINBERG, JOHN CAIRNS during his visit, and perhaps others whom I have forgotten. The next day, MESELSON, obviously shaken by the experience, told me about the party. The celebration began with organized silliness; for example, ILGA, blindfolded, had to use her toes to determine the agar content of the medium in several petri dishes, and ANN and JOHN had to step into a closet and recombine five of their "phenotypes" (articles of clothing) (Figure 2). The party ended with a water fight that drenched everything in the Prufrock House. The recipe for a Phage Course graduation celebration generally included generous quantities of agar, vodka, and water.

In 1960, I myself had a chance to teach the Phage Course at Cold Spring Harbor. ROBERT EDGAR was an Assistant Professor at Caltech at the time. CSH Director ARTHUR CHOVNICK invited EDGAR to teach the Phage

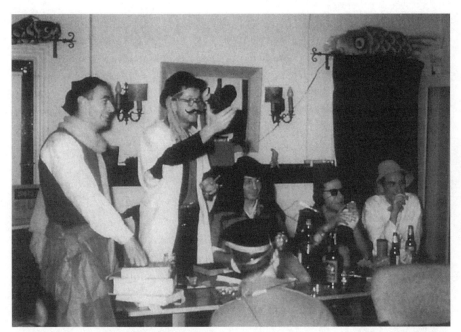

FIGURE 1.—The Board of Examiners at the Phage Course final examination and commencement exercises, held at the Prufrock House, Caltech, 1957. From the left: HARRY RUBIN, MAX DELBRÜCK, RENÉ COHEN, MATTHEW MESELSON, and FRANK STAHL. The person with his back to the camera may be HARRIS BERNSTEIN. (Photograph courtesy of DENNIS BARRETT, University of Denver.)

Course, and EDGAR offered me the opportunity to serve as his assistant. I decided this was a wonderful chance to get some teaching experience and accepted the invitation. For about five weeks that summer, I ate and slept in Blackford Hall at the Cold Spring Harbor Lab and spent most of every day with EDGAR, who was the most meticulous and conscientious of teachers. We pretested every experiment and did not give up until we could be almost certain that the experiment would work. In class, EDGAR was loud, eager, and vigilant. His pre-lab lectures were pep talks—simple, clear, well organized, and illustrated by poorly drawn diagrams with frequently misspelled labels. (The class skit featured EDGAR giving a spirited talk on the use of a spoon, which looked in the drawing like a butternut squash and was labeled "spone.") He ran a group experiment as if he were a coach training a football team. He shouted out the time in kinetics experiments, strictly and noisily enforced the rules of sterile technique, endlessly circled the room to check that the surfaces of the soft-agar plates were smooth as glass. I did learn a lot about teaching that summer and, to the extent that my more timid personality allows it, I continue to imitate EDGAR when I teach students how to do a one-step growth experiment.

EDGAR taught the portion of the lab course that dealt with virulent phages, and ED LENNOX covered the temperate phages. I believe LENNOX arrived at the Lab only a few days before his section of the course began. I remember looking forward to meeting the ingenious fellow who had used the power of phage biology to demonstrate that individual antibody-producing cells could produce one, and only one, antibody. Since LENNOX was on the scene, I find it surprising that I was the one who lectured on the kinetics of phage neutralization by antibodies. However, I remember vividly that I did give that lecture, since it was done impromptu during a class break, when EDGAR suddenly, and without prior notice, asked me if I could explain the mathematics of "one-hit" phage inactivation. Fortunately, he chose a topic that my Caltech training had prepared me to discuss. We were at the time deeply immersed in inactivation kinetics.

The able archivist at Cold Spring Harbor, CLARE BUNCE, has found the lists of instructors, students, and seminar speakers for every one of the Phage Courses from 1945 to 1970. The *only* records that have eluded the archivist's investigatory skills are the ones for the summer of 1960, when I assisted EDGAR and LENNOX. My memories of that summer at Cold Spring Harbor have faded. We had roughly 20 students, and I spent a lot of time with them, but the only ones I can name with confidence are NOBORU SUEOKA, ULF HENNING, IRWIN RUBENSTEIN, and FRED FRANKEL. SUEOKA is memorable because he was such a gifted experimentalist and had such a sharp eye. For example, he could always spot the 0.2-ml pipette in the can of 0.1-ml pipettes or the pin-point colony on a supposedly sterile petri dish, and he let us know gently that we had to prepare materials more carefully if we wanted the experiments to work. Other members of the class have become indistinguishable in my mind from the dozens of people with whom I talked and ate and swam, summer after summer, at the annual Cold Spring Harbor Phage Meetings.

I recall two notable scientific discussions that I had with BOB EDGAR that summer. The first sticks in my mind because it turned out to have damaging relevance to my own work. When we first arrived at Cold Spring

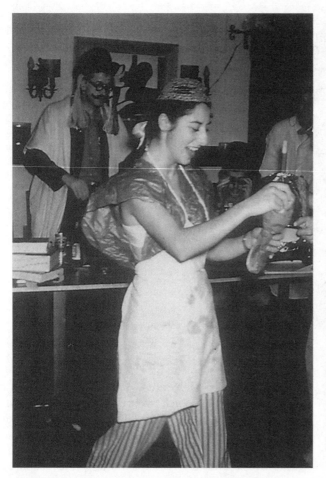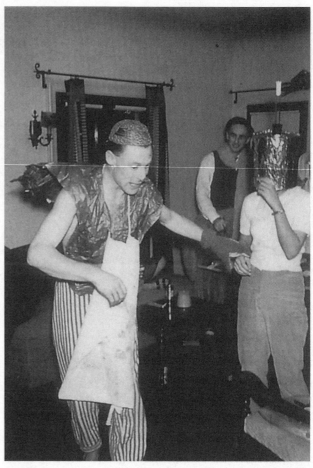

FIGURE 2.—The Recombination Test, in which ANN ROLLER (left panel) was required to exchange five phenotypes (articles of clothing) with JOHN CAIRNS. When they emerged from the recombination closet (right panel), CAIRNS (left) was dressed as ROLLER, and ROLLER (right, with culture apparatus over her head) was dressed as CAIRNS. The gentleman in the derby hat in the left panel is DELBRÜCK; the gentleman in the beret and muffler in the right panel is RUBIN. (Photographs courtesy of DENNIS BARRETT, University of Denver.)

Harbor that summer, EDGAR met with GEORGE STREI-SINGER and discussed several experiments on which they might collaborate. One of these, EDGAR told me, was a mapping experiment to test for circularity of the linkage map of phage T4. This, EDGAR believed, was a long shot, but if *E. coli* could have a circular linkage map, why not T4? Their decision to test this unlikely hypothesis could not have come at a worse time for me. My thesis research at Caltech was aimed at determining the size of the mating group in T4 (*i.e.*, how many phage chromosomes could participate in a single crossover event). The experiment was based on the STEINBERG-STAHL mating theory, which in turn was based on the assumption that phage chromosomes were linear. While I was writing my Ph.D. thesis, STREISINGER, ED-GAR, and GETTA HARRAR-DENHARDT (1964) were doing experiments that demonstrated the circularity of the T4 linkage map and simultaneously demolished the theoretical underpinnings of my thesis. The discovery that the map was circular was exciting in itself and led, over the next few years, to marvelous revelations about the

complex life cycle of phage T4 (see, for example, MOSIG 1983). For me, a graduate student working on the last draft of my Ph.D. thesis, the news that T4 had a circular map was worrisome. The Fates had arranged for me to defend my thesis dressed in the Emperor's new clothes! Fortunately, MAX was willing to let me get a degree on the basis of my suddenly obsolete work because he found my thesis interesting, and his sole test for an acceptable Ph.D. thesis was that it be "either interesting or original—not necessarily both." *Reality* was not on his list of criteria. After all, MAX never really believed any experimental demonstration of anything.

The second discussion I had with BOB EDGAR took place on the beach overlooking the outer harbor. I was sunning with BOB and his wife, LOIS GLASS EDGAR, when he told me that he had been thinking about changing directions in his research when we got back to Pasadena. He might give up studying the mechanisms of recombination in phage and start looking for a new class of mutants, mutants that were unable to grow at elevated temperatures. HOROWITZ AND LEUPOLD (1951) had done experiments like that with *Neurospora* and *E. coli* and had shown that such mutations occurred in exactly the same genes that had already been identified by looking for other, more gene-specific phenotypes. The advantage of "temperature" mutations was that they were lethal only if the temperature was elevated. Why not try to isolate mutants like that in T4? BOB asked me to keep his plan a secret and, in particular, not to tell CHARLEY STEINBERG about it, because he was certain that CHARLEY would consider it ridiculous and would think of so many excellent reasons *not* to do the experiment that the project would be abandoned before the first plate was poured. Of course, BOB *did* do the mutant hunt when we got back to Caltech—in a locked room, safely out of CHARLEY STEINBERG's ken—and the *ts* mutants became a treasure that BOB shared freely with the phage world (EDGAR and LIELAUSIS 1964).

The Phage Course of 1960 ended with the traditional commencement ceremony. The featured speaker for the Class of 1960 was the bombastic "DR. PLOTCHKISS," played, of course, by ROLLIN D. HOTCHKISS, who himself had been a member of the very first phage class. DR. PLOTCHKISS wore, I believe, a mortar board over an abundant and unruly mass of hair. He carried an enormous, accordion-folded scroll of paper on which his "speech" was written. He delivered 10 or 15 minutes of loud, scholarly nonsense, and, as he spoke, his academic gown somehow fell open to reveal an impressive, spherical belly on which was painted a huge red target.

JOHN CAIRNS, who had been my classmate in the 1957 Phage Course, became the Director of the Cold Spring Harbor Lab and invited me to be the Instructor for the summer course in 1966. He asked me to suggest candidates for the second Instructor position, and I immediately named FRANCES WOMACK, who was at Vanderbilt University. I had never met FRANCES, but I was greatly impressed by her published work on the role of phage heterozygotes in recombination in phage T4. She had done single-burst experiments using so many closely linked markers that her resolution of recombination events seemed almost the equivalent of molecular sequencing (WOMACK 1963). Since DNA sequencing was not possible in 1966, FRANCES' work seemed wonderful to me—a combination of brute strength and brilliant analysis. I figured that anyone with the patience and energy to do crosses involving nine markers or more could be counted on to carry more than a fair share of the work that needed to be done in teaching the Phage Course. I was right. FRANCES was a perfect partner for the job. She was smart, full of fun, and happy to take on big jobs. She was, however, hard to get started in the morning, and her son and daughter, who were up with the birds, would arouse FRANCES by serving her a breakfast of Coca Cola in bed.

FRANCES seemed to be fueled by Coca Cola and almost always had a bottle of it in her hand.

BARBARA and I and our two sons, then 4 and 8 years old, stayed in the Firehouse, which once housed the Cold Spring Harbor fire department. In 1930, it was moved by barge across the harbor to the grounds of the Biology Lab [and it has moved once more since we stayed in it (WATSON 1991)]. When RIC DAVERN, who was associate director of the Lab, showed us to our quarters, he seemed a bit apologetic, but we were comfortable in the small apartment, and the location was perfect. Right next door was Davenport Laboratory, where the Phage Course was taught; I could commute from home to work in two minutes, and so could my sons, who frequently came running into the lab while an experiment was in progress to announce exciting news of one sort or another. The class skit that summer made much of my older son's appearance one day with a huge horseshoe crab that he had captured while it was spawning. The boys loved Cold Spring Harbor and seemed extraordinarily energized by the sea, the enormous grounds, the numerous places to climb and to hide. I have often thought that BOB HASELKORN and his family, who lived beneath us in the Firehouse, must have had mixed feelings about their accommodation that summer. They could hardly have failed to notice the stomping of the two little boys upstairs.

Here are the students in the class that FRANCES and I taught in 1966. I cannot resist offering this list because, like all teachers, I take pride in the accomplishments of my students. (The degrees and institutions shown on this list are copied from the original course roster.) ANDREW J. BECKER, Ph.D., Albert Einstein College of Medicine; FLORENCE CAHN, B.A., MIT; JOHN H. CASTER, B.S., St. Louis University School of Medicine; ANANDA M. CHAKRABARTY, Ph.D., University of Illinois-Urbana; STANLEY N. COHEN, M.D., Albert Einstein College of Medicine; DAVID B. FANKHAUSER, B.A., Johns Hopkins University; MARIA C. GANOZA, Ph.D., NIH; MAX E. GOTTESMAN, Ph.D., The Rockefeller University; THEODORE GURNEY, JR., Ph.D., MIT; JOST KEMPER, Ph.D., Cold Spring Harbor Laboratory of Quantitative Biology; STANLEY P. LIEBO, Ph.D., Oak Ridge National Laboratory; DANIEL H. LEVIN, Ph.D., Lab of Biophysics, Beth Israel Medical Center; LEON J. LEWANDOWSKI, B.S., Wistar Institute; CARL R. MERRIL, M.D., NIH; WIM J. MÖLLER, Ph.D., Johns Hopkins University School of Medicine; HAROLD C. NEU, M.D., Columbia University College of Physicians and Surgeons; JOHN W. QUIGLEY, M.S., Rutgers University; WOOLLCOTT K. SMITH, M.S., Johns Hopkins University; HIROKO WATANABE, M.D., Royal Victoria Hospital, Montreal; ROBERT YUAN, B.S., Albert Einstein College of Medicine.

Readers will, of course, recognize many names on this list. It was, like all the other Phage Course classes, a collection of gifted people. Yet many of them had never flamed a pipette, isolated a bacterial colony, or seen a phage plaque. A few members of the class were unfamiliar with semi-log graph paper, and we had to explain to them how and why such paper is used. FRANCES taught them to recognize plaques arising from phage HETs (single phage particles that give rise to a mixed progeny of r and r⁺ phages). She explained how to do spot tests for complementation and recombination of rII mutants; she herself had done zillions of such tests. We did a big single-burst experiment, another of FRANCES' specialties. I prepared the class for experiments that required mathematics—serum inactivation, UV inactivation, nitrous acid induction of mutations, and mapping. The math was essentially the same for most of the labs; only the notation changed. In addition, I tried, probably unsuccessfully, to get the class excited about the STEINBERG-STAHL mating theory. And, following the DELBRÜCK tradition, I derived the Poisson distribution for the class. One cannot do phage biology without the Poisson distribution. Like MAX, I mischievously used a tank of tiny fish to illustrate the derivation, thus creating an uncertainty in the minds of my listeners concerning the origin of the "poisson" in the name of the distribution.

I will mention here only two of the students in this engaging and brilliant class. STAN COHEN stood out because he was so busily involved in a research project that was in progress at Einstein. He made two or three phone calls a day from the wall phone on the South wall of the Davenport Lab. He scribbled numbers on his note pad, gave urgent instructions for the next experiment, and always set up the time for the next contact. FRANCES and I wondered why he had come to Cold Spring Harbor when he was so intensely concerned about work that was going on elsewhere. He was, however, an apt student and seemed genuinely interested in the work he was doing in our course. I remember ANANDA CHAKRABARTY because he seemed so interested in working on exotic organisms that grew on odd substrates and smelled bad. Why would you want to work on organisms that ate asphalt when you had access to well-behaved organisms that ate carbohydrates?

Students participating in the Phage Course carried home a great deal more than a handful of useful techniques. They felt that they had been initiated into the community of biologists. The course featured seminars by leaders in the field, and the students could sit and drink beer with them on the porch at Blackford Hall or chat with them on the beach. When FRANCES and I taught the course, the seminar series included talks by C. A. THOMAS, F. FRANKEL, D. J. MCCORQUODALE, R. HASELKORN, A. SKALKA, C. RADDING, E. KELLENBERGER, E. GOLDBERG, J. KARAM, G. MOSIG, and R. S. EDGAR. It was worth a student's trip to Cold Spring

Harbor just to meet the scientists who worked year round in the labs there; that included BARBARA MCCLINTOCK and AL HERSHEY. I remember with special fondness PAUL MARGOLIN, who showed me the elaborate model train layout that he constructed during the winter months, when the social life at Cold Spring Harbor went into hibernation. In the summer, students could spend their evenings talking molecular biology with JIM WATSON, GEORGE STREISINGER, MAURICE FOX, and a host of other visitors who were drawn to the place year after year.

The pleasures of Cold Spring Harbor come not only from the science, which is wonderful, but also from the place, which is enchanting. The rhythm of the Phage Course often fell into harmony with the rhythm of the sea. We would schedule labs in the very early morning in order to be able to dig clams in the afternoon. On a hot day, when the beach was especially inviting, we would delay an experiment until late afternoon and head for the outer harbor. I remember one night when BOB EDGAR hunted me down and took me to the water's edge. A school of bioluminescent ctenophores surrounded the boat dock in the inner harbor. I scooped one of them into my palm. That simple blob of a creature has stuck in my memory; it was one of the most beautiful things I have ever seen. That is what the Phage Course and Cold Spring Harbor are all about—the wonder and the elegance of life.

LITERATURE CITED

EDGAR, R. S., and I. LIELAUSIS, 1964 Temperature-sensitive mutants of bacteriophage T4: their isolation and genetic characterization. Genetics **49**: 649–662.

HOROWITZ, N. H., and U. LEUPOLD, 1951 Some recent studies bearing on the one gene-one enzyme hypothesis. Cold Spring Harbor Symp. Quant. Biol. **16**: 65–72.

LURIA, S. E., 1966 Mutations of bacteria and of bacteriophage, pp. 173–179 in *Phage and the Origins of Molecular Biology*, edited by J. CAIRNS, G. S. STENT and J. D. WATSON. Cold Spring Harbor Laboratory of Quantitative Biology, Long Island, NY.

MAALØE, O., 1966 The relation between nuclear and cellular division in *Escherichia coli*, pp. 265–272 in *Phage and the Origins of Molecular Biology*, edited by J. CAIRNS, G. S. STENT and J. D. WATSON. Cold Spring Harbor Laboratory of Quantitative Biology, Long Island, NY.

MOSIG, G., 1983 Relationship of T4 DNA replication and recombination, pp. 120–130 in *Bacteriophage T4*, edited by C. K. MATHEWS, E. M. KUTTER, G. MOSIG and P. B. BERGET. American Society for Microbiology, Washington, DC.

STEINBERG, C., and F. STAHL, 1958 The theory of formal phage genetics. Cold Spring Harbor Symp. Quant. Biol. **23**: 42–46.

STREISINGER, G., R. S. EDGAR and G. HARRAR-DENHARDT, 1964 Chromosome structure in phage T4: I. Circularity of the linkage map. Proc. Natl. Acad. Sci. USA **51**: 775–779.

VISCONTI, N., and M. DELBRÜCK, 1953 The mechanism of genetic recombination in phage. Genetics **38**: 5–33.

WATSON, E. L., 1991 *Houses for Science: A Pictorial History of Cold Spring Harbor Laboratory*. Cold Spring Harbor Laboratory Press, Cold Spring Harbor, NY.

WOMACK, F. C., 1963 An analysis of single-burst progeny of bacteria singly infected with a bacteriophage heterozygote. Virology **21**: 232–241.

Vicious Circles
Looking Back on Resistance Plasmids

Julian Davies

Department of Microbiology and Immunology, University of British Columbia, Vancouver, B. C. V6T 1Z3, Canada

DURING the past few years, the popular press has often made play with lurid articles describing the rise in appearance of "superbugs" and emphasizing the menace posed by multiply antibiotic-resistant bacterial pathogens, such as the Gram-negative *Pseudomonas aeruginosa* or Gram-positive *Staphylococcus aureus* and *Enterococcus faecalis*. At medical conventions, infectious-diseases experts regale audiences with descriptions of their pet "Andromeda strain," the drug-resistant bacterial species that causes the most serious and difficult-to-treat infections. *Trends in Microbiology* prepared a special issue entitled "Drug Resistance: The New Apocalypse?" TV and radio shows have echoed these grim stories that dramatize the end of the antibiotic era. What is not realized by the lay public is that these supposed exposés are reporting nothing new; they are simply describing the continuing manifestations of a phenomenon that was first evident in the 1950s and has increased ever since. The sad commentary is that so little has been done to try to avoid the problem.

The rapid development of antibiotic resistance in bacteria, now well recognized, first came as a series of events that evoked both surprise and disbelief. At the beginning of the antibiotic era in the early 1950s, microbial geneticists were more involved in discussions of the controversial topic of the mechanism of acquired antibiotic resistance in bacteria than in considerations of the clinical significance of this resistance. Many symposia and publications were concerned with hot debate on the subject of mutation *vs.* adaptation in the generation of antibiotic-resistant phenotypes in bacteria. Resistance to antibiotics in bacterial pathogens during the course of treatment of infectious diseases was considered by bacterial geneticists to be an event of low probability, and the notion of multiple drug resistance was heretical. Although this period was the heyday of studies on the nature of bacterial conjugation and the role of the F factor in this process, it was considered unlikely, at the time, that sexual mechanisms would contribute to any extent in the development of antibiotic resistance in bacteria. Coincidentally, however, in war-torn Japan, serious outbreaks of dysentery due to *Shigella*

dysenteriae were responding with decreasing effectiveness to sulfonamides, the principal antibacterial treatment available at the time. By 1952, more than 80% of *Shigella* isolates in Japan were sulfonamide-resistant; it is of interest to note that the sulfonamide drugs are not, strictly speaking, antibiotics, since they do not occur naturally. When antibiotics such as streptomycin, tetracycline, and chloramphenicol became available, it was found that their efficacy was temporary, resistant strains developing in the afflicted population as these drugs were used clinically. By 1955 there were reports of the isolation of *S. dysenteriae* strains resistant to as many as four different antibiotics; the first publication of this phenomenon was apparently that of KITAMOTO *et al.* (1956). Numerous other reports confirmed that multiple antibiotic resistance in bacteria was not a rare, unusual observation in Japan; it was epidemic. The papers describing these developments have been widely referenced but very rarely read in the West, since the majority were published in Japanese journals.

Not long after, in 1959–60, it was found that the multiple antibiotic resistance of *Shigella dysenteriae* strains could be transferred to other Enterobacteriaceae, simply by mixing liquid cultures of resistant and sensitive bacteria and plating on solid medium containing the appropriate antibiotics as selective agents (OCHIAI *et al.* 1959; AKIBA *et al.* 1960). The mechanism by which the transfer occurred was revealed when the laboratories of S. MITSUHASHI (HARADA *et al.* 1960), R. NAKAYA (NAKAYA and NAKAMURA 1960a), and T. WATANABE (WATANABE and FUKUSAWA 1960a) all showed that cell-to-cell contact was required for resistance-gene transfer, indicating that bacterial conjugation was involved. This was subsequently confirmed by experiments that showed that blending (agitation) interfered with transfer and that acridine orange treatment of multiply resistant strains caused loss of the resistance determinants. Since HIROTA (1960) had shown previously that bacteria could be "cured" of the F plasmid by this treatment, a functional similarity between F plasmids and resistance factors was established; resistance factors were correctly deduced to be episomes. Most of this work was published in Japanese journals, and it was only in late 1960 that two papers describing the phenomenon of transferable multiple antibiotic resistance appeared in *Biochemical and Biophysical Research Communications*. The publication of these studies was greeted with considerable skepticism; in fact, NAKAYA's paper was under review for nearly six months after submission, and it was (apparently) the receipt of WATANABE's manuscript that led the editors to the realization that the scientific basis for these observations was valid; NAKAYA *et al.* (1960b) and WATANABE and FUKUSAWA (1960b) were published back-to-back. WATANABE became the person most closely identified with the early work on R factors, publishing a long series of papers in *Medical Biology* (in Japanese) and subsequently the *Journal of Bacteriology* (in English) over many years; he wrote the first comprehensive summary of all the work done on R factors in Japan for *Bacteriological Reviews* (WATANABE 1963). A more detailed account of the early history of R factors is given by STANLEY FALKOW (1975).

In the United Kingdom in 1959, NAOMI DATTA initiated her studies of multiple antibiotic resistance by identifying clinical isolates of *Salmonella typhimurium* that were resistant to three antibiotics, only one of which had been used to treat the patients! On seeing the NAKAYA and WATANABE papers, DATTA tested her isolates for cell-to-cell transfer of resistance determinants and confirmed that gene transfer, dependent on cell contact, was involved in the spread of resistance among the bacterial species she was studying. This was the earliest demonstration of transmissible resistance outside Japan. Like the Japanese workers, DATTA encountered opposition to her findings; however, she had the advantage of working in Hammersmith Hospital next door to the bacterial genetics unit of BILL HAYES, who in NAOMI's words "looked at her plates" and gave her confidence in what she was doing. DATTA's results were published in 1962 in the *Journal of Hygiene*—hardly a high-impact journal by today's ratings. Other microbiologists working with multiple antibiotic resistance bacteria had similar experiences with skeptical colleagues, perhaps none so difficult as those of G. LEBEK, who obtained evidence for transferable, multiple antibiotic resistance in *Salmonella typhimurium* and *Escherichia coli* isolated from children in 1960. The presentation of his results was met with "harsh and unpleasant" criticism (his words) in Munich and LEBEK was dismissed. He was unemployed for several months and then accepted a position in Bern, Switzerland. A report of his work was eventually published (LEBEK 1963).

However, additional reports of multiple antibiotic resistance followed worldwide; with the paper of DAVID SMITH (1966) describing the isolation of transferable drug resistance in hospitals in Boston, the concept was generally recognized and the study of R-plasmid biology was on its way.

The number of different antibiotic-resistance determinants increased greatly as multiply antibiotic strains were studied in different countries; there were indications that the resistance determinants often reflected the geography of antibiotic usage. Subsequent studies led to characterization of a variety of types of R factors, many of which were detected outside the Enterobacteriaceae, in pseudomonads, staphylococci, streptococci, *etc.*; very few bacterial species do not possess endogenous plasmids. The magnitude of the clinical problems raised by antibiotic resistance was clearly identified by those working in the field, who often spoke out against the indiscriminate use of antibiotics in the treatment of common human diseases and the massive use of antibiotics in agriculture and as animal growth promotants. Into the 1980s, only about 50% of the antibiotics produced were employed for human use, and this is probably true today. Press coverage of the threat and its consequences was less evident thirty years ago, and even today the subject of antibiotic resistance is brought to the attention of the general public in daily newspapers only briefly, when news of other disasters is lacking.

The problem of antibiotic resistance is now an established fact of life in the clinical treatment of infectious diseases. Microbes have survived almost fifty years of onslaught by millions of tons of toxic agents by employing the processes of gene acquisition and gene transfer on a scale that is still not fully appreciated.

My interest in the subject of transmissible antibiotic resistance began in 1962 upon joining B. D. DAVIS' laboratory as a postdoctoral fellow to work on the mechanism of action of streptomycin. I was intrigued by antibiotic resistance and began to study the biochemical basis of streptomycin resistance in mutants of *E. coli* isolated in the laboratory. This work demonstrated that the structural components of ribosomes were altered by these mutations, which were the first genetic markers identified for these organelles. I met T. WATANABE in 1963 and read his review, but it was not until 1965 when I went to Paris to work with FRANÇOIS JACOB that transmissible antibiotic resistance caught my interest. YUKINORI HIROTA was in JACOB's laboratory, and he described in great detail (usually over a bottle of wine) the background to the R-factor problem in Japan. HIROTA gave me an *E. coli* strain carrying R plasmid NR-1 (variously known as R222 and R100), and JACOB agreed to let me study the resistant strains with HIROTA's help as a sideline to my primary research on genetic studies of *lac* regulation. We found that the ribosomes of the resistant strains remained sensitive to streptomycin, but that incubation of the antibiotic with cell-free extracts from the resistant strain led to inactivation of the antibiotics. Incidentally, although antibiotic-resistant clinical isolates had been isolated (in France) in 1954, it was not until 1968 that they were shown to carry transferable R plasmids. On my move to Wisconsin in 1967, more extensive biochemical studies with TAKESHI YAMADA and DONALD TIPPER (who knew how to do electrophoresis) showed that streptomycin was inactivated by O-adenylyl-ation in the strains carrying plasmid NR1 (YAMADA *et al.* 1968). This unusual modification prompted analysis of other R-factor-mediated antibiotic resistance mechanisms, and some eight biochemically distinct mechanisms have now been identified in bacteria.

The covalently closed circular form of isolated R-plasmid DNA was demonstrated in the late 1960s, which led to extensive physical mapping of the plasmids from a variety of sources. Although plasmid biology (as such) is little discussed in modern courses (many students, if asked to name a plasmid, being likely to mention one of the popular cloning vectors), the discovery of R plasmids revolutionized thinking about gene acquisition and gene exchange in nature, with important consequences for an understanding of the evolution of bacterial genomes. In addition, bacterial resistance plasmids have played a seminal role in the development of recombinant DNA technology and its applications. The study of plasmid-determined resistance in bacteria has been of enormous benefit to molecular science, both fundamental and applied. It is not possible to describe all of these studies, but some are worthy of mention. In 1972, STANLEY COHEN *et al.* successfully transformed competent *E. coli* with R-plasmid DNA. This demonstrated the ability of *E. coli* not only to take up DNA, but also to serve as a useful host strain for the expression of plasmid-encoded genes, converting a laboratory tool into an important industrial microorganism. This experiment also anticipated the development of plasmid replicons as cloning vectors and the use of resistance determinants as markers in the transfer of recombinant plasmids from one bacterial host to another. R plasmids and their bacterial components have played a seminal role in the development of genetic engineering and biotechnology in other ways; many of the restriction endonucleases currently used are plasmid-encoded.

Another highly significant characteristic of R-plasmid structure came to light in 1973. BOB HEDGES, working in NAOMI DATTA's laboratory, was carrying out compatibility tests with R plasmids. On introducing two different R plasmids into the same strain of *E. coli*, he recovered a "recombinant plasmid" from an event in which the ampicillin resistance gene of one plasmid had seemingly jumped onto the other plasmid; no other kind of recombinant was formed. HEDGES and ALAN JACOB carried out more extensive studies of this phenomenon and in 1974 proposed the existence of "transposons" in bacteria (HEDGES and JACOB 1974).

In the following year, several groups characterized a variety of transposable antibiotic resistance genes and demonstrated transposition between bacterial replicons; the molecular nature of "transposons" was established. Subsequent studies confirmed that most R-factor-encoded antibiotic resistance genes (in both Gram-negative and Gram-positive bacteria) are components of transposable elements. Parenthetically, in early experiments on the transduction of multiple antibiotic resistance carried out in Japan, it was found that the resistance genes were not subsequently transferable by conjugation. The stable transconjugants may well have been the products of transposition! Recent studies of the fine structure of transposable elements have provided clues to the mechanism by which resistance genes can be acquired by plasmids and so disseminated within the bacterial population. Resistance-gene cassettes (of unknown origin) are acquired by a mechanism of integrase-catalyzed, site-specific integration into an element named an integron. Integrons are natural, broad-host-range gene-expression cassettes in which transcription and translation of any inserted open reading frame(s) can be effected (STOKES and HALL 1989).

Thus, by use of a combination of different replicons, recombination systems, and gene transfer mechanisms, bacteria have access to an enormous pool of antibiotic resistance genes in the environment that are on tap when needed. Nonetheless, it is now clear that mutation also plays an important role in the development and evolution of antibiotic resistance in bacteria. The appearance of multiple antibiotic resistance in *Mycobacterium tuberculosis* is the result of point mutations, as is resistance to the newer fluoroquinolone antibiotics in pathogens such as *P. aeruginosa* and *S. aureus*, to give just two examples. The evolution of extended β-lactamases in Enterobacteriaceae is largely the result of a series of point mutations in plasmid-encoded resistance genes, showing that extensive natural protein engineering to change enzyme characteristics is yet another strategy that permits bacteria to evade the unwelcome appearance of novel antibiotic analogs.

Finally, after many years, methicillin-resistant *S. aureus* (MRSA), one of the earliest and most resilient of resistant bacterial lines, has been characterized biochemically. MRSA was discovered in 1960, one year after the introduction of penicillinase-resistant antibiotics into clinical practice, and has now become a pathogen of global importance with an incidence of more than 80% in some hospitals. These strains appear to have descended from a single clone of *S. aureus* which acquired the *mec*A gene, encoding a methicillin-insensitive enzyme involved in cell-wall biosynthesis, by chromosomal insertion (DE LENCASTRE *et al.* 1994). The source of the *mec*A gene remains a mystery and, in fact, the resistance genes of all R factors are due to acquisition of DNA encoding novel functions from unknown sources (DAVIES 1994).

In conclusion, while I do not support the "doom and gloom" approach of the popular press, one must recognize that a serious problem exists as a result of the inheritance of antibiotic resistance genes by bacterial pathogens. Bacteria are survivors, and no matter what novel antimicrobial substance is introduced into clinical practice, they resist and thrive. One has to marvel at the ability of microbes to thwart our best efforts to control or eliminate them, but after all, bacteria have inhabited the earth and resisted many hostile environments for close to four billion years, so we can hardly expect to get rid of them in a mere half century of effort.

I thank the community of plasmidologists for their fellowship over many years and many meetings and acknowledge the National Institutes of Health and the National Science Foundation for generous financial support from 1962 to 1980. In addition, ROSARIO BAUZON and DOROTHY DAVIES are thanked for their help in preparing the manuscript.

LITERATURE CITED

AKIBA, T., K. KOYAMA, Y. ISHIKI, S. KIMURA and T. FUKUSHIMA, 1960 On the mechanism of the development of multiple-drug-resistant clones of *Shigella*. Nihon Iji Shimpo **1866:** 45–50.

COHEN, S. N., A. C. Y. CHANG and L. HSU, 1972 Nonchromosomal antibiotic resistance in bacteria: genetic transformation of *E. coli* by R-factor DNA. Proc. Natl. Acad. Sci. USA **69:** 2110–2114.

DATTA, N., 1962 Transmissible drug resistance in an epidemic strain of *Salmonella typhimurium*. J. Hygiene **60:** 301–310.

DAVIES, J., 1994 Inactivation of antibiotics and the dissemination of resistance genes. Science **264:** 375–382.

DE LENCASTRE, H., B. L. M. DE JONGE, P. R. MATTHEWS and A. TOMASZ, 1994 Molecular aspects of methicillin resistance in *Staphylococcus aureus*. J. Antimicrob. Chemother. **33:** 7–24.

FALKOW, S., 1975 *Infectious Multiple Drug Resistance*. Pion Ltd., London.

HARADA, K., M. SUZUKI, M. KAMEDA and S. MITSUHASHI, 1960 On the drug resistance of entire bacteria. 2. Transmission of the drug resistance among *Enterobacteriaceae*. Jpn. J. Exp. Med. **30:** 289–299.

HEDGES, R. W., and A. JACOB, 1974 Transposition of ampicillin resistance from RP4 to other replicons. Mol. Gen. Genet. **132:** 31–40.

HIROTA, Y., 1960 The effect of acridine dyes on mating type factors in *Escherichia coli*. Proc. Natl. Acad. Sci. USA **46:** 57–64.

KITAMOTO, O., N. KASAI, K. FUKAYA and A. KAWASHIMA, 1956 Drug sensitivity of the *Shigella* strains isolated in 1955. J. Jpn. Assoc. Infect. Dis. **30:** 403–404.

LEBEK, G., 1963 Über die Enstehung mehrfachresistanter Salmonellen. Ein experimenteller Beitrag. Zbl. Bakt., Abt. I, Orig. **188:** 494–499.

NAKAYA, R., and A. NAKAMURA, 1960a Mechanism of acquisition of drug resistance by prevalent strains of *Shigella*. Presented at the 13th Meeting of the Kanto Branch of the Society of Japanese Bacteriologists.

NAKAYA, R., A. NAKAMURA and Y. MURATA, 1960b Resistance transfer agents in *Shigella*. Biochem. Biophys. Res. Commun. **3:** 654–659.

OCHIAI, K., T. YAMANAKA, K. KIMURA and O. SAWADA, 1959 Studies on inheritance of drug resistance between *Shigella* strains and *Escherichia coli* strains. Nihon Iji Shimpo **1861:** 34–46.

SMITH, D. H., 1966 *Salmonella* with transferable drug resistance. N. Engl. J. Med. **275:** 626–630.

STOKES, H. W., and R. M. HALL, 1989 A novel family of potentially mobile DNA elements encoding site-specific gene-integration functions: integrons. Mol. Microbiol. **3:** 1669–1683.

WATANABE, T., 1963 Infective heredity of multiple drug resistance in bacteria. Bacteriol. Rev. **27:** 87–115.

WATANABE, T., and T. FUKUSAWA, 1960a Episomic resistance factors in *Enterobacteriaceae*. 1. Transfer of resistance factors by conjugation among *Enterobacteriaceae*. Med. Biol. **56:** 56–59.

WATANABE, T., and T. FUKUSAWA, 1960b "Resistance transfer factor" an episome in *Enterobacteriaceae*. Biochem. Biophys. Res. Commun. **3:** 87–115.

YAMADA, T., D. TIPPER and J. DAVIES, 1968 Enzymatic inactivation of streptomycin by R factor-resistant *Escherichia coli*. Nature **219:** 288–291.

May 1995

LODs Past and Present

Newton E. Morton

Human Genetics, University of Southampton, Princess Anne Hospital, Southampton SO16 5YA, United Kingdom

INFORMATION on linkage in the human is accumulated as a succession of samples, each of which may be small relative to the amount of data required to detect linkage. Analysis within a sample of pedigrees may be complex, with untested individuals, incomplete penetrance, and multiple loci. Despite these obstacles, several hundred disease loci have been mapped, in many cases with sufficient accuracy to permit positional cloning of a gene whose product was unknown. Now polygenic disease is being attacked with some success in maps that include hundreds of markers per chromosome and that pave the way for sequencing large parts of the genome. These developments testify to the power of intellectual curiosity to overcome intractable problems and may rank among the most significant applications of genetics to human welfare.

Linkage before LODs: FELIX BERNSTEIN was one of the pioneers in what is now called genetic epidemiology (CROW 1993). He is perhaps best known for his analysis of the *ABO* locus and bioassay of racial admixture, but he was also the first to realize that linkage could be detected in human pedigrees by taking the product of frequencies that must be in coupling or repulsion, whatever the phase of linkage (BERNSTEIN 1931). Various modifications of this method were made by WIENER (1932), HOGBEN (1934), and HALDANE (1934), but they were superseded by the maximum likelihood *u* scores of FISHER (1935) and FINNEY (1940). Although this elegant method is fully efficient in the limit for loose linkage, it has several disadvantages. Only the asymptotic distribution is known, but many linkage samples are small. FISHER's scores are difficult to compute except in simple two-generation cases and do not accommodate matings of known phase. They are not efficient for close linkage and do not give a good estimate of the recombination fraction. Finally, insufficient attention was paid to the low prior probability that two random loci are linked, which implies that a conservative significance level must be used to provide reasonable assurance that a statistically significant linkage is real. For these reasons the *u*-score approach was abandoned in the fifties.

Another approach was pioneered by PENROSE (1935) for sib pairs with unspecified parents. This did not become popular in the search for major loci because it neglects information in the phenotypes of parents and relatives, does not give an estimate of recombination, and is unreliable when multiple pairs are drawn from the same sibship. However, sib-pair methods have recently been revived for complex inheritance and for disease of late onset where the parents are rarely available.

In this early period only three autosomal linkages were discovered: between the Lutheran blood group (*LU*) and ABH secretion (*SE*) by MOHR (1951); one form of ellipticytosis (*EL1*) and the Rhesus blood group (*RH*) by LAWLER (1954); and the nail patella syndrome (*NPS1*) with the *ABO* blood group (RENWICK and LAWLER 1955; RENWICK and SCHULZE 1965). All these markers had high penetrance, precise diagnosis, and good survival, so that large pedigrees could be collected. Blood groups were markers of choice, despite dominance of antigenic factors. The next period would be characterized by markers with codominance and by analysis based on calculated probabilities.

LODs before linkage: Since its introduction by NEYMAN and PEARSON (1928), the likelihood ratio has been accepted as the optimal basis for statistical decisions. It is defined on the ith sample S_i as $\lambda_i = P(S_i|H_1)/P(S_i|H_0)$, where H_0 and H_1 are alternative hypotheses. The likelihood ratio is to statistics as the microscope is to cytogenetics. Because probabilities for independent samples are multiplicative and a likelihood ratio may be called *odds*, it was natural for BARNARD (1949) to introduce the logarithm of the likelihood ratio and to call this quantity a LOD (logarithms of odds). Therefore, if $z_i = \log \lambda_i$ is the LOD for the ith sample, then the LOD for a set of independent samples is $Z = \sum_{i=1}^{n} z_i$. In this formulation of LODs, the probabilities are conditional and the prior probabilities are unspecified. BARNARD was also interested in "average LODs" in which $\Pi\lambda_i$, the product of the λ_i, is integrated over a prior distribution under H_1 to give a weighted mean Λ that loses the convenience of additivity but appeals to Bayesians (SMITH 1959). In genetics the term "LOD" invariably refers to the z_i, which are often called *LOD* *scores* to contrast them with other scoring procedures. They have three useful properties. First, for any pre-specified alternative H_1 they give a conservative estimate of significance,

$$P(Z > \log A \mid H_0 < 1/A). \tag{1}$$

Second, if common logarithms are used (as they are by convention in genetics) and if H_1 differs from H_0 by m efficiently estimated parameters, then in the limit for large samples under H_0

$$(2 \ln 10)Z = \chi^2 \quad (\text{d.f.} = m) \tag{2}$$

(NEYMAN and PEARSON 1928). Third, if H_0 and H_1 are jointly exhaustive and mutually exclusive and if the prior distribution is correctly specified, the posterior probability of H_1 is

$$P(H_1 \mid S) = \frac{\Lambda[P(H_1)/P(H_0)]}{1 + \Lambda[P(H_1)/P(H_0)]} \tag{3}$$

where $P(H_1)/P(H_0)$ is called the prior (or "forward") odds (BARNARD 1949).

These three properties have led to different applications of LODs. One of these was a consequence of World War II, during which a refugee from the Nazis undertook to optimize the statistical procedure by which a consignment of bombs was selected or rejected by test explosion of a random sample. If the sample were too large, too few bombs would be left for the war. If the sample were too small, men and planes would be wasted on duds. This led ABRAHAM WALD to sequential analysis, whereby two hypotheses specifying acceptable and nonacceptable parameters are discriminated with tolerable errors by the smallest mean number of observations. Military secrecy delayed publication of his work until 1947 (WALD 1947), the year in which HALDANE and SMITH (1947) first applied LODs to analysis of linkage.

Linkage before DNA: Two developments in the fifties accelerated linkage mapping. The first was the application of starch gel electrophoresis to detect genetic variation in proteins (SMITHIES 1955, 1995). Many of these systems were polymorphic, and codominance of alleles was the rule. The laboratories in London and Copenhagen that had initially dominated studies of human linkage adopted isozymes and continued to lead the field. The Galton Laboratory had been headed by R. A. FISHER, who saw the promise of blood groups as linkage markers (FISHER 1935). He was succeeded by LIONEL PENROSE, with J. B. S. HALDANE as Weldon Professor. Younger members of the Galton Laboratory included C. A. B. SMITH, SYLVIA LAWLER, JAMES RENWICK, and later PETER COOK and SUSAN POVEY, all of whom shared enthusiasm for linkage. Their close collaborators included R. R. RACE and RUTH SANGER in blood groups and PATRICIA JACOBS in cytogenetics. ELIZABETH ROBSON provided a bridge between these enthusiasts and the isozyme research of HARRY HARRIS, the next Galton professor, whom she succeeded.

JAN MOHR (1951) at the Institute for Human Genetics in Copenhagen was the discoverer of the first autosomal linkage, of the Lutheran blood group to the Lewis blood group, that was subsequently shown to be an interaction between the *LE* and *SE* loci (the latter being the marker he detected). German and Scandinavian law on child support favors genetic markers that can be used in paternity cases, and so there was a strong tradition of blood grouping and later isozyme typing in Denmark. The head of the Institute, TAGE KEMP, was a pioneer in human population genetics, and the institute provided a stable base for the long-term linkage studies that MOHR undertook after he succeeded KEMP. It is unlikely that the patience required for such research with no immediate payoff (like the work of WATSON and CRICK at the same time) would be supported by research grants today.

The increasing volume of linkage data demanded a method of analysis that would escape the limitations of *u* scores, of which I first became aware when confronted by pedigrees of Pelger-Huet anomaly and elliptocytosis in Japan (MORTON *et al.* 1954; FUJII *et al.* 1955) and to which I was attracted as my interests shifted from Drosophila to human genetics. During this time and my years at the University of Wisconsin, JAMES CROW was a fount of encouragement and stimulation. One of my colleagues in the Atomic Bomb Casualty Commission was JAMES RENWICK, seconded from the medical corps that served the Commonwealth army of occupation and their troops at war in Korea. On our return from Japan we became more interested in linkage, leading RENWICK to join the Galton Laboratory and me to write a Ph.D. thesis on LODs (MORTON 1955), at that time a subject of great interest among statisticians because of WALD's (1947) book on sequential analysis, and among human geneticists because of a paper by HALDANE and SMITH (1947) on linkage of colorblindness and hemophilia. The appeal of sequential analysis was its simplicity and efficiency, conjoined with the fact that linkage detection often depended on a succession of samples, after each of which linkage could be accepted, rejected, or subjected to further test. This corresponded exactly with a sequential sampling rule to accept H_1 for $Z > \log A$ and to accept H_0 for $Z < \log B$, where H_1 specifies a probability in terms of recombination frequency $\theta < 0.5$ and H_0 assumes no linkage ($\theta = 0.5$). Increasing the size of a sample makes the test more conservative and the average sample size larger. For simplicity, WALD developed his theory in terms of a preassigned value of θ, and for many years some statisticians assumed that his bound on the type I error applied to every value of θ except the one that maximizes the likelihood (CHOTAI 1984), but this misunderstanding has been laid to rest (COLLINS and MORTON 1991). The first paper derived a number of LODs for two-generation families and tabulated the z scores (MORTON 1955). In a short time LODs were used to

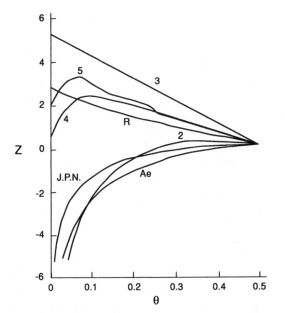

FIGURE 1.—LODs for elliptocytosis and *RH*. Pedigrees 3, 4, 5, and R are *EL1*, closely linked to *RH*. Pedigrees 2, Ae and J.P.N. are unlinked *EL2* and *EL3*.

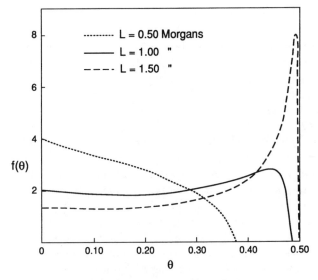

FIGURE 2.—The distribution of the recombinant fraction θ for chromosomes of length L.

disprove earlier claims of autosomal and partial sex linkage, the two reports from the Galton Laboratory were confirmed (MORTON 1957), and elliptocytosis was shown to involve dominant alleles at different loci in different pedigrees (MORTON 1956). One locus, close to *RH*, determines the protein band 4.1, while the others are α spectrin (*SPTA1*) and β spectrin (*SPTB*). These proteins are essential for the integrity of the erythrocyte membrane. Linkage heterogeneity of this type due to one of several mechanisms is common for human disease. To demonstrate the first example (Figure 1), I used the chi-square test derived from Equation 2, $(2 \ln 10)(\sum_{n=1}^{m} \hat{z}_i - \hat{Z})$, where $\hat{z}_i$ is the maximum LOD in the *i*th sample, $\hat{Z}$ is the maximum LOD overall, and there are $m - 1$ d.f. The α test of C. A. B. SMITH (1963) is more powerful. It takes the likelihood ratio as

$$\lambda_i = \frac{\alpha P(S_i | H_1) + (1 - \alpha) P(S_i | H_0)}{P(S_i | H_0)}$$

$$= \alpha P(S_i | H_1) / P(S_i | H_0) + 1 - \alpha \tag{4}$$

where α is the proportion of families linked to the marker. Because θ and α are both estimated, it is necessary to make some allowance when testing linkage for the extra degree of freedom (LANDER and LINCOLN 1988; RISCH 1989).

There is nothing in likelihood ratio theory that mandates a particular choice of logarithms. Following SMITH (1953), I used common logarithms (base 10) that are now universally accepted. Some mathematicians have expressed a preference for natural logarithms (base e), but the advantage of a factor of 2 over a factor of 4.6 is too tenuous to counterbalance the confusion that such a change would cause in a practice that has lasted for forty years.

Early studies presented a standard LOD table with values of θ from 0 to 0.5, from which the likelihood could be recovered. As the volume of data grew this became impractical, and today it is usual to report only the maximum likelihood estimate θ and corresponding LOD if $\theta \neq 0.5$, but otherwise a smaller value (usually 0.3), so that the equivalent number of meioses and recombinants can be estimated. Thus the distinction between sequential and nonsequential tests has diminished but may be reinforced for polygenic traits, where one sample is usually insufficient to assert linkage.

SMITH (1954) and RENWICK (1968) were the first to recognize the importance of sex differences in recombination, which are greater in the human than in the mouse, and to develop methods to factor LODs by sex. Because of their work, it is now usual and should be mandatory to present sex-specific LODs, so that maps may be constructed for both sexes and their differences studied in relation to condensation, coiling, protein binding, and other factors. Sex differences affect risks in genetic counseling and optimal analysis for high-resolution mapping.

The Galton Laboratory has maintained a strong interest in Bayesian statistics, the impact of which has been equivocal. HALDANE and SMITH (1947) suggested "chiefly from a comparison with the known linkage values of Drosophila" that the recombination fraction for linked genes has a nearly uniform distribution from 0 to 0.5. No assumption was or need be made about the distribution on the physical map, but it is now known that regions of high recombination tend to have a high density of CpG islands. Analytic treatment shows that the distribution is only roughly uniform, with an excess of small values of θ if the chromosome is small (Figure 2). At a time when there were no data in the human and the chromosome number was thought to be 48, I suggested that the prior probability of synteny for two random autosomal loci was about 0.05 (MORTON 1955), and subsequent data refined this to 0.054 (RENWICK 1969). With the uniform approximation or a more exact one, the average odds Λ may be calculated, leading to inference about the posterior probability of linkage that appeals strongly to Bayesians. Alternatively, if $\rho(\theta)$ is the power of the test when the true recombination value is θ and $g(\theta)$ is the prior probability of θ given synteny, then $\int_0^{1/2} g(\theta)\rho(\theta)\,d\theta$ is the expected value of Λ, which can be used to select a significance level that is "reasonable" in the sense that a large proportion of statistically significant results will be true (MORTON 1955). The approach is more appealing to frequentists, who distrust Bayesian assumptions. For two random loci a value of $Z > 3$ and therefore $\alpha < 0.001$ is appropriate if sample size is adequate to detect close linkage. However, in smaller samples (such as most single pedigrees) this condition is not met (SKOLNICK et al. 1984; RISCH 1991), and therefore the Bayesian calculation may be favored. However, if there is linkage in some families, the prior probability does not correspond to a uniform distribution but more closely to Equation 4, and so the calculations are error-prone (GÉNIN et al. 1995). Although R. A. FISHER thought he had annihilated Bayesians, he was wrong. They continue to be dissatisfied with significance tests and to defend some formulation of posterior probability that may be useful in some cases. There is even a computer program (SIGMA) that attempts to construct maps from subjective probabilities, exploding the linear chromosome into a tree diagram that purports to give subjective order free of genetic and physical distances (BISHOP 1994; POVEY et al. 1994).

The success of LOD scores has obscured the seminal paper of C. A. B. SMITH (1953), which was largely concerned with probabilities for sib pairs and extension of FISHER's scores to pedigrees, with one section devoted to autozygosity mapping. LODs were introduced and their advantages were noted, but application was limited to matings of known phase and to trios and pairs of sibs with untested parents for the special case of a rare gene and a codominant marker. He was concerned about the computation of LODs, a problem of the utmost seriousness in Britain from 1950 to 1975 because of the protection afforded to computers manufactured in the United Kingdom. Unfortunately, domestic computers seldom worked and had poor compilers. A generation of researchers was sacrificed to protectionism, and scientific computing in Britain still suffers from the check to confidence and originality suffered in that period. Under this stimulus, RENWICK did his linkage computing in Baltimore (RENWICK and BOLLING 1967), and JOHN EDWARDS turned to New York (FALK and EDWARDS 1970). The first portable computer program for computing LODs in general pedigrees (LIPED) was developed by OTT (1974).

By the end of the seventies gene mappers were accustomed to meet every two years at workshops. About 300 loci had been assigned to the human autosomes (HUMAN GENE MAPPING 1979), and there were LODs for about half of them. Linkage had been complemented by expression of a human protein in somatic cell hybrids and in situ hybridization of radioactive probes (RUDDLE et al. 1972), although these physical methods gave lower resolution. Linkage maps were constructed by multiple pairwise LODs, in the most favorable case spanning 13 loci (RAO et al. 1979). Integration of genetic and physical data was crude and largely subjective. A database of LODs had been published (KEATS 1981), but the database on physical assignment was a card index with no linkage data. The stage was set for an advance that would strain these resources to the breaking point.

The DNA revolution: SOUTHERN (1975) demonstrated that specific DNA sequences could be separated by gel electrophoresis. This soon led to use of restriction fragment length polymorphisms as linkage markers (SOLOMON and BODMER 1979; BOTSTEIN et al. 1980), succeeded by markers defined on the polymerase chain reaction (PCR). The Centre d'Etude du Polymorphisme Humain (CEPH) provided DNA from large families to international collaborators, and soon they had linkage data on thousands of markers (DAUSSET et al. 1990). Several multilocus computer programs were developed to handle these samples and pedigrees of disease genes, all based on the assumption of no interference or typing errors (OTT 1991). Despite continued improvement, these programs cannot cope with strong interference, substantial error frequencies, dense maps, and innumerable datasets that can be summarized by LODs. It has been shown that multiple pairwise LODs give more accurate maps in the presence of typing errors (BUETOW 1991). The LODSOURCE database has been incorporated into a location database that includes locus content, clonal and other physical data, and can integrate all these sources into a summary map (MORTON et al. 1992), which the genome database (GDB) cannot do (PEARSON et al. 1991). In desperation, gene mappers have turned to consensus reports of single-chromosome workshops that practice electoral science. Therefore, the current standard of the Human Genome Initiative is a consensus map in which the position of each locus is supported by at least one member of a workshop, but the evidence (if any) on which this location is based is not accessible to other scientists. LODs provide a vehicle to summarize linkage data from unlimited numbers of pedigrees, formats, and data files.

Although linkage is not capable of high resolution, it is the best method to give connectivity to physical maps and to assign an approximate position to disease loci that can be refined by allelic disequilibrium and physical maps, prior to cloning and sequencing. Much of the information on linkage markers generated through disease mapping is neither published nor made public through Internet, but could be captured through LODs, and locus-oriented multiple pairwise mapping can cope with thousands of loci per chromosome. There is no longer any motive to reconstruct the map by crude seriation or stepwise addition, nor to select by necessarily subjective criteria a small set of gold star loci for an index map. Instead, map integration must be used to improve dense but locally unreliable maps by reference to a location database that includes accumulated LODs as well as physical data. Only in this way can an enormously expensive mapping effort be used efficiently to characterize disease genes and to validate YAC and other contigs preparatory to sequencing.

An interesting recent development has been the resurrection of nonparametric sib-pair methods for polygenic inheritance, one of which is based on the asymptotic distribution (Equation 2) of a LOD for identity by descent (RISCH 1990; HOLMANS 1993). This and other nonparametric methods are robust to ascertainment bias (and therefore lend themselves to meta-analysis of multiple samples), but are less reliable than conventional LODs in small samples or with related sib pairs (COLLINS and MORTON 1995). Some investigators use weak significance levels to continue sampling, on the basis of their intuition that power is less than for major loci but the likely number of minor genes is great. The resultant error rate has not been determined, and the power of nonparametric methods against an appropriate genetic model is unknown.

Among genetic models the two-allele, two-locus model has seen greatest use, with a linked "major" locus and an unlinked "modifier" that is a surrogate for more complex inheritance (MORTON et al. 1992). Allelic association is represented by coupling frequencies: if c_i is the coupling frequency for the ith allele A_i with frequency p_i, then $p_i c_i$ is the frequency of haplotypes bearing A_i and an allele at the major locus for disease susceptibility, the total frequency of susceptibility alleles at that locus being $q = \Sigma p_i c_i$. Therefore, a single model tests both linkage and allelic association. To do this within the framework of statistical tests requires that Equations 1 and 2 be extended: if a genetic model specifies m nuisance parameters Ω_0 under H_0 describing gene frequencies and genotypic effects and $m + r$ parameters Ω_1 under H_1, and if the parameters are efficiently estimated under each hypothesis, then Equation 1 holds with $r = 1$, while Equation 2 holds for all r.

This approach and alternatives are being discussed vehemently, as is the optimal sampling strategy. The more the search for polygenes depends on replicate samples, the more closely it conforms to sequential sampling. The LODs that were proposed to detect linkage forty years ago, when the human gene map was only a dream, have proven their fitness to survive in a changed environment. It rests with alternatives to demonstrate equal viability.

LITERATURE CITED

BARNARD, G. A., 1949 Statistical inference. J. R. Stat. Soc. **B11:** 115–139.

BERNSTEIN, F. 1931 Zur Grundlegung der Vererbung beim Menschen. Z. indukt. Abstammungs. Vererbungsl. **57:** 113–138.

BISHOP, M. J. (Editor) 1994 *Guide to Human Genome Computing*. Academic Press, London.

BOTSTEIN, D., R. L. WHITE, M. SKOLNICK and R. W. DAVIS, 1980 Construction of a genetic linkage map in man using restriction fragment length polymorphisms. Am. J. Hum. Genet. **32:** 314–331.

BUETOW, K. H. 1991 Influence of aberrant observations on high-resolution linkage analysis outcomes. Am. J. Hum. Genet. **49:** 985–994.

CHOTAI, J., 1984 On the lod score method in linkage analysis. Ann. Hum. Genet. **48:** 359–378.

COLLINS, A., and N. E. MORTON, 1991 Significance of maximal lods. Ann. Hum. Genet. **55:** 39–41.

COLLINS, A., and N. E. MORTON, 1995 Nonparametric tests for linkage with dependent sib-pairs. Hum. Hered. (in press).

CROW, J. F., 1993 FELIX BERNSTEIN and the first human marker locus. Genetics **133:** 4–7.

DAUSSET, J., H. CANN, D. COHEN, M. LATHROP, J. M. LALOUEL et al., 1990 Centre d'Etude du Polymorphisme Humain (CEPH): collaborative genetic mapping of the human genome. Genomics **6:** 575–577.

FALK, C. T., and J. H. EDWARDS, 1970 A computer approach to the analysis of family genetic data for detection of linkage. Genetics **64:** s18.

FINNEY, D. J., 1940 The detection of linkage. Ann. Eugen. **10:** 171–214.

FISHER, R. A., 1935 The detection of linkage with "dominant" abnormalities. Ann. Eugen. **6:** 187–201.

FUJII, T., W. C. MOLONEY and N. E. MORTON, 1955 Data on linkage of ovelocytosis and blood groups. Am. J. Hum. Genet. **7:** 72–75.

GÉNIN, E., M. MARTINEZ and F. CLERGET-DARPOUX, 1995 Posterior probability of linkage and maximal lod score. Ann. Hum. Genet. **59:** 123–132.

HALDANE, J. B. S., 1934 Methods for the detection of autosomal linkage in man. Ann. Eugen. **6:** 26–65.

HALDANE, J. B. S., and C. A. B. SMITH, 1947 A new estimate of the linkage between the genes for haemophilia and colour-blindness in man. Ann. Eugen. **14:** 10–31.

HOGBEN, L. T., 1934 The detection of linkage in human families. Proc. R. Soc. Lond. **B114:** 340–363.

HOLMANS, P., 1993 Asymptotic properties of affected sib-pair analysis. Am. J. Hum. Genet. **52:** 362–374.

HUMAN GENE MAPPING 5, 1979 Cytogenet. Cell Genet. **25:** 1–236.

KEATS, B. J. B., 1981 *Linkage and Chromosome Mapping in Man*. University of Hawaii, Honolulu.

LANDER, E. S., and S. E. LINCOLN, 1988 The appropriate threshold for declaring linkage when allowing sex-specific recombination rates. Am. J. Hum. Genet. **43:** 396–400.

LAWLER, S. D., 1954 Family studies showing linkage between elliptocytosis and the Rhesus blood group system. Proc. Int. Congr. Genet., IX, Caryologia Suppl., p. 1199.

MOHR, J., 1951 A search for linkage between the Lutheran blood group and other hereditary characters. Acta Pathol. Microbiol. Scand. **28:** 207–210.

MORTON, N. E., 1955 Sequential tests for the detection of linkage. Am. J. Hum. Genet. **7:** 277–318.

MORTON, N. E., 1956 The detection and estimation of linkage between the genes for elliptocytosis and the Rh blood type. Am. J. Hum. Genet. **8:** 80–96.

MORTON, N. E., 1957 Further scoring types in sequential linkage tests, with a critical review of autosomal and partial sex linkage in man. Am. J. Hum. Genet. **9:** 55–75.

MORTON, N. E., W. C. MOLONEY and T. FUJII, 1954 Linkage in man. Pelger's nuclear anomaly, taste, and blood groups. Am. J. Hum. Genet. **6:** 38–43.

MORTON, N. E., A. COLLINS, A. LAWRENCE and D. C. SHIELDS, 1992 Algorithms for a location database. Ann. Hum. Genet. **56:** 223–232.

NEYMAN, J., and E. S. PEARSON, 1928 On the use and interpretation of certain test criteria for purposes of statistical reference. Biometrika **20A:** 175–240, 263–294.

OTT, J. 1974   Estimation of the recombination fraction in human pedigrees—efficient computation of the likelihood for human linkage studies. Am. J. Hum. Genet. **26:** 588–597.

OTT, J., 1991   *Analysis of Human Genetic Linkage,* revised. Johns Hopkins University Press, Baltimore.

PEARSON, P. L., B. MAIDAK, M. CHIPPERFIELD and R. ROBBINS, 1991   The human genome initiative: do databases reflect current progress? Science **254:** 214–215.

PENROSE, L. S., 1935   The detection of autosomal linkage in data which consist of pairs of brothers and sisters of unspecified parentage. Ann. Eugen. **6:** 133–138.

POVEY, S., J. ARMOUR, P. FARNDON, J. L. HAINES, M. KNOWLES *et al.,* 1994   Report on the third international workshop on chromosome 9. Ann. Hum. Genet. **58:** 177–250.

RAO, D. C., B. J. B. KEATS, J. M. LALOUEL, N. E. MORTON and S. YEE, 1979   A maximum likelihood map of chromosome 1. Am. J. Hum. Genet. **31:** 680–696.

RENWICK, J. H., 1968   Ratio of female to male recombination fraction in man. Bull. Eur. Soc. Hum. Genet. **2:** 7–12.

RENWICK, J. H., 1969   Progress in mapping human autosomes. Br. Med. Bull. **25:** 65–73.

RENWICK, J. H., and D. R. BOLLING, 1967   A program-complex for encoding, analysis and storing human linkage data. Am. J. Hum. Genet. **19:** 360–367.

RENWICK, J. H., and S. D. LAWLER, 1955   Genetical linkage between the ABO and nail-patella loci. Ann. Hum. Genet. **19:** 312–331.

RENWICK, J. H., and J. SCHULZE, 1965   Male and female recombination fraction for the nail-patella:ABO linkage in man. Ann. Hum. Genet. **28:** 379–392.

RISCH, N., 1989   Linkage detection tests under heterogeneity. Genet. Epidemiol. **6:** 473–480.

RISCH, N., 1990   Linkage strategies for genetically complex traits.

III. The effect of marker polymorphism on analysis of affected relative pairs. Am. J. Hum. Genet. **46:** 242–253.

RISCH, N., 1991   A note on multiple testing procedures in linkage analysis. Am. J. Hum. Genet. **48:** 1058–1064.

RUDDLE, F., F. RICCIUTI, F. S. MCMORRIS, J. TISCHFIELD, R. CREAGAN *et al.,* 1972   Somatic cell genetic assignment of peptidase and the RH linkage group to chromosome A-1 in man. Science **176:** 1429–1431.

SKOLNICK, M. H., E. A. THOMPSON, D. T. BISHOP and L. A. CANNON, 1984   Possible linkage of a breast cancer-susceptibility locus to the ABO locus: sensitivity of LOD scores to a single new recombinant observation. Genet. Epidemiol. **1:** 363–373.

SMITH, C. A. B., 1953   The detection of linkage in human genetics (with discussion). J. R. Stat. Soc. **B14:** 153–192.

SMITH, C. A. B., 1954   The separation of the sexes of parents in the detection of human linkage. Ann. Eugen. **18:** 278–301.

SMITH, C. A. B., 1959   Some comments on the statistical methods used in linkage investigations. Am. J. Hum. Genet. **11:** 289–304.

SMITH, C. A. B., 1963   Testing for heterogeneity of recombination fraction in human genetics. Ann. Hum. Genet. **27:** 175–182.

SMITHIES, O., 1955   Zone electrophoresis in starch gels: group variations in the serum proteins of normal human adults. Biochem. J. **61:** 629–641.

SMITHIES, O., 1995   Early days of gel electrophoresis. Genetics **139:** 1–4.

SOLOMON, E., and W. F. BODMER, 1979   Evolution of sickle variant gene. Lancet **ii:** 923.

SOUTHERN, E. M., 1975   Detection of specific sequences among DNA fragments separated by gel electrophoresis. J. Mol. Biol. **98:** 503–517.

WALD, A., 1947   *Sequential Analysis.* Wiley, New York.

WIENER, A. S., 1932   Method of measuring linkage in human genetics, with special reference to blood groups. Genetics **17:** 335–350.

See also page 705 in Addenda et Corrigenda.

Quarreling Geneticists and a Diplomat

James F. Crow

Genetics Department, University of Wisconsin–Madison, Madison, Wisconsin 53706

IN the 1950s the hydrogen bomb was new; it was also fearsome. Some of the test explosions produced debris that was dispersed by high-altitude winds, dropping radioactive fallout over an entire hemisphere. Some geneticists feared that mutations induced by the radiation would constitute a significant genetic hazard to future generations. Other people argued that the tests were a necessary part of the Cold War. Above-ground testing became a divisive political issue and played a large role in the presidential campaign between DWIGHT EISENHOWER and ADLAI STEVENSON, STEVENSON calling for cessation.

Responding to calls for a scientific evaluation, the President of the National Academy of Sciences, D. W. BRONK, appointed six committees to study the question. Collectively they were called the Committee on Biological Effects of Atomic Radiations (BEAR). Because of the very low individual doses, most effects of the fallout were thought to be unimportant. Cancer risks were not regarded as significant, because at that time it was generally assumed that somatic effects, cancer in particular, occurred only above a threshold dose much higher than any individual would receive from peacetime nuclear applications. In contrast, geneticists believed that each dose, however small, carried a correspondingly small but nevertheless real risk of mutation induction. And a tiny dose to billions of people added up to an enormous number of ionizations.

The genetics committee included some of the best known geneticists of the classical period: MULLER, WRIGHT, STURTEVANT, BEADLE, DEMEREC, SONNEBORN, and LITTLE.[1] Human genetics was represented by JIM NEEL, who was studying the children of the bomb survivors in Hiroshima and Nagasaki. BILL RUSSELL, from Oak Ridge, brought the latest information from his megamouse experiments. BENTLEY GLASS, as rapporteur, had the tedious job of taking notes. A man with the patience of JOB, he only once asserted his independence and asked for an adjournment to ease his writer's cramp.

In what at first appeared to be a strange decision, BRONK appointed as chairman of the genetics committee, not a geneticist but a mathematician, WARREN WEAVER. The decision turned out to be providential. After a distinguished mathematical career at the University of Wisconsin, WEAVER had joined the Rockefeller Foundation in 1928, becoming director for natural sciences in 1932 and remaining in this position until 1959. He had an enormous influence on the direction of biological research. One of his early decisions was to shift Rockefeller funds away from the physical sciences and toward biology, particularly those areas that made the greatest use of physics, chemistry, and mathematics. He was quick to recognized the importance of FLEMING's discovery that the mold Penicillium had antibiotic properties, and he vigorously supported FLOREY and CHAIN in the isolation and purification of penicillin. He also supported the war-time search for mutations that increased yields and the development of techniques to produce penicillin on a large scale. In the words of GLASS (1991), "If the Rockefeller Foundation had done nothing more in its entire first century than support the inauguration of the age of antibiotics in medicine, would that not be enough to justify its record of humanitarian accomplishments?" For a follow-up discussion on bacterial resistance to antibiotics, see DAVIES (1995).

Another example of WEAVER's foresight was the decision to support LINUS PAULING in his work on structural chemistry. WEAVER recognized PAULING's genius and the future biological possibilities from his discoveries. He also supported the work of BEADLE and TATUM in the development of biochemical genetics in Neurospora. In fact, this project would have been closed down during the war years were it not for WEAVER's backing. And not least, in 1938 he coined the expression "molecular biology." In his own view, nothing that he did was

---

[1] The members of the Genetics Committee were: WARREN WEAVER (Chairman), H. BENTLEY GLASS (Rapporteur), GEORGE W. BEADLE, JAMES F. CROW, M. DEMEREC, G. FAILLA, ALEXANDER HOLLAENDER, B. P. KAUFMANN, C. C. LITTLE, H. J. MULLER, JAMES V. NEEL, W. L. RUSSELL, T. M. SONNEBORN, A. H. STURTEVANT, SHIELDS WARREN, and SEWALL WRIGHT. CHARLES COTTERMAN was appointed but was an early dropout.

as important as realizing the importance of the structure and properties of large biological molecules and supporting research in this area. Even though few knew its origin, molecular biology became not just a catchword, but a guide to the kind of thinking that led to the molecular revolution. The Rockefeller Foundation provided financial support for the BEAR Committee.

WEAVER turned out to be a magnificent chairman, steering a group of contentious geneticists through their rancorous disputes to a consensus, all with the skill worthy of a TALLEYRAND. According to GLASS (1991), "Weaver's contribution to this momentous scientific report remains, I believe, the very greatest scientific contribution of his own life." Surely this was *one* of his greatest, although my vote for *the* greatest accomplishment goes to his early realization of the importance of molecular biology and coining the expression.

The first BEAR Committee meeting took place at Princeton University in November, 1955, and after several more meetings, the report was published in June, 1956 (BEAR 1956). In the early stages, the Committee leaned heavily on the advice of H. J. MULLER. MULLER, in his earliest papers describing X-ray production of mutations, had cautioned against any unnecessary radiation that might reach the germ cells. The principles that were established by 1955, mostly from Drosophila research, were as follows: the overwhelming proportion of mutations whose effects can be detected are harmful; ionizing radiation enhances the mutation rate; most "recessive" mutations are partially dominant; the effect is independent of dose rate; and the number of mutations produced is strictly proportional to the dose, so that there is no "safe" dose. Thus, to MULLER, the total dose to germ-line cells during the pre-reproductive years was all that mattered. Dose-rate dependence was not discovered until after the report was published, and of course, such things as repair mechanisms were not known. Tissue, cell, and sex differences were largely unexplored. In 1956 the problem appeared simpler than it did later, or does now, for that matter.

The amount of radiation required to produce a number of mutations equal to those that occur spontaneously (the doubling dose) was estimated at 5–150 roentgens (r). (In those days radiation was measured in roentgens and rems, rather than the 100-fold greater current units, grays and sieverts.) The doubling dose could hardly be less than 5 r, for the estimated average radiation received in the first 30 years of life from natural sources (cosmic and ground radiation) was estimated as 4–5 r. A doubling dose this low would imply that all mutations are caused by natural radiation. This was known not to be the case in Drosophila, and there was indirect evidence for its not being true in humans either. The Committee consensus was that the value probably lay between 30 and 80 r, based mostly on comparison of radiation-induced rates at selected loci in

the mouse with crude estimates of spontaneous rates in humans. It had recently been discovered that the induced mutation rate per roentgen was considerably higher in the mouse than in Drosophila, and some had worried that the human rate might be still higher. The data on possible indicators of mutations among children in Hiroshima and Nagasaki were not statistically significant, but could be used to set an upper limit on human susceptibility. They provided some assurance that human genes are not grossly more mutable than those of mice.

On all this the Genetics Committee members were in essential agreement. The division arose over a desire to be quantitative about the societal impact of an increased mutation rate. MULLER (1950) was deeply impressed by the principle, first enunciated by HALDANE (1937), that each mutation, however mild, has the same average effect on the fitness of the population. The reason is that mild mutations persist more generations in the population and affect a correspondingly larger number of individuals. In MULLER's terminology, each mutation in a stable population leads to one gene extinction, or "genetic death;" in a growing population the number is correspondingly larger. He realized that recessiveness and, especially, epistasis could reduce the impact, since several mutations could be picked off in a single genetic death. But he did not think that this would make a substantial change; the current emphasis on truncation selection as a load-reducing mechanism was not part of the thinking in those days. MULLER argued forcefully that the genetic death principle was the only way to get at the total impact of a mutation; to measure only tangible effects was to ignore the submerged part of the iceberg. Here is a description of the concept, in WEAVER's lucid prose: "One way of thinking about this problem of genetic damage is to assume that all kinds of mutations on the average produce equivalent damage, whether as a drastic effect on one individual who leaves no descendants because of this damage, or a wider effect on many. Under this view, the total damage is measured by the number of mutations induced by a given increase in radiation, this number to be multiplied in one's mind by the average damage from a typical mutation."

Strong objections to this came from WRIGHT. He argued, and most Committee members agreed with him, that it is not meaningful to equate all genetic deaths. A mutation causing early embryonic death or failure to reproduce could have no appreciable effect on human welfare, in contrast to one causing a severe physical or mental impairment that could have devastating effects on both the individual and the family. Yet each leads to one genetic death.

Furthermore, WRIGHT said, a natural population contains many isoalleles, indistinguishable by ordinary means, and each having an extremely minute effect.

Such alleles were the stuff of human quantitative traits, he argued, and most such traits had an intermediate value as the fitness optimum. Too much or too little of almost anything is bad, he said. At that time the existence of molecular polymorphism at many loci was not known, but WRIGHT was confident that this would one day be revealed. In emphasizing nearly neutral isoalleles, WRIGHT anticipated the "infinite allele model" (KIMURA 1983), which later played such a large part in discussions of molecular polymorphism. Furthermore, WRIGHT emphasized that the HALDANE-MULLER principle did not apply to heterotic and frequency-dependent loci. Thus, the fraction of deleterious mutations might not be nearly as high as MULLER argued. And, as was his wont, WRIGHT provided a detailed analysis, full of equations.

STURTEVANT for the most part sided with MULLER. In particular, he did not like WRIGHT's analysis. STURTEVANT argued that, although indistinguishable isoalleles may well constitute a large part of the genetic variability of natural populations and be of great importance for human welfare and for evolution, they were not the kinds of mutations observed in radiation experiments in Drosophila and mice, which provided the basis for the Committee estimates. He also noted that STADLER had provided evidence that ionizing radiation produces mainly deletions and other products of broken chromosomes. In this regard he differed from MULLER, who had maintained that radiation more or less mimicked spontaneous mutations. Viewed through a 1995 retrospectroscope, STURTEVANT's view looks very good, the best of the three. In any case, the view that mutations were harmful prevailed in the Committee. The report was careful to say, however, that among mutations *with a detectable effect*, the overwhelming majority are harmful. This seemed to gain everyone's acquiescence, if not enthusiastic approval.

This difference was largely reconciled, at least as far as the wording of the report was concerned. But the biggest stumbling block remained. The argument was over genetic deaths and the applicability of the HALDANE-MULLER principle. And MULLER and WRIGHT dug in their heels. (Since I had been associated with both MULLER and WRIGHT and was familiar with their views, my role was to explain these to WEAVER, who, needless to say, was a quick study. I am sure he found the mathematical arguments quite elementary, but he liked the elegance and simplicity of the HALDANE-MULLER principle.) MULLER argued vehemently that his was the only way to assess the total impact; the uncertainties of interpreting genetic deaths in terms of human suffering, he said, were not as fatal as dealing with only tangible effects and sweeping the uncertainties under the rug. MULLER was both stubborn and forceful. He oversimplified, he overstated, and he brought up every possible argument. As he argued, I kept thinking what a great

trial lawyer he would have been. But as a politician, he was far less effective. He never learned that argumentative overkill is not the best way to win converts.

WRIGHT was no less stubborn, and he was longer-winded. He stressed the importance of isoalleles, heterosis, and intermediate optima. He talked at enormous length, arguing, sometimes repetitively, that we must try to make distinctions among the different phenotypic effects of mutations as to their societal impact. He classified people by their cost to society and their contribution. Most people, he said, cost society little and contribute little. Others, such as professionals, cost society a great deal in education and high living standard, but also contribute substantially. Some people make great contributions with little cost—selfless individuals with a social conscience. Others cost heavily, but contribute little—charlatans, criminals, inheritors of wealth. And so on. He tried to determine which classes have a significant mutational component. WRIGHT's seemingly endless monologues did not please everybody. During one of them STURTEVANT whispered to me, "What would it be like if there were two WRIGHTs?"

Only a few days before the release date for the report, MULLER objected violently to a paragraph that had been put in to please WRIGHT, and said he would not sign the report if these sentences were included. At this point WEAVER's diplomatic skills again came into play. He wrote a statement giving both views, softening each somewhat, and in a long telephone conversation persuaded MULLER to accept it. Then he was fearful that WRIGHT might not go along and sent a letter to me (WRIGHT and I worked in the same building and saw each other daily), which I here reproduce.

June 8, 1956

PERSONAL AND CONFIDENTIAL

Dear Jim:

I am sending you herewith a copy of the material which is replacing pages 14 and 15 of the report. It has not been changed since I read it to you on the telephone. I was simply horrified to receive yesterday a telegram from Muller stating that he was unwilling to sign the report if it included "Wright's paragraph alleging great differences in total damage per mutation or its equivalent."

I am taking the position that it would be a scientific and social tragedy if this report cannot receive the unanimous backing of the group. It would create an absolutely false impression, and it would be in fact really ridiculous, if any member fails to stand by the report at this stage because of disagreement over some relatively minor aspect.

I am mailing to Professor Wright a copy of the new version of pages 14 and 15, with a very short note saying that I hope he is reasonably happy with it. I am writing this confidential letter to you so that you will know the background if, by any foul chance, Professor Wright should be disturbed over the way in which I rewrote and incorporated this material. If that happens you could make clear to him that I went just as far as I possibly could, for I talked with Muller on the phone yesterday afternoon, and by reading him this actual version and arguing with him, I have gotten him to agree to accept it. I don't think that he would accept anything that is anything closer to Wright's original wording.

Very sincerely yours,
Warren Weaver

Although he wasn't entirely happy, WRIGHT was willng to go along and I so informed WEAVER. At last, only days before its release date, the report finally carried a unanimous endorsement, to the relief of the Committee members, the National Academy of Sciences, and especially WEAVER. For those who are curious, WEAVER's words may be found in section (7) of the report (BEAR 1956), starting on page 17.

Yet there is a supreme irony. The whole rancorous debate had no effect on the specific recommendations. The Committee recommended: "Keep the dose as low as you can." It used the natural background radiation level, thought to be about 4–5 r per 30-year generation, as the quantitative standard. It recommended that a uniform national standard for man-made radiation be such that the average accumulated gonadal dose from conception to age 30 be less than 10 r. At the time the Committee thought that about half this amount would come from medical radiation, mostly diagnostic. (Therapeutic radiation, although given in much greater individual amounts, produces less genetically significant radiation to the population.) The amount from fallout was much less. The Committee estimated that if weapons testing continued at the current rate, the genetic dose from this source would be less than 0.1 r. Nevertheless, a very small amount of individual radiation from bomb testing, since it spread over much of the world, affected an enormous number of people. Curiously, a study designed to consider the effect of bomb testing ended up showing a much greater contribution from medical radiation. As a result, a number of radiation-reducing procedures were introduced into the practice of diagnostic radiology and are now standard.

The general viewpoint of the Committee members was that, since mankind has survived millions of years with background radiation, increases of the same magnitude are not likely to have any disastrous effect. Furthermore, if the doubling dose is 30–80 r, the increase from 10 r would be a small fraction of the spontaneous rate. In WEAVER's words, the 10 r limit is "reasonable (not <u>harmless</u>, mind you, but <u>reasonable</u>)." The entire genetics section was written in WEAVER's informal, easy to read, conversational style, and I believe that a large part of its quick acceptance and influence is owed to this.

The recommendations were quickly adopted by the National Committee on Radiation Protection and soon

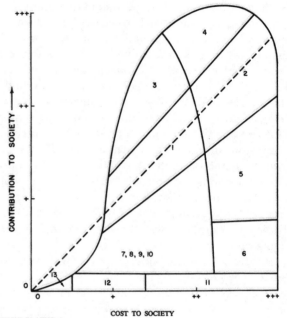

PHENOTYPIC CLASSES:
1. Contribution = cost at low level
2. Contribution = cost at high level
3. Contribution > cost at low level
4. Contribution > cost at high level
5. Contribution < cost because of unearned wealth, etc. (playboy type)
6. Contribution < cost because of antisocial career
7. Contribution < cost because of subnormal physical constitution
8. Contribution < cost because of subnormal mentality
9. Contribution < cost because of interruption of career by physical breakdown
10. Contribution < cost because of interruption of career by mental breakdown
11. No contribution, high cost because of complete incapacity from childhood (long life)
12. No contribution, moderate cost because of death before maturity
13. No contribution, little cost because of pre- or perinatal death

FIGURE 1.—WRIGHT's societal contribution-cost analysis.

became the basis for national policy. The major innovation was to regard the population average as the controlling consideration. Previously, all radiation protection standards had been based on observed somatic harm to the individual, and therefore involved much higher doses. The National Academy of Sciences at that time had not done this kind of policy-setting report. It has done many since, but this one was outstanding in the way it immediately and permanently changed public policy in radiation protection. Since that time there have been studies by the United Nations, the National Council on Radiation Protection and Measurements, the International Committee on Radiation Protection, and the National Academy of Sciences. These are much more detailed, but have not caused a major change in public policy, although acceptable radiation dosages continued to decrease.

What happened to the material that WRIGHT wrote? After 1956, the Committee continued under the chairmanship of BEADLE and with the addition of TH. DOBZHANSKY, who added his debating skills to WRIGHT's arguments. The old divisiveness reappeared. WRIGHT had reworked his analysis and it finally appeared in a second report (BEAR 1960). But whereas the first report (BEAR 1956) was front-page news and widely discussed, the second one passed largely unnoticed and WRIGHT's analysis was buried with it.

WRIGHT's analysis is reproduced here as Figure 1. For the purpose of a societal analysis, he classified people into 13 groups. With typical breadth and thoroughness, he tried to classify phenotypes on the basis of cost and benefit, cost to society *vs.* contribution to society. For most of the population these approximately balance, around the 45° line (provided that society is static; overall improvements would raise the slope). WRIGHT concluded that categories 7–13, in which the costs to society outweigh the benefits, all have a significant genetic component. But he was careful to say that the contribution of mutation to the incidence remains in much doubt, as of course it still does. It is easy to understand that, although this was regarded as a thoughtful analysis, the Committee members generally agreed that it was not needed in the report. It was included as an appendix. JIM NEEL was also on the committee and has written about some of his memories of both reports (NEEL 1994).

A 35-year retrospective look at WRIGHT's diagram is revealing. From the present, when the emphasis is on people's entitlements from society and not on their obligations, it is refreshing to look back on WRIGHT's unabashed balancing of people's contributions to society against their costs. As far as I know, WRIGHT never discussed this again, but it epitomizes his way of thinking.

Recent years have brought two major changes. Shortly after the 1956 report was issued, a new view of somatic effects began to be taken seriously. It was argued by several—E. B. LEWIS, of *Bithorax* fame, was particularly effective—that malignancies may, like mutations, have no threshold. Hence the assumption of linearity at low doses, down to dose zero, began to be applied to cancer risks. Since this affects the current population, not descendants who may be several generations removed, it soon became the item of major concern. Policy debates over radiation protection standards now center mainly on assessment of somatic risks.

The second change concerns chemical mutagens. The BEAR Committee did not consider chemicals. This may seem surprising, in view of the fact that AUERBACH's discovery of the mutagenicity of mustard gas was already well known (BEALE 1993). MULLER regarded any discussion of chemical mutagenesis as likely to dilute his efforts to protect the public from radiation effects. A second and more important reason was that at that time the only known chemical mutagens were highly toxic substances, like mustard gas. Any public exposure would be accidental (or a possible consequence of war). It was several years later, after microbial and molecular techniques became much better, that geneticists found all sorts of compounds that were highly mutagenic, yet not overtly toxic. The 1960 report did discuss chemical mutagens, but they did not receive the emphasis that they would later, when they largely displaced radiation as a matter for health concern.

MULLER didn't have his way with much of the wording of the Committee report. But his major practical recommendation—that the standard be set low, in the vicinity of the natural background level, and that it be based on a population average, not an individual dose—prevailed. In the years immediately following the BEAR report there were numerous discussions, committees, and Congressional hearings. PAULING joined MULLER and was a forceful advocate. Radiation protection became a major concern and, among other consequences, above-ground bomb testing was ended. MULLER certainly won the day. In my view, he and PAULING, along with others much less visible (including me), oversold the dangers and should accept some blame for what now seems, to me at least, to be an irrational emphasis by the general public and some regulatory agencies on low-level radiation in comparison to greater risks.

The National Academy of Sciences continued to issue reports periodically. As information accumulated, the reports were modified. The approach (*e.g.*, BEIR 1972) was that of neither MULLER nor WRIGHT. Like WRIGHT, the Committee dealt with phenotypes and emphasized effects on early generations, rather than counting genetic deaths as MULLER had advocated. But the phenotypes were classified by assumed mode of inheritance, with no attempt to quantify societal costs and benefits. Assuming a doubling dose of 20–200 rem, based mainly on mouse data, the 1972 Committee estimated the first generation and equilibrium numbers of affected persons in a population of one million exposed to 5 rem per generation. The traits were classified as dominant, recessive, X-linked, cytogenetic, physical anomalies, and constitutional and degenerative diseases. There are still no reliable data from which to estimate the human radiation-induced mutation rate. It is still necessary to depend on the mouse and on the upper confidence limits of nonsignificant human effects (NEEL 1994).

As I mentioned earlier, the 1956 report was presented at a press conference and received wide publicity. Then still another problem arose. Most of the report was technical and not controversial; only the genetics section, thanks to WEAVER, was written for the general public. Writers from the *Scientific American* were co-opted to write a popular version of the report, and they proceeded to change some of the hammered-out wording of the genetics section. WEAVER again came to the rescue, persuading these writers to leave this section largely alone, and undoubtedly averted another crisis with MULLER or WRIGHT, or both.

WEAVER had done a great job, but he had had his fill. The press conference was held on June 12, 1956 and he resigned the next day.

I should like here to acknowledge my personal indebtedness to WARREN WEAVER in another regard. The next year, on his recommendation, the Rockefeller Foundation supported me on a trip to Japan to spend the summer of 1957 working with MOTOO KIMURA.

LITERATURE CITED

BEALE, G., 1993 The discovery of mustard gas mutagenesis by Auerbach and Robson in 1941. Genetics **134**: 393–399.

BEAR, 1956 *The Biological Effects of Atomic Radiation. Summary Reports.* National Academy of Science-National Research Council, Washington, D.C.

BEAR, 1960 *The Biological Effects of Atomic Radiation. Summary Reports from a Study by the National Academy of Sciences.* National Academy of Science-National Research Council, Washington, D.C.

BEIR, 1972 *The Effects on Populations of Exposure to Low Levels of Ionizing Radiation.* National Academy of Science-National Research Council, Washington, D.C.

DAVIES, J., 1995 Vicious circles: looking back on resistance plasmids. Genetics **139**: 1465–1468.

GLASS, H. B., 1991 The Rockefeller Foundation: Warren Weaver and the launching of molecular biology. Quart. Rev. Biol. **66**: 303–308.

HALDANE, J. B. S., 1937 The effect of variation on fitness. Am. Nat. **71**: 337–349.

KIMURA, M., 1983 *The Neutral Theory of Molecular Evolution.* Cambridge University Press, Cambridge.

MULLER, H. J., 1950 Our load of mutations. Am. J. Hum. Genet. **2**: 111–176.

NEEL, J. V., 1994 *Physician to the Gene Pool.* John Wiley & Sons, New York.

Galton and Identification by Fingerprints

Stephen M. Stigler

Statistics Department, University of Chicago, Chicago, Illinois 60637

THE history of true fingerprints, or as they are sometimes redundantly referred to, dermal fingerprints, gives an interesting background to current discussion of the use of DNA "fingerprints" as a tool for forensic identification. History may not repeat itself; it may only, as Mark Twain said, rhyme, but some of the issues that have arisen in consideration of the forensic use of DNA have striking parallels a century ago.

Fingerprints as a device for personal identification were not widely used before they were introduced in a district in India in the 1870s by Sir WILLIAM HERSCHEL, grandson of the astronomer of the same name. In 1880, HERSCHEL and, independently, HENRY FAULDS brought them to public attention in England as a potential method for identifying criminals, but it was only in 1890–95 with the work of FRANCIS GALTON (CROW 1993) that the use of fingerprints acquired a scientific basis.

In his 1892 book *Finger Prints* and in two subsequent books (1893, 1895), GALTON identified and studied the basic issues that must be addressed in order that fingerprints be an efficient and reliable method of criminal identification. An individual fingerprint is a marvelously complex pattern. Someone who has not looked closely at a fingerprint might suppose that identification would be accomplished by a subjective evaluation of the gross pattern, for example, the type (arch, loop, or whorl) together with an almost artistic sensitivity to notions of shape. But while these gross features were indeed useful for rough classification, GALTON stressed that identification was accomplished precisely only through attention to the *minutia* of the prints—tiny islets and forks in the ridges (Figure 1).

The basic issues GALTON addressed in his study of fingerprints are also important with "DNA fingerprints," but two of them are not matters of current dispute:

An individual's prints must be persistent over time. From examples furnished by HERSCHEL and others he gathered himself, GALTON was able to establish that human fingerprints were remarkably stable from early youth to advanced age, even to after death. They changed size

with growth, but (with one small exception) they did not change in their minutia. The single exception of several hundred features studied was a minute feature in one boy's print, a slight gap between two ridges that closed between ages $2^{1}/_{2}$ and 15.

A scheme for classification must be devised that permits efficient filing and retrieval of prints. GALTON devised taxonomic methods starting with a set of basic patterns, a method that permitted pigeonhole storage in a way that survived to the computer age.

However, two other issues GALTON raised and dealt with are at the center of current discussions:

The question, were fingerprints unique or at least sufficiently distinguishable to be used for evidence, had to be addressed convincingly. GALTON invented an ingenious probability argument to argue for near-uniqueness.

The heritability of fingerprints and their relationship within families and among ethnic or racial groups needed study. GALTON found, from sib and twin studies, that fingerprints were heritable, but not to a degree that would preclude identification, and he found only small racial differences.

GALTON's assessment of the probability of a match: GALTON took as his goal to attempt "to appraise the evidential value of finger prints by the common laws of Probability, paying great heed not to treat variations that are really correlated, as if they were independent" (1892, p. 10). In order to break a single fingerprint into components, he posed the question: if a small square were dropped onto a fingerprint at random, hiding all the portion of the pattern that lay beneath the square, and an experienced analyst attempted to reconstruct by guesswork the hidden portion based on what was observed outside the small square, how large should the square be for the probability of a successful guess to be $^{1}/_{2}$? From experiment he found that a square with a side about the width of six ridges would do the trick—actually, from 75 trials GALTON estimated that the average chance of a successful guess with a six-ridge square would be about $^{1}/_{3}$. He believed that a five-ridge square would be nearer to the size sought, but he took the six-ridge square in order to err "on the safe side."

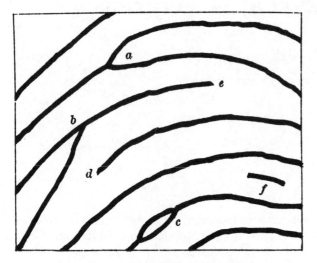

Characteristic peculiarities in Ridges

FIGURE 1.—GALTON's illustration of the characteristic peculiarities in fingerprint ridges, showing the principal types of minutia (from his *Finger Prints*, 1892, Plate 3).

A full fingerprint consisted of 24 six-ridge squares, and GALTON then claimed, "These six-ridge-interval squares may thus be regarded as independent units, each of which is equally liable to fall into one or other of two alternative classes, when the surrounding conditions are alone known" (1892, p. 109). Thus, given that each square was guessed with full knowledge of the surrounding territory, he calculated the chance of a successful composite guess at $1/2^{24}$, a value he regarded as an overestimate. In words that pre-echo those of many who have applied probability in assessing the force of DNA evidence, he wrote, "It is hateful to blunder in calculations of adverse chances, by overlooking correlations between variables, and to falsely assume them independent, with the result that inflated estimates are made which require to be proportionately reduced. Here, however, there seems to be little room for such an error" (1892, p. 109).

GALTON completed his calculation by assessing the chances that he would guess the correct conditions for reconstructing each square. He took as $1/2^4$ the chance that he would have guessed correctly "the general course of the ridges adjacent to each square," and he estimated the chance that he would have correctly guessed the numbers of ridges entering and leaving each square as $1/2^8$. Both numbers were taken as gross overestimates. This gave him an overall assessment of the chance that a random fingerprint would match a specified one as $1/2^{24} \times 1/2^8 \times 1/2^4 = 1/2^{36}$, "or 1 to about sixty-four thousand millions. The inference is, that as the number of the human race is reckoned at about sixteen thousand millions, it is a smaller chance than 1 to 4 that the print of a *single* finger of any given person would be exactly like that of the same finger of any other member of the human race" (1892, pp. 110–111). (In testimony in 1893, reprinted in GALTON 1895,

p. 35, he corrected his figure for the population to 1.6 billion, which would give odds of 1 to 39. GALTON characterized the chance of two individuals' fingerprints not being identical as "enormously greater than what in popular language begins to rank as certainty.")

To be accepted today, GALTON's modeling would require more detail, but with minor qualifications (and acceptance of GALTON's personal experience with fingerprint patterns as an adequate basis upon which to form estimates) it can be rigorously defended as correct and conservative. He also computed the allowance that should be made if two prints should match in all but one, two, or more of 35 minutiae. If prints of two or three fingers were available, GALTON would square or cube his probability, assuming the developmental equivalent of linkage equilibrium. He concluded, "Whatever reductions a legitimate criticism may make in the numerical results . . . , the broad fact remains, that a complete or nearly complete accordance between two prints of a single finger, and vastly more so between the prints of two or more fingers, affords evidence requiring no corroboration, that the persons from whom they were made are the same" (1892, pp. 112–113).

GALTON's study of the heritability of fingerprints and of racial differences: GALTON's interest in fingerprints had initially been aroused in connection with his studies of heredity, and he investigated these topics in the later chapters of his 1892 book. He focused here on the gross patterns of the prints, since he had found that even the closest relatives could be distinguished on the basis of the minutiae of their fingerprints. Indeed, present research shows that even monozygotic twins are not identical in fingerprints.

GALTON started with the association in gross pattern in sib pairs, using the simplest classification into arches, loops, and whorls. His goal was in close parallel to current studies that test for Hardy-Weinberg equilibrium by testing for excess homozygosity in tables of counts of alleles. GALTON formed a table of counts from 105 sib pairs (Figure 2), giving particular attention to the diagonal entries. But how to evaluate this table? How to decide whether the diagonal elements are too large? His solution was a nice precursor to the chi-squared test, which KARL PEARSON would introduce only eight years later. How, GALTON asked, would the counts be arrayed if the individuals classified were independent? He explained how to form such a table by dividing the product of marginal totals by the grand total, so that the expected number of Arch-Arch pairs among 105 with these marginal totals would be $(19 \times 10)/105$. He noted that all three of the diagonal counts exceeded these "random" expectations, even though they fell far short of the maximum counts achievable with these marginal totals, namely 10, 61, and 25. He repeated this study with 150 fraternities and a much finer classification of 53 gross patterns. The results were essentially the same: the total of the observed diagonal counts was

TABLE XXII.

Observed Fraternal Couplets.

B children.	A children.			Totals in B children.
	Arches.	Loops.	Whorls.	
Arches . . .	5	12	2	19
Loops . . .	4	42	15	61
Whorls . . .	1	14	10	25
Totals in A } children	10	68	27	105

FIGURE 2.—A reconstruction of GALTON's table describing sib couplets (GALTON 1892, p. 175).

TABLE XXX.

Frequency of Arches in the Right Fore-Finger.

No. of Persons.	Race.	No. of Arches.	Per Cents.
250	English	34	13·6
250	Welsh	26	10·8
1332	Hebrew	105	7·9
250	Negro	27	11·3
	Hebrews in detail——		
500	Boys, Bell Lane School . .	35	7·0
400	Girls, Bell Lane School . .	34	8·5
220	Boys, Tavistock St. & Hanway St.	18	8·2
212	Girls, Hanway Street School .	18	8·5

FIGURE 3.—A reconstruction of GALTON's table describing frequencies of arches (GALTON 1892, p. 194).

larger than under a "random" hypothesis, but far short of the greatest possible number. He gave as a measure of fraternal resemblance the relative position of the observed count on a centesimal scale, measuring as parts of 100° the distance of the observation on a scale between the "Random" (0°) and the "Utmost feasible" (100°). In his examples, his measures tended to fall between 10° and 20°, values he interpreted as affirmative evidence that there was a "decided tendency to hereditary transmission" (1892, p. 189).

GALTON found even closer similarities in 17 sets of twins. He did not differentiate between monozygotic and dizygotic twins, but in none of 17 sets of twins did he find near identity in the minutiae, although PEARSON (1930, Plate XVIII) reproduced a set of prints from GALTON's collection of twins that show remarkable similarity in pattern. GALTON also examined the relative contributions of the parents, and he thought he detected a slight tendency for the maternal influence on pattern to exceed the paternal, although the uncertainty in the figures (the effect was present for only the middle finger of the three he studied) led him "to reserve an opinion as to their trustworthiness" (1892, pp. 190–191). If valid, this would be a curious example of imprinting.

GALTON expected to find racial differences in fingerprint patterns, but when he investigated this, he was surprised at the result. He used data gathered from children in schools in London, Cardiff, and Niger, with the willing—even eager—assistance of the headmasters. He found (Figure 3) slight "statistical" differences, but concluded nonetheless that "it may emphatically be said that there is no *peculiar* pattern which characterises persons of the above races" (1892, pp. 192–193).

The acceptance of fingerprints as evidence: GALTON's analysis is at least superficially similar to current assessments of the probability of a match with DNA

profiles—a profile is broken down into components, and probabilities for the components are estimated and cautiously multiplied, at all stages erring on the side of over-estimation to ensure a safe margin. But whether this analysis had any impact upon the adoption and general acceptance of fingerprints as evidence is another matter. The first, and for many years the standard, text on the application of fingerprints was E. R. HENRY's *Classification and Uses of Finger Prints* (1900). HENRY included a brief probability calculation of his own. But it was far less satisfactory than GALTON's, and HENRY put more weight on a few striking court cases where fingerprints had been used with dramatic success than he did on theory. HENRY did allow that "It may happen that circumstantial evidence of apparently overwhelming completeness will sometimes lead to a mistaken judgment, but every Court has to act upon probabilities, for if certain evidence, in the strict meaning of the words, were required, no punishments could be inflicted" (p. 58). Other texts and documents took the effective uniqueness for granted. SCOTLAND YARD (1904) did admit to the need to guard against laboratory error, though: "One or two instances having come to notice in which the names of the wrong prisoner had inadvertently been recorded on the slips sent for record, it became necessary to provide an effective check against this source of error" (pp. 10–11).

HENRY's discussion, including at least some probability-based argument for the force of fingerprint evidence, persisted at least through his 7th edition (1934), but in other texts the uniqueness of fingerprints was simply taken for granted. For example, in J. A. LARSON's *Single Fingerprint System* (1924), we find "No two fingerprints are identical in pattern" (p. 2), and WALTER R. SCOTT (1951, p. 9) wrote in a handbook, "A normal person has ten fingers, each finger has its own individual and distinctive ridge pattern or trademark. No two are alike." The F.B.I. handbooks of the 1930s sometimes helpfully provided citations to court cases where fingerprints were admitted as definitive proof of identity, but offered no argument for uniqueness, being content to describe them as "a certain and quick means of identification" (HOOVER 1939, p. 1). The claim was generally presented with no more support than MARK TWAIN had given in *Life on the Mississippi* (1883, p. 345): "When I was a youth, I knew an old Frenchman who had been a prison-keeper for thirty years, and he told me that there was one thing about a person which never changed, from the cradle to the grave—the lines in the ball of the thumb; and he said that those lines were never exactly alike in the thumbs of any two human beings."

Fingerprints were occasionally challenged, as in *Finger-Prints Can Be Forged*, by A. WEHDE and J. N. BEFFEL (1924), but even then the challenge was based on the allegation that prints could be "lifted" and transferred, not that they were unreliable as tools for identification.

How did fingerprints come to be so universally accepted? GALTON's calculation of 1 chance in 64 billion was quoted ceremonially in the decades following his book, but it seems fair to say that by the late 1920s the basis for their acceptance was neither scientific argument nor well-documented empirical study. Rather, a plausible surmise is that it was (i) the striking visual appearance of fingerprints in the court, (ii) a few dra-

matically successful cases, and (iii) a long period in which they were used without a single case being noted where two different individuals exhibited the same pattern. It seems equally plausible that, while the acceptance of DNA evidence may be hastened by scientific argument, it will cease to be a contentious issue only after a similarly long record accumulates of successful use without notable contradiction.

LITERATURE CITED

CROW, J. F., 1993   FRANCIS GALTON: count and measure, measure and count. Genetics **135**: 1–4.

GALTON, F., 1892   *Finger Prints*. Macmillan, London.

GALTON, F., 1893   *The Decipherment of Blurred Finger-Prints*. Macmillan, London.

GALTON, F., 1895   *Fingerprint Directories*. Macmillan, London.

HENRY, E. R., 1900   *Classification and Uses of Finger Prints*. Routledge, London.

HOOVER, J. E., 1939   *Classification of Fingerprints*. FBI, Washington, DC.

LARSON, J. A., 1924   *Single Fingerprint System*. D. Appleton, New York.

PEARSON, K., 1930   *The Life, Letters and Labours of Francis Galton*, Volume IIIA. Cambridge University Press, Cambridge.

SCOTLAND YARD, 1904   *Memorandum on the Working of the Finger Print System of Identification*. HMSO, London.

SCOTT, W. R., 1951   *Fingerprint Mechanics*. C. C. Thomas, Springfield, IL.

TWAIN, M., 1883   *Life on the Mississippi*. James R. Osgood, Boston.

WEHDE, A., and J. N. BEFFEL, 1924   *Finger-Prints Can Be Forged*. Tremonia, Chicago.

Two Genes, No Enzyme
A Second Look at Barbara McClintock and the 1951 Cold Spring Harbor Symposium

Nathaniel C. Comfort

Cold Spring Harbor Laboratory, Cold Spring Harbor, New York 11724 and Department of History,
State University of New York, Stony Brook, New York 11794

"I didn't understand a word of it, but if BARBARA said it, it must be true!" With these words, the great Drosophila geneticist ALFRED STURTEVANT reportedly gave his opinion of BARBARA MCCLINTOCK's first public presentation of transposable elements, at the 1951 Cold Spring Harbor Symposium (GREEN 1992). A legend has sprung up around MCCLINTOCK's presentation, according to which she gave her talk with great expectation of acceptance and interest, only to be ridiculed and ignored by her colleagues. The subtext is that MCCLINTOCK was discriminated against, whether because of her views or her sex. In her biography of MCCLINTOCK, EVELYN FOX-KELLER writes that MCCLINTOCK's talk "was met with stony silence. With one or two exceptions, no one understood. Afterward, there was mumbling—even some snickering—and outright complaints. It was impossible to understand. What was this woman up to?" (KELLER 1983, p. 139).

MEL GREEN, writing in the 1992 Festschrift for MCCLINTOCK, *The Dynamic Genome*, seeks to redress the legend: "There is a widely extant viewpoint that BARBARA's research was much unappreciated and appropriate recognition was too long delayed. . . . I believe this viewpoint to be a half-truth" (GREEN 1992, p. 117). Some of the legend springs from MCCLINTOCK's own lips. In an interview with KELLER, MCCLINTOCK said, "It was just a surprise that I couldn't communicate; it was a surprise that I was being ridiculed, or being told that I was really mad" (KELLER 1983, p. 140). Unexplained, MCCLINTOCK's cool reception supports the idea that her colleagues were obtuse in failing to see the truth and beauty of her discovery, or worse, that they refused to accept her results because MCCLINTOCK was outside the geneticists' old boys' network.

Some of the legend seems to stem from scientists wishing to squelch it. The quote at the beginning of this essay is attributed by GREEN (1992) to ALFRED STURTEVANT, who, GREEN says, had attended the Symposium. Yet the only STURTEVANT listed as a participant in 1951 is one FRANK STURTEVANT, of Northwestern University! The error is quite excusable; while his is the only published version, this story has been repeated many times by many people, and doubtless in many versions. It is part of the legend, a mythology that continues to grow, even among demythologizers.

A re-examination of the 1951 Symposium can help replace the myth with a more rational explanation of the reaction to MCCLINTOCK's paper. It also shows how data and scientific theory are intertwined with the culture of science. MCCLINTOCK was not a passive recipient of her colleagues' judgments. She defiantly and deliberately challenged the paradigm view of the gene—a gutsy move, but one that brought upon herself some of the confusion that so distressed her.

It is certainly true that MCCLINTOCK's work was highly respected by the time she presented her data on transposable elements. Since the 1920s she had published paper after important paper on maize cytogenetics. With HARRIET CREIGHTON at Cornell, MCCLINTOCK produced the first visual evidence of crossing-over, just barely beating out CURT STERN's similar work on Drosophila. Subsequent work took her ever deeper into genomic instability and chromosome structure. First she showed the existence of ring chromosomes. Then she showed that ring chromosomes were a special case of broken chromosomes, one in which the ends became "sticky" and fused to each other. In 1936 MCCLINTOCK moved to the University of Missouri, where she was hired by LEWIS STADLER, who with R. A. EMERSON, MCCLINTOCK's mentor at Cornell, was one of the reigning lions of maize genetics. At Missouri, MCCLINTOCK discovered the "breakage-fusion-bridge" cycle, a further extension of her observations of chromosomal instability. The breakage-fusion-bridge cycle led MCCLINTOCK to two important conclusions, one a prediction

Address for correspondence: Cold Spring Harbor Laboratory, 1 Bungtown Road, Cold Spring Harbor, NY 11724.

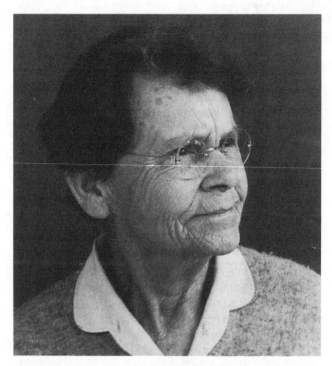

BARBARA MCCLINTOCK

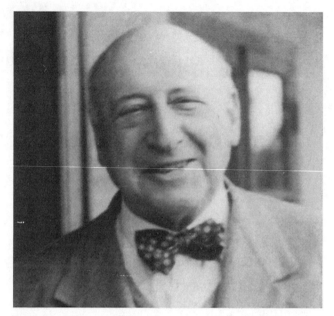

RICHARD GOLDSCHMIDT

and the other her most profound discovery. The observation of the "stickiness" of the broken ends of chromosomes led MCCLINTOCK to the prediction of special structures on the ends of chromosomes needed to maintain the stability lost when the chromosomes broke. She called them telomeres, the study of which today is undergoing rapid growth. When MCCLINTOCK left Missouri for Cold Spring Harbor in 1941, she took with her strains of maize that underwent the breakage-fusion-bridge cycle. From them MCCLINTOCK deduced the existence of transposable elements. The first set of experiments in which she observed transposition were done in 1944 (MCCLINTOCK 1984). She spent the next six years pursuing, confirming and verifying her results.

By 1951 MCCLINTOCK was among the best-respected cytogeneticists in the country. Even ten years earlier, when the director of the Carnegie Department, MILISLAV DEMEREC, told staff scientist E. CARLETON MACDOWELL that he had succeeded in hiring MCCLINTOCK, MACDOWELL "jumped up in the air and said, 'We should mark today's date with red letters in the Department calendar!' That expresses the feeling that is general among our members" (DEMEREC 1942). In 1939 she was elected vice-president, and in 1945 president, of the Genetics Society of America. By 1951 she had received the Achievement Award of the Association of University Women, been awarded two honorary degrees, and been a member of the National Academy of Sciences for seven years. "The influence of her early work is greater than that of any of her peers, with the possible exception of ALFRED STURTEVANT," wrote NINA FEDOROFF and DAVID BOTSTEIN. "Had she done no

more [before transposons], MCCLINTOCK would have become a major figure in the history of genetics" (FEDOROFF and BOTSTEIN 1992).

The 1951 Symposium took place in the years between OSWALD AVERY's demonstration that the transforming principle in Pneumococcus was DNA, and the double revelations of ALFRED HERSHEY and MARTHA CHASE's "blender experiment" and WATSON AND CRICK's model of the DNA double helix. The nature of the gene was the central question in many biologists' minds. Bacteriophage and bacteria were the model systems of choice, with Neurospora and Drosophila close behind. Scientists working with these organisms were heavily invested in the classical T. H. MORGAN model of the gene. MORGAN's group had shown the enormous intellectual productivity of viewing genes as unitary, particulate structures, arranged linearly and statically along the chromosomes. BEADLE AND TATUM's one-gene one-enzyme hypothesis, first developed in the early 1940s, lay atop this foundation. It confirmed that genes were unitary by showing they had unitary effects on metabolic pathways. MILISLAV DEMEREC, director of the Cold Spring Harbor Biological Laboratory and organizer of the 1951 Symposium, acknowledged that the gene concept had been unraveling in recent years. Genes, DEMEREC said, "are regarded as much more loosely defined parts of an aggregate, the chromosome, which in itself is a unit and reacts readily to certain changes in the environment" (DEMEREC 1951). Whatever the gene's precise molecular nature, the working model of the gene was of a unitary entity that acted independently to produce a physiologically active molecule. While many at the time recognized that it was an oversimplification, the view of the genome as a static, linear series of particulate, independently acting genes proved so successful in explaining genetic observations and generating new experiments that few had cause to doubt it.

One who did doubt it was RICHARD GOLDSCHMIDT. For decades, GOLDSCHMIDT had been a gadfly to the genetics community. Brilliant and cantankerous, GOLDSCHMIDT delighted in challenging assumptions and pointing out logical inconsistencies in the evolving genetic theory. Since 1938, GOLDSCHMIDT had been arguing against the theory of the gene. His observations of *Bar eye* in Drosophila led him to conclude that the chromosome, not the gene, was the unitary element of heredity (GOLDSCHMIDT 1938; DUNN 1965). GOLDSCHMIDT argued from translocation data that the position of a locus on the chromosome determined its function. When a locus moved to a different site, its function changed. GOLDSCHMIDT argued in 1938 that "the whole conception of the gene" was "obsolete." GOLDSCHMIDT and BEADLE took up opposing sides in a debate that lasted over a decade. GOLDSCHMIDT's was a dynamic genome, not a static one. By playing the devil's advocate, GOLDSCHMIDT forced geneticists to reconsider their assumptions. Though his style was combative and his views extreme, position effects have been supported by molecular analyses. To be sure, GOLDSCHMIDT seemed to set up a straw man; his notion of the prevailing gene concept seemed to be a globular molecule situated on the chromosome, an almost literal "bead on a string." This caricature doubtless made it easier for him to ridicule the gene theory, but it also made his alternative impossible for most geneticists to accept.

For all his crotchetiness, GOLDSCHMIDT was and is an important figure in genetics. DEMEREC gave GOLDSCHMIDT the honor of presenting the opening talk of the 1951 Symposium in a special session entitled "Theory of the Gene." The session was filled out by MCCLINTOCK herself, LEWIS J. STADLER, who also critiqued the gene model, but in a way less infuriating to geneticists, and N. H. HOROWITZ and URS LEUPOLD, speaking on new evidence for and implications of the one-gene one-enzyme theory. The "Theory of the Gene" session thus had three scientists critical of the standard model and one supportive of it. Much of the rest of the meeting was given over to the microbial geneticists. Three sessions were devoted entirely to bacteriophage and bacteria, with many more papers on microbial genetics sprinkled throughout the remaining sessions. Most of the remainder concerned Drosophila or Neurospora. On both sides of the podium, discussion was dominated by classical genetics, microorganisms, and the one-gene one-enzyme vision of genetic function.

In the opening paper of the Symposium, GOLDSCHMIDT revisited the arguments many had heard before. He had new evidence to support it, however. He took on BEADLE's model early on, accusing BEADLE of "extrapolation from the mutant action to the existence of the original gene" (GOLDSCHMIDT 1951, p. 1). Though he cited examples drawn from work on mutable genes in Drosophila and other organisms, prominent among GOLDSCHMIDT's remarks are several glowing mentions of MCCLINTOCK's description of the *Ac/Ds* system in maize. For GOLDSCHMIDT, transposable elements provided a shining example of position effects and a dynamic genome. He referred to transposable elements as "invisible" (*i.e.*, submicroscopic) rearrangements and position effects. To his full satisfaction, MCCLINTOCK had proved that in Zea, "mutable loci are actually position effects produced by genetically controlled and repeating transpositions and translocations" (GOLDSCHMIDT 1951, p. 4). GOLDSCHMIDT waxed poetic in his analogy for how genetic function derived from position: "If the A-string on a violin is stopped an inch from the end the tone C is produced. Something has been done to a locus in the string, it has been changed in regard to its function. But nobody would conclude that there is a C-body at that point" (GOLDSCHMIDT 1951, p. 7). MCCLINTOCK's data must have seemed a godsend to GOLDSCHMIDT, an example tailor-made to support his attack on the gene concept.

In her own paper, directly following GOLDSCHMIDT's in the Symposium volume, MCCLINTOCK returned the favor. Both implicitly and explicitly, she repeatedly aligned herself with GOLDSCHMIDT. Twenty-three pages into her paper, she said, "It will be noted that use of the term gene has been avoided in the foregoing discussion of instability" (MCCLINTOCK 1951, p. 36). She went on to say that this "does not imply a denial of the existence within chromosomes of units or elements having specific functions. The evidence for such units seems clear." But the gene concept, she said, "stems from studies of mutation." She then made the link with GOLDSCHMIDT explicit: "The author agrees with Goldschmidt that it is not possible to arrive at any clear understanding of the nature of a gene, or the nature of a change in a gene, from mutational evidence alone" (MCCLINTOCK 1951, p. 36). MCCLINTOCK invoked GOLDSCHMIDT again in her conclusion: "Evidence, derived from Drosophila experimentation, of the influences of various known modifiers on expression of phenotypic characters has led Goldschmidt (1949, 1951) to conclusions that are essentially similar to those given here" (MCCLINTOCK 1951, p. 46). In the battle between GOLDSCHMIDT and BEADLE, it could not have been more plain with whom MCCLINTOCK allied herself.

It is clear what appealed to MCCLINTOCK in GOLDSCHMIDT's work. Like MCCLINTOCK, GOLDSCHMIDT was arguing for a dynamic genome, a self-regulating system defined by the interactions among its parts. To both, the static concept of linear beads on a string, though it had enormous predictive value, was a vast oversimplification. Yet MCCLINTOCK undersold herself somewhat by aligning herself so closely with GOLDSCHMIDT. Her model was considerably more sophisticated than GOLDSCHMIDT's. Unlike GOLDSCHMIDT, MCCLINTOCK believed in genes; she just didn't believe they were the entire story. Her "controlling elements" were presented as a new sort of genetic material, not genes but regulators of genes. While GOLDSCHMIDT denied the BEADLE and TATUM model, MCCLINTOCK was working outside of it.

Equally clear, however, is why MCCLINTOCK's work would have received a cool reaction from the assembled audience. The differences between MCCLINTOCK's and GOLDSCHMIDT's views would have been obscured by their obvious mutual admiration. Hadn't MCCLINTOCK avoided even the use of the term gene for the first two thirds of her talk? Hadn't she concluded by saying GOLDSCHMIDT's conclusions were essentially the same as her own? To an audience full of Neurosporists, Drosophilists and phageologists, it must have seemed that they had just had to endure their second GOLDSCHMIDT talk!

Although many geneticists were relaxing their concept of the gene, all were employing it. Whatever a gene was, it was unitary and it acted independently. Eleven papers in the Symposium concerned the mutagenic effects of radiation and chemicals. Further, "mutation" and "gene" were defined in ways that were internally consistent but entirely self-contained. A mutation disrupted a gene. In his paper on pseudoallelism and crossing over, E. B. LEWIS defined the gene as a physical unit within which there is no crossing over. A static, discrete unit was inherent in his definition: "The definition of any particulate unit must be in terms of its indestructibility by some breakage or splitting process" (LEWIS 1951, p. 174). LEWIS's concept of a gene complex became a paradigm in Drosophila developmental genetics, but the regulation of the bithorax complex by chromosomal components has proved to be a key element in understanding its operation. While GOLDSCHMIDT and MCCLINTOCK's 1951 vision of genetic regulation differs from the modern conception, the parallels are in many ways more striking than the differences. MCCLINTOCK's controlling elements were non-genes, genetic particles outside the framework of one-gene one-enzyme biochemical genetics.

MCCLINTOCK did not go unnoticed in the Symposium. Several speakers in later sessions referred to her work, either in their papers or in the reprinted discussion that followed many of the papers. STADLER, of course, cited her graciously, though he did so nonanalytically. JACK SCHULTZ cited her 1933 work on association of nonhomologous chromosomes during prophase of meiosis and NORMAN GILES cited her seminal 1945 paper on the cytology of Neurospora. Two others referred to MCCLINTOCK's work on transposons. ALFRED MARSHAK, commenting on DAVID BONNER's paper on gene-enzyme relationships in Neurospora, cited MCCLINTOCK's work in connection with observations that nuclei contain a pentosenucleoprotein that continually releases polynucleotide into the cytoplasm. This polynucleotide, presumably RNA, was presented in the context of the one-gene one-enzyme theory as direct evidence that unitary genes have discrete, independent effects in the cytoplasm. MARSHAK suggested that MCCLINTOCK's Activator was involved with the formation of nucleoproteins from raw histones and polynucleotides, much like a conventional gene. MCCLINTOCK's data, he says, are

readily explained on the basis of the hypothesis if we suppose that Ds and the other similar factors represent chromosome segments containing greater amounts of DNA than those which were previously associated with the locus in question. . . . If the "activator" is involved in the production of the pentosenucleoprotein[,] as for example from raw materials such as histones and polynucleotides stored in the nucleolus[,] an alteration in the amount of the substance we have assumed to govern the rate of activity of the locus will result and hence a mutated condition: or if the intensity of the activator action varies, in a mutable condition. In this connection it appears significant that the simultaneous presence in the genome of a Ds or Ds-like region together with an "activator" results in a "fusion-breakage event" which further suggests involvement of transport and utilization of nucleolar materials (MARSHAK 1951, p. 157).

In this rather convoluted passage, MARSHAK attempts to explain MCCLINTOCK's observations from a BEADLE-and-TATUM point of view. Although MCCLINTOCK emphasized that Ac and Ds were not conventional genes, MARSHAK's explanation hinges on Ac being involved in the production of nucleic acids—in short, acting like a gene. Significantly, MARSHAK says that "while other interpretations may seem equally plausible, this one . . . is amenable to being tested experimentally," suggesting that MCCLINTOCK's interpretation is not.

In their paper on chemically induced mutations in Neurospora, K. A. JENSEN, INGER KIRK, G. KOLMARK, and M. WESTERGAARD offer a different interpretation of MCCLINTOCK's results. They cite MCCLINTOCK's controlling elements as evidence for their theory that mutable genes might result from unstable precursors accumulating in the nucleus, the result of blocked steps in a BEADLE and TATUM-style biochemical pathway:

We know from the work on biochemical mutants of Neurospora that when a specific intermediate step in the synthesis of a vitamin or an amino acid is blocked by mutation, a precursor may accumulate in the cells. We also know that some of these precursors are highly stable and may be extracted from the mycelium, and that others are very unstable and are converted into by-products, like the purple pigment in our adenineless strain, whereas others disappear completely. We want to suggest that some of the unstable precursors may act as mutagens during the decomposition. This would be a very specific type of mutagens [sic], since, as primary gene products, they may be produced within the nucleus. It does not seem improbable that some of these precursors would be so unstable that they may only react over a very short distance, thus inducing mutations in loci only within a short distance from the "blocked" gene. The so called unstable or mutable loci now under investigation by McClintock (1950) may be due to such an "unstable precursor" mechanism (Jensen et al. 1951, p. 258).

Neither Marshak nor Jensen et al. ignored McClintock's work; neither, however, accepted her interpretation of her data. Marshak and Jensen were working within the dominant paradigm of the Beadle and Tatum model, and attempted to jam McClintock's anomalous controlling elements into that prevailing and familiar conceptual framework. These examples neither illustrate cloddishness on the part of Marshak or Jensen, nor demonstrate that Marshak and Jensen "misunderstood" McClintock's work. Rather, they suggest scientists who listened to and believed McClintock's data but thought her interpretation overly speculative and even untestable. E. B. Lewis had a similar reaction. He said of McClintock, "Everybody recognized her as a great scientist. You could trust what she found out experimentally, but it was the speculation that got out of hand. This reinforced her mystical ideas. You just couldn't fit it into the standard genetic theory" (E. B. Lewis, personal communication). Lewis even suggests that McClintock and Goldschmidt may have been seen as supporting the anti-genetic stance of T. D. Lysenko—a view McClintock and Goldschmidt would have found absurd, but one that illustrates how far out they seemed to mainstream geneticists. McClintock's peers were struggling to re-interpret anomalous data into terms with which they were comfortable.

Other factors doubtless also contributed to the confusion about and lack of acceptance of McClintock's conclusions. Her model system may have had some alienating effect, but it would seem to have been small. True, Stadler was the only other maize geneticist on the program, yet there were several other plant geneticists and several cytologists. And although maize was becoming an unfashionable organism in genetics, it wasn't so far out of style as to be incomprehensible. McClintock's presentation may have been something of a barrier, however. Non-trivial, surely, was her paper's considerable length. It filled 35 pages in the Symposium volume and was by far the longest of any at the meeting. McClintock presented a welter of data, with long sections of background on each important mutation and detailed descriptions of her crosses. Her talk was essentially historical in structure, rather than the more conventional format of Introduction, Results and Conclusion, so it tended to ramble. Also, she used highly unconventional language. Beyond dispensing with the word "gene," she invented new terms to describe her new phenomena. In addition to "activators" and "dissociators"—terms that even those scientists who tackled her data handled with verbal kid gloves, such as quotation marks and "so-calleds"—she spoke of "altered states," "out-of-phase timing," and "controlling

systems." She wrote that "it was the pattern of behavior, rather than the change in expression of the particular phenotypic character, that was obviously of importance" (McClintock 1951, p. 43). She felt it was necessary "to consider these various widely different levels of unitary control and how they may operate in the working nucleus, and also to consider the nature of the changes that can affect their operation" (McClintock 1951, p. 37). This was pretty cosmic stuff to a biochemical geneticist or phage group member.

The controversy between the McClintock/Goldschmidt view of the gene and the Beadle/Tatum view was resolved with the advent of modern molecular techniques. As is often the case, both sides were partly right. Transposition became widely accepted in the 1970s as Saedler, Starlinger, Shapiro, Botstein, Fink, Fedoroff and others identified transposable elements in microbial and animal systems and elucidated the mechanism of transposition. It became clear that transposable elements can encode proteins that regulate other genes. Ac was shown to encode transposase, which activates Ds. Genome instability, position effects, and genomic regulation have become hot topics as molecular techniques allow confirmation and modification of McClintock's ideas. McClintock's vision of biology needed to be filtered through the accepted methodology and language of genetics and molecular biology in order for it to significantly influence our understanding of the gene. Further, the new techniques made it possible to confirm what had seemed speculations, and to do it in multiple species.

McClintock was universally admired as an experimentalist, but to some she seemed to be extrapolating too much from her data. Those unfamiliar with her work probably associated her paper with the one preceding it and considered McClintock just another Goldschmidtian. McClintock herself encouraged this perception by explicitly aligning herself with the notoriously controversial Goldschmidt. And Goldschmidt was, in fact, the closest to McClintock in his concept of the gene. But unlike Goldschmidt, McClintock didn't refute the paradigm—she stepped outside it. Among those who knew and respected her, some tried to squeeze her findings into their conception of the gene, while some, like Sturtevant—or whoever it was—didn't understand a word of what she said.

Thanks to Rob Martienssen for critical reading and discussion of the manuscript, to Carol Greider for critical reading and more, and to Clare Bunce for archival research. The portraits of Barbara McClintock and Richard Goldschmidt were provided by the Cold Spring Harbor Laboratory Research Library Archives.

LITERATURE CITED

Demerec, M., 1942 Letter to W. M. Gilbert, Executive Director of the Carnegie Institution of Washington, 6 April 1942. McClintock file, Cold Spring Harbor Laboratory Archives.

DEMEREC, M., 1951   Foreword. Cold Spring Harbor Symp. Quant. Biol. **16**: v.

DUNN, L. C., 1965   *A Short History of Genetics.* McGraw-Hill, New York.

FEDOROFF, N., and D. BOTSTEIN, 1992   Introduction, pp. 1–4 in *The Dynamic Genome: Barbara McClintock's Ideas in the Century of Genetics,* edited by N. FEDOROFF and D. BOTSTEIN. Cold Spring Harbor Laboratory Press, Cold Spring Harbor, NY.

GOLDSCHMIDT, R., 1938   *Physiological Genetics.* McGraw-Hill, New York.

GOLDSCHMIDT, R., 1951   Chromosomes and genes. Cold Spring Harbor Symp. Quant. Biol. **16**: 1–11.

GREEN, M., 1992   Annals of mobile DNA elements in Drosophila. The impact and influence of Barbara McClintock, pp. 117–122 in *The Dynamic Genome: Barbara McClintock's Ideas in the Century of Genetics,* edited by N. FEDOROFF and D. BOTSTEIN. Cold Spring Harbor Laboratory Press, Cold Spring Harbor, NY.

JENSEN, K. A., I. KIRK, G. KOLMARK and M. WESTERGAARD, 1951   Chemically induced mutations in Neurospora. Cold Spring Harbor Symp. Quant. Biol. **16**: 245–261.

KELLER, E. F., 1983   *A Feeling for the Organism.* W. H. Freeman, New York.

LEWIS, E. B., 1951   Pseudoallelism and gene evolution. Cold Spring Harbor Symp. Quant. Biol. **16**: 159–174.

MARSHAK, A., 1951   Discussion. Cold Spring Harbor Symp. Quant. Biol. **16**: 156–157.

MCCLINTOCK, B., 1951   Chromosome organization and genic expression. Cold Spring Harbor Symp. Quant. Biol. **16**: 13–47.

MCCLINTOCK, B., 1984   The significance of responses of the genome to challenge. Science **226**: 792–801.

September 1995

Emil Heitz (1892–1965)
Chloroplasts, Heterochromatin, and Polytene Chromosomes

Helmut Zacharias

Windmühlenberg 6, D-24631 Langwedel, Germany

TANGLED nuclear threads: EMIL HEITZ is frequently said to have discovered, together with HANS BAUER, polytene chromosomes in Diptera. What is incorrect in this statement is the word "discovered." Priority for this should go to BALBIANI (1881). But at that time the phenomenon was understood as a tangled continuous thread, called *spireme* (TÄNZER 1922; KAUFMANN 1931). An early suspicion that the oversized structure might consist of individual chromosomes was coupled to the idea of a constant number of elements (RAMBOUSEK 1912; for review, BEERMANN 1962). This postulate could not be tested as long as tissues containing giant nuclei were cut into microslices. The difficulty was overcome when the technique of tissue squashing was applied by a botanist at Hamburg University. Heterochromatin could now be studied as a general property of chromosomes.

It is fitting to discuss the history of ideas about heterochromatin at the present time. There has been a recent resurgence of interest in heterochromatin, as molecular methods provide a way to study the subject at a deeper level. This is also evidenced by several recent articles in GENETICS, including one by LE *et al.* in this issue.

The Heitz method: Avoiding the time-consuming use of a microtome, HEITZ (1926, 1928a,b, 1933a) fixed plant material in two parts of alcohol and one part of acetic acid. He then stained it in carmine acetic acid (45%) and prepared, with needles, a single cell layer. STEVENS (1908) and BELLING (1926) had introduced similar methods. However, to obtain the best metaphase spreads free of cytoplasm, HEITZ applied gentle pressure to the cover slip. Thus, the specimen was attached to the slide and was prevented from being carried off when the slide was thoroughly boiled. Later, the more delicate Dipteran tissues were not boiled but cautiously heated. "The described preparation can be done within a moment after some practice. Within half an hour, 4-6 specimens can be produced" (HEITZ 1933b, p. 726; 1936). This technique, nicknamed *hei(t)zen* (heating), was adopted first at the Kaiser-Wilhelm Institute in Berlin-Dahlem (STERN 1931; GEITLER 1962; G. MELCHERS,

personal communication) and at Würzburg University (HAUPT 1932; J. GREHN, personal communication).

The longitudinal differentiation of mitotic chromosomes became apparent, and the terms euchromatin and heterochromatin were coined (HEITZ 1928b). Chromatin is the substance that transforms into chromosomes during mitosis (BOVERI 1904). According to this view, euchromatin is chromatin proper, the chromosomes that are structurally altered during telophase so that their individuality is not recognized in the nucleus. Heterochromatin behaves differently from euchromatin in morphogenesis; specific (parts of) chromosomes do not participate in telophase reorganization (HEITZ 1935).

Heterochromatin in Bryophyta: Using the liverwort *Pellia epiphylla* (*Jungermaniidae*) and exploiting prophases, metaphases and telophases as well as interphase nuclei, HEITZ found evidence that identical chromosome sections are constantly heterochromatic (heteropycnotic). Heterochromatin was found without exception in all genera of acrogynic liverworts (HEITZ 1928b, p. 796), whereas in anacrogynic species the heterochromatin of autosomes depends on the presence of a heteropycnotic *minute* chromosome (p. 801). "With 70 species of true mosses from 20 families, always one chromosome behaves differently. It does not disappear in telophases as do the other chromosomes" (p. 815). HEITZ provided evidence that heteropycnosis is not an artifact. "Initially, it was expected that it must also be observed in vivo, at least in resting nuclei (in interphase). Nuclei of fully grown cells lying at the outer cell wall and not greatly obscured by chloroplasts show the heterochromatin very well" (p. 790). "The cause of heteropycnosis can only lie in the concerned chromosomes themselves" (p. 815).

"It may arouse amazement that the outlined facts were up to now overlooked. However, without the boiling method I would not have visualized the regularity of the phenomenon so soon. The advantage of my method, apart from saving time, is that only chromatin becomes intensely stained, whereas plasma and above all the nucleoli scarcely take color. Thus, one need not search for the right degree of differentiation, since any properly prepared specimen is, by itself, correctly *differentiated*" (p. 802). Boiling in aceto-carmine had produced the first C-banding patterns (PASSARGE 1979).

Heterochromatin "in plants and in substantial details also in animals was hitherto an unknown phenomenon" (HEITZ 1928b). Therefore, he started a series of cytological investigations searching for heteropycnosis in somatic cell nuclei of Diptera.

Heterochromatin in Drosophila: *The Physical Basis of Heredity* by THOMAS HUNT MORGAN (1919) became well known in Germany through an authorized translation by HANS NACHTSHEIM (MORGAN 1921). The book and contact with the "genetics community" (HARWOOD 1993) stimulated EMIL HEITZ (1933b) to breed at least five Drosophila species in the greenhouse. *Drosophila funebris* was caught in the Botanical Institute Hamburg. The species was easily recognized, from the chromosomes. *D. melanogaster* was received from CURT STERN, Kaiser Wilhelm Institute for Biology in Berlin-Dahlem. *D. simulans* was from the Institute for Experimental Biology in Moscow, mailed by Fräulein Dr. FROLOWA (1925). *D. hydei* and *D. virilis*, "originally from the United States," were from RUDOLF GEIGY, Zoological Institution at Basel.

The first attempt was made with the MORGAN fly. HEITZ (1930) was surprised that cells from different organs of larvae and adults gave pictures similar to those known in true mosses. He saw one and sometimes two vacuolated and intensely stained blobs of chromatin during interphase.

Since *D. melanogaster* appeared "rather unfavorable with respect to cytology," HEITZ (1933b) continued with *D. funebris*. Its karyotype was known to contain two remarkably large chromosomes of similar length in both sexes (METZ 1916, 1926). However, while one of these chromosomes (the *Y*) was totally heteropycnotic, the other was differentiated into a euchromatic half and a proximal heterochromatic section. With the finding of partial heteropycnosis in the *X*, a new "structural type" of sex chromosome was detected. This was in contrast to the known "quantitative type" where *X* and *Y* are of different sizes.

After these preliminary examinations, HEITZ (1934a) returned to *D. melanogaster* and added *D. virilis*. The sex chromosomes of these species likewise were of the structural type just described for *D. funebris*. Furthermore, partial heteropycnosis characterized the autosomes. The fact that heterochromatin is proximally localized in any autosome was termed "equilocal heterochromacy." Figure 1 summarizes the findings on heterochromatin distribution in somatic nuclei of the three Drosophila species.

Introductory remarks (HEITZ 1933b) described the main research impetus. (i) Chromosomes are the material substratum of genes. (ii) The genes are linearly arranged according to MORGAN's conclusions from transmission genetics. Now, for the first time, the new technique demonstrated a longitudinal differentiation in cytological entities, euchromatin and heterochromatin. Heteropycnosis characterized not only sex chromosomes (SHOWALTER 1928) but likewise autosomes. Furthermore, heterochromatin was a phenomenon of general biology occurring in both animals and plants. Therefore, Professor WINKLER (who had coined the term *genome* in 1920) "generously put at my disposal the resources of the Botanical Institute for these studies."

HEITZ (1929, 1932) had imagined that "euchromatin is genically active, heterochromatin genically passive. Heterochromatic chromosomes or pieces of chromosomes contain no genes or somehow passive genes." However, the results from MORGAN's laboratory (MORGAN *et al.* 1925; MULLER and STONE 1930; MULLER and PAINTER 1932) forced a revision: "My ideas are not correct, because genes which lie within the heterochromatin do intervene in the developmental process of an organism. Nevertheless, the density of genes in a chromosome is related to the longitudinal differentiation in euchromatin and heterochromatin. Euchromatic pieces are rich, whereas heterochromatic ones are at least poor in genes. One has to suppose further that the genes are evenly and linearly distributed within the euchromatin" (HEITZ 1934a, p. 266). Interestingly, he discussed whether the Drosophila genes *light* and *rolled* are within the euchromatic or heterochromatic environment (p. 264).

Polytene chromosomes: HEITZ was promoted from *Privatdozent* to extraordinary professor in July, 1932. At that time, BAUER worked as a postdoctoral fellow and scientific volunteer in the Institute for Marine and Tropical Diseases at Hamburg. There he became acquainted with the Feulgen procedure as being specific for the chromosomal substance (BAUER 1932). HEITZ (1931) also was aware of this, but he preferred boiling in carmine acetic acid because he could not discriminate heterochromatin and euchromatin with the Feulgen technique (HEITZ 1935, p. 409). A joint venture had been started with a very convenient subject contributed by HERMANN WEBER (1933), a recognized entomologist at Danzig. The results from the black "hairy garden midge" were considered so important that the manuscript was submitted on July 31, 1932. Thus, "Evidence for the chromosomal nature of nuclear loops in the tangled nuclei of *Bibio hortulanus* L." (HEITZ and BAUER 1933) appeared ahead of the Drosophila papers.

The authors had followed their standard procedure of chromosome analysis: first of all, one has to investigate mitotic prophases and metaphases, after which polytene structures can be analyzed. Somatic mitoses were obtained from neuroblasts and follicular epithelium of ovaries. Prophases in *B. hortulanus* showed five pairs of chromosomes that separated into 10 metacentric elements in metaphase (p. 69).

Tangled nuclei were found in salivary glands, midgut,

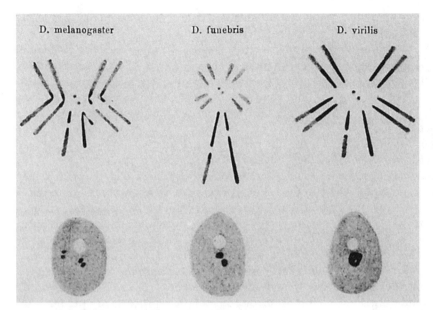

FIGURE 1.—Schematic summary of chromatin structures from three Drosophila species. Longitudinal differentiation in euchromatin and proximal heterochromatin is evident in metaphase configuration. The heteropycnotic material is associated with one or two chromocenters in interphase nuclei (HEITZ 1934a, Figure 9; 1935, Figure 7).

Malpighi tubes, and occasionally in the brain. Especially from the Malpighi tubes it became clear that the large nuclei did not contain a continuous thread. There were always five clearly separated thread sections, each double and different in length. Furthermore, structural features (nucleolus and terminal peculiarities) were not randomly distributed but were found characterizing the individual nuclear loops. Last but not least, they were Feulgen-positive. The results led to the conclusion that the giant threads are twin chromosomes in haploid number (p. 72). The synapsis of homologous chromosomes was later employed extensively as a simple way to detect heterozygous chromosome rearrangements (PAINTER and STONE 1935).

Contest for priority: "The most striking recent development in cytology is the discovery of the chromosomal nature of the long known giant structures in the nuclei of the salivary glands of Diptera. This discovery, made with Bibio (Heitz and Bauer 1933), was extended to Drosophila by Painter in 1934" (STURTEVANT AND BEADLE 1939, p. 364). In Hamburg, both authors were aware of their achievement. "Heitz and Bauer (1933) have provided the final evidence with *Bibio hortulanus* and thus for Diptera generally that there exist enormously enlarged chromosomes" (HEITZ 1933b, p. 727).

No earlier than December, *Science* published a provocative statement by THEOPHILUS SHICKEL PAINTER (1933b) on polytene chromosomes in *D. melanogaster.* "It has long been known that in the functioning salivary glands of many dipteran larvae the chromosomes show an elongated and annulated structure." HEITZ immediately and harshly commented, "Almost one year after the publication of our investigations with *Bibio hortulanus* and shortly after the appearance of the said work (on *D. melanogaster*), Painter reports preliminarily (not less than three times, December 1933, 1933, 1934) and in greater detail (1934, here giving reference to our

work) on a 'new method' for the qualitative analysis of *Drosophila melanogaster* chromosomes. Painter's statement 'It has long been known . . .' was not correct at all. Evidence for the chromosomal nature of nuclear loops was demonstrated initially by our work. Clear objections must be raised to the mode of Painter's account" (HEITZ 1934b, p. 588; see also PAINTER 1933a, 1934b,c, 1935).

It is noteworthy that the "greater details" had already been submitted to GENETICS in May, 1933, but unfortunately appeared one year later (PAINTER 1934a).

The objections obviously were taken into account, and the rephrased sentence reads, "All cytologists have known for a long time that in the salivary glands and other tissues of the larvae of Diptera in general there occurs what has been called a 'permanent spireme.' In the nuclei of such tissues structures called chromosomes are very large and show very conspicuous bands" (PAINTER 1934c). Troubles came not only from PAINTER but also from the young co-author. HEITZ (1933b, p. 723) complained in a footnote, "Bauer (1933) has just reported on partial heteropycnosis in the oocyte nuclei of *Dytiscus marginatus*. My assessments on partial heteropycnosis in *Drosophila funebris, D. melanogaster* and *Scatophila unicornis* were made earlier than those of Bauer with Dytiscus which is not quite obvious from his account."

A burst of research in the new field of cytogenetics had been initiated (HEITZ 1935, p. 429). LOTHAR GEITLER (1934) reported on polytene chromosomes in Simulium, KING and BEAMS (1933, 1934) dealt with Chironomus, and METZ and GAY (1934a,b) with Sciara. KLAUS PÄTAU (1935) focussed on *D. simulans*, and C. C. TAN (1935) did so on *D. pseudoobscura*. THEODOSIUS DOBZHANSKY (1935) recognized that *D. miranda* was different from the sibling species *D. pseudoobscura*, as shown by the banding in polytene elements.

Natural banding pattern: The constant structural characters of polytene chromosomes were already apparent in the first approaches. Especially the discontinuously banded pattern of the giant nuclear loops was recognized, proving the individuality of the chromosome pairs. "The loci of these chromomere-like disks are not randomly distributed but constant. This constitutes new evidence that chromosomes possess a constant differentiation in the direction of their longitudinal axis" (HEITZ and BAUER 1933, pp. 78, 81).

The constancy of polytene bands was also detailed in a following paper (HEITZ 1934b), and the transatlantic success was acknowledged: "The usefulness of giant chromosomes of Diptera for localizing exactly the (Mendelian) factors was shown for the first time by Painter (1933, 1934), who had collected rich material for investigation" (HEITZ 1935, p. 433). Further, "One has to emphasize the work of Bridges (1935), who has carried forward the analysis of longitudinal differentiation in this species (*D. melanogaster*) so far that it is difficult to beat. Furthermore, Bridges has established a very useful system of assignment" (p. 430).

Multistranded elements: The size of the novel chromosomes was initially described as "magnified" and "giant" while the term "polytenic" was introduced by KOLTZOFF (1934). GÜNTHER HERTWIG (1935) noted that the gigantic dimensions are achieved by real growth, *i.e.*, by multiple doubling of the genome: "Thus, any gene is present in the salivary gland chromosomes of *D. melanogaster* at least 256-fold or 512-fold, and not only 8 times as Koltzoff (1934) and Bridges (1935) recently thought.... A substantial point in the discovery of Heitz is that not the number, but only the size of the chromosomes is increased in the salivary gland nuclei. These giant chromosomes lie in enormously enlarged nuclei."

Also HEITZ (1935, p. 430) refers to these papers: "Bridges (1935) and Koltzoff (1934) independently have explained the giant size of these chromosomes this way: There is not a single and strongly enlarged chromonema. The thickness is brought about when the multiplied chromonemata remain in mutual connection between each other." (Nowadays we prefer the word chromatid instead of chromonema.)

An explanation of the extraordinary size must connect the giant structure with the "normal" chromosome. In this view, BAUER (1937, p. 72) has summarized, "Thus, the giant chromosome is a bundle of identically built fibrils of which the homologous parts are at the same level."

Heterochromatin under-represented: Because *D. virilis* possesses some 50% mitotic heterochromatin, it was assessed as especially suitable for investigating chromosome development in the soma. "While euchromatic sections of the chromosomes increase to gigantic size during the growth of the nuclei, the heterochromatic sections, united in a collective chromocenter, are not

able to do this ... The heterochromatin proper is named α-heterochromatin from now on. The adjacent heterochromatin, like the former, does not reveal any differentiation in chromomeres, but has the capability of growing in common with the euchromatin. This β-heterochromatin, as it might be called from now on, possesses only a minor extension and cannot be recognized as such in somatic prophases, while the α-heterochromatin makes up half of the rod-shaped chromosomes" (HEITZ 1934b, p. 596).

Contemporaneous researchers had explained that chromosomal growth is caused by chromatid multiplication. Thus, the original definition of α-type heterochromatin corresponded to suspension from endoreplication rather than to condensation. However, PAINTER (1933b, p. 586) had discussed alternative mechanisms: "Either the inert material of both the X and Y has been eliminated during ontogeny (of *D. melanogaster*), by diminution or some similar process, or this material exists in the salivary nuclei in some unrecognized form not visibly connected with the chromosomes." The idea of elimination probably goes back to Würzburg where PAINTER had spent several months in 1913–14 with THEODOR BOVERI (WAGNER 1970; BOVERI 1910). But HEITZ (1935, p. 433) remained persistent: "The heterochromatin of the Drosophila species is also present at the giant chromosomes. Painter, who believed earlier (1934) that the inert region would be eliminated in the loop-containing nuclei, as he could not find an equivalent, has recently (1935) joined my opinion."

The HEITZ hypothesis of under-replication in larger somatic nuclei was also attacked by BAUER (1936, p. 217), then a research fellow at the California Institute of Technology in Pasadena: "Observations in Chironomidae led me to the conclusion that heterochromatic regions of salivary gland chromosomes are composed of the same number of chromonemata as the euchromatic strands, the difference between them being due to the structure of the single chromomeres." Regarding *D. pseudoobscura*, Figure 5 in his paper is a diagram presenting the two types of chromomeres without local under-representation of chromatids.

HEITZ dismissed: Looking back, shortly after his seventieth birthday, HEITZ wrote to CURT KOSSWIG, then Dean of the Faculty of Mathematics and Sciences, "It is for me a special honor to be made an honorary doctor by the Faculty of the University of Hamburg because I actually have made my most essential works at the Institute for General Botany there." He had joined the staff in November, 1926.

However, on February 4, 1937, EDGAR IRMSCHER, the curator at the Institute for General Botany and thus a close colleague of HEITZ, wrote an official letter to the Rector of the Hamburg University. IRMSCHER did so as the *Gaudozentenführer* of the National Socialistic German Labor Party. He reported to the Rector, Prof. ADOLF REIN, "that Prof. Heitz who, under the law, has to be regarded as non-Aryan, will give a lecture on heredity." The Nazi official recommended cancellation of this lecture, otherwise certain circles might make trouble for the University (ROLAND HEITZ, personal communication; Hamburg Staatsarchiv 1937). The Rector immediately conferred with HANS WINKLER, director of that institute. Because of this intervention, HEITZ changed his lecture title to "General Genetics" for the rector's files, although the former title "Introduction to Heredity" had already been printed in the lecture timetable (Hansische Universität 1936).

More serious consequences arose from the notice that HEITZ was not pure Aryan. His maternal grandfather, Dr. MORITZ SCHWALB (1833–1916), had been Jewish and a protestant clergyman. From 1867 to 1894, he served as an elected parish priest in Bremen and became known for his critical and liberal sermons (SCHWALB 1884; HUNTEMANN 1969).

The German Public Servant Law had just been amended on January 26, 1937. According to §25, an official as well as the spouse had to be of German or related blood. Thus, even partially Jewish descendants were not allowed to teach at German universities (BRAND 1937). A cascade of documents, produced by the university and the government, culminated in a claim for the dismissal of HEITZ as nonpermanent extraordinary professor (Figure 2). However, the academic grade *Doctor habilitatus* expressly remained untouched.

A letter written by HEITZ pointed out that he was ³/₄ Aryan. His paternal grandfather, also named EMIL HEITZ (1885), had been rector of Strassbourg University. His father was a recognized German publisher (PAUL HEITZ 1902). The family had owned the Strassbourg University Press for generations (BURGUN and RAY 1984). His own service as a volunteer and sergeant with the German artillery during World War I was also mentioned. As in many similar cases, the Minister for Science, Teaching, and National Education made a final decision in Berlin. According to §18 of the Imperial Habilitation Rule (Reichs-Habilitations-Ordnung of December 13, 1934), HEITZ was to be removed from the register of professors by August 17, 1937. His last salary was to be paid in October of that year.

This was a shock to a family with four children, ROLAND (then 12 years old), THOMAS (10), ELISABETH (9) and SEBASTIAN (4). Probably Mrs. ELISABETH HEITZ (née STAEHELIN) took the initiative to move to her Swiss native town Basel where her mother MARTHA STAEHELIN-LINDER bought a house for the refugees.

Fate and science: JOHANN HEINRICH *EMIL* HEITZ was his full name. He was born in Strassbourg on October 29, 1892. In the fall of 1912 he went to Munich where he attended 22 lectures on hereditary science by RICHARD GOLDSCHMIDT (1913). Two semesters (1913/1914) were spent at Strassbourg University. World War I (1914–1918) interrupted his course of studies.

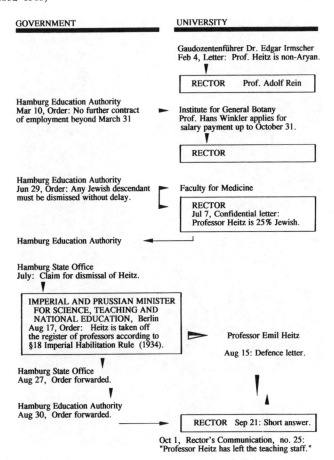

FIGURE 2.—Dismissal of HEITZ from Hamburg University during 1937 (Hamburg Staatsarchiv, Hochschulwesen 1937).

After the war, he met ELISABETH STAEHELIN (1896–1979) when both were students of biology at Basel University. HEITZ moved to Heidelberg and became a Ph.D. student of the plant physiologist LUDWIG JOST. Final examinations were held June 7, 1921, and his thesis on division of chloroplasts came out the following year (HEITZ 1922). He spent nine months as a postdoctoral fellow at Tübingen; during this time ELISABETH and EMIL married. From June, 1922 to May, 1924, HEITZ was scientific assistant to FRIEDRICH BOAS, Institute for Fermentation Physiology at Weihenstephan, Bavaria. A further interval (June, 1924 to September, 1926) was spent at the Prussian University at Greifswald. There, he not only did the job of a botanist but also took advantage of a working place at the Zoological Institute with PAUL BUCHNER.

Giving his inaugural lecture on the problem of speciation on November 3, 1926, HEITZ made a splendid start in Hamburg. "It was here that he spent the most fruitful 11 years of his scientific life" (FLÁVIO RESENDE 1962).

At Basel University, he was also made an extraordinary professor for Botany. RESENDE visited him in 1938 and "found out that his salary was less than that of a tram conductor of that city. The situation improved later, but was never very good." LEWIS J. STADLER in-

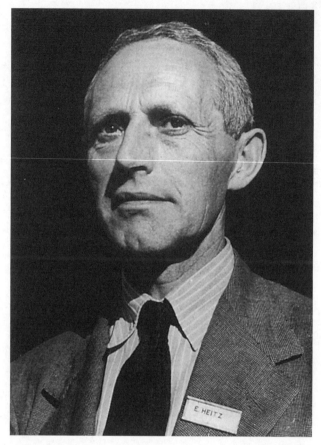

FIGURE 3.—EMIL HEITZ (age 56) at the Eighth International Congress of Genetics, July 7–14, 1948, in Stockholm (BONNIER and LARSSON 1949). Portrait by ESKO SUOMALAINEN (Helsinki).

vited HEITZ to join the University of Missouri, and the family prepared for the move (ROLAND HEITZ, personal communication). The passage was prevented when Germany declared war against the United States on December 11, 1941. Later, in 1947, HEITZ received Swiss nationality and was visiting professor at the University of Missouri from February to June (HEITZ 1955). "However, he did not like the American way of life. Even Hamburg was strange to him. He wrote me a letter from Missouri full of nostalgia that made me quite sad. He returned to Basel" (RESENDE 1962).

These unhappy circumstances changed in 1948 in consequence of the Eighth International Congress of Genetics (Figure 3). There, in Stockholm, EEVA THERMAN learned of the bad situation and informed GEORG MELCHERS (personal communication). The latter provided a laboratory in his department at the Max Planck Institute for Biology and HEITZ became visiting professor at Tübingen University in 1952. On April 1, 1955, EMIL HEITZ became a scientific fellow of the Max Planck Society. This was a final realization of a plan of FRIEDRICH WETTSTEIN (1895–1945), who in 1937 had intended for HEITZ to be in the Kaiser Wilhelm Institute for Biology in Berlin-Dahlem (MELCHERS 1987; HENNING and KAZEMI 1993). After August 30, 1955, HEITZ

was honorary professor of cytology at Tübingen. He did not return to active chromosome research but followed his interest in the ultrastructure of chloroplasts (HEITZ 1960). He retired on October 31, 1961, moved with his wife to Basel, and spent some time in his summer house, *Casa rossa*. In 1962, he received honorary doctorates from the universities of Berlin, Cologne and Hamburg.

EMIL HEITZ died at Lugano, Switzerland, on July 8, 1965, as a result of a broken thigh bone, and was buried in Basel.

Encouragement and information were given by WOLFGANG O. ABEL (Hamburg), HILDE ATZLER (Tübingen), FRANZ BRABEC (Hamburg), HEINRICH EITZEN (Kiel), JOSEF GREHN (Wetzlar), ELISABETH GÜNTHER (Greifswald), ELISABETH HAUSCHTECK-JUNGEN (Zürich), ROLAND HEITZ (Zürich), MARION KAZEMI (Berlin), ROLAND MALY (Kriens), GEORG MELCHERS (Tübingen), CLAUS PELLING (Tübingen), GÜNTER REUTER (Halle), ARMIN SPILLER (Berlin), DAVID STADLER (Seattle), the late ESKO SUOMALAINEN (Helsinki), VIT TASEVSKI (Sydney), RAYLA G. TEMIN (Madison), EEVA THERMAN (Madison), RENATE ULLMANN née DÖRMER (Tübingen), and STEFAN WULF (Hamburg).

LITERATURE CITED

BALBIANI, E. G., 1881 Sur la structure du noyau des cellules salivaires chez les larves de Chironomus. Zool. Anz. **4:** 637–641.

BAUER, H., 1932 Die Feulgensche Nuklealfärbung in ihrer Anwendung auf cytologische Untersuchungen. Z. Zellforsch. mikrosk. Anat. **15:** 225–247.

BAUER, H., 1933 Die wachsenden Oocytenkerne einiger Insekten in ihrem Verhalten zur Nuklealfärbung. Z. Zellforsch. mikrosk. Anat. **18:** 254–298.

BAUER, H., 1936 Structure and arrangement of salivary gland chromosomes in Drosophila species. Proc. Natl. Acad. Sci. USA **22:** 216–222.

BAUER, H., 1937 Neue Ergebnisse der Cytogenetik. Ber. phys. med. Ges. Würzburg, NF **61:** 70–81.

BEERMANN, W., 1962 *Riesenchromosomen*. Protoplasmatologia, Vol. 6D, edited by M. ALFERT, H. BAUER and C. V. HARDING. Springer, Vienna.

BELLING, J., 1926 The iron-acetocarmine method of fixing and staining chromosomes. Biol. Bull. **50:** 160–162.

BONNIER, G., and R. LARSSON (editors), 1949 *Proceedings of the Eighth International Congress of Genetics: 7th–14th of July, 1948, Stockholm.* Hereditas, Suppl. Berlingska Boktryckeriet, Lund.

BOVERI, T., 1904 *Ergebnisse über die Konstitution der chromatischen Substanz des Zellkerne.* Fischer, Jena.

BOVERI, T., 1910 Die Potenzen der Ascaris-Blastomeren bei abgeänderter Furchung. Zugleich ein Beitrag zur Frage qualitativ-ungleicher Chromosomen-Teilung, pp. 131–214 in *Festschrift R. Hertwig*, Vol. 3. Fischer, Jena.

BRAND, A. (editor), 1937 *Das deutsche Beamtengesetz (DBG) vom 26. Januar 1937 mit der amtlichen Begründung, den Durchführungs-, Ausführungs- und Ergänzungsvorschriften.* Julius Springer, Berlin.

BRIDGES, C. B., 1935 Salivary chromosome maps with a key to the banding of the chromosomes of Drosophila melanoaster. J. Hered. **26:** 60–64.

BURGUN, R., and D. RAY, 1984 Heitz: Frédérique-Charles, Jean-Henri-Emile, Paul, p. 3817 in *Encyclopedie de l'Alsace*. Volume 6: *Frey-Hematologie*, edited by A. ACKER, F. BECKER, V. BEYER, R. BURGUN, R. CARBIENER *et al.* Editions Publitotal, Strasbourg.

DOBZHANSKY, TH., 1935 *Drosophila miranda*, a new species. Genetics **20:** 377–391.

FROLOWA, S., 1925 Normale und polyploide Chromosomengarnituren bei einigen Drosophila-Arten. Z. Zellforsch. mikrosk. Anat. **3:** 682–694.

GEITLER, L., 1934 Die Schleifenkerne von Simulium. Zool. Jahrb., Abt. Allg. Zool. Physiol. Tiere **54:** 237–248.

GEITLER, L., 1962 Über die weite Anwendbarkeit der Heitz'schen Essigkarminmethode. Portug. Acta Biol. Ser. A **6:** 373–378.

GOLDSCHMIDT, R., 1913 *Einführung in die Vererbungswissenschaft in zweiundzwanzig Vorlesungen für Studierende, Ärzte, Züchter.* 2nd ed. Wilhelm Engelmann, Leipzig, Berlin.

Hamburg Staatsarchiv: Hochschulwesen, 1937 *Heitz, Emil 29.10.1892.* Dozenten- und Personalakten IV/384, Hamburg.

Hansische Universität, 1936 *Personal- und Vorlesungsverzeichnis: Wintersemester 1936/37, Sommersemester 1937.* Universität, Hamburg.

HARWOOD, J., 1993 *Styles of Scientific Thought: The German Genetics Community 1900–1933.* University of Chicago Press, Chicago, London.

HAUPT, G., 1932 Beiträge zur Zytologie der Gattung Marchantia (L.): I. Z. indukt. Abst. Vererbungslehre **62:** 367–428.

HEITZ, E., 1885 *Zur Geschichte der alten Strassburger Universität: Rede, gehalten am 1. Mai 1885, dem Stiftungstage der Kaiser Wilhelms-Universität zu Strassburg, bei Antritt des Rectorats.* Strassburg.

HEITZ, E., 1922 *Untersuchungen über die Teilung der Chloroplasten nebst Beobachtungen uber Zellgrösse und Chromatophorengrösse: Inaugural-Dissertation zur Erlangung der Doktorwürde einer unter naturwissenschaftlich-mathematischen Fakultät der Rupprecht-Karls-Universität zu Heidelberg.* Heidelberg: Naturwiss.-math. Diss. v. 18. März 1921. Oscar Brandstetter, Leipzig.

HEITZ, E., 1926 Der Nachweis der Chromosomen: Vergleichende Studien über ihre Zahl, Grösze und Form im Pflanzenreich, I. Z. Bot. **18:** 625–681.

HEITZ, E., 1928a Der bilaterale Bau der Geschlechtschromosomen und Autosomen bei *Pellia fabbroniana, P. epiphylla* und einigen anderen Iungermanniaceen. Planta **5:** 725–768.

HEITZ, E., 1928b Das Heterochromatin der Moose, I. Jahrb. wiss. Bot. **69:** 762–818.

HEITZ, E., 1929 Heterochromatin, Chromocentren, Chromomeren (Vorläufige Mitteilung). Ber. Dtsch. Bot. Ges. **47:** 274–284.

HEITZ, E., 1930 Der Bau der somatischen Kerne von *Drosophila melanogaster.* Z. indukt. Abstammungs- Vererbungsl. **54:** 248–249.

HEITZ, E., 1931 Die Ursache der gesetzmäszigen Zahl, Lage, Form und Grösze pflanzlicher Nukleolen. Planta **12:** 775–844.

HEITZ, E., 1932 Geschlechtschromosomen bei einem Laubmoos (Vorläufige Mitteilung). Ber. Dt. Bot. Ges. **50:** 204–206.

HEITZ, E., 1933a Die Herkunft der Chromocentren: Dritter Beitrag zur Kenntnis der Beziehung zwischen Kernstruktur und qualitativer Verschiedenheit der Chromosomen in ihrer Längsrichtung. Planta **18:** 571–636.

HEITZ, E., 1933b Über totale und partielle somatische Heteropyknose, sowie strukturelle Geschlechtschromosomen bei *Drosophila funebris* (Cytologische Untersuchungen an Dipteren, II). Z. Zellforsch. mikrosk. Anat. **19:** 720–742.

HEITZ, E., 1934a Die somatische Heteropyknose bei *Drosophila melanogaster* und ihre genetische Bedeutung (Cytologische Untersuchungen an Dipteren, III). Z. Zellforsch. mikrosk. Anat. **20:** 237–287.

HEITZ, E., 1934b Über α- und β-Heterochromatin sowie Konstanz und Bau der Chromomeren bei Drosophila. Biol. Zbl. **54:** 588–609.

HEITZ, E., 1935 Chromosomenstruktur und Gene. Z. indukt. Abstammungs- Vererbungsl. **70:** 402–447.

HEITZ, E., 1936 Die Nukleal-Quetschmethode. Ber. Dtsch. Bot. Ges. **53:** 870–878.

HEITZ, E., 1955 Über die Struktur der Chromosomen und Chloroplasten: Vortrag auf der Jahresversammlung der "Leopoldina" anläszlich des Empfanges der Schleiden-Medaille 1955 am 13. November 1955 in Halle. Nova Acta Leopold. NF **17:** 517–540.

HEITZ, E., 1960 Zur Kenntnis des lamellaren Musters in ausgewachsenen und der Kristallgitterstruktur in jungen Chloroplasten. Experientia **16:** 265–270.

HEITZ, E., and H. BAUER, 1933 Beweise für die Chromosomennatur der Kernschleifen in den Knäuelkernen von *Bibio hortulanus* L. (Cytologische Untersuchungen an Dipteren, I). Z. Zellforsch. mikrosk. Anat. **17:** 67–82.

HEITZ, P., 1902 *Les filigranes des papiers contenue dans les archives de la ville Strasbourg.* Heitz, Strasbourg.

HENNING, E., and M. KAZEMI, 1993 Dahlem - Domäne der Wissenschaft: Ein Spaziergang zu den Berliner Instituten der Kaiser-Wilhelm-/Max-Planck-Gesellschaft im "deutschen Oxford." Max-Planck-Ges. Ber. Mitt.: 1–144.

HERTWIG, G., 1935 Die Vielwertigkeit der Speicheldrüsenkerne und -chromosomen bei *Drosophila melanogaster.* Z. indukt. Abstammungs- Vererbungsl. **70:** 496–501.

HUNTEMANN, G., 1969 Schwalb, Moritz, Dr. theol., Pastor, pp. 479–

480 in *Bremische Biographie: 1912–1962,* edited by W. LÜHRS, F. PETERS and K. H. SCHWEBEL. Hauschild, Bremen.

KAUFMANN, B. P., 1931 Chromosome structure in Drosophila. Am. Nat. **65:** 555–558.

KING, R. L., and H. W. BEAMS, 1933 Somatic synapsis in Chironomus. Anat. Rec. Suppl. **57:** 89–90.

KING, R. L., and H. W. BEAMS, 1934 Somatic synapsis in Chironomus, with special reference to the individuality of the chromosomes. J. Morphol. **56:** 577–591.

KOLTZOFF, N. K., 1934 The structure of the chromosomes in the salivary glands of Drosophila. Science **80:** 312–313.

LE, M.-H., D. DURICKA and G. H. KARPEN, 1995 Islands of complex DNA are widespread in Drosophila centric heterochromatin. Genetics **141:** 283–303.

MELCHERS, G., 1987 Ein Botaniker auf dem Wege in die Allgemeine Biologie auch in Zeiten moralischer und materieller Zerstörung und Fritz von Wettstein 1895–1945 mit Liste der Veröffentlichungen und Dissertationen (Persönliche Erinnerungen). Ber. Dtsch. Bot. Ges. **100:** 373–405.

METZ, C. W., 1916 Chromosome studies on the Diptera, II: the paired association of chromosomes in Diptera, and its significance. J. Exp. Zool. **21:** 213–280.

METZ, C. W., 1926 Observations on spermatogenesis in Drosophila. Z. Zellforsch. mikrosk. Anat. **4:** 1–28.

METZ, C. W., and C. H. GAY, 1934a Chromosome structure in the salivary glands of Sciara. Science **80:** 595–596.

METZ, C. W., and C. H. GAY, 1934b Organization of salivary gland chromosomes in Sciara in relation to genes. Proc. Natl. Acad. Sci. USA **20:** 617–621.

MORGAN, T. H., 1919 *The Physical Basis of Heredity.* J. B. Lippincott, Philadelphia, London.

MORGAN, T. H., 1921 *Die stoffliche Grundlage der Vererbung:* Vom Verfasser autorisierte deutsche Ausgabe von Hans Nachtsheim. Borntraeger, Berlin.

MORGAN, T. H., C. B. BRIDGES and A. H. STURTEVANT, 1925 The genetics of Drosophila. Bibliogr. Genetica **2:** 1–262.

MULLER, H. J., and T. S. PAINTER, 1932 The differentiation of the sex chromosomes of Drosophila into genetically active and inert regions. Z. indukt. Abstammungs- Vererbungsl. **62:** 316–365.

MULLER, H. J., and W. S. STONE, 1930 Analysis of several induced gene rearrangements involving the X-chromosome of Drosophila. Anat. Rec. **47:** 393–394.

PAINTER, T. S., 1933a A method for the qualitative analysis of the chromosomes of *Drosophila melanogaster.* Anat. Rec. Suppl. **57:** 90.

PAINTER, T. S., 1933b A new method for the study of chromosome rearrangement and the plotting of chromosome maps. Science **78:** 585–586.

PAINTER, T. S., 1934a A new method for the study of chromosome aberrations and the plotting of chromosome maps in *Drosophila melanogaster.* Genetics **19:** 175–188.

PAINTER, T. S., 1934b The morphology of the X chromosome in salivary glands of *Drosophila melanogaster* and a new type of chromosome map of this element. Genetics **19:** 448–469.

PAINTER, T. S., 1934c Salivary chromosomes and the attack on the gene. J. Hered. **25:** 465–476.

PAINTER, T. S., 1935 The morphology of the third chromosome in the salivary gland of *Drosophila melanogaster* and a new cytological map of this element. Genetics **20:** 301–326.

PAINTER, T. S., and W. Stone, 1935 Chromosome fusion and speciation in Drosophilae. Genetics **20:** 327–341.

PASSARGE, E., 1979 Emil Heitz and the concept of heterochromatin: longitudinal chromosome differentiation was recognized fifty years ago. Am. J. Hum. Genet. **31:** 106–115.

PÄTAU, K., 1935 Chromosomenmorphologie bei *Drosophila melanogaster* und *Drosophila simulans* und ihre genetische Bedeutung. Naturwissenschaften **23:** 537–543.

RAMBOUSEK, F., 1912 Cytologische Verhältnisse der Speicheldrüsen der Chironomus-Larve. Sitzungsber. königl. böhm. Ges. Wiss.: Math.-naturw. Klasse.

RESENDE, F., 1962 Reminiscing on my friendship with Prof. E. Heitz. Portug. Acta Biol. Ser. A **6:** I–V.

SCHWALB, M., 1884 Luther's Entwicklung vom Mönch zum Reformator, pp. 205–236 in *Sammlung gemeinverständlicher wissenschaftlicher Vorträge,* edited by R. VIRCHOW and F. VON HOLTZENDORFF. Carl Habel, Berlin.

SHOWALTER, A. M., 1928   The chromosomes of *Pellia Neesiana.* Proc. Natl. Acad. Sci. USA **14:** 63–66.

STERN, C., 1931   Zytologisch-genetische Untersuchungen als Beweise für die Morgansche Theorie des Faktorenaustausches. Biol. Zbl. **51:** 547–587.

STEVENS, N. M., 1908   A study of the germ cells of certain Diptera, with reference to the heterochromosomes and the phenomena of synapsis. J. Exp. Zool. **5:** 359–374.

STURTEVANT, A. H., and G. W. BEADLE, 1939   *An Introduction to Genetics.* Reprint 1962: Dover Publications, New York.

TAN, C. C., 1935   Identification of the salivary gland chromosomes in *Drosophila pseudoobscura.* Proc. Natl. Acad. Sci. USA **21:** 200–202.

TÄNZER, E., 1922   Die Zellkerne einiger Dipterenlarven und ihre Entwicklung. Z. wiss. Zool. **119:** 114–153.

WAGNER, R. P., 1970   Theophilus Shickel Painter 1889–1969. Genetics Suppl. **64:** s87–s88.

WEBER, H., 1933   *Lehrbuch der Entomologie.* G. Fischer, Jena, Stuttgart.

WINKLER, H., 1920   *Verbreitung und Ursache der Parthenogenesis im Pflanzen- und Tierreiche.* Fischer, Jena.

The Amber Mutants of Phage T4

Franklin W. Stahl

Institute of Molecular Biology, University of Oregon, Eugene, Oregon 97403–1229

A MAJOR effort of today's biology is the analysis of development by genetic methods, an approach so successful that previously unimaginable insights have become commonplace. A major moment in the growth of these studies was the discovery and analysis by DICK EPSTEIN and his colleagues of the amber mutants of phage T4.

The discovery of the ambers has been touched upon elsewhere (EDGAR 1966). The present history is a fuller account, offering perspectives not previously detailed. The story is very much of the Rochester T4 Group, headed by GUS DOERMANN, during the period from 1953 to the early 1960s. GUS's group was deeply involved in phage radiobiology, a discipline whose practitioners hurled poorly characterized reagents at invisible targets and hoped for interpretable responses.

LURIA (1947) and LURIA and DULBECCO (1949) observed that bacterial cells infected by more than one UV-irradiated phage particle produced a burst of viable progeny phage with a higher probability than expected if the irradiated phage survived independently of each other. This "multiplicity reactivation" demonstrated that irradiated phage particles could cooperate to come back to life. LURIA and DULBECCO offered a simple, well defined hypothesis for the phenomenon. They proposed that T2 phage (a close relative of T4) are made of functionally distinct subunits of equal UV sensitivity. A phage particle is "killed" by UV when any one of its subunits is "hit." An infected cell will produce progeny phage if, among the several infecting particles, there is at least one un-hit subunit of each type.

DULBECCO (1952) later recognized that a "critical test" of the subunit hypothesis required data collected at higher UV doses. At such doses, the model required that the survival curve for multiply infected cells (multicomplexes) become exponential, with a slope the same as that seen for singly infected cells (monocomplexes). He noted that the survival curve for multicomplexes did become exponential at high dose, but the slope was only about 0.2 of that seen with monocomplexes. Accordingly, DULBECCO rejected the uniform-sensitivity subunit model. In 1956, HARM did similar experiments

with the related phage T4 and showed that the high-dose slope of multicomplexes was 0.4 of that for mono-complexes.

BARRICELLI (1956; see HARM 1956) proposed that the subunit theory for multiplicity reactivation be modified such that part of the phage was composed of largish subunits ("vulnerable centers"), while the remainder of the phage was composed of many small subunits. The sensitivity of a single infecting phage would be a measure of hits anywhere in it. Since one would rarely hit all copies of any given small subunit in any multicomplex, the survival of the multicomplexes would be determined primarily by the vulnerable centers. The quasi-final slope of the multicomplex survival curve would tell the fraction of a phage particle that was composed of vulnerable centers, while the shape of the shoulder of the curve would provide a count of the number of vulnerable centers. By this analysis, 40% of T4 was composed of about three vulnerable centers.

Beginning about 1952, DOERMANN and MARTHA CHASE, working with T4, conducted crosses between single particles of UV-irradiated phage and several particles of genetically marked, nonirradiated phage ("cross-reactivation experiments"). They found that the fraction of multicomplexes that produced phage did not fall with increasing UV doses, but that the probability that any given genetic marker from the irradiated parent would appear in the progeny did decrease. Analysis of these data showed that markers, unless very close to each other, were independently eliminated from the yields of the individual multicomplexes (DOERMANN et al. 1955). DOERMANN hoped that this kind of "probing" would help him in his efforts to get a fuller description of the T4 genome than was possible using the few plaque-morphology mutants that were available. He hoped that UV lesions would serve as generic markers that could be placed at high density throughout the genome. The problem, of course, was that the placing of these lesions was certain to be different from particle to particle, limiting their usefulness as "markers."

SEYMOUR BENZER (1955) used the rII mutants of T4 to examine genetic fine structure, exploiting the inability of *rII* mutants to grow on λ lysogens, which do support growth of wild-type T4. DOERMANN exploited the selective-growth property of these mutants to extend his cross-reactivation analysis to high doses. He found that a wild-type allele of any conventional point mutation *rII* marker was "knocked out" (*i.e.*, not transmitted into a live phage particle) at high doses with a sensitivity that was 1/180 of that of the plaque-forming ability of a phage particle (DOERMANN 1961). This high resistance of individual markers suggested that the bit of genome transferred from a UV-killed phage to an unirradiated coinfecting phage in an individual act of "cross-reactivation" could be as small as 0.0056 of the genome.

In genetically mixed infections of λ lysogens, the wild type is dominant and phage are produced. DAVE KRIEG, a student in the DOERMANN group, exploited this dominance of the *rII*⁺ allele to assess the sensitivity of gene functions to UV inactivation (KRIEG 1959). He UV-irradiated wild-type T4 and adsorbed them to a λ lysogen at low multiplicity along with several particles of *rII* mutant phage. He plated the complexes before lysis on a host that was permissive for both *rII* and *rII*⁺ phage in order to measure, as a function of UV dose, the fraction of mixedly infected cells that could produce phage. KRIEG found that the UV sensitivity for the *rIIA* function was 10% of the sensitivity of the plaque-forming ability of T4, while for the smaller *rIIB* cistron the sensitivity was 5% of the plaque-forming ability. These values were comparable to the estimated sensitivity for a vulnerable center (40%/3 ≈ 13%). Other experiments by KRIEG had shown that, for phage production in the lysogen, the *rII*⁺ function must be provided early in infection.

Putting KRIEG's radiobiological analysis of gene function together with DOERMANN and CHASE's cross-reactivation experiments provided a semi-molecular model for multiplicity reactivation. This model supposed that vulnerable centers are genes specifying early functions that must be expressed before the onset of genetic recombination, which in T4 is so frequent that one damage-free chromosome can almost always be assembled from damaged ones as long as the functions for doing it have survived (BARRICELLI 1956). This view received support from the thesis work of DICK EPSTEIN (1958), also a student in DOERMANN's group. DICK conducted multiplicity reactivation experiments in which infection was made by a mixture of two genetically marked parents. Qualitatively, an expectation of the model was realized: at high dose, each productive cell gave a burst composed primarily of one genotype, which was often recombinant for the markers employed. More on EPSTEIN's work later.

BOB EDGAR, who, as a student with DOERMANN, had identified localized negative interference in T4, arrived as a postdoc in MAX DELBRÜCK's Caltech lab shortly before I (also a DOERMANN student) left my postdoc

spot at Caltech for a faculty job in Missouri. EPSTEIN arrived at Caltech soon thereafter, and in late 1959 visited us in Eugene, where I had landed after fleeing from Missouri.

During the Oregon visit, EPSTEIN and I discussed the state of UV radiobiology in T4 and identified a paradox. As mentioned above, *rII* gene function is required in λ lysogens but not in nonlysogens. The lysogen in standard use in GUS's lab was the *Escherichia coli* K12 derivative K12S(λ). The nonlysogen was *E. coli* B, the standard host for T-phage experiments. From KRIEG's work, described above, the *rII* gene functions appear to be vulnerable centers in K12S(λ). As part of his thesis work, EPSTEIN had carried out multiplicity reactivation experiments in that strain, comparing the survival of wild-type T4 multicomplexes with multicomplexes made of a complementing mixture of *rIIA* and *rIIB* mutants. These experiments supported the view that the *rII* genes act as vulnerable centers in K12S(λ). The argument underlying that conclusion was laid out in a review I wrote while at Caltech (STAHL 1959). However, the *rII* genes should not act as vulnerable centers in strain B, because null mutants of *rII* grow well in strain B. During his visit to Eugene, EPSTEIN remarked that his recent experiments showed that the multiplicity reactivation curves for T4 in those two hosts were not distinguishable. They should have been! The requirement for *rII* function in K12S(λ) should have increased both the high-dose slope of the multiplicity reactivation curve and the estimate of the number of vulnerable centers. We realized that the paradox could be resolved by proposing that T4 had two genes whose functions were required in B but not in K12S(λ), and that the functions of these two genes were about as UV-sensitive as were the functions of the *rII* genes.

Eventually, EPSTEIN returned from Oregon to Caltech, where he shared an apartment with graduate student CHARLEY STEINBERG. Referring to an event in early 1960, CHARLEY (personal communication) writes, "Dick brought up the *rII* mirror gene hypothesis several times, and I was not enamored of it. I just found it difficult to take radiobiology that seriously. . . . One evening at supper, with wine, he brought the hypothesis up yet again . . . and I said with considerable irritation, 'Dick, you don't believe that cockamamie idea any more than I do. If you did, you would have long ago started to hunt for mutants in those genes. You don't do it because you know you won't find any mutants.' Dick was taken aback by my fury and said that he would do it that very night after supper. I felt morally obliged to help him . . ."

DICK writes (personal communication), "Charley, of course, was an essential partner, but I do not remember his encouragement to do the experiments as being angry and impatient. It isn't Charley's style [and] he was agreeable to picking 2000 plaques in the first try. . . . We managed . . . to convince Harris [BERNSTEIN,

Caltech graduate student] to help us and offered the dubious reward of naming the mutants after him. Harris . . . had the nickname Immer Wieder Bernstein (*i.e.,* Forever Amber) . . .''

That night, several apparent B-specific mutants were isolated (''amber'' mutants, of course). However, additional mutant isolations plus complementation tests revealed about 20 genes rather than the two that were anticipated. CHARLEY writes, ''When I told Max [DELBRÜCK] about all the genes we were finding, his response was 'How dull!' ''

Obviously, the original motivation for looking for B-specific genes was no longer useful, but the reality of an abundance of B-specific mutations was now undeniable. DICK writes, ''. . . we fairly quickly grasped that the mutants might open the way to a characterization of the genes of T4, and some primitive physiological studies . . . were among our first efforts . . .''

BOB EDGAR (personal communication) writes, ''[When I heard of DICK's mutants], I was filled with envy and wanted my own genes. So [I looked for and] found the [temperature-sensitive mutants of T4]. I was led to that during a conversation with [ALLAN] Campbell at Cold Spring Harbor about his [host-defective mutants] and Dick's *amber*s, which led us to the notion of conditional lethals . . .'' EPSTEIN writes (personal communication) that it was through JEAN WEIGLE that the Caltech group became aware of the possible relevance of CAMPBELL's work to the understanding of the ambers. CAMPBELL, who was DOERMANN's successor at Rochester, has reviewed (1993) the history of the host-defective (*hd*) mutants of λ and of his interactions with WEIGLE and the T4 group.

A satisfactory explanation for the specificity of the amber mutations was obtained by comparing the plating properties of these mutants with the plating properties of the *hd* (later called *sus*) mutants (CAMPBELL and BALBINDER 1958; CAMPBELL 1959, 1961) and of ''ambivalent'' *rII* mutants (BENZER and CHAMPE 1961). Those hosts that plated *hd* mutants and some of those λ lysogens on which ambivalent *rII* mutants made plaques also plated the *amber* mutants. Apparently, K12S(λ) and many other strains of *E. coli* could suppress the mutant phenotype of certain alleles of any gene (BRENNER and STRETTON 1964). *E. coli* B could not suppress the phenotypes of those alleles. BRENNER and STRETTON decreed that all such suppressible mutants be called *amber*. As envisioned (dimly) by YANOFSKY and ST. LAWRENCE (1960) and (more clearly) by BENZER and CHAMPE (1962), the subsequent identification of chain-termination triplets and of mutant tRNAs that can read those triplets as if they stood for certain amino acids provided a satisfying molecular explanation for these suppressible mutants.

EPSTEIN, in the meantime, had moved to UCLA, where he undertook studies on the function of his various mutants in collaboration with two students, HIL-

LARD BERGER and FRED EISERLING, and with LURIA and MARIE-LOUISE DIRKSEN at MIT. EPSTEIN soon after moved to Geneva, where he continued studies to determine the stage in the life cycle at which each of his amber mutants was blocked. EDOUARD KELLENBERGER, who made possible the early electron microscope studies of amber-infected cells, soon exploited the mutations for the analysis of particle morphogenesis. At Caltech, EDGAR and BILL WOOD later conducted such studies *in vitro*, with results that opened the way to the analysis of complex assembly pathways using *in vitro* complementation. In Geneva, BEN HALL, PETER GEIDUSCHEK, BRUCE ALBERTS, and others were influential in initiating new biochemical studies of the mutants. For PETER and for BRUCE, contact with the amber mutants led to career investigations of T4 transcription and DNA replication, respectively.

EPSTEIN's and EDGAR's parallel studies on ambers and *ts* mutants became more intense when BOB discovered that his *ts* mutants were, for the most part, in the genes that were identified by DICK's ambers. At the 1963 Cold Spring Harbor Symposium, the paper by DICK EPSTEIN, TOINON BOLLE, CHARLEY STEINBERG, EDOUARD KELLENBERGER, E. BOY DE LA TOUR, R. CHEVALLEY (Geneva), and BOB EDGAR, MILLARD SUSMAN, GETTA DENHARDT and ALEX LIELAUSIS (Pasadena) introduced the world to the awesome power of conditional-lethal mutations (EPSTEIN *et al.* 1964). The appearance of this publication implied that it was plausible to undertake a complete developmental analysis of a sophisticated biological system.

The amber mutants and their *ts* cousins, found by graduates of the DOERMANN group at Rochester as spin-off from their radiobiological analyses, provided the phage group with generic, genome-wide markers that could do for phage genetics what random radiation damages could never accomplish (and what RFLPs and SSRs now accomplish for human genetics). They provided a convincing demonstration of the circularity and dimension of the T4 linkage map (STAHL *et al.* 1964; STREISINGER *et al.* 1964), revealed the remarkable clustering of its genes according to function (EPSTEIN *et al.* 1964), and provided the material for an elegant demonstration of the colinearity of a gene and its polypeptide product (SARABHAI *et al.* 1964). More importantly, the steadfast pursuit of an explanation for multiplicity reactivation led to the discovery of mutants that freed the phage field from the genetic and radiobiological formalisms of the time by opening the door to studies of development that employed direct means for analyzing gene function.

ALLAN CAMPBELL offered helpful criticisms. DICK EPSTEIN, CHARLEY STEINBERG and BOB EDGAR added both accuracy and vitality through their responses to my early efforts; DICK helped polish my final draft.

LITERATURE CITED

BARRICELLI, N. A., 1956 A ''chromosomic'' recombination theory for multiplicity-reactivation in phages. Acta Biotheor. **11**: 107–120.

BENZER, S., 1955 Fine structure of a genetic region in bacteriophage. Proc. Natl. Acad. Sci. USA **41:** 344–354.

BENZER, S., and S. P. CHAMPE, 1961 Ambivalent rII mutants of phage
   T4. Proc. Natl. Acad. Sci. USA **47:** 1025–1038.

BENZER, S., and S. P. CHAMPE, 1962 A change from nonsense to
   sense in the genetic code. Proc. Natl. Acad. Sci. USA **48:** 1114–
   1121.

BRENNER, S., and A. O. W. STRETTON, 1964 The *amber* mutation. J.
   Cell. Comp. Physiol. **64** Suppl. 1: 43–50.

CAMPBELL, A., 1959 Ordering of genetic sites in bacteriophage λ by
   the use of galactose-transducing defective phages. Virology **9:**
   293–305.

CAMPBELL, A., 1961 Sensitive mutants of bacteriophage. Virology
   14: 22–32.

CAMPBELL, A., 1993 Thirty years ago in GENETICS: prophage insertion into bacterial chromosomes. Genetics **133:** 433–438.

CAMPBELL, A., and E. BALBINDER, 1958 Properties of transducing
   phages. Carnegie Inst. Wash. Year Book, pp. 386–389.

DOERMANN, A. H., 1961 The analysis of ultraviolet lesions in bacteriophage T4 by cross reactivation. J. Cell. Comp. Physiol. **58**
   Suppl. 1: 79–94.

DOERMANN, A. H., M. CHASE and F. W. STAHL, 1955 Genetic recombination and replication in bacteriophage. J. Cell. Comp. Physiol.
   45 Suppl. 2: 51–74.

DULBECCO, R., 1952 A critical test of the recombination theory of
   multiplicity reactivation. J. Bacteriol. **63:** 199–207.

EDGAR, R. S., 1966 Conditional lethals, pp. 166–170 in *Phage and
   the Origins of Molecular Biology*, edited by J. CAIRNS, G. S. STENT
   and J. B. WATSON. Cold Spring Harbor Laboratory Press, Cold
   Spring Harbor, New York.

EPSTEIN, R. H., 1958 Ph.D. Thesis, University of Rochester, Rochester, New York.

EPSTEIN, R. H., A. BOLLE, C. M. STEINBERG, E. KELLENBERGER, E. BOY
   DE LA TOUR, R. CHEVALLEY, R. S. EDGAR, M. SUSMAN, G. H.
   DENHARDT and A. LIELAUSIS, 1964 Physiological studies of conditional lethal mutants of bacteriophage T4D. Cold Spring Harbor Symp. Quant. Biol. **28:** 375–394.

HARM, W., 1956 On the mechanism of multiplicity reactivation in
   bacteriophage. Virology **2:** 559–564.

KRIEG, D. R., 1959 A study of gene action in ultraviolet-irradiated
   bacteriophage T4. Virology **8:** 80–98.

LURIA, S. E., 1947 Reactivation of irradiated bacteriophage by transfer of self-reproducing units. Proc. Natl. Acad. Sci. USA **33:** 253–
   264.

LURIA, S. E., and R. DULBECCO, 1949 Genetic recombinations leading to production of active bacteriophage from ultraviolet inactivated bacteriophage particles. Genetics **34:** 93–125.

SARABHAI, A. S., A. O. W. STRETTON, S. BRENNER and A. BOLLE, 1964
   Co-linearity of the gene with the polypeptide chain. Nature **201:**
   13–17.

STAHL, F. W., 1959 Radiobiology of bacteriophage, pp. 353–385 in
   The Viruses, Vol. 2, edited by F. M. BURNET and W. M. STANLEY.
   Academic Press, New York.

STAHL, F. W., R. S. EDGAR and J. STEINBERG, 1964 The linkage map
   of bacteriophage T4. Genetics **50:** 539–552.

STREISINGER, G., R. S. EDGAR and G. H. DENHARDT, 1964 Chromosome structure in phage T4. I. Circularity of the linkage map.
   Proc. Natl. Acad. Sci. USA **51:** 775–779.

YANOFSKY, C. and P. ST. LAWRENCE, 1960 Gene action. Annu. Rev.
   Microbiol. **14:** 311–340.

November 1995

Chromosome Behavior in Cell Differentiation
A Field Ripe for Exploration?

Eeva Therman

Department of Medical Genetics, University of Wisconsin–Madison, Madison, Wisconsin 53706

TRADITIONAL chromosome cytology has emphasized the behavior of dividing cells, with their regular mitosis. Yet, in differentiated tissues, regular diploidy is by no means universal. My purpose is to call attention to the variety of chromosomal processes that occur regularly in differentiated cells. A host of problems, frequently of long standing but not familiar to many geneticists, await study by the combination of new molecular techniques with traditional cytological observations. However, most observations made on tissue and cell cultures treated with various substances, bacteria, or viruses have not been included in this presentation.

Interest in the cytogenetics of differentiated cells has been, to say the least, spotty. The best review of the early history of this field was by HEITZ (1953). Before 1933, sporadic observations of polyploidy in differentiated cells were interpreted as cytological peculiarities and were soon forgotten (HEITZ 1953). However, in 1933, HEITZ and BAUER in Germany and, independently, a few months later, PAINTER in Texas realized that the weird structures in Dipteran salivary cells were chromosomes in which the strands had multiplied many times but had remained paired (ZACHARIAS 1995). Cells containing polytene chromosomes were the most thoroughly studied of differentiated cells (BEERMAN 1962). GEITLER (1939) described highly polyploid cells (2,048C) and also a true endomitosis in the water strider, Gerris. In Vienna, studies on differentiated tissues continued in plants, first by GEITLER (reviewed 1953) and then under TSCHERMAK-WOESS (reviewed 1956). This interesting series of papers has been largely neglected, probably because they were written in German. In Germany, NAGL (reviewed 1978) continued the Vienna group's work. D'AMATO and his co-workers have also done important research on differentiated plant tissues (reviewed in D'AMATO 1952, 1977). For elementary background to human chromosomes, see THERMAN and SUSMAN (1993).

I first became interested in the relationship of chromosomal phenomena and cell differentiation in 1951 when studying differentiated cells in onion roots. This interest continued when my student S. KUPILA and I analyzed the cytogenetics of crown gall and genetic tumors in Nicotiana (1955–1974). The many mitotic anomalies in human cancer were studied with S. TIMONEN in 1950–1956, and this work was continued in 1982–1989. The nuclear phenomena in human trophoblast and hydatidiform moles were analyzed with G. E. SARTO during 1982–1986, and those in mouse trophoblast with E. M. KUHN in 1987 and 1988.

Figure 1 shows examples of nuclei discussed in this review: the nucleus in Figure 1f is from a pea root culture; the others are from human female cells. The lower lines suggest possible mechanisms and interpretations.

Tissues can rather arbitrarily be classified in the following groups (THERMAN et al. 1986):

1. Normal dividing diploid cells, as in embryos, germlines, and plant growing points.
2. Normal differentiated tissues.
3. Ephemeral tissues that are not incorporated into the individual, such as plant tapetum cells and endosperm, mammalian trophoblast, insect larval tissues, and Dipteran ovarian nurse cells.
4. Abnormal, but not malignant, tissues; examples include hydatidiform moles in mammals, crown galls in dicotyledons, genetic tumors in Nicotiana, and plant tumors caused by insects.
5. Malignant tumors in mammals, and possibly in other animal groups.

Both the normal tissues in which cells divide and those in which cells are differentiated are governed by the rules of development. In differentiated cells, polyploidy is the chromosomal change most often found. These cells stand out because of the large sizes of the cell nuclei, which are more or less proportional to the degree of polyploidy. In addition to the sizes, nuclear shapes vary greatly from tissue to tissue, from spherical through oblong to elongated and thin. Polyploidy also occurs in ephemeral tissues, but these show other cytogenetic aberrations as well, which vary in closely related species and even in neighboring cells. Nonmalignant tumors contain even more types of aberrations, and

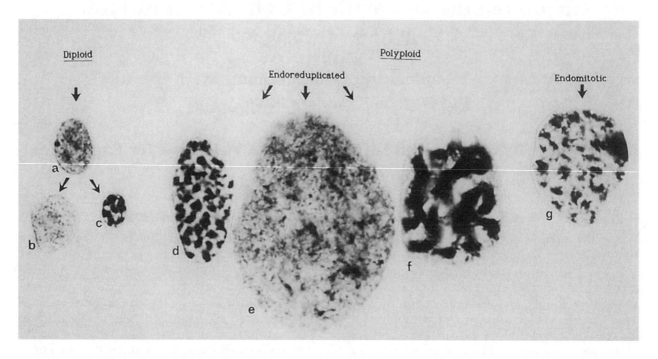

D i p l o i d				P o l y p l o i d		
a: Nucleus with Barr body	b: Nucleus without Barr body	c: Nucleus with chromocenters	d: Large nucleus with chromocenters	e: Giant evenly-stained nucleus	f: Nucleus with polytene chromosomes	g: Endomitotic nucleus
Genes active at different times. Some genes amplified.	X chromosome(s) reactivated.	Some chromosomes inactivated through condensation.	Some chromosomes inactivated through condensation.	Heterochromatin and/or other chromosome parts under-reduplicated. X chromosomes reactivated. Some genes amplified.	Genes active at different times.	Part of each chromosome inactivated through condensation.

FIGURE 1.—Different types of human female nuclei. Feulgen-staining; ×1060. The nucleus in f is from a cultured pea root.

malignant tumors are often veritable samplers of all possible chromosomal aberrations.

Somatic polyploidy: The most common chromosomal change in differentiated cells is somatic polyploidy (endopolyploidy). It has been found in most plant and animal species that have been studied in this respect. In insects, the cells in a tissue usually represent one or a few degrees of ploidy. Plant and mammalian tissues, as a rule, seem to be mosaics containing diploid and a series of differently polyploid cells. For instance, in the embryonic suspensor of the plant *Trepaeolum majus*, mosaicism ranges from 8C to 2,048C (NAGL 1978). However, other tissues of this plant show lower degrees of polyploidy and smaller variations. Very high degrees of polyploidy are found in various glandular cells; for example, about half a million C in the silk glands of the silk worm (GAGE 1974). Lists of organisms in which the cytogenetics of differentiated tissues have been stud-

ied have been published by HEITZ (1953) and by NAGL (1978).

In certain nonmalignant tumors of plants in which anatomical structure is highly irregular—tumors in plants such as crown gall (THERMAN 1956), outgrowths in Nicotiana hybrids (KUPILA and THERMAN 1962), and tumors in an Antirrhinum mutant induced by radium (STEIN 1936)—polyploidy is increased both quantitatively and qualitatively, as seen from the large sizes of nuclei that divide in crown gall and in the snapdragon tumors. Interestingly, the sunflower, which shows no somatic polyploidy in its normal stem, fails to develop polyploidy even in crown gall (KUPILA 1958).

Mechanisms creating polyploidy: Somatic polyploidy is most often created by *endoreduplication*, in which the chromosomes replicate time after time with no chromosome condensation and no mitoses. When polyploid cells of this type divide spontaneously or are induced to divide, the chromosomes appear as diplochromosomes or as bundles of multiple chromatids. If the endoreduplicated sister chromatids remain tightly paired, as in Diptera, they form banded polytene chromosomes. If the chromatids lie more loosely together, as in plants, the polytene chromosomes are not banded (Figure 1f) (TSCHERMAK-WOESS 1956). Although claims have been made that mammalian trophoblast nuclei contain polytene chromosomes, the issue is still somewhat uncertain (ZYBINA et al. 1975; SARTO et al. 1982; VARMUZA et al. 1988).

In *endomitosis*, the chromosomes go through the condensation cycle seen in mitosis, but they do not separate and the nuclear membrane remains intact. This is much rarer than endoreduplication. Endomitosis was first described in the water strider (GEITLER 1939) and later in plant tapetum cells (reviewed in D'AMATO 1977). In human tissues, it was first observed in a cervical cancer (TIMONEN and THERMAN 1956) and, in normal tissues, in the trophoblast (SARTO et al. 1982). In typical endomitosis (GEITLER 1939), a normal-appearing interphase is followed by an ordinary prophase. After this, the chromosomes attached to the nuclear membrane condense, and, in endometaphase, the two sister chromatids lie side by side like a pair of skis (Figure 1g). These separate in endoanaphase, and then the cell returns to interphase. In a variation, some of the chromosomes remain condensed while others replicate (THERMAN et al. 1983b). Human hydatidiform moles, many cancers, and probably some normal tissues grow in size through three mechanisms: mitosis, endomitosis, and endoreduplication (Figure 2) (THERMAN et al. 1986). In human cancer tissues, for instance, these different modes of growth seem to occur in separate strands.

Cell fusion appears to be an extremely rare source of polyploidy and takes place only when at least one of the cells is malignant. Cells of Bloom syndrome patients are an exception; they are able to fuse, although they are nonmalignant (OTTO and THERMAN 1981). Two or more intact nuclei do not fuse; however, if such nuclei divide simultaneously, their spindles may fuse in metaphase or anaphase. How such cells handle the additional centrioles is unclear.

Amitosis, which has been observed in cultured mouse trophoblast, means that a nucleus can simply be constricted into two parts, without the usual condensation and alignment of chromosomes and without the normal formation of a mitotic spindle (KUHN et al. 1991). This can lead to abnormal chromosome constitutions and, possibly rarely, to polyploidy.

A *lack of cell division* of a binucleate cell in which the spindles fuse during mitosis also leads to polyploidy. This occurs in plant tapetum (D'AMATO 1977; OKSALA and THERMAN 1977), many mammalian tissues (NAGL 1978), and malignant tumors (THERMAN and KUHN 1989).

Amplification and underreplication: These are in

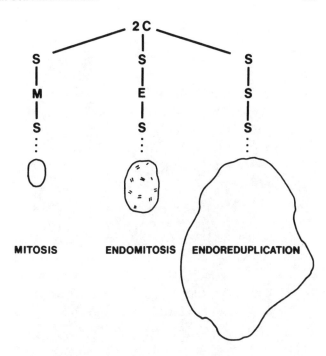

FIGURE 2.—Modes of growth of hydatidiform moles. S, DNA synthesis; M, mitosis; E, endomitosis (THERMAN et al. 1986).

many cases the same phenomenon, looked at from different points of view; some chromosomes (or parts of chromosomes, or apparently even single genes) replicate more times than others. I first encountered this phenomenon when studying onion root tips. The differentiated tissue is a mosaic of diploid and variously polyploid cells (THERMAN 1951). When these cells are induced to divide by plant growth hormones, the chromosomes in the diploid cells are perfectly normal, whereas in the polyploid cells they are broken, forming rings and dicentric or acentric chromosomes. I hypothesized that only those chromosome parts that are needed replicate. When a chromosome consists alternatively of two and of higher multiples of two strands, the chromosomes will break at the low-strand points when they try to divide.

An even earlier example of amplification/underreplication is provided by constitutive heterochromatin in Dipteran polytene chromosomes, in which the heterochromatin is greatly underreplicated (HEITZ and BAUER 1933). The same is true in various tissues of the Coleopteran, *Dermestes maculatus* (FOX 1971). Although the phenomenon has not been systematically studied in mammals, it appears that in both mouse and human the larger the nucleus, the less constitutive heterochromatin it contains (KUHN and THERMAN 1988). In Figure 3, two nuclei from cultured mouse trophoblast are compared. The smaller (inset), probably tetraploid, shows a large number of heterochromatic bodies. (In mouse chromosomes, heterochromatin is situated at the centromere.) The larger nucleus shows considerably fewer pairs of large chromocenters. We assume that only a portion of

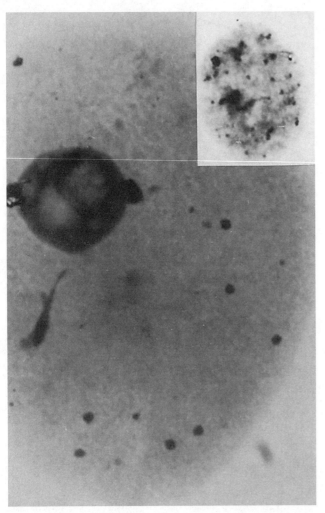

FIGURE 3.—Part of a giant nucleus and a probably tetra-ploid nucleus from cultured mouse trophoblast. The large nucleus has relatively much less constitutive heterochromatin than the tetraploid one; the heterochromatin bodies in the giant nucleus occur pairwise. There was no heterochromatin present in the portion of the giant nucleus that is not shown here. C-staining; ×2500 (KUHN and THERMAN 1988).

the chromosome pairs in this nucleus show heterochromatin. The chromosomes probably consist of some type of multiple bundles of unraveled chromatids attached to the centromere. Since no satisfactory hypothesis exists for the role of constitutive heterochromatin even in normal diploid cells, nothing is known about the significance of its possible underreplication in the various types of polyploid cells. Whether this apparent decrease in heterochromatin depends on its deletion or on a change in condensation and staining properties of constitutive heterochromatin is not known.

When chromosomes or chromosome segments behave like facultative heterochromatin, this naturally means that these chromosomes, or segments, are inactivated. Thus, facultative heterochromatin acts as a regulating mechanism in the cells. The inactivation of all but a single X chromosome in a mammalian cell acts in the same way. In about 20% of cervical tumors, no

Barr body can be seen (THERMAN et al. 1985). Apparently, Barr bodies are absent in some types of normal cells, for instance, in considerable areas of Feulgen squash preparations of human trophoblast (E. THERMAN, unpublished results). The significance of these phenomena is not understood.

The location of chromosomes in nuclei: In intermitotic interphase, the chromosomes occupy limited domains. They also lie in the same position they took in the previous anaphase, the so-called Rabl position. However, in differentiated nuclei, the chromosomes occupy different positions. The condensed chromosomes, endomitotic and variously heterochromatic, can be made visible in the nuclei with C-staining, and the position of the affected chromosomes can be inferred. As a rule, the condensed chromosomes are attached to the nuclear membrane. However, in some types of nuclei they lie at the nucleolus. Thus, MANUELIDIS (1984) showed that the centromeres of different mouse cerebellar cells have characteristic locations. In Purkinje neurons, most of the centromeres are clustered around the central nucleolus, whereas in the granule neurons the more numerous centromere clusters are attached to the nuclear membrane. Even this shows that the internal organization of the nucleus may play an important role in cell differentiation. The telomeres seem, in many cases, also to be attached to the nuclear membrane. This has been observed in Dipteran (MATHOG et al. 1984) and in plant polytene chromosomes (THERMAN and MURASHIGI 1984).

Cancer cells: Strange structures consisting of chromosomal material are visible with Feulgen staining within many giant cancer cells (THERMAN et al. 1983a). Interestingly, large plant cells show similar structures (HASITSCHKA 1956). However, what these features may mean on the chromosomal level is not clear.

Malignant tumors do not actually belong to a discussion of differentiation. However, because all the chromosomal abnormalities mentioned above, as well as several others, may occur in an advanced cancer (reviewed in THERMAN and KUHN 1989), a couple of examples will be mentioned here. An aberration not found in normal tissue is a change in the relative duration of metaphase vs. prophase. The ratio of metaphases to prophases, which is approximately 1 in normal tissue, may reach 30—40 in cancer cells, whereas the proportion of anaphases is not affected. Another feature of malignant tissue, which in untreated normal tissue has been found only in mouse decidua (ILGREN et al. 1983), is the occurrence of multipolar mitoses (THERMAN and TIMONEN 1950; TIMONEN and THERMAN 1950). In cancer tissue, the first of these to appear and the most numerous are tripolar divisions (THERMAN and TIMONEN 1950).

Chromosomes and differentiation: When discussing the relationship of cell differentiation and the various chromosomal changes described above, two possibilities must be considered: (1) that differentiation allows a wide range of phenomena (because cells no longer divide), and (2) that the observed chromosome changes promote or even cause the differentiation. Observations that would permit any conclusions about the correlation of chromosomal phenomena and cell differentiation are too few, and no believable hypotheses have been presented. Such conclusions would need observations on the parameters described above and their correlation with molecular events known to be involved in differentiation of cells.

Since the early observations on insects showed that different tissues fell into limited levels of ploidy, the conclusion was drawn that the polyploidy caused the differentiation (GEITLER 1939; OKSALA 1939). However, because plant and mammalian tissues are mosaics of diploid to high polyploid levels, and because in some plant species diploid, tetraploid, and higher polyploid varieties exist, the idea that polyploidy causes differentiation cannot be generally valid. A more reasonable idea was that, because differentiated cells do not divide, the needed number of genes can be achieved through endoreduplication or endomitosis, while at the same time saving materials and energy (BEERMAN 1962; BARLOW 1978). It is even more economical to amplify only those genes needed in a tissue, as first assumed by THERMAN (1951).

The little information that exists about the positions of chromosomes in differentiated nuclei has been derived mostly from observations on heterochromatin. Now, however, with FISH staining, the positions of individual chromosomes can be determined. In most differentiated cells, heterochromatin and other condensed chromosomes as a rule are attached to the nuclear membrane, or sometimes to the nucleolus. The telomeres are often also attached to the nuclear membrane. The mechanisms that determine arrangement of chromosomes within the nuclei are unknown.

Some of the problems above might be addressed if the results of the following studies were compared in different tissues, or in the same tissue in different organisms. Other comparisons would naturally also be possible. Feulgen staining reveals the size and shape of nuclei, the amount and situation of facultative heterochromatin, including Barr bodies, as well as endomitotic chromosomes. From the same slides, the amount of nuclear DNA can be determined with spectrophotometry. In a limited number of tissues, the chromosomes can be revealed by inducing the cells to divide. The amount and position of constitutive heterochromatin is revealed by C-banding. Electron microscopy might also yield useful information. The arrangement of chromosomes in the nucleus and in relationship to each other is best determined by FISH staining and other molecular techniques. The tools of molecular biology have now given us the means to detect changes in DNA methylation, in DNA-protein interactions, in levels of DNA replication, and in other biochemical processes that are associated with cellular differentiation. The correlation of these molecular phenomena with the cytogenetic phenomena described above should help answer the interesting questions that observations of chromosome behavior have raised. This question will be discussed in a forthcoming *Perspectives* by O. J. MILLER.

The changes that occur in the chromosomes of differentiated cells are striking and varied. The observations are numerous (except in the human), but causal analysis has barely begun. Are these changes a consequence of differentiation, or a cause? I hope I have called attention to enough striking observations to emphasize the possibilities for future study. A combination of classical cytology, new staining methods, and the powerful techniques of molecular biology should usher in a new era of research on the chromosomes of differentiated cells.

For useful suggestions I am grateful to Drs. ORLANDO J. MILLER and MILLARD SUSMAN, and Mrs. BARBARA SUSMAN.

LITERATURE CITED

BARLOW, P. W., 1978 Endopolyploidy: towards an understanding of its biological significance. Acta Biotheor. **27**: 1–18.

BEERMAN, W., 1962 *Riesenchromosomen. Protoplasmatologia 6 D.* Springer, Vienna.

D'AMATO, F., 1952 Polyploidy in the differentiation and function of tissues and cells in plants. Caryologia **4**: 311–358.

D'AMATO, F., 1977 *Nuclear Cytology in Relation to Development.* Cambridge University Press, Cambridge.

FOX, D. P., 1971 The replicative status of heterochromatic and euchromatic somatic DNA in two somatic tissues of *Dermestes maculatus* (*Dermestidae: Coleoptera*). Chromosoma **33**: 183–195.

GAGE, L. P., 1974 Polyploidization of the silk gland of *Bombyx mori.* J. Mol. Biol. **86**: 97–108.

GEITLER, L., 1939 Die Entstehung der polyploiden Somakerne der Heteropteren durch Chromosomenteilung ohne Kernteilung. Chromosoma **1**: 1–22.

GEITLER, L., 1953 *Endomitose und endomitotische Polyploidisierung. Protoplasmatologia 6 C.* Springer, Vienna.

HASITSCHKA, G., 1956 Bildung von Chromosomenbündeln nach Art der Speicheldrüsenchromosomen, spiralisierte Ruhekernchromosomen und andere Struktureigentümlichkeiten in den endopolyploiden Riesenkernen der Antipoden von *Papaver rhoeas.* Chromosoma **8**: 87–113.

HEITZ, E., 1953 Über intraindividuale Polyploidie. Arch. Julius Klaus-Stift. Vererbungsforsch. Sozialanthropol. Rassenhyg. **28**: 260–271.

HEITZ, E., and H. BAUER, 1933 Beweise für die Chromosomennatur der Kernschleifen in den Knäuelkernen von *Bibio hortulanus* L. Z. Zellforsch. Mikrosk. Anat. **17**: 67–82.

ILGREN, E. B., E. P. EVANS and M. D. BURTENSHAW, 1983 Origin of the multinucleate decidual cell of the mouse. Cytologia **48**: 313–322.

KUHN, E. M., and E. THERMAN, 1988 The behavior of heterochromatin in mouse and human nuclei. Cancer Genet. Cytogenet. **34**: 143–151.

KUHN, E. M., E. THERMAN and B. SUSMAN, 1991 Amitosis and endocycles in early cultured mouse trophoblast. Placenta **12**: 251–261.

KUPILA, S., 1958 Anatomical and cytological comparison of the development of crown gall in three host species. Ann. Bot. Soc. Zool. Bot. Fenn. 'Vanamo' **30**: 1–89.

KUPILA, S., and E. THERMAN, 1962 Anatomical observations on genetic tumors and crown gall in amphidiploid Nicotiana glauca × langsdorffii. Ann. Bot. Soc. Zool. Bot. Fenn. 'Vanamo' **32**: 1–25.

MANUELIDIS, L., 1984 Different central nervous system cell types display distinct and nonrandom arrangements of satellite DNA sequences. Proc. Natl. Acad. Sci. USA **81:** 3123–3127.

MATHOG, D., M. HOCHSTRASSER, Y. GRUENBAUM, H. SAUMWEBER and J. SEDAT, 1984   Characteristic folding pattern of polytene chromosomes in *Drosophila* salivary gland nuclei. Nature **308:** 414–421.

NAGL, W., 1978   *Endopolyploidy and Polyteny in Differentiation and Evolution.* North-Holland, Amsterdam.

OKSALA, T., 1939   Über Tetraploidie der Binde- und Fettgewebe bei den Odonaten. Hereditas **25:** 132–144.

OKSALA, T., and E. THERMAN, 1977   Endomitosis in tapetal cells of *Eremurus* (*Liliaceae*). Am. J. Bot. **64:** 866–872.

OTTO, P. G., and THERMAN, E., 1981   Spontaneous cell fusion and PCC formation in Bloom's syndrome. Chromosoma **85:** 143–148.

PAINTER, T. S., 1933   A new method for the study of chromosome rearrangements, and the plotting of chromosome maps. Science **78:** 585–586.

SARTO, G. E., P. A. STUBBLEFIELD and E. THERMAN, 1982   Endomitosis in human trophoblast. Hum. Genet. **62:** 228–232.

STEIN, E., 1936   Durch Radiumbestrahlung erzeugte erbliche Krebsentartung in Pflanzen, pp. 160–167 in *Neuere Ergebnisse auf dem Gebiete der Krebskrankheiten.* Verlag von S. Hirzel, Leipzig.

THERMAN, E., 1951   The effect of indole-3-acetic acid on resting plant nuclei. I. *Allium cepa.* Ann. Acad. Sci. Fenn. Ser. A IV Biol. **4:** 1–40.

THERMAN, E., 1956   Dedifferentiation and differentiation of cells in crown gall of *Vicia faba.* Caryologia **8:** 325–348.

THERMAN, E., and E. M. KUHN, 1989   Mitotic modifications and aberrations in cancer. CRC Crit. Rev. Oncogen. **1:** 293–305.

THERMAN, E., and T. MURASHIGI, 1984   Polytene chromosomes in cultured pea roots (*Pisum, Fabaceae*). Plant Syst. Evol. **148:** 25–33.

THERMAN, E., and M. SUSMAN, 1993   *Human Chromosomes—Structure, Behavior, and Effects.* Springer-Verlag, New York.

THERMAN, E., and S. TIMONEN, 1950   Multipolar spindles in human cancer cells. Hereditas **36:** 393–405.

THERMAN, E., G. E. SARTO and D. A. BUCHLER, 1983a   The structure and origin of giant nuclei in human cancer cells. Cancer Genet. Cytogenet. **9:** 9–18.

THERMAN, E., G. E. SARTO and P. A. STUBBLEFIELD, 1983b   Endomitosis: a reappraisal. Hum. Genet. **63:** 13–18.

THERMAN, E., C. DENNISTON, U. NIEMINEN, D. A. BUCHLER and S. TIMONEN, 1985   X chromatin, endomitoses, and mitotic abnormalities in human cervical cancer. Cancer Genet. Cytogenet. **16:** 1–11.

THERMAN, E., G. E. SARTO and E. M. KUHN, 1986   The course of endomitosis in human cells. Cancer Genet. Cytogenet. **19:** 301–310.

TIMONEN, S., and E. THERMAN, 1950   The changes in the mitotic mechanism of human cancer cells. Cancer Res. **10:** 431–439.

TIMONEN, S., and E. THERMAN, 1956   Endomitotic nuclear growth in a human cervical carcinoma. Ann. Chir. Gynaecol. Fenn. **45:** 237–244.

TSCHERMAK-WOESS, E., 1956   Karylogische Pflanzenanatomie. Protoplasma **46:** 798–834.

VARMUZA, S., V. PRIDEAUX, R. KOTHARY and J. ROSSANT, 1988   Polytene chromosomes in mouse trophoblast giant cells. Development **102:** 127–134.

ZACHARIAS, H., 1995   Emil Heitz (1892–1965): chloroplasts, heterochromatin, and polytene chromosomes. Genetics **141:** 7–14.

ZYBINA, E. V., M. V. KUDRYAVTSEVA and B. N. KUDRYAVTSEV, 1975   Polyploidization and endomitosis in giant cells of rabbit trophoblast. Cell Tiss. Res. **160:** 525–537.

Remembering Sturtevant

E. B. Lewis

Biology Division, California Institute of Technology, Pasadena, California 91125

ALFRED HENRY STURTEVANT (1891–1970) was the youngest of six children of ALFRED HENRY and HARRIET (MORSE) STURTEVANT. His grandfather, JULIAN STURTEVANT, was a Yale graduate, a Congregational minister, and one of the founders and later president of Illinois College in Jacksonville, Illinois. STURTEVANT's father taught mathematics for a while at that college, but later took up farming, first in Illinois and later in southern Alabama, where the family moved when STURTEVANT was seven years old. STURTEVANT went to a one-room country school and later to a public high school in Mobile.

At the age of 17, STURTEVANT entered Columbia University, where his brother EDGAR, who was 16 years older, was teaching at Barnard College. EDGAR and his wife took the young STURTEVANT into their family, and ALFRED lived with them while attending the University. EDGAR was a scholar who later became a professor of linguistics at Yale and an authority on the Hittite language. STURTEVANT said that he learned the aims and standards of scholarship and research from EDGAR. It was a great pleasure for STURTEVANT when he and EDGAR were awarded honorary degrees at the same Yale commencement many years later. Also present at the ceremony were STURTEVANT's nephew, JULIAN (EDGAR's son), Professor (now Emeritus) of Organic Chemistry at Yale, and STURTEVANT's elder son, WILLIAM, then a graduate student in Yale's department of anthropology and now curator of anthropology at the Smithsonian Institution in Washington.

STURTEVANT said that he became interested in genetics as the result of tabulating the pedigrees of his father's horses. He continued this interest at Columbia and also collected data on his own pedigree. At EDGAR's suggestion he went to the library and read some books on heredity, with the result that he read the textbook on Mendelism by PUNNETT.

STURTEVANT saw at once that Mendelism could explain some of the complex patterns of inheritance of coat colors in horses that he and others before him had observed. EDGAR encouraged STURTEVANT to write an account of his findings and take it to MORGAN, who at that time was Professor of Zoology at Columbia, and from whom STURTEVANT had taken a course in zoology during his freshman year. MORGAN encouraged STURTEVANT to publish the paper, and it was submitted to the *Biological Bulletin* in June, 1910, at the end of his sophomore year. The paper appeared that same year (STURTEVANT 1910). The connection between the genetics of horses and that of Drosophila will be familiar to readers of this column from the *Perspectives* by SNELL and REED (1993) on the mouse geneticist W. E. CASTLE.

The other result of STURTEVANT's interest in the pedigrees of horses was that he was given a desk in the famous fly room at Columbia University where, only three months before, MORGAN had found the first white-eyed fly. These stories and more about the early days at Columbia, when modern genetics was in a very real sense born, are a matter of record, especially in the writings of STURTEVANT himself (1965a,b).

STURTEVANT once wrote that he knew of no one else at the time who was so thoroughly committed to the experimental approach to biological problems as was MORGAN. It was MORGAN's aim to produce a mechanistic, as opposed to a purposive, interpretation of biological phenomena. A great deal of this approach clearly rubbed off on STURTEVANT.

STURTEVANT had a remarkable memory. It was as if his memory were composed of a plethora of matrices waiting to be filled with any data that lent themselves to classification into discrete categories. The data might be in the form of numbers and kinds of bristles missing in a mutant fly; numbers of snails with a right-handed coil *vs.* a left-handed coil, the genetics of which STURTEVANT was the first to explain; the relation between inversion sequences in different species; or the host of other characteristics he investigated not only in Drosophila, but in irises, evening primroses, snails, moths, and many other creatures, including human beings. Whatever form the data took, the observations fell into the appropriate matrix in his memory, from which they were readily retrievable to a degree that was truly phenomenal. STURTEVANT liked to refer to this as the "blockhead" approach.

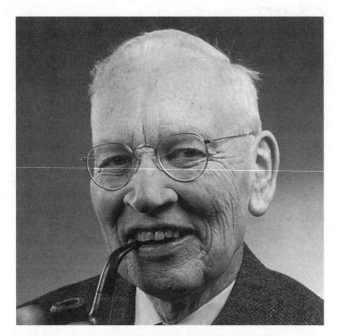

A. H. STURTEVANT

The Caltech period was a time of collaboration, especially with STERLING EMERSON, THEODOSIUS DOBZHANSKY, GEORGE BEADLE, and JACK SCHULTZ. It was STURTEVANT's style, at least after he came to Caltech in 1928 with MORGAN and BRIDGES, to spend his mornings doing experiments. Afternoons were spent in the biology library checking on any incoming journals, few of which in any phase of biology he did not at least dip into. The pace of science was not so frenetic as it is nowadays, so there was time for extended afternoon tea sessions at which STURTEVANT might bring up a paper he had read that afternoon and that had attracted his attention. These sessions were very stimulating for the graduate students in genetics and embryology who usually attended them; among the faculty in genetics, SCHULTZ, EMERSON AND DOBZHANSKY were likely to be present in addition to STURTEVANT, and in embryology, ALBERT TYLER, who was working on the biochemistry of fertilization. Although a rift had developed between STURTEVANT and DOBZHANSKY, there was no sign of it in front of the graduate students.

STURTEVANT taught the undergraduate course in genetics at Caltech for many years. From time to time he also gave a course for undergraduates in entomology, complete with a field laboratory session. His lectures on topics in advanced genetics were scholarly reviews of special areas of genetics, often dealing with organisms with bizarre genetics, such as the protozoa. His lectures were especially valuable because he covered areas of research not ongoing at Caltech. The elementary course in genetics that STURTEVANT taught was based on a textbook that he and GEORGE BEADLE wrote (1939). It was not so widely used as perhaps it should have been, probably because it was considered too difficult for the average student. It was tailored for Caltech

students, and the problems especially were a challenge, even for Caltech undergraduates.

STURTEVANT and BEADLE planned to revise the textbook, but the pressure of other work and the rapidity of developments that followed the discovery of the role of DNA prevented the revision. STURTEVANT also liked to point out that both he and BEADLE found after writing the book that each had used the term "gene" differently. For example, the *white* gene to STURTEVANT was the specific *white* mutant, but to BEADLE it represented the constellation of *white* alleles including the wild-type allele. STURTEVANT facetiously blamed their inability to get out a second edition on this difference in thinking about the gene. Characteristically, he would ask each geneticist whom he met how he or she used the term, and he then promptly catalogued such persons according to whether they thought of the gene the way he did or the way BEADLE did. The person asked did not, of course, need to worry about his answer being in good company in either case.

STURTEVANT read widely and kept abreast of many topics of current interest, especially politics. He would, for example, read the Sunday *New York Times* and the *Manchester Guardian Weekly* virtually from cover to cover. He was especially happy if he could do the crossword puzzle in the *Guardian* at one sitting. Those who know those puzzles will understand that only a very special breed of person attempts them, let alone solves them in one sitting. In the evening he would browse through the *Encyclopedia Britannica*, which was shelved next to his easy chair. He complained one time, and he was not bragging, that he had difficulty in finding an article which he had not already read.

STURTEVANT was fascinated with puzzles of all kinds, especially puzzles involving three-dimensional objects. When ANNE ROE (1953) made a study of what makes scientists tick, she chose STURTEVANT as one of her subjects. He was not only flattered, but overjoyed at the opportunity to take the tests, which he viewed simply as a new set of puzzles to work out.

STURTEVANT would develop a topic logically and succinctly, whether he was publishing a paper or giving a formal lecture. In private conversation, however, he always seemed to assume that the listener was at least as well versed in the subject as he was, so he would leave out the preliminaries and get right to the point. This could be mystifying to some. For others it was a challenge to try to become sufficiently versed to profit by listening to his ideas or tapping the tremendous store of information at his fingertips on almost any topic of substance. His papers were so well written that one would assume that he had labored over each word. His penciled manuscripts rarely contained more than a few minor changes inserted into the original draft, which was done in longhand on foolscap. When asked how he did this, he told me that he usually spent many days mulling the paper over in his mind until all the words fell into place, and then all he had to do was write it down from memory.

Sturtevant developed a keen interest in the history of science; his book, *A History of Genetics* (1965a), is a classic. His main purpose in writing it, I believe, was to give credit where he thought it was due, always a difficult task, and at the same time to trace the history of the ideas underlying scientific discoveries. I believe he would have decried a tendency in some quarters to relate scientific discoveries to the socio-political views of the discoverers themselves. His fascination with pedigrees, including his own, led him to compile an appendix that contained a series of "intellectual" pedigrees. Sturtevant, of course, was a direct descendant of T. H. Morgan and of E. B. Wilson, another eminent biologist who was a contemporary and friend of Morgan's at Columbia. Morgan and Wilson were, in turn, direct descendants of Martin and Brooks, two men who were at Johns Hopkins University where Morgan had obtained his doctorate; Martin was descended from T. H. Huxley and Brooks from Louis Agassiz; and so it went.

Sturtevant had a fund of aphorisms and anecdotes that he liked to spring whenever an occasion arose. Three of his favorites were from Morgan: "Establish a point and publish it;" or, when trying to overcome the difficulty in starting to write a paper, "Compose a flowery introduction, then throw it away and write the paper;" or, when a Drosophila experiment gave a totally unexpected result, "They will fool you every time." Sturtevant had one that pertained to his own marriage to Phoebe Reed Sturtevant and to that of a number of their friends, namely, "Marriages are made in heaven but there is a branch office in Woods Hole." A few were deliberately outrageous in order to make a subtle point: "Too bad graduate students are people;" or "Vertebrates are a mistake and should never have been invented." He liked to deflate pomposity whenever he ran across it and referred to pompous persons as "stuffed shirts." Echoing his contempt for profundity, he would say, "Something is profound if it reaches conclusions which I like by methods I don't understand."

Sturtevant's love for all living things, including people, was expressed in many ways. For example, in 1954 he gave the presidential address before the Pacific Division of the American Association for the Advancement of Science, where he warned of the potential hazards to human beings of the fallout from the atmospheric testing of atomic bombs. What had provoked Sturtevant was a strong statement issued by the executive branch of the government that the fallout levels from testing were far below any that could cause damage to human beings. This assumption, that there is a threshold for damage from ionizing radiation, had no evidence to support it and clearly was being used to justify testing of nuclear weapons.

Although I know that some assumed that the only purpose of Sturtevant's remarks was a desire to see a halt to bomb testing, this was not the case. He took a neutral stance and, although he felt there might be a need for testing, the public should be given the best estimate that scientists could make about the nature of the danger to the unborn from fallout levels of radiation. In "Quarreling Geneticists and a Diplomat," Crow (1995) has described in more detail the ways in which Sturtevant and other geneticists interacted in assessing radiation risks to the germ plasm.

I am indebted to Sturtevant's son, William, for pointing out in a personal communication that his father "had deep disdain for eugenics and a strong contempt for all forms of social discrimination," sentiments that perfectly sum up Sturtevant's position on these matters. Indeed, most of the chapter on the "Genetics of Man" in Sturtevant's *History of Genetics* (1965a) is devoted to a balanced treatment of the nature-nurture question.

Sturtevant's scientific accomplishments have been reviewed elsewhere, by himself (1965a); by Sterling Emerson (1971), who first became acquainted with him in 1922; by G. W. Beadle (1970), who first came to Caltech in 1931 as a National Research Council Fellow; and by me (1976). Some of his most important papers were reprinted in a book, *Genetics and Evolution* (1961), on the occasion of his 70th birthday. Sturtevant was invited to make addenda to those papers as he saw fit; characteristically, he made only the briefest possible ones.

In a *Perspectives*, J. F. Crow (1988) stressed Sturtevant's remarkable contributions to virtually every branch of genetics. One of Sturtevant's most enduring scientific interests was that of evolutionary theory and how to approach it experimentally. One of his first contributions relevant thereto was his discovery and analysis of hybrids between *Drosophila melanogaster* and *D. simulans*, for which there is a valuable *Perspectives* by W. F. Provine (1991).

Sturtevant's research style was to let the experiments lead the way. In this respect he was not restrained by having to write grant proposals, and a decline in his rate of publishing after 1945 might have resulted in a low score anyway. Bateson is often cited for having said, "Treasure your exceptions." I believe Sturtevant's admonition would be, "Analyze your exceptions," for it is his remarkable analytical ability that shines through all his work.

For Sturtevant, science must have been an exciting and rewarding journey into the unknown. It was fortunately a long journey, with detours to many realms, and I am sure he savored every minute of it.

LITERATURE CITED

Beadle, G. W., 1970 Alfred Henry Sturtevant (1981–1970), Year Book of The American Philosophical Society, pp. 166–171.

CROW, J. F., 1988 A diamond anniversary: the first chromosome map. Genetics **118:** 1–3.

CROW, J. F., 1995 Quarreling geneticists and a diplomat. Genetics **140:** 421–426.

EMERSON, S., 1971 Alfred Henry Sturtevant (November 21, 1891–April 6, 1970). Annu. Rev. Genet. **5:** 1–4.

LEWIS, E. B., 1976 Sturtevant, Alfred Henry, pp. 133–138 in *Dictionary of Scientific Biography,* vol. 13, edited by C. C. GILLISPIE. Charles Scribner's Sons, New York.

PROVINE, W. B., 1991 ALFRED HENRY STURTEVANT and crosses between *Drosophila melanogaster* and *Drosophila simulans.* Genetics **129:** 1–5.

ROE, A., 1953 *The Making of a Scientist.* Dodd, Mead & Co., New York.

SNELL, G. D., and S. REED, 1993 WILLIAM ERNEST CASTLE, pioneer mammalian geneticist. Genetics **133:** 751–753.

STURTEVANT, A. H., 1910 On the inheritance of color in the American harness horse. Biol. Bull. **19:** 204–216.

STURTEVANT, A. H., 1961 *Genetics and Evolution: Selected Papers of A. H. Sturtevant,* edited by E. B. LEWIS with a foreword by G. W. BEADLE. W. H. Freeman, San Francisco.

STURTEVANT, A. H., 1965a *A History of Genetics.* Harper & Row, New York.

STURTEVANT, A. H., 1965b The "fly room." Am. Sci. **53:** 303–307.

STURTEVANT, A. H., and G. W. BEADLE, 1939 *An Introduction to Genetics.* W. B. Saunders Co., Philadelphia.

January 1996

Embryonic Transcription and the Control of Developmental Pathways

Eric Wieschaus

Department of Molecular Biology, Princeton University, Princeton, New Jersey 08544

It appears that the initial steps up to the [sea urchin] blastula stage are independent of the quality of the nuclear substance, even though it is essential that the nuclear substance be of a kind capable of existing in the egg. The necessity for particular chromosomes becomes apparent first with the formation of the primary mesenchyme and from then on shows up in all processes as far as development can be observed.... With respect to those characters in which we are able to recognize individual variations, the nuclear substance and not the cytoplasmic cell substance imposes its specific character on the developing trait.

... Earlier stages, for which according to our results, specific chromosomes are not necessary, demonstrate a purely maternal character.... I would like to ascribe to the cytoplasm of the sea urchin egg only the initial and simplest properties responsible for differentiation... it provides the most general basic form, the framework within which all specific details are filled in by the nucleus.   THEODOR BOVERI 1902

EVEN before the molecular nature of the gene was understood, embryos were known to get the products they need from two different sources. In modern terms, the unfertilized egg contains large stores of maternal RNA and protein that are derived from transcription during oogenesis. Initially, these proteins provide the basic machinery for all cellular events. At some point these maternally supplied products are supplemented by transcription from the embryo's own genome (the "nuclear substance" in BOVERI's formulation). This occurs at different stages in different organisms, but significant transcription is usually detected by the blastula or blastoderm stage. Maternal gene products persist after this point, however, and most processes during embryogenesis involve both maternal and zygotic components.

As the quote from BOVERI's classic paper indicates, embryologists at the turn of the century were aware of both maternal and zygotic contributions to embryonic development. They even considered the possibility that maternal components might play different roles in development than zygotic components. In the eighty years that followed BOVERI's work, it became clear that certain zygotically active genes play major controlling roles. Landmark studies were POULSON's (1940) analysis of chromosomal deletions in the *Notch* region and LEWIS' (1978) characterization of the Bithorax complex.

In the following pages, I will address the generality of a hypothesis only partly implied by the BOVERI quote, namely that in organisms where zygotically required gene activities are rare, all such activities have been selected to play unique, controlling roles in development. In this admittedly extreme reformulation of BOVERI's observation, I will restrict consideration to those genes whose products *must* be supplied zygotically and to organisms that have minimized their transcriptional requirements during embryogenesis. I will first present reasons why such a division of labor makes teleological sense and then examine the data from Drosophila to determine the extent to which gene activity actually obeys these expectations. Then I will discuss the exceptions, *i.e.*, certain well-characterized cases where particular Drosophila genes are supplied zygotically but do not seem to play controlling roles. Lastly, the Drosophila data will be compared to that from other organisms.

The simple model: In organisms where embryonic development is rapid and occurs with no increase in size before hatching from the egg, it will be advantageous to maximize maternal contributions, because the duration of oogenesis is often much longer than embryogenesis and the ovary provides a more sophisticated and efficient synthetic machinery. Evolutionary selection for efficiency will maximize such maternal contributions. One major limitation to maternal supplies is the duration of embryonic development. Maternal supplies must be sufficient to last until a larva hatches and can obtain additional nutrients from the environment. In principle, maternal contributions might consist only of nutrient material ("yolk") that could be converted by the embryo to a wide variety of gene products. It may be more efficient, however, that the "nutrients" include RNA directly encoding the individual components of most biological processes, including the cellular machinery required for transcription, translation, energy utilization and basic cell structure.

On the other hand, all embryos have been shown to require certain RNAs supplied by transcription of their own genome. Early indications of this requirement came from the seminal work of BOVERI, as well as species hybridization experiments and actinomycin and α-amantin studies (reviewed in DAVIDSON 1986). If supplying gene products maternally is so advantageous, what can zygotic transcription do that just storing maternal transcribed gene products can't? One possibility is that zygotic transcription allows much more precise expression, putting particular gene products in one cell but not in its immediate neighbors. Such precision is probably not necessary for most gene products. If a gene product is needed in some cells but not others, it may be sufficient (although profligate) to supply it uniformly to the whole egg. A patterned expression only becomes important when the *absence* of a particular gene product is as significant as its presence. This might be the case if the gene product is used as a developmental switch, such that its expression in one cell causes that cell to assume a fate different from its neighbors. While it is possible to localize maternal gene products to particular regions of the egg cytoplasm, local transcription may allow more precision, and may therefore be more useful as spatial patterns become complex.

This view has certain practical consequences. Over the course of evolution, the efficiencies of maternal contribution will reduce zygotic transcription to a minimum. That minimum will define a set of genes, each of which is limiting for a specific process, such that its presence or absence determines when and where in the embryo that process takes place. Not all controlling elements will be zygotic; a process could be initiated by a localized maternal RNA or ligands (ST JOHNSTON and NÜSSLEIN-VOLHARD 1992). However, if there is a zygotic component in a process, its expression is likely to play a controlling role in all events downstream to it. In this view, selection during evolution has solved the research agenda of a large fraction of developmental biologists: in a complex process involving many gene products, it has sorted out which one actually plays the controlling role. Therefore, to understand how a particular process is controlled in the embryo, good candidate genes would be those whose products need to be supplied zygotically. For organisms where genetic analyses are possible, identification of candidates is relatively straightforward; if the genes are removed by mutation, homozygous mutant embryos will develop abnormally.

Consistent with behavior as controlling elements, genes that must be supplied zygotically represent only a small fraction of the Drosophila genome: The mutagenesis screens that CHRISTIANE NÜSSLEIN-VOLHARD, GERD JURGENS and I began more than fifteen years ago in Heidelberg offered an initial opportunity to test whether the expectations outlined above apply to Drosophila (NÜSSLEIN-VOLHARD and WIESCHAUS 1980; JURGENS *et al.* 1984; NÜSSLEIN-VOLHARD *et al.* 1984; WIESCHAUS *et al.* 1984). Of the 18,000 lethal mutations induced in those screens, only about 4500 (25%) cause death during embryogenesis, and only 580 cause alterations in visible morphology sufficient to allow homozygous embryos to be distinguished from their heterozygous siblings. These 580 mutations were assigned to 139 complementation groups with an average hit frequency of 4.2. Identification of mutants in the Heidelberg screens was based on examination of the larval cuticle. Later screens using other aspect of general morphology (EBERL and HILLIKER 1988) or using molecular markers to follow the development of specific organ systems (SEEGAR *et al.* 1993; VAN VACTOR *et al.* 1993; HARBECKE and LENGYEL 1995) identified additional genes, although their number is not large. The major conclusion

from all these studies is that only a small number of loci need be transcribed in the embryo itself to establish normal morphology. Even if the Heidelberg screens detected only half the zygotically important loci, the number of such genes would increase only to 300, fewer than 2% of the estimated 20,000 molecularly defined transcription units and only a small fraction of the transcripts and proteins found in the embryo. The remainder of these proteins and RNAs, and thus the majority of the components involved in any particular embryonic process, must be supplied maternally.

If early acting, zygotically transcribed genes are rare, it should be possible to delete large portions of the genome with little effect on early stages of development. We tested this possibility by examining the development of embryos homozygous for various cytologically defined deletions, and eventually used translocations and chromosomal rearrangements to generate embryos deleted for overlapping regions spanning the entire Drosophila genome (MERRILL *et al.* 1988; WIESCHAUS and SWEETON 1988). In general, such deficiency embryos show phenotypes that could be explained by point mutations previously located to the deleted regions. There are exceptions, notably a group of seven early acting genes required for cellularization at the onset of cycle 14. Ongoing work in my lab suggests the existence of certain regions with previously undescribed effects on gastrulation and early morphogenetic movements (E. WIESCHAUS, unpublished results). In general, however, such newly discovered loci have been rare, confirming the preponderance of maternal gene products and scarcity of gene products that must be supplied by zygotic transcription.

Transcripts that must be supplied to the embryo zygotically appear to play special roles in development: Most of the mutations identified in the Heidelberg screens produce discrete phenotypes, such that differentiation of most structures is normal and defects are limited to specific cell types or regions. Also, most phenotypes are locus-specific (*i.e.,* there is only one locus in the genome that can be mutated to produce that phenotype). Subsequent molecular analyses suggest that this specificity is often reflected in their expression patterns during embryogenesis. On the X chromosome, for example, where 14 of the 20 loci have been cloned, 11 show patterns of transcription corresponding to where the gene products are required in the embryo. Genes that show uniform phenotypes affecting all cells at a particular stage (the early acting cellularization genes *nullo, srya* and *bottleneck*) show uniform transcript distribution, but are only expressed in a short period immediately preceding cellularization (JAMES and VINCENT 1986; ROSE and WIESCHAUS 1992; SCHEJTER and WIESCHAUS 1993).

Another feature of these genes that suggests specialized functions is that their transcription is generally not required during oogenesis. This behavior is different from most genes in Drosophila and is best illustrated by examination of the X chromosome, where the wild-type activities associated with many random lethal loci have been studied using germ-line clones (PERRIMON *et al.* 1984, 1989). Most of these lethals (35/48 and 133/211 in two separate surveys) cause blocks during oogenesis or abnormalities in embryogenesis that cannot be corrected by zygotic transcription. In contrast, only three of the 19 Heidelberg loci that have been tested are required during oogenesis (JIMENEZ and COMPOS-ORTEGA 1982; ZUSMAN and WIESCHAUS 1985; WIESCHAUS and NOELL 1986; EBERL *et al.* 1992). For the remaining 16 loci, a single zygotic allele is sufficient to ensure normal development of the embryo, even when all maternal activity is removed by producing germline clones. In several cases (*mys, exd, fog*) alterations in the development of the resultant progeny suggests that the wild-type genes may normally be transcribed during oogenesis. Unlike the average vital gene, however, such transcription is not necessary for embryonic survival, as long as the embryo has at least one normal copy of the gene.

The precision of these expression patterns might simply reflect an economy of synthesis, the embryo only making gene products where it needs them. In a few cases this possibility has been excluded by expressing the gene ectopically. This was initially accomplished for the *ftz* segmentation gene using a heat-shock promoter (STRUHL 1985), but alternative systems such the Gal4/UAS system of BRAND and PERRIMON (1993) have been designed to produce more specific patterns of expression. If the presence of a particular gene product directs a cell into a fate different from that of its neighbors, then it should be possible to direct its neighbor (or any other cell) into the same fate by forcing expression of the same gene product. Although only a few genes have been tested, the results have confirmed the significance of most of the spatial expression patterns associated with genes affecting all three levels of segmentation (PARKHURST and ISH-HOROWICZ 1991; CAPOVILLA *et al.* 1992; MANOUKIAN and KRAUSE 1992; NOORDEMEER *et al.* 1992; TSAI and GERGEN 1994), as well as neuronal development (RHYU *et al.* 1994), cell proliferation (ED-GAR and O'FARRELL 1990) and gastrulation (P. MORIZE, M. COSTA, S. PARKS and E. WIESCHAUS, unpublished results). One potential exception (*patched*) is discussed below.

Do all zygotically required genes play controlling roles? The observations presented above suggest that most transcriptionally required genes play specific regulatory roles in the Drosophila embryo. There are exceptions, of course, but many of the apparent exceptions can be integrated into the model with little modification. As mentioned above, some of these genes are also transcribed during oogenesis. In many such cases, the maternal products appear to be supplied in insufficient quantities, so that patterned zygotic transcription still provides the critical difference in establishing cell be-

havior (WIESCHAUS and NOELL 1986). Such maternal transcripts may bring all cells close enough to the threshold so that small differentials in zygotic transcription between neighboring cells can make an immediate difference.

At the other end of the spectrum are gene products required throughout embryonic development in such large quantities that maternal supplies are not sufficient and additional zygotic transcription is required by later stages in development. Such genes may represent the bulk of embryonic-lethal mutations that make it through the last major morphological events of Drosophila embryonic development (dorsal closure and head involution), but die before hatching with no obvious visible defects, a class that we found represented about 25% of all lethal genes. In some cases the requirement for additional zygotic transcription may set in earlier, so that mutations cause visible defects in late embryonic processes. The major cytoplasmic myosin gene (*zipper*) may provide an example (YOUNG *et al.* 1993). Although cytoplasmic myosin is required throughout development, mutations that block zygotic transcription cause abnormalities only during dorsal closure and head involution. Zygotic transcription of *zipper* does not appear to play a regulatory role; *zipper* transcripts are uniformly distributed in normal embryos, and the mutant defect can be rescued by ubiquitous *zipper* transcripts supplied from a heat-shock promoter (YOUNG *et al.* 1993). Presumably the early normal development of homozygous mutants reflects maternal myosin RNA and protein that begin to run out shortly before dorsal closure.

More puzzling, however, are cases where the absence of zygotic transcription produces an early phenotype (within the first two hours after the blastoderm stage), yet the relevant gene product is transcribed uniformly in the embryo. Examples include *arm* (RIGGLEMAN *et al.* 1990), *Notch* (JOHANSEN *et al.* 1989), *exd* (RAUSKOLB *et al.* 1993) *odd-paired* (BENEDYK *et al.* 1994) and *flb/DER* (LEV *et al.* 1985; ZAK *et al.* 1990). The uniform distribution of these transcripts makes it difficult to see how their transcription could play a controlling role in choosing between pathways. Some of these genes (*Notch, flb/DER*) encode cell surface receptors or (*armadillo*) other molecules required for the response of cells to local signals. Many of these signals are known; they are encoded by other zygotically active genes that are expressed in restricted patterns, such as *wingless* (BAKER 1987). It is natural to assume that it is the expression of these latter genes that controls cell fate. The early stage of development when signalling is required makes it hard to understand why their receptors could not be supplied maternally.

In some cases, a large supply of maternal receptor protein may be disadvantageous if that receptor can cross-react with or interfere with processes that involve similar components. The Drosophila EGF receptor (*flb/*

DER), for example, is required in the follicle cells but not in the oocyte during oogenesis (SCHÜPBACH 1987). It also utilizes many of the same downstream elements (*e.g.*, Ras, Raf) as certain maternally supplied receptor tyrosine kinases (torso) that pattern the embryo during cleavage; see DUFFY and PERRIMON (1994). To avoid cross-reactions, it may be simplest for the organism not to express *flb/DER* transcripts in maternal germ cells. This would explain why *flb/DER* is not expressed maternally and only expressed zygotically after the blastoderm stage. This notion could be tested by determining whether maternally supplied *flb*/DER product has deleterious effect on development or, alternatively, can rescue mutant embryos. In any case, it is more difficult to apply such explanations to genes like *armadillo*, which act early and are expressed in abundant quantities maternally and yet are also expressed zygotically.

Potentially more damaging to the model are genes that behave like the segment polarity gene *patched*. *patched* transcripts are not supplied maternally and zygotic transcripts accumulate in complicated patterns (NAKANO *et al.* 1989), consistent with a controlling role in development. However, no effects are observed when these patterns are altered by ectopic expression (INGHAM *et al.* 1991; SAMPEDRO and GUERRERO 1991). One possibility is that the informational content of the expression patterns is redundant. Various genes in the segment polarity subgroup are expressed in overlapping patterns and final cell fates are regulated by cell interactions that occur continuously throughout development. This means that patterned expression of a single component may contribute to the efficiency with which the final pattern is achieved, but does not function as an absolutely essential determinant of that pattern. Effects of ectopic expression may therefore be very subtle or transient.

In summary, limited expression patterns seem to play an important role in many of the gene activities that must be supplied to the embryo by zygotic transcription. In the majority of cases, gene products are transcribed in spatial patterns. In many cases where they have been tested, misexpression leads to at least transient abnormalities in development. This behavior is consistent with a role for their expression in controlling where and when specific developmental pathways are initiated. While real and significant exceptions exist, they are rare. In many of the exceptional cases it is not clear whether the analysis was sufficient to exclude subtle roles for the expression pattern, particularly when temporal as well as spatial aspects are considered.

How much is this extrapolatable to other species? In principle, one might expect similar selective pressures to maximize maternal contributions in all organisms that develop rapidly with little growth or increase in size before larval stages. Many organisms fit this description, including *Caernorhabditis elegans*, frogs, sea urchins and fish. The obvious exceptions are mammals and plants, both of which undergo substantial increases in size during early stages when spatial patterns are being established. The model would predict that the average gene in mammals or plants would show substantial transcriptional requirements in the embryo, because the increase in size makes it impractical to supply any gene product in sufficient quantities from purely maternal sources. In contrast to Drosophila, most random lethal mutations would cause death during embryogenesis; see JURGENS *et al.* (1991) and ROSSANT and HOPKINS (1992) for a discussion of this point. In the other organisms, transcription would still be required for only a few genes, but these would be predicted to play controlling roles in specific developmental processes.

It was the discrete phenotypes produced in sea urchin embryos when particular chromosomes were eliminated that led BOVERI to conclude that "the nuclear substance imposes its specific character on the developing trait." (In fact, had the early zygotic defects not been specific, BOVERI would not have been able to conclude that individual chromosomes carry distinct developmental properties.) His observations suggest that the model may apply to sea urchins and other marine organisms. A more concerted genetic approach is possible in other invertebrates, such as nematodes. In a survey of temperature-sensitive lethal mutations, HIRSH *et al.* (1978) identified 25 ts mutants affecting genes required for normal embryogenesis. The mutations had not been selected based on their morphological phenotypes and can be assumed to represent a random sample of gene activities required during that period. In 22 of the 25 cases, a wild-type allele in the mother was sufficient to rescue homozygous mutant embryos, arguing for the numerical predominance of maternal gene products in that organism. The three loci whose products must be supplied zygotically do not represent a very large sample; still, it would be interesting to know whether their zygotic phenotypes suggest specific roles in development. In any case, concerted mutagenesis screens for genes whose transcription is strictly required in *C. elegans* embryos should eventually identify all genes with specific morphological effects in that organism.

In vertebrates, less is known genetically about maternal *vs.* zygotic requirements. In frogs, maternal contributions appear to be substantial. Although few mutants are known, embryos homozygously deleted for ribosomal DNA develop to young tadpoles, even though new rRNA normally begins to be made at the blastula stage (BROWN and GURDON 1964). This indicates that rRNA and probably many cellular components are maternally supplied in quantities sufficient to last the duration of embryogenesis. Data for other vertebrates are not much more extensive. In principle, zebrafish has all the hallmarks of a species that should have minimal and therefore regulatory zygotic transcription. Development is rapid, the basic form being established in 48 hours (KIMMEL 1989). The volume of the embryo increases only after hatching. Zygotically active mutations are known that significantly alter the pattern of the embryo. The real test will involve comparing the frequency of such mutations with the general behavior of random lethals. If the situation in zebrafish is like Drosophila, one would predict that only a small fraction of vital genes have transcripts that must be supplied to the embryo by its own transcription. Such genes should produce discrete phenotypes suggestive of specific roles in development. Results from the ongoing zebrafish screens (MULLINS et al. 1994; SOLNICA-KREZEL et al. 1994) will be interesting in this respect.

However, the major advantage of any mutagenesis screen is not the characterization of general behaviors of genes and their relative maternal and zygotic contributions. The real reason anyone does a screen is to identify interesting genes that offer entry points into studying complex phenomena. In the preceding pages, I have argued for the special advantage of screens directed at zygotic activity in the embryo. Under certain circumstances, those screens are particularly likely to identify controlling elements and will thus be particularly informative about how development is regulated. A second and unemphasized advantage of such screens is their simplicity, because phenotypes produced in early homozygous-mutant embryos are not complicated by later requirements for the same gene. Although chemical mutagenesis with point mutagens like EMS or ENU may only be possible in organisms where large numbers of stocks can be inbred over a number of generations, early acting, zygotically required genes can also be detected by deleting whole regions of the genome (as BOVERI showed in his classic paper). Because deletion embryos can be obtained in a reproducible fashion as meiotic segregants of crosses involving translocations, they can be generated in any organism where a substantial number of translocation chromosomes exist. This might allow an analysis of zygotic activity in mice, where many translocations are known and characterized, and surveys of transcriptional activity in any organisms where translocations can be isolated from natural populations.

LITERATURE CITED

BAKER, N. E., 1987   Molecular cloning of sequences from wingless, a segment polarity gene in Drosophila: the spatial distribution of transcripts in embryos. EMBO J. 6: 1765–1773.

BENEDYK, M. J., J. R. MULLEN and S. DINARDO, 1994   odd-paired: a zinc finger pair-rule protein required for the timely activation of engrailed and wingless in Drosophila embryos. Genes Dev. 8: 105–117.

BOVERI, T., 1902   On the multipolar mitosis as a means of analysis of the cell nucleus. Verhandlungen der physikalisch-medizinischen Gesellschaft zur Wurzburg. Neue Folge 35: 67–90. Translated from the original German, 1964 in Foundations of Experimental Embryology, edited by B. H. WILLIER and J. M. OPPENHEIMER. Prentice Hall, Englewood Cliffs, NJ.

BRAND, A., and N. PERRIMON, 1993   Targeted gene expression as a means of altering cell fates and generating dominant phenotypes. Development 118: 401–415.

BROWN, D. D., and J. B. GURDON, 1964   Absence of ribosomal RNA synthesis in the anucleolate mutant of Xenopus laevis. Proc. Natl. Acad. Sci. USA 51: 139–146.

CAPOVILLA, M., E. ELDON and V. PIROTTA, 1992   The giant gene of Drosophila encodes a b-ZIP DNA-binding protein that regulated the expression of other segmentation genes. Development 114: 99–112.

DAVIDSON, E., 1986   Gene Activity in Early Development. Academic Press, Orlando, FL.

DUFFY, J. B., and N. PERRIMON, 1994   The torso pathway in Drosophila: lessons on receptor tyrosine kinase signalling and pattern formation. Dev. Biol. 166: 380–395.

EBERL, D. F., and A. J. HILLIKER, 1988   Characterization of X-linked recessive lethal mutations affecting embryonic morphogenesis in Drosophila melanogaster. Genetics 118: 109–120.

EBERL, D. F., L. A. PERKINS, M. ENGELSTEIN, A. J. HILLIKER and N. PERRIMON, 1992   Genetic and developmental analysis of polytene section 17 of the X chromosome of Drosophila melanogaster. Genetics 130: 569–583.

EDGAR, B. A. and P. H. O'FARRELL, 1990   The three postblastoderm cell cycles of Drosophila embryogenesis are regulated in G2 by string. Cell 62: 469–480.

HARBECKE, R., and J. A. LENGYEL, 1995   Genes controlling posterior gut development in the Drosophila embryo. Wilhem Roux's Arch. Dev. Biol. 204: 308–329.

HIRSH, D., W. B. WOOD, R. HECHT, S. CARR and R. VANDERSLICE, 1978   Expression of genes essential for early development in the nematode, pp. 347–356 in Molecular Approaches to Eukaryotic Genetic Systems. ICN-UCLA Symposia on Molecular and Cellular Biology Vol. VIII, edited by J. ABELSON, G. WILCOX and C. F. FOX, Academic Press, New York.

INGHAM, P. W., A. M. TAYLOR and Y. NAKANO, 1991   Role of the Drosophila patched gene in positional signalling. Nature 353: 184–187.

JAMES, A. A., and A. VINCENT, 1986   The spatial distribution of a blastoderm stage-specific mRNA from the serendipity locus of Drosophila melanogaster. Dev. Biol. 118: 474–479.

JIMENEZ, F., and J. A. COMPOS-ORTEGA, 1982   Maternal effects of zygotic mutants affecting early neurogenesis in Drosophila. Wilhem Roux's Arch. Dev. Biol. 191: 191–201.

JOHANSEN, K. M., R. G. FEHON and S. ARTAVANIS-TSAKONAS, 1989   The Notch gene product is a glycoprotein expressed on the cell surface of both epidermal and neuronal precursor cells during Drosophila development. J. Cell Biol. 109: 2427–2440

JURGENS, G., H. KLUDING, C. NUSSLEIN-VOLHARD, and E. WIESCHAUS, 1984   Mutations affecting the pattern of the larval cuticle in Drosophila melanogaster. II. Zygotic loci on the third chromosome. Wilhem Roux's Arch. Dev. Biol. 193: 283–295.

JURGENS, G., U. MAYER, R. TORRES RUIZ, T. BERLETH and S. MISERA, 1991   Genetic analysis of pattern formation in the Arabidopsis embryo. Development Suppl. 1: 27–38.

KIMMEL, C. B., 1989   Genetics and early development of zebrafish. Trends Genet. 5: 283–288.

LEV, Z., B. Z. SHILO and Z. KIMCHIE, 1985   Developmental changes in expression of the Drosophila melanogaster epidermal growth factor receptor gene. Dev. Biol. 110: 499–502.

LEWIS, E. B., 1978   A gene complex controlling segmentation in Drosophila. Nature 276: 565–570.

MANOUKIAN, A. S., and H. M. KRAUSE, 1992   Concentration-dependent activities of the even-skipped protein in Drosophila embryos. Genes Dev. 6: 1740–1751.

MERRILL, P. T., D. SWEETON and E. WIESCHAUS, 1988   Requirements for autosomal gene activity during precellular stages of Drosophila melanogaster. Development 104: 495–509.

MULLINS, M. C., M. HAMMERSCHMIDT, P. HAFFTER and C. NUSSLEIN-VOLHARD, 1994   Large-scale mutagenesis in the zebrafish: in search of genes controlling development in a vertebrate. Curr. Biol. 4: 189–202.

NAKANO, Y., I. GUERRERO, A. HIDALGO, A. TAYLOR, J. R. S. WHITTLE et al., 1989   The Drosophila segment polarity gene patched encodes a protein with multiple potential membrane spanning domains. Nature 341: 508–513.

NOORDEMEER, J., P. F. JOHNSTON, F. RIJSEWIJK, R. NUSSE and P. LAWRENCE, 1992   The consequences of ubiquitous expression of the wingless gene in the Drosophila embryo. Development 116: 711–719.

NÜSSLEIN-VOLHARD, C., and E. WIESCHAUS, 1980   Mutations affecting segment number and polarity in *Drosophila*. Nature **287:** 795–801.

NÜSSLEIN-VOLHARD, C., E. WIESCHAUS and H. KLUDING, 1984 Mutations affecting the pattern of the larval cuticle in *Drosophila melanogaster*. I. Zygotic loci on the second chromosome. Wilhem Roux's Arch. Dev. Biol. **193:** 267–282.

PARKHURST, S. M., and D. ISH-HOROWICZ, 1991 Mis-regulating segmentation gene expression in *Drosophila*. Development **111:** 1112–1135.

PERRIMON, N., L. ENGSTROM and A. P. MAHOWALD, 1984 The effects of zygotic lethal mutations on female germline functions in *Drosophila*. Dev. Biol. **105:** 404–414.

PERRIMON, N., L. ENGSTROM, and A. P. MAHOWALD, 1989 Zygotic lethals with specific maternal effect phenotypes in *Drosophila melanogaster*. I. Loci on the *X* chromosome. Genetics **121:** 333–352.

POULSON, D. F., 1940 The effects of certain X-chromosomal deficiencies on the embryonic development of *Drosophila melanogaster*. J. Exp. Zool. **83:** 271–325.

RAUSKOLB, C., M. PEIFER and E. WIESCHAUS, 1993 *extradenticle*, a regulator of homeotic gene activity, is a homolog of the homeobox-containing human proto-oncogene *pbx1*. Cell **74:** 1101–1112.

RHYU, M., Y. N. JAN and L. JAN, 1994 Asymmetric distribution of numb protein during division of the sensory organ precursor cell confers distinct fates to daughter cells. Cell **76:** 477–491.

RIGGLEMAN, B., P. SCHEDL and E. WIESCHAUS, 1990 Spatial expression of the Drosophila segment polarity gene *armadillo* is posttranscriptionally regulated by *wingless*. Cell **63:** 549–560.

ROSE, L. S., and E. WIESCHAUS, 1992 The *Drosophila* cellularization gene *nullo* produces a blastoderm-specific transcript whose levels respond to the nucleocytoplasmic ratio. Genes Dev. **6:** 1255–1268.

ROSSANT, J., and N. HOPKINS, 1992 Of fin and fur: mutational analysis of vertebrate embryonic development. Genes Dev. **6:** 1–13.

SAMPEDRO, J., and I. GUERRERO, 1991 Unrestricted expression of the *Drosophila* gene *patched* allows a normal segment polarity. Nature **353:** 187–190.

SCHEJTER, E. D., and E. WIESCHAUS, 1993 *bottleneck* acts as a regulator of the microfilament network governing cellularization of the Drosophila embryo. Cell **75:** 373–385.

SCHÜPBACH, T., 1987 Germ line and soma cooperate during oogenesis to establish the dorsoventral pattern of egg shell and embryo in Drosophila melanogaster. Cell **49:** 699–707.

SEEGAR, M. A., G. TEAR, D. FERRES-MARCO and C. S. GOODMAN, 1993 Mutations affecting growth cone guidance in Drosophila: genes necessary for guidance toward or away from the midline. Neuron **10:** 409–426.

SOLNICA-KREZEL, L., A. F. SCHIER and W. DRIEVER, 1994 Efficient recovery of ENU-induced mutations from the zebrafish germline. Genetics **136:** 1401–1420.

ST JOHNSTON, D., and C. NÜSSLEIN-VOLHARD, 1992 The origin of pattern and polarity in the Drosophila embryo. Cell **68:** 201–219.

STRUHL, G., 1985 Near-reciprocal phenotypes caused by inactivation or indiscriminate expression of the *Drosophila* segmentation gene *ftz*. Nature **318:** 667–680.

TSAI, C., and J. P. GERGEN, 1994 Gap gene properties of the pairrule gene *runt* during *Drosophila* segmentation. Development **120:** 1671–1683.

VAN VACTOR, D., H. SINK, D. FAMBROUGH, R. TSOO and C. S. GOODMAN, 1993 Genes that control neuromuscular specificity in Drosophila. Cell **73:** 1137–1153.

WIESCHAUS, E., and E. NOELL, 1986 Specificity of embryonic lethal mutations in *Drosophila* analyzed in germ line clones. Wilhem Roux's Arch. Dev. Biol. **195:** 63–73.

WIESCHAUS, E., and D. SWEETON, 1988 Requirements for X-linked zygotic gene activity during cellularization of early *Drosophila* embryos. Development **104:** 483–493.

WIESCHAUS, E., C. N;AUUSSLEIN-VOLHARD, and G. JURGENS, 1984 Mutations affecting the pattern of the larval cuticle in *Drosophila melanogaster*. III. Zygotic loci on the X-chromosome and the fourth chromosome. Wilhem Roux's Arch. Dev. Biol. **193:** 296–307.

YOUNG, P. E., A. M. RICHMAN, A. S. KETCHUM and D. P. KIEHART, 1993 Morphogenesis in *Drosophila* requires nonmuscle myosin heavy chain function. Genes Dev. **7:** 29–41.

ZAK, N. B., R. J. WIDES, E. D. SCHEJTER, E. RAZ and B. Z. SHILO, 1990 Localization of the DER/*flb* protein in embryos: implications on the *faint little ball* lethal phenotype. Development **109:** 865–874.

ZUSMAN, S., and E. WIESCHAUS, 1985 Requirements for zygotic gene activity during gastrulation in *Drosophila melanogaster*. Dev. Biol. **111:** 359–371.

February 1996

The "Genesis of the White-Eyed Mutant" in *Drosophila melanogaster*
A Reappraisal

M. M. Green

Section of Molecular and Cellular Biology, University of California, Davis, California 95616

THE science of genetics is, in all probability, unique among the biological sciences in that it is possible to pinpoint precisely the date of its inception. The rediscovery of MENDEL's laws in 1900 independently by DE VRIES, CORRENS, and VON TSCHERMAK marks the start. During the subsequent decade, the universality of MENDEL's laws among plants and animals was demonstrated, the Danish geneticist JOHANNSEN gave the name *gene* to MENDEL's factors, and the British geneticist BATESON coined the term *genetics*. However, while the arithmetic of Mendelian genetics was quickly established, the cellular mechanism was unclear. Without experimental evidence, SUTTON and MONTGOMERY each independently speculated on the correlation between meiotic chromosome disjunction and gene segregation. *Sensu stricto,* modern genetics began in 1910 with the discovery of the white-eyed mutant in *Drosophila melanogaster* by T. H. MORGAN and his demonstration of the correlation between the inheritance of this mutation and the transmission of the *X* chromosome. Experimental proof for the linkage between gene and chromosome came with the publication in 1916 (in Volume 1, page 1 of GENETICS) of BRIDGES' monumental doctoral dissertation on nondisjunction of the *D. melanogaster X* chromosome.

The recent publication of a detailed, instructive, and valuable history of the roots and proliferation of Drosophila genetics by ROBERT E. KOHLER, intriguingly titled *Lords of the Fly*, has reopened two issues of historical interest. When exactly was the *white* mutation in *D. melanogaster* discovered, and did MORGAN really find this mutation?

When considering the first question, it is important to note that the first sentence in MORGAN's seminal publication describing the inheritance of *white*, published July 22, 1910 in *Science*, reads as follows: "In a pedigree culture of Drosophila which had been running for nearly a year through a considerable number of generations, a male appeared with white eyes." No date of discovery is given, nor is the finder specifically named, although presumably this must have been MOR-

GAN because he is the sole author of the brief paper, only a bit more than three pages long. It should be noted that the paper is dated July 7, 1910. In his discussion of MORGAN's first mutation experiment with *D. melanogaster*, KOHLER emphasizes the discovery of a putatively first mutation called *with* ("with trident") in which a pigmented triangular area appears on the thorax just anterior to the adult fly's scutellum. The following quotation (pp. 41–42) is relevant: "Ross Harrison recalled visiting Morgan's lab in the first days of January, 1910. 'There's two years work wasted,' he (Morgan) exclaimed, having his hand on rows of bottles on shelves. 'I've been breeding these flies for all that time and have gotten nothing out of it.' But, just a few days later, Morgan observed a few flies with a darker pattern than any he had seen before. Inbreeding quickly produced a mutant strain, *with*, which had a distribution of pigment that was distinctly darker than wild type which further selection did not alter . . . Visiting his wife and newborn daughter in the hospital in the second week of January, Morgan could talk of nothing but his new mutant." Was MORGAN really talking about *with* or was he talking about *white*? Three pages later in his narrative, KOHLER writes, "When Lillian (*sic*) Morgan recalled her husband's visit to the hospital in January, 1910, she remembered him talking about the *white* mutant. It must have been *with*, since *white* turned up in May!" While it is not always necessary for historians of science to understand the intricacies of the sciences about which they write, there are instances when some comprehension is useful in interpreting or explaining relevant historical events. Had KOHLER appreciated fully the vagaries of the *with* phenotype, he probably would not have dismissed Mrs. MORGAN's recollection out of hand. Accordingly, several compelling reasons militate against the May, 1910 date and support a date in January, 1910.

In describing the *with* mutation, KOHLER wrote, "It was just what Morgan expected the process of speciation would look like!" By and large, almost every neophyte Drosophila geneticist used to make an attempt at delineating the genetics of *with* but gave it up as a hopeless task. The reason is simple: the *with* phenotype is variable, overlaps wild type, and is precisely the kind of mutant phenotype not readily amenable to Mendelian analysis. In fact, in the first compilation of the mutants of *D. melanogaster* by MORGAN, BRIDGES, and STURTEVANT (1925), the linkage, map position, and phenotype of *with* are described as follows: "With III 48±. M. (B and M '23). Semi-dominant dark trident pattern on thorax. Discarded." (Note: M = MORGAN; B and M = BRIDGES and MORGAN.) It hardly seems possible that MORGAN would discard a mutant with the qualities KOHLER describes. More importantly, those who knew LILIAN MORGAN knew that she was a superb Drosophila geneticist in her own right, the discoverer of the famous attached-X female, and certainly one who would not confuse *with* and *white*. In this connection, it is interesting to relate here the following anecdotal story concerning the white eye mutant, extant in the MORGAN family and disclosed during a visit my colleague C. M. RICK and I recently made to the home of Mrs. LILIAN M. SCHERP, the MORGAN daughter whose birth was noted above as January, 1910. In the course of our lively conversation, Mrs. SCHERP was asked whether she knew anything about the Drosophila white eye mutation. She related the following story, paraphrased here. At the time of her birth, obstetricians commonly mildly anesthetized women in labor in order to ease the pain of delivery. When Mrs. MORGAN recovered from the ether, her first words were, "Oh, I do hope the white-eyed fly is still alive." This story was confirmed by her older sister, Mrs. EDITH WHITAKER, also participating in the conversation. Taking this story together with the quotation from KOHLER, apropos Mrs. MORGAN and the white mutant (see above), *white*, not *with*, was the crucial mutation of January, 1910.

What is the source of the date "May, 1910" noted by KOHLER? In the first catalog of *D. melanogaster* mutations (MORGAN *et al.* 1925), the origin of *white* is given only as 1910. In their 1916 compendium of sex-linked inheritance in *D. melanogaster*, MORGAN and BRIDGES date the finding of *white* as May, 1910. (It should be noted here that this monograph includes a table of sex-linked mutants found up to that time in the MORGAN laboratory. Here, it is explicitly stated that the white-eyed mutant was found by MORGAN.) Subsequently, BRIDGES and MORGAN (1923), in describing the third-chromosome eye-color mutation *pink*, wrote,."The first eye-color, and the character *first* clearly recognized as a sharp mutation was 'white', found in *April* 1910, by Morgan" (emphasis mine). Note the date and note, too, the statement that *white*, not *with*, was the first sharp mutation! There is yet another good reason to believe that neither May nor April is correct and that the actual date is January. The data contained in the 1910 paper involve four generations of flies. Under optimal culture conditions, the generation time for *D. melanogaster* is two weeks. As de-

scribed by KOHLER, conditions in the MORGAN lab in 1910 were hardly optimal. Thus, for MORGAN to find the mutant in May, complete and score the crosses, prepare the manuscript, and move the family and menagerie from New York City to Woods Hole between, at the earliest, May 1 and July 7, is highly unlikely. An April date is possible but, for the same reasons, improbable. However, the discovery of *white* in January satisfies all necessary conditions. Can the April and/or May dates be rationalized with January? It is only possible to speculate, but one possibility is that the date of origin as April or May was given for the time the genetic analysis was completed, not the specific day the mutant male was found.

Did MORGAN find the first *white* mutant? Although not stated in his 1910 paper, the discovery of the *white* mutant was attributed to MORGAN and first explicitly so stated by MORGAN on page 63 of his 1913 book, *Heredity and Sex*, as follows: "In my culture, a male appeared that had white eyes." (No date of origin is given.) The attribution was brought into question with the publication in 1941 of a book by F. E. LUTZ entitled *A Lot of Insects: Entomology in a Suburban Garden*. In this book, LUTZ describes the insects collected in the garden surrounding his residence and includes the following statement, which occurs on page 238 and is quoted verbatim: "Meanwhile, something far more worthwhile happened, more worthwhile even if my results are not to be explained by wild flies 'contaminating' my 'pure line' of pedigreed Drosophila. Professor T. H. Morgan visited the station and I told him that a white-eyed Drosophila had appeared in one of the pedigreed strains, but that I was too busy with abnormal veins to attend to it. *He took live descendants of this white-eyed 'sport' and bred them. Eventually, he got the white eye back*" (emphasis mine). Thus, LUTZ asserts that it was he who found the white mutant, and MORGAN isolated white-eyed flies from among the progeny of the wild flies given to him. The situation is confounded further by a review of the LUTZ book by RAMSEY SPILLMAN, which appeared in the *Journal of Heredity* (1942). In his review, SPILLMAN wrote as follows, again verbatim: "It is surely of scientific historic interest that, while studying Drosophila for variations in the wing veins, Dr. Lutz found a white-eyed mutant, but having his hands full with the wing-vein problem, gave over five descendants of the white-eyed sport to Professor T. H. Morgan." In a brief note in the *Journal of Heredity* entitled "Genesis of the White-Eyed Mutant," MORGAN (1942) rebuts SPILLMAN by noting first that SPILLMAN's statement is not quite what LUTZ wrote. He notes further, "It is not obvious from this statement that the flies Lutz gave me were the descendants of the 'white-eye sport' since it was dead when found, unless the bottle had contained a virgin female and the white-eyed male. Moreover, if it had mated before death to a female, many white-eyed males would have appeared in the next generation which was not the case." On equivalent genetic grounds, MORGAN points to the inconsistency in SPILLMAN's statement. Finally, as MORGAN emphasizes, the *white* mutation occurs frequently, and the white-eyed male he found is independent of LUTZ's dead male. In this connection, it is important to note that MORGAN was quite correct in the matter of *white* mutations. Between March, 1915 and April, 1942, the independent occurrence of 27 white-eyed mutants is recorded in the second published catalog of *D. melanogaster* mutants (BRIDGES and BREHME 1944). This number is in all likelihood an underestimate because not all such mutants are reported. Thus, conceivably LUTZ did find a white-eyed mutant which, however, left no progeny. Without progeny, there is no genetics! Whether LUTZ's observation alerted MORGAN to be on the lookout for the white-eye mutation is a question that cannot be answered.

Finally, it should be noted that *white* was not the first sex-linked mutation discovered. In the currant moth Abraxus, DONCASTER and RAYNOR (1906) described a trait called *lacticolor* segregating among wild females but not among males. The sex-linked, recessive inheritance of *lacticolor* was not understood until it was recognized that, in Abraxus and other Lepidoptera, the female is the heterogametic sex, not the male (BRIDGES 1916).

To sum up: the beginning of modern genetics can best be dated to January, 1910 with the discovery by T. H. MORGAN of a white-eyed *D. melanogaster* male.

For the science of genetics, the portent of the white mutation was enormous. Quickly, additional sex-linked mutants were discovered by MORGAN and his students. By 1913 STURTEVANT, with unsurpassed intuition, constructed the first linear genetic map of the X chromosome, followed by BRIDGES' (1916) cytogenetic proof of the chromosome theory, already cited. Crucial for the demonstration of *D. melanogaster* as the genetic organism par excellence was MULLER's (1918) establishment of the principle of balanced lethals, the implementation of which made routine the recovery, maintenance, and analysis of all classes of mutations, genic and chromosomal. By 1925 the vast amount of information accumulated by MORGAN and his students in less than 15 years was summarized in the monograph *The Genetics of Drosophila*. Documented therein are those fundamental principles of genetics derived from the study of Drosophila, principles that have withstood the test of time and that are included in all contemporary textbooks of genetics.

Readers of this series may note the irony that has been identified by LEWIS (1995): A. H. STURTEVANT and G. W. BEADLE found that they could not agree whether the *white* gene was the specific *white* mutant (STURTEVANT) or the entire set of alleles including wild-type (BEADLE).

I am indebted to my colleagues C. H. LANGLEY, J. H. GILLESPIE, M. TURELLI and J. J. SEKELSKY for critical comments on the manuscript. They bear no responsibility for the opinions and conclusions rendered therein.

LITERATURE CITED

BRIDGES, C. B., 1916 Nondisjunction as proof of the chromosome theory of heredity. Genetics **1**: 1–52, 107–163.

BRIDGES, C. B., and K. S. BREHME, 1944 The mutants of *Drosophila melanogaster*. Carnegie Inst. Washington, Publ. 552, p. 253.

BRIDGES, C. B., and T. H. MORGAN, 1923 The third-chromosome group of mutant characters in *Drosophila melanogaster*. Carnegie Inst. Washington, Publ. 327, p. 251.

DONCASTER, L., and G. H. RAYNOR, 1906 Breeding experiments with Lepidoptera. Proc. Zool. Soc. Lond. Part 1: 125–133.

KOHLER, R. E., 1994 *Lords of the Fly*, p. 321. University of Chicago Press, Chicago.

LEWIS, E. B., 1995 Remembering STURTEVANT. Genetics **141**: 1227–1230.

LUTZ, F. E., 1941 *A Lot of Insects: Entomology in a Suburban Garden*, p. 304. G. P. Putnam and Sons, New York.

MORGAN, T. H., 1910 Sex-limited inheritance in Drosophila. Science **32**: 120–122.

MORGAN, T. H., 1913 *Heredity and Sex*, p. 282. Columbia University Press, New York.

MORGAN, T. H., 1942 Genesis of the white-eyed mutant. J. Hered. **31**: 91–92.

MORGAN, T. H., C. B. BRIDGES and A. H. STURTEVANT, 1925 The genetics of Drosophila. Bibliogr. Genet. **2**: 1–262.

MULLER, H. J., 1918 Genetics variability, twin hybrids and constant hybrids in a case of balanced lethal factors. Genetics **3**: 422–499.

SPILLMAN, R., 1942 Are insects people? J. Hered. **31**: 23–24.

STURTEVANT, A. H., 1913 The linear arrangement of six sex-linked factors in Drosophila as shown by their mode of association. J. Exp. Zool. **14**: 43–59.

Lancelot Hogben, 1895–1975

Sahotra Sarkar

Dibner Institute, Massachusetts Institute of Technology, Cambridge, Massachusetts 02139
and Department of Philosophy, McGill University, Montréal, P. Q. H3A 2T7, Canada

LANCELOT HOGBEN, whose birth centennial was last December, was one of the most versatile biologists of his generation. In genetics he made methodological contributions to human and medical genetics and provided an analysis of the nature-nurture dispute that was influential in its time. In zoology he was a pioneer of comparative (and evolutionary) physiology. He helped found the Society for Experimental Zoology. He invented what was, for 15 years, the standard pregnancy test. He made significant contributions to medical statistics in the United Kingdom and drew on that experience to write an incisive philosophical work on the foundations of statistics. He wrote four books on linguistics.

Although overshadowed by J. B. S. HALDANE, HOGBEN was like him in being one of the most successful popularizers of science of his generation. One of his books, *Mathematics for the Million* (HOGBEN 1936), went through four editions and sold more than half a million copies during his lifetime. It was translated into fifteen languages and remains in print. In his early years, he was a self-proclaimed socialist; in later years he called himself a scientific humanist. During World War I he was briefly imprisoned as a conscientious objector. Under the influence of his first wife, the mathematician ENID CHARLES, he was an active feminist. In the 1920s, unlike some geneticists, he did not succumb to racial prejudice. During a stay in South Africa (1927–30), he actively fought racial prejudice and discrimination to such an extent that he felt compelled to leave.

Childhood and education: LANCELOT THOMAS HOGBEN was born in the Portsmouth suburb of Swansea on 9 December 1895, two months prematurely. His father, THOMAS HOGBEN, was a fundamentalist (Plymouth Brethren) evangelist. His mother, MARGARET ALICE HOGBEN (*neé* PRESCOTT), was similarly religious—HOGBEN's "miraculous" premature birth prompted her to vow that he would be a medical missionary. In an intel-

lectually austere family environment, made more austere by poverty, HOGBEN was brought up with that end in mind. He was encouraged to read secular textbooks of botany and zoology. These helped him develop a scientific interest in biology independent of the missionary hopes of his parents.

In 1905 the HOGBENs moved to London. HOGBEN attended Tottenham County School, where he pursued biology systematically and demonstrated exceptional academic abilities. He struck up many friendships with working-class boys of the neighborhood. This began a lifelong left-wing political orientation. At 16 he passed the University of London's External Intermediate Examinations. At 17 he became the first student from a London County Council secondary school to win a scholarship to Cambridge (Trinity College). In later life, when eugenists such as L. DARWIN attacked these scholarship schemes for allegedly being dysgenic and a waste of public resources (because students from poor families were genetically inferior), HOGBEN would remember his origins and rise to their defense.

By the time HOGBEN arrived at Cambridge in 1913, he had already graduated from the University of London. He found Cambridge intellectually stimulating and learned much from the physiologists W. M. FLETCHER, A. V. HILL, and K. LUCAS. He was influenced by BERTRAND RUSSELL, who was lecturing at Cambridge, especially on the philosophy of science. An additional influence were the writings of A. R. WALLACE, co-discoverer of natural selection and also an avowed socialist. HOGBEN's first significant publication, in 1918, was a journalistic account of WALLACE's life and work. During his Cambridge period HOGBEN became convinced that he would pursue a career in science instead of medicine. Socially, HOGBEN found Cambridge decrepit. Though he was an active member of the (left-leaning) student Fabian Society, which he moved further to the left, HOGBEN otherwise found it difficult to associate with the generally upper-class Cambridge students or to appreciate their predominantly extracurricular interests.

In 1914 HOGBEN found himself opposed to World

Corresponding author: Department of Philosophy, McGill University, 855 Sherbrooke St. W., Montreal, P.Q. H3A 2T7, Canada.
E-mail: sahotra@philo.mcgill.ca

War I. By this point he had fulfilled his academic requirements for a degree. He was left with only his residency requirements, which could be satisfied through war service. HOGBEN volunteered for noncombatant roles in two Quaker organizations. However, when conscription was introduced in 1916, he chose not to use this work to exempt himself from military service. Rather, encouraged by RUSSELL's public pronouncements on the issue, he returned to Cambridge and refused to serve on conscientious grounds. During his subsequent interrogation, he refused to be medically examined or to appeal to religious convictions. He was imprisoned but discharged on medical grounds before the completion of his initial three-month sentence. His convictions remained unchanged. When RUSSELL was himself imprisoned, HOGBEN wrote to him, "I am writing . . . to tell you how splendid I think your stand has been. Being an ex-convict I understand a little at what cost you have been true. It is inspiring to us who are younger men and who see so many of our friends succumbing to cynical indifference or academic preoccupation to know that there is at least one of the Intellectuals of Europe who have not allowed the life of the mind to kill the life of the spirit" (RUSSELL 1968, p. 83).

Early professional career: After his release, HOGBEN barely supported himself in London through journalism. In 1917 he was appointed a lecturer in zoology at Birbeck College. During this period he met ENID CHARLES, an organizer for the women's wing of the Trade Union Movement. CHARLES had a degree in mathematics, economics, and social sciences from Liverpool and was a committed feminist and socialist. They began living together almost immediately and were married shortly before the birth of their first child. HOGBEN moved to Imperial College in 1918 and wrote his only paper on paleontology (HOGBEN 1919). He attended the mathematical lectures of H. LEVY and developed his mathematical competency. In 1920 and 1921 he published six papers on experimental cytology, which earned him a D.Sc. from the University of London. His most important result was that cockroach chromosomes exhibited parasynapsis, rather than telosynapsis as was then generally believed (HOGBEN 1920a,b). This observation provided support for the MORGAN school's model of linkage and crossing over (WELLS 1978).

This cytological work led F. A. E. CREW to offer HOGBEN a position at the new Animal Breeding Research Laboratory in Edinburgh. However, HOGBEN's research had shifted to comparative endocrinology, which is what he pursued at Edinburgh. He studied the role of internal secretions in amphibian metamorphoses and color changes. HOGBEN (1923) was the first to describe hypophysectomy by the ventral approach (WARING 1963). His primary interest remained evolutionary and comparative. *The Pigmentary Effector System* (HOGBEN 1924) reviewed what was known about color changes

in all groups of animals. HOGBEN and WINTON (1924) and HOGBEN (1926, 1927a) published systematic reports of these comparative studies. During this period, HOGBEN, HALDANE, JULIAN HUXLEY, and CREW founded the *Journal of Experimental Biology* and the Society for Experimental Biology to back the new journal (WELLS 1976). Financial support for the journal came partly from H. G. WELLS.

In 1925, HOGBEN left Edinburgh for Montréal to become Assistant Professor of Medical Zoology at McGill University. The post was short-lived. He left for South Africa in 1927 to his first appointment to a Chair (in zoology) at the University of Cape Town. HOGBEN's major innovations were to introduce experimental work in the department and to replace samples from the United Kingdom with local fauna. Outside the university he lectured to school teachers who were being trained in biology. Out of these lectures emerged *Mathematics for the Million* (HOGBEN 1936), his most popular book. In his research he concentrated mainly on Xenopus, particularly *Xenopus laevis* (the clawed toad). HOGBEN noted that female *X. laevis* laid eggs after being injected with anterior pituitary extract. CHARLES collaborated in this work (HOGBEN *et al.* 1931). At that time the active hormone in this extract was believed to be identical to the gonadotrophic substance in the urine of pregnant women (WELLS 1978). After protocols for maintaining reproductively healthy *X. laevis* stocks in the laboratory were worked out, in HOGBEN's laboratory and elsewhere (see LANDGREBE 1939), this observation led to what CREW (1939) named the "HOGBEN pregnancy test."

Except for the Montréal interlude, HOGBEN remained politically active throughout this period. In London he tried left-wing labor organizing. In Edinburgh he hosted meetings of the students' Socialist Society. In Cape Town he was confronted by the racism that eventually led to apartheid. Many years later, in *Dangerous Thoughts*, HOGBEN (1939b) recorded that there was a universal consensus among South African whites, even in relatively liberal Cape Town, about the racial inferiority of Africans, Coloureds, and Indians. "Chromatocracy" was his description of South Africa. In his classes, and in his social life, he challenged the chromatocracy. In *Principles of Evolutionary Biology* (HOGBEN 1927b), based on his classroom lectures, he extensively quoted MORGAN (1925) and BATESON (1913) on the fallacy of assuming the genetic superiority of one race over another. He dismissed eugenics, claiming that it had "no enthusiastic supporters among the leading investigators in genetics" (HOGBEN 1927b, p. 100). He admitted colored students in his classes and welcomed them to his home. South African whites did not appreciate this racial apostasy. By 1929 HOGBEN felt uncomfortable in South Africa. It was lucky for him that, right at this juncture, the London School of Economics (LSE) created a new Chair of Social Biology. HOGBEN was appointed to it in 1930.

By this time, HOGBEN's basic philosophical views were set. As a physiologist in the 1920s, just like J. B. S. HALDANE (see SARKAR 1992a), HOGBEN was accosted by a dominant holist epistemology, barely different from "vitalism" and propounded most forcefully by HALDANE's father, the physiologist J. S. HALDANE. HOGBEN (1930) provided a vigorous defense of mechanistic explanation. However, he separated the private from the public sphere—scientific questions, as well as issues of metaphysics and epistemology, occurred only in the latter. Religious and political beliefs, ethical commitments, and aesthetic preferences, all belonged to the former. The main function of this distinction was that it permitted HOGBEN to declare the ethical neutrality of science. HOGBEN rejected eugenics because it violated this distinction; moreover, in the private sphere of politics and ethics, it was offensive to his egalitarian principles. However, this left open the pursuit of a value-neutral human genetics that could potentially be put to medical and social use. This is the task that he set for himself in his new position at the LSE.

Human genetics: R. A. FISHER was among those over whom HOGBEN was preferred for the Chair at LSE (see BENNETT 1983, pp. 112–113). Ironically, when HOGBEN turned to human genetics as a way of fulfilling the mandate of his new position, it was FISHER's seminal work that provided the point of departure. *Genetic Principles in Medicine and Social Sciences* (HOGBEN 1931b) summarized his agenda. It was a critical look at the practice of human genetics up to that point. The first chapter gave a careful analysis of twin studies, how they can reveal genetic origins of phenotypic differences, and how they are prone to misinterpretation by both sides in the nature-nurture dispute. The second chapter attempted a rigorous treatment of segregation analysis. The sixth chapter contained the first systematic account of HALDANE's work on selection in the 1920s, which FISHER (1930) had completely ignored (SARKAR 1992b). However, the third chapter was the most important. It drew attention, for the first time to an English-speaking audience, to the important work done by BERNSTEIN (1931) on the detection of linkage (MAZUMDAR 1992). Let *Aa Bb, aa bb, etc.,* represent the frequencies of the genotypes in a two-locus/two-allele model (*A* and *a* are the alleles at the first locus, *B* and *b* at the second). Bernstein had invented the statistic $y = (Aa\ Bb + aa\ bb)(Aa\ bb + aa\ Bb)$, which does not depend on the linkage phase (*cis* or *trans*), but increases monotonically with the recombination fraction, in order to detect linkage from the mating *Aa Bb* × *aa bb* (see CROW 1993). The invention of this statistic was a crucial step in human linkage studies—HOGBEN had immediately recognized its importance.

The last two chapters, as HOGBEN clearly indicated, were political rather than scientific. HOGBEN's implicit

target was the controversial last chapters of FISHER's (1930) *Genetical Theory of Natural Selection*. The same topics were treated but, whereas FISHER emphasized heredity and pushed for eugenics, HOGBEN attempted to dissect hereditarian claims. He opted for social renewal and continued his campaign against eugenics. The suggestion of LEONARD DARWIN (1926), CHARLES DARWIN's son, that scholarships to poor children be discontinued because they were obviously dysgenic met with particular scorn—HOGBEN was clearly recalling his own origins. The book was well received and, during the 1930s, was probably HOGBEN's most influential work (MAZUMDAR 1992). In *Eugenics Review,* HUXLEY (1932), though extremely critical of HOGBEN's anti-eugenic ideas, nevertheless commended the book as "an important contribution to human biology, and one which it will be extremely salutary for eugenists to read." In *Nature,* HALDANE (1932) opined that "Hogben's book is at least the herald of a more scientific epoch" of human genetics. Needless to say, DARWIN was less pleased. "I ... should enjoy giving him one in the eye!!" he confided to FISHER in a letter (29 March 1932; see BENNETT 1983, p. 153).

Much of HOGBEN's work on mathematical human genetics consisted of extensions of methods discussed in *Genetic Principles.* HOGBEN (1931a, 1932a–c) developed more rigorous methods for segregation analysis. HOGBEN *et al.* (1932) used these methods to establish, rigorously, the dependence of alkaptonuria on a single recessive gene, which GARROD (1902) had suggested immediately after the rediscovery of MENDEL's laws. HOGBEN (1932d,e) worked out the correlation of relatives for sex-linked inheritance, extending FISHER's (1918) classic treatment. CHARLES (1933) extended these results. HOGBEN (1934a,b) turned to the detection of linkage. He corrected and extended BERNSTEIN's (1931) analysis. HALDANE (1934) provided other extensions. In 1935, FISHER (1935) showed that maximum likelihood methods were more efficient than the *y* statistic. However, computing FISHER's *u*-scores was very laborious, as HALDANE and SMITH (1947) pointed out—instead, they applied LODs to linkage analysis (see MORTON 1995). Between maximum likelihood and LOD methods, BERNSTEIN's and HOGBEN's attempts are now only of historical interest.

HOGBEN's attempt to clarify and analyze the nature-nurture dispute, also initiated during this period, has been of more lasting interest. His basic argument was for the "relativity" (HOGBEN 1933a) or "interdependence" (HOGBEN 1933b) of nature and nurture. He emphasized the interaction of nature and nurture. While the calculation of correlation coefficients could be used to show the genetic or the environmental origin of differences in traits such as IQ (HERRMAN and HOGBEN 1933; HOGBEN 1939a), it could not be used to ascribe definite values to the relative importance of these factors. Such techniques (and all others that could be

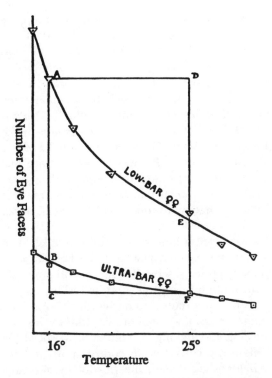

16°   25°
Temperature

FIGURE 1.—Modified from HOGBEN (1933a, p. 384). The graphs, as indicated, are for the *low-Bar* and *ultra-Bar* genotypes. Ordinate, number of eye facets; abscissa, temperature during development. The data are from KRAFKA (1920). For a full discussion, see the text.

derived from the analysis of variance) were only quantitatively meaningful when relativized to a specified environment. Using KRAFKA's (1920) data on development in Drosophila, HOGBEN (1933a) drew a figure (see Figure 1) to show the interaction of nature and nurture. Two mutants, *low-Bar* and *ultra-Bar*, both have many fewer facets in the compound eye than the nonmutant. The graph shows the number of facets as a function of the temperature at which the strains were cultured. Assuming the same frequency (0.5) for both mutants, HOGBEN calculated the (total) phenotypic means and variances for facet numbers to be (120.5, 4692.5) at 15° and (49.5, 600.25) at 25°. Neither estimate is preferred, he argued, and this shows that it is unjustified to try to use these parameters to assign a quantitative value to genetic or environmental influences in general, independent of a specified environment. HOGBEN emphasized that situations similar to that depicted in Figure 1 were routine rather than exceptional.

This argument was repeated in *Nature and Nurture* (HOGBEN 1933b). Throughout his career, HOGBEN continued to devise better didactic methods for a recognition of nature-nurture interactions (see, *e.g.,* HOGBEN 1951). Though it eventually became standard, in the 1930s HOGBEN's argument was greeted by silence. HALDANE (1936, 1946) devised an alternative argument to demonstrate nature-nurture interaction. Even FISHER was circumspect. "I think I see your point now. You are

on the question of non-linear interaction of environment and heredity," he wrote to HOGBEN (25 February 1933; see BENNETT 1983, p. 218). "[t]he main point is that you are under no obligation to analyze variance into parts if it does not come apart easily, and its unwillingness to do so naturally indicates that one's line of approach is not very fruitful."

However, to J. A. F. ROBERTS, FISHER wrote more confidently, "There is one point in which Hogben and his associates are riding for a fall, and that is in making a great song about the possible, but unproved, importance of non-linear interactions between hereditary and environmental factors. J. B. S. Haldane seems tempted to join in this" (18 January 1935; see BENNETT 1983, p. 260). Over 60 years later, for human traits, the dispute remains unresolved. (Graphs showing nonlinear interactions are routinely found for many traits in animal populations. However, because of the obvious experimental difficulties, any such graphs are not only not available for human populations, but nature-nurture interactions have proven difficult to detect.)

Medical statistics: In 1936 HOGBEN was finally elected to the Royal Society. In 1937 he left LSE to become Regius Professor of Natural History at the University of Aberdeen. Though he continued some of his work in endocrinology, from this point on any active interest in genetical research seems to have waned. It was replaced by a newfound interest in linguistics, which continued for the rest of his life. In March, 1940 HOGBEN went to Norway to lecture on Nazi theories of racial superiority. While he was there, Germany invaded Norway. HOGBEN and his daughter escaped to Sweden, but were unable to return to the United Kingdom by any direct route. They flew to Moscow, crossed the Soviet Union on the Trans-Siberian Railway, and traveled by ship to Japan and finally to San Francisco. The trip reinforced HOGBEN's dislike for the Soviet Union, but, strangely, largely on aesthetic grounds (HOGBEN 1940).

HOGBEN's family assembled in America. CHARLES was already working in Ottawa; their eldest son, ADRIAN, was a student at the University of Wisconsin. HOGBEN accepted a one-semester Visiting Professorship there and lectured on mathematical genetics. These lectures were eventually published as *An Introduction to Mathematical Genetics* (HOGBEN 1946). It included what was then the most detailed discussion of the problem of relating theoretical results (such as the Hardy-Weinberg ratios) with population data. Those in his class were impressed by his convivial manner, his personal interest in his students, and his ability to present mathematical arguments in a clear and easily comprehensible way. The Wisconsin appointment provided HOGBEN with sufficient funds to return to the United Kingdom; CHARLES remained in Canada. Back at Aberdeen, he was irritated by suggestions that he had not returned there as soon as possible. In any case, his laboratory staff had been dispersed by World War II, and HOGBEN left in 1942 to become Professor of Zoology at the University of Birmingham.

At Birmingham, HOGBEN studied comparative temperature regulation in mollusks, earthworms, amphibians, and reptiles (HOGBEN and KIRK 1944; KIRK and HOGBEN 1946), as well as sensory responses in Drosophila (BEGG and HOGBEN 1946). He also continued writing political tracts. However, his health deteriorated owing to thyroid problems, and he underwent thyroidectomy in 1943. After a partial recovery, he began war work under CREW (while refusing to wear a uniform). Most of his work was statistical and consisted of a revision of army medical documentation followed by therapeutic trials. An important result was a demonstration that indiscriminate prophylactic use of antibiotics leads to the selection of resistant strains of disease-causing microorganisms (WELLS 1978). To publicize the work that emerged from these statistical studies, the *British Journal of Social Medicine* was founded by the British Medical Association, with HOGBEN as its first Editor.

After the war, HOGBEN continued work in medical statistics, though with less success. Perhaps the most important offshoot of this work was his searching examination of the foundations of statistical theory (and practice), which remains relevant today. HOGBEN (1957) was skeptical of the mathematical basis for the methods for inference introduced by FISHER, while also doubting the NEYMAN-PEARSON methods and WALD's decision theory (WELLS 1978). However, he had no alternative framework to present. Meanwhile, his marriage had ended. In 1947 CHARLES had returned from Canada, but she and HOGBEN never readjusted to living together after their six-year separation. In 1953 CHARLES left for East Asia. They were divorced in 1957 so that HOGBEN could marry SARAH EVANS, a Welsh school teacher and local political activist. After their marriage, they settled in Wales, where HOGBEN had bought a riverside cottage. Throughout this phase of his career, HOGBEN's most significant interest was in linguistics. *The Loom of Language* (BODMER 1944), which HOGBEN supervised, dealt with the evolution of language and proposed the creation of an auxiliary language for international communication. It sold over 130,000 copies (WELLS 1978).

Retirement: HOGBEN retired from the University of Birmingham in 1961. In 1963 the premier of British Guyana, C. JAGAN, invited him to become the Vice-Chancellor of a new University of Guyana. HOGBEN visited Georgetown for a month in 1963 and accepted the position. He reorganized the plans for the University to make it more directly responsive to local economic needs and interests (rather than being a liberal arts college affiliated with the University of the West Indies). He spent much of 1963 raising funds for the new university. For the 1963–64 academic year, HOGBEN served as Vice-Chancellor. However, an extended strike and political instability made his short tenure uncomfortable. After ensuring that sufficient financial support was assured to the University, he resigned in 1964.

Returning to Wales, HOGBEN continued his work on linguistic subjects. HOGBEN's *The Vocabulary of Science* (1969) is an analysis of scientific vocabulary in all European languages. He continued his popular scientific writing and prepared the fourth edition of *Mathematics for the Million* (1967). He also wrote some intriguing philosophical pieces. However, the last decade of his life (from 1965 to 1975) was unhappy. Both his and EVANS' health deteriorated progressively. EVANS died in 1974, after the ultimate failure of an earlier mastectomy to remove a malignant tumor. HOGBEN died on 22 August 1975.

HOGBEN lived a long and varied life. Like his more famous contemporary, HALDANE, he became involved in so many projects, scientific, social, and political, that his contribution to any one was diminished. As a result, there is no important finding by which we remember his name. Instead, we memorialize him for his breadth of interest, his lifelong commitment to social justice, and his not inconsiderable contributions to such diverse fields as social medicine, physiology, and genetics. He should also be remembered as a superb popularizer of science, one who could make scientific matters alive for any audience he chose. Mindful of his great emphasis on interactions, we can note that the totality of his contributions is not properly measured by summing the component parts.

No detailed scientific biography of LANCELOT HOGBEN exists. Biographical details for this piece were mostly gleaned from WELLS (1978), who provides personal information and a very useful chronology. WERSKEY (1978) provides an interpretation of HOGBEN's political development (along with those of J. D. BERNAL, J. B. S. HALDANE, H. LEVY, and J. NEEDHAM). The historical research on which this piece is based was partly funded by the National Institutes of Health (grant HG-00912).

LITERATURE CITED

BATESON, W., 1913 *Mendel's Principles of Heredity.* Cambridge University Press, Cambridge.

BEGG, M., and HOGBEN, L., 1946 Chemoreceptivity of Drosophila melanogaster. Proc. R. Soc. Lond. B Biol. Sci. **133:** 1–19.

BENNETT, J. H. (Editors), 1983 *Natural Selection, Heredity, and Eugenics: Including Selected Correspondence of R. A. Fisher with Leonard Darwin and Others.* Clarendon Press, Oxford.

BERNSTEIN, F., 1931 Zur Grundlegung der Vererbung beim Menschen. Z. Indukt. Abstammungs. Vererbungsl. **57:** 113–138.

BODMER, F., 1944 *The Loom of Language—A Guide to Foreign Languages for the Home Student.* Allen and Unwin, London.

CHARLES, E., 1933 Collateral and ancestral correlations for sex-linked transmission irrespective of sex. J. Genet. **27:** 97–104.

CREW, F. A. E., 1939 Biological pregnancy diagnosis tests—a comparison of the rabbit, the mouse and the "clawed toad" (Xenopus laevis) as the experimental animal. Br. Med. J. 15 April 1939, p. 766.

CROW, J. F., 1993 FELIX BERNSTEIN and the first human marker locus. Genetics **133:** 4–7.

DARWIN, L., 1926 *The Need for Eugenic Reform.* J. Murray, London.

FISHER, R. A., 1918 The correlation between relatives on the supposition of Mendelian inheritance. Trans. R. Soc. Edinb. **52:** 399–433.

FISHER, R. A., 1930 *The Genetical Theory of Natural Selection*. Clarendon Press, Oxford.

FISHER, R. A., 1935 Eugenics, academic and practical. Eugen. Rev. **27:** 95-100.

GARROD, A., 1902 The incidence of alkaptonuria: a study in chemical individuality. Lancet, December 13, pp. 1616-1620.

HALDANE, J. B. S., 1932 A programme for human genetics [review of HOGBEN (1931b)]. Nature **129:** 345-346.

HALDANE, J. B. S., 1934 Methods for the detection of autosomal linkage in man. Ann. Eugen. **6:** 26-65.

HALDANE, J. B. S., 1936 Some principles of causal analysis in genetics. Erkenntnis **6:** 346-357.

HALDANE, J. B. S., 1946 The interaction of nature and nurture. Ann. Eugen. **13:** 197-205.

HALDANE, J. B. S., and C. A. B. SMITH, 1947 A new estimate of the linkage between the genes for hemophilia and colour-blindness in man. Ann. Eugen. **14:** 10-31.

HERRMAN, L., and L. HOGBEN, 1933 The intellectual resemblance of twins. Proc. R. Soc. Edinb. Sect. B (Biol.) **53:** 105-129.

HOGBEN, L., 1918 *Alfred Russel Wallace: The Story of a Great Discoverer.* Society for Promoting Christian Knowledge, London.

HOGBEN, L., 1919 The progressive reduction of the jugal in mammals. Proc. Zool. Soc. Lond. **1919:** 71-78.

HOGBEN, L., 1920a Studies on synapsis. I. Oogenesis in the hymenoptera. Proc. R. Soc. Lond. B Biol. Sci. **91:** 268-293.

HOGBEN, L., 1920b Studies on synapsis. II. Parallel conjugation and prophase complex in Periplaneta with special reference to the premeiotic telophase. Proc. R. Soc. Lond. B Biol. Sci. **91:** 305-329.

HOGBEN, L., 1923 A method of hypophysectomy in adult frogs and toads. Q.J. Exp. Physiol. **13:** 177-179.

HOGBEN, L., 1924 *The Pigmentary Effector System.* Oliver & Boyd, Edinburgh.

HOGBEN, L., 1926 *Comparative Physiology.* Sedgwick and Jackson, London.

HOGBEN, L., 1927a *The Comparative Physiology of Internal Secretion.* Cambridge University Press, Cambridge, United Kingdom.

HOGBEN, L., 1927b *Principles of Evolutionary Biology.* Juta & Co., Cape Town.

HOGBEN, L., 1930 *The Nature of Living Matter.* Kegan-Paul, London.

HOGBEN, L., 1931a The genetic analysis of familial traits. I. Single gene substitutions. J. Genet. **25:** 97-112.

HOGBEN, L., 1931b *Genetic Principles in Medicine and Social Science.* Williams and Norgate, London.

HOGBEN, L., 1932a The genetic analysis of familial traits. II. Double gene substitutions, with special reference to hereditary dwarfism. J. Genet. **25:** 211-240.

HOGBEN, L., 1932b The genetic analysis of familial traits. III. Matings involving one parent exhibiting a trait determined by a single recessive gene substitution with special reference to sex-linked conditions. J. Genet. **25:** 293-314.

HOGBEN, L., 1932c The factorial analysis of small families with parents of undetermined genotype. J. Genet. **26:** 75-79.

HOGBEN, L., 1932d Filial and fraternal correlations in sex-linked inheritance. Proc. R. Soc. Edinb. Sect. B (Biol.) **52:** 331-336.

HOGBEN, L., 1932e The correlation of relatives on the supposition of sex-linked transmission. J. Genet. **26:** 417-432.

HOGBEN, L., 1933a The limits of applicability of correlation technique in human genetics. J. Genet. **27:** 379-406.

HOGBEN, L., 1933b *Nature and Nurture.* W. W. Norton, New York.

HOGBEN, L., 1934a The detection of linkage in human families. I.

Both heterozygous genotypes indeterminate. Proc. R. Soc. Lond. B Biol. Sci. **114:** 340-352.

HOGBEN, L., 1934b The detection of linkage in human families. II. One heterozygous genotype indeterminate. Proc. R. Soc. Lond. B Biol. Sci. **114:** 353-363.

HOGBEN, L., 1936 *Mathematics for the Million: A Popular Self-Educator.* Allen & Unwin, London.

HOGBEN, L., 1939a Genetic variation and human intelligence, pp. 147-153 in *Proceedings of the Seventh International Genetical Congress*, edited by R. C. Punnett. Cambridge University Press, Cambridge, UK.

HOGBEN, L., 1939b *Dangerous Thoughts.* Allen & Unwin, London.

HOGBEN, L., 1940 *Author in Transit.* Norton, New York.

HOGBEN, L., 1946 *An Introduction to Mathematical Genetics.* W. W. Norton, New York.

HOGBEN, L., 1951 The formal logic of the nature-nurture issue. Acta Genet. Stat. Med. **2:** 101-140.

HOGBEN, L., 1957 *Statistical Theory: An Examination of the Contemporary Crisis in Statistical Theory from a Behaviourist Viewpoint.* Allen & Unwin, London.

HOGBEN, L., 1967 *Mathematics for the Million*, 4th ed. Allen & Unwin, London.

HOGBEN, L., 1969 *The Vocabulary of Science.* Heinemann, London.

HOGBEN, L., and R. L. KIRK, 1944 Studies on temperature regulation. I. The pulmonata and oligochaeta. Proc. R. Soc. Lond. B Biol. Sci. **132:** 239-252.

HOGBEN, L., and F. R. WINTON, 1924 *An Introduction to Recent Advances in Comparative Physiology.* Collins, London.

HOGBEN, L., E. CHARLES and D. SLOME, 1931 Studies on the pituitary. VIII. The relation of the pituitary gland to calcium metabolism and ovarian function in Xenopus. J. Exp. Biol. **8:** 345-354.

HOGBEN, L, R. L. WORRALL and I. ZIEVE, 1932 The genetic basis of alkaptonuria. Proc. R. Soc. Edinb. Sect. B (Biol.) **52:** 265-295.

HUXLEY, J., 1932 Eugenics [review of HOGBEN (1931b)]. Eugen. Rev. **23:** 341-344.

KIRK, R. L., and L. HOGBEN, 1946 Studies on temperature regulation. II. Amphibia and reptiles. J. Exp. Biol. **22:** 213-220.

KRAFKA, J., 1920 The effect of temperature upon facet number in the bar-eyed mutant of Drosophila. J. Gen. Physiol. **2:** 409-464.

LANDGREBE, F. W., 1939 The maintenance of reproductive activity in Xenopus laevis for pregnancy diagnosis. J. Exp. Biol. **16:** 89-95.

MAZUMDAR, P. M. H., 1992 *Eugenics, Human Genetics and Human Failings: The Eugenics Society, Its Sources and Its Critics in Britain.* Routledge, London.

MORGAN, T. H., 1925 *Evolution and Genetics.* Princeton University Press, Princeton, NJ.

MORTON, N., 1995 LODs past and present. Genetics **140:** 7-12.

RUSSELL, B., 1968 *The Autobiography of Bertrand Russell,* Vol. 2. Allen & Unwin, London.

SARKAR, S., 1992a Science, philosophy, and politics in the work of J. B. S. Haldane, 1922-1937. Biol. Philos. **7:** 385-409.

SARKAR, S., 1992b Haldane and the emergence of theoretical population genetics, 1924-1932. J. Genet. **71:** 73-79.

WARING, H., 1963 *Color Change Mechanisms of Cold-Blooded Vertebrates.* Academic Press, New York.

WELLS, G. P., 1976 The early days of the S. E. B., pp. 1-6 in *Perspectives in Experimental Biology*, Vol. 1, edited by P. S. DAVIES. Pergamon, London.

WELLS, G. P., 1978 Lancelot Thomas Hogben. Biogr. Mem. Fellows R. Soc. Lond. **24:** 183-221.

WERSKEY, G., 1978 *The Visible College: The Collective Biography of British Scientific Socialists of the 1930's.* Holt, Rinehart and Winston, New York.

Worm Spadework

Robert K. Herman

Department of Genetics and Cell Biology, University of Minnesota, St. Paul, Minnesota 55108

I fell in love with *Caenorhabditis elegans* in the summer of '72. Our relationship was cemented four years later, 20 years ago now, by the publication of a paper in GENETICS on *C. elegans* chromosome rearrangements (HERMAN *et al.* 1976). My pleasant assignment here is to describe the beginnings of that work and to relate it to current worm cytogenetics and chromosome mechanics.

In 1972 my research experience had been limited to *Escherichia coli* genetics, but I was caught up in the prevailing restless mood of many phage and bacterial geneticists who were thinking about switching to eukaryotes. SYDNEY BRENNER's plans for the worm first became known to me in 1971 from a brief but intriguing news account in *Nature* of a talk he gave to the Royal Society. [For a description of the beginnings of *C. elegans* work, see HODGKIN (1989).] I had been learning genetics in the best possible way, by teaching it, and the idea of starting over on the classical genetics of a model eukaryote was very appealing, so I jumped at the chance to take a three-week summer course on *C. elegans* at Cold Spring Harbor Laboratory in August of 1972 (the only time the course was given). There were eight students, including GÜNTER VON EHRENSTEIN, who became converted to worm research, and CHRIS GUTHRIE, who did not. The instructors were DICK RUSSELL, who had learned about *C. elegans* as a postdoctoral fellow working mostly on phage and bacteria with BRENNER, and RUTH PERTEL, who had been trained as a more traditional nematologist. (Sadly, VON EHRENSTEIN died in 1980, RUSSELL in 1994.) Our teaching assistant was DAVE DUSENBERY, with whom I shared a home town (Vancouver, Washington) and training in biophysics. In course exercises, we induced Dumpy and Uncoordinated mutants with ethyl methanesulfonate, conducted simple crosses (we were unaware of any genetic maps), and did Feulgen staining of nuclei. Apart from the graduation ceremony presided over by MAX DELBRÜCK in what I took to be an archbishop's costume (see SUSMAN 1995), the high point of the three weeks was a mini-symposium on the last day, attended by many visitors, including several from the BRENNER lab at the MRC Laboratory of Molecular Biology in Cambridge, England.

I wrote to BRENNER in the fall of '72 proposing to spend a sabbatical furlough in his laboratory and suggested working on extragenic suppressors, genetic mosaics, or mutations affecting gametogenesis. He put me off until 1974–75. Meanwhile, I did a little worm genetics in my lab at Minnesota, while two graduate students continued their *E. coli* work. An important influence at the time was the Drosophila work of JUDD *et al.* (1972), which suggested that it took only about 5000 genes to make a fly, and I vaguely hoped that it might some day be possible to study the cell-by-cell effects of mutations in essential genes in *C. elegans* (something I am now doing, using genetic mosaics). A pilot screen showed that it was fairly easy to identify Sterile mutants, but it quickly became obvious that chromosome balancers, standard equipment in Drosophila genetics, would be very useful. I found pairs of loosely linked mutations that conferred visible phenotypes and ran one unsuccessful screen for X-ray-induced crossover suppressors before going with my family to Cambridge in the fall of 1974.

My timing could not have been luckier. BRENNER's famous 1974 GENETICS paper came out that summer, assigning 300 mutations to 100 genes, mapping them onto six linkage groups, and describing how to do worm hermaphrodite genetics. Also available was JONATHAN HODGKIN's newly completed Ph.D. thesis, which contained useful lore on mutagenesis, suppression, and meiotic *X* chromosome nondisjunction. My goal was to develop some of the genetic tools that had proved so useful in Drosophila genetics. PETER LAWRENCE directed me to some fly literature; he clearly appreciated the genetic tools available to fly workers, but I think he was surprised that someone would want to do spadework.

My first experiment in Cambridge, suggested by BRENNER, yielded a useful chromosome rearrangement, an X-ray-induced duplication of the right end of the X

Author e-mail: bob-h@biosci.cbs.umn.edu

chromosome that was translocated to chromosome *V*. This was equivalent to a half translocation; the scheme used in identifying it, which involved following the transmission of an unlinked *X* duplication from irradiated father to son, precluded recovery of the other half. Clearly it was BRENNER's new genetic map and the large collection of mapped mutants that made this work possible. I was surprised to find that the duplication, now called *mnDp1(X;V)*, showed no detectable recombination with the homologous region of the *X*. It was also homozygous inviable. These features meant that it could be used rather handily to balance lethal mutations, including a set of overlapping deletions that could be used for rapid complementation mapping of point lethals, in the corresponding region of the *X* chromosome. P. MENEELY was later to use *mnDp1* as a balancer of this sort in his Ph.D. thesis work (MENEELY and HERMAN 1981). Additional balancer chromosomes, involving different kinds of chromosome rearrangement, have since been collected by us and by others (EDGLEY *et al.* 1995). For example, ROSENBLUTH and BAILLIE (1981) discovered that one of BRENNER's original uncoordinated mutants contained a reciprocal translocation that dominantly suppressed recombination over large regions of chromosomes *III* and *V*. Over half of the genome is now covered by balancers, but more good balancers are still needed. A curious feature of balancers, probably related to the nature of chromosome pairing, is that one end of each chromosome seems to be much more susceptible to crossover suppression than the other (ZETKA and ROSE 1995).

None of the next four *X* duplications I recovered seemed to be linked to anything. My suspicion that these might be chromosome fragments or free duplications, unattached to any other chromosome, was confirmed when DONNA ALBERTSON, my Cambridge labmate who had been staining *C. elegans* chromosomes with the fluorescent dye Hoechst 33258, looked at oocytes of animals carrying one of the unlinked duplications: she often saw a small fragment in addition to the normal six bivalents (HERMAN *et al.* 1976).

Cytogenetics: NIGON (1949) had much earlier shown that *C. elegans* hermaphrodites have six pairs of chromosomes (males have five pairs and a single *X*), all small, featureless, and about the same size. BRENNER's six linkage groups corresponded properly to the cytological chromosome number, but it was impossible to assign a particular linkage group to a particular chromosome. It was nice to be able to see the small free duplications cytologically, but the only benefit was in confirming that they were free. Some other rearrangements—insertional translocations and asymmetric reciprocal translocations—have also resulted in distinctive karyotypes, but deletions, inversions, and many other translocations have not. *C. elegans* cytogenetics at this stage was obviously primitive compared with the cytogenetics of Drosophila. What finally cured our envy of polytene chromosomes was the development by JOHN SULSTON,

ALAN COULSON and colleagues of the *C. elegans* physical map, consisting of overlapping cosmid and YAC clones of genomic DNA [reviewed by COULSON *et al.* (1995)]. Cytogenetics helped reciprocally in the early development of the physical map: ALBERTSON (1985) used cytologically detectable chromosome rearrangements to map cosmid clones to particular chromosomal regions within about 20% of a chromosome length, by *in situ* hybridization and fluorescence microscopy (FISH). Now that the physical map is essentially complete, cloned DNA is positioned on the map more directly. Indeed, a filter spotted with a grid of worm DNA cloned as yeast artificial chromosomes and selected for coverage of the genome is called a "polytene" filter because it is used in the same way that Drosophila polytene chromosomes are used to map cloned DNA by *in situ* hybridization.

The physical map has made it possible to do *C. elegans* cytogenetics at high resolution: ALBERTSON (1993) has used FISH to locate chromosome rearrangement breakpoints within specific cosmids on the physical map. She has also used FISH to localize specific interphase chromosomes by "painting" (CHUANG *et al.* 1994; ALBERTSON *et al.* 1995) and to study meiotic chromosome pairing and segregation (see below).

Centromeres: The free duplications described in our 1976 paper seemed to segregate faithfully during most mitotic divisions, as if they had centromeric function. Either we were lucky to pick a region that contained the *X* centromere or the *X* does not have a single localized centromere. Centromeric constrictions were not apparent cytologically, and free duplications of other regions of the *X* were later obtained. It had been suggested earlier that certain nematodes have diffuse centromeres (TRIANTAPHYLLOU 1971), as do certain other animals, plants, and protozoa (WHITE 1973). Some members of the nematode family Ascaridae had long been known to have atypical centromeres. BOVERI showed over 100 years ago that in the somatic cells of *Parascaris equorum*, the ends of each chromosome are cast off into the cytoplasm, where they ultimately degenerate, and the central segments split into many small chromosomes, each of which retains centromere function; at the same time, the large unfragmented germline chromosomes appear to have multiple spindle attachment points (WHITE 1973). *C. elegans* chromosomes do not undergo chromatin diminution and fragmentation (EMMONS 1988), but ALBERTSON and THOMSON (1982) showed by serial section microscopy that they are holocentric: the microtubules of the mitotic spindle attach to kinetochores that extend along the entire lengths of the condensed chromosomes (each of which is only about 1–2 μm long). It is unclear whether kinetochore formation requires specific centromeric DNA sequences sprinkled along the lengths of the chromosomes. The fact that DNA of apparently any sequence injected into the hermaphrodite gonad forms extrachromosomal arrays that behave much like free duplications cytologically and genetically

(STINCHCOMB *et al.* 1985) suggests that specific centromeric sequences may be unnecessary. On the other hand, differences in mitotic stability among various free duplications and extrachromosomal arrays (see below) suggest that centromere function may be affected by *cis*-acting DNA sequences.

Meiotic centromeres seem wholly unrelated to the mitotic ones. No meiotic kinetochores are apparent in electron micrographs: the spindle microtubules appear to project directly into the chromatin (ALBERTSON and THOMSON 1993). The meiotic chromosomes also orient differently on the metaphase plate. The chromatids of the meiotic bivalent are held together in an end-to-end association, which may be generated by the terminalization of chiasmata. ALBERTSON and THOMSON (1993) showed by FISH that for any given bivalent, the ends that are associated can be either the left or right ones as defined by the genetic map. Furthermore, each bivalent appears to orient with its axis perpendicular to the metaphase I plate; the attached ends are on the plate prior to disjunction, with the opposite ends of each pair of sister chromatids pointing toward the spindle poles. The spindle pole proximal ends then provide the centromeric function of leading the way to the poles at anaphase I. They also appear to keep sister chromatids attached until disjunction at anaphase II (just as classical centromeres do), at which time the opposite ends of the chromatids appear to lead the way to the poles (ALBERTSON and THOMSON 1993; D. ALBERTSON, personal communication). Thus, it seems that at meiosis I either end of a chromosome may act as the centromere, and at meiosis II the opposite end is the centromere! The chromosomes are very compact at both meiotic anaphases, however, so that the chromosome "end" centromeres do not seem very localized and might be defined simply by their proximity to the spindle poles. The molecular mechanisms of meiotic centromere function are obviously quite mysterious.

Free duplications and genetic mosaics: We presented suggestive evidence in the 1976 paper that free duplications were subject to loss during the premeiotic divisions of the hermaphrodite germline, and we mentioned the possibility of using the somatic loss of free duplications to generate genetic mosaics. But the only genetic markers at that time known to be covered by free duplications were loci that conferred an overall uncoordinated phenotype, and we couldn't see how to go about using them to identify mosaic worms. Our inspiration for wanting to generate mosaics of course came from Drosophila: the power of mosaic analysis had been amply demonstrated earlier in flies (for example, STERN 1968; HOTTA and BENZER 1972).

I returned to this problem on my second sabbatical furlough to Cambridge, in 1981–82. By then, additional markers were known. Particularly useful were mutations that ED HEDGECOCK had shown affected the uptake in living animals of the fluorescent dye FITC by groups of chemosensory neurons in the head and tail (PERKINS *et al.* 1986). By using a combination of genetic markers, I showed that the spontaneous somatic loss of free duplications carrying wild-type alleles of genes that were otherwise homozygous mutant did generate genetic mosaics and that such mosaics yielded information about the cell or tissue specificity of gene function (HERMAN 1984). Crucial to the interpretation of these experiments and all subsequent mosaic analyses was the essentially invariant and completely known cell lineage (SULSTON *et al.* 1983), which made it possible to figure out where in the lineage a duplication was lost. I was proud of one experimental design in which somatic loss at a specific cell division of a duplication carrying two visible markers resulted in a phenotypic recombinant, which could be readily identified among the many non-mosaic siblings. For this design to work, the foci of action of the two genes must be different. If, for example, gene a^+ is needed in motor neurons and gene b^+ is needed in body muscle, then a mosaic in which the a^+b^+ duplication is present in motor neurons and absent in muscle would be phenotypically wild-type with respect to a and mutant with respect to b. Mosaicism in the animal could then be confirmed by scoring the dye-filling phenotype conferred by a third marker, and transmission of the duplication to the germline could also be monitored by scoring self progeny. When I described this scheme to HEDGECOCK, he wondered why it had taken me so long to come up with it. Of course, the trick was in finding the markers that made it work; one of the critical ones came from GREENWALD and HORVITZ (1980).

In 1985 an abstract by HEDGECOCK that appeared in *The Worm Breeder's Gazette* gave mosaic analysis a big boost. *The Worm Breeder's Gazette* was founded by BOB EDGAR in 1975 and has been used by *C. elegans* workers ever since to communicate preliminary findings, work in progress, and other news about *C. elegans* to everyone else in the field. HEDGECOCK reported that a mutation in the gene he called *ncl-1* results in enlarged nucleoli, is cell autonomous, and makes it possible to score, by Nomarski microscopy, nearly every cell in a living animal for the presence or absence of an *ncl-1(+)*-bearing duplication. I learned to score *ncl-1* mosaics during my third sabbatical leave, 1989–90, in HEDGECOCK's laboratory at Johns Hopkins. *ncl-1* has been used as a duplication marker in the mosaic analysis of many genes [reviewed by HERMAN (1995)]. It has also been useful in clarifying the nature of spontaneous somatic duplication loss (HEDGECOCK and HERMAN 1995); for example, most patterns of mosaicism can be traced to duplication loss by a single cell—which often involves nondisjunction, with the sister cell receiving two copies—but occasionally a duplication is transmitted to only a single daughter cell for two or three consecutive cell divisions (a temporary pattern of linear inheritance), after which it recovers and is transmitted to all remaining progeny cells.

Additional advances in mosaic analysis extended

the use of *ncl-1* as a cell-autonomous marker to the study of genes that are not normally present on a *ncl-1(+)*-containing free duplication. For example, a *ncl-1(+)*-bearing duplication can be fused either to an unlinked free duplication (HUNTER and WOOD 1992; HEDGECOCK and HERMAN 1995) or to an extrachromosomal array of cloned DNA carrying a gene of interest (LEUNG-HAGESTEIJN *et al.* 1992). Finally, in what will probably become the most popular technique of all, an extrachromosomal array containing *ncl-1(+)*, at least one visible marker, and the gene to be analyzed can be generated by germline transformation and used as a kind of synthetic free duplication, which yields mosaic animals by somatic extrachromosomal loss (LACKNER *et al.* 1994; L. MILLER, D. WARING and S. KIM, personal communication).

Different free duplications can exhibit very different frequencies of spontaneous mitotic loss (HEDGECOCK and HERMAN 1995). Duplication size affects mitotic stability, as does a chromosomal mutation that affects chromosomal segregation, but other factors affecting duplication stability—and perhaps, concomitantly, normal chromosome stability—also seem to be important, but remain to be elucidated. Finally, we do not understand why free duplications acquire deletions at very high rates ($>10^{-3}$ per generation) during germline transmission.

Conclusion: *C. elegans* cytogenetics and chromosome mechanics have turned up unexpected and interesting findings concerning the behavior of holocentric chromosomes and free duplications. But I think the most important contribution of work in this area has been to facilitate the analysis of developmental and behavioral mutants. The wonderful progress that the *C. elegans* field as a whole has enjoyed, which has relied heavily on mutant analysis, has amply justified the genetic spadework that has been done—and should justify continued spadework.

I thank DONNA ALBERTSON, JONATHAN HODGKIN, and JOCELYN SHAW for helpful comments, and I thank the National Institutes of Health for support (GM-22387).

LITERATURE CITED

ALBERTSON, D. G., 1985 Mapping muscle protein genes by *in situ* hybridization using biotin-labeled probes. EMBO J. **4:** 2493–2498.

ALBERTSON, D. G., 1993 Mapping chromosome rearrangement breakpoints to the physical map of *Caenorhabditis elegans* by fluorescent *in situ* hybridization. Genetics **134:** 211–219.

ALBERTSON, D. G., and J. N. THOMSON, 1982 The kinetochores of *Caenorhabditis elegans*. Chromosoma **86:** 409–428.

ALBERTSON, D. G., and J. N. THOMSON, 1993 Segregation of holocentric chromosomes at meiosis in the nematode, *Caenorhabditis elegans*. Chromosome Res. **1:** 15–26.

ALBERTSON, D. G., R. M. FISHPOOL and P. S. BIRCHALL, 1995 Fluorescence *in situ* hybridization for the detection of DNA and RNA, pp. 340–364 in *Caenorhabditis elegans: Modern Biological Analysis of an Organism*, edited by H. F. EPSTEIN and D. C. SHAKES. Academic Press, San Diego.

BRENNER, S., 1974 The genetics of *Caenorhabditis elegans*. Genetics **77:** 71–94.

CHUANG, P.-T., D. G. ALBERTSON and B. J. MEYER, 1994 DPY-27: a chromosome condensation protein homolog that regulates C. elegans dosage compensation through association with the X chromosome. Cell **79:** 459–474.

COULSON, A., C. HUYNH, Y. KOZONO and R. SHOWNKEEN, 1995 The physical map of the *Caenorhabditis elegans* genome, pp. 534–550 in *Caenorhabditis elegans: Modern Biological Analysis of an Organism*, edited by H. F. EPSTEIN and D. C. SHAKES. Academic Press, San Diego.

EDGLEY, M., D. L. BAILLIE, D. L. RIDDLE and A. M. ROSE, 1995 Genetic balancers, pp. 148–184 in *Caenorhabditis elegans: Modern Biological Analysis of an Organism*, edited by H. F. EPSTEIN and D. C. SHAKES. Academic Press, San Diego.

EMMONS, S. W., 1988 The genome, pp. 47–79 in *The Nematode Caenorhabditis elegans*, edited by W. B. WOOD. Cold Spring Harbor Laboratory Press, Cold Spring Harbor, NY.

GREENWALD, I. S., and H. R. HORVITZ, 1980 *unc-93(e1500)*: a behavioral mutant of *Caenorhabditis elegans* that defines a gene with a wild-type null phenotype. Genetics **96:** 147–164.

HEDGECOCK, E. M., and R. K. HERMAN, 1995 The *ncl-1* gene and genetic mosaics of *Caenorhabditis elegans*. Genetics **141:** 989–1006.

HERMAN, R. K., 1984 Analysis of genetic mosaics of the nematode *Caenorhabditis elegans*. Genetics **106:** 165–180.

HERMAN, R. K., 1995 Mosaic analysis, pp. 123–146 in *Caenorhabditis elegans: Modern Biological Analysis of an Organism*, edited by H. F. EPSTEIN and D. C. SHAKES. Academic Press, San Diego.

HERMAN, R. K., D. G. ALBERTSON and S. BRENNER, 1976 Chromosome rearrangements in *Caenorhabditis elegans*. Genetics **83:** 91–105.

HODGKIN, J., 1989 Early worms. Genetics **121:** 1–3.

HOTTA, Y., and BENZER, S., 1972 Mapping of behaviour in *Drosophila* mosaics. Nature **240:** 527–535.

HUNTER, C. P., and W. B. WOOD, 1992 Evidence from mosaic analysis of the masculinizing gene *her-1* for cell interactions in *C. elegans* sex determination. Nature **355:** 551–555.

JUDD, B. H., M. W. SHEN and T. C. KAUFMAN, 1972 The anatomy and function of a segment of the X chromosome of *Drosophila melanogaster*. Genetics **71:** 139–156.

LACKNER, M. R., K. KORNFELD, L. M. MILLER, H. R. HORVITZ and S. K. KIM, 1994 A MAP kinase homolog, *mpk-1*, is involved in *ras*-mediated induction of vulval cell fates in *Caenorhabditis elegans*. Genes Dev. **8:** 160–173.

LEUNG-HAGESTEIJN, C., A. M. SPENCE, B. D. STERN, Y. ZHOU, M.-W. SU *et al.*, 1992 UNC-5, a transmembrane protein with immunoglobulin and thrombospondin type 1 domains, guides cell and pioneer axon migrations in C. elegans. Cell **71:** 289–299.

MENEELY, P., and R. K. HERMAN, 1981 Suppression and function of X-linked lethal and sterile mutations in *Caenorhabditis elegans*. Genetics **97:** 65–84.

NIGON, V., 1949 Les modalités de la reproduction et le déterminisme de sexe chez quelques Nématodes libres. Ann. Sci. Natl. Zool. **2:** 1–132.

PERKINS, L. A., E. M. HEDGECOCK, J. N. THOMSON and J. G. CULOTTI, 1986 Mutant sensory cilia in the nematode *Caenorhabditis elegans*. Dev. Biol. **117:** 456–487.

ROSENBLUTH, R. E., and D. L. BAILLIE, 1981 The genetic analysis of a reciprocal translocation, *eT1(III;V)*, in *Caenorhabditis elegans*. Genetics **99:** 415–428.

STERN, C., 1968 *Genetic Mosaics and Other Essays*. Harvard University Press, Cambridge.

STINCHCOMB, D. T., J. E. SHAW, S. H. CARR and D. HIRSH, 1985 Extrachromosomal DNA transformation of *Caenorhabditis elegans*. Mol. Cell. Biol. **5:** 3484–3496.

SULSTON, J. E., E. SCHIERENBERG, J. G. WHITE and J. N. THOMSON, 1983 The embryonic cell lineage of the nematode *Caenorhabditis elegans*. Dev. Biol. **100:** 64–119.

SUSMAN, M., 1995 The Cold Spring Harbor phage course (1945–1970): a 50th anniversary remembrance. Genetics **139:** 1101–1106.

TRIANTAPHYLLOU, A. C., 1971 Genetics and cytology, pp. 1–34 in *Plant Parasitic Nematodes*, Vol. 2, edited by B. M. ZUCKERMAN, W. F. MAI and R. A. RHODE. Academic Press, New York.

WHITE, M. J. D., 1973 *Animal Cytology and Evolution*, 3rd ed. Cambridge University Press, Cambridge.

ZETKA, M., and A. ROSE, 1995 The genetics of meiosis in *Caenorhabditis elegans*. Trends Genet. **11:** 27–31.

The Sixtieth Anniversary of Biochemical Genetics

N. H. Horowitz

Biology Division, California Institute of Technology, Pasadena, California 91125

MAY, 1996 marks 60 years since the publication in GENETICS of the paper that opened modern biochemical genetics (BEADLE and EPHRUSSI 1936). The authors, GEORGE W. BEADLE and BORIS EPHRUSSI, had published some preliminary reports of their experiments on the transplantation of imaginal discs in Drosophila, but this was their first full paper on the subject. A direct line leads from this publication to the production of nutritional mutants in Neurospora and bacteria and to all that followed from that.

The two authors, both in their thirties, had met at Caltech in 1934 and had agreed to launch this investigation in order to throw light on the mechanisms of gene action in development. The original plan had been to transfer imaginal discs from Drosophila larvae to a tissue culture medium, where, it was hoped, the discs would continue to develop. With this idea in mind, the site of the investigation was moved from Caltech to EPHRUSSI's laboratory at the Institut de Biologie in Paris, which was equipped for tissue culture studies (Figure 1). The discs did not do well *in vitro*, however, and the two researchers decided instead to transplant them to the body cavity of other larvae, a technique that had been used successfully in the moth Ephestia by CASPARI (1933). In the larval environment, the discs developed and yielded the results to be described below.

The inspiration for these experiments was an early observation by STURTEVANT (1920), who found that, in gynandromorphs of Drosophila, genetically *vermilion* eyes behaved nonautonomously, *i.e.*, they developed not *vermilion*, but wild-type, eye color, if the other parts of the fly were genetically wild type for the *vermilion* gene. This nonautonomy, with its hint that in some cases the phenotypic defect of a mutant could be rectified, suggested to BEADLE and EPHRUSSI that the transplantation method might be applied to the study of gene action in Drosophila. It is not clear how much influence CASPARI's earlier findings with Ephestia had on this decision, but there was probably some.

Interest in the biochemistry of gene action appeared shortly after the rediscovery of Mendelism and led to some notable early researches. The best known and most brilliant of these were by LUCIEN CUÉNOT and ARCHIBALD GARROD, who, respectively, studied inherited traits in mice and men. These authors were the first to link gene mutations to specific biochemical defects (see WAGNER 1989). Their work was followed by studies by others on the inheritance of coat colors in mammals and anthocyanins in plants (for references, see STURTEVANT 1965). These early investigations had been largely forgotten by geneticists by the time BEADLE and EPHRUSSI began their work. This neglect was due only partly to the fact that genetics took a different turn after the highly fruitful chromosome theory came into existence. At least as important must have been the fact that higher animals and plants, with their long generation times and inherent complexities, were too difficult and unpromising a material for studies of the biochemistry of gene action. Even Drosophila, as we shall see, was only marginally useful for this purpose. It was not until geneticists discovered microorganisms that a science of biochemical genetics could come into existence.

In their 1936 paper, BEADLE and EPHRUSSI studied the fate of eye discs from 26 different eye-color mutants of Drosophila after their implantation into the body cavity of larvae of the same or a different genotype. The discs developed into adult eyes, which, because they were detached from the optic nerve, failed to evert, but which were otherwise normal eyes. Their pigmentation, in particular, developed normally.

Of the 26 mutants, just two, *vermilion* and *cinnabar*, proved to be nonautonomous, *i.e.*, they developed wild-type pigmentation when grown in a wild-type host. The authors inferred that, in both cases, a diffusible substance needed for production of normal pigmentation was supplied by the host to the mutant disc. The effect of the mutation had been to prevent formation of the substance. They found, furthermore, that a different substance was required by each mutant. This was shown by reciprocal implants in which a *cn* disc developing in a *v* host remained *cn*, but a *v* disk in a *cn* host became wild type. This result showed that *cn* mutants produce what they called the v^+ substance, but *v* mutants do not

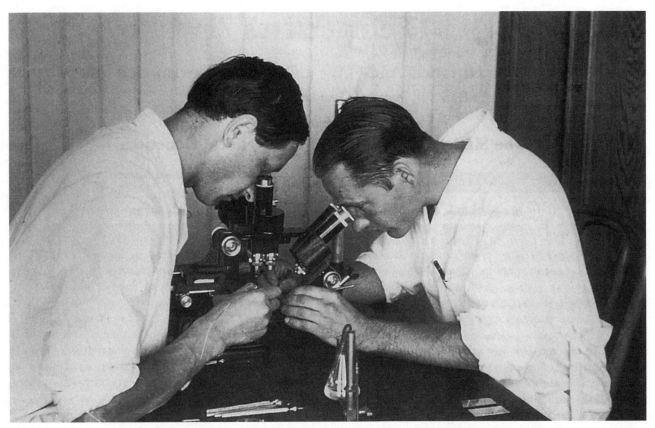

FIGURE 1.—BORIS EPHRUSSI (left) and GEORGE W. BEADLE (right) transplanting imaginal discs; Paris, 1935. Courtesy of the Archives, California Institute of Technology.

make the cn^+ substance. A simple explanation of these facts, they suggested, assumes that the v^+ substance is a precursor of the cn^+ substance in a reaction chain, so that a block in the synthesis of the former (a mutation from v^+ to v) also blocks synthesis of the latter. Mutation from cn^+ to cn, however, blocks only the synthesis of the cn^+ substance.

In later papers, they often referred to the two substances as "hormones" because in implanted flies they are formed in one place and used in another. As will be seen, it was eventually found that the two substances are actually precursors of the brown component of the Drosophila eye pigment. The other component is red. The duplex nature of the pigment was shown by German workers in the late 'thirties.

In their 1936 paper, BEADLE and EPHRUSSI also included the claret gene in the reaction sequence, as a precursor of the v^+ substance. Thus,

$$\rightarrow ca^+ \text{ substance} \rightarrow v^+ \text{ substance} \rightarrow cn^+ \text{ substance}$$

The evidence for a ca^+ substance was indirect, since claret eye discs develop autonomously in wild type. It derived from the observation that wild-type eye discs transplanted to *claret* develop "*claret*-like" pigmentation. This was interpreted to mean that the eye needs a factor made elsewhere in the fly to develop full wild-type coloration. *claret* lacks this factor; hence, the ca^+ substance.

This interpretation soon led to logical difficulties that increasingly required *ad hoc* explanations for newer observations. The latter included the findings that the *claret* effect was variable in degree and that it was observed in implants to mutants other than *claret*, in particular those known to be deficient in the v^+ substance. Before long, the existence of the ca^+ substance was called into question (BEADLE *et al.* 1938), and finally the idea was abandoned (CLANCY 1942). The *claret* story illustrates difficulties that are perhaps inevitable when critical judgements are based on visual estimates of subtle differences in shades of color.

The validity of the *vermilion* and *cinnabar* findings was not affected by the difficulties with *claret*, and it became the goal of the BEADLE and EPHRUSSI groups to identify the v^+ and cn^+ substances. EPHRUSSI was still in Paris, and BEADLE was now at Stanford University, where he had been joined by EDWARD TATUM. The two groups succeeded in their quest, but the story has a curious ending, as will be seen.

Several discoveries made in the two laboratories greatly facilitated the identification. It was found that v^+ substance was effective when fed to larvae or injected into them, making it no longer necessary to implant eye discs. Then it was found that addition of tryptophan to the fly food led to partial restoration of the brown pigment; in other words, tryptophan supplied in this way showed v^+ activity. Next it was discovered that the effect of tryptophan was caused by bacteria growing in cultures to which this amino acid had been added. TATUM then isolated a Bacterium sp. that produced large amounts of a substance with v^+ activity from tryptophan. He set about isolating the active factor and by 1940 had obtained a crystalline preparation which he identified as a compound of L-kynurenine with sucrose (TATUM and HAAGEN-SMIT 1941). The compound showed high v^+ activity; acid hydrolysis removed the sucrose and left all the activity in the kynurenine moiety. This, then, was the long-sought substance.

The odd twist to the story is that kynurenine had been identified as the v^+ substance some months earlier by BUTENANDT et al. (1940), German chemists who had been studying insect eye colors. Learning that the active compound was a bacterial product formed from tryptophan, they simply tested known metabolites of the amino acid for v^+ activity. L-kynurenine was active. The paper by TATUM and HAAGEN-SMIT confirmed this finding. BUTENANDT's group later found that the cn^+ substance is 3-hydroxy-L-kynurenine (BUTENANDT et al. 1949), and they eventually showed that the brown pigment is formed by condensation of two molecules of hydroxykynurenine. The v^+ and cn^+ substances are thus precursors of the pigment.

In subsequent investigations, the enzymes determined by the vermilion and cinnabar genes were identified. Their activities are missing from the respective mutants (see GHOSH and FORREST 1967). Further interesting details of this work are reviewed in a later publication by COCHRAN (1975).

The vermilion-cinnabar case differed importantly from the mutations studied earlier by CUÉNOT and GARROD in that it involved sequential steps in a reaction chain. Each step was determined by its own gene and, presumably, its own enzyme. This was a strong hint of things to come. Eventually, it led to the one-gene-one-enzyme hypothesis, fully documented in Neurospora. At the time, no more along this line could be done with Drosophila owing to the scarcity of nonautonomous mutants. Beyond that, however, BEADLE was conscious of the years of effort that he, TATUM, and many others had expended on the identification of the vermilion and cinnabar substances. A different, more effective way was needed. It occurred to him that "it ought to be possible to reverse the procedure we had been following and instead of attempting to work out the chemistry of known genetic differences we should be able to select mutants in which known chemical reactions were blocked. Neurospora was an obvious organism ..." (BEADLE 1966). This idea—to search for nutritional (i.e., nonautonomous) mutants in a genetically understood microorganism growing on a synthetic medium— was, as I have said more than once before, a stroke of genius. It created the science of biochemical genetics and made bacterial genetics possible.

In a curious article with some relevance to the present subject that has appeared in these pages, COMFORT (1995) gives a historian's view of the 1951 Cold Spring Harbor Symposium on Genes and Mutations. It is this author's belief that the 1951 Symposium was the occasion for a major confrontation between what he calls the MCCLINTOCK-GOLDSCHMIDT (or "dynamic") view of the gene and the BEADLE-TATUM (or "static") view. [In language and outlook, COMFORT's article strongly resembles EVELYN FOX KELLER's biography of BARBARA MCCLINTOCK (KELLER 1983).] COMFORT's picture of events rests, in part, on the fact that he misdates the acceptance by geneticists of the one-gene-one-enzyme idea. This idea, first intimated in the paper by BEADLE and EPHRUSSI commemorated here, was proposed formally by BEADLE in 1945, but it was not accepted by geneticists until they were compelled to do so by advances in the understanding of DNA and the genetic code made in the 'fifties and 'sixties. The Neurospora findings were widely admired, but the prevailing view in 1951 was that the conclusion BEADLE had drawn from them was a vast oversimplification. (This resistance was not found among microbiologists and biochemists, who welcomed the idea.) BEADLE (1966) wrote that after reading the 1951 Symposium volume, he had the impression that supporters of one-gene-one-enzyme "could be counted on the fingers of one hand, with a couple of fingers left over."

Unaware of the state of affairs, and apparently not noticing that the paper I gave at the Symposium (HOROWITZ and LEUPOLD 1951; HOROWITZ 1995) was a defense of one-gene-one-enzyme against its most influential critic—a Cold Spring Harbor frequenter named MAX DELBRÜCK—COMFORT assumes that BEADLE's hypothesis was already part of the entrenched genetic canon. This allows him to construct the scenario referred to above in which the "static" gene is opposed by the "dynamic" one. GOLDSCHMIDT's contribution to the "dynamic" gene at the 1951 Symposium consisted of some elegantly phrased but predictably implausible thoughts on genes and chromosomes, while MCCLINTOCK's was an account of her discovery of transposable elements.

COMFORT's article has a certain operatic quality, with arias and golden duets by MCCLINTOCK-GOLDSCHMIDT alternating with dark basso rumblings from the BEADLE-TATUM side, the villain's role being assigned to E. B. LEWIS. Unlike most operas, however, this one ends happily. "As is often the case," COMFORT says, "both sides were partly right." By this he means that MCCLINTOCK's findings were confirmed in diverse species, but transposable elements were found to encode proteins, just as do "static" genes. He does not tell us that no biological function has yet been established for these elements. It is still an open question whether, if one or all of an organism's transposable elements could be removed, the organism would be harmed or benefited. (A defensible guess is that the organism would benefit, but the species would suffer from loss of a source of genetic variability.)

I attended McClintock's lecture in 1951. There was great interest in it. She gave it twice, owing to the fact that the small lecture hall was overfilled at the morning session. Before she began, M. Demerec, director of the laboratory, arose to announce that McClintock would repeat the lecture after dinner for those unable to find seats. I attended the evening session, heard the talk and, like many others, was mystified. I did not see Barbara as a character in a drama, however, but as an old friend. We had first met in 1944, when Beadle invited her to come to Stanford to straighten out the cytogenetics of Neurospora. She spent ten weeks in the lab, and I got to know her as a coworker. She was knowledgeable and intense, a perfectionist, with a sense of humor that revealed itself in a deep, hearty laugh, startling coming from a tiny woman. I can easily imagine her laughing that laugh on being told that 45 years after the 1951 Symposium, people would still be debating the significance of transposable elements and trying to find a role for them.

LITERATURE CITED

BEADLE, G. W., 1945 Biochemical genetics. Chem. Rev. 37: 15–96.

BEADLE, G. W., 1966 Biochemical genetics: some recollections, pp. 23–32 in *Phage and the Origins of Molecular Biology*, edited by J. CAIRNS, G. S. STENT and J. D. WATSON. Cold Spring Harbor Laboratory of Quantitative Biology, Cold Spring Harbor, NY.

BEADLE, G. W., and B. EPHRUSSI, 1936 The differentiation of eye pigments in Drosophila as studied by transplantation. Genetics 21: 225–247.

BEADLE, G. W., R. L. ANDERSON and J. MAXWELL, 1938 A comparison of the diffusible substances concerned with eye color develop-

ment in Drosophila, Ephestia and Habrobracon. Proc. Natl. Acad. Sci. USA 24: 80–85.

BUTENANDT, A., W. WEIDEL and E. BECKER, 1940 Kynurenin als Augenpigmentbildung auslösendes Agens bei Insekten. Naturwissenschaften 28: 63–64.

BUTENANDT, A., W. WEIDEL and H. SCHLOSSBERG, 1949 3-Oxykynurenin als cn^+-Gen-ahhängiges Glied im intermediären Tryptophan-Stoffwechsel. Z. Naturfosch. 4b: 242–244.

CASPARI, E., 1933 Über die Wirkung eines pleiotropen Gens bei der Mehlmotte *Ephestia kühniella* Zeller. Arch. Entwicklungsmech. Org. (Wilhelm Roux) 130: 353–381.

CLANCY, C. W., 1942 The development of eye colors in *Drosophila melanogaster*. Further studies on the mutant claret. Genetics 27: 417–440.

COCHRAN, D. G., 1975 Excretion in insects, pp. 177–281 in *Insect Biochemistry and Function*, edited by D. J. CANDY and B. A. KILBY. Chapman and Hall, London.

COMFORT, N. C., 1995 Two genes, no enzyme: a second look at BARBARA McCLINTOCK and the 1951 Cold Spring Harbor Symposium. Genetics 140: 1161–1166.

GHOSH, D., and FORREST, H. S., 1967 Enzymatic studies on the hydroxylation of kynurenine in *Drosophila melanogaster*. Genetics 55: 423–431.

GOLDSCHMIDT, R., 1951 Chromosomes and genes. Cold Spring Harbor Symp. Quant. Biol. 16: 1–11.

HOROWITZ, N. H., 1995 One-gene-one-enzyme: remembering biochemical genetics. Protein Sci. 4: 1017–1019.

HOROWITZ, N. H., and U. LEUPOLD, 1951 Some recent studies bearing on the one gene-one enzyme hypothesis. Cold Spring Harbor Symp. Quant. Biol. 16: 65–74.

KELLER, E. F., 1983 *A Feeling for the Organism*. W. H. Freeman and Company, New York.

McCLINTOCK, B., 1951 Chromosome organization and genic expression. Cold Spring Harbor Symp. Quant. Biol. 16: 13–47.

STURTEVANT, A. H., 1920 The vermilion gene and gynandromorphism. Proc. Soc. Exp. Biol. Med. 17: 70–71.

STURTEVANT, A. H., 1965 *A History of Genetics*. Harper & Row, New York.

TATUM, E. L., and A. J. HAAGEN-SMIT, 1941 Identification of Drosophila V⁺ hormone of bacterial origin. J. Biol. Chem. 140: 575–580.

WAGNER, R. P., 1989 On the origins of the gene-enzyme hypothesis. J. Hered. 80: 503–504.

June 1996

A Metabolic Basis for Dominance and Recessivity

Peter D. Keightley

Institute of Cell, Animal and Population Biology, University of Edinburgh, West Mains Road, Edinburgh, EH9 3JT, Scotland

THE reasons for the existence of genetic dominance have provoked much debate in the literature, starting with FISHER's (1928) paper on a possible evolutionary explanation for dominance. Any theory for the basis of dominance and recessivity, whether evolutionary or physiological, should explain three patterns in dominance relationships of the diploid phenotypes. The first is MENDEL's observation that the heterozygote is often indistinguishable in phenotype from one or the other of the homozygotes, and we now know that in the vast majority of cases the wild type is dominant over the mutant. Second, in the few cases where measurement of degrees of dominance for mutations of small phenotypic effect has been carried out, it appears that the heterozygote phenotype is on average close to intermediate (CROW and SIMMONS 1983). Third, there are several interesting series of mutations at the same locus that produce different phenotypes, *e.g.,* the *albino* series of mutants in rodents. In such cases, heterozygotes between "lower" mutant alleles of the series are usually intermediate in phenotype, whereas the wild type is usually dominant over all of them.

In 1981 H. KACSER and J. A. BURNS published in GENETICS an explanation for dominance based on properties of metabolic systems that can account for each of the above phenomena. They showed that dominance of the wild type over null alleles is an *inevitable* consequence of the kinetic properties of metabolic systems, and their theory has become widely accepted as the explanation of dominance of the wild type over the mutant for the majority of cases. Sadly, HENRIK KACSER died on March 13, 1995, ending his scientific career which for more than 40 years was focused on the kinetic properties of living systems. I first met HENRIK in 1981 as an undergraduate student and can well recall his great satisfaction at having published this paper. Although some of the basic ideas concerning dominance in metabolic systems appeared much earlier (KACSER 1963), the 1981 paper with BURNS was the culmination of years of experimental and theoretical effort directed toward understanding the consequences of changes of enzyme activity on properties of metabolism.

Evolutionary and physiological explanations for dominance: FISHER (1928) proposed a general explanation for dominance based on selection of alleles that increase dominance of the wild type. FISHER noted that heterozygotes far outnumber mutant homozygotes, so the selection pressure acting on heterozygotes to change the phenotype toward wild type would be much stronger than that acting on homozygotes. He argued that an intermediate phenotype for heterozygotes must have been the "original" state for new mutations in the history of a species and concluded that an evolutionary explanation for dominance of the wild type was necessary. In reaching this conclusion, FISHER seems to have been particularly impressed by the pattern found for series of mutant alleles at the same locus in which heterozygotes between the mutants produce intermediate phenotypes, while dominance of the wild type is typical.

WRIGHT (1934) challenged FISHER's theory of the evolution of dominance by selection at modifier loci by showing that the selection coefficients of dominance-modifier alleles would be extremely small, of the order of the mutation rate, and selection would be swamped by the random process of mutation. WRIGHT put forward an alternative explanation for the general prevalence of recessivity, but also emphasized that there would need to be different explanations in different cases. He envisaged a "chain of processes" linking genes with phenotypes and placed particular emphasis on enzymes whose importance in intermediary metabolism had become known. WRIGHT considered the relationship between the activity of one enzyme in a metabolic pathway and the steady-state rate of production of the product of the pathway (the pathway flux). The pathway consisted of a chain of nearly irreversible monomolecular transformations in which the rate of each step was proportional to the product of enzyme activity and substrate concentration. Because the product of one step was the substrate for the next, the effect of changing one enzyme's activity depended on the activities of all the others. WRIGHT predicted a hyperbolic

Author e-mail: p.keightley@edinburgh.ac.uk

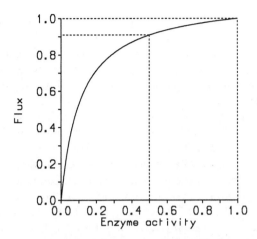

FIGURE 1.—Flux (arbitrary units) as a function of the activity of one enzyme in a pathway of monomolecular reactions with 10 steps catalyzed by unsaturated enzymes with equivalent activities. A reduction in the activity of one enzyme by 50% leads to only a 9% reduction in flux.

relationship between enzyme activity and flux. Thus, if the wild-type enzyme activity is usually at the plateau of the flux-enzyme curve and the enzyme activity of the heterozygote is intermediate, null mutants tend to be recessive (Figure 1). Although WRIGHT did not agree with FISHER's argument about the evolution of dominance modifier alleles, he still invoked an evolutionary mechanism by arguing that the wild-type activity would tend to lie on the plateau of the curve owing to selection for a "safety factor," an argument also used by HALDANE (1930).

Development of theory of the control of metabolic processes: KACSER and BURNS' explanation of the underlying basis for dominance and recessivity rests upon global properties of complex metabolic systems, which result in the control of flux being shared among many enzymes, and upon analysis of the behavior of some simple model metabolic pathways. KACSER's ideas for the control of metabolic processes and his kinetic approach to biological phenomena came directly from his background in physical chemistry, which he studied at Queen's University, Belfast. He came to the University of Edinburgh in 1951 to take a Diploma course at the Institute of Animal Genetics. This course was set up specifically to attract students into genetics from other fields. C. H. WADDINGTON, the Professor of Animal Genetics at the Institute, was particularly keen on an interdisciplinary approach to problems in genetics (WADDINGTON 1969) and appointed KACSER to the staff of the Institute in 1955. KACSER was very amused to tell the story of how he was appointed to the academic staff: during a chance conversation, WADDINGTON asked him what he would be doing next, to which KACSER replied he didn't know. WADDINGTON asked him if he would like a tenured position at the Institute and that, apparently, was that!

BURNS came to the Institute of Animal Genetics with

a background in physics to take a post in the Epigenetics Research Group in 1962, and went on to do a Ph.D. with KACSER. He studied the relationship between phenotype and genotype in multienzyme systems, and began by setting up model metabolic systems on an analog computer. BURNS soon noted that increases of one enzyme's activity often produced little effect on a pathway flux, and this led naturally to the idea of "control coefficients" (earlier called sensitivity coefficients), which have analogies in engineering and economics, and were also studied in the context of control of metabolism by HIGGINS (1965). The control coefficient, C, is defined as the fractional response of a systemic property of a metabolic system such as a flux (J) to a fractional change in the activity of one enzyme (E_i)

$$C_i^J = \frac{\partial J/J}{\partial E_i/E_i} \tag{1}$$

In their landmark 1973 paper, KACSER and BURNS laid down a logically consistent framework for measuring the extent to which elements of a metabolic system exert control over systemic properties such as fluxes or metabolite concentrations. This metabolic control analysis is having an increasingly important influence in biochemistry (reviewed by FELL 1992). Terms such as "rate limiting step," "key enzyme," or "pacemaker enzyme" have dogged the logical analysis of the control of metabolism, and KACSER was energetically against the use of such terms, as many of his students will remember with amusement. KACSER and BURNS's (1973) analysis of rate control of biological processes was published almost at the same time as an analysis of the same problem by HEINRICH and RAPOPORT (1974), working in Berlin. For any metabolic system of any complexity at steady state in which the rates of reaction are proportional to enzyme concentration and enzymes are parameters rather than variables of the system, the Edinburgh and Berlin groups independently showed that the sum over all enzymes of control coefficients for a flux is unity:

$$\sum C_i^J = 1 \tag{2}$$

The summation property was observed by BURNS, who was conducting empirical investigations of the kinetic properties of model metabolic systems by solving the nonlinear equations for the fluxes with an analog computer. It is valid for complex systems involving nonlinearities such as saturation and feedback inhibition. The summation property constrains the extent to which different enzymes control flux. Experiments involving the individual modulation of the enzymes controlling a flux have since provided evidence for the validity of the summation theorem (GROEN et al. 1982; SALTER et al. 1986).

A metabolic explanation for dominance and recessivity: In common with WRIGHT's (1934) analysis, KACSER

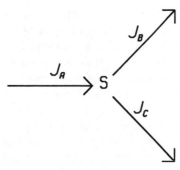

FIGURE 2.—A branched metabolic pathway in which competition for a common substrate, S, occurs at the branch point. At steady-state the flux in the common branch (J_A) is the sum of the fluxes in the competing branches (J_B) and (J_C).

and BURNS (1981) emphasized the central importance of the enzymes among classes of gene product. Measurable phenotypes of metabolism are fluxes, flux time integrals, or substrate pool concentrations, and traits more usually observed are functions of these. (Enzyme activity itself can be considered as a trait, but heterozygotes are usually intermediate in activity.) In simple model metabolic systems similar to those investigated by WRIGHT, they showed that the curve relating flux with enzyme activity tends to have the form of a rectangular hyperbola. Numerous studies, many from KACSER's own laboratory, in which the activity of an enzyme can be varied from zero to the wild-type activity, support this. There will usually be several enzymes in a given metabolic pathway, so the summation property (2) implies that the majority of control coefficients will be small, and as there is a hyperbolic relationship between flux and enzyme activity, recessivity of null mutants is an automatic consequence (Figure 1). The lack of dominance between lower members of allelic series can also be explained by such arguments: these mutants have low enzyme activities, so have flux control coefficients approaching unity and a linear relationship between the three phenotypes. Thus, KACSER and BURNS used models similar to WRIGHT's to illustrate their point, but their key conclusion was that the wild-type enzyme activity lies on the plateau of the flux-enzyme curve as an inevitable consequence of the kinetic properties of metabolic systems, and evolutionary mechanisms such as the evolution of "safety factors" as invoked by WRIGHT are not needed. While selection to decrease the sensitivity of flux with respect to one enzyme is possible (HARTL et al. 1985), the summation property implies a consequent increase in sensitivity with respect to the other enzymes in the pathway.

The arguments become more complicated for branched pathways for which an increase of enzyme activity in a competing pathway leads to a decrease in flux and hence to negative control coefficients (Figure 2). LAPORTE et al. (1984) investigated the circumstances in which a flux can become highly sensitive to variation

of enzyme activity in a competing branch. One situation where this can occur is when a competing flux is large relative to the flux being measured. Because of the summation property, the presence of negative control coefficients implies that the sum of positive control coefficients elsewhere in the system will be greater than unity. KACSER and BURNS argued that the majority of flux control coefficients will be positive (i.e., increases in enzyme activity will generally lead to increases in flux); there may be negative control coefficients owing to branched pathways, but these coefficients will tend to be small. It turns out, however, that the relationship between flux in a branch and the activity of an enzyme in the same branch is a rectangular hyperbola, and the sum of control coefficients of the flux with respect to the enzymes in the branch is less than unity. It follows that if there are several enzymes in the branch, recessivity for the flux is expected for null mutants. Furthermore, degrees of dominance are the same for all fluxes and metabolite pool concentrations in the system, so recessivity for null mutants is the expectation for all "metabolic traits" despite the possible presence of high positive or negative control coefficients (KEIGHTLEY and KACSER 1987; KEIGHTLEY 1996).

Further evidence against selection theories: Two of the most telling arguments against an evolutionary explanation for dominance are due to CHARLESWORTH (1979) and ORR (1991).

CHARLESWORTH (1979) analyzed a model of the evolution of dominance by selection of modifier alleles and showed that such a model predicts no relationship between effects of mutant alleles on fitness and their degrees of dominance. However, experiments in which spontaneous mutations are allowed to accumulate in Drosophila second chromosomes show that lethals and mutations of major effect on viability tend to be nearly recessive, while minor viability mutations tend to be additive or slightly recessive (MUKAI et al. 1972). The model of dominance based on metabolic pathways predicts such a pattern.

ORR (1991) surveyed dominance relationships of mutations in the alga Chlamydomonas reinhardtii, which, apart from a brief diploid phase, normally spends almost all its life as a haploid. Diploid cells also occur spontaneously at a low frequency, allowing dominance of mutations to be measured. ORR showed that mutations are as often recessive in Chlamydomonas as in Drosophila. The evolution of dominance of the wild type therefore seems unlikely for this predominantly haploid organism, as the diploid is rare in nature and the opportunity for selection is small (assuming its ancestors were also haploid). ORR also found a prevalence of recessivity for mutations affecting the flagellum, which is not present at all in the nonflagellate diploid cell.

Dominant mutations: KACSER and BURNS' "molecular basis of dominance" is formulated in terms of the

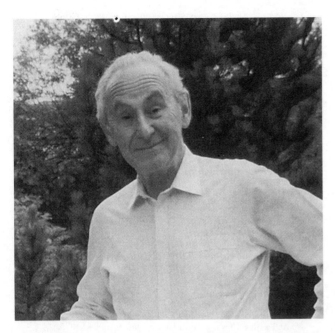

FIGURE 3.—Photograph of HENRIK KACSER (1918–1995) taken in the summer of 1994.

theory of the behavior of complex metabolic systems (which predicts in general a diminishing-returns relationship between flux or substrate pool and enzyme activity) and the summation property with the majority of control coefficients positive. A requirement of the theory is that the majority of enzymes in a pathway are not close to saturation, which can lead to dominant mutations (CORNISH-BOWDEN 1987), but KACSER (1987) argues that this is unlikely. An implicit assumption of their theory is that the relationship between the measured phenotype and the flux is not strongly nonlinear, as this can also produce dominance of the mutant.

The analysis clearly does not apply to gene products involved in the timing or tissue specificity of gene expression, or to hormone/receptor systems. It is not known what proportion of expressed genes encode enzymes or, perhaps more relevantly, what fraction of mutations known from classical genetics is at genes encoding enzymes. KACSER and BURNS (1981) do not claim that their analysis applies to genes encoding nonenzyme products. While cases of dominant or semi-dominant mutations are far outnumbered by recessives, the biological basis of dominant mutations is often interesting, and these are more frequently at structural or regulatory genes than at enzyme loci. WILKIE (1994) has extensively reviewed the molecular basis of dominant mutations and has shown that many of the underlying mechanisms fall far outside the KACSER and BURNS framework. Two broad categories for the mechanisms of dominant mutations are haploinsufficiency and gain of function. For example, haploinsufficient mutations occur at loci encoding the structural protein collagen, which is needed in large quantities (WILLING et al. 1992). Huntington's disease is one of five currently

known dominant hereditary neurodegenerative diseases caused by expansion of trinucleotide CAG repeats, resulting in translation of a lengthened polyglutamine stretch. It is suggested that in diseases such as Huntington's, the expanded polyglutamine stretch results in a gain of function that leads to neuronal death (NASIR et al. 1995). HODGKIN (1993) has highlighted some of the more unusual processes that can lead to dominant mutations. There are several examples of dominant gain-of-function mutations in which the mutant produces a toxic gene product. For example, mutant alleles at the murine *brown* locus (whose product is an enzyme involved in melanin biosynthesis) are mostly recessive, but there are rare examples of dominant alleles. One is a missense mutation that leads to the disruption of the melanosome and the release of poisonous products into the cytoplasm (JOHNSON and JACKSON 1992).

Simultaneous changes of several enzyme activities: The treatment of fluxes or substrate concentrations as characters and of enzymes as their genetic determinants has also been applied to the problem of the nature of epistatic interactions. In general, mutations that decrease enzyme activity at different loci will tend to generate antagonistic epistasis for flux, because a decrease in the activity of one enzyme in a pathway makes flux less sensitive to changes in the activities of enzymes in other parts of the pathway (KEIGHTLEY 1989). Synergistic epistasis is more likely for cases where traits are nonlinear functions of flux or pool levels (SZATHMARY 1993).

NIEDERBERGER et al. (1992) conducted a detailed experimental investigation of the consequences of simultaneous changes of activities of several enzymes affecting the same flux in the tryptophan biosynthesis pathway in yeast. In experiments with tetraploid yeast containing between zero and four copies of different *TRP* genes, flux to tryptophan is insensitive to downmodulation of individual enzyme activities to as low as 25%, but null alleles abolish tryptophan synthesis. In a series of upmodulation experiments in which multicopy vectors were used to increase activities of single enzymes by factors of between 10 and 50, increases in flux of only about a factor of 1.2 were observed. However, with *simultaneous* increases in activities of four of the enzymes in the pathway, flux increased by a factor of 8, much more than expected by summing the increases from independent changes. Such synergistic epistasis is exactly as predicted by metabolic control theory: increases of an enzyme activity sensitize flux to changes of other enzyme activities in a pathway (see also DYKHUIZEN et al. 1987).

KACSER later worked with J. R. SMALL and L. ACERENZA on predicting the effects of simultaneous finite changes of several enzyme activities on flux and metabolite pool concentrations. This is of practical importance because experimentalists are rarely able to detect effects of small perturbations of metabolism, but metabolic control theory is concerned with such small changes. They devised a "universal method" for achieving increases in the production of an *in vivo* metabolite by manipulating a limited number of enzyme activities without perturbing fluxes and metabolite concentrations elsewhere in metabolism, a procedure with implications for industrial biosynthesis where overproduction of single metabolites is sometimes the objective (KACSER and ACERENZA 1993). KACSER's contributions to the understanding of the control of metabolism were increasingly recognized during his later years. His unique approach to science and original thinking profoundly influenced many students and colleagues at Edinburgh and elsewhere, and he is greatly missed by all.

I thank D. J. BOND, J. A. BURNS, A. CABALLERO, A. CORNISH-BOWDEN, D. S. FALCONER, W. G. HILL, and S. A. KNOTT for helpful discussions.

LITERATURE CITED

CHARLESWORTH, B., 1979   Evidence against Fisher's theory of dominance. Nature **278**: 848–849.

CORNISH-BOWDEN, A., 1987   Dominance is not inevitable. J. Theor. Biol. **125**: 333–338.

CROW, J. F., and M. J. SIMMONS, 1983   The mutation load in Drosophila, pp. 1–35 in *The Genetics and Biology of Drosophila*, Vol. 3C, edited by M. ASHBURNER, H. L. CARSON and J. N. THOMPSON. Academic Press, London.

DYKHUIZEN, D. E., A. M., DEAN and D. L. HARTL, 1987   Metabolic flux and fitness. Genetics **115**: 25–31.

FELL, D. A., 1992   Metabolic control analysis—a survey of its theoretical and experimental development. Biochem. J. **286**: 313–330.

FISHER, R. A., 1928   The possible modification of the response of the wild type to recurrent mutations. Am. Nat. **62**: 115–126.

GROEN, A. K., R. J. A. WANDERS, H. V. WESTERHOFF, R. VAN DER MEER and J. M. TAGER, 1982   Quantification of the contribution of various steps to the control of mitochondrial respiration. J. Biol. Chem. **257**: 2754–2757.

HALDANE, J. B. S., 1930   A note on Fisher's theory of dominance. Am. Nat. **63**: 87–90.

HARTL, D. L., D. E. DYKHUIZEN and A. M. DEAN, 1985   Limits of adaptation: the evolution of selective neutrality. Genetics **111**: 655–674.

HEINRICH, R., and T. A. RAPOPORT, 1974   A linear steady state treatment of enzyme chains. Eur. J. Biochem. **42**: 89–102.

HIGGINS, J., 1965   Dynamics and control in cellular reactions, pp. 13–46 in *Control of Energy Metabolism,* edited by B. CHANCE, R. K. ESTABROOK and J. R. WILLIAMSON. Academic Press, New York.

HODGKIN, J., 1993   Fluxes, doses and poisons—molecular perspectives on dominance. Trends Genet. **9**: 1–2.

JOHNSON, R., and I. J. JACKSON, 1992   *Light* is a dominant mouse mutation resulting in premature cell death. Nat. Genet. **1**: 226–229.

KACSER, H., 1963   The kinetic structure of organisms, pp. 25–41 in *Biological Organisation at the Cellular and Supercellular Level,* edited by R. J. C. HARRIS. Academic Press, New York and London.

KACSER, H., 1987   Dominance not inevitable but very likely. J. Theor. Biol. **126**: 505–506.

KACSER, H., and L. ACERENZA, 1993   A universal method for achieving increases in metabolite production. Eur. J. Biochem. **216**: 361–367.

KACSER, H., and J. A. BURNS, 1973   The control of flux. Symp. Soc. Exp. Biol. **27**: 65–104.

KACSER, H., and J. A. BURNS, 1981   The molecular basis of dominance. Genetics **97**: 639–666.

KEIGHTLEY, P. D., 1989   Models of quantitative variation of flux in metabolic pathways. Genetics **121**: 869–876.

KEIGHTLEY, P. D., 1996   Metabolic models of selection response. J. Theor. Biol. (in press).

KEIGHTLEY, P. D., and H. KACSER, 1987   Dominance, pleiotropy and metabolic structure. Genetics **117**: 319–329.

LAPORTE, D. C., K. WALSH and D. E. KOSHLAND, Jr., 1984   The branch point effect. J. Biol. Chem. **259**: 14068–14075.

MUKAI, T., S. I. CHIGUSA, L. E. METTLER and J. F. CROW, 1972   Mutation rate and dominance of genes affecting viability in *Drosophila melanogaster*. Genetics **72**: 333–355.

NASIR, J., S. B. FLORESCO, J. R. O'KUSKY, V. M. DIEWERT, J. M. RICHMAN et al., 1995   Targeted disruption of the Huntington's disease gene results in embryonic lethality and behavioral and morphological changes in heterozygotes. Cell **81**: 811–823.

NIEDERBERGER, P., R. PRASAD, G. MIOZZARI and H. KACSER, 1992   A strategy for increasing an *in vivo* flux by genetic manipulations. Biochem. J. **287**: 473–479.

ORR, H. A., 1991   A test of Fisher's theory of dominance. Proc. Natl. Acad. Sci. USA **88**: 11413–11415.

SALTER, M., R. G. KNOWLES and C. I. POGSON, 1986   Quantitation of the importance of individual steps in the control of aromatic amino acid metabolism. Biochem. J. **234**: 635–647.

SZATHMARY, E., 1993   Do deleterious mutations act synergistically? Metabolic control theory provides a partial answer. Genetics **133**: 127–132.

WADDINGTON, C. H., 1969   *Towards a Theoretical Biology*. Edinburgh University Press, Edinburgh.

WILKIE, A. O. M., 1994   The molecular basis of genetic dominance. J. Med. Genet. **31**: 89–98.

WILLING, M. C., C. J. PRUCHNO, M. ATKINSON and P. H. BYERS, 1992   Osteogenesis imperfecta type I is commonly due to a COL1A1 null allele of type I collagen. Am. J. Hum. Genet. **51**: 508–515.

WRIGHT, S., 1934   Molecular and evolutionary theories of dominance. Am. Nat. **68**: 24–53.

July 1996

Alexander Hollaender
Myth and Mensch

R. C. von Borstel[*,†] and Charles M. Steinberg[*]

*Basel Institute for Immunology, CH4058 Basel, Switzerland; and
†160 Department of Genetics, University of Alberta, Edmonton, Alberta T6G 2E9, Canada

SCIENCE is not kind to the memories of its former practitioners. We were gently reminded of this brutal fact by the editors of the *Perspectives* section of GENETICS after they read the original version of this essay on ALEXANDER HOLLAENDER. While the insiders, those who had known ALEX, those who had been at Oak Ridge, might find our essay amusing and perhaps even enlightening, they are a dying breed. These days, most of the readers of GENETICS would have never even heard of HOLLAENDER, and as a consequence, would have no motivation even to try to understand what we wanted to say. Upon reflection, we had to agree with the editors. Mentioning a name as illustrious as BRIDGES draws a blank stare from most of our young colleagues. MORGAN's name recognition is a bit better, but after all, a centimorgan is a unit.

ALEXANDER HOLLAENDER was a radiation biologist. His scientific interest was mutation research. SETLOW (1987) and VON BORSTEL (1987), in their obituaries of HOLLAENDER, described his numerous scientific contributions. The most important of these was that the action spectrum for UV-induced mutation of spores of the ring-worm fungus *Trichophyton mentagrophytes* resembled the absorption spectrum of nucleic acids (EMMONS and HOLLAENDER 1939; HOLLAENDER 1941; HOLLAENDER and EMMONS 1941). Thus, HOLLAENDER realized that genes were made of nucleic acids at a time when most of his contemporaries were sure that they were made of proteins. No, most of their contemporaries did not change their views because of the work by HOLLAENDER and EMMONS, nor the work by KNAPP *et al.* (1939); they either explained it away or ignored it. As KUHN (1962) would have put it, the time was not yet ripe for a scientific revolution. But eventually the paradigm did change. In retrospect, it is clear that HOLLAENDER fired one of the first shots in the molecular biological revolution.

HOLLAENDER's other major scientific contribution is known as the "oxygen effect" (HOLLAENDER *et al.* 1951). Most, perhaps all, of the biological effects of ionizing radiation are dramatically reduced in the ab-

sence of molecular oxygen. In one sense, this contribution was bad news. It meant that the cells in the center of large tumor masses, which are often anoxic, would be resistant to radiation therapy. The good news, however, was that the biological effects of radiation could be modulated to achieve desirable results, a possibility that was not so widely recognized at the time. The oxygen effect was actually an old and forgotten discovery by HOLTHUSEN (1921), which HOLLAENDER realized could be put to practical use. Many people date the beginning of research on DNA repair as 1958 when RUTH HILL discovered radiation-sensitive strains of bacteria. More than 20 years earlier, however, HOLLAENDER and CURTIS (1935) had aired the possibility of a mechanism for the recovery of cells from the effects of ultraviolet radiation, and seven years prior to 1958 HOLLAENDER had been pushing people at Oak Ridge to study organic "radical traps" as a potential way of protecting against the effects of ionizing radiation.

These are solid scientific achievements. However, it is a moral certainty that were HOLLAENDER "just" a scientist, we would not have been invited to write this essay. ALEX achieved greatness as a scientific impresario, as the founder and first director of the Biology Division at Oak Ridge National Laboratory (ORNL). The enormity of this assertion may not sink in immediately, for there have been many great directors of institutions devoted to biological research. But JIM WATSON, for instance, did not become great because he was director of the Cold Spring Harbor Laboratory; WATSON had already achieved greatness before he became director. In our opinion, ALEXANDER HOLLAENDER was a unique example in this regard. Had he been recognized as a great scientist, he might have been offered a professorship at Harvard or Stanford. Had he been recognized as a great organizer of science, he might have been offered the presidency of MIT or Caltech. In any event, he would have found a more likely venue to demonstrate his talents than that God-forsaken hundred square miles bounded by the Clinch River and the Black Oak Ridge.

What was so great about Oak Ridge? In one sense, great means large. In this day of genome projects, biotechnology conglomerates and university megalabs, no one is likely to be impressed by the size of the Biology Division, which was never more than roughly 200 doctoral-level scientists. In the early sixties, however, that was big biology if not Big Science, a phrase coined by the then-director of ORNL, ALVIN WEINBERG. Despite the best laid plans of the Atomic Energy Commission (AEC; the predecessor of the Department of Energy), plans predicated on the assumption that real research would not thrive in a national laboratory not closely associated with a major university, HOLLAENDER reared a Biology Division devoted to basic research that was larger than those at Brookhaven, Argonne and Los Alamos combined. As would be expected in a federal laboratory, there was much programmatic research done by relatively large groups. While even ALEX was unable to ensure that all of the large-scale efforts were of the highest quality, we would not want to denigrate them. Indeed, some, such as the mouse mutation project, were national assets. As would also be expected in an environment dominated by engineers, there was much technical research. This, too, we do not wish to denigrate; indeed, we were involved in some of it ourselves (transmutation of ^{33}P from ^{33}S). But the answer to the question posed at the beginning of this paragraph is that Oak Ridge was a great place to do basic research. HOLLAENDER conjured up this research paradise out of thin air.

In addition to his scientific contributions and presiding over the ORNL Biology Division, HOLLAENDER was famous as an organizer of scientific symposia on a grand scale. His first venture into this field, which was an attempt to mitigate the isolation imposed by the location of Oak Ridge and by its security gates, is described in detail below. But these activities soon expanded beyond the confines of East Tennessee and the North American continent. Organizing symposia became his preferred method of biotechnology transfer to the second and third worlds, and he continued doing it to the end of his life. He personally initiated more than 40 such symposia after his retirement as Director of the Biology Division.

This essay was written at the Basel Institute for Immunology (BII). One of us (C.M.S.) moved there from Oak Ridge when the BII was founded some 25 years ago. The other author (R.C.vB.) has spent two sabbatical years at the BII and is a persistent visitor. NIELS JERNE always claimed that Caltech was the model for the BII. Maybe so, but the BII is far closer to being Oak Ridge Europe than it is to being Caltech East. Some day, perhaps, we shall write an essay on "NIELS JERNE: Myth and Mensch." What is interesting in the present context is how the two directors with polar opposite public images—HOLLAENDER the autocrat and JERNE the democrat—created such similar institutions. Obviously the Mensch is more important than the Myth.

HOLLAENDER moved to Oak Ridge in 1947 to become Director of the Biology Division of the ORNL. The conditions were right. The AEC was planning a nuclear energy future for the United States, the budget was expanding, and scientific fields were not yet crowded with individuals who had chosen science as a high-salaried occupation (a state of affairs created by Sputnik) rather than as an area of intense interest. From the way the Biology Division came to be structured, a case can be made that HOLLAENDER's vision for biology placed genetics at the core, with the rest of the biological sciences radiating outward. During the decade of the fifties, the Biology Division was unique for the variety of organisms used for genetic experiments. Genetics was needed to carry out the *raison d'être* of the Biology Division, that of determining the fundamental actions of ionizing and nonionizing radiation on cells and organisms and of determining what the findings might imply for human health in the new age of atomic energy. A competent cadre of young scientists was assembled, and the interactions among them created a center of excellence during the 1950s and 1960s. Eventually the Division reached a size of about 180 principal investigators, with postdoctoral fellows and visiting investigators bringing the total to over 200 scientists during HOLLAENDER's heyday. At that time, only the summer gatherings of scientists at Woods Hole were comparable in number, and research on biology at the ORNL lasted all year round.

In one respect, however, conditions were far from ideal. Oak Ridge was far from the lights of any big city, and until the summer of 1952 not only the laboratory but the town itself remained behind locked gates.

How did HOLLAENDER accomplish this in a small town in the foothills of the Cumberland Mountains? To answer that question, we need to consider ALEX the Mensch and ALEX the Myth. These two HOLLAENDERS may overlap, but they do not coincide. Personally, we have a great affection for ALEX the Mensch. Thus, although we have tried hard to avoid it, we may have created a few new myths of our own here.

The allocator of research problems: *Myth:* ALEX assigned to each scientist the research projects he wanted done and told them which experiments to do.

Mensch: The Myth and the Mensch here are exactly 180 degrees out of phase. ALEX's method was simply to hire scientists who wanted to do the sort of research he wanted done. In an approach like that of the immune system, ALEX realized that selection is superior to instruction as a way to achieve a desired result. He hired the best scientists he could in a certain field and gave them complete freedom for research. He encouraged adventurous science by providing equipment, supplies, and a technician for each investigator and placed more than one scientist in each laboratory so that collaborations could flourish. Because universities in the late 1940s and 1950s found it difficult to acquire advanced equipment and supplies and required much teaching, a scientific career at the Biology Division of the ORNL was an opportunity to spend time in a scientific paradise.

No one was exempt from ALEX's badgering for publications. He was always telling each staff member to publish more. One could feel satisfied, with a new paper just appearing in *Nature*, the *Proceedings of the National Academy of Sciences* or GENETICS, a manuscript in press in another of these journals, and another in the editorial office, yet ALEX would say, "I know you got some more stuff," and as every investigator knows, he was usually right. He kept everyone on the edge of defensiveness about publications, and all of them kept publishing as much as they could muster. After a while, each staff member became pretty good at it.

The financial wizard: *Myth:* ALEX was a good administrator who attended to business so closely that the Biology Division thrived. He was a penny pincher, so the Division operated efficiently.

Mensch: The first axiom from which ALEX worked was, "They've got lots of money, and we've got to help them spend it wisely." ALEX was the biggest-spending penny pincher east of Texas, at least when he was spending someone else's money.

His first problem was to get the money to make the Biology Division grow. The fuel to keep the Division expanding came from paying scientists about 10% less than the average for ORNL. In the late 1940s and 1950s, the salaries paid young biologists in universities were even less than those paid by ALEX, so he could easily convince individuals about the good deal they were getting. Moreover, the cost of living in East Tennessee was the lowest in the country. The target budget for each division of ORNL was calculated on the average salary per person. Thus, by paying the biologists less, ALEX could hire more young scientists, which in turn justified a still higher budget for the next year. Because salaries consumed about 90% of all funds, the average growth of the Biology Division was close to 10% per year. This simple bootstrap operation worked for about 15 years.

After that, ALEX's skills as a fund-raiser began to show in other ways. He began making deals with the National Institutes of Health and the National Aeronautics and Space Administration to sell the expertise in the Biology Division to solve problems for these agencies. This research was carried out at the Biology Division, despite the strict AEC policy that subcontractors were not allowed to obtain funds from any other federal agency. The AEC and their administrative subclasses were afraid that growth, spending, and vision might get out of their control, and that is precisely what ALEX wanted.

The public relations expert: *Myth:* ALEX relied on ORNL policy and its public relations department to develop a national presence and to give itself visibility.

Mensch: ALEX was convinced that in order to thrive in the Cumberland foothills, he had to make himself visible nationally. He did his best to keep the Biology Division in the minds of biologists everywhere. For example, when he arrived in Oak Ridge, ALEX began a small weekly bulletin for the Biology Division, listing the travels and seminars of the staff members and the names of everyone who visited the laboratory, and each issue listed references that staff members had checked in incoming journals. Since he had built such a superb library, there were many articles to be checked. ALEX sent this little bulletin to friends and acquaintances in hundreds of colleges and universities, who came to welcome each issue. Anyone who requested it could receive the bulletin at no cost. He also sent out yearly lists of the papers published by Biology Division staff, with the offer to send any reprints that might interest the reader.

ALEX wanted everyone to visit Oak Ridge as speaker, adviser and rumor-monger to keep the staff informed about what was going on in cutting-edge science everywhere else. So he publicized the Biology Division both by bringing in many speakers from everywhere and by traveling to see scientists all over the globe. All of these were mentioned in the weekly bulletin and added to the mailing list.

Far from relying on ORNL policy, ALEX did his best to circumvent it. He worked relentlessly to open the Biology Division for all to visit. From the 1940s to the end of the 1960s, Oak Ridge tried to hide itself from view. Everyone in Oak Ridge had to have Q-clearance and visitors were regarded with suspicion. The security division of the AEC could and would prevent even the investigators at the laboratory from knowing what was going on simply by classifying everything "Confidential." Even so, this didn't stop the Soviet Union from exploding hydrogen bombs. From the 1960s, the gate to the Biology Division was the only gate at X-10, Y-12, and K-25 unguarded by a security officer. (These were code names, taken from the map coordinates for the three major AEC installations in Oak Ridge.)

Even before ALEX turned to other agencies for funds to run his continually growing Biology Division, he had found ways to extend the Biology Division operation extracurricularly by using other peoples' money. He initiated a small program of sending young staff scientists to visit Southern colleges and universities to present seminars about their work as well as to tout the wonders of the Biology Division. The traveling scientists were asked to size up people at these colleges and universities and invite the interested ones to come to Oak Ridge to work during the summer months. When this program was successfully under way, it was managed by the Oak Ridge Institute of Nuclear Studies (ORINS), an organization originally set up in the early 1950s that provided predoctoral fellowships for graduate students interested in radiation studies. ORINS saw the utility of the program and extended this idea to all Divisions of the

ORNL. Other investigators in other divisions were recruited by ORINS to travel to Southern schools, but the Biology Division always was the power user.

The apolitical politician: *Myth:* ALEX HOLLAENDER was apolitical. He steered clear of the liberal-conservative whirlpools that stirred the country in the post-World War II period.

Mensch: ALEX did not steer clear of the liberal-conservative polarity; he used the situation to his own advantage. ALEX started an annual symposium at Oak Ridge on various topics related to work being carried out in the Biology Division. For the 1954 symposium, he wanted to have LINUS PAULING as a speaker. LEWIS STRAUSS, the Chairman of the AEC, talked to ALEX, trying to dissuade him of his choice of PAULING as a visitor to Oak Ridge, because those were the days of JOSEPH MCCARTHY. J. EDGAR HOOVER apparently thought that LINUS PAULING was a security risk, and LEWIS STRAUSS did not want to get the AEC into trouble with MCCARTHY. ALEX persisted relentlessly. Finally, the Chairman of the Commission, out of frustration, offered to pay to have the symposium held outside of Oak Ridge. ALEX was ready and immediately suggested Gatlinburg. Thus the Gatlinburg Symposia were born, and thereafter many scientific divisions at Oak Ridge copied ALEX's example.

LINUS PAULING was invited to attend the 1954 Gatlinburg Symposium, but he never appeared.

ORNL and the other two operations at Oak Ridge had only a small base of political clout, amounting to two senators from Tennessee and the congressman representing the district where Oak Ridge was located. ALEX improved this clout for the Biology Division by the simple ploy of assigning to each research group a suitable scientific consultant. The consultants were usually from different states, and they usually were eminent enough in their own state to be listened to. Whenever ALEX needed a little persuasion in Washington, he would ask one or more of the consultants to send a little note to their senators and/or congressmen to explain the problem. In this way, the Biology Division was represented by about 30 or 40 members of the House and Senate.

The traveler: *Myth:* ALEX liked to travel.

Mensch: Here Myth and Mensch coincide exactly. ALEX did like to travel. He devised ways to travel internationally while helping others to "spend money wisely."

After sending MARY ESTHER GAULDEN to South America as a scout in 1959, he initiated the Latin American Symposia, which the National Science Foundation (NSF) assisted in financing. The NSF funds were usually matched by the host nation, and every European country paid to send at least one scientist to speak at the symposia in "third-world countries" as they then were called. The annual Latin American Symposia always were arranged by Biology Division staff scientists, by one or two of the leading scientists in the chosen field

from outside, and by the hosts who had agreed to hold the symposium in their country.

ALEX didn't stop there. He decided that South Asia would be his next target, and so the South Asian Symposia were born. Here he exhibited his true genius in helping people spend their money wisely. The U.S. Agency for International Development raised most of its funds by having nations provide their own currency to pay for goods, like wheat, that were "given" to these nations in times of famine and for other needs. These local currencies were used mostly by the Central Intelligence Agency (CIA) for information collecting and other, more distasteful uses. Somehow, ALEX was able to convince someone in the federal hierarchy that some of these funds should be used to support the International Symposia. It never approached one part per million of the sums used by the CIA, but ALEX certainly did much more for international relations than the CIA ever did. In addition to promoting international relations, the symposia provided a lot of publicity for the Biology Division.

The domineering director: *Myth:* ALEX dominated others by the force of his personality and character. He collected and discarded scientific talent helter-skelter.

Mensch: There is no doubt that ALEX frightened those who could be frightened easily, but this was not how he operated. He never feared surrounding himself with individuals who had more intellectual ability than he had himself. A few of these were real intellectual giants, and several others were creative technical wizards with breadth of vision. These alone could provide the scope, the ideas, and the dynamism of the Biology Division for which ALEX, as Director, could take full credit.

Moreover, ALEX was indeed a collector of scientific talent, but a collector with exquisite taste. He collected potentially capable young scientists and urged them to collaborate with more experienced individuals. In the Oak Ridge of ALEX's day, the independent postdoctoral fellow was not an oxymoron. If a person did not take off on his own, he or she was shuffled into a highly successful laboratory. If those persons then failed either to integrate or to take off on their own initiative, ALEX found academic positions for them. He was proud of his ability never to fire anyone, but to find suitable positions for everyone. If they departed, it wasn't for lack of publications; ALEX had already seen to that.

The art collector: *Myth:* HENRIETTA HOLLAENDER had the artistic sensibility and the good taste for whatever art that ALEX and HENRIETTA acquired.

Mensch: ALEX and HENRIETTA were strong promoters of all the arts in Oak Ridge, and he was the first President of an Arts Council that brought together the symphony, the art gallery, the chamber music group, the theater, and the choral society as a strong voice in community affairs.

When ALEX emigrated to the United States after

World War I, his most prized possession was a drawing by OSKAR KOKOSCHKA. He and HENRIETTA collected the art of talented young artists with skill and insight. For example, ALEX happened to walk by an art dealer's window when he saw and purchased on the spot the first painting that FRIEDENSREICH HUNDERTWASSER ever sold. ALEX purchased perhaps the best painting that ASGER JORN had ever done. As was often the case, this painting was done during a transitional period of the artist.

HENRIETTA and ALEX did work together on buying art, but ALEX was always in charge. HENRIETTA would say, "Alex, I can't choose between these two." ALEX would reply, "We take this one." At another studio, ALEX would say, "Henrietta, take one of these three." Then HENRIETTA would make her choice. There was the occasional failure. HENRIETTA put it best: "We went back to Rome to see how that young genius was developing . . . and he had become a poet!"

The HOLLAENDERS' collection had paintings and lithographs by nearly every important artist in the 20th Century. The range and variety of their collection of the Cobra artists (Copenhagen, Brussels, Amsterdam) was unparalleled in the United States at the end of the 1960s; the first Cobra show in the United States was held in Oak Ridge with but one picture from outside their own collection.

The HOLLAENDERS were approached to leave their art collection in Oak Ridge. But when ALEX's postretirement consultantship with the Biology Division was canceled, HENRIETTA announced that she wouldn't leave anything in "this village." Their art collection now resides in the Elvehjem Museum at the University of Wisconsin.

Moreover, ALEX collected fossils from the nearby Cumberland Mountains where he hiked every Sunday. These he gave away as gifts to visiting scientists from around the world, whether or not they had room in their luggage.

The perfectionist: *Myth:* ALEX never made a mistake.

Mensch: ALEX was skilled at blaming others for his mistakes, and he nearly always succeeded in convincing them it really was their fault. The rewriting of unwritten history was a powerful weapon in his arsenal. This ability made administrators tread lightly around him. ALEX's memory wasn't better than theirs; he was just more alert and pragmatic than they were. For example, in the mid-1960s it came to the attention of the AEC administrators in Washington, D.C., that assimilation of heavy isotopes in the bones could constitute a hazard. ALEX immediately reminded them that when he had come to Oak Ridge in 1947 he would have liked to set up a large group to study the problem, but he had been told that the effect of radiation on cells and tissues was enough for him to take on. He rubbed it in, elaborating more and more on why and how they had failed to heed his

advice and why they would never have gotten into such a mess if they had listened to him. Since nearly all of the administrators had changed in the 20 years since ALEX had moved to Oak Ridge, they had to take his verbal punishment lying down. Back at the Division, ALEX was asked if he thought his remonstrances would bring in any more money. He replied, "No, they know me too well."

ALEX conveniently forgot that he had insistently urged people to write proposals for the Biosatellite program. When the investigators who were canvassed argued strongly and loudly that it was a waste of time and money, he simply replied, "Yes, but we need the money." So, for reasons of loyalty, a number of investigators complied. Then, several years later, when a news article in *Nature* by JOHN TOOZE quoted JIM WATSON as saying, "Biosatellites are a waste of money," ALEX went around to tell the investigators that they "should never have gotten into this program."

The psychiatrist and probation officer: *Myth:* ALEX did not understand people and their needs very well.

Mensch: He understood the capabilities of people extremely well. At meetings where someone would make a snide remark or give praise about one of the staff members at Oak Ridge, he would add this knowledge to his intracranial database, and through a continual assessment process he would integrate all the information until he knew exactly how each individual in the Biology Division was regarded by the scientific community as a whole. Moreover, because he knew how each staff member thought, he used them for advice. He knew who was usually right, who was usually wrong, who was overly enthusiastic, who was overly cynical, and who had unusual views of problems that should be taken into account. Then he would act and take credit if things went well. If they did not go well, he would seek out the people who had given him wrong advice and tell them that they were to blame. ALEX had an unusual capacity for integrating information obtained from others, far beyond that of any other administrator that we have known. But even he occasionally was fooled by sycophants who would agree with him and carry out his ideas unthinkingly. Like all administrators everywhere, he was susceptible to believing they must be highly intelligent if they agreed to do everything he suggested.

Nevertheless, ALEX's suspiciousness and perspicacity of capability bore to the center of the souls of the staff members of the Biology Division, and he knew how best to develop and use the talents of the first, second, and third class scientists in the Biology Division, whether it was by punishment and reward, flattery of egos, or increases of salary. He never showed mercy for wasted resources. For example, if a person wasn't particularly interested in money, he was not rewarded with an increase in salary. ALEX knew there are multiple ways to massage vanities, and he never misused the best way. When people had done some excellent work, he put them on display. He carefully arranged ways for the scientists to be better appreciated, through seeing to it that they were invited to local, national, and international seminars, meetings, and symposia, but only when they had something interesting to say.

ALEX told each person what he had arranged for them, but many of the staff already knew how the world worked and assumed their invitation had been his doing. Nevertheless, there were always those who assumed their gift must have come from a chance reading by a symposium organizer of their latest papers. ALEX kept better control when everyone knew that the goodies of this world had come from him. The one time that ALEX didn't get a chance to mention it was the day when W. K. ARNOLD learned he had been made a member of the U.S. National Academy of Sciences. Before ALEX could say anything, BILL ARNOLD came up to ALEX and said, "You must have done a lot of work to get me admitted." ALEX just grinned and congratulated him.

The Optimist: *Myth:* ALEX was too realistic to be optimistic.

Mensch: ALEX's iron rule was *be optimistic at all times.* No matter how many large problems were looming, ALEX's smile always gave courage to everyone. From his smile, we believed he had every situation well in hand, and only he knew the real truth.

The only times that his optimism grew thin, and pragmatism set in fast, was at the end of the fiscal year when deficits were beginning to loom. When the extent of the short-fall of the budgeted funds could be seen, ALEX might even send out a panicky order to the staff to stop buying everything from stores. He would have to sign every order of five dollars or more. The store was always prepared, ready to dole out plastic petri dishes in $4.95 lots. In those last few weeks or months before the next budget came through, whenever something larger was needed from stores in order to keep the scientific show going, platinum crucibles were returned to the stores for which full value could be obtained. Objects made of noble metals had been purchased by different research groups for their own needs, usually during the years of excess funds, when the money had to be spent before the fiscal year ended. In that way "funds" were available to order badly needed consumables in dire times. This was a real saving in money for the U.S. government.

Also, platinum weighed less per dollar and took up less space than the heavy water that the physicists hoarded and sold back to the stores for about a dollar a gram.

Epilogue: This short account cannot list all of the facets that constituted the man named ALEXANDER HOLLAENDER. A book could be written about his administrative methods, and another could be written based on the anecdotes told by everyone who knew him. All his investigators respected him, and some feared him. And many have attempted to imitate ALEX's wonderful accent. Only KIM ATWOOD had perfect mimicry, and he often used it by telephone or by a voice coming from around a corner to gain the sudden, startled attention of the more fearing of the scientific staff members of the Biology Division.

The Basel Institute for Immunology was founded and is supported by F. Hoffmann-La Roche, Basel, Switzerland. The research of R. C. VON BORSTEL at the University of Alberta is supported by an Operating Grant from the Natural Science and Engineering Research Council of Canada.

LITERATURE CITED

EMMONS, C. W., and A. HOLLAENDER, 1939   The action of ultraviolet radiation on dermatophytes. II. Mutations induced in cultures of dermatophytes by exposure of spores to monochromatic radiation. Am. J. Bot. **26:** 467–475.

HILL, R., 1958   A radiation-sensitive mutant of *Escherichia coli.* Biochim. Biophys. Acta **30:** 636–637.

HOLLAENDER, A., 1941   Wave-length dependence of the production of mutations in fungus spores by monochromatic ultra-violet radiation (2180–3650 A). Proc. Seventh International Genetical Congress (23–30 AUGUST 1939), J. Genet. (Suppl.): 153–154.

HOLLAENDER, A., and J. T. CURTIS, 1935   Effect of sublethal doses of monochromatic ultraviolet radiation on bacteria in liquid suspensions. Proc. Soc. Exp. Biol. Med. **33:** 61–62.

HOLLAENDER, A., and C. W. EMMONS, 1941   Wavelength dependence of mutation production in the ultraviolet with special emphasis on fungi. Cold Spring Harbor Symp. Quant. Biol. **9:** 179–186.

HOLLAENDER, A., W. K. BAKER and E. H. ANDERSON, 1951   Effect of oxygen tension and certain chemicals on the X-ray sensitivity of mutation production and survival. Cold Spring Harbor Symp. Quant. Biol. **16:** 315–326.

HOLTHUSEN, H., 1921   Beiträge zur Biologie der Strahlenwirkung. Untersuchungen an Askarideneiern. Pflueg. Arch. Gesamte Physiol. Menschen Tiere **187:** 1–24.

KNAPP, E., A. REUSE, O. RISSE and H. SCHREIBER, 1939   Quantitative Analyse der mutationsauslösenden Wirkung monochromatischen UV-Lichtes. Naturwissenschaften **27:** 304.

KUHN, T. S., 1962   *The Structure of Scientific Revolutions.* University of Chicago Press, Chicago.

SETLOW, R. B., 1987   ALEXANDER HOLLAENDER (1898–1986). Genetics **116:** 1–3.

VON BORSTEL, R. C., 1987 Alexander Hollaender, In Memoriam. Mutageneses **2:** 149–150.

August 1996

Sewall Wright's "Systems of Mating"

William G. Hill

Institute of Cell, Animal and Population Biology, University of Edinburgh, West Mains Road, Edinburgh, EH9 3JT, Scotland

NINETEEN ninety-six marks the 75th anniversary of the publication in this journal of the series of five papers by SEWALL WRIGHT (1921a–e) on "Systems of Mating." The definitions, methods, and results he presented in these and two other papers published at about the same time (WRIGHT 1920, 1922) have had a major and lasting effect on the theory and application of population genetics. My aim in this paper is to review the work in these papers and to consider their influence mostly, but not exclusively, on animal improvement, but without being comprehensive in either topics or references. Indeed, were I to cite only WRIGHT's works that developed ideas from his 1921 papers, there would be a long bibliography, and it is easy to see why the reference lists in WRIGHT's own papers looked so egocentric. PROVINE's (1986) excellent biography provides a full review of WRIGHT's role in genetics and evolutionary biology, while WRIGHT's (1968–1978) four-volume treatise describes much of his work and views.

Background: WRIGHT had a broad training in biology and came into genetics as a graduate student of Castle at the Bussey Institute of Harvard University. He worked mainly on coat color patterns in guinea pigs for his Ph.D., which stimulated among other things his interest in multilocus inheritance and interactions. His first job, from 1915, was as Senior Animal Husbandman at the U.S. Department of Agriculture in Washington, with a particular remit to analyze extensive data on traits such as color and body weight collected by ROMMEL on inbred lines of guinea pigs to test the value, or otherwise, of using inbreeding in animal improvement programs. WRIGHT also undertook a substantial amount of biometrical work and a widespread correspondence on animal breeding. It was, therefore, important that he could interpret data on quantitative traits from both inbred lines and livestock populations. These and other problems he tackled in the "Systems of Mating" series while still with the U.S. Department of Agriculture.

The Mendelian theory of inheritance had become widely accepted for discrete characters, but controversy remained as to the basis of variation in continuous traits (PROVINE 1971). WEINBERG (1910), FISHER (1918), and WRIGHT (ignorant of the work of the other two) set what became the accepted framework. WRIGHT also successfully addressed the problem of how genotype frequencies change in populations as a result of nonrandom mating based on relationship or performance. Previous analysis of, for example, full-sib mating had involved the laborious evaluation of genotype probabilities, whereas WRIGHT's methods were computationally simple and general. They were then and are still not easy to understand, partly because of his use of path coefficients with analysis in terms of continuous variables rather than genotypes and partly because critical points were dealt with very tersely.

WRIGHT had invented and used path coefficients before the 1921 papers. The initial steps in their development, to describe general and specific size factors influencing bone size of rabbits, had been taken while he was a graduate student. He had computed all partial correlations, but found that such an analysis provided no understanding of causation. By computing the path coefficients, which in statistical terms are standardized partial regression coefficients, he aimed to describe the effect of causal components. In 1918 WRIGHT published his first version of the method of path coefficients (although not calling them such), partitioning variation in length of an individual bone to independent hereditary causes including general size, length of leg bones, length of hind limbs, and an independent term.

In the first paper in which he undertook a genetic analysis of a quantitative trait, WRIGHT (1920) used path coefficients to analyze data on the proportion of white color in spotted guinea pigs, and attributed variation to three principal causes: heredity (h), environment common to litter mates (e), and other factors, largely "ontogenic irregularity" or developmental noise (d). The quantity h is the path coefficient from genotype to phenotype and equals the correlation between them. WRIGHT shows that h^2 is the proportion of variance attributable to heredity; this is, of course, the heritability,

Address for correspondence: William G. Hill, Institute of Cell, Animal and Population Biology, University of Edinburgh, West Mains Rd., Edinburgh EH9 3JT, Scotland. E-mail: w.g.hill@ed.ac.uk

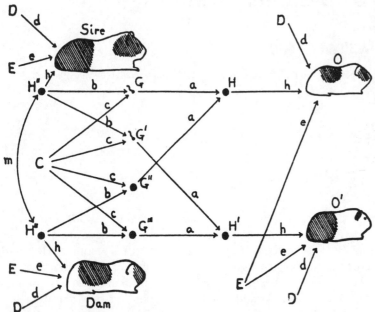

FIGURE 1.—WRIGHT's famous diagram from his 1921 papers. The original legend is included.

FIGURE 2.—A diagram illustrating the relations between two mated individuals and their progeny. *H, H', H''* and *H'''* are the genetic constitutions of the four individuals. *G, G', G''* and *G'''* are four germ-cells. *E* and *D* represent tangible external conditions and chance irregularities as factors in development. *C* represents chance at segregation as a factor in determining the composition of the germ-cells. Path coefficients are represented by small letters.

a term that he did not coin (see BELL 1977 for a discussion). In his partition of variation, WRIGHT had a term for common environment of sibs but not dominance, whereas FISHER (1918) had one for dominance but not common environment. WEINBERG (1910) had already included both (see translation by MEYER in HILL 1984), but had been ignored!

The "Systems of Mating" series: Although the path diagram for coat color in guinea pigs first appears in the 1920 paper, it returns in part I of the better known "Systems of Mating" the following year with one significant change, which took WRIGHT beyond the work of WEINBERG and FISHER, the addition of a term (*m*) describing the correlation of the parents, which enabled him to analyze the effects of nonrandom mating. The figure from WRIGHT (1921a), surely one of the best known diagrams in biological science, is reproduced here (Figure 1). Important definitions in the 1921 paper are indeed obscure. He introduced and defined *f* (called the inbreeding coefficient in a later paper) as follows (p. 118):

> If there is assortative mating from any cause, there will be some correlation between the gametes which unite. Represent this correlation by *f*.

Later (p. 119) he introduces *m*:

> The correlation between the egg and the sperm depends on that between the parental formulae which we will represent by *m*. . . . The correlation between the parents is greater or less than that between their genetic constitutions, depending on whether the assortative mating is based on somatic resemblance or consanguinity.

For these two cases he gives formulas relating *f* to *m*,

thereby setting the basic framework for the analysis of the effects of inbreeding and assortative mating on the correlation among relatives. In particular, WRIGHT computes how, for a locus with two equally frequent alleles, the frequency with which *A* alleles unite with *A*, *a* with *a*, and *A* with *a* depends on the correlation *f* and shows that the percentage of heterozygosis is $p = (1 - f)/2$. The result is then used to show how h^2 depends on heterozygosity and thus *f*. WRIGHT thereby made the critical transitions from a correlation *f* of continuous variables to a function *p* of frequencies of discrete genotypes and back to another quantitative measure h^2.

Subsequently (p. 121), WRIGHT defines *m* more explicitly as "the correlation between the genetic constitutions of the parents" and provides many formulas, including that for the correlation between full sibs when there is nonrandom mating, *i.e., m ≠* 0. [Unfortunately, his results for dominance were incorrect and were corrected subsequently (WRIGHT 1931 and by hand on the reprinted copy of the 1921 papers issued by Iowa State College Press). FISHER (1918) had given the right formulas for the dominance contribution to the sib correlation.] WRIGHT also points out that if an expression can be provided for *m*, the correlations and path coefficients in each generation can be expressed in terms of those in the previous generation.

This he does in the second paper (WRIGHT 1921b), initially deriving results for repeated brother-sister matings: "As the reader may feel some doubt as to the validity of the method of analysis used here, it will be well to begin with a case in which the results have already been determined by direct methods. . . . In this case the correlation between mates is simply that between a brother and sister, produced by the preceding generation." He gives a recurrence formula for m, which he shows can be written in terms of f in preceding generations (f' and f'') as the now familiar result $f = (1 + 2f' + f'')/4$. WRIGHT provided such recurrence formulas for a range of repeated mating systems and thereby essentially solved the problem of computing the consequences on genotype frequencies for mating systems based on consanguinity.

The third paper deals with assortative mating based on phenotype, in which WRIGHT (1921c) showed that, in contrast to mating of relatives, the consequences depend on the number of loci affecting the trait. Although there may be little increase in homozygosity when the nonrandom mating is continued, the variance in the population can increase greatly with very strong positive assortative mating. The fourth paper is on selection; although the mathematical results have had less influence than those in the first three papers, significant conclusions are drawn. For example, he introduces the idea of selecting for an intermediate fixed phenotype and shows this does not lead to a substantial reduction in variability of the trait, just as for perfect negative assortative mating, even if the trait is completely heritable (WRIGHT 1921d). The final paper comprises a review and a summary (WRIGHT 1921e, pp. 177–178) of the series:

> It will be seen that all of the systems of mating have their advantages and disadvantages. Close inbreeding automatically brings about fixation of type and prepotency. Intermediate types are fixed as readily as extremes. It is the only method of bringing to light hereditary differences in characters which are determined largely by factors other than heredity. On the other hand, close inbreeding is likely to lead toward reduced fertility, size and vigor.
>
> Matings between relatives more remote than first cousins have little significance as inbreeding, except in so far as there is continued breeding within a population of small size.
>
> Assortative mating and selection can lead to fixation of extreme types only and are not very efficient in this respect. Selection, however, is the only means of permanently changing the relative proportions of the various genes present in the original stock. It is an essential adjunct of the other systems as means of improvement.
>
> Assortative mating leads to the greatest diversification of the population as a whole, and thus is practically always accompanied by selection either in nature or in live-stock breeding. Under conditions such that all progeny are to be saved for breeding, this diversification of the population is a disadvantage. Disassortative mating is the method which best holds the whole population together, pending the fixation of the average type by close inbreeding.

Inbreeding and relationship: In the following year, WRIGHT (1922) formally defined the correlation of uniting gametes, f, as the inbreeding coefficient and extended the ideas to relationship, defining the coefficient of relationship of two individuals as the correlation between them. He is not explicit as to what measure on the individuals is being taken, but the formulas imply it is the sum of values of the gametes, regarded as quantitative traits, of an individual. Hence the relationship is referred to by LUSH (1948) as the correlation of genic values. The relationship r_{sd} between sire (S) and dam (D) in terms of their own and their offspring's (O) inbreeding coefficient is given by

$$r_{sd} = 2f_o/\sqrt{(1 + f_s)(1 + f_d)}$$

and the numerator of the expression (to which we shall return) is the covariance of genic values. WRIGHT (1922) showed how to compute the inbreeding coefficient of O from a general pedigree by the now famous formula

$$f_o = \sum (1/2)^{n + n' + 1}(1 + f_a)$$

where summation is over all paths, of length n and n' from the parents of O to the common ancestor A with inbreeding coefficient f_a [Subsequently, WRIGHT (1951) changed the algorithm but not the result by simply counting the total number, $n + n' + 1$, of *zygotes* in the path, a form that can also be applied to sex-linked loci.] These formulas are sufficient to enable inbreeding and relationship to be computed for all pedigrees, and in the 1922 paper WRIGHT used them to compute the inbreeding coefficients for animals of the Shorthorn breed, finding one bull, Comet, with an inbreeding coefficient of 0.47. The impact that high values such as this had on WRIGHT's ideas on both animal breeding and evolution is discussed later. WRIGHT subsequently contributed further both to methods of calculating the inbreeding coefficient, showing how it could be estimated by sampling rather than taking all paths back in the pedigree (WRIGHT and MCPHEE 1925), which was useful in analysis of livestock breeds, and to its prediction for specified mating systems.

In the "Systems of Mating" and associated papers, WRIGHT had made major advances: he had introduced the ideas of path coefficients and of the inbreeding coefficient, given a formal definition to relationship, shown how to compute changes in inbreeding and heterozygosity, quantified the effects of assortative mating, and more. These are fundamental to any modern population genetics course and were a great achievement. WRIGHT's inbreeding coefficient, both as a concept and, as he showed, an easily computed quantity, is arguably his most important, widely used, and lasting single technical contribution to population genetics, even though alternative definitions and derivations were obtained subsequently and FISHER (1949) wrote a whole book on *The Theory of Inbreeding* without citing WRIGHT. Further, the inbreeding coefficient was noncontroversial, in contrast to some of WRIGHT's later ideas such as the shifting balance theory.

Influences on animal breeding: I now take up some threads from the papers. I shall deal mainly with implications for animal improvement, where his ideas and methods had ready application, and in some circumstances WRIGHT's definitions led to more natural application than others. Further, his work on animal breeding also had an impact on his views on evolutionary biology, on which he concentrated after his appointment to the University of Chicago in 1926. The photograph of WRIGHT (Figure 2) was taken in 1928, shortly after his move.

Although WRIGHT never had a significant research group, he greatly influenced JAY L. LUSH of Iowa State College (later University) who became the leading figure in the genetics of livestock improvement and perhaps WRIGHT's most important disciple. LUSH had previously corresponded with WRIGHT and then attended his classes in Chicago immediately after moving to Iowa in 1930. LUSH established a major school at Ames, where he and colleagues trained many who were to become influential in animal breeding in the United States and abroad. LUSH's book *Animal Breeding Plans* (1937 and later editions) was nontechnical but had a big impact on thinking. He prefaced it, "The ideas in this book have been drawn freely from the published works of many persons, I wish to acknowledge especially my indebtedness to Sewall Wright for many published and unpublished ideas upon which I have drawn, and for his friendly counsel." LUSH's (1948) mimeograph *The Genetics of Populations,* which was widely read but unpublished until recently (1994), included a formal exposition of much of WRIGHT's work, particularly that relating to animal improvement. "Systems of Mating" and other important papers were reprinted in 1949 and 1958 by Iowa State College Press with a preface by LUSH and some handwritten corrections by WRIGHT.

The quantitative genetics and animal breeding group in Edinburgh were also influenced directly by WRIGHT (see FALCONER 1993). ALAN ROBERTSON spent some time with him in 1947 while converting from chemist to geneticist. Subsequently WRIGHT visited Edinburgh for a year (1949–1950) and taught a course, much of it summarized in a review paper (WRIGHT 1952) that was a forerunner to his treatise published later.

The method of path coefficients was used almost exclusively by LUSH, but now is little used in animal breeding research. It was developed at almost the same time as FISHER (1918) invented the analysis of variance to partition variability between hereditary and nonhereditary causes. The path diagram provides a nice picture of the model and many quantitative problems can be solved with the method, and it is featured in LI's (1955) text on population genetics. Unless people were schooled in path coefficients to the exclusion of variance/covariance methods, however, they generally used the latter. Indeed, at Ames, applied statistics was taught by SNEDECOR from his book, and the more fun-

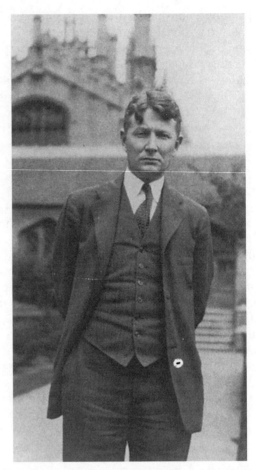

FIGURE 2.—SEWALL WRIGHT in 1928, shortly after moving to the University of Chicago.

damental genetic statistics by KEMPTHORNE, both of whom were very much committed to use of the analysis of variance. KEMPTHORNE (1957) included, however, an expository chapter on path coefficients in *An Introduction to Genetic Statistics.* Path coefficient methods did not feature significantly in the 1940s to 1960s in other centers of quantitative genetics and animal breeding research and teaching: Berkeley (LERNER, DEMPSTER), Birmingham (MATHER, JINKS), Edinburgh (ROBERTSON, FALCONER, REEVE), Ithaca (HENDERSON), Raleigh (COMSTOCK, ROBINSON, COCKERHAM). In what is probably the most widely used text on quantitative genetics, FALCONER (1960 *et seq.*) makes no use of path coefficients.

Definitions of inbreeding and relationship: WRIGHT's definition of inbreeding coefficient (variously f or F) in terms of a correlation is obscure to population geneticists not used to thinking in terms of quantitative traits. What he did was to attach implicit values to each gamete, which are sums of the effects of the genes on some arbitrary trait, essentially assuming what has become known as the infinitesimal model (BULMER 1980) or, alternatively, attaching to an arbitrary locus assigned allelic values of 1 and 0. For this reason, MALÉCOT's (1948) definition of inbreeding as probability of identity by descent is less opaque to population geneticists or students. Both alternatives have specific useful features, however: WRIGHT's can naturally take negative values, for example, when parents are less related than random, which leads on to his partition of the correlation of uniting gametes using his F statistics (WRIGHT 1951). MALÉCOT's but not WRIGHT's is readily extended to include mutation, for example, to compute heterozygosity for infinite alleles (KIMURA and CROW 1964), and to more than one locus, for example, the probability that alleles are identical by descent at both of a pair of loci. This is important in computing covariances among relatives in which contributions from epistasis (see KEMPTHORNE 1957) are included. Similarly, such higher-order terms are essential when computing probabilities of identity and correlations among inbred relatives (COCKERHAM and WEIR 1972).

Prediction of breeding value: There are various threads to developments in animal breeding that date back to or rely heavily on the "Systems of Matings" papers. Perhaps that of greatest current utilization is in breeding value prediction, to which WRIGHT's definitions of inbreeding and relationship in terms of covariances and correlations transfer directly. In livestock improvement, the objective is to select animals expected to have the highest performing offspring, so that accurate prediction of breeding value is of fundamental importance. The problem is, however, that selection may have to be practiced among animals that are not directly comparable on performance either in space or time and have different amounts of information available on them or their relatives. In dairy cattle, bulls are used in artificial insemination unequally over many herds, and cows to rear the next generation of bulls have to be chosen among herds. Furthermore, it is necessary to combine information on several traits of different economic importance. These problems were seen by LUSH (see 1937, 1948 for details) among others. He showed how records from different individuals, *e.g.*, the animal itself, its sibs and progeny, differed in their information content and how a progeny mean should be regressed to allow for different numbers of records. His colleague HAZEL (1943) showed how information on multiple traits should be combined into a selection index, basing his arguments on a path coefficient approach to multiple traits.

The problem of comparisons of dairy sires having daughters distributed unequally over many herds required both statistical and computational input. This was first provided through the contemporary comparison (ROBERTSON 1953), in which environmental effects were eliminated in a cross-classified structure by assuming that sires of contemporaries were randomly sampled. The problem of simultaneously estimating the breeding value of all animals to take account of nonrandom usage became more important as progeny test results became used by breeders. The principles of mod-

ern procedures are due to HENDERSON, initially in his 1949 Ph.D. thesis while a student of LUSH at Ames, where he saw how to simultaneously estimate fixed effects (*e.g.*, environmental groups) and predict random effects (*e.g.*, breeding values); he elaborated later in the context of dairy cattle (HENDERSON 1974). The method, which he called best linear unbiased prediction (BLUP), became applied to dairy sire evaluation in the 1970s, but with computing kept to a minimum by predicting breeding values only of sires and ignoring other relationships.

The additive genetic contribution to the variances and covariance of all animals in a population can be described by the numerator term in WRIGHT's definition of relationship. This could be readily evaluated in a sequential manner to construct a table or matrix. (In 1963 I attended LUSH's course at Ames based on *The Genetics of Populations*, in which he illustrates the computation of the genic covariance. He described the construction of a "covariance chart," which he used extensively, for one is so labeled in my handwritten notes and there is a separate mention that it is a covariance matrix.) It is more commonly described, to follow HENDERSON's usage, as the *numerator relationship matrix*. For example, the covariance of records of a pair of half sibs, otherwise unrelated, is $V_A/4$, and the variance of inbred individuals is $(1 + f) V_A$, where V_A is the additive genetic (or genic) variance. In general, using, as is the animal breeding custom, **A** to denote the matrix and a_{ij} its elements, the (co)variance of the performance of two individuals is $a_{ij} V_A$. [The numerator relationship is twice the *coefficient de parenté* of MALÉCOT (1948).] HENDERSON showed how this covariance matrix featured in a simple way in generalizations of his mixed model or BLUP equations. Evaluation of the equations requires the inverse of the numerator relationship matrix, which needs major computation to get from **A** if many animals are being evaluated. HENDERSON (1976) found, however, that the elements of $\mathbf{A}^{-1}$ could be evaluated by simple steps directly from the pedigree. This enabled the computations for the so-called animal model, which includes an equation for each animal, to be undertaken with all the data, even for dairy populations of millions of animals. The methodology is widespread and standard for breeding programs of most species of livestock and has spread into improvement of trees. Thus, WRIGHT's concept of relationship and inbreeding in quantitative genetic terms corresponds directly to the animal model BLUP framework, and the pedigree of the method was undoubtedly from WRIGHT to LUSH to HENDERSON.

Current methods of estimating genetic variance components, heritabilities and correlations are based on maximum likelihood, specifically on restricted maximum likelihood (REML) developed primarily by THOMPSON (1973 *et seq.*) for quantitative genetic application, although there is increasing use of Bayesian ideas. In these methods, general data structures including information on animals of different generations are handled by using the numerator relationship matrix to specify the covariance between all observations. Critically, as for the development of BLUP, increased computing power has facilitated the utilization of theoretical developments.

Population size: WRIGHT had a great interest in the importance of the size and mating structure within populations on the opportunities for and rates of genetic improvement by artificial selection and the beneficial and harmful effects inbreeding might have. In the "Systems of Mating" series (1921b), he computed rates of inbreeding for different fixed mating structures in closed populations and subsequently used his methods to estimate levels and rates of inbreeding in livestock populations, an activity that persists to this day. The schemes he computed, such as quadruple second cousin matings, are what have become known as maximum avoidance schemes, in that inbreeding is delayed for as many generations as possible but at the expense of higher long-term rates of loss of heterozygosity when family sizes are equal (KIMURA and CROW 1963; CABALLERO 1994).

WRIGHT later (1931 *et seq.*) developed the idea of effective population size (N_e) and showed how to compute it for a range of breeding structures. WRIGHT's N_e has, like his f (or F), become a standard for comparison among breeding programs. While WRIGHT found very high levels of inbreeding in some of the breeds he studied, there was concern among breeders in the 1950s and subsequently that the concentration of genes possible with the introduction of artificial insemination would lead to an increase in rates. This did not happen initially because a wider pool of breeding stock was tested in artificial insemination than in traditional pedigree programs; but as selection has become more intense and international movement of livestock more common, rates of increase in average relationship are rising in the world's major breeds of dairy cattle, with inbreeding lagging by avoidance of mating relatives. In particular, the high weight given to family information in modern breeding programs through the use of selection indices or BLUP means that rates of inbreeding are likely to be much higher than with selection on individual phenotype. ROBERTSON (1961) initially identified the effects of selection on rates of inbreeding, and formulas have been developed recently by WRAY, THOMPSON, WOOLLIAMS, and colleagues to give more precise answers and to allow for selection using combinations of individual and relatives' performance (see CABALLERO 1994 for a review). There is a conflict in that maximizing rates of short-term response leads to increasing rates of inbreeding and loss of heterozygosity, thereby reducing long-term improvement from within population selection.

Breeding structure and shifting balance: The analyses of breeding structure that WRIGHT conducted while working for the Department of Agriculture had a very significant influence on his views not only on animal improvement but also on the evolutionary process, for the shifting balance theory was developed before he moved to Chicago and published "Evolution in Mendelian Populations" (WRIGHT 1931). Many years later, WRIGHT (1978) recalled that he was impressed by four observations: the large responses obtained by CASTLE to high and low selection for extent of color in the coats of hooded rats, which showed the power of mass selection but also revealed unfavorable correlated responses in mortality and fecundity; the results of his Ph.D. thesis on the interaction among genes for color and pattern in the coat of guinea pigs, which indicated that an organism must be viewed as a vast network of interacting systems; the great variation found for many traits among inbred strains of guinea pigs, which showed the effectiveness of simple genetic sampling in creating diversity; and the high levels of inbreeding and high relationship to particular animals found in the Shorthorn breed of cattle, which "yielded the proper balance between the extreme plasticity of the original heterogeneous Shorthorn stock and the more complete fixation of the characters which would have resulted from closer inbreeding." These observations led him to suggest both the shifting balance theory of adaptive evolution and the way to improve livestock breeds. Improvement would occur most rapidly in small populations, where favorable new epistatic combinations of genes would arise, and these would spread by migration or between-line selection. For further discussion, see HILL (1989) and CROW (1990).

In animal improvement programs, there are many cases in which a subset of a population has improved rapidly and others have caught up by introgression. For example, North American Holstein cattle originated from Europe 100 years or so ago, but underwent more rapid improvement for milk production than the European populations and have, over the last two decades, largely replaced the latter. There is little or no evidence that this or any other example is conferring benefits through epistatic interactions; what is striking is the almost complete lack of detectable interactions among, for example, sire families when tested in the United States or abroad in different populations and environments, so that there is a major international trade in dairy cattle semen.

There have been a number of laboratory experiments to evaluate improvement programs by use of WRIGHT's ideas on population structure. These have not usually been effective, in that simple mass selection in a large population has typically outperformed a program of selection in small lines with subsequent between-line selection, at least partly because the experiments have used mainly additive traits (see HILL and CABALLERO 1992 for review). Direct experimental evaluation of the shifting balance theory by interdemic selection and migration has, however, revealed some response indicative of nonadditive effects (WADE and GOODNIGHT 1991).

There was much interest in the 1940s and 1950s in inbreeding and crossbreeding programs in animals to utilize heterosis following their success in hybrid maize, with the most obvious potential application being in poultry breeding for table egg production. The low reproductive rate of even this species compared with maize and the long number of generations required to obtain high levels of inbreeding implied that each round of selection was slow and expensive, and selection intensities were low. While there is extensive use of crossbreeding to utilize heterosis and different properties of breeds, *e.g.*, specialized sire and dam lines with high performance for traits of growth and reproduction, respectively, there is not much use of inbreeding and between-line selection in animal improvement programs.

Thus, it is the case that, for one reason or another, animal improvement has been in recent decades and still is very much based on additive genetic change. Consider, for example, broiler chickens, where intense selection on juvenile growth has been practiced for many decades. In a recent comparison of "1957" broilers, available as an unselected control stock, and 1992 broilers, HAVENSTEIN *et al.* (1994) found that at 8 weeks of age the modern strain was almost four times heavier. Nor is there evidence that levels of heritability are declining appreciably because of selection and inbreeding. Therefore, the ideas of WRIGHT's shifting balance theory, which he elucidated at least in part to explain the apparent success of breeding programs, have, as far as I know, had little impact on livestock improvement as practiced by professional geneticists and the companies they advise (but, of course, details of programs in commercial companies are not public). Furthermore, I have surmised (HILL 1989) that had WRIGHT known of the effectiveness of direct selection in large populations of livestock, he would not have arrived at and championed the shifting balance theory.

Concluding remarks: Even if WRIGHT had done nothing else in his long research career, his standing would be recognized for the major technical impact he made in his series on "Systems of Mating." Who cannot have wished to invent something so simple and important as the inbreeding coefficient? No doubt someone else would have developed it later, but he was first.

I thank NICK BARTON, ARMANDO CABALLERO, DOUGLAS FALCONER, GENE FREEMAN, PETER KEIGHTLEY, WILL PROVINE, and particularly JIM CROW for helpful comments. The errors that remain are mine.

LITERATURE CITED

BELL, A. E., 1977 Heritability in retrospect. J. Hered. **68:** 297–300.

BULMER, M. G., 1980 *The Mathematical Theory of Quantitative Genetics.* Clarendon Press, Oxford.

CABALLERO, A., 1994 Developments in the prediction of effective population size. Heredity **73:** 657–679.

COCKERHAM, C. C., and B. S. WEIR, 1972 Descent measures for two loci with some applications. Theor. Popul. Biol. **4:** 300–330.

CROW, J. F., 1990 Sewall Wright's place in twentieth century biology. J. Hist. Biol. **23:** 57–89.

FALCONER, D. S., 1960 *Introduction to Quantitative Genetics.* Oliver and Boyd, Edinburgh.

FALCONER, D. S., 1993 Quantitative genetics in Edinburgh: 1947–1980. Genetics **133:** 137–142.

FISHER, R. A., 1918 The correlation between relatives on the supposition of Mendelian inheritance. Trans. R. Soc. Edinb. **52:** 399–433.

FISHER, R. A., 1949 *The Theory of Inbreeding.* Oliver and Boyd, Edinburgh.

HAVENSTEIN, G. B., P. R. FERKERT, S. E. SCHEIDLER and B. T. LARSON, 1994 Growth, livability, and feed conversion of 1957 *vs.* 1991 broilers when fed 'typical' 1957 and 1991 broiler diets. Poult. Sci. **73:** 1785–1794.

HAZEL, L. N., 1943 The genetic basis for constructing selection indices. Genetics **28:** 476–490.

HENDERSON, C. R., 1974 General flexibility of linear model techniques for sire evaluation. J. Dairy Sci. **57:** 963–972.

HENDERSON, C. R., 1976 A simple method for computing the inverse of a numerator relationship matrix used in prediction of breeding values. Biometrics **32:** 69–83.

HILL, W. G., 1984 *Benchmark Papers in Quantitative Genetics. Part. I. Explanation and Analysis of Quantitative Variation.* Van Nostrand Rheinhold, New York.

HILL, W. G., 1989 Sewall Wright and quantitative genetics. Genome **31:** 190–195.

HILL, W. G., and A. CABALLERO, 1992 Artificial selection experiments. Annu. Rev. Syst. Ecol. **23:** 287–310.

KEMPTHORNE, O., 1957 *An Introduction to Genetic Statistics.* John Wiley, New York.

KIMURA, M., and J. F. CROW, 1963 On the maximum avoidance of inbreeding. Genet. Res. **4:** 399–415.

KIMURA, M., and J. F. CROW, 1964 The number of alleles that can be maintained in a finite population. Genetics **49:** 725–738.

LI, C. C., 1955 *Population Genetics.* University of Chicago Press, Chicago.

LUSH, J. L., 1937 *Animal Breeding Plans.* Iowa State College Press, Ames, Iowa. (3rd ed., 1945).

LUSH, J. L., 1948 *The Genetics of Populations.* Mimeograph.

LUSH, J. L., 1994 *The Genetics of Populations*, edited by A. B. CHAPMAN and R. R. SHRODE, with an addendum by J. F. CROW. Iowa State Univ. Press, Ames.

MALÉCOT, G., 1948 *Les Mathématiques de l'Hérédité.* Masson et Cie., Paris.

PROVINE, W. B., 1971 *The Origins of Theoretical Population Genetics.* University of Chicago Press, Chicago.

PROVINE, W. B., 1986 *Sewall Wright and Evolutionary Biology.* University of Chicago Press, Chicago.

ROBERTSON, A., 1953 The use and interpretation of progeny tests in livestock improvement. Proc. Br. Soc. Anim. Prod. pp. 3–16.

ROBERTSON, A., 1961 Inbreeding in artificial selection programmes. Genet. Res. **2:** 189–194.

THOMPSON, R., 1973 The estimation of variance and covariance components with an application when records are subject to culling. Biometrics **29:** 527–550.

WADE, M. J., and C. J. GOODNIGHT, 1991 Wright's shifting balance theory: an experimental study. Science **253:** 1015–1018.

WEINBERG, W., 1910 Further contributions to the theory of inheritance. Arch. Rassen. Ges. Biol. **7:** 35–49.

WRIGHT, S., 1918 On the nature of size factors. Genetics **3:** 367–374.

WRIGHT, S., 1920 The relative importance of heredity and environment in determining the piebald pattern of guinea pigs. Proc. Natl. Acad. Sci. USA **6:** 320–332.

WRIGHT, S., 1921a Systems of mating. I. The biometric relations between offspring and parent. Genetics **6:** 111–123.

WRIGHT, S., 1921b Systems of mating. II. The effects of inbreeding on the genetic composition of a population. Genetics **6:** 124–143.

WRIGHT, S., 1921c Systems of mating. III. Assortative mating based on somatic resemblance. Genetics **6:** 144–161.

WRIGHT, S., 1921d Systems of mating. IV. The effects of selection. Genetics **6:** 162–166.

WRIGHT, S., 1921e Systems of mating. V. General considerations. Genetics **6:** 167–178.

WRIGHT, S., 1922 Coefficients of inbreeding and relationship. Am. Nat. **56:** 330–338.

WRIGHT, S., 1931 Evolution in Mendelian populations. Genetics **16:** 97–159.

WRIGHT, S., 1951 The genetical structure of populations. Ann. Eugen. **15:** 323–354.

WRIGHT, S., 1952 The genetics of quantitative variability, pp. 5–41 in *Quantitative Inheritance,* edited by E. C. R. REEVE and C. H. WADDINGTON. Her Majesty's Stationary Office, London.

WRIGHT, S., 1968, 1969, 1977, 1978 *Evolution and the Genetics of Populations,* Volumes 1–4. University of Chicago Press, Chicago.

WRIGHT, S., 1978 The relation of livestock breeding to theories of evolution. J. Anim. Sci. **46:** 1192–1200.

WRIGHT, S., and H. C. MCPHEE, 1925 An approximate method of calculating coefficients of inbreeding and relationship from livestock pedigrees. J. Agric. Res. **31:** 377–383.

September 1996

Recollections of Howard Temin (1934–1994)

John W. Drake* and James F. Crow†

*Laboratory of Molecular Genetics, National Institute of Environmental Health Sciences, Research Triangle Park, North Carolina 27709;
and †Laboratory of Genetics, University of Wisconsin–Madison, Madison, Wisconsin 53706

IN 1960 HOWARD TEMIN finished a postdoctoral year at Caltech and moved to the University of Wisconsin. His brilliance was evident to his Caltech associates, but as to promise he got mixed reviews. GEORGE BEADLE and RAY OWEN both recognized HOWARD's ability but differed in their assessment of his future. RAY was confident, BEETS not so sure. They decided to bet a fifth of whiskey on whether HOWARD would do something important within five years of graduation. After five years he had a publication record that was respectable but not unusual, and he had kept plugging away at an heretical idea. RAY was particularly impressed by one of HOWARD's papers and thought his accumulated work good enough to win the bet, but BEETS demurred. A few years later he reluctantly conceded and the bet was paid off (a bottle of Old Crow, we are told). Of course, if they had waited until the discovery of reverse transcriptase in 1970, there would have been no question.

HOWARD was honest, strongly individual, and willing to state and stand by his convictions. These traits were evidenced at his graduation from Swarthmore, where he had had a disagreement with a college policy and refused to dress for the graduation ceremony. (Years later, after he became famous, Swarthmore awarded him an honorary degree; this time he donned cap and gown.) His outspokenness was also evident at the 1975 Nobel Prize banquet in Stockholm, when he shocked the audience by expressing his outrage that the one known major cause of cancer, cigarette smoking, was so blithely overlooked, even at the event itself. At a gathering of Nobel laureates in 1991, one speaker said that if the world were more loving, many social problems would be solved and world tensions lessened. HOWARD, with AIDS in mind, used his turn to shock an international television audience by saying, "If you love, use a condom." Perhaps the most characteristic example was his steady belief in and defense of the provirus theory during a time when the transfer of information from RNA to DNA was unthinkable.

HOWARD MARTIN TEMIN was born on December 10, 1934, in Philadelphia. He was bracketed by two brothers, MICHAEL (now an attorney) and PETER (now a professor of economic history). His father HENRY was an attorney, his mother ANNETTE (née LEHMANN) was what we might now call a volunteer. Both were strongminded and voluble. HENRY conducted a diverse one-man legal practice; at home he held high expectations of those around him. ANNETTE had wanted to be a physicist but found that world closed to women. A bright and busy person, she founded a Citizens' Committee for Public Education in Philadelphia and a free summer camp for children who would otherwise be denied that experience. She was active in both Hadassah and the synagogue, where she chaired the School Committee. Thus, whatever may have been the genetic contributions to his abilities, HOWARD also benefited from an environment in which both analysis and action reigned.

As an undergraduate at Swarthmore, HOWARD studied biology. He quickly became a practicing scientist, participating in two summers of research at the Jackson Laboratory. His first paper, dealing with the genetics of congenital anomalies (INGALLS et al. 1953), was based on work done there. His final oral examination in 1955 for an honors degree at Swarthmore is well remembered at that institution, because his thoughtful and far-seeing responses elicited a vigorous debate among the external examining committee that soon subverted the examination into a professorial exchange.

There have been numerous tributes to and reviews of HOWARD's life in science (e.g., COOPER et al. 1995). Here, instead, are personal accounts by two of us who knew him well, but at different times and in different ways. The first deals with his virology and his Caltech years, the second with his life in Wisconsin.

Caltech and virology (J.W.D.): HOWARD initiated his Caltech graduate work in 1955. He settled first into the laboratory of ALBERT TYLER, a kindly, scholarly developmental biologist who was interested in fertilization and early development. I had been working in the same lab, both of us having arrived at Caltech with an interest in embryology. We were impatient, however, and saw no

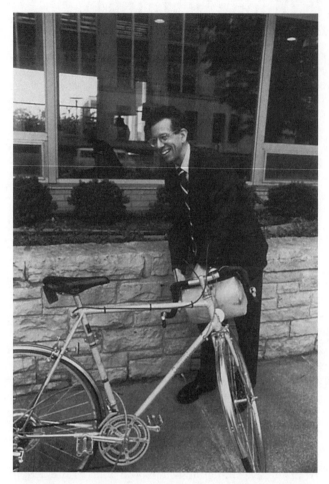

FIGURE 1.—HOWARD in 1977 with his favorite mode of transportation in Madison.

way to advance the field, the probes of the time often being no better understood than their target tissues.

After a while, as word of our frustrations spread, JIM WATSON intervened. He was a visiting scientist at the time, fresh off DNA and an object of considerable local curiosity. He decided that we might profitably work with RENATO DULBECCO, a virologist who had recently invented plaque assays for animal viruses and was about to apply the attack mode of the Phage School to these previously intractable viruses. DULBECCO agreed that we could work in his lab and introduced us to the members of his group who were to become our daily mentors. These included MARGUERITE VOGT, who was in charge of overall operations and was intimately familiar with the technical procedures involved in the plaque assays. Another was HARRY RUBIN, a senior research fellow, an adventuresome thinker, and a singer and guitar player much in demand at parties.

Probably because of perceived parallels between developmental processes and the cellular modifications wrought by tumor viruses, HOWARD took up Rous Sarcoma Virus (RSV), which had been discovered by PEYTON ROUS in 1911 and was the canonical "cancer virus." HOWARD spent most of his subsequent career

exploring this and related retroviruses. At Caltech he promptly engaged in a vigorous collaboration with HARRY RUBIN. Their first success was the development of an RSV assay suggested by the then-recent results of MANAKER and GROUPÉ (1956). This "focus" assay was a hybrid between a virus-induced plaque and a cell colony, in which RSV-transformed cells locally out-proliferate their contact-inhibited siblings (TEMIN and RUBIN 1958). Just as with the invention of the phage and the animal virus plaque assays, the focus assay brought all the analytical power of quantitation to bear on the question of virus-induced cell transformation.

1950–1959 was a decade of great excitement in biology. There was much discussion at Caltech about the still mysterious prophage state in lysogenic bacteria. By the middle 1950s it had become clear that the prophage was so closely associated with the bacterial chromosome that it behaved like a bacterial marker. Thus, HOWARD's mind was soon steeped in the powerful concept of the chromosomal prophage, and he began to imagine "lysogeny" by an RSV "provirus." He later found an RSV variant that produced a variant morphology in transformed chicken cells, further strengthening the analogy with bacterial lysogeny.

In 1960 HOWARD moved to the University of Wisconsin, where he remained for the rest of his life. He continued to probe the nature of the RSV-transformed cell and began to advocate in print the notion that a provirus state could be achieved by an RNA tumor virus (e.g., TEMIN 1963, 1964a). He surmised that the RNA of the virus would have to be copied into the DNA of the provirus and that progeny virus could result from transcription of this provirus. However, in addition to assuming a different shape and becoming tumorigenic, most or all RSV-transformed cells continuously release virus without dying. This was very different from the prophage → phage transition so elegantly elucidated by ANDRÉ LWOFF a few years earlier in which an occasional cell suddenly bursts, releasing many phage particles.

In support of his hypothesis, HOWARD found that blocking transcription with actinomycin D stopped virus production (TEMIN 1963), whereas transformed cells continued to make virus in the presence of inhibitors of DNA replication such as fluorodeoxyuridine, aminopterin, and cytosine arabinoside (TEMIN 1964b). Then, using hybridization techniques, he demonstrated sequence homology between RNA from the virus and DNA from transformed cells (TEMIN 1964c). However, these studies are more persuasive in retrospect than they were when first described, in part because of complexities in some of the results and universal uncertainties in the interpretation of inhibitor studies, but probably more because of the novelty of the hypothesis.

HOWARD's prophage model required that viral single-stranded RNA be copied into double-stranded DNA and that the latter be integrated into the host DNA. Early attempts to find an enzymatic activity to catalyze

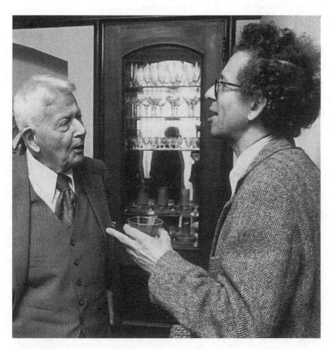

FIGURE 2.—HOWARD TEMIN and SEWALL WRIGHT in an animated discussion in 1980.

these steps in infected cells produced only negative results. Only several years later did he find the requisite activity, reverse transcriptase, which turned out to be sequestered in the virus particles themselves. The enzyme was simultaneously discovered by DAVID BALTIMORE (BALTIMORE 1970; TEMIN and MIZUTANI 1970). For this discovery, TEMIN and BALTIMORE received the 1975 Nobel Prize in Physiology or Medicine (along with DULBECCO for his pioneering work with virulent animal viruses).

The power of the provirus hypothesis and its implied biochemistry was attractive to some of HOWARD's associates. However, the notion was less compelling to most virologists, and the walk to consensus was very much uphill. This is a period for which close scrutiny might contribute interestingly to the history of science, particularly to the problem of how scientists come to accept a radical notion. Much was made of the apparent contradiction between the provirus hypothesis and CRICK's "Central Dogma" of the unidirectional flow of information from DNA (through RNA) to protein. The streak of antireligious humor that turned a paradigm into a dogma was unfortunate, for CRICK had later to clarify that his dictum did not preclude information flow from RNA to DNA but stressed instead the impossibility of information flow from protein to nucleic acid. An attractive but far less explicit alternative hypothesis for HOWARD's results, and one under vigorous examination in those days, was that of a "carrier" state, an ill-defined association between viruses and infected cells. Work on the carrier state produced a bin full of arcane phenomenology that could be interpreted in many ways without embracing the TEMIN hypothesis. Although then still

undiscovered, RNA plasmids might have offered an even more compelling (albeit incorrect) hypothesis to explain the carrier state. By standing firm, HOWARD later gained praise for his courage in the face of widespread disbelief of his thesis.

HOWARD did a great deal of virology during his decades in Madison, publishing some 276 research and review articles on the subject in addition to his Caltech output and training several-score graduate students and postdoctoral fellows. Starting even before Madison, he repeatedly wrote on the role of viruses in cancer, a vexing question before the discovery of oncogenes, and he argued for the origins of retroviruses from cellular transposons.

HOWARD became steadily more interested in the problem of viral variation. Even in the Caltech years it had been obvious that RNA viruses mutate rapidly, frustrating attempts to obtain stable genetic markers. From the middle 1970s onwards he worked on this problem. He showed that reverse transcriptases exhibit high error rates (MIZUTANI and TEMIN 1976) and that viral mutations not only occur at high rates (ZARLING and TEMIN 1976; DOUGHERTY and TEMIN 1986) but are sometimes bizarre (PATHAK and TEMIN 1990a,b). He also showed that the two retrovirus genomes that are packaged together in the typical particle recombine at a high rate (HU and TEMIN 1990a,b), further enhancing viral variability. This high rate of variation complicates both the prevention and the treatment of RNA-virus infections.

The Wisconsin years (J.F.C.): I first noticed HOWARD in seminars. Upon his arrival in the fall of 1960, he immediately started his life-long custom of sampling widely in several departments. His breadth of knowledge and depth of insight were apparent in the frequent questions he asked, always to the point. At about the same time there began an active discussion group devoted to peace. Most of those attending were motivated to control nuclear weapons and prevent war, but HOWARD stood out. He had a detailed technical knowledge of arms control, weapons, and military strategies. He more than any other kept the group from degenerating into vacuous do-goodism.

My next notice of HOWARD, some months later, was the increasing attention he was paying to my graduate student, RAYLA GREENBERG. They met in 1961, RAYLA having returned from a year spent in Edinburgh with CHARLOTTE AUERBACH. RAYLA and HOWARD married in May of 1962. I didn't lose RAYLA; I gained HOWARD.

HOWARD was recognized for his knowledge and intelligence. Yet, his provirus hypothesis was received with skepticism, if not downright hostility. His move up the academic ranks was not rapid: four years as assistant professor, five as associate. His promotion to full professor came only a year before his discovery of reverse transcriptase in 1970 made him instantly famous. While serving as Acting Dean, I obtained some unexpected funds and used them to increase the salaries of a few people who seemed particularly promising. One was HOWARD, but my action led to a complaint from HAROLD RUSCH, then Chairman of the Department of Oncology. RUSCH had a detailed schedule of salaries for his faculty and my move had thrown the plan out of balance.

Scientifically, the years from 1960 to 1970 were frustrating ones for HOWARD. Although he was eager to explain his ideas to anyone who was able to understand them, and did this with vigor and patience, he was generally greeted with disbelief. MICHAEL BISHOP (1995) describes listening in on a long discussion between HOWARD and the skeptics at a Gordon Conference in 1968. The argument was "strong, even vitriolic." HOWARD met all the arguments with reasoned answers, but his was the lone voice of support among the many dissenters, and he failed to convince.

In 1964 HOWARD gave me a manuscript reporting that virus-infected cells contained DNA that was complementary to RNA from the virus, whereas uninfected cells did not. This seemed to HOWARD like the evidence he was seeking and I communicated it to the PNAS (TEMIN 1964c). I was innocent of any detailed technical knowledge, but greatly respected HOWARD's judgment. The paper was widely regarded as unconvincing. Hybridization techniques then were not what they are now, and the presence of other retroviral genomes, unsuspected at the time, interfered. But HOWARD steadfastly continued to view this paper as an important part of his argument.

Is there a lesson to be learned from this? HOWARD's critics found each experiment wanting in some important respect, yet the several separate lines of evidence all pointed in the same direction. HOWARD accepted this (DULBECCO 1995), but the novelty of his hypothesis caused many to continue to doubt. In much of biology, there is rarely a single definitive experimental result. Evidence grows from a number of sources, none perhaps singly conclusive, but impressive in their cumulative impact. In retrospect, HOWARD was right. I wonder how much farther along the biology of retroviruses would be now if his work had gained acceptance in 1964 rather than only after reverse transcriptase was demonstrated chemically six years later. Would our ideas of an RNA basis of early life, our understanding of retrotransposons, our concepts of HIV activity, and our biotechnology be six years farther along?

In any case, the definitive evidence came in 1970. In that summer I was in Japan. HOWARD mailed me a copy of his paper along with a letter of thanks for my confidence in him when the theory was in great disrepute. He was finally vindicated. It was characteristic of HOWARD to take the trouble to write a letter of thanks.

HOWARD became instantly famous. His standing on the Wisconsin campus changed accordingly, and when the Nobel Prize came in 1975 nobody was surprised.

He began to publish more, partly because of a plethora of writing invitations. Nevertheless, paper after paper was full of new data. In the decade of the 1960s he published 27 papers; by contrast, in the 1970s there were 93 and in the 1980s, 104.

He immediately set to work to discover whether reverse transcriptase (which he preferred to call RNA-dependent DNA polymerase) was a normal cell constituent and found that indeed it was. RNA transposons were not only present, but abundantly so. Although he contributed to numerous symposium volumes, he kept up his laboratory work and with his students produced a steady stream of important papers. In addition, he became even more involved in political and social affairs. He was eager to lower the town-gown barrier, taking time to talk with legislators and inviting the Governor to his lab. Yet, he was always in active contact with his laboratory and was involved in the day-to-day work. Increasingly he was drawn into the AIDS question, and one of his last papers presented a novel strategy for developing a vaccine (TEMIN 1993).

On the Wisconsin campus, HOWARD played an increasingly influential role right up to the time of his death. When DONNA SHALALA came to the University as Chancellor, she relied heavily on HOWARD's judgment about University policies, especially research policies. This kind of behind-the-scenes, thoughtful, informal advice was HOWARD's style. His influence was felt in many ways, and no doubt wiser decisions emerged from the Chancellor's office thanks to his input. When SHALALA moved to Washington as Secretary of Health, Education and Welfare, she continued to rely on HOWARD for advice. It was on his suggestion that she invited HAROLD VARMUS to become Director of the National Institutes of Health, an exemplary choice. In Washington as a member of the National Cancer Advisory Board, HOWARD was a strong advocate of investigator-initiated research. He was an outspoken opponent of the Vietnam war, using an occasion during the Stockholm festivities to make his point publicly. He opposed too much expansion of cancer research, citing other needs with higher priority and promise. He got involved in trying to define and cope with scientific dishonesty. I remember a lawn party in which he conducted a poll, systematically asking each of his guests for an opinion.

Despite his heavy schedule of research and the innumerable demands on his time, HOWARD was somehow able to take all this in his stride. He liked to bicycle to work and did so when the Madison weather permitted; when it didn't, he walked. He took great interest in his garden and flowers, and kept detailed, computerized records. He met with his students every Friday afternoon at a conference known as the "confession session." He avoided having too many students and postdocs and was always acquainted in detail with what each was doing. He met for lunch Monday and Tuesday each week with like-minded colleagues for an always-stimulating discussion of science and public affairs. HOWARD liked to teach and felt it his responsibility to do so. For more than 30 years he taught in the basic virology course that he had organized. Despite national and international commitments, he was in Madison and easily available most of the time. A call to his phone was usually answered by him personally.

HOWARD's Jewish heritage meant a great deal to him, and he regularly attended Sabbath services. Always an avid reader, he had an extensive library of Judaism. He loved reading the Torah and often had a copy with him. He enjoyed discussions with his Rabbi and was especially interested in Jewish history and archeology.

HOWARD had a strong institutional loyalty. He naturally received offers of other positions, but he preferred to stay in Madison. Part of the reason was that he and his family liked their home and their life. HOWARD was close to his wife, RAYLA, and their two daughters, SARAH and MIRIAM. He spent many hours with them, and their interests took highest priority in his schedule. He was respectful of his daughters' feminism and political activism, and joined them in symbolically expressing sympathy for AIDS victims at a White House ceremony; the occasion was HOWARD's receipt of the National Medal of Science in 1992.

HOWARD liked to travel, and after each trip his friends were invited to his home to hear about it and see the numerous colored slides that he brought back. A trip for HOWARD was often a working trip, reading books in advance and giving seminars and visiting labs while there. After touring China in 1977 as part of a trade mission, he wrote a report on the state of biological research (TEMIN 1978). Most memorable was a trip to Russia in 1976. He took with him several forbidden items, including Hebrew books and recent scientific journals. Before leaving, he obtained lists of scientists, especially refuseniks and dissidents. He prepared for the trip by learning the Cyrillic alphabet and bringing a pocket flashlight; these enabled him to find apartments at night. In this way he was able surreptitiously to meet dissidents and refuseniks and to attend their clandestine "Sunday Seminar." Notably, he obtained and brought back a recording taped at the apartment of ANDREI SAKHAROV along with a message to the outside world from SAKHAROV himself. These evening expeditions were made in considerable fear, both for himself and those he was visiting. The distressing details of the life of dissident Russian scientists are spelled out in a diary of his visit (TEMIN 1977). HOWARD brought back valuable information for such groups as Amnesty International. The Madison evening when he told his guests about the trip was especially poignant for one attendee, my newly acquired graduate student, ALEXANDER GIMELFARB, recently a refusenik himself.

HOWARD's final illness, premature, unexpected, and ironic, was a body blow to the Wisconsin community. This man, Wisconsin's best known scientist, the indis-

pensable faculty member, was stricken by the very disease that he had devoted his life to. To add to the irony, the cancer started in the lung, although HOWARD had been a lifelong nonsmoker; however, his was an adenocarcinoma, not associated with smoking. His treatments, many of them experimental, were devastating. But he was determined and stoic. To the extent humanly possible—superhumanly, it seemed—he carried on with research conferences, writing, and advising policymakers. He published 15 papers in the short period, a little over a year, between his diagnosis and his death. HOWARD had always been a voracious reader, and in his last days he read more than ever, especially biographies. One of my last contacts with HOWARD was lending him a biography of R. A. FISHER. His last public talk was in October, 1993 at a Chicago symposium celebrating the fortieth anniversary of the WATSON-CRICK model of DNA (TEMIN 1995). His death came on February 9, 1994 at the age of 59.

In planning the remainder of his life, HOWARD assisted in organizing a 60th birthday symposium featuring his former students and postdocs. Alas, he did not live to attend the symposium, which was held in October, 1994. The resulting published book includes several of HOWARD's key papers along with contributions from former students and associates, a fitting memorial (COOPER et al. 1995).

HOWARD is survived by his wife RAYLA GREENBERG TEMIN and two daughters, SARAH and MIRIAM. RAYLA carried out several studies on the concealed viability and sterility loads in natural populations of Drosophila. More recently, she has turned her attention to the *Segregation Distortion* phenomenon and, among other things, demonstrated the independent distorting activity of the *Enhancer* locus, $E(SD)$. She is an unusually conscientious teacher and regularly offers an introductory genetics course; she is held in great admiration and affection by her students.

We thank RAYLA TEMIN and BILL SUGDEN for carefully reading an early draft and offering thoughtful suggestions. RAYLA provided documents and shared personal memories that have enriched this article. We thank RAY OWEN for his recollections and MATT MESELSON and FRANK STAHL for their critical comments.

LITERATURE CITED

BALTIMORE, D., 1970 Viral RNA-dependent DNA polymerase in virions of RNA tumor viruses. Nature **226:** 1209–1211.

BISHOP, M., 1995 Viruses, genes, and cancer: a lineage of discovery, pp. 81–94 in *The DNA Provirus: Howard Temin's Scientific Legacy*, edited by G. M. COOPER, R. G. TEMIN and B. SUGDEN. American Society for Microbiology, Washington.

COOPER, G. M., R. G. TEMIN and B. SUGDEN, 1995 *The DNA Provirus: Howard Temin's Scientific Legacy*. American Society for Microbiology, Washington, DC.

DOUGHERTY, J. P., and H. M. TEMIN, 1986 High mutation rate of a spleen necrosis virus-based retrovirus vector. Mol. Cell. Biol. **6:** 4387–4395.

DULBECCO, R., 1995 Howard M. Temin (10 December 1934–9 February 1994). Proc. Am. Philos. Soc. **139:** 452–462.

HU, W.-S., and H. M. TEMIN, 1990a Genetic consequences of packaging two RNA genomes in one retroviral particle: pseudodiploidy and high rate of genetic recombination. Proc. Natl. Acad. Sci. USA **87:** 1556–1560.

Hu, W.-S., and H. M. Temin, 1990b Retrovirus recombination and reverse transcription. Science **250:** 1227–1233.

Ingalls, T. H., F. R. Avis, F. J. Curley and H. M. Temin, 1953 Genetic determinants of hypoxia-induced congenital anomalies. J. Hered. **44:** 185–194.

Manaker, R. A., and V. Groupé, 1956 Discrete foci of altered chicken embryo cells associated with Rous sarcoma virus in tissue cultures. Virology **2:** 838–840.

Mizutani, S., and H. M. Temin, 1976 Incorporation of noncomplementary nucleotides at high frequencies by ribodeoxyvirus DNA polymerases and *Escherichia coli* DNA polymerase I. Biochemistry **15:** 1510–1516.

Pathak, V., and H. M. Temin, 1990a Broad spectrum of *in vivo* forward mutations, hypermutations, and mutational hotspots in a retroviral shuttle vector after a single replication cycle: substitutions, frameshifts, and hypermutations. Proc. Natl. Acad. Sci. USA **87:** 6019–6023.

Pathak, V., and H. M. Temin, 1990b Broad spectrum of *in vivo* forward mutations, hypermutations, and mutational hotspots in a retroviral shuttle vector after a single replication cycle: deletions and deletions with insertions. Proc. Natl. Acad. Sci. USA **87:** 6024–6028.

Temin, H. M., 1963 The effects of actinomycin D on growth of Rous sarcoma virus *in vitro*. Virology **20:** 577–582.

Temin, H. M., 1964a Malignant transformation in cell culture. Health Lab. Sci. **1:** 79–83.

Temin, H. M., 1964b The participation of DNA in Rous sarcoma virus production. Virology **23:** 486–494.

Temin, H. M., 1964c Homology between RNA from Rous sarcoma virus and DNA from Rous sarcoma virus-infected cells. Proc. Natl. Acad. Sci. USA **52:** 323–329.

Temin, H. M., 1977 Moscow diary. Sciences **17**(4): 26–27.

Temin, H. M., 1978 China diary. Sciences **18**(4): 27–28.

Temin, H. M., 1993 A proposal for a new approach to a preventive vaccine against human immunodeficiency virus type I. Proc. Natl. Acad. Sci. USA **90:** 4419–4420.

Temin, H. M., 1995 Genetics of retroviruses. Ann. N.Y. Acad. Sci. **758:** 161–165.

Temin, H. M., and S. Mizutani, 1970 RNA-dependent DNA polymerase in virions of Rous sarcoma virus. Nature **226:** 1211–1213.

Temin, H. M., and H. Rubin, 1958 Characteristics of an assay for Rous sarcoma virus and Rous sarcoma cells in tissue culture. Virology **6:** 669–688.

Zarling, D. A., and H. M. Temin, 1976 High spontaneous mutation rate of an avian sarcoma virus. J. Virol. **17:** 74–84.

Genetic Recombination in *Escherichia coli*
Disputation at Cold Spring Harbor, 1946–1996

Joshua Lederberg[1]

The Rockefeller University, New York, New York 10021

THE Cold Spring Harbor Symposium in July, 1946 was a celebration of the postwar reunion of international genetic science. It was devoted to the genetics of microorganisms; apart from the phytopathogenic fungi (MOULTON 1940), this was virtually *terra incognita* before World War II. Only within the most recent few years had any geneticists schooled in the main-line organisms (Drosophila, maize) made any serious contact with the microbes. One of those, importantly, was MILISLAV DEMEREC, who had found drug- and phage-resistance mutations in *Escherichia coli* to be ideal for his own favorite interests in chemically induced mutation. As Director of the Cold Spring Harbor Laboratory, he had given great nurturance to LURIA and DELBRÜCK and, among other newly rising stars, to EVELYN WITKIN. He was also the organizer of the symposium. The international contingent numbered such celebrities as EPHRUSSI, F. KAUFFMANN, LATARJET, LWOFF, MONOD, PIRIE, PONTECORVO, and M. J. D. WHITE. Scarcely any American even remotely interested in the area was absent; I can only think of G. W. BEADLE, who was just moving to Caltech and whose work in Neurospora biochemical genetics was represented by his recent collaborators, EDWARD L. TATUM and DAVID BONNER.

ED TATUM (LEDERBERG 1990), just recently moved from Stanford to Yale, had been my own lab chief since mid-March, when I had come up from Columbia to join him at the behest of FRANCIS RYAN. My status at Yale was a temporary research fellow (of the Jane Coffin Childs Fund), a medical student on brief elective leave from Columbia Medical School (P&S) after the grinding schedules of wartime education under the Navy V-12 training program.

Since the summer of 1945 I had been working with RYAN on a fanciful project, namely the search for sexual processes in bacteria, more precisely genetic recombination in *E. coli*. This had been motivated by the 1944 report from the Rockefeller Institute (AVERY *et al.* 1944) on transformation in pneumococcus mediated by DNA. To my mind, that report had all the earmarks of being the foundation of a new molecular genetics, as indeed turned out to be the case (LEDERBERG 1994). One catch was, could one really speak of "genes" in bacteria when there was no experimental procedure to see them segregate and reassort, no Mendelian paradigm? Among those who thought about the matter at all, there were plenty of skeptics who took a more holistic view of the bacterium, including such giants as HINSHELWOOD (1946) and HUXLEY (1942) who saw no reason to impute more fine-grained genetic structure within the bacterial cell. It was looked upon as a dynamic reaction network. Mendelian genetics was a battleground of political ideologies as well, with its suppression in the Soviet Union under the banner of LYSENKO, enforced by STALIN's police state, who nevertheless found many sympathizers among intellectuals not actively involved in experimental genetics research.

After a half-hearted and for then futile effort to achieve transformation in Neurospora with extracts (which may or may not have had any DNA aboard), I concluded that these investigations with DNA would have to be pressed with bacteria. I searched the historic literature, but found no compelling evidence, pro or con, to reject sexuality as part of the life history of bacteria. Never mind that LEEUWENHOEK and most reputable microscopists since had failed to see any couplings of the kind readily observable, *e.g.*, with Paramecium; and never mind that the class name "Schizomycetes" virtually defined bacteria by their chastity. In this agnosticism, I was greatly encouraged by RENÉ DUBOS's (1945) extraordinarily insightful *The Bacterial Cell*, which fulfilled the expectations of its title in offering a very broad biological perspective on bacteria as organisms, not merely as malicious agents of putrefaction and disease. In this work, which appeared late in the summer of 1945, he remarks, "If bacteria do really reproduce by sexual methods, it should be possible to cross closely related species and strains and

Dedicated to the memory of ANDRÉ LWOFF, 1902–1994 (see JACOB 1994).

[1] Sackler Foundation Scholar.

to determine something of their genetical behavior . . . . most workers have reported only failure . . . it has not yet been proven that the inheritance of characters in bacteria follows the Mendelian pattern." I took this as strong encouragement that the question was still open, and a bolstering of the experiments I had already begun with RYAN's critical oversight.

Furthermore, looking at the natural history of bacteria, I was struck by the combinatorial patterning of the cell envelope and the flagellar antigens in Salmonella serovars (KAUFFMANN 1941); this would have its most ready explanation if some mechanism of genetic exchange did operate in that genus. We were helped by the mystique that denominated each new serovar with a new species name, like *S. durban, S. newport*, etc., occasioning a formal published report and periodic recompilation of the names already apportioned. My expectations were also bolstered by the experience I had under RYAN's tutelage with the life history of Neurospora, and my reading of the complex life histories, including sexual stages, of many other microfungi, algae, and protozoa (CALKINS 1926; HARTMANN 1943). They were reinforced by my personal experience as a parasitology technician in a naval hospital, where my main duty was to diagnose malaria (*Plasmodium falciparum vs. P. vivax*) in blood smears from the First Division Marines returned from Guadalcanal in 1943.

My proposed experimental design was derivative of my experiments with RYAN on auxotrophic mutants of Neurospora, that these could be subjected to stringent selection for reverse mutations by plating large numbers of cells in minimal medium (RYAN and LEDERBERG 1946). Similar things happen with mutants of *E. coli*; but could one nevertheless find additional outcomes from the interaction of two complementary strains? I felt that could only be settled by using pairs of double mutants, each strain then being pragmatically perfectly stable even when billions of cells were subjected to stringent selection. The trouble was, with the methods of those days, mutants were hard to come by, and needed a lot of tedious handpicking of colonies. But ED TATUM had made that investment—he already had gotten on to using presterilized toothpicks, which saved the step of flaming a nichrome wire needle—and he had already reported getting double auxotrophs (TATUM 1945).

I wrote to TATUM asking if he had exercised those double mutants in the direction of seeking recombination; if not, might he either make them available to me or, my even fonder hope, allow me to work on the project in his own laboratory. TATUM knew RYAN well, from the latter's postdoctoral experience at Stanford in 1941–1942, prior to his return to Columbia to find me (an eager sophomore) camped on his doorstep imploring him for a place in his lab. So RYAN's recommendation carried a lot of weight. Many years later, after RYAN's early death in 1963 (RAVIN 1976), a mutual

friend told me of one of RYAN's deeper motives in arranging that liaison, in behalf of my long-term academic career interests. He foretold I would face serious obstacles as a brash New Yorker, and a Hebraic one to boot, without an established champion. An Ivy League stamp might help ameliorate that. In fact, in his letters of recommendation for my first academic position, TATUM took pains to argue that my research qualifications far outweighed the impediments "of . . . personality and . . . race."

So I did arrive via the New York-New Haven-Hartford railroad on the 18th of March. The first question was to find an affordable place to live. I doubt if it had anyone's formal approval, but I was able to camp in the medieval tower of the Osborn Botanical Laboratory, a ladder's climb up from the third-floor laboratory bench assigned to me. For a couple of weeks, I was glad to have the company in my encampment of ART GALSTON, just arrived from Caltech and looking for an apartment so that his family could join him in his appointment to the Yale faculty. ART still chides me for my ravings about crossing bacteria, when he was trying to get some rest. It was pretty lonely there after he left, but the Tower was a convenient location for getting in two or three shifts of experiments a day with zero distractions.

I felt the main task was to get all of the controls in place, before I dared do a crossing experiment. I was worried about syntrophy or cross-feeding of complementary auxotrophs, an interchange of metabolites through the medium which might confuse a finding of interchange of genes between cells (LEDERBERG 1946). Single mutants would often do this, as could be shown by the diffuse growth seen when agar layers heavily seeded with one mutant were superimposed with the other. BERNIE DAVIS made very constructive use of asymmetrical syntrophy in ordering metabolic pathways (DAVIS 1955). As expected, this was greatly reduced with double mutants. It was also important to isolate more mutants, and I worked out an elementary way to do this: just look for the small colonies, or the late-appearing ones, on marginally supplemented agar medium. Most of these were phenocopies, but it did reduce the tedious picking of thousands of bacterial colonies at random. There was still plenty of motivation to develop more efficient procedures later on (LEDERBERG and ZINDER 1948; LEDERBERG 1989). Above all, I remonstrated with myself, be sure that the double mutants live up to their reputation and show no measurable reversion to wild type (prototrophs), imputedly a two-step process, even under stringent selection of large populations (10^8 or 10^9 at one blow).

My notebooks show the first clear-cut positive finding on Sunday, June 2, 1946. By the 19th I had already repeated it a dozen times, and while visiting HARRIETT TAYLOR, later EPHRUSSI (RAVIN 1968) at the Rockefeller Institute, I wrote, "Still working to clinch the evidence . . . it may take another week more." (HARRIETT had been an important herald at Columbia of the work in AVERY's lab at the Rockefeller; and it was her reprint of the 1944 paper that actually propelled me on the trail.) And on the 21st, I had written to Dean AURA E. SEVERINGHAUS pleading for a more extended leave from medical school, and excusing it in the following terms: "compelling evidence not as yet conclusive for the existence of a primitive sexuality in bacteria . . . importance epidemiology, chemotheraphy, . . . gene action and growth in general."

I had had one false start: shaken, aerated cultures did not work well. I could not anticipate how fragile the mating pairs were, as was beautifully exploited later by JACOB and WOLLMAN (1961), nor that aeration that promotes vegetative growth actually inhibits the fertility function. In fact, the simplest design worked beautifully: just spread a drop each of broth cultures of the two parents on a minimal agar plate. The residual nutrient carry-over is negligible, may even be helpful, and there is a high enough cell density to allow for undisturbed mating contacts.

By the end of June, three and a half months after arrival, I had also incorporated unselected, segregating markers into the crosses, namely resistance to phage T1 as well as additional auxotrophies. It was reassuring that a variety of recombinant types for unselected markers could be found among the selected prototrophs. To use today's terminology, *bio met ton* × *thr leu* gave prototrophs, some *ton*, some *ton*$^+$. In other experiments where biotin selection was relaxed, one could also find *bio*$^+$ *ton* and *bio ton*$^+$ among recombinants selected as *met*$^+$ *thr*$^+$ *leu*$^+$. This was feasible because *met* proved to be absolutely stable against reversion (probably a deletion).

So these lab results came to a head just as the Cold Spring Harbor symposium loomed. ED TATUM had been scheduled to give a talk on chemical and ultraviolet mutagenesis in *E. coli* (TATUM 1946); he helped me get into the audience as a graduate student. Somewhat archly, he mentioned, "The main attribute lacking in bacteria which would make them ideal material for combined genetic and biochemical investigation is their apparent lack of a sexual phase . . ." We were just not sure whether the time was ripe for the announcement of my recent findings. CARL LINDEGREN did pick up the cautious wording about "apparent lack," saying "[Tatum] was somewhat more cautious than Dr. Dubos, Dr. Lwoff, and Dr. Luria all of whom deplored the fact that 'there is no sexual mechanism in bacteria'." He then voiced the parable that the sexual phase of a red bread mold (namely Neurospora) was unknown for a hundred years. TATUM's discussion did then refer to my experiments, and he negotiated with DEMEREC for an exception from the published program to permit me to present them. We were also motivated by A. D. HERSHEY's (1946) presentation of the first data on genetic recombination in bacteriophage. TATUM's care to

be sure that I would get full credit (or blame?) was characteristic of his fairness and generosity to his younger colleagues. I was grateful that he did append his name, for that surely enhanced the credibility of a 21-year-old making his first appearance before the scientific establishment.

So, there was a presentation, by LEDERBERG and TATUM (1946a), entitled "Novel genotypes in mixed cultures of biochemical mutants of bacteria." Besides the publication and my own recollections, I have no written record of that day. The date was probably Thursday, July 11, and I would be most grateful (as I have asked before) for any more detailed documentation.

I do recall most vividly a protracted debate, notably with ANDRÉ LWOFF, who was not at all convinced that I had demonstrated prototrophy in single-cell clones despite my care with conventional plating, and the bolstering evidence of some clones being *ton*, some *ton*$^+$. I rejoined that, in addition to my repeated replatings, a *ton*$^+$ clone, fully sensitive to phage T1, could hardly be a mixture. LWOFF had been an early pioneer in bacterial nutrition and had discovered the requirements for hemin and for nicotinamide on the part of various Hemophilus species (LWOFF 1971). He was well aware, as indeed I was, of a prototypic example of syntrophy, the cross-feeding of *Hemophilus canis* and *H. parainfluenzae* (VALENTINE and RIVERS 1927). Perhaps my "prototrophs" were no more than cross-feeding mixtures. I insisted I had taken full account of that possibility; he persevered. After a while we were talking past each other, and MAX ZELLE offered to assist in the technology of single-cell isolation to put the matter to rest. The opportunity for that critical debate was a boon I did not appreciate for many years (ZUCKERMAN and LEDERBERG 1986; LEDERBERG 1987a). Hard questions had been fully argued in front of an informed audience; that forum undoubtedly led to an earlier acceptance among geneticists than simply floating a publication, which would have allowed a diffuse skepticism or diffidence. One could not have participated in that critical discourse, amongst so many peers, without reaching a conclusion one way or another.

The term "sex" does not appear in the Cold Spring Harbor paper: several experiments remained to be done to show that the genetic recombinants entailed a cell-to-cell interaction, which would be a hallmark of any process that deserved the term sexual.

There was one hiccup: LURIA promptly tried to emulate the findings, using phage resistance markers in *E. coli* strain B. He failed, and it soon became apparent that *E. coli* K-12 was an especially lucky selection; only about one strain in twenty would have worked with the protocol used (LEDERBERG 1951). This is just one more example of ED TATUM's notorious serendipity. But LURIA's failure was made much of at Caltech, though greatly mitigated later when AARON NOVICK and LEO SZILARD at Chicago were able to advise the grapevine that they had no trouble reproducing my results with the K-12 strains I had furnished them. LURIA himself was wholly congenial and encouraged me to stand up to the few old-timers whose critical rationality, he said, might be complicated by envy. And I have similar, warmest recollections of avuncular encouragement from TRACY SONNEBORN, CURT STERN, and H. J. MULLER, not to mention my prime mentor FRANCIS RYAN. I have been so fortunate: I could name dozens of others who have stood as wonderful role models of science as a sharing community devoted to truth, and supportive even of the callowest youngsters.

The main competitor to a sexual model was that of DNA-mediated transformation, as in the pneumococcus, though our knowledge of this was still confined to the single marker for the polysaccharide capsule (LEDERBERG 1994). After the symposium, that was the first order of business. Sterile filtrates of single and of mixed cultures had no gene transfer capability. The symposium itself would not be published for many months, so in mid-September we submitted a paper for *Nature*, "Gene recombination in *Escherichia coli*," a far less reticent title (LEDERBERG and TATUM 1946b). And this did recite "cell fusion" and "sexual process" as the prime candidates of interpretation. This was published on October 19, 1946, and was the first exposure in print of these claims. Subsequently, thanks to MACLYN McCARTY, I could test his crystalline deoxyribonuclease and found it had no influence on genetic exchange. Then BERNARD DAVIS introduced the "bundling board," a sintered glass filter separating the cultures of would-be mating cells; this did frustrate genetic exchange and lent further credence to cell-cell interactions (DAVIS 1950).

Beguiled by copulating paramecia and gamete fusion in yeast, I was, however, wrong about "cell fusion." As we know from the later work of JACOB and WOLLMAN (1961), the transfer of DNA is progressive. It may take up to 100 minutes for the entire chromosome to be transmitted, and the process is easily disrupted by mechanical shaking, greatly simplifying the construction of linkage maps. While "sex pili" play an indispensable role in the cohesion of mating cells, the fine structural details of the DNA transfer remain enigmatic (FIRTH *et al.* 1996).

Most of the following year was devoted to the recruitment of additional markers, notably *lac*, and the elaboration of the first linkage maps (LEDERBERG 1987b). This work was retrospectively designated as my Ph.D. dissertation, and armed with that credential, I had to face the agonizing decision whether to complete my medical studies or embark on a new academic research position at the University of Wisconsin. This would not have happened without the staunch support of the late R. A. BRINK (OWEN and NELSON 1986), heading the Genetics Department there, who had to overcome many ramparts of prejudice in sponsoring a New Yorker, 22 years old, in a new branch of genetics, and bringing no farm experience whatsoever, for an appointment as assistant professor in a college of agriculture.

The wisdom of my choice for the latter option in September, 1947 was warmly confirmed when an editor of this series, JAMES F. CROW, joined the same faculty; so I have the occasion to commemorate a 50-year friendship as well.

In later years, I came to wonder why such simple experiments as came to fruition in 1946 had not been concocted, say in the wake of the rediscovery of MENDEL's laws in 1900. That might have set microbiology ahead by a half-century. In pondering this issue, HARRIET ZUCKERMAN's sociological and historical insights have been invaluable. We have jointly posited a class of what we term "postmature discoveries" (ZUCKERMAN and LEDERBERG 1986). This may be a bit like asking why evolution took four billion years, not three, to come up with *Homo sapiens*; others might marvel or lament that it could have that consummation at all. Indeed, earlier history of science was vastly less saturated with the expertise and energy than prevail today. We concluded nevertheless that the differentiation of disciplines played a crucial role: bacteriology was mainly the province of medically oriented people, whose task was the eradication of evil infection. In this task, the long way round, the surest way, is getting involved with the target organism and understanding pathogenetic mechanisms as part of its way of making a living. Among historic figures in bacteriology, we could locate very few candidates who might have transcended the disciplinary boundaries. MARTIN BEIJERINCK was one, but he was busy enough as one of the pioneers of bacterial physiology. Today's academic and grantmaking structures still propagate that constraint. The joint M.D.-Ph.D. curriculum is one rare counter-avenue towards achieving a broader interdisciplinary education. But it is immensely costly in time and in money, for both the student and the school. With a truncated *de facto* experience, I got the best of both worlds at a far more affordable price. However, no university would countenance that as a designed plan.

Another impediment is the fallacy of the name. In a wonderful taxonomic clarification, FERDINAND COHN categorized the Class Schizomycetes, distinguishing bacteria from other microbes. But in labeling them "fission fungi" he institutionalized the perception that they must lack a sexual phase.

Finally, it may be argued that science today is so much more densely populated—some regions are a highly competitive jungle—that no stone will be left unturned. But who dares today to undertake risky experiments, even for high stakes, when interruption of external grant support is tantamount to the guillotine, and our universities are on too tight a tether to provide their own shelter? We can foresee many wonderful fruits from the rather obvious and virtually risk-free paths of exploration of the human genome, with industrial as well as governmental enthusiasm—and the more highly automated the better. Will we ever know whatever still more revolutionary redirections we will have missed, or will they eventually be recounted as the postmature discoveries of another era?

LITERATURE CITED

AVERY, O. T., C. M. MACLEOD and M. MCCARTY, 1944 Studies on the chemical nature of the substance inducing transformation of pneumococcal types. J. Exp. Med. **79:** 137–158.

CALKINS, G. N., 1926 *The Biology of the Protozoa.* Lea & Febiger, Philadelphia.

DAVIS, B. D., 1950 Nonfiltrability of the agents of recombination in *Escherichia coli.* J. Bacteriol. **60:** 507–508.

DAVIS, B. D., 1955 Biochemical explorations with bacterial mutants. Harvey Lectures, Series L, 1954–1955, pp. 230–257.

DUBOS, R. J., 1945 *The Bacterial Cell.* Harvard University Press, Cambridge, MA.

FIRTH, N., K. IPPEN-IHLER and R. A. SKURRAY, 1996 Structure and function of the F factor and mechanism of conjugation, pp. 2377–2401 in *Escherichia coli and Salmonella typhimurium: Cellular and Molecular Biology,* Vols. 1 and 2, Ed. 2, edited by F. C. NEIDHARDT, American Society of Microbiology, Washington, DC.

HARTMANN, M., 1943 *Die Sexualität.* Gustav Fischer Verlag, Jena.

HERSHEY, A. D., 1946 Spontaneous mutations in bacterial viruses. Cold Spring Harbor Symp. Quant. Biol. **11:** 67–77.

HINSHELWOOD, C. N., 1946 *The Chemical Kinetics of the Bacterial Cell.* Clarendon Press, Oxford.

HUXLEY, J. S., 1942 *Evolution: The Modern Synthesis.* Harper Press, New York.

JACOB, F., 1994 André Lwoff (1902–1994). Nature **371:** 653.

JACOB, F., and E. L. WOLLMAN, 1961 *Sexuality and the Genetics of Bacteria.* Academic Press, New York.

KAUFFMANN, F., 1941 *Die Bakteriologie der Salmonella-Gruppe.* Munksgaard, Copenhagen.

LEDERBERG, J., 1946 Studies in bacterial genetics. J. Bacteriol. **53:** 503.

LEDERBERG, J., 1951 Prevalence of *Escherichia coli* strains exhibiting genetic recombination. Science **114:** 68–69.

LEDERBERG, J., 1987a Genetic recombination in bacteria: a discovery account. Annu. Rev. Genet. **21:** 23–46.

LEDERBERG, J., 1987b Gene recombination and linked segregations in *Escherichia coli.* Genetics **117:** 1–4.

LEDERBERG, J., 1989 Replica plating and indirect selection of bacterial mutants: isolation of preadaptive mutants in bacteria by sib selection. Genetics **121:** 395–399.

LEDERBERG, J., 1990 Edward Lawrie Tatum. Biographical Memoirs, National Academy of Sciences **59:** 357–386.

LEDERBERG, J., 1994 The transformation of genetics by DNA: an anniversary celebration of AVERY, MACLEOD and MCCARTY (1944). Genetics **136:** 423–426.

LEDERBERG, J., and E. L. TATUM, 1946a Novel genotypes in mixed cultures of biochemical mutants of bacteria. Cold Spring Harbor Symp. Quant. Biol. **11:** 113–114.

LEDERBERG, J., and E. L. TATUM, 1946b Gene recombination in *Escherichia coli.* Nature **158:** 558.

LEDERBERG, J., and N. D. ZINDER, 1948 Concentration of biochemical mutants of bacteria with penicillin. J. Am. Chem. Soc. **70:** 4267–4268.

LWOFF, A., 1971 From protozoa to bacteria and viruses. Fifty years with microbes. Annu. Rev. Microbiol. **25:** 1–22.

MOULTON, F. R. (Editor), 1940 *The Genetics of Pathogenic Organisms.* Science Press, Lancaster, PA.

OWEN, R. D., and O. E. NELSON, JR., 1986 ROYAL ALEXANDER BRINK (1897–1984). Genetics **112:** 1–10.

RAVIN, A. W., 1968 HARRIETT EPHRUSSI-TAYLOR. April 10, 1918–March 30, 1968 Genetics **60,** Suppl. **24** (unpaginated).

RAVIN, A. W., 1976 FRANCIS JOSEPH RYAN (1916–1963). Genetics **84:** 1–15.

RYAN, F., and J. LEDERBERG, 1946 Reverse-mutation and adaptation in leucineless Neurospora. Proc. Natl. Acad. Sci. USA **32:** 163–173.

TATUM, E. L., 1945 X-ray induced mutant strains of *E. coli.* Proc. Natl. Acad. Sci. USA **31:** 215–219.

TATUM, E. L., 1946 Induced biochemical mutations in bacteria. Cold Spring Harbor Symp. Quant. Biol. **11:** 278–284.

VALENTINE, F. C. O., and T. M. RIVERS, 1927 Further observations concerning growth requirements of hemophilic bacilli. J. Exp. Med. **45:** 993–1001.

ZUCKERMAN, H. A., and J. LEDERBERG, 1986 Forty years of genetic recombination in bacteria. Postmature scientific discovery? Nature **324:** 629–631.

See also page 705 in Addenda et Corrigenda.

A Golden Anniversary
Cattle Twins and Immune Tolerance

James F. Crow

Laboratory of Genetics, University of Wisconsin–Madison, Madison, Wisconsin 53706

OCCASIONALLY a chance observation jump-starts a whole field of science. The discovery of immune tolerance and the recognition of self and non-self is such an event. It started with a 1944 letter from a cattle breeder in Maryland to the University of Wisconsin immunogenetics laboratory, reporting a curious pair of twin calves, unusual in having different fathers. RAY OWEN, a postdoctoral fellow in the laboratory and already interested in blood groups of cattle twins, thought they would provide an interesting opportunity for blood group analysis, so blood samples were sent to him.

In the thirties and forties, the genetics of blood cell antigens was an active field for investigation. It was then a popular view among geneticists that antigens, because of their simple inheritance, might be immediate gene products. For this reason, they might provide an insight into the nature of that maddeningly elusive entity, the gene. In pursuit of this possibility, new blood types were actively sought in various species, including *Homo sapiens* and *Bos taurus*. By the early 1940s, 40 different antigenic specificities had been identified in cattle.

The world leader in cattle blood groups was the immunogenetics laboratory at the University of Wisconsin, founded by L. J. COLE and M. R. IRWIN (OWEN 1989). There was sometimes uncertainty about paternity in cattle, and when valuable animals were involved, that could be an important economic issue. Breeders and breed associations welcomed blood groups as a foolproof way of identifying sires. The immunogenetics laboratory provided valuable information and the breed associations provided financial support, vitally important in those pre-NIH/NSF days. It was a win-win situation.

The events that led to the letter involved a Guernsey cow with twin calves. She had been properly mated to a Guernsey bull, but shortly afterward a lustful Hereford escaped from a neighboring area and got into the act. The color patterns of the calves showed clearly that the twins had different fathers. Blood analysis revealed that the cow carried (among many others) antigen G. The Guernsey bull had antigens S and X_2, while the Hereford bull had R and I'.

The big surprise came with the calves. They had identical blood groups. This could not be explained by their being identical twins, for they were of different sexes to say nothing of having different fathers. Furthermore, *each* twin had antigens from the mother and from *both* sires, G S X_2 R I'. Why should nonidentical twins be identical for these blood groups (and for several others)? How could a calf inherit blood groups from both fathers?

RAY OWEN soon did a differential hemolysis, destroying cells of certain genotypes, and thereby demonstrated that each twin indeed had two kinds of red blood cells. One cell type was G S X_2 and the other was R I', which made genetic sense. RAY was familiar with the peculiar uterine anatomy of cattle, which facilitates cross-connections between the extra-embryonic blood vessels of the twins (LILLIE 1916). These anastomoses provide a ready opportunity for exchange of blood between the two embryos.

RAY, with his rural background, had long known about "freemartins." These are frequently found when a female calf is born twin to a male. Such a female develops into a sterile, intersex-like adult, totally useless to breeders and dairy farmers. Long before, LILLIE (1916) had demonstrated the union of circulatory systems of twin cattle embryos and postulated that hormones from the male suppressed the normal sexual development of his sister. The blood group admixture showed that more than hormones were exchanged.

The study was soon extended to a large number of twins, and most of the time they were found to share identical blood groups (OWEN 1945). There were no regular proportions of the two types of cells, but whatever the proportion, it was similar in both twins. Thus, the vessels must be broadly connected so that the blood cells of the twins are thoroughly mixed. Are embryonic germ cells exchanged? Possibly yes, but one twin sired 20 progeny yet failed to transmit those antigens that he had gotten from his co-twin. Thus, the mixing of blood cells did not, at least in this case, extend to any mixing of germ cells. RAY's most spectacular example was a set of cattle quintuplets born on a farm in Nebraska (OWEN

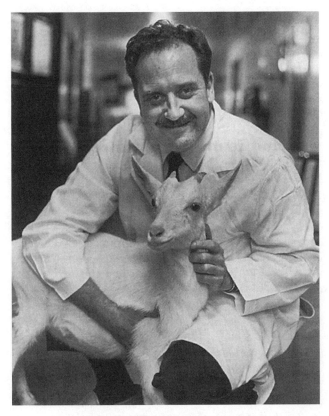

FIGURE 1.—RAY OWEN around 1960.

et al. 1946). Four calves were male, one was female, and all had identical blood groups. Each quint had three identifiable kinds of blood cells representing at least three genotypes; very likely there were five.

An immediate practical consequence of this work was that freemartins could be identified as very young calves. If opposite-sexed twins showed mixed blood types, the consequence of fused vessels (which occurred about 90% of the time), the female calf could be predicted to develop into a freemartin. The breeder could sell this one for veal and save the costs of feeding a calf that would turn out to be sterile. For many years the immunogenetics laboratory at Wisconsin offered a valuable freemartin-identifying service to cattle raisers.

Another feature of the blood mixtures was quickly noted. The chimerism persisted far beyond the maximum life of blood cells. Therefore, what had been exchanged between the twins included blood cell precursors, not just the blood cells themselves. In fact, the antigenic phenotype persisted throughout the animals' lives.

The blood admixture challenged a fundamental immunological tenet. Ordinarily, transfusion of blood from one individual to another leads to a specific, often severe transfusion reaction. Yet, somehow, each twin had survived and thrived, despite a massive transfusion of incompatible cells from the co-twin. Why should this embryonic exchange be exempt from the regular rules of blood transfusion?

RAY wrote a longer paper discussing this question and foreseeing the possibility of what was later to be called immune tolerance. Unfortunately, the paper was rejected and only a much shorter one was published (OWEN 1945). It included only an explanation of the exchange, with no discussion of possible immunological implications. Alas, no copy of the first, unpublished paper can be located. It would be a great find for historians.

A few years later, another serendipitous discovery was made, this time on the other side of the Atlantic. The late HUGH DONALD, who did research on animal breeding in Edinburgh, was looking for identical twin calves. A genetically identical twin provides the perfect control for many kinds of experiments. The statistical gain to be gotten from reducing the between-twin variance was well understood, and identical twin calves were eagerly sought by researchers. The problem was, and is, that identical twins are rare in cattle. Also, especially in pure breeds with uniform color, it is often quite difficult to distinguish the two types of twins in newborn calves. In their search, DONALD and his colleagues (1951) had made a rare find: identical quadruplets, identified as identical by exhaustive phenotypic analysis. I am sure the experimenters wished for many more; it would have been a statistical bonanza.

At the 1948 International Genetics Congress in Stockholm, DONALD encountered by chance PETER MEDAWAR, who at the time was working on tissue transplants in mice. MEDAWAR—over a cocktail, it is said—was certain that skin grafting would be an easy, certain way to distinguish between identical and fraternal twins. So he and his colleagues began an extensive grafting experiment in cattle. To their amazement, skin grafts were accepted by almost all the twin pairs, including those of the opposite sex.

On still another continent, F. MACFARLANE BURNET and FRANK FENNER in Australia were developing the concept of self and non-self in antigen recognition (BURNET and FENNER 1949). Their book included a reference to OWEN's work. According to MEDAWAR, he read this, and the solution to the mystery was quickly apparent and soon published (ANDERSON *et al.* 1951; BILLINGHAM *et al.* 1952, 1953). Another version is that the connection with OWEN's work was first noticed by DONALD. Whatever the exact sequence of recognition, the explanation for the graft acceptance was immediately clear, and the new science of immune tolerance was born.

Still a third party was involved at about the same moment, this time in Czechoslovakia. MILAN HAŠEK was a follower of LYSENKO and MICHURIN (KLEIN 1985). Impressed by the graft-hybrid results in plants claimed by LYSENKO, HAŠEK decided that double-yolked eggs and parabiotic twins in chickens and between chickens and ducks would be an elegant way to demonstrate such effects in animals. The vascular connections seemed an excellent avenue for Lamarckian inheritance. He clearly showed the exchange of blood cells and the failure of antibody production. The paper, published in 1953, was written in Russian and the interpretation was in accord with Soviet orthodoxy. In 1955 HAŠEK met MEDAWAR and BRENT, who told him of their interpretation in terms of immune tolerance. HAŠEK's views changed and he later adopted Mendelism. He became a leading figure, heading a large, productive laboratory in Prague. Thanks to his leadership, Prague became a world center in immunology. This didn't last, however, for under the 1968 Soviet putsch in Czechoslovakia he became *persona non grata*. He was deposed, his laboratory and assistants were taken away, his co-workers were dispersed, and his subsequent personal life was a series of crises. He died in 1984.

Remember that the cattle twin work was done in the dark ages of immunology. It was still believed that antibodies were molded by protein-folding on an antigen template. Shortly after, BURNET and others formulated the clonal selection hypothesis, and the research target changed from antigen to antibody (see EDELMAN 1994). This was a much more fruitful direction, and the field of immunology was poised to explode; the immune tolerance discovery helped light the fuse.

In 1960 the Nobel Prize in Physiology or Medicine was awarded to BURNET and MEDAWAR for the discovery of acquired immunological tolerance. MEDAWAR assigned much of the credit to his colleagues, BRENT and BILLINGHAM. Some have suggested that HAŠEK should have shared the prize. MEDAWAR, however, thought of OWEN, who after all was there first. In a letter to RAY, MEDAWAR said that he should have been included in the award, a statement that does honor to both men. Others—not including RAY—have also noted his absence from the Nobel Prize list and have wondered why. Yet, how much better this is than to have received the award and have people wonder why, as has been suggested in some instances.

MEDAWAR got into the field of transplants while working with severely burned patients during World War II. He realized that skin grafts from other areas of the same person were permanently accepted, while those (homografts) from another person were eventually rejected (although they might persist long enough to be clinically useful). But, significantly, he found that a second homograft from the same donor was rejected very quickly. This, to him, was strong evidence for the immune nature of graft rejection. He went on to study mice and was involved with this work when the cattle twin question arose.

MEDAWAR was a man of many parts, a twentieth century renaissance man. He was an opera buff (as is RAY OWEN). He studied mathematical logic and mastered the symbols needed to read the RUSSELL-WHITEHEAD *Principia*. He did experiments on such diverse topics as allometry and diffusion, and a number of other subjects (small experiments, he called them). He was fascinated by the transformation of Amphioxus from a highly asymmetric larva into a symmetrical adult and published an article on the evolutionary implications.

MEDAWAR's best known work, aside from immunology, is on the evolution of senescence. He wrote two semi-popular essays on the subject (reprinted in MEDAWAR 1957) that have been widely heralded as the beginning of modern evolutionary theories of aging (*e.g.*, STEARNS 1992, p. 200). Noting that post-reproductive (or post-progeny rearing) selection against deleterious mutations is weak at most, he suggested the accumulation of such mutations as one explanation. A second explanation, now called antagonistic pleiotropy, notes that selection can increase mutations that are favorable at early ages even if they are deleterious later. Although many other geneticists had similar ideas, MEDAWAR set them forth explicitly. He used FISHER's (1930) reproductive value as a measure of age-specific selection intensity. This intuitively appealing idea has been largely replaced by other measures due to HAMILTON (1966), which can more readily be interpreted in terms of gene-frequency change or probability of fixation (CHARLESWORTH 1994, pp. 197ff). But MEDAWAR was clearly on the right track. The relative importance of the two processes is still not clear and is being actively researched (ROSE 1991; CHARLESWORTH and HUGHES 1996).

Like his friends JULIAN HUXLEY and J. B. S. HALDANE, MEDAWAR enjoyed popular writing. He was a fluent writer of gracefully worded, easily understood essays, and many have been republished in book form. An example is a series of Sunday evening lectures broadcast by the BBC in 1959 and published under the title *The Future of Man* (MEDAWAR 1959). His breadth of knowledge is impressive (as is the high level of programming of the BBC). As he said, "A human biologist must be a demographer, geneticist, anthropologist, historian, psychologist and sociologist all in one;" he came close. His mastery of English prose shows on every page. The book led to one minor disagreement. This was with H. J. MULLER, who thought that MEDAWAR overemphasized the importance of overdominant loci for quantitative traits and was therefore too pessimistic about the effectiveness of selection.

Late in life, MEDAWAR suffered a stroke that slowed his physical activity, but not his restless, wide-ranging mind. He continued to read, work (but not with his hands), and dictate essays and books. He published a charming autobiography with the intriguing title, *Memoir of a Thinking Radish* (MEDAWAR 1986). Death came in 1987 at age 72.

RAY OWEN was born the same year as MEDAWAR (1915) and grew up on a Wisconsin dairy farm. For eight grades, he attended a two-room school. Then and through high school, he did his farm chores each day before and after classes. Following graduation from Carroll College, he began graduate studies at Wisconsin with L. J. COLE and worked mainly with birds. His thesis

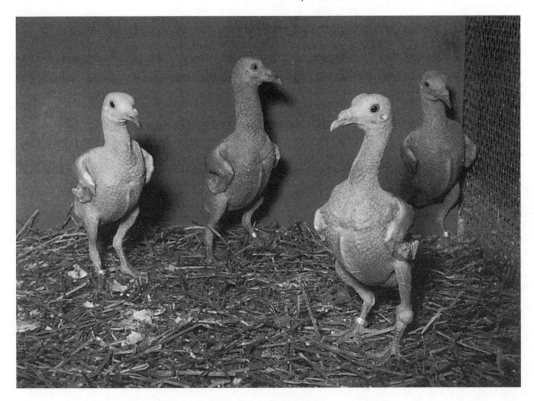

FIGURE 2.—Naked pigeons. These four had 13 normal sibs from a mating between two heterozygous parents.

was on the sterility of species hybrids. The observation of germ-cell migration alerted him to the possibility of such events as were later observed in the twin calves.

One of RAY's early papers—a favorite among his friends—describes "naked" pigeons (COLE and OWEN 1944). These birds, because of a recessive mutant gene, are completely featherless (Figure 2). The paper, largely written by RAY, was published in the *Journal of Heredity*. In those days science was less competitive and publications less crowded, and the editor, R. C. COOK, encouraged humorous, informal, clever writing (and contributed some himself). Here are some choice passages; those who know RAY will recognize the style. "Pigeon courtship, with its strutting, cooing and puffing out of feathers is an interesting performance. When there are no feathers to puff or to clothe the performer, it becomes a ludicrously macabre travesty... Although their wings are almost useless organs, these birds seem unable to learn to regard them as such. Placed on a table, they will hopefully take off into space, beating their wings vigorously, as though confident of a controlled landing which, however, ends in a 'crash'... They are also active and aggressive lovers. Inadequate attire produces no inferiority complex in them; they strut and coo, puff and bow as if arrayed in the finest of raiment." Alas, matings required artificial insemination and the fertility was low. Keeping the mutant gene by mating heterozygotes proved too laborious, and the strain was lost. "The perpetuation of the strain is so tedious that it will be a long time before the housewife can buy her squabs gene-plucked."

RAY's immunogenetic work was done as a postdoc-

toral fellow. In 1947 he left Wisconsin for Caltech. The venue changed from cattle barns to rodent labs. Although the emphasis was always on immunogenetics, the organisms were strikingly varied. He and his students studied, in addition to rats and mice, viruses, ciliates, goldfish, birds, and humans. Always a popular teacher, he devoted considerable time to it. Along with ADRIAN SRB, he wrote a pathbreaking textbook (SRB and OWEN 1952) that started a trend in presenting genetics as an active, evolving subject. It quickly became a best seller.

RAY's later record shows a diminished number of scientific papers with his name attached, and there is a reason. In the 1960s, he decided no longer to permit his name to appear on papers by his students when they had done most of the laboratory work. But he continued to suggest problems and to offer assistance and guidance. His helpfulness to students, his and others', is a Caltech legend. RAY is never too busy to help with a problem, be it scientific or personal. Nor is he too busy to accept a difficult administrative task, and this became a large part of his life. At Caltech he has become the students' friend and advocate, and in many ways contributed to the conscience of the institution.

Having recently passed his eightieth birthday anniversary, RAY has been the recipient of well-justified praise by former Caltech students and scientific colleagues. In the summer of 1996 a symposium in his honor was held at the University of Wisconsin. It was an exciting event, marred only by the death a few days earlier of GEORGE SNELL, another pioneering transplant geneticist. The symposium was an intellectual feast. The latest theories and observations were on display. The contrast between what was known in 1946 and the state of the science in 1996 is amazing. It seems especially so to those, like me, who have viewed the subject with continued interest, but always from the outside. What a difference a half-century makes!

I should like to thank RAY OWEN for helping me with a number of historical details. As a consequence there are far fewer errors than there would otherwise have been.

LITERATURE CITED

ANDERSON, D., R. E. BILLINGHAM, G. H. LAMPKIN and P. B. MEDAWAR, 1951 The use of skin grafting to distinguish between monozygotic and dizygotic twins in cattle. Heredity **5:** 379–397.

BILLINGHAM, R. E., G. H. LAMPKIN, P. B. MEDAWAR and H. L. WILLIAMS, 1952 Tolerance to homografts, twin diagnosis, and the freemartin condition in cattle. Heredity **6:** 201–212.

BILLINGHAM, R. E., L. BRENT and P. B. MEDAWAR, 1953 Actively acquired tolerance of foreign cells. Nature **172:** 603–606.

BURNET, F. M., and F. FENNER, 1949 *The Production of Antibodies.* Macmillan, London.

CHARLESWORTH, B., 1994 *Evolution in Age-Structured Populations,* 2nd ed. Cambridge University Press, Cambridge.

CHARLESWORTH, B., and K. A. HUGHES, 1996 Age-specific inbreeding depression and components of genetic variance in relation to the evolution of senescence. Proc. Natl. Acad. Sci. USA **93:** 6140–6145.

COLE, L. J., and R. D. OWEN, 1944 Naked pigeons. J. Hered. **35:** 1–7.

DONALD, H. P., W. S. BIGGAR and D. M. LOGAN, 1951 Monozygotic bovine quadruplets. Heredity **5:** 135–142.

EDELMAN, G. M., 1994 The evolution of somatic selection: the antibody tale. Genetics **138:** 975–981.

FISHER, R. A., 1930 *The Genetical Theory of Natural Selection.* Clarendon Press, Oxford.

HAMILTON, W. D., 1966 The moulding of senescence by natural selection. J. Theor. Biol. **12:** 12–45.

KLEIN, J., 1985 In memoriam. Immunogenetics **21:** 105–108.

LILLIE, F. R., 1916 The theory of the free-martin. Science **43:** 611–613.

MEDAWAR, P. B., 1957 *The Uniqueness of the Individual.* Basic Books, New York.

MEDAWAR, P. B., 1959 *The Future of Man.* Methuen and Co., London.

MEDAWAR, P. B., 1986 *Memoir of a Thinking Radish.* Oxford University Press, Oxford.

OWEN, R. D., 1945 Immunogenetic consequences of vascular anastomoses between bovine twins. Science **102:** 400–401.

OWEN, R. D., 1989 M. R. IRWIN and the beginnings of immunogenetics. Genetics **123:** 1–4.

OWEN, R. D., H. P. DAVIS and R. F. MORGAN, 1946 Quintuplet calves and erythrocyte mosaicism. J. Hered. **37:** 291–297.

ROSE, M., 1991 *The Evolutionary Biology of Aging.* Oxford University Press, Oxford.

STEARNS, S. C., 1992 *The Evolution of Life Histories.* Oxford University Press, Oxford.

SRB, A. M, and R. D. OWEN, 1952 *General Genetics.* W. H. Freeman, San Francisco.

Dobzhansky, Bateson, and the Genetics of Speciation

H. Allen Orr

Department of Biology, University of Rochester, Rochester, New York 14627

That essential bit of evolutionary theory which is concerned with the origin and nature of *species* remains utterly mysterious.   W. BATESON (1922)

SIXTY years ago, THEODOSIUS DOBZHANSKY (1936) took a large step towards solving "the Species Problem." He published his seminal work on the genetics of speciation in these pages, an analysis of hybrid sterility between two sibling species, *Drosophila pseudoobscura* (then called "race A") and *D. persimilis* ("race B"). This work is renowned among evolutionary geneticists for several reasons. Most important, DOBZHANSKY showed that the genetics of species differences—even reproductive isolation itself—could be studied with the same genetic tools that had been wielded so successfully *within* species. In doing so, he was quickly able to put several popular theories of speciation to the sword. (Indeed, some of these hypotheses were so thoroughly dispatched that their very existence is now forgotten.) DOBZHANSKY's paper also lent strong support to an alternative view of speciation that he and H. J. MULLER are usually credited with introducing. This view—that hybrid sterility and inviability are caused by sets of interacting "complementary genes"—laid the foundation for nearly all subsequent work in the genetics of speciation, including the recent explosion of papers in this journal.

Despite the fact that DARWIN left the species problem largely unsolved (see below), geneticists made few forays into speciation before the 1930s. There were two reasons for this neglect. For one thing, there was simply too much else to do in the early years of Mendelism: mutants had to be mapped and chromosome mechanics untangled. But speciation also posed serious technical problems. The study of, say, hybrid sterility was invariably foiled by the very phenotype under study; sterile flies do not, after all, afford the most promising material for genetics. This simple problem had stopped dead in its tracks the only previous serious venture into speciation, STURTEVANT's (1920) work on *D. melanogaster*–*D. simulans* hybrids. All of the hybrids were sterile or inviable, and little could be done.

Author e-mail: haorr@darwin.biology.rochester.edu

But all this changed in 1922. In that year, DONALD LANCEFIELD, working in MORGAN's lab at Columbia, found a stock of what was then called *D. obscura* that produced sterile males when crossed to all other stocks. But the hybrid females (and this was the important part) remained fertile. With LANCEFIELD's discovery of what came to be called *D. persimilis* (the new stock) and *D. pseudoobscura* (the old stocks), the door swung open on the genetic study of speciation. Here were beasts that both thrived in Drosophilists' vials and that yielded sterile hybrids *and* some fertile hybrids upon crossing.

But as PROVINE (1981) recounts in his careful history of this period, DOBZHANSKY grew frustrated by LANCEFIELD's slow progress. A long ten years after LANCEFIELD's initial discovery, DOBZHANSKY had had enough and announced his intent to start his own work on *D. pseudoobscura*. DOBZHANSKY published several brief reports on hybrid sterility in 1933 and 1934, but he dropped the bomb in his 1936 paper, a work that was far more complete and far more convincing than any preceding it.

DOBZHANSKY's approach was simple enough. In a forerunner to quantitative trait locus (QTL) analysis, he crossed *D. pseudoobscura* carrying mapped visible markers (one to three per chromosome) to *D. persimilis*. By backcrossing the fertile F_1 females to males from either of the pure species, he recovered backcross hybrids carrying many combinations of chromosomes from the two species. By scoring the fertility of these hybrids, which he assessed by measuring testis size, DOBZHANSKY could see which chromosome regions, if any, caused hybrid sterility. As LEWONTIN (1981) has rightly emphasized, here, finally, was a study of speciation that looked a good deal like genetic studies within species: crosses were made, balancer chromosomes were used, and *XO* males were characterized, all on material that was by then cytologically well known.

The nucleus *vs.* the cytoplasm: DOBZHANSKY's greatest finding is today the most easily overlooked: hybrid sterility is caused by genes. This fact was far from obvious in the 1930s. Debate over the cause of hybrid sterility had raged for decades and, as always, vague speculation proliferated in inverse proportion to the number of experiments. Although lumping these speculations is tricky, several did share a common theme: species differences, it was claimed, are not caused by Mendelian genes. Instead, something unique, some novel process or novel kind of factor, causes speciation and the differences seen among species. This reluctance to render unto MENDEL what (it turned out) was clearly MENDEL's appeared in two forms, one saner than the other.

First, a surprisingly large number of biologists held that, while Mendelism might explain the trivial and uninteresting differences seen within species, Morganist genes could never explain species differences. These "fundamental" or specific differences were instead due to the cytoplasm. This view was especially popular among European embryologists (*e.g.,* LOEB and BRACHET), but even luminaries like JOHANNSEN (1923) claimed that "the Problem of [the Evolution of Species] does not seem to be approached seriously through Mendelism." Although members of this "cytocentric" camp were mostly concerned with morphological species differences, there was a strong suspicion that Mendelian genes could not explain *any* sort of difference between species. Indeed, SAPP (1987) argues that the well known failure of breeders to produce "good" species drove many biologists to the cytocentric view, for as HUXLEY and BATESON had emphasized, breeders had succeeded in duplicating virtually every evolutionary phenomenon *except* good species that produced sterile hybrids.

Second (and, to modern ears, more reasonably), many geneticists asserted that hybrid sterility resulted not from ordinary changes in ordinary genes, but from large chromosome rearrangements. These rearrangements allegedly disrupted chromosome pairing in hybrids, derailing meiosis. This view gained support from two lines of evidence: chromosome pairing problems clearly *were* the frequent cause of sterility in plants and, more important, meiotic chromosomes failed to pair in some sterile animal hybrids.

DOBZHANSKY's work falsified both the cytoplasmic and the rearrangement hypotheses. As he noted elsewhere, the "cytocentric" view was absurdly vague anyway: "It was only said that the latter [variation within races or species] is clearly genic, while the former [differences between races or species] was alleged to be non-Mendelian and to be due to some vague principle which assiduously escapes all attempts to define it more clearly" (DOBZHANSKY 1937a). Arguing that "the mechanisms isolating species from each other must be considered the only true specific differences, if the expression 'specific character' is to have any real meaning," DOBZHANSKY (1937a) set out to determine if reproductive isolation itself was Mendelian. His results were unambiguous.

Sterility of *D. pseudoobscura-D. persimilis* hybrids mapped to chromosomes. In backcrosses to *D. pseudoobscura*, for example, males carrying all three *X*-linked markers from *D. persimilis* were often sterile, while those carrying all three markers from *D. pseudoobscura* were almost always fertile. The effect was large and unquestionable. Moreover, recombination analysis showed that factors causing sterility resided on both the left and right arms of *X*. Similar results recurred at all the chromosomes: most of DOBZHANSKY's markers were associated with hybrid sterility. Any lingering hope for a fundamental role of the cytoplasm (maybe the chromosomes and the cytoplasm together cause hybrid sterility?) were shattered by DOBZHANSKY's next result: "Backcross males having only race A chromosomes are fertile irrespective of whether they have the cytoplasm derived from race A or from race B. Backcross males having only race B chromosomes are likewise fertile irrespective of the source of their cytoplasm." Ironically, DOBZHANSKY found that the fertility of one hybrid genotype did vary with its cytoplasm, but he quickly showed that this was due to a maternal effect (depending on the mother's nuclear genotype), not to some autonomous force lurking in the cytoplasm. In sum, "no indication ... of an inherent difference between the cytoplasms of the two races is apparent" (DOBZHANSKY 1936, p. 126) (although we do now know that intracellular endosymbionts such as Wolbachia sometimes cause hybrid lethality, though not sterility, in insects.) Two years later, in a review entitled "The nature of interspecific differences," J. B. S. HALDANE (1938) announced that Mendelian genes also explained *morphological* differences between species, and the cytocentric hypothesis sank into well-deserved obscurity.

Genes *vs.* chromosome rearrangements: Although this "sterility is due to chromosomes" result was anticipated by the previous work of LANCEFIELD (1929) and KOLLER (1932) (indeed, DOBZHANSKY barely found the cytoplasmic hypothesis worthy of mention by 1936), DOBZHANSKY's paper went far beyond its predecessors. DOBZHANSKY showed not only that hybrid sterility is due to chromosomes, but that this effect is in turn due to genes, not to large rearrangements. Although *D. pseudoobscura* and *D. persimilis* differed by six inversions and although meiotic chromosomes failed to pair in hybrids, several lines of evidence proved that the rearrangements were not to blame. For one thing, four of the inversion differences were *X*-linked and so could play no role in hybrid *male* sterility. DOBZHANSKY (1936) further showed that hybrid sterility often mapped to regions that were *not* heterozygous for rearrangments in hybrid males, *e.g.,* both arms of the *X* and the fourth chromosome. Indeed the *X*-linked factors had the largest effect on hybrid fertility.

Last, DOBZHANSKY had previously shown that structural differences between species did not even cause the pairing problems seen in hybrids, much less sterility *per se.* DARLINGTON (1932) had earlier discovered a remarkable pattern proving that hybrid sterility in plants involves chromosome rearrangement: while diploid hybrids often display univalents at meiosis and are sterile, tetraploid hybrids between the same species display bivalents and are fertile. Because all chromosomes have perfect pairing partners in tetraploid hybrids, the simple availability of unrearranged partners clearly rescues fertility. DOBZHANSKY (1933), in what, for my money, stands among the cleverest experiments in evolutionary genetics, showed that DARLINGTON's rule is *not* obeyed in animals. Sidestepping the fact that one can't make tetraploid males, DOBZHANSKY compared the frequency of pairing failure in diploid *vs.* tetraploid hybrid *spermatocytes* (tetraploid cells being fairly common in *D. pseudoobscura–D. persimilis* hybrid testes). Remarkably, he found that chromosomes fail to pair just as often in tetraploid cells, where all chromosomes have perfect pairing partners, as in diploid cells. Hybrid meiotic problems were not due to structural incompatibilities.

DOBZHANSKY would drive the message home in his book, *Genetics and the Origin of Species* (1937b): while hybrid sterility in plants is often due to chromosome rearrangements, hybrid sterility in animals is not. Although exceptions surely occur here and there, this conclusion has been largely confirmed in the recent burst of work on the genetics of speciation in Drosophila: hybrid sterility typically maps to genes.

Complementary genes: DOBZHANSKY's 1936 paper is best remembered for yet another reason: it provided the best evidence yet that speciation occurred by what is now called the "DOBZHANSKY-MULLER" model. It is hard to overestimate the importance of this simple model. Indeed, it resolved a paradox that had stared down evolutionists for half a century: how could something as patently maladaptive as the evolution of sterility or inviability be allowed by natural selection? Although DARWIN obviously did not subscribe to the modern biological species concept, he was painfully aware of the problem posed by hybrid sterility. He recognized that he asked his readers to believe both that most evolution is due to natural selection and that sterility of hybrids routinely evolves. Indeed, DARWIN spent an entire chapter of the *Origin of Species* trying to explain away this paradox, but his attempt was less than overwhelmingly successful. Hence the common (and correct) charge that the *Origin of Species* neglected to explain the origin of species.

To see DARWIN's paradox, consider the simplest possible scenario: a single gene causes hybrid sterility. One species has genotype *AA* and the other *aa*. While each species is fertile, *Aa* hybrids are sterile. Now consider how these species could evolve from a common ancestor, say, *AA*. They can't. Starting with two allopatric *AA* populations, one simply remains *AA* while the other must become *aa*. But how can it? The *a* mutation, like any mutation, has the unfortunate property of arising in the heterozygous state. But the resulting *Aa* individual *is* the sterile hybrid genotype, and the line comes crashing to an end.

DOBZHANSKY's solution was simple. Hybrid sterility, he said, involves an interaction between at least *two* genes. To see this, let our allopatric populations begin with an *aabb* genotype. An *A* mutation appears and gets fixed in one population; the *Aabb* and *AAbb* genotypes are perfectly fertile. Indeed *A* may be selectively favored. A *B* mutation appears and gets fixed in the other population; the *aaBb* and *aaBB* genotypes are also fertile. And, again, *B* may be favored. The critical point is that, although *B* is compatible with *a*, it hasn't been "tested" with *A*. We simply have no guarantee that *A* and *B* can work together. Indeed, *AaBb* hybrids may be sterile. The point is deceptively simple: if hybrid sterility is caused by epistatic incompatibilities *between* loci, Darwin's paradox is resolved. Speciation can occur and two taxa can become separated by an adaptive valley even though *no genotype ever passed through the valley*.

This model is very simple. In fact, it has proved too simple for many evolutionary biologists, who have offered countless elaborate ways of getting populations across adaptive valleys, explaining speciation. (We evolutionists have a long track record of preferring fancy over simple theories, dating from our infamous reluctance to surrender GALTON in the face of Mendelism. Surely something as *déclassé* as 3:1 ratios were not to be preferred to GALTON's sophisticated and seductive mathematics.) Alas, the simple theory has once again proved right. Although geneticists dissecting the basis of postzygotic isolation continue to squabble over many details, we *all* agree that hybrid sterility and inviability in animals is caused by sets of complementary genes (WU and BECKENBACH 1983; COYNE 1992; ORR 1995).

DOBZHANSKY's paper provided the clearest evidence yet for this new model of speciation. DOBZHANSKY beautifully showed not only that the *X* from *D. persimilis* and the second chromosome from *D. pseudoobscura* caused hybrid sterility, but that sterility resulted from an *interaction* between these (and other) chromosomes, and hence between different loci. Evolutionists were no longer free to imagine that hybrid sterility was typically caused by heterozygote disadvantage or by inversions and translocations (although many continued to do so, *e.g.,* KING 1993).

DOBZHANSKY was not the first to find complementary incompatibilities in hybrids. Several hybrid complementary systems were known by the 1930s (BELLAMY 1922; HOLLINGSHEAD 1930). DOBZHANSKY gets credit because he, unlike his peers, saw that complementary sterility was more than a technical curiosity: he saw that, unlike single-gene sterility, two-gene sterility resolved DARWIN's paradox. DOBZHANSKY first hinted at this idea in an absurdly obscure paper in 1934, noting that, while the distinction between complementary *vs.* single genes isn't important as far as the physiology of sterility is concerned, it is "obviously important as far as the way of the establishment of the genetic differences of this kind in a wild population is concerned" (DOBZHANSKY

1934). This is (uncharacteristically modest) code-talk for "complementary genes can explain the origin of species." DOBZHANSKY again hinted at this message on the first page of his 1936 paper and finally spelled it out in his book, where the model is laid out step by step with some fanfare. In the end, then, DOBZHANSKY's title was considerably less misleading than DARWIN's: *Genetics and the Origin of Species* really did explain the origin of species.

BATESON's forgotten role: While DOBZHANSKY seemed content to present the gist of the complementary gene model, H. J. MULLER gave it its most careful treatment. MULLER (1940, 1942) considered the evolution of hybrid sterility in two classic papers. His 1942 essay, "Isolating mechanisms, evolution, and temperature," is an especially remarkable and insightful work. (The odd title reflects the fact that the paper was delivered at a session ostensibly devoted to temperature; MULLER insisted on speaking about speciation instead and his paper makes only a few strained references to temperature.) In this paper, MULLER offered a number of important refinements of the complementary model.

He showed that complementary lethals and steriles could evolve between species even when all substitutions occurred in one lineage (a fact that is still often misunderstood). He showed that, in Drosophila, complementary incompatibilities are often "complex," involving interactions between triplets, etc., not pairs, of genes. He speculated on the biochemical basis of hybrid incompatibilities: do hybrid problems involve genes that act as poisons or as loss-of-function alleles on a "foreign" genetic background? And, most important, he considered X linkage and offered an explanation of HALDANE's rule (the preferential sterility or inviability of the hybrid XY sex) which, in slightly modified form, could well be right (TURELLI and ORR 1995).

DOBZHANSKY and MULLER's views of the complementary model differed subtly (*e.g.,* MULLER's emphasis on "transfer of function"). Consequently, each later tended to preferentially cite his own formulation of the idea. As it turns out, their concern with precedent was utterly beside the point: I recently discovered that WILLIAM BATESON offered the "DOBZHANSKY-MULLER" model in 1909, just nine years after the rediscovery of Mendelism and a good quarter-century before DOBZHANSKY or MULLER. And when I say that BATESON offered the model, I do not mean that he obliquely alluded to it. Rather, BATESON spells it out, step by step, presenting it as the likely "secret of interracial sterility" (BATESON 1909).

BATESON's 1909 discussion appears in a forgotten essay, "Heredity and variation in modern lights," in an equally forgotten volume, *Darwin and Modern Science.* (To appreciate how long ago BATESON's essay appeared, consider that its preface was penned by DARWIN's longtime associate, J. D. HOOKER.) Midway through his essay, BATESON asks what discovery would most advance our understanding of evolution, and concludes that he'd most like to see hybrid sterility laid bare. After all, as noted above, hybrid sterility remained the sole evolutionary phenomenon not duplicated among artificially selected varieties.

BATESON's explanation of how sterility could evolve between varieties is identical to that later offered by DOBZHANSKY and MULLER. He first notes that "when two species, both perfectly fertile severally, produce on crossing a sterile progeny, there is a presumption that the sterility is due to the development in the hybrid of some substance which can be formed only by the meeting of two complementary factors." He then explains, in a remarkably prescient passage, how such factors evolve (p. 98, italics in original):

> Now if the sterility of the cross-bred be really the consequence of the meeting of two complementary factors, we see that the phenomenon could only be produced among the divergent offspring of one species by the acquisition of at least *two* new factors; for if the acquisition of a single factor caused sterility the line would then end. Moreover each factor must be separately acquired by distinct individuals, for if both were present together, the possessors would by hypothesis be sterile. And in order to imitate the case of species each of these factors must be acquired by distinct breeds. The factors need not, and probably would not, produce any other perceptible effects . . . Not till the cross was actually made between the two complementary individuals would either factor come into play, and the effects even then might be unobserved until an attempt was made to breed from the cross-bred.

BATESON even proposes a way of testing his conjecture. Noting that the pair of factors causing sterility between two closely related varieties might not yet be fixed in either line, he suggests obtaining "a pair of parents [one from each breed] which are known to have had any sterile offspring, and to find the proportions in which these steriles are produced. If, as I anticipate, these proportions are found to be definite, the rest is simple." In short, he expects such crosses will show that sterility is due to Mendelizing factors and, further, to *pairs* of interacting factors: "My conjecture therefore is that in the case of sterility of cross-breds we see the effect produced by a complementary pair of such factors." Although BATESON stumbles in a few places (*e.g.,* he thinks his model explains hybrid sterility but not hybrid inviability), he clearly foresaw the simple "secret of interracial sterility." Why, then, has his role been forgotten?

The chief reason is that neither DOBZHANSKY nor MULLER acknowledged BATESON's precedent. (They, of course, occasionally cite BATESON, but, as far as I can tell, never this essay, and never for this idea.) There are good reasons for thinking neither DOBZHANSKY nor MULLER knew of BATESON's model. For one thing, BATESON unveiled his model in a less-than-visible place, although his essay was reprinted in 1928 in *William Bateson, Naturalist,* a posthumous collection. More important, BATESON apparently never repeated his argument. While my search has not been exhaustive, BATESON does not offer his model in his more popular writings, even when discussing speciation. In *Problems of Genetics* (1913), his most widely read work, BATESON devotes his entire last chapter to hybrid sterility. While he suggests that hybrid sterility results from "complementary factors" (p. 238), he never explains why this is important nor how such factors can evolve. Indeed, the book ends with a depressing confession that once-confident evolutionists "no longer see how varieties give rise to species." By 1922, BATESON was reduced to admitting that "When students of other sciences ask us what is now currently believed about the origin of species we have no clear answer to give. Faith has given place to agnosticism." [And there is no doubt that by "species" BATESON more or less meant biological species: the "chief attribute of species [is] that the product of their crosses is frequently sterile" (BATESON 1922).] Two years before his death, BATESON lamented that "no general principles governing the incidence of interspecific sterility have been ascertained" and thus that "of the origin of specific distinctions we have . . . no acceptable account" (BATESON 1924). BATESON, to put it mildly, suffered a few doubts about his earlier solution to DARWIN's "mystery of mysteries." Indeed, as the years wore on, he grew increasingly obsessed and depressed by Darwinism's failure to crack the Species Problem which, to BATESON, meant the origin of hybrid sterility.

There is, of course, one other reason why DOBZHANSKY and MULLER may not have known of BATESON's precedent. BATESON, as the most vocal champion of Mendelism, harbored deep reservations about natural selection. To DOBZHANSKY and MULLER, BATESON surely represented an ancient (and somewhat unfriendly) regime that was irredeemably confused about evolution. BATESON was, to some extent, one of the enemies battled against during the modern synthesis. The inevitable lack of communication between the Mendelian old-guard and the modern synthetic upstarts probably had something to do with DOBZHANSKY and MULLER's oversight. Indeed, only HALDANE seems to have followed BATESON's evolutionary work (see especially HALDANE 1958, his fond assessment of BATESON).

By recalling BATESON's precedent in a commemoration of DOBZHANSKY's 1936 paper, it may seem that I give to DOBZHANSKY with one hand while taking away with the other. But this is not my intent. It is, after all, one of the virtues of science that those who differ on larger issues, as BATESON and DOBZHANSKY surely did, can nonetheless arrive at the same conclusion. Recent work on speciation renders this coincidence all the happier: for BATESON and DOBZHANSKY not only arrived at the same conclusion, but at the right conclusion.

I thank JERRY COYNE, CORBIN JONES and JAMES CROW for helpful discussions and comments.

LITERATURE CITED

BATESON, B., 1928 *William Bateson, Naturalist.* Cambridge University Press, Cambridge.

BATESON, W., 1909 Heredity and variation in modern lights, pp. 85–101 in *Darwin and Modern Science,* edited by A. C. SEWARD. Cambridge University Press, Cambridge.

BATESON, W., 1913 *Problems of Genetics.* Yale University Press, London.

BATESON, W., 1922 Evolutionary faith and modern doubts. Science **55:** 55–61.

BATESON, W., 1924 Progress in biology. Nature **113:** 644–646.

BELLAMY, A. W., 1922 Breeding experiments with the viviparous teleosts *Xiphophorus helleri* and *Platypoecilus maculatus.* Anat. Rec. **23:** 98–99.

COYNE, J., 1992 Genetics and speciation. Nature **355:** 511–515.

DARLINGTON, C. D., 1932 The control of the chromosomes by the genotype and its bearing on some evolutionary problems. Am. Nat. **66:** 25–51.

DOBZHANSKY, T., 1933 On the sterility of the interracial hybrids in *Drosophila pseudoobscura.* Proc. Natl. Acad. Sci. USA **19:** 397–403.

DOBZHANSKY, T., 1934 Studies on hybrid sterility. I. Spermatogenesis in pure and hybrid *Drosophila pseudoobscura.* Z. Zellforsch. Mikrosk. Anat. **21:** 169–221.

DOBZHANSKY, T., 1936 Studies on hybrid sterility. II. Localization of sterility factors in *Drosophila pseudoobscura* hybrids. Genetics **21:** 113–135.

DOBZHANSKY, T., 1937a Genetic nature of species differences. Am. Nat. **71:** 404–420.

DOBZHANSKY, T., 1937b *Genetics and the Origin of Species.* Columbia University Press, New York.

HALDANE, J. B. S., 1938 The nature of interspecific differences, pp. 19–94 in *Evolution,* edited by G. R. DE BEER. Clarendon Press, Oxford.

HALDANE, J. B. S., 1958 The theory of evolution, before and after Bateson. J. Genet. **56:** 1–17.

HOLLINGSHEAD, L., 1930 A lethal factor in *Crepis* effective only in interspecific hybrids. Genetics **15:** 114–140.

JOHANNSEN, W., 1923 Some remarks about units of heredity. Hereditas **4:** 133–141.

KING, M., 1993 *Species Evolution.* Cambridge University Press, Cambridge.

KOLLER, P. C., 1932 The relation of fertility factors to crossing-over in the *Drosophila obscura* hybrid. Z. Indukt. Abstammungs-Vererbungsl. **60:** 137–151.

LANCEFIELD, D. E., 1929 The genetic study of crosses of two races or physiological species of *Drosophila obscura.* Z. Indukt. Abstammungs-Vererbungsl. **52:** 287–317.

LEWONTIN, R. C., 1981 The scientific work of Th. Dobzhansky, pp. 93–115 in *Dobzhansky's Genetics of Natural Populations,* edited by R. C. LEWONTIN, J. A. MOORE, W. B. PROVINE, and B. WALLACE. Columbia University Press, New York.

MULLER, H. J., 1940 Bearing of the *Drosophila* work on systematics, pp. 185–268 in *The New Systematics,* edited by J. S. HUXLEY. Clarendon Press, Oxford.

MULLER, H. J., 1942 Isolating mechanisms, evolution, and temperature. Biol. Symp. **6:** 71–125.

ORR, H. A., 1995 The population genetics of speciation: the evolution of hybrid incompatibilities. Genetics **139:** 1805–1813.

PROVINE, W. B., 1981 Origins of the Genetics of Natural Populations series, pp. 1–85 in *Dobzhansky's Genetics of Natural Populations,* edited by R. C. LEWONTIN, J. A. MOORE, W. B. PROVINE and B. WALLACE. Columbia University Press, New York.

SAPP, J., 1987 *Beyond the Gene.* Oxford University Press, New York.

STURTEVANT, A. H., 1920 Genetic studies on *Drosophila simulans.* I. Introduction. Hybrids with *Drosophila melanogaster.* Genetics **5:** 488–500.

TURELLI, M., and H. A. ORR, 1995 The dominance theory of HALDANE's rule. Genetics **140:** 389–402.

WU, C.-I., and A. T. BECKENBACH, 1983 Evidence for extensive genetic differentiation between the sex-ratio and the standard arrangement of *Drosophila pseudoobscura* and *D. persimilis* and identification of hybrid sterility factors. Genetics **105:** 71–86.

Invasions of *P* Elements

William R. Engels

Laboratory of Genetics, University of Wisconsin–Madison, Madison, Wisconsin 53706

SOMEWHERE in Latin America a single *P*-element copy found its way into the genome of *Drosophila melanogaster* from another insect species. Once there, these transposable elements made use of their new hosts' DNA repair mechanism to increase their copy number while transposing to new genomic positions. Within the span of a few decades they spread worldwide to encompass nearly the entire species. The only populations to escape this invasion were the stocks that were maintained in the laboratories of early Drosophila geneticists and were thus reproductively isolated from the rest of the species.

This remarkable scenario (reviewed by ENGELS 1992) was followed by a *P*-element invasion of another kind. Within the last 10 years these elements have become ubiquitous tools for Drosophila geneticists of all stripes and have changed the way Drosophila research is conducted.

The spread of *P* elements through natural populations of *D. melanogaster* went largely unnoticed while it was happening, with the possible exception of some early observations of unstable mutations in the Soviet Union that might have been due to *P* mobility (BERG 1974). It was not until the 1970s that *P* elements were recognized as mobile genetic sequences, and by then the invasion was essentially complete. At that time, Drosophila research itself seemed to be on the wane. Most of the exciting and fundamental work on genetic mechanisms was being done with *Escherichia coli,* and flies were increasingly associated with old-fashioned classical genetics. Only the field of population genetics clung to Drosophila as the experimental organism of choice. Many population genetic experiments involved capturing flies from nature and crossing them to laboratory stocks in order to "extract" chromosomes for fitness measurements or to study variability in other traits such as recombination frequency. It is now known that crosses of this kind provided precisely the conditions needed to mobilize *P* elements and bring them to the attention of experimenters.

Address for correspondence: William R. Engels, Laboratory of Genetics, University of Wisconsin, Madison, WI 53706.
E-mail: wrengels@facstaff.wisc.edu

The first observations now recognized to be associated with *P* elements came from work of this kind by HIRAIZUMI (1971), M. and J. KIDWELL (1975), and SVED (1976). See CROW (1988) for a discussion of the earliest findings of genetic instability. A curious legacy of this history is that in the annual Drosophila meetings, transposable elements are often still categorized in the "Population and Evolution" section, even though many of the talks are entirely mechanistic.

A typical experiment for isolating chromosomes from a natural population of Drosophila starts with a cross of wild-caught males to multiply marked, laboratory-stock females. Sons are then backcrossed to the marker strain to take advantage of the lack of recombination in male meiosis. However, when HIRAIZUMI (1971) tried to do this with wild-caught flies from a Texas population, he consistently found recombination in the premeiotic germline of the sons. The frequency was only 1% that of meiotic recombination in females, but it was high enough to be conspicuous and even troublesome in the experiments.

It was not immediately clear that this male recombination required hybridization with a laboratory stock. A natural assumption was that the same events were occurring within the wild-derived stocks but were not observable without markers. However, other traits such as elevated mutation rates and temperature-sensitive sterility were soon seen to be associated with male recombination. These abnormalities were not seen in the wild-derived lines, but only in the hybrids. Moreover, only one of the two reciprocal crosses, the one with wild-derived males, produced hybrids with these traits (KIDWELL *et al.* 1973; KIDWELL and KIDWELL 1975). The syndrome was named "hybrid dysgenesis" (SVED 1976; KIDWELL *et al.* 1977).

Before the landmark paper by MARGARET and JIM KIDWELL and JOHN SVED (1977), all these observations seemed mysterious and rather chaotic. Most geneticists were happy to write them off as the idiosyncratic behavior of a few unusual Drosophila stocks. After the paper, hybrid dysgenesis still seemed mysterious and chaotic, but never again idiosyncratic. The authors found that all Drosophila strains could be classified neatly (more or less) into two categories they called *P* and *M*, depending on whether they contributed paternally or maternally to make dysgenic hybrids. Moreover, these categories were distributed systematically, with recently derived wild lines being *P* and old laboratory stocks behaving as *M* strains. The global nature of this phenomenon meant it could no longer be ignored, and the split of *D. melanogaster* into two categories with a hint of reproductive incompatibility suggested incipient speciation.

Meanwhile, GREEN (1977) noted that some of the mutations at the *singed* locus from HIRAIZUMI's original male recombination lines were unstable. He pointed out the parallel between this instability and the behavior of insertion mutations in *E. coli*, and suggested that the *singed* mutations were due to insertions of a mobile genetic element. This idea was quite influential, and it became the working hypothesis for most of us in the field. It was confirmed about five years later.

GREEN, however, did not accept the idea that the *singed* instability was part of the vastly wider phenomenon of hybrid dysgenesis. Instead, he approached the problem as though the source of the instability were a single, mappable site, which appeared to lie near the base of chromosome 2 (SLATKO and HIRAIZUMI 1975; SLATKO and GREEN 1980). The mapping data, however, were ambiguous, primarily because of the difficulty of using mutability or low levels of male recombination as a phenotype. A more powerful approach proved to be the use of temperature-sensitive female sterility, which could be observed in the first-generation hybrids themselves, and which had a very distinctive phenotype of missing germline tissues (ENGELS and PRESTON 1979; SCHAEFER *et al.* 1979). When this trait was used for mapping, the results showed that the factors responsible for hybrid dysgenesis resided simultaneously on all of the major chromosomes from a *P* strain, but were nowhere on the *M* chromosomes (ENGELS 1979b). Still more powerful evidence came from the hotspots for chromosome rearrangements that were found in many places of *P*-derived chromosomes (ENGELS and PRESTON 1981). These were hypothesized to be the sites of the transposable elements themselves.

These results led to the suggestion that hybrid dysgenesis was due to a family of transposable elements that existed in many positions throughout the *P* strain genomes, but were lacking in the *M* strains (ENGELS 1979a, 1981). These elements, called "*P* factors" and later generalized to "*P* elements" to include nonautonomous copies, were presumably quiescent within the *P* strains but became mobilized in the hybrid offspring of M-strain females. Molecular work from the the HOGNESS lab (FINNEGAN *et al.* 1978) had already demonstrated the existence of dispersed, mobile elements in many copies in the Drosophila genome. *P* elements were proposed to be another such family, but distin-

guished by their absence in *M* strains and their mobilization in the hybrids.

The game of speculating about the nature of hybrid dysgenesis came to an abrupt end when *P* elements were cloned. The Drosophila *white* gene had recently been cloned by the newly devised strategy of transposon tagging, making use of a *copia* element insertion there (BINGHAM *et al.* 1981). Dysgenesis-induced *white* mutations had been found by SIMMONS and LIM (1980) and proved to contain insertions of a new family of transposable elements (BINGHAM *et al.* 1982; RUBIN *et al.* 1982). Could these be the elements behind hybrid dysgenesis? The answer was not long in coming. Not only did the sequence of the new elements hybridize *in situ* to the breakage hotspots previously identified on *P* chromosomes (ENGELS and PRESTON 1981), but a dramatic Southern blot showed that the elements were present in many variable locations in *P* strains and absent in all but one of the *M* strains tested (BINGHAM *et al.* 1982). It was later found that the one exceptional *M* strain had come from a lab where stocks were regularly outcrossed to wild populations to enhance their vigor. Thus, the newly cloned transposable elements matched precisely the expected properties of *P* elements.

About the same time as the *P*-element story was developing, there were several other observations of unusual genetic behavior that would eventually prove to be due to transposable element mobilization, though unrelated to *P* elements. One such finding was the IR system of hybrid dysgenesis (PICARD and L'HERITIER 1971), which turned out to be caused by an element related to mammalian LINE transposons (BUCHETON *et al.* 1992). A case of unstable lethal mutations studied by LIM (1979) eventually proved to be due to *hobo* transposons (LIM 1988).

Observations of this kind along with the *P*-element findings had a disorienting effect at the time on many geneticists who had been used to a more placid view of the genome. Some who were once skeptical of hybrid dysgenesis now swung to the opposite extreme and seemed to assume that *any* claim about *P* elements, no matter how implausible, must be believed. The old standards of experimental evidence and rigor, like the old rules of heredity, must now be relaxed when *P* elements were involved. *Nature* seemed to embrace this new era with particular enthusiasm. One paper published there purported to show that the hybrid dysgenesis syndrome could be induced merely by injecting *M* strain flies with the ground-up remains of *P* strain flies (SOCHACKA and WOODRUFF 1976) even though the evidence and statistical analysis probably would not have stood up in any other field. Another report alleged that crossing *P* and *M* strains mobilized not only *P* elements, but most other transposable elements as well (GERASIMOVA *et al.* 1984), although the data could readily be explained in terms of pre-existing variability in the stocks. Both of these claims were later debunked (also in *Nature* articles: SVED *et al.* 1978; EGGLESTON *et al.* 1988).

The question of why *P* elements are mobile only in the germline, and only in certain hybrids, has been studied by many groups. Evidence to date shows the existence of a complex web of regulatory mechanisms involving both RNA processing (LASKI *et al.* 1986; RIO 1991; TSENG *et al.* 1991) and transcriptional regulation with a maternally inherited component (LEMAITRE *et al.* 1993; RONSSERAY *et al.* 1993).

Perhaps the most intriguing issue concerning *P* elements throughout the 1980s was the question of why the elements were ubiquitous in nature but absent in old laboratory stocks. For some of us, it was easier to think that the laboratory stocks somehow lost *P* elements from their genomes during a thousand or more generations of artificial conditions, as opposed to the rest of the species acquiring them during the same time span. A specific mechanism for ridding the laboratory stock genomes of *P* elements was suggested by the "stochastic loss" hypothesis (ENGELS 1981). According to this model, transposition and excision cause fluidity in the number of *P*-element copies in a population. Unlike the situation for Mendelian alleles, there is no such thing as fixation of *P* elements since there is essentially an unlimited number of potential insertion sites, and excision can remove elements from occupied sites. However, it is possible for all *P* elements to be lost from a population. Indeed, loss would be the only stable state of a population, and that state should be reached sooner or later. The expected time to reach this stable state would be vastly shorter for small populations, such as laboratory stocks, than for natural populations. Thus, according to this view, *M* strains were populations that have reached the stable state of zero copy number owing to many generations of small populations. For natural populations, the expected time for stochastic loss would be so great that it may never occur in human history.

M. KIDWELL took the alternative view that *P* elements were a new addition to the genome of *D. melanogaster* (KIDWELL 1979). She was impressed by quantitative variability in *P*-element activity between natural populations in different geographical locations; this suggested that *P* elements were not invariant components of the genome even in nature (KIDWELL 1983). Moreover, she thought that if *P* elements were being lost from laboratory stocks, such events should be observed directly, and none was (BINGHAM *et al.* 1982). According to this view, *I* elements, the LINE-like transposons responsible for the IR system of hybrid dysgenesis, also invaded natural populations of *D. melanogaster* in the present century, but did so several years prior to *P* elements, thus explaining the present-day distributions of *P* and *I* (KIDWELL 1983).

The biggest drawback of the rapid invasion hypothesis was that it was hard to explain the coincidence of a transposable element invading the genome of any well-studied species in such an evolutionarily insignificant time span. Transposon invasions can happen only a few times in the history of a species, since there are probably fewer than 100 transposable element families in most genomes. The observation of even one such invasion within the present century would be highly unlikely, and two would seem nearly impossible. Therefore, human intervention was almost certainly involved in some way to cause the schism between *P* and *M* strains and between *I* and *R*.

Many experiments meant to distinguish between recent loss *vs.* recent invasion yielded results that could be explained equally well under either hypothesis. For example, KIDWELL observed that the proportion of laboratory strains that were presently *M* decreased monotonically when plotted against the date of capture (KIDWELL 1983). She interpreted this trend to reflect the global spread of *P* strains in nature during the last few decades, but it could also be explained by noting that the more recently captured laboratory strains have had less time to lose their *P* elements. Just when it began to seem that the question would never be answered without ambiguity, a new kind of data emerged to resolve the issue with breathtaking clarity!

When the genomes of other Drosophila species were probed with *P*-element sequences, it was found that some but not all of these species had *P*-like elements (LANSMAN *et al.* 1985). Significantly, the closest relatives of *D. melanogaster* were without any sequences that would hybridize with the *P* probe, whereas there was strong hybridization from almost all species in the more distant willistoni and saltans species groups (STACEY *et al.* 1986; LANSMAN *et al.* 1987). This observation seemed to indicate that *D. melanogaster* did acquire *P* elements since the divergence from its sibling species, estimated at 2 million years. However, this finding still fell far short of proving that *P* elements invaded within the last 100 years. The denouement came from the sequencing of a specific *P*-like element from the genome of *D. willistoni* (DANIELS *et al.* 1990). This element was selected for analysis because its restriction map appeared to match that of the standard *P* element. The sequence showed that there was only one base pair difference among the 2907 bp of the complete *P* element. Such extreme conservation between sequences, which included three introns, was inconceivable over the estimated 60 million years that *willistoni* and *melanogaster* have diverged. The result could only mean that a very recent horizontal transfer had occurred. Since *P*-like elements were much more variable and widespread in the *willistoni* group than in *melanogaster*, the latter species must have been the recipient.

The near identity between *P*-element sequences in distantly related species would have been a powerful argument for recent horizontal transmission and invasion in any case. However, there was an extra bonus in the form of a plausible explanation for the apparent paradox of why these elements would invade *D. melanogaster* only now after 60 million years of evolution. The willistoni species group is endemic to South America, Central America, and parts of Florida, whereas *D. melanogaster* is common in temperate climates worldwide. This cosmopolitan distribution of *melanogaster* is thought to be a recent development. The species probably evolved in Western Africa (LACHAISE *et al.* 1988) and was introduced into the Americas only in recent historical times through human commercial activity (JOHNSON 1913). Thus, *melanogaster* did not come into contact with *willistoni* and *P* elements until shortly before the *P* invasion occurred. The relatively recent global expansion of *melanogaster* might have provided an opportunity for acquisition of other new transposable elements in addition to *P*, such as the active forms of the *I* factor and *hobo*, but the details are less clear in those cases. One can even speculate that acquiring new transposable elements is a general hazard associated with the expansion of any species into a new ecosystem.

How did *P* elements make the jump from *D. willistoni* to *D. melanogaster,* and how did they spread throughout the new host species so quickly? The first question is difficult because it hinges on what may be a single contamination event that happened in nature many years ago. *P* elements can be moved between species by the injection of purified DNA (BRENNAN *et al.* 1984), but a natural process to accomplish the same thing is a matter of speculation. One suggestion is that parasitic mites played the role of "dirty injection needles" to carry *P*-element DNA from one species to another (HOUCK *et al.* 1991; KIDWELL 1992). Insect viruses have also been suggested as potential vectors for spreading transposons (MILLER and MILLER 1982). Neither process has yet been observed directly. Horizontal movement of transposable elements is probably widespread in the animal kingdom (ROBERTSON 1995), suggesting that multiple mechanisms for their interspecific movement might exist.

The second question, however, is more tractable because the spread of *P* elements through populations is readily observed experimentally (KIDWELL *et al.* 1988; GOOD *et al.* 1989; PRESTON and ENGELS 1989). It is unlikely that this spread is aided by natural selection, since *P* elements confer no apparent advantage to their hosts and even have detrimental effects such as partial sterility. Instead, transposition itself is probably the driving force behind the invasion. *P* elements jump nonreplicatively, leaving behind a double-strand DNA break that is handled by the cell's normal DNA repair pathways (ENGELS *et al.* 1990; GLOOR *et al.* 1991; ENGELS 1996). In most cases, this repair involves replacing the missing sequences with homologous material from the sister chromatid (JOHNSON-SCHLITZ and ENGELS 1993). A *P* element on the sister chromatid is, therefore, copied into the site just vacated by the transposition. The net

result is a gain of one *P*-element copy. This net gain provides a powerful mechanism for the spread of *P* elements through a population, and natural selection would be unable to prevent it. In small populations, rapid invasion of *P* elements usually leads to extinction of the stock, but in larger ones the population usually survives, probably owing to negative regulation of *P*-element transposition activity (PRESTON and ENGELS 1989).

As mentioned above, *P* elements have now become the Swiss army knives of Drosophila genetics (reviewed by KAISER *et al.* 1995). They are used for mutagenesis, transposon tagging, and, most importantly, germline transformation (RUBIN and SPRADLING 1982; SPRADLING and RUBIN 1982). Massive collections of *P*-insertion lines are being built to identify transcription patterns (HARTENSTEIN and JAN 1992) and provide a framework for the Drosophila genome project (SPRADLING *et al.* 1995). New uses for *P* elements are still being found, such as the exploitation of *P*-induced, double-strand breakage to effect gene replacement (GLOOR *et al.* 1991), and the use of *P*-induced recombination to generate duplications and deletions in nearby genes (PRESTON *et al.* 1996). *Drosophila melanogaster* might have dodged a bullet when it survived the acquisition of a highly invasive transposable element in its genome. That same element then helped prevent Drosophila from being abandoned as an important experimental organism and helped usher in a new era of Drosophila research.

LITERATURE CITED

BERG R. L., 1974 A simultaneous mutability rise at the *singed* locus in two out of three *Drosophila melanogaster* populations studied in 1973. Dros. Inf. Serv. **51:** 100–102.

BINGHAM, P. M., R. LEVIS and G. M. RUBIN, 1981 The cloning of the DNA sequences from the *white* locus of *Drosophila melanogaster* using a novel and general method. Cell **25:** 693–704.

BINGHAM, P. M., M. G. KIDWELL and G. M. RUBIN, 1982 The molecular basis of *P-M* hybrid dysgenesis: the role of the *P* element, a *P* strain-specific transposon family. Cell **29:** 995–1004.

BRENNAN, M. D., R. G. ROWAN and W. J. DICKINSON, 1984 Introduction of a functional *P* element into the germ line of *Drosophila hawaiiensis.* Cell **38:** 147–151.

BUCHETON, A., C. VAURY, M. C. CHABOISSIER, P. ABAD, A. PELISSON *et al.,* 1992 *I* elements and the Drosophila genome. Genetica **86:** 175–190.

CROW, J. F., 1988 The genesis of dysgenesis. Genetics **120:** 315–318.

DANIELS, S. B., K. R. PETERSON, L. D. STRAUSBAUGH, M. G. KIDWELL and A. CHOVNICK, 1990 Evidence for horizontal transmission of the *P* transposable element between Drosophila species. Genetics **124:** 339–355.

EGGLESTON, W. B., D. M. JOHNSON-SCHLITZ and W. R. ENGELS, 1988 *P-M* hybrid dysgenesis does not mobilize other transposable element families in *D. melanogaster.* Nature **331:** 368–370.

ENGELS, W. R., 1979a Extrachromosomal control of mutability in *Drosophila melanogaster.* Proc. Natl. Acad. Sci. USA **76:** 4011–4015.

ENGELS, W. R., 1979b Hybrid dysgenesis in *Drosophila melanogaster:* rules of inheritance of female sterility. Genet. Res. Camb. **33:** 219–236.

ENGELS, W. R., 1981 Hybrid dysgenesis in Drosophila and the stochastic loss hypothesis. Cold Spring Harbor Symp. Quant. Biol. **45:** 561–565.

ENGELS, W. R., 1992 The origin of *P* elements in *Drosophila melanogaster.* BioEssays **14:** 681–686.

ENGELS, W. R., 1996 *P* elements in Drosophila, pp. 103–123 in *Transposable Elements*, edited by H. SAEDLER and A. GIERL. Springer-Verlag, Berlin. ⟨http://www.wisc.edu/genetics/CATG/engels/Pelements/⟩

ENGELS, W. R., and C. R. PRESTON, 1979 Hybrid dysgenesis in *Drosophila melanogaster:* the biology of male and female sterility. Genetics **92:** 161–175.

ENGELS, W. R., and C. R. PRESTON, 1981 Identifying *P* factors in Drosophila by means of chromosome breakage hotspots. Cell **26:** 421–428.

ENGELS, W. R., D. M. JOHNSON-SCHLITZ, W. B. EGGLESTON and J. SVED, 1990 High-frequency *P* element loss in Drosophila is homolog-dependent. Cell **62:** 515–525.

FINNEGAN, D. J., G. M. RUBIN, M. W. YOUNG and D. S. HOGNESS, 1978 Repeated gene families in *Drosophila melanogaster*. Cold Spring Harbor Symp. Quant. Biol. **42:** 1053–1063.

GERASIMOVA, T. I., L. J. MIZROKHI and G. P. GEORGIEV, 1984 Transposition bursts in genetically unstable *Drosophila melanogaster*. Nature **309:** 714–716.

GLOOR, G. B., N. A. NASSIF, D. M. JOHNSON-SCHLITZ, C. R. PRESTON and W. R. ENGELS, 1991 Targeted gene replacement in Drosophila via *P* element-induced gap repair. Science **253:** 1110–1117.

GOOD, A. G., G. A. MEISTER, H. W. BROCK, T. A. GRIGLIATTI and D. A. HICKEY, 1989 Rapid spread of transposable *P* elements in experimental populations of *Drosophila melanogaster*. Genetics **122:** 387–396.

GREEN, M. M., 1977 Genetic instability in *Drosophila melanogaster:* de novo induction of putative insertion mutations. Proc. Natl. Acad. Sci. USA **74:** 3490–3493.

HARTENSTEIN, V., and Y.-N. JAN, 1992 Studying Drosophila embryogenesis with P-*lacZ* enhancer trap lines. Roux's Arch. Dev. Biol. **201:** 194–220.

HIRAIZUMI, Y., 1971 Spontaneous recombination in *Drosophila melanogaster* males. Proc. Natl. Acad. Sci. USA **68:** 268–270.

HOUCK, M. A., J. B. CLARK, K. R. PETERSON and M. G. KIDWELL, 1991 Possible horizontal transfer of Drosophila genes by the mite *Proctolaelaps regalis*. Science **253:** 1125–1128.

JOHNSON, C. W., 1913 The distribution of some species of Drosophila. Psyche **20:** 202–204.

JOHNSON-SCHLITZ, D. M., and W. R. ENGELS, 1993 *P* element-induced interallelic gene conversion of insertions and deletions in Drosophila. Mol. Cell. Biol. **13:** 7006–7018.

KAISER, K., J. W. SENTRY and D. J. FINNEGAN, 1995 Eukaryotic transposable elements as tools to study gene structure and function, pp. 69–100 in *Mobile Genetic Elements*, edited by D. J. SHERRATT. IRL Press, Oxford.

KIDWELL, M. G., 1979 Hybrid dysgenesis in *Drosophila melanogaster:* the relationship between the *P-M* and *I-R* interaction systems. Genet. Res. Camb. **33:** 105–117.

KIDWELL, M. G., 1983 Evolution of hybrid dysgenesis determinants in *Drosophila melanogaster*. Proc. Natl. Acad. Sci. USA **80:** 1655–1659.

KIDWELL, M. G., 1992 Horizontal transfer of *P* elements and other short inverted repeat transposons. Genetica **86:** 275–286.

KIDWELL, M. G., and J. F. KIDWELL, 1975 Cytoplasm-chromosome interactions in *Drosophila melanogaster*. Nature **253:** 755–756.

KIDWELL, M. G., J. F. KIDWELL and M. NEI, 1973 A case of high rate of spontaneous mutation affecting viability in *Drosophila melanogaster*. Genetics **75:** 133–153.

KIDWELL, M. G., J. F. KIDWELL and J. A. SVED, 1977 Hybrid dysgenesis in *Drosophila melanogaster:* a syndrome of aberrant traits including mutation, sterility, and male recombination. Genetics **86:** 813–833.

KIDWELL, M. G., K. KIMURA and D. M. BLACK, 1988 Evolution of hybrid dysgenesis potential following *P* element contamination in *Drosophila melanogaster*. Genetics **119:** 815–828.

LACHAISE, D., M. L. CARIOU, J. R. DAVID, F. LEMEUNIER, L. TSACAS *et al.*, 1988 Historical biogeography of the *Drosophila melanogaster* species subgroup. Evol. Biol. **22:** 159–225.

LANSMAN, R. A., S. N. STACEY, T. A. GRIGLIATTI and H. W. BROCK, 1985 Sequences homologous to the *P* mobile element of *Drosophila melanogaster* are widely distributed in the subgenus Sophophora. Nature **318:** 561–563.

LANSMAN, R. A., R. O. SHADE, T. A. GRIGLIATTI and H. W. BROCK,

1987 Evolution of *P* transposable elements: sequences of *Drosophila nebulosa P* elements. Proc. Natl. Acad. Sci. USA **84:** 6491–6495.

LASKI, F. A., D. C. RIO and G. M. RUBIN, 1986 Tissue specificity of Drosophila *P* element transposition is regulated at the level of mRNA splicing. Cell **44:** 7–19.

LEMAITRE, B., S. RONSSERAY and D. COEN, 1993 Maternal repression of the *P* element promoter in the germline of *Drosophila melanogaster:* a model for the *P* cytotype. Genetics **135:** 149–160.

LIM, J. K., 1979 Site-specific instability in *Drosophila melanogaster:* the origin of the mutation and cytogenetic evidence for site specificity. Genetics **93:** 681–701.

LIM, J. K., 1988 Intrachromosomal rearrangements mediated by *hobo* transposons in *Drosophila melanogaster*. Proc. Natl. Acad. Sci. USA **85:** 9153–9157.

MILLER, D. W., and L. K. MILLER, 1982 A virus mutant with an insertion of a *copia*-like element. Nature **299:** 562–564.

PICARD, G., and P. L'HERITIER, 1971 A maternally inherited factor inducing sterility in *Drosophila melanogaster*. Dros. Inf. Serv. **46:** 54.

PRESTON, C. R., and W. R. ENGELS, 1989 Spread of *P* transposable elements in inbred lines of *Drosophila melanogaster*, pp. 71–85 in *Progress in Nucleic Acid Research and Molecular Biology: Hollaender Symposium Proceedings*, Vol. 36, edited by W. COHN and K. MOLDAVE. Academic Press, San Diego.

PRESTON, C. R., J. A. SVED and W. R. ENGELS, 1996 Flanking duplications and deletions associated with *P*-induced male recombination in Drosophila. Genetics **144:** 1623–1638.

RIO, D. C., 1991 Regulation of Drosophila *P* element transposition. Trends Genet. **7:** 282–287.

ROBERTSON, H. M., 1995 The *Tc1-mariner* superfamily of transposons in animals. J. Insect Physiol. **41:** 99–105.

RONSSERAY, S., B. LEMAITRE and D. COEN, 1993 Maternal inheritance of *P* cytotype in *Drosophila melanogaster:* a "pre-*P* cytotype" is strictly extra-chromosomally transmitted. Mol. Gen. Genet. **241:** 115–123.

RUBIN, G. M., and A. C. SPRADLING, 1982 Genetic transformation of Drosophila with transposable element vectors. Science **218:** 348–353.

RUBIN, G. M., M. G. KIDWELL and P. M. BINGHAM, 1982 The molecular basis of *P-M* hybrid dysgenesis: the nature of induced mutations. Cell **29:** 987–994.

SCHAEFER, R. E., M. G. KIDWELL and A. FAUSTO-STERLING, 1979 Hybrid Dysgenesis in *Drosophila melanogaster:* morphological and cytological studies of ovarian dysgenesis. Genetics **92:** 1141–1152.

SIMMONS, M. J., and J. K. LIM, 1980 Site specificity of mutations arising in dysgenic hybrids of *Drosophila melanogaster*. Proc. Natl. Acad. Sci. USA **77:** 6042–6046.

SLATKO, B. E., and M. M. GREEN, 1980 Genetic instability in *Drosophila melanogaster:* mapping the mutator activity of an MR strain. Biol. Zbl. **99:** 149–155.

SLATKO, B. E., and Y. HIRAIZUMI, 1975 Elements causing male crossing over in *Drosophila melanogaster*. Genetics **81:** 313–324.

SOCHACKA, J. H., and R. C. WOODRUFF, 1976 Induction of male recombination in *Drosophila melanogaster* by injection of extracts of flies showing male recombination. Nature **262:** 287–289.

SPRADLING, A. C., and G. M. RUBIN, 1982 Transposition of cloned *P* elements into Drosophila germ line chromosomes. Science **218:** 341–347.

SPRADLING, A. C., D. M. STERN, I. KISS, J. ROOTE, T. LAVERTY *et al.*, 1995 Gene disruptions using *P* transposable elements: an integral component of the Drosophila genome project. Proc. Natl. Acad. Sci. USA **92:** 10824–10830.

STACEY, S. N., R. A. LANSMAN, H. W. BROCK and T. A. GRIGLIATTI, 1986 Distribution and conservation of mobile elements in the genus Drosophila. Mol. Biol. Evol. **3:** 522–534.

SVED, J. A., 1976 Hybrid dysgenesis in *Drosophila melanogaster:* a possible explanation in terms of spatial organization of chromosomes. Aust. J. Biol. Sci. **29:** 375–388.

SVED, J. A., D. C. MURRAY, R. E. SCHAEFER and M. G. KIDWELL, 1978 Male recombination is not induced in *Drosophila melanogaster* by extracts of strains with male recombination potential. Nature **275:** 457–458.

TSENG, J. C., S. ZOLLMAN, A. C. CHAIN and F. A. LASKI, 1991 Splicing of the Drosophila *P* element ORF2-ORF3 intron is inhibited in a human cell extract. Mech. Dev. **35:** 65–72.

Whatever Happened to Paramecium Genetics?

John R. Preer, Jr.

Department of Biology, Indiana University, Bloomington, Indiana 47405-5143

IN the period between 1945 and 1965 the genetics of Paramecium enjoyed its heyday. All introductory college texts on genetics had a section on Paramecium. SRB *et al.* (1965) had the most extensive coverage. Topics considered were the life cycle, infectious heredity (killers), stable states of gene expression (serotypes), the ability of preexisting structure to control the development of new structure (cortical inheritance), and inheritance due to macronuclear differentiation (mating types). At a more advanced level, *The Genetics of Microorganisms* (CATCHESIDE 1951) had a whole chapter on protozoan genetics (almost all on Paramecium), alongside chapters on viral genetics and bacterial genetics.

A perusal of many of today's popular introductory textbooks of genetics reveals that the vast majority, such as GRIFFITHS *et al.* (1993) and RUSSELL (1994) are completely free of all references to Paramecium. Only an occasional text such as KLUG and CUMMINGS (1994) or TAMARIN (1994) presents some of the findings on Paramecium. At the more advanced level, *Genes V* (LEWIN 1994) has only one reference to Paramecium and, alas, it is wrong. In the same book a discussion of deviations from the universal genetic code in ciliates, first discovered in Paramecium, mentions only Tetrahymena and Euplotes.

The facts presented in those early times haven't changed, and, indeed, our knowledge of most of the subjects has been advanced considerably since then. Nevertheless, the work on Paramecium appears either to have been judged inconsequential or else has just been forgotten. This paper is devoted to the question of what happened. Is the work truly inconsequential? Has only a loss of memory occurred? And if the work was forgotten, then why?

In our search for answers to these questions we go back in time. In the early days of T. H. MORGAN in the 1920s, there was somewhat of a battle going on between the "Mendelian-Morgan geneticists" and the "physiol-

ogists." The geneticists had established the chromosome as the basis of heredity and the genes as the units of inheritance. The physiologists maintained that the genes being studied by geneticists all affected rather trivial and superficial characters, which were capable of undergoing mutation. The really important characteristics such as membrane permeability, cell mobility, and cell division were invariant and determined by the cytoplasm, not the genes on chromosomes. Mutations affecting such fundamental traits, they argued, would invariably lead to cell death and were, therefore, inaccessible to the science of genetics. H. S. JENNINGS at Johns Hopkins felt that the argument was worth attention and that the protozoa might well be able to contribute to the answer. For accounts of JENNINGS, see SONNEBORN (1975b) and CROW (1987). Protozoan genetics was a flourishing science at that time, and JENNINGS' (1929) review of the subject had 259 references. While Paramecium was not the only game in town in 1929, it was surely a major one . Moreover, some of that work didn't seem to fit with the notion that all heredity could be explained by assorting genes on chromosomes.

Since that time, much has been learned about the genetics of Paramecium, primarily owing to the work of SONNEBORN and his students. SONNEBORN (PREER 1996) was a giant figure in protozoan genetics, laying the basis for studies on virtually all the subjects now present in the modern work on ciliates. With the advent of WATSON and CRICK's double helix, the focus of research in genetics changed, and the earlier arguments mentioned above have been largely forgotten. We will go back and review the findings that seem pertinent, bringing each topic up to date. Perhaps in this way we will be able to understand what has happened and judge better what the significance of each area is.

The macronucleus: Paramecium, like most other ciliates, has one or more diploid micronuclei and a polyploid macronucleus. The polyploid macronucleus is the metabolically active nucleus, while the genes of the micronucleus are largely unexpressed. At conjugation the micronuclei undergo meiosis, while the old macronucleus starts to degenerate. One of the meiotic products

Address for correspondence: John R. Preer, Jr., Department Of Biology, Indiana University, Bloomington, IN 47405-5143.
E-mail: jpreer@bio.indiana.edu

now divides once to produce a stationary and a migratory haploid nucleus. After migratory nuclei are exchanged, the migratory and stationary nuclei unite to produce a diploid syncaryon, which divides mitotically twice to produce nuclei that develop into new micronuclei and macronuclei. Autogamy is identical except that the process occurs in a single cell, the migratory and stationary nuclei formed in each cell simply fusing to produce the syncaryon. It was always obvious that a knowledge of the fundamental structure of the macronucleus was necessary to understand the genetics of Paramecium. However, the techniques suitable for attacking this problem were not available until fairly recently. It has been known for a very long time that extensive amplification occurs at macronuclear formation, ploidy levels going from diploid to 1000 or more copies. We know now that, in addition to amplification, extensive rearrangements in the DNA also occur.

Two major types of DNA rearrangements are found in ciliates (see the review by PRESCOTT (1994). In the first kind, chromosomes are simply broken (usually with concomitant loss of a few bases), and telomeres are added to the broken ends. The breaks occur at a conserved 15 base pair chromosome breakage sequence in Tetrahymena, where it is estimated that several thousand such breaks occur at the formation of a new macronucleus (YAO 1988). The size of the resulting macronuclear chromosomes varies with the ciliate species, reaching its most extreme case in the hypotrichous ciliates, where the rule is one macronuclear chromosome for one gene. More recently, information is also becoming available about such breaks in *Paramecium tetraurelia* (PREER and PREER 1979; FORNEY and BLACKBURN 1988; PHAN *et al.* 1988; CARON 1992), where each of the many micronuclear chromosomes is broken into an average of about seven new macronuclear chromosomes with an average size of 300–600 kb. We know that there is often variation in the way these events occur and that, once formed, the resulting variations can be constant throughout the life of a given macronucleus (AMAR 1994). Telomeres consist of C4A2 repeats in Tetrahymena and a mixture of C4A2 and C3A3 repeats in Paramecium. Telomerase, the enzyme responsible for telomere addition, is a ribonucleoprotein, with the RNA component containing a complement of C4A2. Surprisingly, the RNA is encoded by a gene that contains only the complement of C4A2 in both Tetrahymena and Paramecium (MCCORMICK-GRAHAM and ROMERO 1994).

In the second kind of chromosome breakage, chromosomes undergo internal deletion. The deleted sections, which never get into the macronucleus and are lost, vary in size from about 20 to several hundred bases and are called internal eliminated sequences (IESs). Such sequences are very numerous and are often found within the coding region of a single gene (STEELE *et al.* 1994). The gene for surface protein A in Paramecium contains seven IESs within the coding region of the gene and two more just upstream. In Paramecium and Euplotes, IESs are bounded by the dinucleotide, TA, and a short consensus sequence within the ends of the IESs has been characterized (KLOBUTCHER and HERRICK 1997). The deletions are made with perfect precision, and the resulting macronuclear genes have intact coding regions. Remarkably, it has been found (see review in PRESCOTT 1994) that in some ciliates the portions of the genes between the eliminated pieces are in a scrambled order in the micronucleus, and during macronuclear formation the sections destined for the macronucleus are miraculously recombined to give properly ordered functional genes. Some of these internal eliminated sequences have homology to transposon-related sequences found in the micronuclei of ciliates (KLOBUTCHER and HERRICK 1995). It is interesting that in ciliates the transposon-like elements are eliminated during macronuclear formation. The transposon-related sequences have also been shown to show sequence homology with well-known transposons found in a variety of organisms (DOAK *et al.* 1993).

The macronucleus is a particularly suitable place to study the many kinds of variation that can occur in DNA.

Amitosis: When cells divide, they do so by mitosis, which ensures that the chromosomes of the parent are precisely reproduced in the daughter cells. When the macronuclei of ciliates divide, however, there is no mitosis and the macronuclei simply pinch into two by amitosis. This process seems to be the only true case of amitosis known. The question of how genic balance is maintained during many cycles of amitosis has never been answered. In the absence of mitosis, random distribution of chromosomes at cell division should lead to drift in the numbers of the different kinds of chromosomes and result in imbalances. If divisions continued long enough, some chromosomes would even be lost altogether. Such drift does occur in Tetrahymena in the case of chromosomes bearing alternative alleles, for heterozygous lines show allelic segregation during continued fissions, eventually producing lines pure for one or the other allele. Although single alleles are segregated out into pure lines, genic balance is maintained permanently among genes at different loci. Evidence obtained in Tetrahymena shows that in lieu of mitosis, some other mechanism must operate in ciliates to maintain balance (see PREER and PREER 1979). It is difficult to conceive of any simple mechanism that might produce proper balance. According to one hypothesis (PREER and PREER 1979; BRUNK 1986), each kind of macronuclear chromosome can sense its own copy number (much like different plasmids in a bacterium) and adjust its replication in such a way that it maintains a constant level. This is an old problem that cries for a solution. The existence of unique sites on macronuclear chromosomes that determine copy number is an exciting possibility.

Caryonidal inheritance: Soon after Tracy SONNEBORN discovered mating types in Paramecium, he began a serious study of the genetics of Paramecium. He first looked at the inheritance of the newly discovered mating types, quickly demonstrated simple Mendelism, and confirmed the essential nuclear events at cell division, conjugation, and autogamy. As already noted, new macronuclei and micronuclei are derived from a single diploid micronucleus. These are segregated to separate cells at the next cell division. SONNEBORN called these lines "caryonides" and found that they were often of different mating type, even though both the nuclei were derived from a single diploid nucleus by mitosis. Caryonidal inheritance was defined as the inheritance of character differences that arise at the time of macronuclear formation and remain constant throughout subsequent vegetative fissions. We now know that variations in the organization of macronuclear DNA often arise when new macronuclei develop from micronuclei (AMAR 1994). Such variations are also inherited caryonidally, and it is likely that caryonidal inheritance of mating type has a similar explanation (ORIAS 1981). DNA processing, that is, the production of variations in DNA, is well known in many organisms (Ascaris, scale insects, development of the immune system in vertebrates). Macronuclear development gives us a unique system in which to study the phenomenon of DNA processing.

Transformation: GODISKA et al. (1987) showed that the macronucleus of Paramecium can be transformed by injecting DNA. The disadvantage of having to inject cells individually is more than offset by very high transformation frequencies (nearly 100% in the hands of some investigators). Telomeres are added directly to the terminal bases of the ends of the injected DNA (GILLEY et al. 1988). Unlike Tetrahymena, Paramecium can apparently add telomeres to any piece of DNA from any source and then provide for its reproduction. Moreover, injected genes derived from Paramecium are transcribed and translated. The DNA is usually replicated at the same level at which it is injected (KIM et al. 1992) and finally is lost at the next autogamy or conjugation. In Tetrahymena, fragments of DNA do not acquire telomeres, but suitable vectors have been produced, and integration of genes into preexisting chromosomes occurs. Thus, transformation produces a macronucleus consisting of a few transformed macronuclear chromosomes mixed with a large number of untransformed. At subsequent vegetative fissions, these types segregate out into pure types and make it possible to carry out gene replacement. These new techniques are proving to be powerful additions to our ability to study the molecular genetics of ciliates.

Macronuclear inheritance: Perhaps the most unusual and intriguing phenomenon in ciliate genetics was discovered many years ago when SONNEBORN was first studying the inheritance of mating type. Although mating type in most strains of Paramecium showed caryonidal inheritance, as described above, in one group of species the caryonidal inheritance was found to be modified by a very strong tendency for the mating type of each caryonide to be like that of its cytoplasmic parent. In other words, cytoplasmic inheritance was involved. SONNEBORN, however, was able to show by an ingenious experiment, using conjugation, cytoplasmic exchange, and regeneration of fragments of the old macronucleus, that the genetic determinants lay in the macronuclei, not in the cytoplasm. Using genetic markers, he was able to recover and distinguish lines whose macronuclei were derived from normally produced syncarya and lines whose macronuclei were derived from regenerating fragments of the old macronucleus. He found that determination of macronuclei occurs only during new macronuclear formation and is usually the same type as the type of the old macronucleus. He concluded that the macronucleus determines the cytoplasm, and the cytoplasm, in turn, determines the type of newly forming macronuclei. Thus, genetic information is transferred by way of the cytoplasm from the old macronucleus to the new macronucleus at conjugation and autogamy. This pattern of inheritance has subsequently been called macronuclear inheritance. Later discoveries have led to considerable advances in our knowledge of the situation.

Most of these advances began with the discovery of a puzzling mutant discovered by EPSTEIN and FORNEY (1984). This mutant appeared in a screen for mutants that were unable to express surface antigen A in stock 51 of *Paramecia tetraurelia*. Although most of the mutants proved to be Mendelian, one, d48, showed a cytoplasmic pattern of inheritance. Since the A gene had been isolated, it was possible to ascertain that the chromosome bearing the A gene, which was near the end of a macronuclear chromosome, had been deleted at a point just upstream of the A gene, eliminating the entire gene from the macronucleus. The genetic results, however, were consistent only with the conclusion that the micronucleus still contained the complete A gene [later proved directly with the isolation of micronuclei in Paramecium (PREER et al. 1992)]. Thus, d48 was a defect in DNA processing. Soon after this discovery, HARUMOTO (1986) found that d48 could be "rescued" (converted to wild type permanently) by injecting into its macronucleus macronuclear material from wild-type cells. This surprising discovery was soon followed by the observation that the injection of the whole of the cloned A gene, or even a small portion of the A gene, sufficed for rescue (KIM et al. 1994; YOU et al. 1994). There is more than one effective region in the A gene, and the longer the region, the more effective it is. It was concluded that the genetic defect in d48 that leads to its apparent cytoplasmic inheritance is only the lack of the A gene in the old macronucleus. If this conclusion is correct, then one should be able to create d48 mutations at will as follows. The micronucleus of a mutant strain containing a micronuclear deletion for the A gene is removed by micromanipulation and then replaced with a micronucleus from wild type. When this experiment was carried out (KOBAYASHI and KOIZUMI 1988), it was found that the new lines were stable through subsequent autogamies and were indistinguishable from d48. This dramatic result confirms that d48 is not inherited as a simple cytoplasmic mutant, but is a macronuclear DNA processing mutation.

The same phenomenon has been shown for the serotype B gene. A d48-like mutation defective in serotype B was constructed by removing the micronuclei from a mutant deficient in its micronucleus for the B gene and transplanting in new micronuclei from wild type (SCOTT et al. 1994). The B gene cannot rescue d48, and A cannot rescue the d48-like no-B mutation, nor will any other DNA serve the purpose. Specificity is complete. No complementary RNAs appear to be produced. The explanation for macronuclear inheritance is totally unknown. One suggestion is that normally, when new macronuclei are formed, small bits of DNA leave the A gene in the old degenerating macronucleus, pass through the cytoplasm, enter the newly forming macronuclei, and serve as an essential element in DNA processing of the regions in and adjacent to the A gene.

Macronuclear inheritance is exhibited not only by mating type and d48 and d48-like mutants, but also by a trichocyst non-discharge mutant studied by SONNEBORN and SCHNELLER (1979) and by reversion of a paranoiac behavioral mutant by RUDMAN and PREER (1996). Mating type has recently been associated with rearrangements in Paramecium (MEYER and KELLER 1996). The generality of macronuclear inheritance is further revealed by a remarkable observation of MEYER (1992). He injected very high amounts of various clones of wild-type DNA into wild-type cells. Surprisingly, he found that offspring of such injected cells carry deletions in their DNA. These occur in the vicinity of the chromosomal location of the sites from which the injected DNA was taken. Moreover, further analysis of these clones shows that the deletions exhibit macronuclear inheritance. These experiments reinforce the conclusion that the DNA of the old macronucleus can influence DNA processing during new macronuclear formation. Elucidation of these remarkable events at the molecular level will give us new insights into the mechanisms that control DNA cutting and splicing.

Killers: SONNEBORN found that, although Mendelian genetics plays the same role in Paramecium as it does in other organisms, it often fails to provide satisfactory explanations for the phenomena he encountered. Not only did caryonidal inheritance, amitosis, and the life cycle present problems, but every other trait that he examined seemed to show some sort of non-Mendelian behavior. This was true of antigenic variation, cell

shape, and, most dramatically, the inheritance of "killer" paramecia. Killer paramecia constituted the first example of cytoplasmic inheritance in animals, although many cases had been found in plants. Killers liberated a toxin into the medium that killed non-killer (sensitive) paramecia. Crosses showed that the trait was dependent upon a cytoplasmic factor which SONNEBORN designated "kappa." Kappa, in turn, depended upon the presence of the Mendelian gene K. Kappa also rendered the cells in which it was found resistant to the toxin.

At about this time EPHRUSSI was beginning his classic work on yeast that eventually led to our understanding of mitochondrial genetics. S. SPIEGELMAN also found non-Mendelian phenomena in his studies on adaptive enzymes in yeast. When SONNEBORN viewed his own findings on Paramecium in the light of these other discoveries, the "plasmagene theory" (SONNEBORN 1947) was proposed. It was hypothesized that genes could produce messengers with the capacity for self-reproduction. The work on kappa constituted the underpinnings of the plasmagene theory. Later it became increasingly evident that kappa was a symbiotic bacterium, not a self-reproducing gene product. Moreover, the inheritance of enzymatic adaptation in Escherichia coli, which closely resembled that in yeast, was explained in terms of metabolic steady states (NOVICK and WEINER 1957). Plasmagenes were gone even before they had become well known. Moreover, the other phenomena that had led SONNEBORN to the proposal, as we will see, eventually turned out to have different bases.

Subsequent work on kappa revealed many species of bacterial symbionts present in Paramecium (see reviews in PREER and PREER 1984; POND et al. 1989). Each of the symbionts has a restricted cellular location, a few in the micronuclei, some in macronuclei, most in cytoplasm. Some have flagella, some have a thick cell wall. None are capable of culture free of Paramecium. Different strains produce different toxins, each resulting in a different prelethal effect on sensitive paramecia. Some of the toxins are found in the medium in which killers live; some are active only during cell-to-cell contact at conjugation; some produce no toxins at all. The production of toxins has been related to the presence in the symbionts of plasmids in some cases, to defective phages in others. The toxins appear to be insoluble substances and in many cases are found associated with refractile (R bodies) that develop within kappa, minute, tightly wound rolls of proteinaceous ribbons that can unroll and reroll in a fraction of a second in response to certain environmental stimuli. The gene for one type of R body has been found on one of the plasmids found in kappa and has been cloned into E. coli, where it is expressed, thereby making E. coli an R body producer (but not a killer). Each killer strain of Paramecium is resistant to the toxin it produces, and most strains of Paramecium that have been freed of kappa are sensitive to the toxin produced by that strain. The function of the *K* gene, how the toxins kill sensitive paramecia, and the mechanism by which kappa is able to confer resistance on its host present intriguing but unanswered questions. The significance of the kappa story is that free-living organisms can enter cells and become integral parts of the workings of the hosts. Even mitochondria and chloroplasts are presumed to have arisen in this way. The studies on Paramecium symbionts tell us that the borderline between heredity and parasitism can become very blurred.

Serotypes: SONNEBORN found that every clone of Paramecium has a single major antigenic protein on its surface, designated A, B, C, etc. (reviewed in PREER 1986; CARON and MEYER 1989). The serotypes are mutually exclusive, for only a single surface antigen was found on a given cell at a time. The clones are designated serotype A, serotype B, serotype C, etc., and a single genotype can express approximately a dozen serotypes. Although each type is expressed better under one set of environmental conditions than another, most types may be stabilized under a single set of environmental conditions. SONNEBORN was able to find a single set of conditions under which most serotypes will reproduce true to type indefinitely and therefore concluded that the serotypes were inherited. Crosses between any two serotypes under constant conditions reveal cytoplasmic inheritance. Examination of a number of different natural strains shows that there are serologically distinguishable differences between the A serotype in each strain, differences between the B serotypes, etc. Moreover, the between-strain differences are inherited as simple Mendelian factors. The conclusion that SONNEBORN reached is that there is a series of unlinked genes that are expressed in a mutually exclusive fashion depending upon the cytoplasmic state, and that the cytoplasmic state is subject to environmental influence.

At first SONNEBORN interpreted the results on serotypes in terms of the plasmagene theory. At a meeting in Paris on biological units endowed with genetic continuity, DELBRÜCK (1948) suggested that such stable states of gene expression might be explained entirely by a series of mutually exclusive reactions that occurred during antigen synthesis. Although the details of this suggestion were not correct, he was right in pointing out that diverse hereditary states don't necessarily emanate from self-reproducing particles, but might be produced by competing chemical reactions that affect gene expression. This general conclusion was quickly accepted as the most probable explanation for serotype inheritance.

Today the protein antigens, the mRNAs, and the genes have all been isolated (FORNEY *et al.* 1983; RUDMAN *et al.* 1991). Although regulation is usually at the level of mRNA, in some serotype genes it is also regulated posttranscriptionally (GILLEY *et al.* 1990). The region starting approximately 200 bp upstream of the start of translation and extending to the start of translation is necessary for expression (MARTIN *et al.* 1994; LEECK and FORNEY 1996). Most of the region is not transcribed and is thought to contain the promoter. LEEK and FORNEY prepared a hybrid plasmid with the upstream nontranscribed region of the *B* gene ligated to the whole of the transcribed portion of the *A* gene (including the entire A protein coding sequence). They then injected various combinations of this hybrid and complete *A* and *B* genes into a strain containing Mendelian deletions for both *A* and *B*. These co-transformed cells were also subjected to different environments affecting serotype expression (A is favored by high temperature, B by low.) The hybrid antigen gene acted exactly like the complete *A* gene itself, that is, the putative *B* promoter acts exactly like the putative *A* promoter in its response to the environment. Moreover, regulation was at the level of transcription. It was concluded that the upstream nontranscribed region of the gene, while necessary for transcription, is not involved in the mutually exclusive expression seen among serotypes. Mutual exclusion is controlled by the transcribed region of the gene. These results are consistent with hypotheses that assume stable antigen expression involving feedback of immobilization antigens or their mRNA (FINGER *et al.* 1995). Serotype variation in Paramecium tells us that highly stable states of genetic expression can develop, leading to cellular differentiations that can be maintained for hundreds of cell generations. Such stable states appear to operate at the level of transcriptional control and involve feedback loops. Thus, the process of obtaining an understanding of this phenomenon at the molecular level is in progress.

Cytotaxis: By the mid-1950s after SONNEBORN had investigated the inheritance of mating type, killers, and serotypes, he decided to push his research in a different direction. The genetic aspects of the kappa story seemed completed. Although the molecular mechanisms responsible for serotype variation were not known, it appeared that the serotypes were cases of stable changes in gene expression, and the techniques available to understand the mechanisms of such phenomena were also not available at that time. So he decided to turn his attention to cell shape and the nature of the cellular cortex in Paramecium. When paramecia conjugate, they do not always separate, and double animals are sometimes formed that reproduce true to type as double animals. SONNEBORN found that by treating cells with antiserum he could induce double animals at will. He crossed single animals with double animals, and in an ingenious set of experiments he showed that the genetic basis lay not in the micronuclei, not in the macronucleus, and not in the fluid cytoplasm. The only candidate left was the cortical structure itself. In cooperation with J. BEISSON, he found that even a portion of the cortex could become rearranged and act as its own genetic element in inheritance. The influence of preexisting structure on the development of new structure he called cytotaxis. The ciliate cortex and its development has since been extensively studied. It has been suggested that cytotaxis is a fundamental process in cellular development and applies to structures found in all organisms. Microtubule organizing centers and cell membranes are candidates. For a detailed discussion of these problems the reader is referred to FRANKEL (1989) and GRIMES and AUFDERHEIDE (1991).

Behavioral genetics: As a graduate student, CHING KUNG read H. S. JENNINGS' *Behavior of Lower Organisms,* a work better known to psychologists than biologists. He became interested in the behavior of Paramecium. Working as a postdoctoral in SONNEBORN's laboratory in the late 1960s, he developed techniques that enabled him to isolate large numbers of behavioral mutants. Analysis of these mutants soon led to the conclusion that they were largely mutations that affected the electrophysiological properties of the cell membranes in Paramecium by affecting the constitution of membrane channels for Ca^{2+} and other ions. One of these behavioral mutations was found to be in the gene coding for calmodulin. The use of mutants of Paramecium in studying channels presents an unprecedented opportunity, for simple mutants that affect channel function are not available in higher organisms. KUNG has made major contributions to our knowledge of the electrophysiology of membrane transport. More recently he has found that injection of whole cell DNA from wild type into the mutants can restore normal behavior. Injection of DNA prepared from libraries of whole cell DNA also works. Taking advantage of these observations, he and coworkers have recently been able to screen a library using this technique and to isolate the gene that may encode a specific membrane ion channel protein (W. J. HAYNES, Y. SAIMI, and C. KUNG, personal communication). The identification of channel proteins has proved difficult in work on higher organisms. Significant advances in our understanding of membrane ion channel proteins in Paramecium now seem certain.

The life cycle: After conjugation, paramecia typically undergo stages of immaturity, maturity, and senescence. Each of these stages can last as many as several hundred fissions, depending upon the species. Immature cells, while vigorous, cannot mate. Mature cells are vigorous and mate readily. During senescence fission rate and viability both decline, and unless conjugation or autogamy occurs the cells die. Another feature of the life cycle is that species that undergo autogamy will not do so unless a sufficient number of fissions has elapsed since the last autogamy or conjugation. These slow progressive changes seen in the stages of the life cycle were considered to be subjects for genetic analysis by the early workers in the time of JENNINGS and SONNEBORN (see PREER 1968 for a short review of the early

work). Some studies have occurred since those early days and a few are discussed below.

SIEGEL (1961) showed that the genes that determine specificity of mating type are repressed during the immature period in *P. bursaria* and that these genes become active sequentially as the cells enter the period of maturity. HAGA and HIWATASHI (1981) isolated a protein from immature *P. caudatum* called immaturin that is able to transform mature cells into immature cells when injected. It is likely that passage from immaturity to maturity involves changes in stable states of gene repression and gene activation. Immaturin appears to be a regulatory protein. The way is now open to find the gene for immaturin. Perhaps the time has now come to make progress on the molecular biology of immaturity and maturity.

Two recent studies on Paramecium shed light on the problem of aging. AUFDERHEIDE (1987), working on Paramecium, has shown us where the primary site of aging is located. By transferring cytoplasm between young and aging cells by microinjection and by doing the same for nuclear material, he was able to show that the primary cause for aging is located within the macronucleus, not within the cytoplasm. In the field of aging, where almost nothing seems certain, this is a solid finding as well as a promising beginning for further studies. Another interesting study is a test of the theory that aging stems from changes in telomere length (GILLEY and BLACKBURN 1994). They established that senescence is not due to changes in telomere length in Paramecium, for telomere length does not vary significantly during the life cycle. They also noted a great decrease in the size of macronuclear chromosomes during aging.

Nevertheless, the way that Paramecium counts its fissions, what controls the programmed changes in gene expression leading to maturity, and the nature of senescence are not much better understood today than when these fascinating problems were first encountered.

So what did happen to the genetics of Paramecium? We conclude that the facts about Paramecium genetics that we knew in its period of high visibility many years ago are still valid today. We also have reviewed what we consider to be some fascinating new advances in Paramecium genetics as well as some very bright opportunities for future discoveries. We proceed by considering why Paramecium has become, in the words of CHING KUNG, an "endangered genetic species."

Possibility no. 1: One of my colleagues, presumably with tongue in cheek, suggested that autogamy is just too complicated for geneticists to understand. Having seen the blank looks on the faces of many non-Paramecium geneticists at the mention of autogamy, I have concluded that this possibility should be taken seriously. During autogamy all but one of the products of a typical meiosis are lost, and the one remaining haploid nucleus divides, the two nuclei recombine to give a homozygous diploid nucleus, and this then divides mitotically to produce the new micronuclei and macronuclei. On reflection, I just don't believe that geneticists who seem to be capable of understanding meiosis, recombination, interference, and sex determination in Drosophila are unable to comprehend autogamy. This possibility must be rejected.

Possibility no. 2: Paramecium is too difficult to culture. There is a little more truth to this possibility. It may, indeed, account for the fact that Tetrahymena appears to be replacing Paramecium in ciliate laboratories, for Tetrahymena is quite happy with a solution of just Difco protease peptone. Nevertheless, workers in the 1800s made no such complaints, and judging from the smells and boiling pots I sense as I go past Drosophila kitchens, I cannot give much credence to this possibility.

Possibility no. 3: With the advent of molecular genetics, there are too many really important things to cover, and there isn't any room for Paramecium genetics any more. I don't think so. The few pages that are included in the present essay have covered far more about Paramecium than need be covered in a student's introduction to modern genetics and would scarcely increase the thickness of such books.

Possibility no. 4: Paramecium is just too queer, and nothing that happens in Paramecium is relevant to what happens in other organisms. Well, this isn't everyone's opinion. I can still remember the administrator of my NIH study section in Washington noting that such and such projects on various weird organisms were especially valuable, for they provided much-needed evolutionary diversity to the NIH-sponsored research programs. Of course, I don't know how many people believe that Paramecium is too queer. I am not one of them. SONNEBORN always quoted BATESON in saying, "Treasure your exceptions." They often provide the key to the usual.

Possibility no. 5: Funding for research on ciliates has not been available. This possibility has certainly been important in Great Britain, where the decision was made many years ago to put research funds for biology only into areas of clear economic importance. The ciliate workers there have left for other fields of research, several to Plasmodium, a difficult organism, indeed, in which to study genetics. In this country, in spite of attacks from various sources, the prevailing view still seems to be that the advance of science is best served by supporting all kinds of basic research. Most panels that influence funding consist of workers on the currently popular organisms, and hence might be suspected of bias. Nevertheless, I do not believe that the proposals for work on Paramecium that have been rejected are any better than the rejected proposals for work on organisms popular at the present time such as Drosophila, yeast, worms, etc.

Possibility no. 6: Most of SONNEBORN's students later turned to studies on other organisms. For example, DAVE NANNEY left Paramecium for Tetrahymena, RICHARD SIEGEL left Paramecium for Drosophila, MYRON LEVINE and DAVID SKAAR left Paramecium for bacteria. Now, with two or three laboratories in Europe and not many more in the United States, Japan seems to be the only place where Paramecium is not in danger of disappearing altogether. Perhaps SONNEBORN so dominated the field that others left to prevent being smothered; perhaps they just wanted to spread his gospel to other fields. NANNEY did just that with Tetrahymena, laying the basis for all the current genetic work on that organism (see NANNEY 1980). Perhaps others thought that Paramecium was just too queer.

Possibility no. 7: SONNEBORN is not around any more. There is a lot to this possibility. TRACY was a giant among experimentalists. The richness of the knowledge he gave us about the life cycle of Paramecium and how to exploit this knowledge with useful genetic techniques was truly amazing. Moreover, TRACY thought deeply about his research and explored the relevance of all our knowledge of Paramecium to the broad problems in biology of his day. His enthusiasm knew no bounds, and he had to tell everyone about it. He did it by attending all meetings, participating in the workings of many societies, becoming president of the Genetics Society of America, of the American Society of Naturalists, of the American Institute of Biological Societies, participating in symposia without end, becoming a Sigma Xi Lecturer, and giving innumerable named lectures. Many graduate students and postdoctorals from around the world came to his laboratory in Bloomington, Indiana, the Mecca for ciliate studies. Moreover, his enthusiasm was infectious. Undergraduates and graduates alike in his classes were found to have cultures of the organisms he happened to be lecturing about surreptitiously hidden around their rooms. Students could hardly keep from following him from his lectures back to his laboratory to find out the result of some current experiment he had told them about. He is irreplaceable.

Possibility no. 8: Paramecium is just irrelevant today. This just has to be wrong, for where could one find an organism so full of possibilities? Cells are infected with a rich flora of all kinds of symbiotic microorganisms that will only grow in Paramecium, many with plasmids or phages that are involved in the killing and also the resistance of the hosts to the toxin they produce. Some traits are due to mitochondria (BEALE 1969). Gene activity or gene inactivity is passed on to the progeny in the case of surface antigens. There is one set of mating types determined by a biological clock that regularly switches from one type to the other every morning and every evening (BARNETT 1966). The arrangement of surface structures is inherited, but how is not known. Macronuclei pass on many of their characteristics to new macronuclei, by an unknown and mysterious mechanism. A simple gene sequencing demonstrates a variation in the "universal" genetic code (CARON and MEYER 1985; PREER *et al.* 1985). All injected DNA multiplies, and new telomeres attach to any sequence. It is an organism that continues to offer intriguing puzzles to be solved. Almost every natural character leads to some kind of inheritance unknown elsewhere. I don't think Paramecium is irrelevant today. But then I still work on Paramecium!

LITERATURE CITED

AMAR, L., 1994 Chromosome end formation and internal sequence elimination as alternative genomic rearrangements in the ciliate *Paramecium.* J. Mol. Biol. **236:** 421–426.

AUFDERHEIDE, K. J., 1987 Clonal aging in *Paramecium tetraurelia.* II. Evidence of functional changes in the macronucleus with age. Mech. Aging Dev. **37:** 265– 279.

BARNETT, A., 1966 A circadian rhythm of mating type reversals in *Paramecium multimicronucleatum*, syngen 2, and its genetic control. J. Cell. Physiol. **67:** 239–270.

BEALE, G. H., 1969 A note of the inheritance of erythromycin-resistance in *Paramecium aurelia.* Genet. Res. **14:** 341–342.

BRUNK, C. F., 1986 Genome reorganization in *Tetrahymena.* Int. Rev. Cytol. **99:** 49–83.

CARON, F., 1992 A high degree of macronuclear chromosome polymorphism is generated by variable DNA rearrangements in *Paramecium primaurelia* during macronuclear differentiation. J. Mol. Biol. **225:** 661–678.

CARON, C. F. and E. MEYER, 1985 Does *Paramecium primaurelia* use a different genetic code in its macronucleus? Nature **314:** 185–188.

CARON, F. and E. MEYER, 1989 Molecular basis of surface antigen variation in paramecia. Annu. Rev. Microbiol. **43:** 23–42.

CATCHESIDE, D. G., 1951 *The Genetics of Microorganisms.* Pittman, London.

CROW, J. F., 1987 Seventy years ago in *Genetics:* H. S. JENNINGS and inbreeding theory. Genetics **115:** 389–391.

DELBRÜCK, M., 1948 In discussion of paper by SONNEBORN, T. M. and G. H. BEALE. Influence des gènes, des plasmagènes et du milieu dans le déterminisme des caracteres antigéniques chez Paramecium aurelia (variété 4), pp. 33–34 in Unités Biologiques douees de continuite Génétique. Centre National Recherche Scientifique, Paris.

DOAK, T. G., F. P. DOERDER, L. JAHN and G. HERRICK, 1993 A proposed superfamily of transposase genes: transposon-like elements in ciliated protozoa and a common "D32E" motif. Proc. Natl. Acad. Sci. USA **91:** 942–946.

EPSTEIN, L. M., and J. D. FORNEY, 1984 Mendelian and non-Mendelian mutations affecting surface antigen expression in *Paramecium tetraurelia.* Mol. Cell. Biol. **4:** 1583–1592.

FINGER, I., A. LYNN and M. BERNSTEIN, 1995 Identification of regulators of *Paramecium* surface antigen expression and of regulator-antigen complexes. Arch. Protistenkd. **146:** 207–218.

FORNEY, J. D., and E. H. BLACKBURN, 1988 Developmentally controlled telomere addition wild-type and mutant paramecia. Mol. Cell. Biol. **8:** 251–258.

FORNEY, J. D., L. M. EPSTEIN, L. B. PREER, B. M. RUDMAN, D. J. WIDMAYER *et al.,* 1983 Structure and expression of genes for surface proteins in *Paramecium.* Mol. Cell. Biol. **3:** 466–474.

FRANKEL, J., 1989 *Pattern Formation: Ciliate Studies and Models.* Oxford University Press, New York.

GILLEY, D. and E. H. BLACKBURN, 1994 Lack of telomere shortening during senescence in *Paramecium.* Proc. Natl. Acad. Sci. USA **91:** 1955–1958.

GILLEY, D., J. R. PREER, JR., K. J. AUFDERHEIDE and B. POLISKY, 1988 Autonomous replication and addition of telomere-like sequences to DNA microinjected into *Paramecium tetraurelia* macronuclei. Mol. Cell. Biol. **8:** 4765–4772.

GILLEY, D., B. M. RUDMAN, J. R. PREER, JR. and B. POLISKY, 1990 Multi-level regulation of surface antigen gene expression in Paramecium tetraurelia. Mol. Cell. Biol. **10:** 1538–1544.

GODISKA, R., K. J. AUFDERHEIDE, D. GILLEY, P. H. HENDRIE, T. FITZWATER *et al.,* 1987 Transformation of Paramecium by microin-

jection of a cloned serotype gene. Proc. Natl. Acad. Sci. USA **84:** 7590–7594.

GRIFFITHS, A. J. F., J. H. MILLER, D. T. SUZUKI, R. C. LEWONTIN and W. M. GELBART, 1993 *An Introduction to Genetic Analysis.* W. H. Freeman and Co., New York.

GRIMES, G. W., and K. J. AUFDERHEIDE, 1991 *Cellular Aspects of Pattern Formation: The Problem of Assembly.* Basel, New York.

HAGA, N. and K. HIWATASHI, 1981 A protein called immaturin controlling sexual maturity in *Paramecium.* Nature **289:** 177–179.

HARUMOTO, T., 1986 Induced change in a non-Mendelian determinant by transplantation of macronucleoplasm in *Paramecium tetraurelia.* Mol. Cell. Biol. **6:** 3498–3501.

JENNINGS, H. S., 1929 Genetics of the protozoa. Bibliogr. Genet. **5:** 105–330.

KIM, C. S., J. R. PREER, JR. and B. POLISKY, 1992 Bacteriophage lambda DNA fragments replicate in the *Paramecium* macronucleus: absence of active copy number control. Dev. Genet. **13:** 97–102.

KIM, C. S., J. R. PREER, JR. and B. POLISKY, 1994 Identification of DNA segments capable of rescuing a non-Mendelian mutant in Paramecium. Genetics **136:** 1325–1328.

KLOBUTCHER, L. A., and G. HERRICK, 1995 Consensus inverted terminal repeat sequence of *Paramecium* IESs: resemblance to termini of Tc1-related and *Euplotes* Tec transposons. Nucleic Acids Res. **23:** 2006–2013.

KLOBUTCHER, L. A., and G. HERRICK, 1997 Developmental genome reorganization in ciliated protozoa: the transposon link. Prog. Nucleic Acid Res. Mol. Biol. (in press).

KLUG, W. S. and M. R. CUMMINGS, 1994 *Concepts of Genetics.* Prentice Hall, Englewood Cliffs, NJ.

KOBAYASHI, S., and S. KOIZUMI, 1988 Characterization of non-Mendelian and Mendelian mutant strains by micronuclear transplantation in *Paramecium tetraurelia.* J. Protozool. **37:** 489–492.

LEEK, C. L., and J. D. FORNEY, 1996 The 5 coding region of Paramecium surface antigen genes controls mutually exclusive transcription. Proc. Natl. Acad. Sci. USA **93:** 2838–2843.

LEWIN, B., 1994 *Genes V.* Oxford University Press, New York.

MARTIN, L. D., S. POLLACK, J. R. PREER, JR. and B. POLISKY, 1994 DNA sequence requirements for the regulation of immobilization antigen A expression in Paramecium tetraurelia. Dev. Genet. **15:** 443–451.

McCORMICK-GRAHAM, M., and D. P. ROMERO, 1994 A single telomerase RNA is sufficient for the synthesis of variable telomeric DNA repeats in ciliates of the genus *Paramecium.* Mol. Cell. Biol. **16:** 1871–1879.

MEYER, E., 1992 Induction of specific macronuclear developmental mutations by microinjection of a cloned telomeric gene in *Paramecium primaurelia.* Genes Dev. **6:** 211–222.

MEYER, E., and A.-M. KELLER, 1996 A Mendelian mutation affecting mating-type determination also affects developmental genomic rearrangements in Paramecium tetraurelia. Genetics **143:** 191–202.

NANNEY, D. L., 1980 *Experimental Ciliatology. An Introduction to Genetic and Developmental Analysis in Ciliates.* Wiley, New York.

NOVICK, A., and M. WEINER, 1957 Enzyme as an all-or-none phenomenon. Proc. Natl. Acad. Sci. USA **43:** 553–566.

ORIAS, E., 1981 Probable somatic DNA rearrangements in mating type determination in *Tetrahymena thermophila:* a review and a model. Dev. Genet. **2:** 185–202.

PHAN, H. L., J. FORNEY and E. H. BLACKBURN, 1988 Analysis of *Paramecium* macronuclear DNA using pulsed field gel electrophoresis. J. Protozool. **36:** 402–408.

POND, F. R., I. GIBSON, J. LALUCAT and R. L. QUACKENBUSH, 1989 R-body-producing bacteria. Microbiol. Rev. **53:** 25–67.

PREER, J. R., JR., 1968 Genetics of the Protozoa, pp. 129–278 in *Research in Protozoology,* edited by T.-T CHEN. Pergamon Press, Oxford.

PREER, J. R., JR., 1986 Surface antigens of Paramecium, pp. 301–339 in *The Molecular Biology of Ciliated Protozoa,* edited by J. G. GALL. Academic Press, NY.

PREER, J. R., JR., 1996 Tracy M. Sonneborn 1905–1981. Biogr. Mem. Natl. Acad. Sci. **69:** 3–26.

PREER, J. R. JR., and L. B. PREER, 1979 The size of macronuclear DNA and its relationship to models for maintaining genic balance. J. Protozool. **26:** 14–18.

PREER, J. R., JR., and L. B. PREER, 1984 Endosymbionts of Protozoa, pp. 795–811 in *Bergey's Manual of Systematic Bacteriology*, Vol. 1. N. R. KRIEG, editor. Williams & Wilkins, Baltimore.

PREER, J. R. JR., L. B. PREER, B. M. RUDMAN and A. J. BARNETT, 1985 Deviation from the universal code shown by the gene for surface protein 51A in *Paramecium*. Nature **314:** 188–190.

PREER, L. B., G. HAMILTON and J. R. PREER, JR., 1992 Micronuclear DNA from *Paramecium tetraurelia*: serotype 51 A gene has internally eliminated sequences. J. Protozool. **39:** 678–682.

PRESCOTT, D. M., 1994 The DNA of ciliated protozoa. Microbiol. Rev. **58:** 233–267.

RUDMAN, B. M., and J. R. PREER, JR., 1996 Non-Mendelian inheritance of revertants of paranoiac in *Paramecium*. Eur. J. Protistol. **32** (Suppl. i): 141–146.

RUDMAN, B. M., L. B. PREER, B. POLISKY and J. R. PREER, JR., 1991 Mutants affecting processing of DNA in macronuclear development in *Paramecium*. Genetics **129:** 47–56.

RUSSELL, P. J., 1994 *Fundamentals of Genetics*. Harper-Collins, New York.

SCOTT, J., K. MIKAMI, C. LEECK and J. FORNEY, 1994 Non-Mendelian inheritance of macronuclear mutations is gene specific in *Paramecium tetraurelia*. Mol. Cell. Biol. **14:** 2479–2484.

SIEGEL, R. W., 1961 Nuclear differentiation and transitional cellular phenotypes in the life cycle of *Paramecium*. Exp. Cell Res. **24:** 6–20.

SONNEBORN, T. M., 1947 Experimental control of the concentration of cytoplasmic genetic factors in Paramecium. Cold Spring Harbor Symp. Quant. Biol. **11:** 236–255.

SONNEBORN, T. M., 1975a *Paramecium aurelia*, pp. 469–594 in *Handbook of Genetics*, Vol. 2, R. KING, editor. Plenum, New York.

SONNEBORN, T. M., 1975b Herbert Spencer Jennings 1868–1947. Biogr. Mem. Natl. Acad. Sci. **47:** 142–223.

SONNEBORN, T. M., and M. V. SCHNELLER, 1979 Dev. Genet. **1:** 21–46.

SRB, A. M., R. D. OWEN and R. E. EDGAR, 1965 *General Genetics*. W. H. Freeman, San Francisco.

STEELE, C. J., G. A. BARKOCY-GALLAGHER, L. B. PREER and J. R. PREER, JR., 1994 Developmentally excised sequences in micronuclear DNA of *Paramecium*. Proc. Natl. Acad. Sci. USA **91:** 2255–2259.

TAMARIN, R. H., 1994 *An Introduction to Genetic Analysis*. W. H. Freeman, New York.

YAO, M.-C., 1988 Site-specific chromosome breakage and DNA deletion in ciliates. In *Mobile DNA*, D. BERG and M. HOWE, editors. American Society of Microbiology Press, Washington, DC.

YOU, Y., J. SCOTT and J. FORNEY, 1994 The role of macronuclear DNA sequences in the permanent rescue of a non-Mendelian mutation in *Paramecium tetraurelia*. Genetics **136:** 1319–1324.

Reassessing Forty Years of Genetic Doctrine
Retrotransfer and Conjugation

Robert G. Ankenbauer

Pfizer Central Research, Groton, Connecticut 06340

SCIENTISTS exhibit great respect and deference to established doctrine. Paradoxically, they also hope to topple this authority and, in so doing, make a name for themselves. Thus, scientists are ambivalent *iconoclasts* (*i.e.,* image breakers), recognizing and adhering to scientific authority while simultaneously desiring to destroy it. This apparent dichotomy in the scientific mindset, the simultaneous advocacy and denunciation of orthodoxy, has led many individuals studying the history, philosophy, and sociology of science to question the impartiality of the scientific process (KUHN 1962; COHEN 1985; GRINNELL 1996). Despite these real concerns about the objectivity of the scientific process, scientists can strive for impartiality by the use of opposing hypotheses, modeling, and empirical testing. The philosophy of scientific falsification promulgated by KARL POPPER (1959), although currently considered out of favor as a method of scientific progress (KUHN 1962; COHEN 1985), is perhaps the most dispassionate method for the testing of established scientific doctrine. The identification of potentially contradictory data, the construction of divergent hypotheses, and the empirical resolution between competing models provide an exquisitely discriminating method for the test.

The recent debate surrounding bacterial conjugation and retrotransfer provided the opportunity for the testing of a long-standing doctrine of bacterial genetics, unidirectional transfer. The combined efforts of several investigators, ostensibly adversaries, united in a set of experiments that put two distinct and mutually exclusive models of conjugation on trial. Featured in several high-profile journals, this episode serves as an exemplary illustration of model testing at its finest.

WILLIAM HAYES and unidirectional transfer: In a 1952 report consisting of six paragraphs, WILLIAM HAYES fortuitously erected the scientific framework for the detailed study of bacterial genetics, plasmid biology, and horizontal gene transfer as we know them today (HAYES 1952). The nature of bacterial recombination proposed by HAYES served as an essential catalyst for the subsequent advances made not only in the genetics of a potentially irrelevant prokaryote, *Escherichia coli*, but in the genetics of virtually all biological systems. The importance of this publication to the field of genetics is difficult to overestimate. In view of its lasting repercussions, HAYES' discovery was called an "intellectual bombshell" by SILVER *et al.* (1995) in a tribute to their former mentor. In his book *The Emergence of Bacterial Genetics*, THOMAS BROCK goes so far as to delineate two phases of research in bacterial genetics: pre-HAYES and post-HAYES (BROCK 1990).

Although the phenomenon of bacterial mating had been discovered by LEDERBERG and TATUM in 1946 (LEDERBERG and TATUM 1946), the mechanism of mating was unknown, and the field of bacterial genetics had become hampered by the persistent tendency to interpret bacterial mating in the light of sexual reproduction of eukaryotes. Independent work by both LEDERBERG and CAVALLI showed that the ability to mate was not universal among *E. coli* strains, but the ability to differentiate between the sexual phenotypes of specific strains had not been realized (see BROCK 1990 for a detailed account).

During studies on the kinetics of bacterial matings, HAYES stumbled upon a result that served to clear away much of the confusion involved in interpreting the data obtained from bacterial matings. Working with a fertile pair of *E. coli* K-12 derivatives, 58-161 and W677, HAYES demonstrated that the two strains were phenotypically distinct and not equivalent in the mating process. One of the strains, 58-161, could be streptomycin poisoned for up to 18 hours prior to mating with W677 and still generate recombinants. In contrast, matings in which W677 was streptomycin poisoned invariably failed to produce recombinants. The fact that 58-161 could be inviable but nevertheless required for prototroph formation indicated that this strain possessed some unique genetic capacity that allowed the transfer of genetic material to W677, while the inability of streptomycin-poisoned W677 to yield recombinants demonstrated its lack of this fertility factor. In his discovery of unidirec-

Address for correspondence: Robert G. Ankenbauer, Pfizer Central Research, Bldg. 118N-N103B, Box 1222, Eastern Point Road, Groton, CT 06340. E-mail: bob_ankenbauer@groton.pfizer.com

tional transfer of genetic material, HAYES deduced the inequality between the strains and identified 58-161 as a donor and W677 as a recipient.

Nearly 45 years later, HAYES appears remarkably prescient as he foretold the essential features of horizontal plasmid transfer (conjugation) with his experiments on the unidirectional transfer of genetic markers in *E. coli*. In the absence of any knowledge of the existence of F as a plasmid, the streptomycin-poisoning experiments revealed the existence of a specific donor phenotype exhibited by those strains bearing F. HAYES' work provided the insight to consider participants unequal in the mating and to regard them as "males" and "females" or, more recently, "donors" and "recipients." While utilizing such anthropomorphic terms as conceptual aids, this work succeeded in displacing other inappropriate Mendelian terms from the bacterial genetics lexicon.

Subsequent research with a variety of physical, radiological, and genetic approaches provided support for the unidirectional model (SKAAR and GAREN 1955; LEDERBERG 1957; WOLLMAN and JACOB 1957; ANDERSON 1958; SILVER 1963). The empirical evidence and resultant predictive power of the unidirectional model resulted in its virtual enshrinement as doctrine in the succeeding decades (for example, see various textbooks: HAYES 1968; STENT and CALENDAR 1978; GLASS 1982; HARDY 1986; STREIPS and YASBIN 1991).

The advent of retrotransfer: Questions about the universality of the unidirectional model of conjugation arose from work published by MAX MERGEAY and his colleagues during the mid-1980s. Initial reports (THIRY *et al.* 1984; MERGEAY *et al.* 1985) described the ability of IncP1, IncM, and IncN plasmids to mediate "back transfer" or "back mobilization," the movement of a mobilizable (Tra⁻ Mob⁺) plasmid from a recipient into the donor in canonically defined matings. In contrast, other incompatibility groups (*e.g.,* IncW plasmids) were not observed to mediate such "back transfer." A subsequent paper reported that the chromosome-mobilizing IncP derivative pULB113 promoted inheritance of recipient chromosomal markers in the plasmid-bearing donor strain at an anomalously high frequency (MERGEAY *et al.* 1987). This inheritance took the form of both recombinants or R-prime plasmids and was at least as frequent as the transfer of donor markers to recipients. The similarities of these frequencies indicated that the transfer of recipient chromosomal markers to the donor was unaffected by surface exclusion. These observations led to the birth of a novel conjugative phenomenon designated 'retrotransfer." A short report by TOP *et al.* (1991) reiterated the exclusive ability of retrotransfer to specific plasmid incompatibility groups and indicated that retrotransfer of a mobilizable plasmid occurred as rapidly as canonical conjugation.

In a more theoretical presentation of the phenomenon, TOP *et al.* (1992) proposed two mechanistically

distinct models for retrotransfer, the one-step and the two-step. In the one-step (or bidirectional) model, retrotransfer is a single event during which DNA moves freely in two directions between a cell bearing a Tra⁺ plasmid and a cell carrying a Tra⁻ Mob⁺ plasmid. By contrast, the two-step (or unidirectional) model involved two transfer events, the first step being the transfer of the Tra⁺ plasmid from the donor to the recipient, and the second step, the transfer of the Tra⁻ Mob⁺ plasmid back to the original donor. Mathematical representations of each model were generated by a mass action approach to plasmid transfer kinetics. With data sets obtained from brief matings, the kinetics of retrotransfer correlated well with the bidirectional model. The correspondence of the data points with the bidirectional equations led TOP *et al.* to conclude that retrotransfer was distinct from canonical conjugation and mobilization.

RAMOS-GONZALEZ *et al.* (1994) described the ability of the IncP9 TOL plasmid pWW0 to retrotransfer chromosomal markers, a property earlier characterized for pULB113 (MERGEAY *et al.* 1987). In addition to extending the retrotransfer capacity to another plasmid incompatibility group, RAMOS-GONZALEZ *et al.* provided the best evidence for the bidirectional model to date. In triparental mating assays employing a Nal^R donor bearing the conjugative plasmid pWW0, a "substrate" strain carrying a chromosomally encoded kanamycin resistance marker as the mobilizable substrate, and a Rif^R recipient, it was demonstrated that the generation of retrotransconjugants (Nal^R Km^R cfu) occurred more rapidly than did that of triparental transconjugants (Rif^R Km^R cfu). Since triparental mating is nothing more than two successive rounds of unidirectional transfer (FIGURSKI and HELINSKI 1979), the kinetic differentiation between retrotransfer and triparental mating led to the conclusion that retrotransfer is the result of a single conjugational event.

Throughout these reports, the term retrotransfer evolved from a primarily descriptive designation to one more mechanistically explicit. Phrases in these papers reveal the transformation from the mundane "back transfer" (THIRY *et al.* 1984; MERGEAY *et al.* 1985) to the aggressive "gene capture" and "gene recruitment" (TOP *et al.* 1990; RAMOS-GONZALEZ *et al.* 1994). Although never fully developed, the bidirectional model of retrotransfer received perhaps its most detailed exposition in two papers from MERGEAY's lab (MERGEAY *et al.* 1987; TOP *et al.* 1992). From this entire body of work, the bidirectional model of retrotransfer emerged with the following characteristics: (i) retrotransfer is a one-step process of bidirectional DNA transfer consisting of a single conjugative event during which DNA flows freely between donor and recipient; (ii) retrotransfer is mechanistically distinct from canonical conjugation and mobilization; (iii) retrotransfer is not dependent upon the transfer of the Tra⁺ plasmid to the recipient;

(iv) the time required for retrotransfer is indistinguishable from that required for canonical conjugation; (v) retrotransfer is unaffected by surface exclusion; and (vi) the ability to retrotransfer is a property possessed by an exclusive set of plasmid incompatibility groups.

The dissection of retrotransfer: The citing of the bidirectional model of retrotransfer in a number of recent reviews on conjugation (AMABILE-CUEVAS and CHICUREL 1992; AMABILE-CUEVAS 1993; FROST 1992; GUINEY 1993) indicated that the long-standing doctrine of exclusively unidirectional transfer in conjugation was being slowly modified and supplanted by the bidirectional model of retrotransfer. Although an explicit molecular mechanism for the bidirectional model of retrotransfer was not proposed, it was unlikely that this doctrinal revision would escape careful scrutiny.

Indeed, recent studies from the laboratories of J. A. HEINEMANN and D. H. FIGURSKI have subjected the phenomenon of retrotransfer to an in-depth genetic and molecular dissection. Exploiting the exquisite sensitivity of detection afforded by the retrotransfer assays devised by MERGEAY's group (MERGEAY et al. 1985; TOP et al. 1992), the HEINEMANN and FIGURSKI labs carried out an array of experiments submitting both the unidirectional and bidirectional models to highly stringent and rigorous testing. Recognizing the localization of the Tra$^+$ plasmid as the crux of the retrotransfer controversy, most of the attention has been focused on that aspect.

Taking a page (or perhaps a paragraph) directly from HAYES, HEINEMANN subtly modified HAYES' streptomycin-poisoning experiment by using a recipient bearing a mobilizable (Tra$^-$ Mob$^+$) plasmid and then assaying for retrotransfer (HEINEMANN and ANKENBAUER 1993a). Streptomycin poisoning of the recipient prevented retrotransfer and demonstrated the need for protein expression in the recipient for retrotransfer to occur. By employing the constitutively mobilized plasmid pMS2260 (PANSEGRAU et al. 1990) in the recipient, HEINEMANN obviated concerns about the inability of the streptomycin-poisoned recipient to express necessary mobilization genes in response to potential intercellular mating signals received from the Tra$^+$ donor. This experiment indicated that the Tra$^+$ plasmid must first be transferred to, and its genes expressed in, the recipient to allow retrotransfer. In other words, retrotransfer is dependent upon the recipient's first being converted into a donor. In the same paper, it was demonstrated that both IncW and IncF plasmids were capable of mediating retrotransfer, albeit at 100- to 1000-fold lower frequency than IncP plasmids. The depression in frequency of retrotransfer was the consequence of the intense entry exclusion phenotype exerted by both IncW and IncF plasmids. In contrast, IncP plasmids exhibited virtually no entry exclusion and, therefore, very high retrotransfer frequencies. These results provide an explanation for the apparent lack of retrotransfer

observed earlier with IncW plasmids (THIRY et al. 1984; MERGEAY et al. 1985). The fact that surface exclusion is still exerted during retrotransfer suggests that the theorized pore or mating structure is unidirectional, as is the transfer of the Tra$^+$ plasmids.

Retrotransfer received a concise yet severe test at the hands of AYRES SIA et al. (1996). These authors constructed an oriT mutant of RK2 by site-directed mutagenesis of the nic site; such a mutation should result in a Tra$^+$ plasmid wild type in all its abilities except for self-transfer. As expected, the RK2 oriT mutant was severely depressed in self-transfer but nevertheless mobilized coresident IncQ or mini-IncP oriT$^+$ plasmids in trans at high efficiency. In retrotransfer assays, the RK2 oriT mutant was incapable of retromobilizing the Tra$^-$ Mob$^+$ plasmid carried by the recipient. Similar to HEINEMANN's deduction from the streptomycin-poisoning experiment (HEINEMANN and ANKENBAUER 1993a), AYRES SIA et al. concluded that retrotransfer requires the recipient to acquire the self-transferable (Tra$^+$) plasmid and the donor phenotype before retrotransfer can occur.

A recent paper in GENETICS from the HEINEMANN laboratory presents several experiments that conclude the painstaking analysis of retrotransfer (HEINEMANN et al. 1996). An isogenic pair of oriT/oriT$^+$ plasmids were used to ascertain the necessity of this cis-required mobilization locus in retrotransfer. Recipients bearing these plasmids were able to retrotransfer only the oriT$^+$ plasmid, thereby providing support for the requirement of intracellular mobilization predicted by the unidirectional model, in contrast to the intercellular mobilization of the bidirectional model. In another experiment designed to determine whether only a limited subset of plasmid-encoded genes are required for retrotransfer, these investigators employed the extensive collection of F tra amber mutants developed in the laboratory of the late KARIN IPPEN-IHLER (IPPEN-IHLER and MINKLEY 1986). Relying on the differential ability of sup mutants to suppress the F tra^{am} mutations, retrotransfer assays were performed with F$^+$ tra^{am} supC supF donors and a sup^o (nonsuppressing) recipient bearing a mobilizable (Tra$^-$ Mob$^+$) substrate plasmid. Although fully capable of transferring to the sup^o recipient, nine different tra^{am} allelic mutants of F were incapable of mediating retrotransfer. This result established the requirement of the expression of multiple tra genes in the recipient for retrotransfer to occur.

Interspecies matings were used to analyze the effect of restriction barriers on retrotransfer. The bidirectional model predicts that matings of an E. coli hsdS (restriction-negative, modification-negative) donor and a Salmonella typhimurium hsd$^+$ (restriction-positive) recipient should not depress the frequency of retrotransfer while the unidirectional model suggests that retrotransfer in E. coli × S. typhimurium matings would be reduced since genetic conversion of the recipient would be prevented by restriction. In experiments testing these models, *E. coli* × *S. typhimurium* matings yielded a much lower level of retrotransfer than did *E. coli* × *E. coli* matings. In fact, the low observed frequency of retrotransfer of the mobilizable (Tra⁻ Mob⁺) substrate plasmid from *S. typhimurium* to *E. coli* was proportional to that observed for the direct transfer of the Tra⁺ plasmid from *E. coli* to *S. typhimurium*. The effect of restriction barrier on retrotransfer confirms the necessity of conversion of recipients into donors. In a final experiment analyzing the kinetics of canonical conjugation, native donors and recipients simultaneously applied to media selective for transconjugants yielded a small yet reproducible number of colonies (HEINEMANN *et al.* 1996). The selective medium was not only permissible for conjugation (as expected from HAYES' initial streptomycin-poisoning experiments), but also allowed a fraction of the recipients to inherit the plasmid even in the presence of counterselection. In contrast to these results, retrotransfer was never observed without >30 min preincubation on permissive media prior to plating on selective media. The results of this experiment provided the first kinetic differentiation between canonical conjugation and retrotransfer, a distinction previously inaccessible to other assays (TOP *et al.* 1992; RAMOS-GONZALEZ *et al.* 1994).

This series of experiments re-evaluated HAYES' conclusions on unidirectionality to a stringency unimagined by HAYES. HAYES' use of F and his scoring of chromosomal recombinants prevented the detection of retrotransfer. F, although possessing Cma⁺ (chromosome-mobilizing activity), does not exhibit the extremely high levels of Cma⁺ associated with RP4 mini-Mu plasmid derivatives (VAN GIJSEGEM and TOUSSAINT 1982; LEJEUNE *et al.* 1983) such as pULB113, which allowed the initial detection of retrotransfer by MERGEAY *et al.* (1987). Further advances in plasmid biology, especially the development of mobilizable plasmids and techniques such as triparental mating (FIGURSKI and HELINSKI 1979), provided the sensitive assays necessary to qualitatively and quantitatively evaluate retrotransfer (TOP *et al.* 1991, 1992).

The conclusion of this work is the reaffirmation of HAYES' unidirectional (two-step) model of bacterial conjugation. The HEINEMANN and FIGURSKI groups explicitly demonstrated that retrotransfer is mechanistically identical to conjugation and that no novel mechanism of DNA transfer is involved. Retrotransfer is absolutely dependent upon the conversion of a *female* recipient to a *male* donor. These italicized distinctions are not redundant semantics in the retrotransfer debate. The cornerstone of the bidirectional model of retrotransfer was the hypothesized existence of "female donors." Such female donors would merely provide a reservoir of DNA that is accessed or recruited by the male donor without any genetic conversion of the female. Employing an array of genetic and molecular approaches, HEINEMANN and FIGURSKI have, in essence, defined the idea of a "female donor" as an oxymoron. A donor must be male or, as stated by HAYES in 1953: "When the *F* agent was discovered...it soon became apparent that the donor state and the F+ state were synonymous and that acceptor cells were those which did not harbor the *F* agent" and "Cells lacking this agent [f] are restricted to the passive role of recipient" (HAYES 1953).

Did HEINEMANN and FIGURSKI create a "straw man" out of the bidirectional model of retrotransfer merely to knock it down? Were their experiments designed to test hypotheses actually put forth by MERGEAY and TOP, or were the arguments a misrepresentation of the bidirectional model? Certainly, HEINEMANN and FIGURSKI were guilty of the aggressive application of KARL POPPER's falsification approach to scientific theorems (POPPER 1959). In an effort to understand the mechanism of retrotransfer, HEINEMANN and FIGURSKI made explicit the two models put forth by TOP *et al.* (1992). By clarifying the predictive power of the two models, vague and ambiguous statements supporting the bidirectional model were dismissed in favor of high relief, opposing hypotheses. The proponents of the bidirectional model did not unequivocally assert a molecular mechanism for retrotransfer, regarding it as unknown and yet to be determined (MERGEAY *et al.* 1987; TOP *et al.* 1992). However, in a scientifically necessary exercise, HEINEMANN and FIGURSKI made clear and inescapable the distinctions between the unidirectional and bidirectional models and based their experiments on the logical predictions of these well-resolved models. Their acumen led to the design of experiments capable of refuting the full-fledged models of retrotransfer, unidirectional or bidirectional. The overtly severe hypothesizing employed by HEINEMANN and FIGURSKI and subsequent experimental dismantling of the bidirectional model are not mere sophistries, but instead an exhibition of the implicit severity of Popper's scientific philosophy (POPPER 1959).

Whither retrotransfer? Although retrotransfer has proven to be canonical conjugation, in this author's opinion the term "retrotransfer" should be maintained. The term "retrotransfer," despite the inaccurate mechanistic baggage of the bidirectional model, seems to be an accurate term for the phenomenon. Retro signifies return or back, and therefore retrotransfer must mean return transfer or back transfer. Retrotransfer, in and of itself, does not imply a molecular or genetic mechanism. It is primarily descriptive, conveying a behavioral phenomenon of conjugation rather than its inner workings.

Maintaining the designation of retrotransfer serves additional purposes. Retrotransfer underscores the idea of gene flux (AMABILE-CUEVAS and CHICUREL 1992) from recipient to original donor regardless of the mechanism. Furthermore, it communicates the reality of the cascading and amplifying effect of conjugation on the dissemination of genetic units. The depiction of experimentally assigned recipients as exclusively recipient has been put to rest by the work of the proponents of the bidirectional model. The conjugative potential conferred by Tra$^+$ plasmids is much broader and more fluid than the narrow and linear conception of unidirectional transfer that we have inherited from HAYES. The apparent delocalization of the donor phenotype during matings as stressed by the bidirectional model of retrotransfer (MERGEAY et al. 1987) provided a larger, albeit mechanistically erroneous, vision of the radiation and exponential dissemination of conjugative plasmids and genes in general. Coupled with the ability of conjugation to cross the lines of kingdoms (HEINEMANN 1991), such a view has provided further momentum for concepts such as panprokaryota (the absence of circumscribed bacterial species) (SONEA 1988), the biosphere (GHILAROV 1995), and the Gaia hypothesis (LOVELOCK 1979).

The elucidation of the mechanism of retrotransfer unfortunately has not allayed fears about the containment of genetically engineered microorganisms. Retrotransfer and other unusual variations of this procedure have been used by a number of groups to recruit a variety of mobile genetic elements (e.g., mobilizable and self-transferable plasmids) from heretofore unknown reservoirs (TOP et al. 1990, 1994, 1995; SMIT et al. 1993). The generation of transient, irretrievable donor forms of unculturable bacteria provides opportunity for the further dissemination of unsuspected episomal and chromosomal sequences.

The retrotransfer assays developed by MERGEAY and colleagues have provided opportunities to address difficult questions in the area of horizontal DNA transfer. In addition to identifying previously unknown, horizontally mobile elements from soil biota, the use of retrotransfer has also been applied to basic research on conjugation. By successfully demonstrating retrotransfer from maxicells bearing a mobilizable (Tra$^-$ Mob$^+$) substrate plasmid, the HEINEMANN lab provided evidence that self-transferable plasmids encode all the genes necessary and sufficient for conjugation. No specific genetic response by a recipient was required for its conversion to a donor (HEINEMANN and ANKENBAUER 1993b). Retrotransfer allows the detection of extremely early events in conjugation, including reception, inheritance, and conjugal initiation, which have been historically difficult to analyze. Indeed, the streptomycin-poisoning experiments carried out by HAYES underscore the derepressed nature of many Tra$^+$ plasmids (HAYES 1952; DENNISON and BAUMBERG 1975; BRADLEY and WILLIAMS 1982). The extant donor phenotype of cells bearing Tra$^+$ plasmids prevents the analysis of the events involved in the establishment of that phenotype. The retrotransfer assay permits the detection of temporal events in conjugation owing to the controlled in situ generation of new donors.

The inability of streptomycin (HAYES 1952), tetracycline (HEINEMANN et al. 1996), rifampicin (KINGSMAN and WILLETTS 1978), and UV light (HEINEMANN and ANKENBAUER 1993b) to inhibit conjugation from sensitive donors necessitates the re-analysis of the definition of cell death. From HAYES' initial report up to the present, streptomycin-poisoned donors have been repeatedly referred to as "killed," "inactivated," or "dead" (HAYES 1952; HEINEMANN and ANKENBAUER 1993b; SILVER et al. 1995). The maintenance of the conjugative potential for as long as 18 hours after treatment indicates that poisoned donors should be classified as nonviable, metabolically active cells rather than merely dead. Such a reclassification reflects the growing recognition and differentiation of bacterial states other than alive or dead (MASON et al. 1986; HIGGINS 1992; KAPRELYANTS et al. 1993). In contrast to streptomycin-poisoned cells, nonviable, metabolically inert donor cells, such as those treated with arsenate (CURTISS 1969), are not capable of behaving as donors and are considered truly dead.

Regardless of the replicative potential of bacteria, it still takes two to tango. The ability of donor cells to replicate is not a valid indication of the life of cells as far as conjugation is concerned. Antibiotic-poisoned cells preserve pronounced metabolic activity sufficient for the transfer of even large self-transferable plasmids of the IncP and IncF groups. The maintenance of conjugative activity subsequent to antibiotic treatment, initially used by HAYES (HAYES 1952), has been regarded by the scientific community as a mere curiosity of self-transferable plasmids. This unfortunate oversight has delayed the recognition of the resistant nature of the conjugative potential. Many antibiotics, advertised as magic bullets capable of neutralizing prokaryotes, have no effect on the transfer of genetic material by conjugation. The generation of conjugation-proficient, nonviable, metabolically active cells essentially creates a reservoir of transmissible resistance that is invulnerable to further antimicrobial assault. The classic work by HAYES (1952) and subsequent work by others (HEINEMANN and ANKENBAUER 1993a,b; HEINEMANN et al. 1996) emphasize the unexpectedly robust survival mechanisms possessed by plasmids. Plasmids not only commandeer their host for both vertical and horizontal replication, but are also capable of parasitizing the final energy reserves of an irreversibly damaged host and successfully surviving by conjugative transfer to a viable host. Instead of alleviating fears, the debate over retrotransfer and its resolution only heightens our concerns about the adaptive capacity and survival of bacteria, plasmids, and genes.

Re-evaluating doctrine: Re-evaluating long-standing scientific doctrine often generates heated controversy. The debate over adaptive mutagenesis serves as an example of the dissension induced by questioning authority (as described by STAHL 1990). During these intense and passionate disagreements, inadvertent partiality and self-interest in the outcome of investigations can compromise the scientific process. The employment of multiple assays and techniques, the malleability of experimental conditions, the ongoing repetition of experiments, and prejudice in interpretation can lead to the scientist-induced selection of experimental results confirming or contradicting a hypothesis. The analysis of retrotransfer avoided this temptation by the employment of oppositional hypotheses. The common use of a single assertional hypothesis (*e.g.*, "retrotransfer is unidirectional") and the design of experiments to accumulate data in support (or contradiction) of the hypothesis renders science highly susceptible to personal bias. With the construction of opposing hypotheses, two conflicting incompatible models are pitted against each other. Relying upon the distinguishing characteristics of the models, carefully constructed experiments have the capacity to discriminate between the two models. The prospective use of oppositional hypotheses in these experiments and the execution of tests capable of allowing the experimental results to be the arbiter between the two models furnished the retrotransfer controversy with a strong flavor of fairness and objectivity.

Now that the bidirectional model of retrotransfer has been adequately falsified, the scientific community returns once again to the ever-provisional unidirectional model of conjugation proffered by HAYES nearly 45 years ago. The most regrettable outcome of the demise of the bidirectional model of retrotransfer would be if this controversy were considered pointless and unnecessary. The periodic trials that scientific doctrines undergo cannot necessarily be considered "wise" or "foolish" before the fact, nor even after it. The results of such experiments, after all, are not mere human invention but are innate to the biology of the subject.

I thank DAVID FIGURSKI, BARRY GANETZKY, EVERETT ROSEY, SHELLY SHIELDS, and SIMON SILVER for their critical input during the composition of this manuscript.

LITERATURE CITED

AMABILE-CUEVAS, C. F., 1993 *Origin, Evolution and Spread of Antibiotic Resistance Genes*. R. G. Landes Co. Molecular Biology Intelligence Unit, Austin, TX.

AMABILE-CUEVAS, C. F., and M. E. CHICUREL, 1992 Bacterial plasmids and gene flux. Cell **70:** 189–199.

ANDERSON, T. F., 1958 Recombination and segregation in *Escherichia coli*. Cold Spring Harbor Symp. Quant. Biol. **23:** 47.

AYRES SIA, E., D. M. KUEHNER and D. H. FIGURSKI, 1996 Mechanism of retrotransfer in conjugation: prior transfer of the conjugative plasmid is required. J. Bacteriol. **178:** 1457–1464.

BRADLEY, D. E., and P. A. WILLIAMS, 1982 The TOL plasmid is naturally-derepressed for transfer. J. Gen. Microbiol. **128:** 3019–3024.

BROCK, T. D., 1990 *The Emergence of Bacterial Genetics*. Cold Spring Harbor Laboratory Press, Cold Spring Harbor, NY.

COHEN, S. B., 1985 *Revolution in Science*. Harvard University Press, Cambridge, MA.

CURTISS III, R., 1969 Bacterial conjugation. Annu. Rev. Microbiol. **23:** 69–136.

DENNISON, S., and S. BAUMBERG, 1975 Conjugational behaviour of N plasmids in *Escherichia coli* K12. Mol. Gen. Genet. **138:** 323–331.

FIGURSKI, D. H., and D. R. HELINSKI, 1979 Replication of an origin-

containing derivative of plasmid RK2 dependent on a plasmid function provided in *trans*. Proc. Natl. Acad. Sci. USA **76:** 1648–1652.

FROST, L. S., 1992 Bacterial conjugation: everybody's doin' it. Can. J. Microbiol. **38:** 1091–1096.

GHILAROV, A. M., 1995 Vernadsky's biosphere concept: an historical perspective. Quart. Rev. Biol. **70:** 193–203.

GLASS, R. E., 1982 *Gene Function: E. coli and Its Heritable Elements*. University of California Press, Berkeley, CA.

GRINNELL, F., 1996 Ambiguity in the practice of science. Science **272:** 333.

GUINEY, D. G., 1993 Broad host range conjugative and mobilizable plasmids in gram-negative bacteria, pp. 75–103 in *Bacterial Conjugation*, edited by D. B. CLEWELL. Plenum Press, New York.

HARDY, K., 1986 *Bacterial Plasmids*. American Society for Microbiology, Washington, D.C.

HAYES, W., 1952 Recombination in *Bact. coli K* 12: unidirectional transfer of genetic material. Nature **169:** 118–119.

HAYES, W., 1953 The mechanism of genetic recombination in *Escherichia coli*. Cold Spring Harbor Symp. Quant. Biol. **18:** 75–93.

HAYES, W., 1968 *The Genetics of Bacteria and Their Viruses: Studies in Basic Genetics and Molecular Biology*. John Wiley & Sons Inc., New York.

HEINEMANN, J. A., 1991 Genetics of gene transfer between species. Trends Genet. **7:** 181–185.

HEINEMANN, J. A., and R. G. ANKENBAUER, 1993a Retrotransfer in *Escherichia coli* conjugation: bidirectional exchange or de novo mating? J. Bacteriol. **175:** 583–588.

HEINEMANN, J. A., and R. G. ANKENBAUER, 1993b Retrotransfer of IncP plasmid R751 from *Escherichia coli* maxicells: evidence for the genetic sufficiency of self-transferable plasmids for bacterial conjugation. Mol. Microbiol. **10:** 57–62.

HEINEMANN, J. A., H. E. SCOTT and M. WILLIAMS, 1996 Doing the conjugative two-step: evidence of recipient autonomy in retrotransfer. Genetics **143:** 1425–1435.

HIGGINS, N. P., 1992 Death and transfiguration among bacteria. Trends Biochem. Sci. **17:** 207–211.

IPPEN-IHLER, K., and E. G. MINKLEY, JR., 1986 The conjugation system of F, the fertility factor of *Escherichia coli*. Annu. Rev. Genet. **20:** 593–624.

KAPRELYANTS, A. S., J. C. GOTTSCHAL and D. B. KELL, 1993 Dormancy in non-sporulating bacteria. FEMS Microbiol. Rev. **104:** 271–286.

KINGSMAN, A., and N. WILLETTS, 1978 The requirements for conjugal DNA synthesis in the donor strain during F*lac* transfer. J. Mol. Biol. **122:** 287–300.

KUHN, T. S., 1962 *The Structure of Scientific Revolutions*. University of Chicago, Chicago, IL.

LEDERBERG, J., 1957 Sibling recombinants in zygote pedigrees of *Escherichia coli*. Proc. Natl. Acad. Sci. USA **43:** 10–60.

LEDERBERG, J., and E. L. TATUM, 1946 Gene recombination in *Escherichia coli*. Nature **158:** 558.

LEJEUNE, P., M. MERGEAY, F. VAN GIJSEGEM, M. FAELEN, J. GERITS *et al.*, 1983 Chromosome transfer and R-prime plasmid formation mediated by plasmid pULB113 (RP4 mini-Mu) in *Alcaligenes eutrophus* CH34 and *Pseudomonas fluorescens* 6.2. J. Bacteriol. **155:** 1015–1026.

LOVELOCK, J. E., 1979 *Gaia: A New Look at Life on Earth*. Oxford University Press, Oxford.

MASON, C. A., G. HAMER and J. D. BRYERS, 1986 The death and lysis of microorganisms in environmental processes. FEMS Microbiol. Rev. **39:** 373–401.

MERGEAY, M., P. LEJEUNE, G. THIRY and M. FAELEN, 1985 Back transfer: a property of some broad host range plasmids, p. 942 in *Plasmids in Bacteria*, edited by D. HELINSKI, S. N. COTEN, D. B. CLEWELL, D. A. JACKSON and A. HOLLAENDER. Plenum Press, New York.

MERGEAY, M., P. LEJEUNE, A. SADOUK, J. GERITS and L. FABRY, 1987 Shuttle transfer (or retrotransfer) of chromosomal markers mediated by plasmid pULB113. Mol. Gen. Genet. **209:** 61–70.

PANSEGRAU, W., G. ZIEGELIN and E. LANKA, 1990 Covalent association of the *traI* gene product of plasmid RP4 with the 5′-terminal nucleotide at the relaxation nick site. J. Biol. Chem. **265:** 10637–10644.

POPPER, K. R., 1959 *The Logic of Scientific Discovery*. Hutchinson, London.

RAMOS-GONZALEZ, M.-I., M.-A. RAMOS-DIAZ and J. L. RAMOS, 1994 Chromosomal gene capture mediated by the *Pseudomonas putida* TOL catabolic plasmid. J. Bacteriol. **176:** 4635–4641.

SILVER, S. D., 1963 Transfer of material during mating in *Escherichia coli*. Transfer of DNA and upper limits on the transfer of RNA and protein. J. Mol. Biol. **6:** 349.

SILVER, S., J. SHAPIRO, N. MENDELSON, P. BRODA and J. BECKWITH, 1995 William Hayes: pioneering contributions remembered. ASM News **61:** 1720.

SKAAR, D., and A. GAREN, 1955 Transfer of DNA accompanying genetic recombination in *Escherichia coli* K-12. Genetics **40:** 596.

SMIT, E., D. VENNE and J. D. VAN ELSAS, 1993 Mobilization of a recombinant IncQ plasmid between bacteria on agar and in soil via cotransfer or retrotransfer. Appl. Environ. Microbiol. **59:** 2257–2263.

SONEA, S., 1988 A bacterial way of life. Nature **331:** 216.

STAHL, F. W., 1990 If it smells like a unicorn... Nature **346:** 791.

STENT, G. S., and R. CALENDAR, 1978 *Molecular Genetics: An Introductory Narrative.* W. H. Freeman and Company, San Francisco.

STREIPS, U. N., and R. E. YASBIN, 1991 *Modern Microbial Genetics.* Wiley-Liss, New York.

THIRY, G., M. MERGEAY and M. FAELEN, 1984 Back mobilization of Tra⁻ Mob⁺ plasmids mediated by various IncM, IncN and IncP1 plasmids. Arch. Int. Physiol. Biochim. **92:** 6465.

TOP, E., M. MERGEAY, D. SPRINGAEL and W. VERSTRAETE, 1990 Gene escape model: transfer of heavy metal resistance genes from *Escherichia coli* to *Alcaligenes eutrophus* on agar plates and in soil samples. Appl. Environ. Microbiol. **56:** 2471–2479.

TOP, E., M. MERGEAY and D. SPRINGAEL, 1991 Retrotransfer: a specific trait of certain broad-host range plasmids (which allows the host to pick up new genes from other species and genera). Plasmid **25:** 238.

TOP, E., P. VANROLLEGHEM, M. MERGEAY and W. VERSTRAETE, 1992 Determination of the mechanism of retrotransfer by mechanistic mathematical modeling. J. Bacteriol. **174:** 5953–5960.

TOP, E., I. DE SMET, W. VERSTRAETE, R. DIJKMANS and M. MERGEAY, 1994 Exogenous isolation of mobilizing plasmids from polluted soils and sludge. Appl. Environ. Microbiol. **60:** 831–839.

TOP, E. M., W. E. HOLBEN and L. J. FORNEY, 1995 Characterization of diverse 2,4-dichlorophenoxyacetic acid-degradative plasmids isolated from soil by complementation. Appl. Environ. Microbiol. **61:** 1691–1698.

VAN GIJSEGEM, F., and A. TOUSSAINT, 1982 Chromosome transfer and R-prime formation by an RP4 mini-Mu derivative in *Escherichia coli, Salmonella typhimurium, Klebsiella pneumoniae,* and *Proteus mirabilis.* Plasmid **7:** 3044.

WOLLMAN, E. L., and F. JACOB, 1957 Sur les processus de conjugaison et de recombinaison chez *E. coli.* II. La localisation chromosomique du prophage l et les consequences genetiques de l'induction zygotique. Ann. Inst. Pasteur **93:** 323.

Ultraviolet-Induced Mutation
and the Chemical Nature of the Gene

David Stadler

Department of Genetics, University of Washington, Seattle, Washington, 98195–7360

TEXTBOOKS tell us that it was generally believed that genes were made of protein until the demonstration by AVERY, MACLEOD and MCCARTY (1944) that the material that caused bacterial transformation was DNA. Most textbooks fail to note that studies done several years earlier on mutations induced by ultraviolet (UV) radiation also indicated that DNA had genetic activity. And it is often forgotten that neither the UV experiments nor the identification of the transforming principle really convinced scientists that genes were made of DNA.

The first convincing demonstration of the mutagenic action of UV was made in Drosophila by EDGAR ALTENBURG (1934). His close colleague, H. J. MULLER, had shown that X-rays induced mutations in Drosophila, but that natural sources of ionizing radiation could account for only a small fraction of the spontaneous mutations (MULLER and MOTT-SMITH 1930). Therefore, ALTENBURG set about testing other kinds of natural radiation for a possible role. UV seemed to him a good candidate.

ALTENBURG first attempted to monitor UV-induced mutation by treating mature males and scoring sex-linked recessive lethals by MULLER's ClB procedure. He immediately ran into trouble administering the UV to the testes, because so much of the radiation was absorbed by the superficial tissues. (Perhaps this should have forewarned him that UV could not be responsible for much of the spontaneous *germinal* mutation in animals.) ALTENBURG (1934) adopted a procedure developed by GEIGY (1931) for irradiation of Drosophila eggs at the polar cap end; these pole cells are destined to give rise to the germ cells. With this material, ALTENBURG was able to show highly significant frequencies of recessive lethal mutations resulting from UV treatment. However, most of the further work on UV-induced mutations was done, not on Drosophila, but on other forms whose naked germ cells were readily accessible: pollen cells, fungus spores, and bacteria.

During the late 1930s, three separate investigators set up experiments to determine the *action spectrum* of UV-induced mutation. The experiments involved measuring the mutagenic action of monochromatic UV, comparing the effect of the same dose for many different wave lengths. The results could be collected on a graph, plotting wave length *vs.* mutagenicity (see Figure 1). This action spectrum of mutation could then be compared with the UV absorption spectra of substances known to be present in chromosomes (proteins and nucleic acids). The logical assumption was that the substance that produced mutations when it absorbed UV radiation must be the genic material.

Experiments of this type were reported by L. J. STADLER (1939) on mutations induced in maize pollen, by HOLLAENDER (1939) on mutations in spores of the fungus Trichophyton, and by KNAPP and SCHREIBER (1939) on the spermatozoids of the liverwort Sphaerocarpus. All three studies concluded that the most effective wave lengths for the induction of mutations were those with maximum absorption by nucleic acid (and not by protein). It is not known whether any of them was aware of the work of the others before all of them reported their results at the International Congress of Genetics in Edinburgh in 1939, nor whether any of them had known beforehand of an earlier preliminary experiment of the same kind on Antirrhinum pollen by NOETHLING and STUBBE (1936).

The maize experiments have been described in a memoir by ROMAN (1988). This material had the advantage of an extensive set of known genes for endosperm traits that could be scored independently for mutations. This permitted STADLER to note a high frequency of coincident mutations (in the same pollen cell), which meant that some nuclei were receiving a larger dose than others. This alerted him to the unwanted complication that the nuclei were asymmetrically located in the pollen cells and the superficial layers were absorbing much of the incident UV. This required a rather complex correction to convert incident UV to actual dose.

The other two materials were not endowed with known mutable loci, but had the advantage of avoiding the complications of absorption by superficial tissues. The Sphaerocarpus spermatozoids provided especially

Author e-mail: dstad@genetics.washington.edu

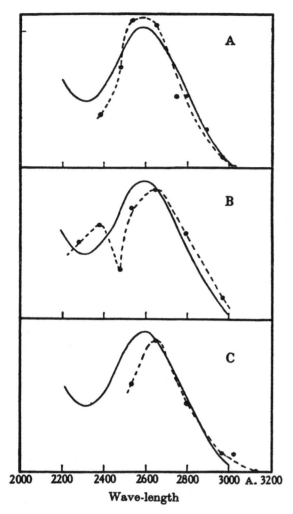

FIGURE 1.—Results of studies on the action spectrum of UV mutation as presented by LEA (1947). The dashed lines show the observed mutation rates in corn pollen (A), fungus spores (B), and liverwort spermatozoids (C). The solid curves show the absorption spectrum of DNA.

good material in this regard, being almost completely naked nuclei (KNAPP and SCHREIBER 1939). The investigators verified that the observed changes were gene mutations by their 2:2 segregations in tetrads.

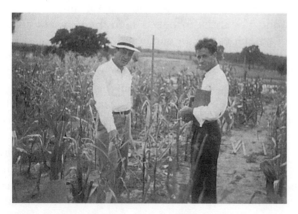

LEWIS STADLER (left) in the cornfield with HERSCHEL RO-MAN, about 1940.

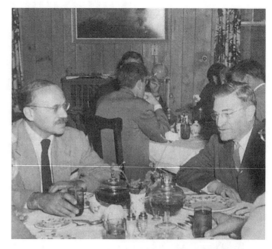

ALEXANDER HOLLAENDER (left) at a Gatlinburg Symposium with the Wisconsin photochemist FARRINGTON DANIELS, 1952. Photo from the University of Wisconsin-Madison Archives.

The mutations scored in the experiments with fungus spores were changes in pigmentation or morphology of the colonies. These studies are discussed in an obituary of HOLLAENDER by SETLOW (1987), who notes that the authors showed extreme caution in their conclusions: "It is probably somewhat dangerous to overemphasize the importance of nucleic acid in the study of radiation effects on living cells. It is very well possible that in radiation produced mutations, the nucleic acid is only the 'absorbant' agent, then transfers the absorbed energy to the protein closely associated with it" (HOLLAENDER and EMMONS 1941). [For more information on HOLLAENDER's career, see the recent memoir by VON BORSTEL and STEINBERG (1996).]

The authors of the other studies were no more bold in their conclusions. STADLER (1939) at first worried that the apparent fit to nucleic acid absorption might be an artifact caused by the superficial absorption: "Unfortunately, the material is not suited to a rigorous physical analysis, and it is to be hoped that similar determinations of genetic effect may be made in material in which the dosage at the chromosomes may be more accurately determined." Later (STADLER and UBER 1942), after further refinements of the analysis still gave the same result, he was slightly more bold: "Considering the various approximations involved, the agreement (to the absorption spectrum of DNA) is surprisingly good and lends further support to the frequently advanced hypothesis that nucleic acid is intimately associated with the functioning of the germinal material."

KNAPP and SCHREIBER (1939), whose experiments with Sphaerocarpus clearly showed a nucleic acid spectrum for mutation induction, concluded "that the absorption of thymonucleic acid has a significant meaning in the mutagenic effect of UV." But they were quick to add, "It does not seem proven that thymonucleic acid is part of the organization of the gene."

JUDSON (1993), in a short, insightful paper that was

part of a symposium observing the 40th anniversary of the WATSON-CRICK paper, notes that AVERY and his colleagues also showed great caution in their conclusions about the genetic role of DNA. And JUDSON tells us the reason this happened: nucleic acids were then believed to be made up of a monotonous series of identical tetranucleotides and thus were incapable of any variety or specificity. They couldn't possibly carry the genetic information. It was only when ERWIN CHARGAFF developed a method for accurate quantitative analysis of the nucleotide content of DNA, that this mistaken view was corrected. CHARGAFF (1950) showed that the four kinds of nucleotides did not have to be present in equimolar amounts and that the DNA of each species had its own nucleotide ratio. JUDSON makes a convincing case that it was this finding that liberated us to think of genes made of DNA. He does not discuss the earlier evidence of genetic activity of DNA that came from the studies of the action spectrum of UV-induced mutation, but he would certainly have made the same argument to explain the modesty of the conclusions of the authors of that work.

JUDSON points out that even for proteins our imagination was limited by the prevailing chemical theory that amino acid sequences were restricted and repetitive because of structural constraints. JUDSON maintains that it was only when SANGER determined the amino acid sequence of bovine insulin and found no sequence restrictions (SANGER and TUPPY 1951) that theorists were liberated to think about a genetic code: sequence equals information.

My own limited recollection of the viewpoint of biologists in the 1940s differs from JUDSON on this point. Biologists of that time didn't know much chemistry and didn't think about the implications of a limit to variability in the primary sequence of proteins. We were much more impressed by their *biological* properties. We knew that, both as enzymes and as antibodies, proteins showed the capacity for amazing diversity, so why not as genes? Besides, we were not then so concerned about the need for a unique *sequence* in every gene. The idea that genetic information comes in a one-dimensional array came to most of us only with the WATSON and CRICK (1953) paper. Before 1953, we could entertain two- and three-dimensional models for gene structures of head-spinning complexity.

I thank HENRY STADLER for helpful discussions and suggestions and REINHARD STÖGER for translating the paper by KNAPP and SCHREIBER.

LITERATURE CITED

ALTENBURG, E., 1934 The artificial production of mutations by ultraviolet light. Am. Nat. **68**: 491–507.

AVERY, O. T., C. M. MACLEOD and M. MCCARTY, 1944 Studies on the chemical nature of the substance inducing transformation in Pneumococcal types. J. Exp. Med. **79**: 137–158.

CHARGAFF, E., 1950 Chemical specificity of nucleic acids and mechanism of their enzymatic degradation. Experientia **6**: 201–209.

GEIGY, R., 1931 Action de l'ultraviolet sur le pole germinal dans l'oeuf de *Drosophila melanogaster*. Rev. Suisse Zool. **38**: 187.

HOLLAENDER, A., 1939 Wave-length dependence of the production of mutations in fungus spores by monochromatic ultra-violet radiation (2180–3650 A). Proc. 7th Int. Congr. Genet., pp. 153–154.

HOLLAENDER, A., and C. W. EMMONS, 1941 Wavelength dependence of mutation production in the ultraviolet with special emphasis on fungi. Cold Spring Harbor Symp. Quant. Biol. **IX:** 179–186.

JUDSON, H. F., 1993 Frederick Sanger, Erwin Chargaff, and the metamorphosis of specificity. Gene **135**: 1923.

KNAPP E., and H. SCHREIBER, 1939 Quantitative Analyse der mutationsauslösenden Wirkung monochromatischen UV Lichtes in Spermatozoiden von Sphaerocarpus. Proc. 7th Int. Congr. Genet., pp. 175–176.

LEA, D. E., 1947 *Actions of Radiations on Living Cells*. Macmillan, New York.

MULLER, H. J. and MOTT-SMITH, L. M., 1930 Evidence that natural radioactivity is inadequate to explain the frequency of "natural" mutations. Proc. Nat. Acad. Sci. **16**: 277–285.

NOETHLING, W., and H. STUBBE, 1936 Neuere botanische Untersuchungen über die Beziehung von Genmutabilität zur Quantität und Qualität kurzwelliger Strahlung. Verhandl. 3rd Int. Kongr. Lichtforsch., pp. 238–246.

ROMAN, H., 1988 A diamond in a desert. Genetics **119**: 739–741.

SANGER, F. and TUPPY, H. 1951 The amino-acid sequence in the phenylalynyl chain of insulin I and II. Biochem. J. **49**: 463–490.

SETLOW, R. B., 1987 Alexander Hollaender 1898–1986. Genetics **116**: 13.

STADLER, L. J., 1939 Genetic studies with ultraviolet radiation. Proc. 7th Int. Congr. Genet., pp. 269–276.

STADLER, L. J., and F. M. UBER, 1942 Genetic effects of ultraviolet radiation in maize. IV. Comparison of monochromatic radiations. Genetics **27**: 84–118.

VON BORSTEL, R. C., and C. M. STEINBERG, 1996 Alexander Hollaender: Myth and Mensch. Genetics **143**: 1051–1056.

WATSON, J. D. and CRICK, F. H. C. 1953 Molecular structure of nucleic acids: a structure for deoxyribose nucleic acid. Nature **171**: 737–738.

Chromosome Changes in Cell Differentiation

Orlando J. Miller

Center for Molecular Medicine and Genetics, Wayne State University, Detroit, Michigan 48201

IN a recent "Perspectives" article, EEVA THERMAN (1995) called attention to a variety of alterations in chromosomes that occur regularly in differentiating cells, have been known for many years, and are still poorly understood. These included *facultative heterochromatinization*, polyploidization by *endoreduplication*, *underreplication* of some sequences in polytene chromosomes, and *gene amplification*. The related programmed DNA loss phenomena called *chromatin diminution* and *chromosome elimination* also belong to this group of highly regulated developmental chromosome changes. Here I shall briefly review these changes, with particular emphasis on the cell and molecular genetic approaches that have provided, or could provide, insights into the signaling pathways and molecular mechanisms involved.

Facultative heterochromatinization during differentiation is widespread in metazoans and is functionally equivalent to programmed DNA loss. The best known examples are mammalian *X* chromosome inactivation (LYON 1961) and the inactivation of the paternally derived set of chromosomes in coccids destined to become males (HUGHES-SCHRADER 1948; BROWN and NELSON-REES 1961). Both involve imprinting, the epigenetic process that leads to differential expression of the two parental alleles at a locus. When the fragmented chromosomes produced by massive doses of ionizing radiation are transmitted from father to son in the mealybug, each fragment undergoes heterochromatinization, suggesting there are multiple *cis*-acting centers of inactivation in these holocentric chromosomes (BROWN and NELSON-REES 1961). These may contain nuclease-resistant, matrix-associated AT-rich fragments (KHOSLA *et al.* 1996). In contrast, there is a single center of *X*-inactivation in mammals, and inactivation is mediated by the *cis*-acting RNA product of the *XIST* gene (BROWN *et al.* 1991).

Centers of inactivation and *cis*-acting RNA products appear to be involved in at least one other type of imprinting. The imprinting of a cluster of four genes on mouse chromosome 7 is mediated by one of the four,

Author e-mail: ojmiller@cmb.biosci.wayne.edu

the *H19* gene. The maternal *H19* allele is expressed, and its *cis*-acting, nontranslatable RNA product inhibits the expression of the maternal alleles of the other three genes, *mash-2*, *Ins-2*, and *Igf2*. The paternal *H19* allele is methylated and not expressed, so the paternal alleles of the other three genes are expressed. Imprinting of the *Ins-2* and *Igf2* genes is disrupted by maternal inheritance of a targeted deletion of the *H19* gene and its flanking sequence, while paternal inheritance has no effect, reflecting the normally silent state of the paternal *H19* allele (LEIGHTON *et al.* 1995). There is also a cluster of several genes on human chromosome 15 that are expressed exclusively on the paternal chromosome; these may play a role in the Prader-Willi syndrome. One of these genes has only an RNA product (WEVRICK *et al.* 1994). It remains to be seen whether such *cis*-acting, nontranslatable RNAs play a more general role in imprinting and facultative heterochromatinization in vertebrates, coccids, or other taxons.

DNA methylation plays a role in imprinting as well as in gene and *X* chromosome inactivation (CHAILLET *et al.* 1995). Histone underacetylation may be an even more general mechanism in imprinting and facultative heterochromatinization (JEPPESEN 1997). While hyperacetylation of histones is characteristic of the DNA in active genes, underacetylation of histones is characteristic of the inactive micronucleus of Tetrahymena, the inactive *X* chromosome of eutherian or metatherian mammals, and the inactive spermatocyte *X* chromosome of the desert locust, *Schistocerca gregaria* (WOLF and TURNER 1996); surprisingly, this may not be the case for the inactive *X* chromosome in the male germline of the mouse (ARMSTRONG *et al.* 1997).

Programmed DNA loss is a common event in metazoan differentiation. It may involve whole chromosomes, large or small segments of chromosomes, or precisely defined short sequences. The earliest examples of programmed DNA loss were chromatin diminution in the nematode Ascaris (BOVERI 1887) and chromosome elimination in the dipteran Sciaridae (METZ 1938). Cell and molecular genetic approaches have provided exciting insights into the mechanisms responsible for each of these, as well as those involved in the V(D)J recombination that assembles diverse functional immunoglobulin and T-cell receptor genes from segments that are separated in the germline genome. This is directed by evolutionarily conserved *cis*-acting heptamer and nonomer recombination signal sequences flanking the segments (TONEGAWA 1983). Recognition and cutting at V(D)J recombination signal sequences requires the B and T lymphocyte-specific expression of two recombination-activating genes, *RAG1* and *RAG2* (MCBLANE *et al.* 1995), but repair of the resultant double-strand breaks (DSBs) uses the same enzyme that all cells use for repairing DSBs, a DNA-dependent protein kinase (BLUNT *et al.* 1995).

Chromatin diminution in Ascaris and Parascaris species involves fragmentation at the third to fifth cleavage divisions of the very large chromosomes then present and elimination of most of the chromatin. The fragmentation occurs at specific chromosome breakage regions (CBRs) and is followed by the addition of 2–4 kb of telomeric TTAGGT repeats (MULLER *et al.* 1991). Chromatin diminution takes place at a specific stage in the early embryo and occurs in all somatic precursor cells. It is prevented in germline cells by cytoplasmic factors close to the vegetal pole and can be induced by chemical treatment of eggs, suggesting that the inhibitory cytoplasmic factors are already present in the zygote (ESTEBAN *et al.* 1995). Chromatin diminution leads to the elimination not only of all detectable heterochromatin but also of some euchromatic genes. Three single-copy genes were identified in *Ascaris suum* that were eliminated from somatic cells by chromatin diminution; each is clearly related to a gene that is retained, leading to the suggestion that chromatin diminution is linked to partial genome duplication (MULLER *et al.* 1996).

Chromatin diminution has been most extensively characterized in ciliates and shows considerable variation among the various taxons (PRESCOTT 1994; YAO 1996; PREER 1997). After conjugation and completion of the sexual phase of its life cycle, hypotrichous ciliates such as Stylonychia or Euplotes transform a mitotic copy of the transcriptionally silent micronucleus into a macronucleus by a process that takes about 4 days. The first half of this period is taken up by endoreduplication and produces polytene chromosomes. An extreme form of precise chromatin diminution then occurs, resulting in loss of more than 90% of the DNA. Early in the process of endoreduplication, abundant long transposon-like elements (Tec1 and Tec2 families in *Euplotes crassus*) are excised; a bit later, short unique DNA sequences called internal eliminated sequences (IES) are excised. Both Tec and IES are bounded by a direct repeat of the TA dinucleotide, and excision is precise, leaving one TA. Excision, presumably by nuclease-mediated staggered cuts, is associated with rejoining of the flanking sequences. After Tec and IES have been eliminated and polytenization is completed, the chromosomes undergo fragmentation to form linear molecules whose ends are then capped by telomeric GGGGTTTT repeats. Additional rounds of DNA replication produce the mature macronucleus (PRESCOTT 1994). In *Tetrahymena thermophila,* the degree of polyploidy is only about 45C, and only some 15% of the micronuclear genome is eliminated during macronuclear development. The deletion process is very precise and involves specific *cis*-acting sequences (YAO 1996). In *Paramecium tetraaurelia,* developmental genomic rearrangements also affect mating type determination (MEYER and KELLER 1996).

Chromosome elimination shares a number of features with chromatin diminution. Both occur at a precise time in early development, both lead to the elimination of a large fraction of the germline genome, both can be involved in sex determination, and both can occur in the same organism, as in several primitive agnathan hagfish species. In one of these, *Eptatretus okinoseanus,* some of the restricted sequences are highly repetitive, and there is variation in the number of germline-restricted chromosomes, leading to the suggestion that some supernumerary (B) chromosomes are germline-restricted chromosomes that have escaped their programmed elimination (KUBOTA *et al.* 1992, 1993). Somatic elimination of supernumerary chromosomes has been described in both plants and animals (DARLINGTON and THOMAS 1941; MELANDER 1950). In the myrmicine ant, *Leptothorax spinosior,* B chromosomes are usually restricted to the germline of the haploid males, although they are rarely seen in the germline of the diploid females (IMAI 1974). Chromosome elimination is common in several genera of gall midges (Diptera: Cecidomyidae), such as Miastor, in which there is weak but suggestive evidence linking chromosome elimination to partial genome duplication (BREGMAN 1975). This point could be clarified with chromosome-specific libraries (painting probes) for *in situ* suppression hybridization (LICHTER *et al.* 1988; PINKEL *et al.* 1988).

Chromatin diminution and chromosome elimination have repeatedly led to the evolution of organisms in which the germline contains DNA sequences not present in somatic cells. Since germline-restricted DNA sequences are subject only to selective forces operating on the germline and gametes, mutations in them will inactivate any genes not expressed in the germline and will drive the evolution of separate germline-specific and soma-specific genomes, whether interspersed on the same chromosomes or carried by different chromosomes. As a result, the germline may transcribe a partially or completely different set of genes than does the soma. Some genes essential in both compartments might be present in two copies, one germline-specific, the other soma-specific. These might arise by partial genome duplication, as suggested by MULLER *et al.* (1996) for some genes in Ascaris, or by polyploidy, with elimination of unwanted chromatin or chromosomes only from somatic cells and capture of these by the germline to serve as its own set of genes.

Chromosome elimination in the dipteran fungus

gnat *Sciara coprophila* is particularly interesting. All zygotes contain three *X* chromosomes and several large L (limited) chromosomes. The L chromosomes are lost from all somatic cells by anaphase lag at the fifth or sixth cleavage division. Shortly thereafter, a single paternal *X* chromosome is lost to produce *X/X* or *X/X′* females, or two paternal *X* chromosomes are successively lost to give rise to *X/O* males. In male meiosis the maternal chromosome set plus the paternal L chromosomes proceed to the single pole of the monopolar spindle; the rest of the paternal set is lost. The two chromatids of the *X* chromosome fail to separate at the second meiotic division. Thus, each primary spermatocyte yields only one sperm, and it contains all the L chromosomes and two *X* chromosomes as a result of nondisjunction (METZ 1938). HELEN CROUSE (1960) found that a *cis*-acting controlling element near the centromere of the *X* chromosome was responsible for *X* nondisjunction. When this element was translocated to an autosome, the translocation chromosome was lost during male meiosis.

How does such regular, or programmed, nondisjunction of both limited and *X* chromosomes occur? Confocal laser scanning microscopy combined with fluorescence *in situ* hybridization (FISH) with an *X*-specific painting probe has provided some insight into this, showing that the long arms of the sister chromatids fail to separate completely, although the centromeres are attached to the spindle and progress towards the poles. The chromosome remains at the metaphase plate and is lost. The sister chromatids of the *X*-autosome translocation chromosome also fail to separate, and L chromosomes are lost by the same mechanism (DE SAINT PHALLE and SULLIVAN 1996).

The molecular mechanisms involved in anaphase separation of sister chromatids are beginning to be worked out. In general, two types of enzyme activity are required: topoisomerase II, to separate interlocked DNA strands, and proteolysis. The role of topoisomerase II in sister chromatid separation is best understood in yeast (HOLM *et al.* 1989), but in mammals chemical inhibition of topoisomerase II causes prolonged mitosis and anaphase separation is completely prevented, although the cells still attempt cleavage. With lower concentrations of the inhibitor, abnormalities of chromosome segregation are seen (DOWNES *et al.* 1991). In Drosophila, chromatid segregation at anaphase requires the product of the *barren* gene, a protein that associates with topoisomerase II throughout mitosis and activates topoisomerase activity. In homozygous *barren* mutants, centromeres move apart as anaphase begins, but sister chromatids fail to separate (BHAT *et al.* 1996). Separation of sister chromatids requires specific proteolysis of gene products such as *PDS1* in budding yeast, *CUT2* in fission yeast, *pimples* in Drosophila, and *CENP-E* in mammals. Proteolysis of the first two, and possibly the others, is mediated by the anaphase-promoting

complex (APC), which also degrades cyclins (KING *et al.* 1996).

Endoreduplication: Polyploidization during somatic cell differentiation is extremely widespread in both plant and animal kingdoms. I shall limit my discussion to polyploidy arising by endoreduplication rather than by endomitosis, failed cytokinesis after telophase, or cell fusion. Endoreduplication is highly regulated. It occurs only at certain stages of differentiation in specific cell lineages and reaches ploidy levels that are specific to the tissue, the species, or the inbred strain within a species. In addition, one or more genes or segments of the genome often show greater or lesser degrees of amplification than expected from the ploidy level. The formation of polytene chromosomes by endoreduplication in plants and animals involves repeated rounds of DNA replication without intervening mitotic cell divisions. This requires bypassing or suppressing cell cycle mechanisms that block further replication until mitosis has occurred.

Cell cycle progression depends upon a coordinated system in which unstable regulatory subunits, called cyclins because of their changing abundance throughout the cell cycle, activate specific CDKs (NASMYTH 1996). For example, in animal cells, S phase is induced by CDK2 complexed with S phase cyclins of E or A type, and M phase, mitosis, is induced by CDK1 complexed with M phase cyclins of A or B type. The maturation- or M-phase promoting factor, MPF, is an activated M phase CDK. It is found in late G2 or M phase cells and is capable of inducing nuclear disruption and chromosome condensation in G1, S, or G2 cells.

In Drosophila, the switch from mitotic cycles to endoreduplication (endocycles) is associated with the loss of the mitosis-promoting cyclins A and B and the continued periodic expression of the S phase-promoting cyclin E (SAUER *et al.* 1995; LILLY and SPRADLING 1996). Endocycles are composed of alternating S and Gap phases and do not require the product of the *cdc25^string* gene, a key regulator of normal mitotic cycles (SMITH and ORR-WEAVER 1991). Endoreduplication in maize endosperm involves changes similar to those seen in Drosophila. The onset of mitosis is blocked by the induction of an inhibitor of MPF, and S phase-promoting protein kinases are induced (GRAFI and LARKINS 1995). A change also occurs in the level and state of phosphorylation of the Rb105-like protein ZmRb, a negative regulator of cell cycle progression. ZmRb can be phosphorylated *in vitro* by an S phase protein kinase from endoreduplicating endosperm cells (GRAFI *et al.* 1996).

DNA replication in eukaryotic nuclear genomes generally begins at specific origins and proceeds bidirectionally. Origins in yeast are very short, well-characterized sequences, while those in metazoans are less well defined; *e.g.,* that of a salivary secretory protein gene in *S. coprophila* is contained within a 2-kb region of the gene (GERBI *et al.* 1993), and that of the Chinese hamster dihydrofolate reductase gene within a 0.45-kb region (BURHANS et al. 1990). Initiation of replication requires the assembly at origins of a prereplication (pre-RC) complex composed of a fairly stable origin replication complex (ORC), a Cdc6p-type protein, and a minichromosome maintenance (Mcm) complex. ORCs are bound to origins for most of the cell cycle. The other proteins bind at origins in the G1 phase, when Cdc6p is synthesized. The binding of Cdc6p is essential for the binding of the Mcm complex and the formation of a pre-RC.

Activated S phase, cyclin-dependent kinases (CDKs) initiate replication only from origins with pre-RCs, and replication is followed by dissociation of pre-RCs. Both S phase and M phase CDKs phosphorylate a component of the Mcm complex, thus inhibiting the de novo assembly of pre-RCs and preventing any new pre-RCs from forming between late G1 and anaphase, when M phase cyclins are degraded by the proteolytic anaphase-promoting complex (APC). This prevents origins from firing more than once during normal cell cycles (KING et al. 1996; NASMYTH 1996). In fission yeast, overexpression of the Cdc18 gene, the homologue of Cdc6 in budding yeast, leads to multiple rounds of replication and the formation of giant nuclei (NISHITANI and NURSE 1995). In Drosophila, a member of the Mcm family of replication factors, the disc proliferation abnormal (dpa) gene product, is essential for mitotic replication but is not required for endoreduplication (FEGER et al. 1995). Perhaps an as yet unrecognized Mcm family member is required for pre-RC formation or stabilization in endoreduplicating chromosomes.

Studies in mammalian cells have added to our understanding of the signaling pathways in endoreduplication. One of my former associates, MENASHE MARCUS, produced a temperature-sensitive mutant Chinese hamster cell line, ts41. At the nonpermissive temperature, the DNA content of these cells rose from 2C to 16C (HIRSCHBERG and MARCUS 1982). These cells replicate normally, but after completing S phase they skip G2, M, and G1 phases and go directly into S again (HANDELI and WEINTRAUB 1992). Thus, the ts41 gene product appears to couple S phase to M phase, blocking entry into S and fostering entry into G2 and mitosis. Is this gene turned off during the normal induction of polyploidy in megakaryocytes or placental trophoblasts, and does a homologous gene play a similar role in endoreduplication in other animals or plants?

The differentiation of bone marrow precursor cells into platelet-producing giant megakaryocytes is associated with a low degree of polyploidization. The DNA content, or ploidy level, in megakaryocytes is slightly higher in mice of the C3H inbred strain than in those of the C57BL6 strain, reaching at most 128C. The DNA content is intermediate in F_1 mice and shows a continuous rather than bimodal distribution in backcrosses to either parental strain, suggesting that several genes influence ploidy level. Furthermore, the female parent has a greater influence on ploidy level than the male

parent, suggesting a role for imprinting (MCDONALD and JACKSON 1994). The genes influencing endoreduplication in this system might be mapped to short regions within the genome by the quantitative trait loci (QTL) approach (LANDER and SCHORK 1994) with a large number of the murine microsatellite markers now available. Any genes known to be involved in signal transduction or cell cycle control that have been mapped to one or more of these locations would be likely candidates as regulators of megakaryocyte polyploidy, but additional genes in the regulatory pathway might also be identified by this positional cloning approach.

Identification of the genes involved in megakaryocyte differentiation would permit a detailed molecular analysis of the signaling pathways for polyploidization. Attention might be directed first to the genes for receptors or ligands known to be involved in megakaryocyte differentiation. Thrombopoietin, the ligand of the lymphokine receptor c-mpl, is a good candidate. It acts synergistically with erythropoietin, stem cell factor, and interleukin-11 to increase murine megakaryocyte colony growth and ploidy level in mouse cell cultures, as shown by flow cytometric analysis (BROUDY et al. 1995). Erythropoietin alone can yield ploidy levels up to 16C, but with thrombopoietin 30% of the cells achieve a 64C level. The rho gene product, a small molecular weight GTP-binding protein, is also involved in polyploidization in a megakaryocyte cell line (TAKADA et al. 1996).

The differentiation of polyploid megakaryocytes can be mimicked in human erythroleukemia cells by exposure to a phorbol ester such as TPA. Mitosis is arrested because cdk1 protein level falls markedly and cyclin B1 is modified so it cannot physically associate with cdk1. Thus, even though the expression of cyclin B1 is elevated and sustained, there is a lack of cdk1/cyclin B1-associated H1-histone kinase activity, i.e., a failure to form MPF, so the completion of S phase does not trigger mitosis (DATTA et al. 1996). This is similar to the elevation of S-phase-related protein kinases and inhibition of MPF activity seen during endoreduplication in maize endosperm (GRAFI and LARKINS 1995).

Trophoblast cells of the rodent placenta attain ploidy levels of 512C or higher. Chromosomes are not easily visualized in these giant cells, leaving some question as to whether they have arisen by endoreduplication or endomitosis (THERMAN 1995). However, in the rat, polyploid trophoblast cells from females always contain a single giant sex chromatin body, whereas those from males have none (NAGL 1972). Multiple inactive X chromosomes in a cell do not fuse together (THORLEY et al. 1967), so a giant sex chromatin body is unlikely to represent fusion of endomitotic inactive X chromosomes. It is much more likely that endoreduplication is the process involved and that all the polytene sister chromatids of the inactive X chromosome have remained tightly apposed.

Cell and molecular genetic approaches generally support the occurrence of tight bundling of sister chromatids during endoreduplication in trophoblast cells. *In situ* hybridization with probes for transgene integration sites on two different chromosomes showed only one site of hybridization for each probe in 16C-512C nuclei from mice heterozygous for a tandemly repetitive transgene inserted at a single site and two sites of hybridization in comparable nuclei from homozygotes. A class I MHC probe gave comparable results. Thus, endoreduplication appears to be involved in the formation of polyploid trophoblastic cells, with all the newly replicated strands of both chromatids of a chromosome remaining closely apposed, but no pairing of the homologous chromosomes (VARMUZA *et al.* 1988). In situ hybridization to the endogenous alpha-1 antitrypsin locus gave similar results, but with less strand clustering in this chromosome region (BOWER 1987).

Four of the five loci tested with molecular probes showed tight clustering of the amplified copies. Is this representative of the entire genome? The most efficient approach to answering this question would require visualizing all the chromosomes in polyploid megakaryocytes. VARMUZA *et al.* (1988) suggested treating the cells with Xenopus egg extract, which induces premature chromosome condensation (PCC) in diploid interphase cells. A much more informative approach would be to use *in situ* hybridization with whole chromosome painting probes (PINKEL *et al.* 1988) to evaluate the looseness or compaction of each chromosome at every point throughout its length during polyploidization. In seeking the mechanism of polyploidization, one might first determine whether the phorbol ester TPA will induce polyploidy in trophoblasts, as it does in megakaryocyte precursors and whether the same changes in cdk1 and MPF occur during polyploidization of trophoblasts as occur in mammalian megakaryocytes and maize endosperm.

Under-replication: An eclectic range of transcribed as well as nontranscribed DNA sequences are under-represented in Drosophila cells that have undergone endoreduplication. EMIL HEITZ (1934) noted that cytologically visible heterochromatin is markedly reduced in polytene chromosomes and used this as a basis for distinguishing α-heterochromatin (under-represented) from β-heterochromatin (still present). The various satellite DNAs of α-heterochromatin in *Drosophila melanogaster* and *D. virilis* are virtually totally unreplicated in salivary polytene DNA (GALL *et al.* 1971). A surprising number and type of genes are also under-represented in Drosophila polytene DNA, *e.g.*, 18S+28S rRNA genes (rDNA; HENNIG and MEER 1971), histone genes, and the 3′ end of the 100-kb Ultrabithorax (*Ubx*) gene, but not its distant 5′ end (LAMB and LAIRD 1987). Are other sequences also under-represented in polytene chromosomes? Comparative genomic hybridization (CGH) provides a general method that might answer this question, as it enables the visualization of minimally under-

or over-represented regions on a chromosome (KALLIONIEMI *et al.* 1992).

The process leading to under-representation of some sequences in polytene chromosomes is unclear. Chromatin diminution, analogous to that seen in nematodes (BOVERI 1887), was suggested by PAINTER (1933) and more recently by KARPEN and SPRADLING (1990), who suggested it as one cause of position-effect variegation. While there is no convincing cytological or molecular evidence for chromatin diminution in Drosophila, its occurrence early in polytenization in the macronucleus of hypotrichous ciliates such as *Euplotes crassus* (PRESCOTT 1994) provides an attractive model. An alternative mechanism, under-replication of heterochromatin, was suggested by HEITZ (1934), and this term is the one generally used when referring to under-representation of particular sequences. Recently, LILLY and SPRADLING (1996) have provided evidence that appears to favor the under-replication model. They identified a hypomorphic mutant of the Cyclin E gene. Mutant polyploid ovarian nurse cells in Drosophila had a reduced level of Cyclin E, with altered cyclical oscillation in this level. The mutant polyploid cells failed to show the usual under-representation of satellite DNA, and, in contrast to wild-type cells, had a late S pattern of bromodeoxyuridine incorporation similar to that in mitotic cells, presumably reflecting the presence of abundant heterochromatin in both cases. Their results support the idea that oscillating levels of Cyclin E control the endocycle S-phase and may indicate the absence of a checkpoint ensuring S-phase completion. This would permit incomplete replication of late-replicating sequences such as satellite DNA during endocycles, but this could occur only if the S-phase in at least some of the endocycles is too short for late-S sequences to complete their replication. Does the mutation in the Cyclin E gene prolong the S-phase? Do histone and rRNA genes replicate late enough in endocycle S-phases for this mechanism to account for their under-representation? Do the regions of the under-represented histone and ultrabithorax genes that are closest to an origin of replication show the least under-representation? Alternatively, the firing of late-replicating origins may be suppressed in endocycles, leading to a shorter S phase and more efficient increase in copy number of expressed genes.

Whatever the mechanism of under-representation of some sequences in Drosophila, it acts not long after endoreduplication begins. In the first two rounds of endoreduplication in ovarian follicle cells, DNA content doubles each time, but in the next few rounds the DNA content falls below that expected (MAHOWALD *et al.* 1979). The DNA content at stages corresponding to ploidy levels of 16C to 1024C increases at a rate comparable to that expected if 25% of the genomic DNA were unreplicated and 75% of the DNA were undergoing endoreduplication. Satellite 1.703 DNA, rDNA, and histone DNA all replicate normally during the last one or two rounds of salivary endoreduplication

(HAMMOND and LAIRD 1985). After one round of endoreduplication, Drosophila hindgut cells have a ploidy level of only 3.4C rather than 4C, representing an under-replication of about 30% of the genome (SMITH and ORR-WEAVER 1991). If chromatin diminution is involved, rather than under-replication of particular sequences, it may be restricted to a narrow window, say the third to fifth rounds of replication (the relative copy number would provide an estimate of the time of chromatin diminution). Diminution would have to spare some copies of any under-represented but still amplified sequence; for example, it might act only on the paternal set of chromosomes, owing to imprinting. Alternatively, imprinting of these sequences in the germline of one parent might modify their origins of replication and prevent their firing during endoreduplication.

Under-representation involves primarily the interspersed, intron-containing, generally nonfunctional copies of rDNA in polytene nuclei of Drosophila (ENDOW and GLOVER 1979). This is also true in the highly polyploid nurse cells of *Calliphora erythrocephala*; in which there is no under-replication of intronless rDNA; interestingly, most of the amplified rDNA is in extrachromosomal micronuclei (BUCKINGHAM and THOMPSON 1982). There is no under-representation of rDNA in the polytene salivary cells of the dipteran Rhynchosciara, which, like the fungus gnat, *S. coprophila*, has a much smaller amount of rDNA, all intron-free. Again, there are abundant rDNA-containing micronucleoli in these cells, suggesting that there may be under-replication of rDNA in the polytene chromosomes themselves, and compensatory extrachromosomal rDNA replication (GERBI 1971). The amplification of rDNA is apparently unique in another way: usually only one of the two rDNA clusters participates in endoreduplication and there is a dominance hierarchy, controlled by a factor associated with the rDNA itself, or even the number of rRNA genes in the cluster (ENDOW 1983).

The massive endoreduplication of silk gland DNA in *Bombyx mori*, which exceeds a 500,000C DNA level, is not associated with under-representation of repetitive sequences, rRNA genes or tRNA genes, on the basis of analysis of reassociation kinetics (GAGE 1974). Comparative genomic hybridization might reveal sites of under-represented sequences missed by the less sensitive earlier method. It could also answer the question of whether under-replication or chromatin diminution occurs during endoreduplication in vertebrates. All that is known so far is that satellite sequences are not under-represented in the giant cells of mouse trophoblast (LEJEUNE *et al.* 1982). Thus, the apparent scarcity of visible heterochromatin in large trophoblast cells (THERMAN 1995) must have another cause.

Amplification: In some organisms, endoreduplication is accompanied by even greater amplification of a few specific genes. DNA amplification involves escape from the usual requirement that each origin of replica-

tion fire once, and only once, during each S phase. The first example of such amplification was the DNA puffs seen in salivary glands of Sciarid flies in the last (fourth) larval instar (CROUSE and KEYL 1968). The level of amplification in DNA puffs in *S. coprophila* is 16-fold higher than that of the polytene chromosomes in which they occur. Puff II/9A contains two amplified transcription units with quite similar sequences; they are separated from each other by a 2.5-kb spacer (GERBI *et al.* 1993). What induces DNA puffing? HELEN CROUSE (1968) showed it was the steroid molting hormone, ecdysone. The molecular mechanisms involved in this signal transduction pathway might be clarified by cloning the genes whose expression is activated by ecdysone. Some will have steroid response elements in the promoter region, as GERBI *et al.* (1993) found in a DNA puff II/9A gene. However, genes whose products are used for pupation are unlikely to be the ones that initiate further rounds of DNA replication. Novel members of gene families involved in cell cycle regulation would be more likely candidates, and might be identified by this approach.

The two pairs of chorion genes in Drosophila ovarian follicle cells provide another example of intrachromosomal DNA amplification. During oogenesis the gene pair on the X chromosome is amplified about 16-fold, and the pair on chromosome 3 about 60-fold. The two genes of each pair, and the 1-kb spacer between them, are amplified equally, while the flanking sequences show a gradient of decreasing amplification extending for 40–50 kb in each direction. This suggests that additional rounds of replication are specifically initiated within the central, gene-containing region and are followed by bidirectional replication in the absence of discrete termination sites (SPRADLING 1981). Two-dimensional (2-D) gel studies have demonstrated the expected replication intermediates, and in the proper abundance (HECK and SPRADLING 1990). Direct visualization of amplifying chorion genes supports this onionskin model of DNA amplification from nested replication forks (OSHEIM *et al.* 1988). Several *cis*-acting DNA sequence elements have been identified that regulate chorion gene amplification. An important one, ACE3 (amplification control element from the third chromosome), is only 440 bp long, and amplification begins within it (CARMINATI *et al.* 1992).

GERBI's group mapped the origin of replication of the DNA puff II/9A gene in *S. coprophila*, using two different 2-D gel methods, and showed that here, too, replication proceeds bidirectionally from the origin (GERBI *et al.* 1993). Thus, intrachromosomal amplification of DNA puff and chorion genes does not occur by the rolling circle type of replication responsible for the extrachromosomal amplification of ribosomal genes in Drosophila (HOURCADE *et al.* 1973). It is interesting that both the DNA puff II/9A genes and the chorion genes that undergo endoreduplication consist of gene pairs with quite similar sequences. Perhaps this facilitates the formation of easily amplifiable structures. Is a specific sequence involved, such that substitution of an origin from a chorion or DNA puff gene could lead to amplification of a different gene?

The degree of amplification of chorion and DNA puff genes is fairly extreme. Do equal or lesser degrees of intrachromosomal amplification occur at other sites in these or other genomes, and is polytenization a necessary precondition? These questions might be answered with techniques such as comparative genomic hybridization (KALLIONIEMI *et al.* 1992), a computer-assisted fluorescence *in situ* hybridization technique that can produce a map of DNA sequences with increased (or decreased) copy number as a function of chromosomal location throughout the genome.

Endoreduplication in dipteran insects is associated with a very high level of production of a limited number of proteins, those encoded by the transcriptionally hyperactive genes in the RNA puffs found in virtually all polytene chromosomes and the DNA puffs found in those of Sciarid flies. The overproduction of poly $(A)^+$ RNA by DNA puffs in *S. coprophila* enabled DiBARTO-LOMEIS and GERBI (1989) to clone two tandem transcription units for salivary secretory proteins from DNA puff II/9A from a fourth instar salivary gland cDNA library. Differential display of mRNAs (LIANG and PARDEE 1992) by a PCR-based method to detect and clone overproduced (or underproduced) messages might be particularly useful for identifying additional overexpressed genes in the various tissues that undergo endoreduplication in species of interest.

Studies incorporating modern concepts and methods of cell and molecular biology have greatly enriched our understanding of some of the chromosome changes that occur regularly in cell differentiation. The many unsolved problems of classical genetics and cytogenetics will continue to present a challenge for investigators, and a source of interesting avenues of research.

LITERATURE CITED

ARMSTRONG, S. J., M. A. HULTEN, A. M. KEOHANE and B. M. TURNER, 1997 Different strategies of X-inactivation in germinal and somatic cells: histone H4 underacetylation does not mark the inactive X chromosome in the mouse male germline. Exp. Cell Res. **230:** 399–402.

BHAT, M. A., A. V. PHILIP, D. M. GLOVER and H. J. BELLEN, 1996 Chromatid segregation at anaphase requires the *barren* product, a novel chromosome-associated protein that interacts with topoisomerase II. Cell **87:** 1103–1114.

BLUNT, T., N. J. FINNIE, G. E. TACCIOLI, G. C. M. SMITH, J. DEMENGEOT *et al.*, 1995 Defective DNA-dependent protein kinase activity is linked to V(D)J recombination and DNA repair defects associated with the murine SCID mutation. Cell **80:** 813–823.

BOVERI, T., 1887 Über Differenzierung der Zellkerne während der Furchung des Eies von *Ascaris megalocephala*. Anat. Anz. **2:** 688–693.

BOWER, D. J., 1987 Chromosome organization in polyploid mouse trophoblast nuclei. Chromosoma **95:** 76–80.

BREGMAN, A., 1975 Q-, C-, and G-banding patterns in the germ-line and somatic chromosomes of *Miastor sp.* (Diptera: Cecidomyidae). Chromosoma **53:** 119–130.

BROUDY, V. C., N. L. LIN and K. KAUSHANSKY, 1995 Thrombopoietin (c-mpl ligand) acts synergistically with erythropoietin, stem cell factor, and interleukin-11 to enhance murine megakaryocyte col-

ony growth and increases megakaryocyte ploidy in vitro. Blood **85:** 1719–1726.

BROWN, S. W., and W. A. NELSON-REES, 1961 Radiation analysis of a lecanoid genetic system. Genetics **46:** 983–1007.

BROWN, C. J., A. BALLABIO, J. L. RUPERT, R. G. LEFRENIERE, M. GROMPE *et al.*, 1991 A gene from the region of the human X inactivation centre is expressed exclusively from the inactive X chromosome. Nature **349:** 38–44.

BUCKINGHAM, K., and N. THOMPSON, 1982 Under-replication of intron⁺ rDNA cistrons in polyploid nurse cell nuclei of *Calliphora erythrocephala*. Chromosoma **87:** 177–196.

BURHANS, W. C., L. T. VASSILIEV, M. S. CADDLE, N. H. HEINTZ and M. L. DE PAMPHILIS, 1990 Identification of an origin of bidirectional DNA replication in mammalian chromosomes. Cell **62:** 955–965.

CARMINATI, J. L., C. G. JOHNSTON and T. L. ORR-WEAVER, 1992 The Drosophila ACE3 chorion element autonomously induces amplification. Mol. Cell. Biol. **12:** 2444–2453.

CHAILLET, J. R., D. S. BADER and P. LEDER, 1995 Regulation of genomic imprinting by gametic and embryonic processes. Genes Dev. **9:** 1177–1187.

CROUSE, H. V., 1960 The controlling element in sex chromosome behavior in Sciara. Genetics **45:** 1429–1443.

CROUSE, H. V., 1968 The role of ecdysone in DNA-puff formation and DNA synthesis in the polytene chromosomes of *Sciara coprophila*. Proc. Natl. Acad. Sci. USA **61:** 971–978.

CROUSE, H. V., and H. G. KEYL, 1968 Extra replications in the "DNA-puffs" of *Sciara coprophila*. Chromosoma **25:** 357–364.

DARLINGTON, C. D., and P. T. THOMAS, 1941 Morbid mitosis and the activity of inert chromosomes in sorghum. Proc. Roy. Soc. Lond. B **159:** 127–150.

DATTA, N. S., J. L. WILLIAMS, J. CALDWELL, A. M. CURRY, E. K. ASH-CRAFT *et al.*, 1996 Novel alterations in CDK1/cyclin B1 kinase complex formation occur during the acquisition of a polyploid DNA content. Mol. Biol. Cell **7:** 209–223.

DE SAINT PHALLE, B., and W. SULLIVAN, 1996 Incomplete sister chromatid separation is the mechanism of programmed chromosome elimination during early *Sciara coprophila* embryogenesis. Development **122:** 3775–3784.

DIBARTOLOMEIS, S. M., and S. A. GERBI, 1989 Molecular characterization of DNA puff II/9A gene in *Sciara coprophila*. J. Mol. Biol. **210:** 531–540.

DOWNES, C. S., A. M. MULLINGER and R. T. JOHNSON, 1991 Inhibitors of DNA topoisomerase II prevent chromatid separation in mammalian cells but do not prevent exit from mitosis. Proc. Natl. Acad. Sci. USA **88:** 8895–8899.

ENDOW, S. A., 1983 Nucleolar dominance in polytene cells of *Drosophila*. Proc. Natl. Acad. Sci. USA **80:** 4427–4431.

ENDOW, S. A., and D. M. GLOVER, 1979 Differential replication of ribosomal gene repeats in polytene nuclei of Drosophila. Cell **17:** 597–605.

ESTEBAN, M. R., G. GIOVINAZZO and C. GODAY, 1995 Chromatin diminution is strictly correlated to somatic behavior in early development of the nematode *Parascaris univalens*. J. Cell Sci. **108:** 2393–2404.

FEGER, G., H. VAESSIN, T. T. SU, E. WOLFF, L. Y. JAN *et al.*, 1995 *dpa*, a member of the MCM family, is required for mitotic DNA replication but not endoreduplication in *Drosophila*. EMBO J. **14:** 5387–5398.

GAGE, L. P., 1974 Polyploidization of the silk gland of *Bombyx mori*. J. Mol. Biol. **86:** 97–108.

GALL, J. G., E. COHEN and M. L. POLAN, 1971 Repetitive sequences in Drosophila. Chromosoma **33:** 319–344.

GERBI, S. A., 1971 Localization and characterization of the ribosomal RNA cistrons in *Sciara coprophila*. J. Mol. Biol. **58:** 499–511.

GERBI, S. A., C. LIANG, N. WU, S. M. DIBARTOLOMEIS, B. BIENZ-TADMOR *et al.*, 1993 DNA amplification in DNA puff II/9A of *Sciara coprophila*. Cold Spring Harbor Symp. Quant. Biol. **58:** 487–494.

GRAFI, G., and B. A. LARKINS, 1995 Endoreduplication in maize endosperm: involvement of M-phase promoting factor inhibition and induction of S phase-related kinases. Science **269:** 1262–1264.

GRAFI, G., R. J. BURNETT, T. HELENTJARIS, B. A. LARKINS, J. A. DECA-PRIO *et al.*, 1996 A maize cDNA encodes a member of the retinoblastoma protein family: involvement in endoreduplication. Proc. Natl. Acad. Sci. USA **93:** 8962–8967.

HAMMOND, M. P., and C. D. LAIRD, 1985 Chromosome structure and DNA replication in nurse and follicle cells of *Drosophila melanogaster.* Chromosoma **91:** 267–278.

HANDELI, S., and H. WEINTRAUB, 1992 The ts41 mutation in Chinese hamster cells leads to successive S phases in the absence of intervening G2, M, and G1. Cell **71:** 599–611.

HECK, M. M. S., and A. C. SPRADLING, 1990 Multiple replication origins are used during *Drosophila* chorion gene amplification. J. Cell Biol. **110:** 903–914.

HEITZ, E., 1934 Über α- und β-heterochromatin sowie Konstanz und Bau der Chromosomeren bei Drosophila. Biol. Zbl. **54:** 588–609.

HENNIG, W., and B. MEER, 1971 Reduced polyteny of ribosomal RNA cistrons in giant chromosomes of *Drosophila hydei.* Nat. New Biol. **233:** 70–72.

HIRSCHBERG, J., and M. MARCUS, 1982 Isolation by a replica-plating technique of Chinese hamster temperature-sensitive cell cycle mutants. J. Cell. Physiol. **115:** 159–166.

HOLM, C., T. STEARNS and D. BOTSTEIN, 1989 DNA topoisomerase II must act at mitosis to prevent nondisjunction and chromosome breakage. Mol. Cell. Biol. **9:** 159–168.

HOURCADE, D., D. DRESSLER and J. WOLFSON, 1973 Amplification of ribosomal genes involves a rolling circle intermediate. Proc. Natl. Acad. Sci. USA **70:** 2926–2930.

HUGHES-SCHRADER, S., 1948 Cytology of coccids (Coccoidea-Homoptera). Adv. Genet. **2:** 127–203.

IMAI, H. T., 1974 B-chromosomes in the myrmicine ant, *Leptothorax spinsior.* Chromosoma **45:** 431–444.

JEPPESEN, P., 1997 Histone acetylation: a possible mechanism for the inheritance of cell memory at mitosis. BioEssays **19:** 67–74.

KALLIONIEMI, A., O.-P. KALLIONIEMI, D. SUDAR, D. RUTOVITZ, J. W. GRAY *et al.,* 1992 Comparative genomic hybridization for molecular cytogenetic analysis of solid tumors. Science **258:** 818–821.

KARPEN, G. H., and A. C. SPRADLING, 1990 Reduced DNA polytenization of a minichromosome region undergoing position-effect variegation in Drosophila. Cell **63:** 97–107.

KHOSLA, S., P. KANTHETI, V. BRAHMACHARI and H. S. CHANDRA, 1996 A male-specific nuclease-resistant chromatin fraction in the mealybug *Planococcus lilacinus.* Chromosoma **104:** 386–392.

KING, R. W., R. J. DESCHAIES, J.-M. PETERS and M. W. KIRSCHNER, 1996 How proteolysis drives the cell cycle. Science **274:** 1652–1659.

KUBOTA, S., Y. NAKAI, M. KURO-O and S. KOHNO, 1992 Germ line-restricted supernumerary (B) chromosomes in *Eptatretus okinoseanus.* Cytogenet. Cell Genet. **60:** 224–228.

KUBOTA, S., K. MASAKI, S. MIZUNO and S. KOHNO, 1993 Germ line-restricted, highly repeated DNA sequences and their chromosomal localization in Japanese hagfish (*Eptatretus okinoseanus*). Chromosoma **102:** 163–173.

LAMB, M. M., and C. D. LAIRD, 1987 Three euchromatic DNA sequences under-replicated in polytene chromosomes of *Drosophila* are localized in constrictions and ectopic fibers. Chromosoma **95:** 227–235.

LANDER, E. S., and N. J. SCHORK, 1994 Genetic dissection of complex traits. Science **265:** 2037–2048.

LEIGHTON, P. A., R. S. INGRAM, J. EGGENSCHWILER, A. EFSTRATIADIS and S. M. TILGHMAN, 1995 Disruption of imprinting caused by deletion of the H19 gene region in mice. Nature **375:** 34–39.

LEJEUNE, B., J. VAN HOECK and F. LEROY, 1982 Satellite versus total DNA replication in relation to endopolyploidy of decidual cells in the mouse. Chromosoma **84:** 511–516.

LIANG, P., and A. B. PARDEE, 1992 Differential display of eukaryotic messenger RNA by means of the polymerase chain reaction. Science **257:** 967–971.

LICHTER, P., T. CREMER, J. BORDEN, L. MANUELIDIS and D. C. WARD, 1988 Delineation of individual human chromosomes in metaphase and interphase cells by in situ suppression hybridization using recombinant DNA libraries. Hum. Genet. **80:** 224–234.

LILLY, M. A., and A. C. SPRADLING, 1996 The Drosophila endocycle is controlled by Cyclin E and lacks a checkpoint ensuring S-phase completion. Genes Dev. **10:** 2514–2526.

LYON, M. F., 1961 Gene action in the *X* chromosome of the mouse (*Mus musculus* L.). Nature **190:** 372–373.

MAHOWALD, A. P., J. H. CAULTON, M. K. EDWARDS and A. D. FLOYD,

1979 Loss of centrioles and polyploidization in follicle cells of Drosophila. Exp. Cell Res. **118:** 404–410.

MCBLANE, J. F., D. C. VAN GENT, D. A. RAMSDEN, C. ROMEO, C. A. CUOMO *et al.,* 1995 Cleavage at a V(D)J recombination signal requires only RAG1 and RAG2 proteins and occurs in two steps. Cell **83:** 387–395.

MCDONALD, T. P., and C. W. JACKSON, 1994 Mode of inheritance of the higher degree of megakaryocyte polyploidization in C3H mice. I. Evidence for a role of genomic imprinting in megakaryocyte polyploidy determination. Blood **83:** 1493–1498.

MELANDER, Y., 1950 Accessory chromosomes in animals, especially in *Polycelis tenuis.* Hereditas **36:** 19–38.

METZ, C. W., 1938 Chromosome behavior, inheritance and sex determination in *Sciara.* Am. Nat. **72:** 485–520.

MEYER, E., and A.-M. KELLER, 1996 A Mendelian mutation affecting mating type determination also affects developmental genomic rearrangements in *Paramecium tetraaurelia.* Genetics **143:** 191–202.

MULLER, F., C. WICKY, A. SPICKER and H. TOBLER, 1991 New telomere formation after developmentally regulated chromosome breakage during the process of chromatin diminution in *Ascaris lumbricoides.* Cell **67:** 815–822.

MULLER, F., V. BERNARD and H. TOBLER, 1996 Chromatin diminution in nematodes. BioEssays **18:** 133–138.

NAGL, W., 1972 Giant sex chromatin in endopolyploid trophoblast nuclei in the rat. Experientia **28:** 217–218.

NASMYTH, K., 1996 Viewpoint: putting the cell cycle in order. Science **274:** 1643–1645.

NISHITANI, H., and P. NURSE, 1995 p65^{cdc18} plays a major role in controlling the initiation of DNA replication in fission yeast. Cell **83:** 397–405.

OSHEIM, Y. N., O. L. MILLER, JR. and A. L. BEYER, 1988 Visualization of *Drosophila melanogaster* chorion genes undergoing amplification. Mol. Cell. Biol. **8:** 2811–2821.

PAINTER, T. S., 1933 A new method for the study of chromosome rearrangements, and the plotting of chromosome maps. Science **78:** 585–586.

PINKEL, D., J. LANDEGENT, C. COLLINS, J. FUSCOE, R. SEAGRAVES *et al.,* 1988 Fluorescence in situ hybridization with human chromosome-specific libraries: detection of trisomy 21 and translocation of chromosome 4. Proc. Natl. Acad. Sci. USA **85:** 9138–9142.

PREER, J. R., JR., 1997 Whatever happened to Paramecium genetics? Genetics **145:** 217–225.

PRESCOTT, D. M., 1994 The DNA of ciliated protozoa. Microbiol. Rev. **58:** 233–267.

SAUER, K., J. A. KNOBLICH, H. RICHARDSON and C. F. LEHNER, 1995 Distinct modes of cyclin E/cdc2c kinase regulation and S-phase control in mitotic and endoreduplication cycles of *Drosophila* embryogenesis. Genes Dev. **9:** 1327–1339.

SMITH, A. V., and T. L. ORR-WEAVER, 1991 The regulation of the cell cycle during *Drosophila* embryogenesis. Development **112:** 997–1008.

SPRADLING, A., 1981 The organization and amplification of two chromosomal domains containing Drosophila chorion genes. Cell **27:** 193–201.

TAKADA, M., N. MORII, S. KUMAGAI and R. RYO, 1996 The involvement of the *rho* gene product, a small molecular weight GTP-binding protein, in polyploidization of a human megakaryocyte cell line, CMK. Exp. Hematol. **24:** 524–530.

THERMAN, E., 1995 Chromosome behavior in cell differentiation: a field ripe for exploration? Genetics **141:** 799–804.

THORLEY, J., D. WARBURTON and O. J. MILLER, 1967 Absence of somatic pairing of sex chromatin masses (inactivated X chromosomes) in cultured cells from a human XXXXY male. Exp. Cell Res. **47:** 663–665.

TONEGAWA, S., 1983 Somatic generation of antibody diversity. Nature **302:** 575–581.

VARMUZA, S., V. PRIDEAUX, R. KOTHARY and J. ROSSANT, 1988 Polytene chromosomes in mouse trophoblast giant cells. Development **102:** 127–134.

WEVRICK, R. J. A. KERNS and U. FRANCKE, 1994 Identification of a novel paternally expressed gene in the Prader-Willi syndrome region. Hum. Mol. Genet. **3:** 1877–1882.

WOLF, K. W., and B. M. TURNER, 1996 The pattern of histone H4 acetylation on the X chromosome during spermatogenesis of the desert locust *Schistocerca gregaria.* Genome **39:** 854–865.

YAO, M.-C., 1996 Programmed DNA deletions in tetrahymena: mechanisms and implications. Trends Genet. **12:** 26–30.

See also page 705 in Addenda et Corrigenda.

mutS, Proofreading, and Cancer

Edward C. Cox

Department of Molecular Biology, Princeton University, Princeton, New Jersey 08544

"... the tendency to variability is itself hereditary..."
CHARLES DARWIN (1859)

SIEGEL and BRYSON published the first report of *mutatorS* (*mutS*) of *Escherichia coli* in 1964 (SIEGEL and BRYSON 1964). Their more detailed results appeared in 1967, when they demonstrated that most of the mutations induced by *mutS* were transitions, since the majority of them could be reverted by 2-aminopurine and ethylmethane sulfate (EMS; SIEGEL and BRYSON 1967). The next paper on *mutS* was published in GENETICS by myself, DEGNEN, and SCHEPPE (COX *et al.* 1972), and it is the silver anniversary of this article that occasions this essay. Among other things, we showed by reversion analysis that *mutS* did indeed cause AT → GC and GC → AT transitions, and that the transversion mutation rate in *mutS* strains was very close to that of the wild type.

The base-pair specificity of *mutS* was not, however, what we were after. I had noticed in 1967 that an AT pair in a *mutS* background reverted at a high frequency in one location, but not at another. It occurred to me that this might provide a clue to DNA replication, since at that time lagging strand replication was a complete mystery. Indeed, the term "lagging strand" hadn't been invented. It *was* clear that PolI, the DNA polymerase isolated and studied so productively by KORNBERG and his students, extended only from the 3' end of a growing chain, and this presented an obvious paradox. I thought that *mutS* might be the polymerase that extended the 5' end of the complementary strand and that the difference between the two AT pairs was one of error rate and orientation with respect to the replication origin. This was an attractive idea, more so then than it might seem now, because it was known from the work of several labs that there are strong GC biases between the strands of λ bacteriophage (reviewed in DAVIDSON and SZYBALSKI 1971), and it had been proposed that polymerization biases might explain this result (SUEOKA 1962). We set out to test this idea by looking at the *lacZ* gene in two orientations at the same spot on the chromosome in *mutS* backgrounds. Both orientations could be constructed with φ80d*lac* transducing phage (SIGNER and BECKWITH 1966). Alas, the experiments revealed that the differences in AT → GC rates could best be explained by nearest neighbor effects, and it now seems that GC strand biases are due to transcription-associated errors (FRANCINO *et al.* 1996), also associated with *mutS* function (MELLON and CHAMPE 1996).

Proofreading in bacteria: It is now well-known that *mutS* affects just one component of two proofreading machines in *E. coli*, which together push the mutation rate down to ~10^{-10} per base-pair replication (COX 1976). The first proofreading step occurs at the replication fork, involving a balance between chain elongation on the one hand and 3' → 5' exonuclease activity on the other. The exonuclease is associated with either the DNA polymerase itself (PolI), or with the ε subunit of the DNA polymerase PolIII holoenzyme, encoded by the *mutD* (*dnaQ*) gene (SCHEUERMANN and ECHOLS 1984). The second proofreading system is mismatch repair, which detects base-pairing and frame-shift errors that escape the 3' → 5' proofreading exonuclease and is composed of *mutH* and *mutL* in addition to *mutS*. The MutHLS complex recognizes errors in newly replicated DNA, paving the way for their repair (COX 1995). Contributions to accurate replication by base-pairing, proofreading, and mismatch repair have been sorted out in an excellent study of forward mutation rates in the *lacI* gene. As predicted from earlier, somewhat fragmentary work, base pairing accounts for the first five orders of magnitude in fidelity, proofreading the next two, and mismatch repair the next two to three (SCHAAPER 1993). Interestingly, transition mutations are most efficiently edited by MutHLS, and transversions by the PolIII holoenzyme. The observation that both transitions and transversions are elevated two or more orders of magnitude in a *mutD* but otherwise wild-type background suggests either that the mismatch repair system is easily overwhelmed (SCHAAPER and RADMAN 1989) or that the PolIII holoenzyme is responsible for repairing lesions detected by MutHLS (MODRICH and LAHUE 1996).

Corresponding author: Edward C. Cox, Department of Molecular Biology, Princeton University, Princeton, NJ 08544-1014.

Mismatch repair plays a second major role by selecting against mispaired intermediates that arise during recombination, often between different bacterial species (reviewed in COX 1995). Normally, recombination between *E. coli* and Salmonella is rare, but it is common when the Salmonella recipient is also *mutS* (RAYSSIGUIER *et al.* 1989). This failure of mismatch-defective strains to maintain species barriers has assumed dramatic new importance with the discovery that many pathogenic *E. coli* strains are deleted for *mutS* and thus not only mutate to drug resistance at high frequency, but probably also mate promiscuously with distantly related species, some of which are undoubtedly also drug resistant (LECLERC *et al.* 1996).

In addition to *mutD* and the mutHLS system, three mutator loci recognize and destroy 8-oxodG, a common oxidation product in the deoxytriphosphate pool and in DNA itself. Because 8-oxodG pairs with A, as well as C, it specifically elevates AT → CG transversions upon replication, the signature mutation of TREFFERS' mutator, *mutT* (TREFFERS *et al.* 1954; YANOFSKY *et al.* 1966). It is not clear why the ϵ subunit and the mismatch repair complex together cannot discriminate between 8-oxodG:A and G:C pairs. It may be that the mispair frequency is so high that proofreading at the replication fork is swamped, or it may equally well be that MutS simply fails to recognize this mismatch, as with C:C pairs (MODRICH and LAHUE 1996). Wherever the problem lies, MutT functions by destroying 8-oxodGTP in the triphosphate pool, thereby lowering the probability of misincorporation *via* an A:oxodG mispair. *mutT* is backed up by two glycosylases that also recognize 8-oxodG, this time in the DNA, either paired with C (MutM) or paired with A (MutY). In addition, MutY recognizes G:A mispairs, removing the A. If these mispairs replicate, the G:C → T:A transversion rate increases (reviewed in MILLER and MICHAELS 1996).

There are other modifiers of mutation rate in bacteria and phage, most importantly the particular allele fixed at the loci encoding PolI and PolIII (*dnaE*). In fact, the first genetic association of mutators with DNA replication came when SPEYER showed that certain polI mutations in T4 bacteriophage had mutator phenotypes (SPEYER 1965). DRAKE extended this work by demonstrating that other alleles in the same gene could depress the mutation rate below that of the wild type (DRAKE and ALLEN 1968). These genetic results were placed on a firm biochemical footing by BESSMAN and his students, who showed that the ratio of polymerase to proofreading exonuclease activity increases in the series antimutator < wild type < mutator (BESSMAN *et al.* 1974). In *E. coli*, this ratio is governed by interactions between *mutD* (*dnaQ*) and *dnaE*. Thus, dnaQ926 leads to error catastrophe unless combined with an antimutator allele of *dnaE* (FIJALKOWSKA and SCHAAPER 1996).

Mutations increase in bacteria exposed to ultraviolet light and other insults. A common view is that imperfect repair and recombination lead to errors, but the mechanism is not fully understood. It seems likely that there are mechanisms in the cell that actively inhibit proofreading and mismatch repair, at least temporarily. Active suppression of proofreading could be important in bacteria, because new mutations at a high rate are the primary adaptive mechanism for a haploid, largely asexual organism faced with an uncertain and changing environment. This could be accomplished, for example, by inactivating the ϵ subunit, or by modifying MutS. The same goals could also be achieved by linking MutS synthesis to a cell cycle checkpoint. In both *E. coli* and *Saccharomyces cerevisiae*, *mutS* levels are known to be cell cycle dependent (FENG *et al.* 1996; KRAMER *et al.* 1996), and this is highly suggestive.

All in all, *E. coli* has evolved a proofreading system that reduces errors to $\sim 10^{-10}$ per base-pair replication. Thus, in a wild-type population only one cell in a thousand accumulates a single base-pairing error per generation. This is astonishing and difficult to explain by simple selectionist arguments (COX 1976).

Proofreading and cancer: What lessons from the *E. coli* mutator world are relevant to the causes of human cancer? Approximately 30 years after SIEGEL and BRYSON reported on *mutS*, two labs published papers showing a one-to-one correspondence between hereditary nonpolyposis colon cancer (HNPCC), an autosomal dominant disorder, and a defective *hMSH2* gene, a human homologue of *mutS* (FISHEL *et al.* 1993; LEACH *et al.* 1993). Approximately 60% of all HNPCC patients are mutant for *hMSH2* (FISHEL *et al.* 1993; LEACH *et al.* 1993; NYSTROM LAHTI *et al.* 1994). A characteristic feature of HNPCC tumors is microsatellite repeat instability, one of the clues from research in bacteria and yeast that helped focus attention on mismatch repair defects in HNPCC (LEVINSON and GUTMAN 1987; IONOV *et al.* 1993; STRAND *et al.* 1993). This correspondence between instability and mismatch repair has been systematically explored in HNPCC kindreds. There is an excellent, if incomplete, correspondence between instability and defects in the five known human mismatch repair genes (LIU *et al.* 1996).

Mismatch repair in yeast, mice, and humans is clearly much more complex than the MutHLS system in *E. coli* and Salmonella. There appears to be, among other things, specialization in the recognition process, so that there may be, for example, one complex for insertion-deletion recognition and another for single residue mispairing. Subunits may also be interchanged to provide greater specificity for one mismatch over another. There is also a mitochondrial-specific system and evidence that a second system unrelated to MutHLS is active in yeast, although this evidence is inferential and based on activities that remain in mismatch repair null mutants (reviewed in KOLODNER 1996).

Given what we know about proofreading in *E. coli*, we might predict with some confidence that many of the other proofreading pathways described here will be associated with familial cancers. For example, it is very likely that *mutT, M,* and *Y* homologues exist in eukaryotes, because 8-oxodG is unavoidable, and an effective proof-reading system must have evolved to handle it. There is also a large gap in our understanding of mismatch repair in eukaryotes. All mismatch repair systems must distinguish old from new strands; if not, the correction process would be at best 50% efficient, not the two orders of magnitude we observe. In *E. coli* and other bacteria, freshly replicated DNA is hemimethylated at the 6-position of adenine in the sequence GATC (the *dam* methylase that methylates this residue was, in fact, first identified by its mutator phenotype; MARINUS and MORRIS 1974). MutHLS thus recognizes and sets in motion the correction of the base on the undermethylated new strand, and in this way corrects only the incorporation error. How eukaryotes distinguish newly replicated from parental DNA is unknown, but if the lessons learned from bacteria are fruitful here too, we can expect mutator activity in the strand-marking system and microsatellite instability related to these hitherto unidentified loci.

Possibly the most potent mutator in *E. coli* is *mutD*, coding for the ϵ subunit of the PolIII holoenzyme. All classes of mutations, including frame-shifts, are elevated many orders of magnitude in *mutD* mutants (DEGNEN and COX 1974; FOWLER *et al.* 1974). Proofreading activity lies in the ExoI domain of ϵ, which is highly conserved in viral, prokaryote, and eukaryote polymerases (BLANCO *et al.* 1992). As noted above, strong alleles in this region mutate at such high rates that strains rapidly die from error catastrophes (FIJALKOWSKA and SCHAAPER 1996). The first *mutD* allele isolated lies in the ExoI motif (DEGNEN and COX 1974). Other weaker alleles exist. They are dominant, and many are outside the ExoI region (S. THOMAS, D. HORNER and E. C. COX, unpublished data). Thus, it is reasonable to suggest that weak alleles in the ExoI domain of human Polγ polymerase would become fixed and also cause satellite instabilities as well as base-pairing errors in precancerous cells. This possibility has been examined in a colorectal cell line, where substitutions at two positions were detected. However, they were outside the ExoI motif, and the relationship between polymerase structure and the cancerous state in this cell line is uncertain (DA COSTA *et al.* 1995).

Thus, many functions revealed in studies of bacterial proofreading may have counterparts in humans. Since proofreading is incompletely understood, even in bacteria, it is almost certainly the case that we currently know only a fraction of what can be known about proofreading in humans. It reasonably follows that mutators in as yet undiscovered loci will lie at the heart of other familial cancers.

Sporadic tumors: This brief summary of an extensive and rapidly growing literature makes it clear, I hope,

that mismatch repair defects play a major role in the genesis of HNPCC. I have also argued that other components of proofreading are strong candidates for familial cancers, not only those involving microsatellite instabilities. But what of sporadic tumors? LOEB has suggested that selection for high mutation rate is necessary to supply the multiple mutations required on the road to metastasis (LOEB 1991). The difficulty is that this suggestion involves second-order selection, which is almost always very weak: selection operates on the new mutant directly, and not on the agent that caused it. In asexual populations, as LEIGH pointed out many years ago, mutators remain linked to the mutations they cause and can become fixed if the overall fitness of the population is not depressed too far (LEIGH 1970). Experiments with *E. coli mutT1* populations support this view (GIBSON *et al.* 1970). HNPCC mutations are formally autosomal dominant, and thus HNPCC clones can be thought of as essentially asexual populations. By analogy with bacterial populations, we can then ask whether the population is large enough always to contain one new mutator allele arising at the wild-type mutation rate and, if so, whether the new mutation rate is high enough to provide cancer cells that are more fit in the sense that they have escaped cell cycle checkpoints and specific cell-cell adhesion regulation. If the answer to both of these questions is yes, then mutators can arise and go to fixation in sporadic tumors. It is simply a question of population size, mutation rate, and time, since cancerous cells are supremely fit in a wild-type background. Recently TOMLINSON and BODMER have examined this issue by simulation and have arrived at similar conclusions (TOMLINSON *et al.* 1996). Of course, if the mutator phenotype confers higher fitness directly, all bets are off (LEIGH 1970).

At the moment, the data on tumor progression in sporadic tumors that would allow us to address this question are fragmentary, although recent results suggest that new mismatch mutators can appear in sporadic colorectal tumors and that *in vitro* the repair system is defective in mismatch repair as well as microsatellite stability (PARSONS *et al.* 1996). One would very much like to know when during sporadic tumor progression mismatch repair defects first appear. Do they expand clonally with time, suggesting higher fitness for the mutator itself or for the more fit mutants associated with it? In general, are there causal links between the appearance of mutators and the progression of tumor phenotype early during tumorigenesis? Studies of this kind might be modeled after population studies in bacterial mutator populations, where cause and effect can be disentangled by following phenotypic and molecular markers in competing populations (CHAO *et al.* 1983).

Conclusions: Studies begun by SIEGEL and BRYSON for the best reason in science, curiosity, have thus yielded a rich harvest that has contributed in a deep way to our understanding of tumorigenesis. It is not unlikely that other mutators first studied in bacteria and then in yeast will have a similar impact. These are active research areas. What seems to be missing at the moment are studies inspired by the rich population genetic literature on mutagenesis, fitness, selection, and drift. Perhaps here, too, population studies in bacteria have something to offer.

LITERATURE CITED

BESSMAN, M. J., N. MUZYCZKA, M. F. GOODMAN and R. L. SCHNAAR, 1974 Studies on the biochemical basis of spontaneous mutation II. The incorporation of a base and its analogue into DNA by wild-type, mutator and anti-mutator DNA polymerase. J. Mol. Biol. 88: 409–421.

BLANCO, L., A. BERNAD and M. SALAS, 1992 Evidence favouring the hypothesis of a conserved 3'-5' exonuclease active site in DNA-dependent DNA polymerases. Gene 112: 139–144.

CHAO, L., C. VARGAS, B. B. SPEAR and E. C. COX, 1983 Transposable elements as mutator genes in evolution. Nature 303: 633–635.

COX, E. C., 1976 Bacterial mutator genes and the control of spontaneous mutation. Annu. Rev. Genet. 10: 135–156.

COX, E. C., 1995 Recombination, mutation and the origin of species. BioEssays 17: 747–749.

COX, E. C., G. E. DEGNEN and M. L. SCHEPPE, 1972 Mutator gene studies in *Escherichia coli*: the mutS gene. Genetics 72: 551–567.

DA COSTA, L. T., B. LIU, W. EL DEIRY, S. R. HAMILTON, K. W. KINZLER et al., 1995 Polymerase delta variants in RER colorectal tumors. Nat. Genet. 9: 10–11.

DAVIDSON, N., and W. SZYBALSKI, 1971 Physical and chemical characteristics of lambda DNA, p. 792 in *The Bacteriophage Lambda*, edited by A. D. HERSHEY. Cold Spring Harbor Laboratory, Cold Spring Harbor, NY.

DEGNEN, G. E., and E. C. COX, 1974 Conditional mutator gene in *Escherichia coli*: isolation, mapping, and effector studies. J. Bacteriol. 117: 477–487.

DRAKE, J. W., and E. F. ALLEN, 1968 Antimutagenic DNA polymerases of bacteriophage T4. Cold Spring Harbor Symp. Quant. Biol. 33: 339–344.

FENG, G., H. C. TSUI and M. E. WINKLER, 1996 Depletion of the cellular amounts of the MutS and MutH methyl-directed mismatch repair proteins in stationary-phase *Escherichia coli* K-12 cells. J. Bacteriol. 178: 2388–2396.

FIJALKOWSKA, I. J., and R. M. SCHAAPER, 1996 Mutants in the Exo I motif of *Escherichia coli* dnaQ: defective proofreading and inviability due to error catastrophe. Proc. Natl. Acad. Sci. USA 93: 2856–2861.

FISHEL, R., M. K. LESCOE, M. R. RAO, N. G. COPELAND, N. A. JENKINS et al., 1993 The human mutator gene homolog MSH2 and its association with hereditary nonpolyposis colon cancer [published erratum appears in Cell 77: 167, 1994]. Cell 75: 1027–1038.

FOWLER, R. G., G. E. DEGNEN and E. C. COX, 1974 Mutational specificity of a conditional *Escherichia coli* mutator, *mutD5*. Mol. Gen. Genet. 133: 179–191.

FRANCINO, M. P., L. CHAO, M. A. RILEY and H. OCHMAN, 1996 Asymmetries generated by transcription-coupled repair in enterobacterial genes. Science 272: 107–109.

GIBSON, T. C., M. L. SCHEPPE and E. C. COX, 1970 Fitness of an *Escherichia coli* mutator gene. Science 169: 686–688.

IONOV, Y., M. A. PEINADO, S. MALKHOSYAN, D. SHIBATA and M. PERUCHO, 1993 Ubiquitous somatic mutations in simple repeated sequences reveal a new mechanism for colonic carcinogenesis. Nature 363: 558–561.

KOLODNER, R., 1996 Biochemistry and genetics of eukaryotic mismatch repair. Genes Dev. 10: 1433–1442.

KRAMER, W., B. FARTMANN and E. C. RINGBECK, 1996 Transcription of *mutS* and *mutL*-homologous genes in *Saccharomyces cerevisiae* during the cell cycle. Mol. Gen. Genet. 252: 275–283.

LEACH, F. S., N. C. NICOLAIDES, N. PAPADOPOULOS, B. LIU, J. JEN et al., 1993 Mutations of a *mutS* homolog in hereditary nonpolyposis colorectal cancer. Cell 75: 1215–1225.

LECLERC, J. E., B. LI, W. L. PAYNE and T. A. CEBULA, 1996 High mutation frequencies among *Escherichia coli* and *Salmonella* pathogens. Science 274: 1208–1211.

LEIGH, E. G. J., 1970 Natural selection and mutability. Am. Nat. 104: 301–305.

LEVINSON, G., and G. A. GUTMAN, 1987 High frequencies of short frameshifts in poly-CA/TG tandem repeats borne by bacteriophage M13 in *Escherichia coli* K-12. Nucleic Acids Res. 15: 5323–5338.

LIU, B., R. PARSONS, N. PAPADOPOULOS, N. C. NICOLAIDES, H. T. LYNCH et al., 1996 Analysis of mismatch repair genes in hereditary non-polyposis colorectal cancer patients. Nat. Med 2: 169–174.

LOEB, L. A., 1991 Mutator phenotype may be required for multistage carcinogenesis. Cancer Res. 51: 3075–3079.

MARINUS, M. G., and N. R. MORRIS, 1974 Biological functions for 6-methyl adenine residues in the DNA of *Escherichia coli* K12. J. Mol. Biol. 85: 309–322.

MELLON, I., and G. N. CHAMPE, 1996 Products of DNA mismatch repair genes *mutS* and *mutL* are required for transcription-coupled nucleotide-excision repair of the lactose operon in *Escherichia coli*. Proc. Natl. Acad. Sci. USA 93: 1292–1297.

MILLER, J. H., and M. MICHAELS, 1996 Finding new mutator strains of *Escherichia coli*—a review. Gene 179: 129–132.

MODRICH, P., and R. LAHUE, 1996 Mismatch repair in replication fidelity, genetic recombination, and cancer biology. Annu. Rev. Biochem. 65: 101–133.

NYSTROM LAHTI, M., R. PARSONS, P. SISTONEN, L. PYLKKANEN, L. A. AALTONEN et al., 1994 Mismatch repair genes on chromosomes 2p and 3p account for a major share of hereditary nonpolyposis colorectal cancer families evaluable by linkage. Am. J. Hum. Genet. 55: 659–665.

PARSONS, R., G. M. LI, M. J. LONGLEY, W. H. FANG, N. PAPADOPOULOS et al., 1996 Hypermutability and mismatch repair deficiency in RER+ tumor cells. Cell 75: 1227–1236.

RAYSSIGUIER, C., D. S. THALER and M. RADMAN, 1989 The barrier to recombination between *Escherichia coli* and *Salmonella typhimurium* is disrupted in mismatch-repair mutants. Nature 342: 396–401.

SCHAAPER, R. M., 1993 Base selection, proofreading, and mismatch repair during DNA replication in *Escherichia coli*. J. Biol. Chem. 268: 23762–23765.

SCHAAPER, R. M., and M. RADMAN, 1989 The extreme mutator effect of *Escherichia coli* mutD5 results from saturation of mismatch repair by excessive DNA replication errors. EMBO J. 8: 3511–3516.

SCHEUERMANN, R., and H. ECHOLS, 1984 A separate editing exonuclease for DNA replication: the ε subunit of *Escherichia coli* DNA polymerase III holoenzyme. Proc. Natl. Acad. Sci. USA 81: 7747–7751.

SIEGEL, E. C., and V. BRYSON, 1964 Selection of resistant strains of *Escherichia coli* by antibiotics and antibacterial agents: role of normal and mutator strains. Antimicrob. Agents Chemother. 1963: 629–634.

SIEGEL, E. C., and V. BRYSON, 1967 Mutator gene of *Escherichia coli* B. J. Bacteriol. 94: 38–47.

SIGNER, E. R., and J. R. BECKWITH, 1966 Transposition of the Lac region of *Escherichia coli* III. The mechanism of attachment of bacteriophage φ80 to the bacterial chromosome. J. Mol. Biol. 22: 33–51.

SPEYER, J. F., 1965 Mutagenic DNA polymerase. Biochem. Biophys. Res. Commun. 21: 6–8.

STRAND, M., T. A. PROLLA, R. M. LISKAY and T. D. PETES, 1993 Destabilization of tracts of simple repetitive DNA in yeast by mutations affecting DNA mismatch repair [published erratum appears in Nature 368: 569, 1994]. Nature 365: 274–276.

SUEOKA, N., 1962 On the genetic basis of variation and heterogeneity of DNA base composition. Proc. Natl. Acad. Sci. USA 48: 582–592.

TOMLINSON, I. P., M. R. NOVELLI and W. F. BODMER, 1996 The mutation rate and cancer. Proc. Natl. Acad. Sci. USA 93: 14800–14803.

TREFFERS, H. P., V. SPINELLI and N. O. BELSER, 1954 A factor (or mutator gene) influencing mutation rates in *Escherichia coli*. Proc. Natl. Acad. Sci. USA 40: 1064–1071.

YANOFSKY, C., E. C. COX and V. HORN, 1966 The unusual mutagenic specificity of an *E. coli* mutator gene. Proc. Natl. Acad. Sci. USA 55: 274–281.

Recombination and Population Structure in *Escherichia coli*

Roger Milkman

Department of Biological Sciences, The University of Iowa, Iowa City, Iowa 52242

A major focus of population genetics, and now of molecular evolution, is the study of gene lineages. Population genetic parameters usually apply to small chromosomal regions rather than to the genome as a whole, although genes do not always descend independently of their surroundings. The genome of *Escherichia coli* strikes me as an unusually favorable theater in which to observe the lineages of genes and their relationships with the evolutionary processes that operate at the population level.

I should like to trace the developing understanding of *E. coli*'s population genetics in terms of the coexistence of clonality and recombination, the recognition of restriction as important to recombination, and the emerging features of its genomic structure.

When ATWOOD, SCHNEIDER and RYAN (1951) set out to describe *E. coli* population structure, they explicitly excluded recombination, assuming *E. coli* to be a "nonsexual" species, at least outside of the lab. This simplifying assumption laid the groundwork for a clonal selection model, in which a rare, broadly favorable mutation led its entire (haploid) genome to prominence: since linkage was absolute, the entire genome hitchhiked to a high frequency as the new allele responded to selection. This *periodic selection model,* based on a series of experiments with asexual laboratory populations, contradicted my naive view of *E. coli* as having ordinary (read "Drosophila") population genetics but unburdened by diploidy, when I proposed *E. coli* as an organism with which to test the neutral hypothesis of electrophoretic variation in proteins (MILKMAN 1972, 1975; see also MILKMAN 1985). I was not convinced that the model applied to natural populations, but ATWOOD and many others (BRUCE LEVIN and ALLAN WILSON, personal communications; KOCH 1974; KUBITSCHEK 1974) felt that recombination in natural populations of *E. coli* was negligible in this context. Clonality and the frequency of recombination thus became the crucial issues. Addressing these issues and their evolutionary significance required a good look at *E. coli* from nature, and this proved more fruitful than the intended test of neutrality.

With five enzyme loci and a collection of 829 newly isolated strains of diverse natural origins, I found far less allelic electrophoretic variation than the panmictic model predicted, and inferred that the electromorphs were not neutral (MILKMAN 1973, 1975). In a study of 20 electrophoretically variable loci in some 100 of these strains and a few others, however, there were four cases of identical pairs (highly improbable by chance alone!), which clearly argued for a clonal structure of the species (SELANDER and LEVIN 1980; LEVIN 1981). My neutrality test was invalid, and neutral variation was soon addressed and abundantly demonstrated in DNA and elsewhere (MILKMAN 1985; MAYNARD SMITH 1996). Meanwhile, further support for a basic clonal structure of *E. coli* followed from comparative sequencing in the *tryptophan* (*trp*) operon, where 1-kilobase (kb) sequences from K12 (the geneticists' lab strain) and 12 of our new strains, which had diverse enzyme mobility and thermostability at other loci, were classified as follows: three were identical to K12, five were different from K12 by one nucleotide (each unique), three differed from K12 by the same set of 10 nucleotides, and one differed by 44 (MILKMAN and CRAWFORD 1983). But HARTL and DYKHUIZEN (1984) were quick to conjecture, "Conceivably, each small region of the chromosome in a group of strains could have a unique phylogeny, reflecting identity by descent, but the phylogeny might differ according to the region examined." This mosaic structure would be due, of course to recombination in the past, but at a level not remotely approaching that in a panmictic species like *Drosophila melanogaster*. In a panmictic species, individuals undergo random mating and recombination every generation.

Confirmation of the importance of recombination in nature followed in 1986, when DYKHUIZEN and GREEN (1986, 1991) sequenced 770 nucleotides in the *gnd* (6-phosphogluconate dehydrogenase) gene in nine of the 13 strains referred to above, plus the LT strain of *Salmonella typhimurium* (now part of *S. enterica*). The *gnd* gene was already known to be unusually variable (MILKMAN 1973; SELANDER and LEVIN 1980). The sequences were indeed highly varied: some strains that were identical in *trp* were as different from one another as they were from *S. typhimurium* LT. But the striking feature was a tree entirely different from the *trp* tree. A regional mosaic of phylogenies within the genome must reflect recombination in the recent history of *E. coli*, specifically after the formation of the existing group of clones. A small, excited group met to discuss the implied genomic structure. What should we call the segments? DAN HARTL suggested isoancestral segments, which persisted until the shorter (not necessarily better) clonal segments (MILKMAN and STOLTZFUS 1988). Clearly, it was time to begin a systematic comparative molecular analysis of the *E. coli* chromosome. This would benefit greatly from the recent establishment of the ECOR (*E. coli* Reference) collection of 72 strains of diverse natural origin by OCHMAN and SELANDER (1984).

First, a comparison of restriction patterns in a large number of ECOR strains in 15 different sets of 1.5-kb PCR fragments showed a regional mosaic of similarities among strains (MILKMAN and McKANE BRIDGES 1990). Nevertheless, certain groupings were prominent, suggesting that while some of the clonal segments were (remnants of) recombinational replacements, others were directly descended from the most recent ancestor of the clone. These were now called part of the clonal frames. Nine of the sets of PCR fragments were contiguous in and near the *trp* operon [28 min (BERLYN *et al.* 1996)], and the rest were scattered on both sides, leaving about half the chromosome (46 to 93 min) unsurveyed at that time.

The extensive multilocus enzyme electrophoresis (MLEE) studies of the 1980s (CAUGANT *et al.* 1981; WHITTAM *et al.* 1983) were of immense value in documenting extensive genetic variation and providing a basis for a tree-like phenogram defining similarity-based groupings among the ECOR strains (SELANDER *et al.* 1987; HERZER *et al.* 1990) as well as other strains, especially pathogens (SELANDER *et al.* 1996; WHITTAM 1996). The phenogram compiles degrees of difference but does not (in contrast to a true phylogenetic tree) imply genome-wide uniformity of relationships. (see also AVISE 1989.) The resolution of differences at a given locus by enzyme electrophoresis was lower than that indicated by restriction fragment length polymorphism (RFLP), but the effort required was far less for MLEE than for the five to eight digests of PCR fragments. Until more recently, the map locations of many of the enzyme loci were not known.

The restriction survey led to comparative sequencing of K12 and 36 ECOR strains, first for 4.4 kb in the *trp* operon (MILKMAN and McKANE BRIDGES 1993), and eventually for a total of 12.7 kb (MILKMAN and McKANE 1995; Figure 4 in MILKMAN 1996). The sequence comparisons now revealed discontinuities on a small scale: numerous clonal segments were on the order of 1 kb in length. Interestingly, despite the mosaic similarity patterns, the grouping that emerged from the sequenc-

ing closely parallels that of the overall MLEE phenogram of the ECOR strains; this confirms the prominence of DNA descended from common clonal ancestors, the clonal frames. Nevertheless, distinct highly localized phylogenies were obvious. These two patterns are easily reconciled by envisioning the descent of a chromosome in a growing clone. The DNA inherited from the clonal ancestor initially is the clonal frame. Initially, the frame is 100% of the genome, but individual genomes are punctuated progressively by small discrete recombinant replacements from outside the clone. These segments, which often appear in numerous related strains, are inferred to be related by descent and in this sense can still be called clonal segments, too. After some time, as the present situation reflects, the cells descended from an original clonal ancestor—a clonal Eve—still share possession of a large proportion of the ancestral DNA, but these residual clonal frames differ from one another in extent. It now made sense to refer to these descendants, not as a true (genomically uniform) clone, but as a meroclone—a "partial clone" (MILKMAN and McKANE 1995; MILKMAN 1996, 1997). While we are unlikely to calculate back to the time that Eve Coli lived (unless rRNA will serve), we can in principle use the fragmentary clonal frames, each shared by some high proportion of the meroclone, to envision the most recent common ancestor of each meroclone. Clearly, this situation is different from that in sexual eukaryotes.

The three major groups of ECOR strains that emerged from MLEE studies reflected sets of specific correlated alleles at a large number of loci—that is, alleles in linkage disequilibrium. And alleles that follow the overall correlation pattern must be part of the respective clonal frames of the major groups. Similarly, agreement between local restriction site patterns or sequence patterns on one hand and the overall MLEE grouping on the other identifies them with the clonal frames. Disagreements reveal the extent of exogenous clonal segments, which may locally exceed in extent the segments of the clonal frame.

Meanwhile, LEVIN (1986) had presented theoretical and experimental evidence supporting the possibility that bacteriophages in natural populations might impose frequency-dependent selection on *E. coli* favoring rare restriction-modification types, and that this could help maintain clonal diversity. Further, PRICE and BICKLE (1986) proposed that "DNA restriction and modification systems serve to accelerate evolution by stimulating recombination . . . essentially by cleaving the incoming DNA and providing double-stranded DNA ends that are highly recombinogenic." This view, foreshadowed or shared by others (BOYER 1964; PITTARD 1964; ARBER 1965; ARBER and MORSE 1965; DUBOSE *et al.* 1988), led to an interest in reconciling the mosaic patterns (particularly those seen in sequence comparisons) with recombinational events, and possibly restriction. The extensive degree of polymorphism at the *hsd* restriction-modification locus has been documented in detail by MURRAY's group (DANIEL *et al.* 1988; SHARP *et al.* 1992; BARCUS and MURRAY 1995; BARCUS *et al.* 1995).

We began with the analysis of phage P1 transductants from ECOR 47 into a K12 *trp*A strain, in order to see the extent to which the DNA entering the recipient cell was incorporated into its chromosome (McKANE and MILKMAN 1995). P1 transducing particles contain about 80 kb of donor DNA, and we anticipated that after entry into the cell this DNA might be cut by restriction endonucleases and (before or after cutting) shortened by exonucleases. Discrimination between donor and recipient DNA is possible at high resolution because, for example, ECOR 47 and K12 sequences differ by several percent of their nucleotides. With primers for a string of contiguous 1.5-kb PCR fragments (often distinguishable between ECOR 47 and K12 by several restriction sites with a single enzyme), we found donor fragment sizes averaging about 9 kb (much smaller than 80 kb, and much larger than the 1-kb size range of the observed clonal segments). And seven of the 18 transductants had more than one donor fragment. Was this due to restriction? JOHN ROTH (personal communication) had suggested following this cross with a backcross to the K12 recipient on the grounds that, aside from the ECOR 47 DNA in the *trp* region, the transductants would be identical to K12, notably in restriction-modification properties. (For the same reason that bacteria don't cut up their own chromosomes, crosses within a given strain, or between strains with identical R-M systems, are not subject to restriction.) Indeed, the results of two backcrosses, involving a transductant with a 25- or a 20-kb fragment of donor DNA, were dramatically different from those of the original cross: in the two sets of 15 backtransductants, 28 were identical to the donor transductant, and two were shortened but not split. This experimental paradigm has been followed frequently in subsequent transduction and conjugation experiments, always with comparable results. LISE RALEIGH (1987; KELLEHER and RALEIGH 1994) also deleted the known restriction genes from our K12 strain; as a recipient, this version fragmented and shortened the donor DNA far less than ordinary K12 (MILKMAN 1997). And to address the possibility that DNA mismatch plays a major role in the patterns (note that the mismatch is far more extensive in the initial cross than in the backcross), reciprocal conjugations between ECOR 47 and K12 (whose extent of mismatch would be identical) were found to be quite disparate.

Last summer in Woods Hole, I learned from ED ADELBERG that a postdoc in his lab, HERBERT BOYER (1964), had done some backcrosses, too. BOYER wanted to transfer arabinose genes from *E. coli* B into K12; efforts to introduce the K12 Hfr conjugation system into B worked poorly. BOYER wondered whether bacteria might restrict bacterial DNA the way they did viral DNA. His backcross results were superficially similar to ours in that the restriction effects were overcome, and further crosses were successful—for a different reason. K12 Hfr × B progeny were crossed back to the K12 Hfr donor, and it turned out that in some of the initial progeny the K12 restriction-modification genes had been transferred to B. BOYER correctly localized the R-M genes to near the threonine locus, concluded that strain B could be made in this way to behave like K12, and explained the observations in terms of restriction and modification. Finally, in interrupted mating experiments, few markers were successfully transferred until 30 minutes had passed, after which time the linkage of the markers was greatly reduced from normal. He concluded that short pieces of DNA would be digested completely by exonucleases, but longer pieces overloaded the system, and some of them lasted long enough to be incorporated into the recipient chromosome. They had usually been cut into pieces by restriction endonucleases, however, and linkage was therefore reduced. Restriction polymorphism and its role in recombination had to be rediscovered when population genetics arrived in *E. coli*, and, how does that go? Phylogeny recapitulated ontogeny.

In *E. coli* the male sex factors can be carried on a free ("F") plasmid, in which case only they are transmitted in conjugation. But if the plasmid is integrated into the chromosome, the origin of transfer splits the male factors, so that some of them lead a chromosomal strand into the recipient cell, resulting in the high-frequency recombination of chromosomal genes for which the Hfr strains are named.

Chromosomal recombination in *E. coli* (FIRTH *et al.* 1996; LOW 1996; MASTERS 1996; WEISBERG 1996) can be seen as an (actually very infrequent!) two-step process. In transduction or Hfr conjugation, a donor cell (1) transmits a stretch of DNA to one or more recipient cells, after which (2) some of the DNA is incorporated into the recipient chromosome. Its size is influenced by more than the mode of transmission (transduction or conjugation); once it enters the recipient cell, it is subject to the action of restriction endonucleases, which are highly polymorphic in the species, as well as exonuclease activity. This often results in a set of small DNA fragments, which can be incorporated independently into one of one-to-several incipient chromosomes, since chromosome replication is continuous in the life of a growing bacterial cell. This permits the segregation of a small variety of recombinants, whose replacements may often be small enough to avoid containing the grab-bag of changes that might be brought in by a large stretch of DNA. After any phenotypic lag, the new recombinants are promptly exposed to natural selection. Conjugative plasmids are transmitted and are either propagated as free plasmids or, with a very wide range of probabilities, integrated into the chromosome.

Nonconjugative plasmids may be transmitted by transformation (HANAHAN and BLOOM 1996) and integrated or not.

Our reciprocal conjugations and other crosses became possible after PETER KUEMPEL provided us with an F plasmid that contains the Broca 7 (LOW 1996) Hfr origin of transfer and establishes a dynamic equilibrium between free and integrated states (the latter always at the Broca 7 region near 31 min). This plasmid has been useful in several ways: it can be conjugated into various natural isolates (*e.g.*, ECOR strains) and laboratory marker strains, converting them to Hfrs. Indeed, some cells may carry, and transmit, both an integrated origin of transfer with a long stretch of chromosome and also a free plasmid with no chromosomal genes but all the male factors. In such a case, some transconjugants are ready (after integration) to act as Hfrs in a subsequent cross (HEINEMANN *et al.* 1996; ANKENBAUER 1997). Because of the dynamic equilibrium, these Hfrs produce fewer transconjugants than the standard fixed Hfr strains, but relatively few are needed for the intensive analysis of closely linked PCR fragments.

At this point it might appear that the periodic selection model of *E. coli* population structure and dynamics needs only a little random recombinational speckling, spread uniformly over the originally clonal genomes, but this is not entirely true. There are in fact two dramatic exceptions, and they reflect the localized interplay of powerful frequency-dependent selection, recombination, and random genetic drift. PETER REEVES and co-workers (BASTIN *et al.* 1993; REEVES 1993; LIU and REEVES 1994; LAN and REEVES 1996; STEVENSON *et al.* 1996) have described and analyzed the molecular genetics of the polymorphic O antigen, a complex lipopolysaccharide, in Salmonella and in *E. coli*. There are literally hundreds of different O antigens, each determined by a set of sugar synthases and transferases, whose genes have been assembled in a small region of the chromosome. The sets of such genes are not entirely homologous: the antigenic variation results, not from amino acid substitutions, or small deletions/insertions, but from the acquisition of novel genes, evidently by lateral transfer. Apparently the hosts recognize the bacterial O antigens and exercise some restraint over the growth of the cells bearing them. A novel antigen would then have a powerful advantage—as long as it is in very low frequency. Presumably this initial advantage is repeated as each new serotype colonizes host after host, in place after place. Eventually the frequency in the species rises to the level where the O antigen complex is essentially neutral, but new imports evidently continue to arrive and spread.

The pertinent interaction of random genetic drift and powerful, frequency-dependent selection occurs at the first appearance in a species or a population of a novel recombinant. Perhaps the most interesting absolute allele frequency is 1, because a mere ordinary selective advantage does not improve the probability of persistence of a single allele very much. For natural selection to gain the upper hand over drift, the probability in haploids may be about equal to the value of the selection coefficient (difference in fitness) s. If $s = 0.0001$, then this probability may be about 0.0002. [The interpretation of s is not the same as for classical diploid organisms, and the growth and multiplication dynamics of *E. coli* are not clearly isomorphic with a process characterized by random mating and a Poisson distribution of progeny number, upon which the calculation is based (CROW and KIMURA 1970, pp. 425–426).] Thus, short of drug resistance genes, there are very few individual recombinational replacements that have a good chance of becoming established. New O antigen gene complexes seem to have what it takes. In addition, the "JUMPstart" sequences in the O antigen gene complex (HOBBS and REEVES 1994) may increase the probability of the incorporation of foreign DNA there, synergizing with the subsequent action of natural selection.

In any region, the frequency of effective recombinational replacement, including horizontal transfer from phylogenetically distant (but presumably physically close) sources, is the product of the frequency of all replacement times its probability of persisting. Thus, the O antigen gene complex near 45 min may be one of the few regions of the genome that can capitalize on horizontal transfer effectively enough to demonstrate via polymorphism that it occurs at evolutionarily potentially important rates. Halfway around the chromosome, at 98 min, a region containing several restriction loci, including the highly polymorphic *hsd* restriction-modification complex, is the only presently known region with the same property. In both cases, nonhomologous replacements are flanked by regions of unusually high homologous variation stretching a few minutes on each side. The existence of these hypervariable regions (one of which is *gnd*) seems to be due to the occasional importation of valuable novelties in small packages and their redistribution among various strains by the usual processes of transduction and conjugation, by which more extensive, essentially neutral, homologous-but-not-identical substitutions flank the critical novelty (SELANDER *et al.* 1996). For a much broader set of historical inferences of horizontal transfer, not specifying frequency-dependent selection, see LAWRENCE and ROTH (1996) and LAWRENCE and OCHMAN (1997).

The present version of the periodic selection model of *E. coli* population structure/dynamics goes as follows: rare, broadly favorable mutations (*motivating alleles*) occur that carry their respective genomes to high frequencies in the species—these events are called *clonal sweeps,* or *selective sweeps,* a term applied to chromosomal regions in Drosophila and elsewhere as well. No genetic variability is present in a newborn clone. The clones do not reach fixation, owing either to environmental heterogeneity or to the acquisition of one another's motivating alleles. The new clones gradually become randomly speckled with recombinational replacements from other clones. They are thus no longer clones (the genome does not have a single phylogeny applicable uniformly over its entire length), yet they share a high proportion of their common ancestral DNA (*clonal frames*), so they can be called meroclones (*partial clones*).

Finally, the two hypervariable regions resist the clonal sweep by virtue of their novel antigens or restriction systems, which confer their own great advantages, but which lose their advantages as they rise in frequency, so that they themselves can never function as motivating alleles. The two regions are *bastions of polymorphism.*

Now the recent completion of the *E. coli* K12 MG1655 genome sequence (BLATTNER *et al.* 1997) has brought three great benefits to studies of genomic function and variation in the species. For one thing, all the DNA in this strain has been described as an ordered set of sequences presently or potentially described further in terms of functionally specific and other properties such as GC content and Codon Adaptation Index (SHARP and LI 1986). These constitute the complete set of genetic factors responsible, together with its epigenetic history, for the form and function of the organism. Second, in addition to intragenomic comparisons to reveal paralogy, genes may be compared with genes, and genomes with genomes, from other *E. coli* isolates and from other species. And finally, the genome sequence, determined with a high standard of care, is a reference by which to verify individually collected sequences, whose error frequency is presumably greater. Comparisons with genome-standard sequences can often reveal disparities that do not follow the pattern of evolutionary divergence and can thus be retested.

The population structure of *E. coli* also expresses a genomic character. Local sequence variation among the ECOR strains is an example: the tightest group of 10 ECOR strains, plus K12, show no or essentially no RFLP variation over most parts of the genome; but near the two bastions of polymorphism, variation is high and declines with distance (minutes). Thus, one can screen the entire genome for local discontinuities of this type. In *E. coli*, clonal sweeps are major events, and bastions of polymorphism are major structures—not something to be discovered by chance, but inescapable features of the species genome.

LITERATURE CITED

ANKENBAUER, R. G., 1997 Reassessing forty years of genetics doctrine: retrotransfer and conjugation. Genetics **145:** 543–549.

ARBER, W., 1965 Host-controlled modification of bacteriophage. Annu. Rev. Microbiol. **19:** 365–378.

ARBER, W., and M. L. MORSE, 1965 Host specificity of DNA produced by *Escherichia coli.* VI. Effects on bacterial conjugation. Genetics **51:** 137–148.

ATWOOD, K. C., L. K. SCHNEIDER and F. J. RYAN, 1951 Selective mechanisms in bacteria. Cold Spring Harbor Symp. Quant. Biol. **16:** 345–355.

AVISE, J., 1989 Gene trees and organismal histories: a phylogenetic approach to population biology. Evolution **43:** 1192–1208.

BARCUS, V. A., and N. E. MURRAY, 1995 Barriers to recombination: restriction, pp. 31–58 in *Population Genetics of Bacteria,* edited by R. BISHOP. Cambridge University Press, Cambridge, UK.

BARCUS, V. A., J. B. TITHERADGE and N. E. MURRAY, 1995 The diversity of alleles at the *hsd* locus in natural populations of *Escherichia coli.* Genetics **140:** 1187–1197.

BASTIN, D. A., G. STEVENSON, P. K. BROWN, A. HAASE and P. R. REEVES, 1993 Repeat unit polysaccharides of bacteria: a model for polymerization resembling that of ribosomes and fatty acid synthetase, with a novel mechanism for determining chain length. Mol. Microbiol. **7:** 725–734.

BERLYN, M. K. B., K. B. LOW, K. E. RUDD, and M. SINGER, 1996 Linkage map of *Escherichia coli* K12, edition 9, pp. 1715–1902 in *Escherichia coli and Salmonella Cellular and Molecular Biology,* edited by F. C. NEIDHARDT. American Society for Microbiology, Washington, D.C.

BLATTNER, F., G. PLUNKETT III, C. BLOCH, N. T. PERNA, M. RILEY *et al.,* 1997 The complete genome sequence of *Escherichia coli.* Science (in press).

BOYER, H., 1964 Genetic control of restriction and modification in *Escherichia coli.* J. Bacteriol. **88:** 1652–1660.

CAUGANT, D., B. R. LEVIN and R. K. SELANDER, 1981 Genetic diversity and temporal variation in the *E. coli* population of a human host. Genetics **98:** 467–490.

CROW, J. F., and M. KIMURA, 1970 *An Introduction to Population Genetics Theory.* Harper and Row, New York.

DANIEL, A. S., F. V. FULLER-PACE, D. M. LEGGE and N. E. MURRAY, 1988 Distribution and diversity of *hsd* genes in *E. coli* and other enteric bacteria. J. Bacteriol. **170:** 1775–1782.

DUBOSE, R. F., D. E. DYKHUIZEN and D. L. HARTL, 1988 Genetic exchange among natural isolates of bacteria: recombination within the *phoA* gene of *Escherichia coli.* Proc. Natl. Acad. Sci. USA **85:** 7036–7040.

DYKHUIZEN, D. E., and L. GREEN, 1986 DNA sequence variation, DNA phylogeny, and recombination. Genetics **113:** s71.

DYKHUIZEN, D. E., and L. GREEN, 1991 Recombination in *Escherichia coli* and the definition of biological species. J. Bacteriol. **173:** 7257–7268.

FIRTH, N., K. IPPEN-IHLER and R. A. SKURRAY, 1996 Structure and function of the F factor and mechanism of conjugation, pp. 2377–2401 in *Escherichia coli and Salmonella Cellular and Molecular Biology,* edited by F. C. NEIDHARDT. American Society for Microbiology, Washington, D.C.

HANAHAN, D., and F. R. BLOOM, 1996 Mechanisms of DNA transformation, pp. 2449–2459 in *Escherichia coli and Salmonella Cellular and Molecular Biology,* edited by F. C. NEIDHARDT. American Society for Microbiology, Washington, D.C.

HARTL, D. L., and D. DYKHUIZEN, 1984 The population genetics of *Escherichia coli.* Annu. Rev. Genet. **18:** 31–68.

HEINEMANN, J. A., H. E. SCOTT and M. WILLIAMS, 1996 Doing the conjugative two-step: evidence of recipient autonomy in retrotransfer. Genetics **143:** 1425–1435.

HERZER, P. J., S. INOUYE, M. INOUYE and T. WHITTAM, 1990 Phylogenetic distribution of branched RNA-linked multicopy single-stranded DNA among natural isolates of *Escherichia coli.* J. Bacteriol. **172:** 6175–6181.

HOBBS, M., and P. R. REEVES, 1994 The JUMPstart sequence: a 39 bp element common to several polysaccharide gene clusters. Mol. Microbiol. **12:** 855–856.

KELLEHER, J. E., and E. A. RALEIGH, 1994 Response to UV damage by four *Escherichia coli* K-12 restriction systems. J. Bacteriol. **176:** 5888–5896.

KOCH, A. L., 1974 The pertinence of the periodic selection phenomenon to prokaryotic evolution. Genetics **77:** 127–142.

KUBITSCHEK, H. E., 1974 Operation of selection pressure on microbial populations, pp. 105–130 in *Evolution in the Microbial World,* edited by M. J. CARLILE and J. J. SKEHEL. Cambridge University Press, Cambridge.

LAN, R., and P. R. REEVES, 1996 Gene transfer is a major factor in bacterial evolution. Mol. Biol. Evol. **13:** 47–55.

LAWRENCE, J. G., and H. OCHMAN, 1997 Amelioration of bacterial genomes: rates of change and exchange. J. Mol. Evol. **44:** 383–397.

LAWRENCE, J. G., and J. R. ROTH, 1996 Selfish operons: horizontal transfer may drive the evolution of gene clusters. Genetics **143:** 1843–1860.

LEVIN, B. R., 1981 Periodic selection, infectious gene exchange, and the genetic structure of *E. coli* populations. Genetics **99:** 1–23.

LEVIN, B. R., 1986 Restriction-modification immunity and the maintenance of genetic diversity in bacterial populations, pp. 669–688 in *Evolutionary Processes and Theory*, edited by S. KARLIN and E. NEVO. Academic Press, New York.

LIU, D., and P. R. REEVES, 1994 Presence of different O antigen forms in three isolates of one clone of *Escherichia coli*. Genetics **138:** 6–10.

LOW, K. B., 1996 Hfr strains of *Escherichia coli* K-12, pp. 2402–2405 in *Escherichia coli and Salmonella Cellular and Molecular Biology*, edited by F. C. NEIDHARDT. American Society for Microbiology, Washington, D.C.

MASTERS, M., 1996 Generalized transduction, pp. 2421–2441 in *Escherichia coli and Salmonella Cellular and Molecular Biology*, edited by F. C. NEIDHARDT. American Society for Microbiology, Washington, D.C.

MAYNARD SMITH, J. 1996 Population genetics: an introduction, pp. 2685–2690 in *Escherichia coli and Salmonella Cellular and Molecular Biology*, edited by F. C. NEIDHARDT. American Society for Microbiology, Washington, D.C.

MCKANE, M., and R. MILKMAN, 1995 Transduction, restriction and recombination patterns in *Escherichia coli*. Genetics **139:** 35–43.

MILKMAN, R., 1972 How much room is left for Non-Darwinian evolution? pp. 217–229 in *Evolution of Genetic Systems*, edited by H. H. SMITH. Gordon and Breach, New York.

MILKMAN, R., 1973 Electrophoretic variation in *Escherichia coli* from natural sources. Science **182:** 1024–1026.

MILKMAN, R., 1975 Allozyme variation in *E. coli* of diverse natural origins, pp. 273–285 in *Isozymes. IV. Genetics and Evolution*, edited by C. L. MARKERT. Academic Press, New York.

MILKMAN, R., 1985 Two elements of a unified theory of population genetics and molecular evolution, pp. 65–83 in *Population Genetics and Molecular Evolution*, edited by T. OHTA and K. AOKI. Japan Scientific Societies Press, Tokyo.

MILKMAN, R., 1996 Recombinational exchange among clonal populations, pp. 2663–2684 in *Escherichia coli and Salmonella Cellular and Molecular Biology*, edited by F. C. NEIDHARDT. American Society for Microbiology, Washington, D.C.

MILKMAN, R., 1997 Recombination and sequence variation in *E. coli*, pp. 177–189 in *Ecology of Pathogenic Bacteria, Molecular and Evolutionary Aspects*, edited by B. A. M. VAN DER ZEIJST, W. P. M. HOEKSTRA, J. D. A. VAN EMBDEN and A. J. W. VAN ALPHEN. North-Holland, Amsterdam.

MILKMAN, R., and I. P. CRAWFORD, 1983 Clustered third-base substitutions among wild strains of *Escherichia coli*. Science **221:** 378–380.

MILKMAN, R., and M. MCKANE, 1995 DNA sequence variation and recombination in *E. coli*, pp. 127–142 in *Population Genetics of Bacteria*, edited by S. BAUMBERG, J. P. W. YOUNG, E. M. H. WELLINGTON and J. R. SAUNDERS. Cambridge University Press, Cambridge, UK.

MILKMAN, R., and M. MCKANE BRIDGES, 1990 Molecular evolution of the *E. coli* chromosome. III. Clonal frames. Genetics **126:** 505–517.

MILKMAN, R., and M. MCKANE BRIDGES, 1993 Molecular evolution of the *E. coli* chromosome. IV. Sequence comparisons. Genetics **133:** 455–468.

MILKMAN, R., and A. STOLTZFUS, 1988 Molecular evolution of the *Escherichia coli* chromosome. II. Clonal segments. Genetics **120:** 359–366.

OCHMAN, H., and R. K. SELANDER, 1984 Standard reference strains of *E. coli* from natural populations. J. Bacteriol. **157:** 690–693.

PITTARD, J., 1964 Effect of phage-controlled restriction on genetic linkage in bacterial crosses. J. Bacteriol. **87:** 1256–1257.

PRICE, C., and T. A. BICKLE, 1986 A possible role for DNA restriction in bacterial evolution. Microbiol. Sci. **3:** 296–299.

RALEIGH, E., 1987 Restriction and modification *in vivo* by *E. coli* K12. Methods Enzymol. **152:** 130141.

REEVES, P., 1993 Evolution of Salmonella O antigen variation by interspecific gene transfer on a large scale. Trends Genet. **9:** 17–22.

SELANDER, R. K., and B. R. LEVIN, 1980 Genetic diversity and structure in *Escherichia coli* populations. Science **210:** 545–547.

SELANDER, R. K., D. A. CAUGANT and T. S. WHITTAM, 1987 Genetic structure and variation in natural populations of *Escherichia coli*, pp. 1625–1648 in *Escherichia coli and Salmonella typhimurium Cellular and Molecular Biology*, edited by F. C. NEIDHARDT. American Society for Microbiology, Washington, D.C.

SELANDER, R. K., J. LI and K. NELSON, 1996 Evolutionary genetics of *Salmonella enterica*, pp. 2691–2707 in *Escherichia coli and Salmonella Cellular and Molecular Biology*, edited by F. C. NEIDHARDT. American Society for Microbiology, Washington, D.C.

SHARP, P., and W.-H. LI, 1986 An evolutionary perspective on synonymous codon usage in unicellular organisms. J. Mol. Evol. **24:** 28–38.

SHARP, P., J. E. KELLEHER, A. S. DANIEL, G. M. COWAN and N. E. MURRAY, 1992 Roles of selection and recombination in the evolution of type I restriction-modification systems in enterobacteria. Proc. Natl. Acad. Sci. USA **89:** 9836–9840.

STEVENSON, G., K. ANDRIANOPOULOS, M. W. HOBBS and P. R. REEVES, 1996 Organization of the *Escherichia coli* K12 gene cluster responsible for the extracellular polysaccharide colanic acid. J. Bacteriol. **178:** 4885–4893.

WEISBERG, R. A., 1996 Specialized transduction, pp. 2442–2448 in *Escherichia coli and Salmonella Cellular and Molecular Biology*, edited by F. C. NEIDHARDT. American Society for Microbiology, Washington, D.C.

WHITTAM, T. S., 1996 Genetic variation and evolutionary processes in natural populations of ESCHERICHIA COLI, pp. 2708–2720 in *Escherichia coli and Salmonella Cellular and Molecular Biology*, edited by F. C. NEIDHARDT. American Society for Microbiology, Washington, D.C.

WHITTAM, T. S., H. OCHMAN and R. K. SELANDER, 1983 Multilocus genetic structure in natural populations of *Escherichia coli*. Proc. Natl. Acad. Sci. USA **80:** 1751–1755.

See also page 705 in Addenda et Corrigenda.

The Value of Basic Research
Discovery of *Thermus aquaticus* and Other Extreme Thermophiles

○　　　　　　　　　　　　　　　　　　　　　　　○

Thomas D. Brock

E. B. Fred Professor of Natural Sciences Emeritus, Department of Bacteriology, University of Wisconsin–Madison, Madison, Wisconsin 53706

POLYMERASE chain reaction (PCR), the revolutionary technique for DNA research, depends on Taq polymerase, an enzyme from *Thermus aquaticus,* an organism that I first isolated from a hot spring in Yellowstone National Park. The PCR technique is so important that Hoffmann-LaRoche, the giant Swiss pharmaceutical company, paid more than $300 million to acquire world rights for this procedure. Essentially, Hoffmann-LaRoche was acquiring the rights to two patents, those of GELFAND *et al.* (1989) on Taq polymerase and of MULLIS *et al.* (1990) on the PCR technique.

The importance of Taq polymerase was recognized by the White House in 1991. D. ALLAN BROMLEY, the Director of the Office of Science and Technology Policy and the President's chief science advisor, testified before the House of Representatives:

> Different kinds of research and development tend to have different kinds of returns. With basic research—the majority of which is done by individual scientists and small groups of scientists at universities—it is very difficult to predict when, where, and to whom the returns will eventually accrue. Yet even work that can seem highly abstract can have surprisingly immediate impacts. To take just one example, in 1968 Thomas Brock, a microbiologist at the University of Wisconsin, discovered a form of bacteria in the thermal vents of Yellowstone that can survive at very high temperature. From these bacteria an enzyme was extracted that is stable at near-boiling temperatures. Nearly two decades later this enzyme proved to be vital in the process known as the polymerase chain reaction, which is used to duplicate specific pieces of DNA. Today, PCR is the basis of a multimillion dollar business with applications ranging from the rapid diagnosis of disease to forensic medicine.[1]

In 1989 *Science* magazine (December 22, 1989 issue) established a new award called "The Molecule of the Year" award. Taq polymerase from *T. aquaticus* was designated the first awardee.

Discovery of *T. aquaticus*: I began my scientific career in 1951 as a microbial physiologist and did extensive work in molecular biology and microbial genetics through the mid-1960s. Although I found this work satisfying, I had always been interested in the outdoors. In 1963 my professional circumstances were such that I could branch out into new areas of research. It was at this time that I initiated what was to become a long-term research program in microbial ecology.[2] My ecological work focused on the study of microorganisms directly in their natural environments. I worked on a variety of habitats, including marine intertidal pools, freshwater lakes, and soils, but for 10 years I concentrated my research on hot springs and geysers, which I viewed as model systems for basic research in microbial ecology.

My discovery of *T. aquaticus* and other high-temperature bacteria could not have been made without studies directly in the natural environment in Yellowstone National Park. At the time I began this work, thermophilic bacteria were thought to have temperature optima of only 55°, and the upper temperature for life was stated as 73° (KEMPNER 1963). However, I was not initially interested in defining the upper temperature limits of life. My first Yellowstone work involved a study of the distribution of photosynthetic microorganisms (primarily cyanobacteria) along the thermal gradients created by the outflow channels of hot springs. The research was part of a broader study on the thermal control of photosynthesis and primary productivity in natural environments (BROCK and BROCK 1967, 1968). The hot springs were viewed as "steady state" ecosystems or what I came to call "experiments in nature" where critical ecological research could be carried out. High-temperature bacteria were an unexpected discovery.

I did my first research in Yellowstone National Park

Address for correspondence: Thomas D. Brock, 1227 Dartmouth Rd., Madison, WI 53705.

[1] Testimony of D. ALLAN BROMLEY, Director, Office of Science and Technology Policy, before the Committee on Science, Space, and Technology, House of Representatives, February 20, 1991. BROMLEY's statement should be corrected. The discovery was made in 1966 (published in 1969), and I was then at Indiana University in Bloomington.

[2] For background on my career, and how I came to work on thermophilic bacteria, see BROCK (1995a).

in June 1965 when I was Professor of Microbiology at Indiana University. I studied a large group of thermal pools, many of which had good effluents that provided thermal gradients from boiling down to ambient temperature. I was able to show that there was a definite upper temperature for photosynthetic life, at around 70–73°, but higher temperatures were not devoid of life. I observed that in the effluents of certain springs there were masses of filamentous bacteria living at temperatures much hotter than those at which photosynthetic organisms were present. One particular spring, Octopus Spring, had large amounts of pink filamentous bacteria at temperatures of 82–88°. Here were organisms living at temperatures above the reputed "upper temperature for life."

Attempts to cultivate these pink bacteria were initially unsuccessful, but during the next several years, as I continued broader work on the ecology of the Yellowstone springs, I continued to make occasional observations on these bacteria. At that time, I was doing a large amount of work on the photosynthetic microorganisms of Mushroom Spring, a large spring in the Lower Geyser Basin (BROCK 1967a). The source pool of this spring had a temperature of 73°, just at the known upper temperature limit for photosynthetic life. Because of the difficulty I had cultivating bacteria at temperatures above 80°, I decided to study the bacteria in Mushroom Spring that lived at 70–73°. Beginning in the fall of 1966, with undergraduate student HUDSON FREEZE, I began the work that was to lead to the discovery and culture of T. aquaticus. It was from a sample collected from Mushroom Spring on September 5, 1966 that culture YT-1 of T. aquaticus was isolated. This is the culture that is used today as the source of Taq polymerase for PCR and is the culture specified in the Taq polymerase patent (GELFAND et al. 1989).

HUDSON FREEZE and I isolated T. aquaticus culture YT-1 in October 1966. During various travels to study thermal areas in other parts of the world, I isolated a number of other cultures of T. aquaticus. An interesting culture was isolated from the hot water system of a building on the Indiana University campus. Subsequently, I was able to show that T. aquaticus was widespread in artificial hot-water environments, and other workers have isolated it from hot tap water in other parts of the world.

All of the cultures had an optimum temperature for growth at around 70° and were able to grow at temperatures up to 79°. FREEZE also showed that enzymes from T. aquaticus were able to tolerate temperatures higher than the maximum growth temperature, even surviving boiling water (FREEZE and BROCK 1970). Another student in my laboratory, J. GREGORY ZEIKUS, studied aspects of the protein-synthesizing system of T. aquaticus and showed that ribosomes and amino acid-activating enzymes were also active at high temperature (ZEIKUS et al. 1970; ZEIKUS and BROCK 1971).

By the fall of 1968, I had obtained a large number of cultures of T. aquaticus and had characterized them. Most of the thermophilic bacteria that had been described by earlier researchers were members of a group called the spore-forming bacteria (because they produced heat-resistant spores). The new bacterium was definitely not a spore-former, and it was clear that it was a member of a new genus of organisms.

In preparing a paper for publication, I needed to create a name for this new genus. I did an extensive survey of the literature of thermophilic bacteria, listing all the names that had been used over the years. The new name I first selected was Caldobacter trichogenes, reflecting the fact that the organism lived in hot water (caldo is Italian for hot), and under some conditions forms filaments (tricho derives from the Greek for filament or thread). However, after the first draft of the manuscript was written, I decided that this name was too fanciful. I chose instead the name T. balnearius (Thermus referring to heat and balnearius to a spa or thermal bath). Later, for reasons that I no longer remember, I replaced balnearius with aquaticus (aquaticus referring to water, where the bacterium grows). This last name, T. aquaticus, became official when the paper describing this organism was published (BROCK and FREEZE 1969).

The name for Taq polymerase is often abbreviated "Taq" in common usage. Is a name really a trivial matter? The word Taq rolls readily off the tongue and also fits well into molecular biology jargon and advertising copy. I suppose if I had kept my original name, Caldobacter trichogenes, the enzyme might be called "Cat!"

At the time that the paper on T. aquaticus was being written, I also deposited representative cultures of the organism in the American Type Culture Collection in Washington, D.C. Among these cultures was YT-1, the culture later to be used in PCR. Culture YT-1 became ATCC 25104. When DAVID GELFAND of Cetus conceived of the idea of using a thermophile as a source of DNA polymerase for PCR, he tested all of the available cultures of T. aquaticus from the American Type Culture Collection. Strain YT-1 turned out to have the enzyme with the best properties for PCR (D. GELFAND, personal communication).

Long before GELFAND's work on Taq polymerase, biochemists had started work on thermostable enzymes from T. aquaticus. Even before my first papers on T. aquaticus, I had been sending out cultures to biochemists who had seen a feature article I had written in Science (BROCK 1967b). A variety of thermostable enzymes were discovered. One enzyme that worked with DNA was Taq I restriction endonuclease (SATA et al. 1977). Also, JOHN TRELA at the University of Cincinnati described a thermostable DNA polymerase from T. aquaticus (EDGAR et al. 1975). Although there have been some fairly expensive legal arguments about whether TRELA's enzyme is the same Taq polymerase that GEL-

FAND *et al.* (1989) patented, the fact remains that there was a long history of research on thermostable enzymes from *T. aquaticus* before PCR was discovered.

It is fair to say, however, that it was PCR that put *T. aquaticus* on the map, and there has been a veritable "feeding frenzy" among the media on this subject. Television has particularly liked to discuss Taq polymerase in the context of forensic medicine, because footage of Old Faithful erupting can be shown. I have ceased trying to note all references in the popular literature to *T. aquaticus,* but a brief listing through mid-1995 can be found in BROCK (1995a).

In 1991, when I did a retrospective computer search, over 1000 papers on *T. aquaticus* had been published, and the number continues to increase. Truly, one does not know where a research study will lead!

Bacteria in boiling water: Although I had convinced myself in 1965 that bacteria were living at much higher temperatures than had been previously suspected, I had still not realized that they were living in "boiling" water. My ideas had been based only on observations in outflow channels where "visible" accumulations were present (such as the pink bacteria at temperatures above 80° in Octopus Spring). Culture studies on extreme thermophiles are technically difficult, and if I had relied on standard bacteriological isolation procedures I might never have been successful. Here is where the ecologist's approach, study of organisms directly in nature, comes to the fore.

Near the end of the summer of 1967 I started using a sensitive immersion slide technique to demonstrate microscopically the presence of living bacteria in boiling water. This immersion slide technique had been widely used by microbial ecologists studying "normal" environments. With this technique, I was able to show that although there were no visible accumulations of microorganisms in the boiling pools themselves, bacteria were present in microscopic amounts in virtually every boiling pool I looked in.

In 1967 I initiated a systematic search for the presence of bacteria in Yellowstone boiling springs. The experiment was simple: tie one or two microscope slides to a piece of string, drop in the pool, and tie the other end of the string to a log, rock, or nail. Return later, retrieve the slides, and examine under the microscope. The results were dramatic. Virtually every slide, from every boiling or superheated pool, had heavy bacterial growth, readily visible microscopically. In some cases, the density was so heavy that the slides had a film visible to the naked eye. The following summer (1968) THOMAS BOTT did an outstanding job of proving that these bacteria were really growing, by measuring their growth rates *in situ* (BOTT and BROCK 1969).

Because of the altitude, water boils at only 92.5° in Yellowstone. Once I knew that bacteria could live in boiling springs here, it was natural to plan field trips to thermal areas at lower altitudes, where higher tem-

peratures could be found. I made visits to Iceland and New Zealand, where the boiling springs are at low altitudes and temperatures range up to 100° or a little higher in superheated waters. I was able to find bacteria in virtually every boiling spring of neutral or alkaline pH in these areas, thus extending to a somewhat higher value the upper temperature limit for life.

Deep sea vents: For many years my Yellowstone work had seemed somewhat "exotic" to many microbiologists, perhaps because of the presumed restricted distribution on earth of hot springs. This attitude changed after the discovery of the deep sea vents, with their very high temperatures and the associated diverse and flourishing life forms. Deep sea thermal vents are widespread in the oceans, usually associated with volcanic activity and tectonic movements of the earth. After the deep sea vents were discovered in the late 1970s, my Yellowstone work took on broader significance, because it not only made it reasonable to hypothesize that microbes might be present in some of these high temperature systems, it also provided the essential foundation for studies on the microbiology of thermal vents. The techniques and principles that I had developed for proving that bacteria live and reproduce in boiling water could then be applied to the deep sea habitats.

The upper temperature limit for life has still not been completely resolved, but the chance to study microorganisms living in deep sea vents, where temperatures range up to greater than 300°, has opened up a whole new approach. Although it is clear that no organisms exist at such high temperatures (even amino acids are not stable under these conditions), there are also thermal vents in the sea at temperatures between 100 and 150°. The German microbiologist KARL STETTER in particular has done an excellent job of isolating bacteria capable of growth at temperatures above 100° from some of these vents. One microorganism, *Pyrolobus fumarii,* has an optimum temperature for growth of 105° and can still grow at 113° (MADIGAN and MARRS 1997). (This organism finds 90° too cold!)

Microbial prospecting in Yellowstone: Although it was clear when I ended my project in 1975 that there were many interesting organisms with potential practical applications in hot springs, it was not until the advent of PCR that widespread attention really focused on thermophiles. Not only has the biotechnology industry discovered Yellowstone, but the National Park Service itself has finally realized that there is more of biological interest in Yellowstone than grizzly bears and lodgepole pines (MILSTEIN 1994). Dozens of research groups now have permits to collect microbial samples in Yellowstone. Although another discovery as valuable as Taq polymerase may not come out of this work, it is certainly possible that some of these groups may discover organisms of value. Never before has industry profited directly from living creatures taken from a national park, and the Yellowstone administrators are concerned about whether the Park itself should participate in the largess. Yellowstone, of course, has no monopoly on thermophiles, but it provides the most accessible location where a wide variety of thermal habitats are available.

Also, thermophilic bacteria are now just one example of "extremophiles," microorganisms capable of living under extreme conditions. Other extreme habitats where interesting bacteria live are those with high or low pH, high salt, and low temperature. Extremophiles are suddenly "hot" research topics with the biotechnology industry (MADIGAN and MARRS 1997).

EPILOGUE

The work I have discussed here is just a small subset of the various research areas that I have been involved in throughout my career. A more detailed overview is given in my memoir for the *Annual Review of Microbiology* (BROCK 1995a) and in two supplements to this memoir (BROCK 1995b,c). However, of all the work I have been involved with, the Yellowstone project has been the most exciting and has continued to elicit the most interest from others. For 10 years I operated a field research laboratory in West Yellowstone, Montana, which provided facilities for research by a variety of students and postdoctorates, as well as visitors from across the country and around the world. Much of this work is discussed in a book (BROCK 1978) and in over 100 research and review papers (see BROCK 1995c for listing).

Thermostable enzymes were only a small part of this work, since my focus was not on biotechnology but on basic research. However, the new microorganisms that have been discovered in Yellowstone and elsewhere around the world have been made available to the scientific community. Only one of these organisms led to PCR, but others have provided interesting research problems for microbiologists, biochemists, geneticists, evolutionists, geologists, and ecologists.

See also page 703 in Addenda et Corrigenda.

LITERATURE CITED

BOTT, T. L., and T. D. BROCK, 1969 Bacterial growth rates above 90° in Yellowstone hot springs. Science **164:** 1411–1412.

BROCK, T. D., 1967a Relationship between standing crop and primary productivity along a hot spring thermal gradient. Ecology **48:** 566–571.

BROCK, T. D., 1967b Life at high temperatures. Science **158:** 1012–1019.

BROCK, T. D., 1978 *Thermophilic Microorganisms and Life at High Temperatures.* Springer-Verlag, New York.

BROCK, T. D., 1995a The road to Yellowstone—and beyond. Annu. Rev. Microbiol. **49:** 1–28.

BROCK, T. D., 1995b Photographic supplement to "The road to Yellowstone—and beyond." Available from T. D. BROCK, Madison, WI.

BROCK, T. D., 1995c *Bibliography of Thomas D. Brock, Publications 1951–1995.* Available from T. D. BROCK, Madison, WI.

BROCK, T. D., and M. L. BROCK, 1967 The measurement of chlorophyll, primary productivity, photophosphorylation, and macromolecules in benthic algal mats. Limnol. Oceanogr. **12:** 600–605.

BROCK, T. D., and M. L. BROCK, 1968 Measurement of steady-state growth rates of a thermophilic alga directly in nature. J. Bacteriol. **95:** 811–815.

BROCK, T. D., and H. FREEZE, 1969 *Thermus aquaticus* gen. n. and sp. n., a non-sporulating extreme thermophile. J. Bacteriol. **98:** 289–297.

EDGAR, D., A. CHIEN and J. TRELA, 1975 Purification and characterization of a DNA polymerase from an extreme thermophile, *Thermus aquaticus.* Abstracts, Annual Meeting, Am. Soc. Microbiol. **75:** 151.

FREEZE, H., and T. D. BROCK, 1970 Thermostable aldolase from *Thermus aquaticus.* J. Bacteriol. 101: 541–550.

GELFAND, D. H., S. STOFFEL, F. C. LAWYER and R. K. SAIKI, 1989 Purified Thermostable Enzyme, United States patent number 4,889,818, December 26, 1989.

KEMPNER, E., 1963 Upper temperature limit of life. Science **142:** 1318–1319.

MADIGAN, M. T., and B. L. MARRS, 1997 Extremophiles. Sci. Am. April 1997, 82–87.

MILSTEIN, M., 1994 Yellowstone managers eye profits from hot microbes. Science **264:** 655.

MULLIS, K. B., H. A. ERLICH, D. H. GELFAND, G. HORN and R. K. SAIKI, 1990 Process for amplifying, detecting, and/or cloning nucleic acid sequences using a thermostable enzyme. United States patent number 4,965,188, October 23, 1990.

SATA, S., C. A. HUTCHISON and J. I. HARRIS, 1977 A thermostable sequence-specific endo nuclease from *Thermus aquaticus.* Proc. Natl. Acad. Sci. USA **74:** 542–546.

ZEIKUS, J. G., and T. D. BROCK, 1971 Protein synthesis at high temperatures: aminoacylation of tRNA. Biochim. Biophys. Acta **228:** 736–745.

ZEIKUS, J. G., M. W. TAYLOR and T. D. BROCK, 1970 Thermal stability of ribosomes and RNA from *Thermus aquaticus.* Biochim. Biophys. Acta **204:** 512–520.

Birth Defects, Jimson Weeds, and Bell Curves

James F. Crow

Laboratory of Genetics, University of Wisconsin–Madison, Madison, Wisconsin 53706

IN 1959 the word had gotten around that Down syndrome is caused by trisomy of one of the human chromosomes, later designated number 21. This came as a surprise, for although the idea had been proposed several times, the published information was negative. T. S. PAINTER, at the instigation of C. B. DAVENPORT (1932), examined the chromosomes of a person with "mongolism," as the condition was then called, and found no abnormalities. PAINTER had earlier made another error, reporting 48 as the human chromosome number. These may seem like blunders, but early cytologists deserve our sympathetic understanding. Cytological techniques of that time, employing serial sections and with no means for spreading chromosomes apart, were very crude and chromosome counts were correspondingly uncertain. By 1959 the methods were much better. Counts had become reliable, although individual chromosomes could not yet be identified.

After hearing the Down syndrome gossip, KLAUS PATAU and I discussed this over lunch and wondered about looking for other human trisomies. We knew from BLAKESLEE's studies on the Jimson weed that each trisomic type has a distinct phenotype with characteristic multiple anomalies. PATAU reasoned that one phenotype would surely be mental retardation, since this is found with almost any major developmental disturbance. So he decided to look for trisomy in a hospital for mentally retarded. In this population, he looked for a patient with two additional unrelated abnormalities.

Remarkably, the first day's search was successful. PATAU and his group found an infant with polydactyly and cleft lip, along with other anomalies, and it turned out to have an extra representative of what was later designated as chromosome 13 (PATAU et al. 1960). The condition is now called 13 trisomy or Patau syndrome. His good fortune continued, for he found another the next day. This infant also had multiple defects, but they differed from those caused by trisomy 13. The phenotype was discovered independently in another laboratory

and is now known as 18 trisomy, or Edwards syndrome. With two successes in two days it looked as if all 22 autosomal trisomies would be found in another 19 days, and knowledge of human cytogenetics would begin to rival that of the Jimson weed. But that was not to be. Trisomies 13, 18, and 21 were all. The other autosomal trisomies cause prenatal death or occur only as mosaics.

Another of PATAU's ideas was to use partial trisomy, resulting from chromosome breakage, to identify the parts of the chromosome responsible for the individual defects; he immediately set to work on this project and had moderate success (PATAU 1964). Today the results seem exceedingly limited when compared with current cytogenetics, with its chromosome painting and fine structure mapping, but it was a start.

In PATAU's mind were A. F. BLAKESLEE's extensive studies on the Jimson weed, Datura stramonium. Who was BLAKESLEE and why his interest in Datura? BLAKESLEE was a leading figure in the genetics world in the decades before and after World War I. He worked with various plant and animal species, but finally decided on Datura. To farmers it was a stinking, noxious weed. In fact some people were seriously poisoned when they ate tomatoes grown from a scion that had been grafted onto a Jimson weed stock. But to BLAKESLEE, Datura was "the very best plant with which to discover the principles of heredity." He was moved to say this while smarting from a derisive poem by EDNA ST. VINCENT MILLAY, who wrote of the "rank-smelling thorn apple,—and who would plant this by his dwelling?" BLAKESLEE bounded to the defense of his beloved weed, saying that he, for one, delighted in having this plant by his dwelling. But he went on to say that he regretted that he had not used the euphonious "thorn apple" rather than the disparaging "Jimson weed."

The Datura work was for many years the major research project of a man with boundless energy, insatiable curiosity, and great organizational skill. He grew as many as 70,000 plants in a summer, together with winter crops in six greenhouses. He soon identified 12 characteristic phenotypes, affecting the stems, leaves, and seed capsules, corresponding to trisomy for each of the 12

With one exception, I have not included any of the numerous writings of BLAKESLEE. A full list is given in the biography by SINNOTT (1959), which is also the source of much of my information.

chromosomes. Each trisomic was multiply-abnormal, but highly specific and reproducible. BLAKESLEE realized that the abnormal phenotypes were the result of genic imbalance rather than mutation, since the genes themselves were all normal. He ensured this by starting with a doubled haploid and deriving all the trisomics therefrom. Clearly he was dealing with dosage effects. He also noticed that triploids were much more nearly normal than trisomics. From these studies, along with those of others, it was clear that genic balance is crucial; in general, aneuploids are more grossly abnormal than polyploids.

BLAKESLEE also found tetraploids. Crossing them with diploids, he obtained triploids which, although rather infertile, nevertheless produced a few progeny that included many trisomics and other unbalanced chromosome combinations. Crosses among these led not only to all the primary trisomics, but also to "secondary" and "tertiary" types. Datura chromosomes all have a median centromere, and a secondary trisomic carried an isochromosome with the same arm duplicated and the two fused at the centromere. The tertiary trisomics had combinations of nonhomologous chromosomes.

The genus Datura includes several species, of which BLAKESLEE and his associates studied seven. All have the same number of chromosomes, 12. Yet they differ by translocations, which show up as complex meiotic rings in interspecies crosses. BLAKESLEE combined these hybrids in such a way as to produce new artificial species, several of which "bred true." He was able to make such combinations almost at will and speculated that such processes have played a role in speciation.

Datura stramonium is widespread. BLAKESLEE and his associates collected some 550 geographical races. Even within the species there were translocations. The races fell into five groups that appeared identical cytologically, yet involved different translocations, which showed up as chromosome rings at meiosis. He called these nonobvious chromosomal races "cryptic types," since their differences appeared only in the meioses of hybrids.

The first to report that the meiotic rings were due to translocations was BLAKESLEE's associate, JOHN BELLING (1927). This was immediately picked up by those working on other species, especially Oenothera. And it brought a historical insight, showing that the "mutations" of DE VRIES were mostly, if not entirely, the result of aneuploids segregating from complex chromosomal heterozygotes (EMERSON and STURTEVANT 1931). These, of course, are much more striking phenotypically than most gene mutations. It is likely that the mutation theory would ever have been promulgated if DE VRIES had had only gene mutations available. This was not the only time that an important scientific theory has come from erroneous observations.

Today one hears little about Datura in genetics courses, partly because many of the conclusions are now commonplace, having been confirmed in many other species. Yet BLAKESLEE's studies were pioneering in many ways. The haploid strain was particularly interesting, for it dispelled the widely held belief that haploidy *per se* determines the gametophyte state. Whatever determines the distinction between sporophyte and gametophyte is clearly not ploidy. Everybody knows this now, and we tend to forget that it was once an issue.

Chromosome doubling by colchicine was discovered in 1937, and BLAKESLEE immediately plunged into activity. He demonstrated how to get fertile interspecies hybrids by doubling the chromosome numbers. He also studied the dioecious white campion, *Melandrium album*, which has heteromorphic X and Y chromosomes. In contrast to Drosophila, sex is determined by the Y chromosome and X-Y balance. Using colchicine, he and WARMKE produced tetraploids and found that *XXXY* plants are male, rarely intersexes. Therefore, BLAKESLEE and WARMKE had produced a stable dioecious tetraploid strain with *XXXX* females and *XXXY* males. This attracted considerable interest at the time, for tetraploidy in species with two sexes was thought by analogy with Drosophila to be incompatible with the sex-determining system.

Melandrium fell out of fashion, but—rechristened *Silene latifolia*—it is especially suited for quantitative studies of sex dimorphism (MEAGHER 1997). Furthermore, the huge Y chromosome leads to measurable differences in DNA content between the sexes and to the hypothesis that nonrecombining regions of the X and Y serve as a reservoir for repetitive sequences that are responsible for some quantitative variation (MEAGHER and COSTICH 1996).

Almost always the Datura tetraploids arose as mosaics. BLAKESLEE and STURTEVANT had the same idea, to use mosaics to study embryology. Whereas STURTEVANT (1932) employed mutants as cell markers, BLAKESLEE used polyploidy, for polyploid cells could easily be distinguished by their size. Using colchicine to generate polyploid mosaics, he was able to trace cell lineage and determine which meristematic layers led to leaves, sepals, stamens, and pistils. It was a significant advance in angiosperm embryology.

BLAKESLEE soon learned that aneuploid gametes are poorly transmitted through the ovule and hardly ever through the pollen, a fact that had been noted in many species and which is now a commonplace. But with characteristic zeal he set out to bypass this barrier. One trick was to shorten the style by resection, thus making it possible for a poorly growing pollen tube to reach the ovary. Another tack was to use embryo culture, and BLAKESLEE became prominent in this field.

In the course of his years of Datura study, BLAKESLEE identified 541 mutations. Many were mapped to a chromosome or chromosome region, not only by conventional linkage analysis, but by pollen abortion, trisomic segregation, and other cytogenetic trickery.

I have described only part of his voluminous research, but I hope I have conveyed the impression of a remarkably energetic and productive worker, curious about all aspects of genetics, willing to try every new trick as it came along, and never losing his enthusiasm for research. And he never tired of talking about his research or about genetics in general.

Long before the Datura work, while he was still a graduate student at Harvard, BLAKESLEE made a discovery that immediately brought him fame in the world of fungi. He had an assistantship in mycology and undertook a classification of a group of bread molds, the Mucors. These were known to produce conspicuous zygospores, and BLAKESLEE's path-breaking discovery was that zygospores form only by the fusion of opposite mating types. At the time, the discovery of a sexual process in fungi was a sensation and it set off a flurry of research. For his discovery of heterothallism, BLAKESLEE was awarded the Bowdoin Prize at Harvard. His name is perpetuated in the fungal literature by the species *Phycomyces blakesleeanus*. This species attained fame several decades later in another way. In his later years, MAX DELBRÜCK made it the center of his research, and his great influence among molecular biologists brought BLAKESLEE's name to the attention of a new generation. In fact, BLAKESLEE has a still higher honor, if an eponymous genus is regarded as more prestigious than a mere species. The Mucor, *Blakeslea trispora*, has been the subject of research in several labs.

ALBERT FRANCIS BLAKESLEE was born on November 9, 1874, and died 80 years later on November 16, 1954. His ancestors were from New England and he spent most of his youth in East Greenwich, Rhode Island. From childhood he was interested in natural history. On graduating from East Greenwich Academy, of which his father was principal, he entered Wesleyan College. There he was a tennis champion, played football, was elected to Phi Beta Kappa, and won prizes in mathematics and chemistry.

After graduation he spent three years as a teacher in preparatory schools. He loved teaching and planned to make this his career. But after trying graduate work at Harvard, he caught the research virus and went on to get his Ph.D. in 1904, using the Mucor work as a thesis. He was able to spend two years in Germany, where he became proficient in the language and had a chance to indulge his cultural loves, particularly art museums and concerts. He retained a deep interest in the arts throughout his life, and in his final illness he found consolation from records of his favorite classics.

BLAKESLEE's first permanent job began in 1907 at the Connecticut Agricultural College at Storrs, later to become the University of Connecticut. At Storrs the emphasis was on teaching, which BLAKESLEE loved, and on practical agriculture. He did little research during this time and largely abandoned his work on fungi in the belief that it was not sufficiently relevant to agricul-

ture. He wrote a book on trees, based on his studies of ways to identify trees in winter when they lacked foliage. He planned and did much of the work preparing an experimental garden that was used for various courses. He did considerable research on chickens and found, among other things, a negative correlation between yellow pigment on the legs and egg production. He enjoyed a brief success in early selection for egg production by the color of the legs of young chicks. During his years at Storrs he experimented with a large number of plants, and eventually settled on Datura as the most promising species. It was an economically important weed, hence suitable for an institution with an agricultural emphasis. The original package of seeds that he received from the United States Department of Agriculture produced two flower colors, leading him to decide that in addition to its practical importance as a weed, this was a good organism for genetic research.

Although he concentrated on Datura, it was not to the exclusion of other species. He worked with several other plants and, as a curious sideline, got interested in the inheritance of human tasting ability. He found that some people find phenylthiocarbamide (PTC) very bitter, whereas to others it is tasteless; the trait follows simple Mendelian rules. He also studied a number of other taste differences. He liked to invite audience participation in PTC tasting as an attention-getter in his teaching and public lectures. He was a popular teacher and a great showman, part MARK HOPKINS and part P. T. BARNUM.

Another teaching device was a way to generate a normal distribution. He allowed irregularly shaped beans to move down an inclined plane and fall into compartments. Their random changes of direction generated a crude Gaussian distribution. I don't know whether he knew of GALTON's rather similar idea, the *Quincunx* (CROW 1993b). Still another attention-getting device was his colorful use of the maize mutant, "sun-red," in which parts exposed to the sun are red. He used this to dramatize the influence of environment on genetic traits. By wrapping the developing ear in opaque paper and appropriately cutting out spaces, he had red kernels spelling out the word "LIGHT."

In 1915 BLAKESLEE moved to Cold Spring Harbor. The research opportunity was much greater there and he made the most of it, but he missed his teaching. Later, in 1935 he succeeded C. B. DAVENPORT as director of the Cold Spring Harbor Laboratory and remained in this position until his retirement in 1941. Figure 1 shows BLAKESLEE during his Cold Spring Harbor days.

After retiring from Cold Spring Harbor, he was invited to a special professorship at Smith College. Once again he could satisfy his desire to teach, and as always he was a catalyst. With undiminished physical and mental vigor, he quickly got funds for a new greenhouse. He organized a four-college genetics conference, pool-

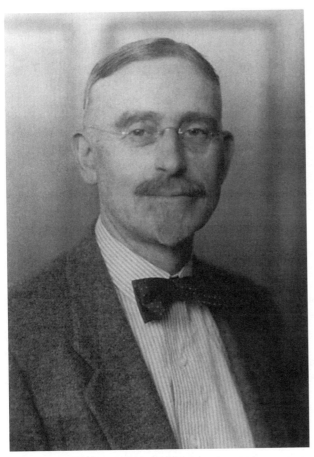

FIGURE 1.—A. F. BLAKESLEE, about 1932.

ing the resources of Smith, Holyoke, Amherst, and the University of Massachusetts, a big boost for genetics in this region. It was during his Smith College period that I became acquainted with him. I accompanied H. J. MULLER, then at Amherst College, on a visit to BLAKES-LEE's lab, and because of MULLER's prestige we got the full treatment. BLAKESLEE was in great form. He took us to the lab where several Smith students were carrying out individual research projects. Like a proud papa, he hovered over each one and served as prompter while she described her research. How he enjoyed it! It would be hard to imagine a retirement life more ideal for a born teacher.

Between 1904 and 1955, BLAKESLEE published 221 articles. The range is astonishing. In the early years most of them dealt with fungi, particularly sexuality in a number of species. Later the emphasis changed to Datura, mainly genetics and cytology, but with other aspects, such as effects of hormones and radiation. He was quick to use neutrons, after the atomic age made these accessible. Always interested in technical innovations, he wrote several papers in which he described new techniques. After one of his honorary degrees he wrote an article on honorary degrees. And always he was the educator. At Connecticut he taught one of the first genetics courses anywhere. Not only was he an

active classroom teacher, but he wrote several articles on teaching, one with the fascinating title "Teachers Talk Too Much." It was based on a talk which he enlivened by passing out papers with PTC for members of the audience to taste. He also advocated research in education. At Cold Spring Harbor he was chairman of the school district. One of his ideas was a school with only identical twins, in which different educational methods could be tested. One twin could be taught by a new experimental method while the other served as a control. He estimated that there were 150 pairs of identical twins in the New York City schools and it should be a simple matter to get them into one experimental school. Even in those days of fewer regulations, this was easier said than done. It was never implemented.

BLAKESLEE was interested in human heredity, particularly the complementary roles of heredity and environment. While in Connecticut he wrote an article entitled, "Corn and Men," in which he showed pictures illustrating the great differences between identical corn strains grown in crowded and uncrowded conditions. At the same time, he pointed out that tall and short varieties show characteristic differences when grown in the same environment. He was interested in variability, genetic and environmental, and with the tendency for quantitative traits to fit the normal distribution. Again he showed his flair for the dramatic. He had the idea of arranging 175 students at Connecticut State College by height so that they formed a good approximation to the normal curve (Figure 2). I don't know how he arranged to get them together and lined up by height, but the students are in army uniforms, so perhaps some military discipline was involved. The picture was reproduced in textbooks and elsewhere, and many of you may recall seeing it. I first encountered it in STERN's widely used textbook of human heredity, published in 1949.

BLAKESLEE noted that the normal, bell-shaped distribution of variability would be found if height were entirely genetic, or entirely environmental, or any mixture. So he followed up by looking into the ancestry of the tallest and shortest students and found, to no surprise, that they came from tall and short families, respectively. Although he was careful not to discount environment, he concluded that genetic factors were much more important. Again, he dramatized his message by having the shortest and tallest students pose with the corn varieties, Tom Thumb (short) and Leaming dent (tall).

Recently, LINDA STRAUSBAUGH decided to update BLAKESLEE's photo. She got a large group of University of Connecticut biology students, along with a few ringers, to line up just as BLAKESLEE had arranged them more than 80 years earlier. For gender-identification she provided two sets of T-shirts. The photo is shown in Figure 3. Since both sexes are included, the distribu-

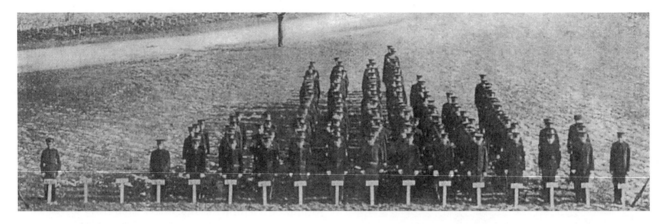

4:10   4:11   5:0   5:1   5:2   5:3   5:4   5:5   5:6   5:7   5:8   5:9   5:10   5:11   6:0   6:1   6:2

FIGURE 2.—A living histogram from Connecticut State Agricultural College (BLAKESLEE 1914). The number of men is 175, the mean height is 67.3 in., and the standard deviation is 2.7 in.

tion is bimodal. It is striking that the men are about 3 inches taller than those in the earlier picture (70.1 vs. 67.3 inches). The average of men and women currently (67.6) is about the same as the men at the earlier time. The variance has hardly changed. What would BLAKESLEE have thought of this? He might have been surprised that the mean shifted by as much as a standard deviation, surely the result of better environment.

BLAKESLEE's article appeared in the *Journal of Heredity* in 1914. (This was the first volume after the name was changed from the *American Breeder's Magazine* to reflect its interest in human genetics in addition to plant and animal breeding.) The state and emphasis of genetics at the time is indicated by the other articles in this volume. One paper advocated growing pigmy hippopotami as meat animals in swampy parts of the Gulf states. Another discussed the increasing problem of Chestnut blight. ALEXANDER GRAHAM BELL, of telephone fame, described his extensive studies of inheritance in sheep, including selection for twinning. DAVENPORT described his overly simple, two-locus theory of human skin color inheritance and independence of skin color and hair

shape. C. C. LITTLE, later to study histocompatibility and establish The Jackson Laboratory, reported on coat-color inheritance in dogs. Another article described crosses between buffalo and cattle. The first generation hybrids were all female, and animals from later crosses were often sterile, but a fertile mixed strain, the "cattalo," was developed. It was said to be superior to cattle as a range animal, being hardier and immune to many cattle diseases. Furthermore, since it was said to get up on its forelegs first rather than the hind legs as cattle do, it was less likely to perish in deep snow.

There was a report of a radish-cabbage hybrid that was completely sterile, but which provided the most extreme example of heterosis that I know of (perhaps *luxuriance* is better). This plant not only reached the top of the greenhouse, but "grew through the ventilator on the roof and was traveling down the roof on both sides" when it finally died. This, of course, was many years before KARPECHENKO's doubling the chromosomes to make a fertile allopolyploid, Raphanobrassica. Alas, KARPECHENKO was one of the earliest victims of the STALIN purge of geneticists (CROW 1993a).

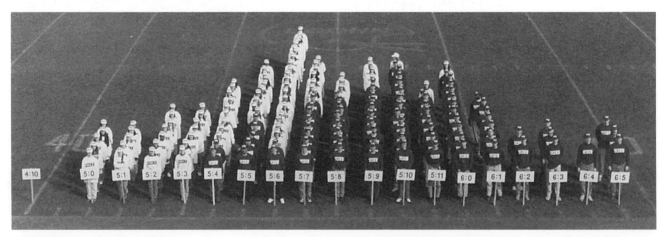

FIGURE 3.—A modern version of Figure 2, from Connecticut State University in 1996. The means and standard deviations in inches are as follows: males, 70.1 ± 3.0; females, 64.8 ± 2.7; combined, 67.6 ± 4.0. Photo from LINDA STRAUSBAUGH.

JOHN BELLING reported a puzzling case of inherited semisterility in bean hybrids. Half the progeny of semisterile plants were semisterile, the others normal. Obviously he had a translocation. This is the same man who first understood translocation rings, but he didn't know about them in 1914. Another article reported the puzzle of seedlessness of domesticated bananas compared with wild varieties with seeds. This is because of triploidy and other odd ploidies in the domestic varieties, but that also wasn't known in 1914.

Finally, the *Journal of Heredity* had many articles on eugenics; this is a good place to read some of the early eugenic stirrings among breeders and geneticists. One author was BELL, and GALTON was liberally quoted throughout the volume. The *Journal* was edited by an active eugenicist, PAUL POPENOE, who later was associated with the Human Betterment Foundation in California and was an active proponent of eugenic sterilization. He was personable and a good speaker. I heard him at a genetics colloquium in the 1930s, by which time his interest had shifted to sex education and birth control. His life parallels the ascent and decline of the American eugenics movement.

Let's give BLAKESLEE the last word. At a time when extreme views of nature versus nurture prevailed, his was a voice of moderation. He called for more knowledge before any hasty action: "A safe watchword is— Information before Legislation." Later in the same 1914 article: "In the garden of human life as in the garden of corn, success is the resultant complex of the two factors, environment and heredity." A commonplace sentiment today, but in 1914 it needed to be said.

I am thankful to HAL KRIDER and LINDA STRAUSBAUGH for letting me know of the current human histogram and providing pictures. DON WALLER told me about the renewed interest in Silene (earlier, Melandrium).

LITERATURE CITED

BELLING, J., 1927 The attachment of chromosomes at the reduction division of flowering plants. J. Genet. **18:** 177–205.

BLAKESLEE, A. F., 1914 Corn and men. J. Hered. **5:** 511–518.

CROW, J. F., 1993a S. I. VAVILOV, martyr to genetic truth. Genetics **134:** 1–4.

CROW, J. F., 1993b FRANCIS GALTON: count and measure, measure and count. Genetics **135:** 1–4.

DAVENPORT, C. B., 1932 Mendelism in man. Proc. 6th Int. Congr. Genet. **1:** 135–140.

EMERSON, S. H., and A. H. STURTEVANT, 1931 Genetic and cytological studies of Oenothera. III. The translocation interpretation. Z. Indukt. Abstammungs-Vererbungsl. **59:** 395–419.

MEAGHER, T. R., 1997 The quantitative genetics of sexual dimorphism, in *Sexual Dimorphism in Plants,* edited by M. GEBER, T. DAWSON and L. DELPH. Springer-Verlag, New York (in press).

MEAGHER, T. R., and D. E. COSTICH, 1996 Nuclear DNA content and floral evolution. Proc. R. Soc. Lond. B Biol. Sci. **263:** 1455–1460.

PATAU, K., 1964 Partial trisomy, pp. 52–59 in *Second International Congress on Congenital Malformations,* edited by M. FISHBEIN. International Medical Congress, New York.

PATAU, K., D. W. SMITH, E. THERMAN, S. L. INHORN and H. P. WAGNER, 1960 Multiple congenital anomaly caused by an extra autosome. Lancet **1:** 790–793.

SINNOTT, E. W., 1959 Albert Francis Blakeslee. *Biographical Memoirs. National Academy of Sciences,* **33:** 1–38. Columbia University Press, New York.

STURTEVANT, A. H., 1932 The use of mosaics in the study of the developmental effects of genes. Proc. 6th Int. Congr. Genet. **1:** 304–307.

Dobzhansky's *Genetics and the Origin of Species*
Is It Still Relevant?

Richard C. Lewontin

Museum of Comparative Zoology, Harvard University, Cambridge, Massachusetts 02138

THE first edition of THEODOSIUS DOBZHANSKY's *Genetics and the Origin of Species* appeared almost precisely 60 years before this issue of GENETICS. It would be hard to find anyone, even envious authors of other *magna opera*, who would disagree with JEFFREY POWELL's 50th anniversary assessment that "it is the most important and influential book on evolution of the twentieth century" (POWELL 1987). It must be remembered, however, that the book was only the concrete form of the Jesup Lectures given the previous year at the invitation of L. C. DUNN and others at Columbia, an invitation that signaled the importance that influential biologists already placed on DOBZHANSKY's previous 10 years of work on genetics and evolution. In an important sense, the publication of the book, to be followed by other Jesup Lectures books by MAYR (1942) and SIMPSON (1944) and eventually STEBBINS (1950), was a manifesto representing a view that was already taking hold.

Nothing would be gained by plagiarizing POWELL's masterful summary of the schism between the communities of genetics and evolutionary biology at the time, and of the highlights of DOBZHANSKY's integration of Mendelism and Darwinism. In this respect, two things that were unique to DOBZHANSKY's book need to be emphasized. First, *Genetics and the Origin of Species* seemed to be essentially a treatise in observational *biology*, speaking in the language and using the biological materials of experimentalists and natural historians. Second, DOBZHANSKY's entire schema began with the origin of variation and culminated with the formation of species, thus seeming to engage DARWIN's outline directly. Some years before, FISHER (1930), WRIGHT (1931), and HALDANE (1932) had already completed syntheses of genetics and evolution at the conceptual level, showing how Mendelism served as a basis for evolutionary change. But their expositions did not rely, as DOBZHANSKY's did, on a large amount of description of observations from nature, and the problem of the origin of species was treated by them only *en passant* (FISHER spent three and a half pages on it), although

Author e-mail: dick@mcz.harvard.edu

WRIGHT's picture of alternative adaptive peaks certainly sidled up to the problem.

One historical viewpoint for an appreciation of DOBZHANSKY's book is that of the observer in 1937 looking retrospectively, seeing how DOBZHANSKY's synthesis succeeded in bringing the full apparatus of genetics and of genetic observations in natural populations to bear on the observable facts of speciation and species diversity. It is this synthetic element that was so compelling to his readers of the time. But, like any major scientific synthesis, *Genetics and the Origin of Species* was not simply a compelling reorganization of existing knowledge into a unified structure. The real test of its importance lay in its prospective aspect, in the implicit program for evolutionary genetics from 1937 into the future. As POWELL pointed out in his essay, the book, especially in later editions (1941, 1951), had an important impact in establishing observational population genetics as a scientific field for investigation. In fact, the entire problematic of evolutionary genetics for the last 60 years, including its detailed formulation at present, flows from the organization and content of DOBZHANSKY's Jesup Lectures and the book that embodied them.

DOBZHANSKY's argument, which every graduate student in Zoology at Columbia in his day was expected to reproduce on the written qualifying examination for the Ph.D., was the skeleton of DARWIN's theory of the origin of species. Species are groups of interbreeding organisms that have been cut off, biologically, from sharing heredity with other species with which they share a common ancestry in the remote past. This reproductive isolation is the final step in divergence between geographically separated populations, geographical races, which were originally kept apart only by geography, but which have acquired during their geographical separation sufficient genetic difference to prevent future interbreeding. But for genetic differences to accumulate between populations, there must be genetic variation within populations to begin with. That is, species evolution is a process of the conversion of the variation present between individuals within populations at a given moment into variation between populations in time and space. This scheme then places the investigation of intrapopulation genetic variation and polymorphism at the very center of the study of evolutionary dynamics. Even the description of differences between populations is in the form of the statistical description of their polymorphisms rather than by characteristic typological differences. This point of view has differentiated population and evolutionary genetics from all other modes of studying evolution. It is the reason that in a book of 321 pages of text, whose ultimate goal is to explain the origin of species, 178 pages at the beginning are taken up with intrapopulation variation. It is the reason that at present so many population geneticists are skeptical of simple *post hoc* optimality explanations of species characteristics, for they are predisposed to consider the contingency of just the right kind of genetic variation to make the stories work. "I can call monsters from the vasty deep" says that ur-adaptationist OWEN GLENDOWER. "Why, so can I and so can any man. But will they come when you do call for them?" replies the doubtful population geneticist HOTSPUR. It is the reason that evolutionary geneticists until recently had so neglected a detailed genetic study of the differences that underlie species divergence. After all, species differences are simply the final disposition of the standing genetic variation within species, so it is the nature of that standing variation and of the forces modulating it that is the real stuff of evolutionary genetics. All else is just developmental and molecular biology.

The degree to which the first edition of *Genetics and the Origin of Species* was the enunciation of a problematic for the future, rather than a synthesis of an already adequate body of fact and theory, can be seen in a comparison between the original and later editions. While so much emphasis was placed on the importance of intrapopulation genetic variation in the first edition, the actual evidence was pretty thin. Aside from the few human blood groups then known, DOBZHANSKY and EPLING's (1944) survey of inversion polymorphism in geographical populations of *Drosophila pseudoobscura*, and a few studies of simple Mendelizing morphological polymorphisms and chromosomal lethals by the Dubinin school (see pp. 42–46 in DOBZHANSKY 1937), virtually nothing was known of the frequencies of Mendelian genetic variations in natural populations. DOBZHANSKY's own famous *Genetics of Natural Population* series began to appear only after the Jesup Lectures. By the time he finished the revised third edition in 1951, twenty papers in that series had appeared, comprising a model for how genetical variation in natural populations could be studied. This included observations of temporal variation and stability in polymorphism, estimates of migration and effective population size, evidence for the existence of selective differences in nature, and the creation of laboratory model populations in which selection could be demonstrated and esti-

mated. The third revised edition of 1951 now could refer to 15 years of data from natural and laboratory populations estimating parameters of selection, migration, and breeding structure. Moreover, large quantities of data were now available on the viability and fertility variation among genomes sampled from natural populations of Drosophila, data made possible by an adaptation of MULLER's *ClB* trick for making chromosomes homozygous. Nor was it DOBZHANSKY's school alone that pursued the program, nor Drosophila alone that was the object of study. As a consequence of the medical demands created by the Second World War, great advances had been made in immunological genetics, resulting in an explosion of information on human blood groups and HLA polymorphisms. The most complete model for how to study a Mendelian polymorphism within and between local populations was LAMOTTE's (1951) monograph on the shell color and banding polymorphisms in *Cepaea nemoralis*. A manifesto had become an industry.

The program, while seemingly prosperous, was, however, in deep difficulties. Aside from the occasional, genetically simple morphological or immunological polymorphism, studies of natural genetic variation were dependent on observations of whole chromosomes rather than single physiological and developmentally defined loci. Inversion polymorphism, while serving as a model object of study, could really give no information about the generality of variation on which the genetical theory of evolution depended. Alternatively, the measurement of viability and fertility variation in nature, surely the stuff of evolutionary change, could be assayed only at the whole chromosome level, providing no real information about how much genic variation existed. DOBZHANSKY had created a field and focused investigation on a problematic that seemed impossible to clarify.

The response to this conundrum was the introduction of a method of investigation, protein electrophoresis, that seemed to cut through the difficulty because it (1) provided a phenotype whose variation was easily observable; (2) did not depend on any assumptions on the physiological or developmental consequences of the variation; (3) would detect a large fraction of the variation at a large fraction of loci, locus by locus; and (4) could be applied to any organism irrespective of its amenability to genetic manipulation (HUBBY and LEWONTIN 1966). While it might be flattering to the self-esteem of those who introduced the technique to think of it as "revolutionizing" the field, the truth is quite the opposite. The immense popularity that electrophoretic studies enjoyed for nearly 20 years after their introduction in 1966 was precisely that they seemed to provide the possibility of at last coming to grips with the problematic that had occupied evolutionary genetics since 1937. Unfortunately, the main strength of the method was its fatal flaw. Its essence was that it allowed the assessment of genetic variation unaffected by the physi-

ological and developmental consequences of that variation. But, by liberating the observations from physiology
and development, the method also guaranteed that,
except in the very extraordinary circumstance that allelic variation at a single locus had a strong marginal
effect on fitness, no inferences about the forces operating on the variation could be tested. The Dobzhanskian problematic was even more frustratingly stymied.
Now we could describe genetic variation quite generally
but seemed barred from explaining it!

The impasse was broken, at least in part, by a lucky
fact of nature: the lack of a one-to-one correspondence
between the DNA sequence and the amino acid sequence of proteins. The degeneracy of the code, the
existence of introns, of transcribed but untranslated
and of nontranscribed DNA, all mean that within the
same small genic region there are classes of nucleotides
with very different relationships to the physiology and
development of the organism. Different patterns of genetic variation of these different classes could then provide *internal* evidence about the cumulative effect of
selection, which should operate differently on the different classes, as opposed to forces of mutation, population structure, and recombination, which should affect
all classes equally. Beginning with the original demonstration by KREITMAN (1983) of the unique power of
DNA sequence studies to detect even very weak natural
selection unambiguously, the central problematic of
evolutionary genetics seemed once again to be accessible. More than a dozen years of population genetics at
the nucleotide level have clearly shown that selective
constraints exist for all classes of nucleotides including
so-called "silent" positions in codons, as well as introns
and flanking sequences. (see, as an example, RICHTER
et al. 1997). Moreover, it has been possible to detect,
in patterns of haplotypes, traces of migration among
populations (RICHTER *et al.* 1997) and the constraints
imposed on variation by differing amounts of recombination (BEGUN and AQUADRO 1992). But, more than
this, the study of nucleotide variation has allowed evolutionary genetics to proceed to the next set of questions
posed by the schema outlined in *Genetics and the Origin
of Species*.

The existence of genetic variation and the modulation of its pattern within a population at any time are
only the beginning of the process of species evolution,
according to DOBZHANSKY. It is not sufficient that local
populations are simply different in gene frequency, for
every population must differ from every other one in
the real world of finite assemblages. Species are not
simply assemblages of organisms that are not interbreeding, but are distinct life forms with distinct relations to the environment, making a living in distinct
ways. Nor can this ecological differentiation commonly
be a process that follows after reproductive isolation
has already occurred, for then we would often observe
that partially reproductively isolated populations would

show no adaptive differentiation. Unless the populations have come to occupy different peaks in the adaptive landscape, the local populations or geographical
races are not likely to be in the preliminary stages in
species formation. This, then, poses a second set of
problems for population genetics: to demonstrate that
natural selection has played a role in population differentiation. It is easy enough to show that strains drawn
from different populations have different norms of reaction and different fertilities and viabilities in different
experimental circumstances. The first edition of *Genetics and the Origin of Species* uses precisely such evidence
to demonstrate genetic differences between local populations. It is a very different matter, however, to link
these divergences to specific genetic differences, to
show that they matter in nature and that they have
been established by some process of adaptive natural
selection.

Because of the evident difficulty of such demonstrations, this critical next element in the Dobzhanskian
program has been the subject of a great deal of talk
but only limited action. The geographical variation of
shell patterns in Cepaea provided the opportunity for
a long struggle between the English school, which explained all variation as a consequence of local variations
in environmental conditions (see, for example, CAIN
and SHEPPARD 1950), and the French school, which
interpreted the results as a consequence of genetic drift
(LAMOTTE 1951). During the heyday of electrophoretic
studies, a number of cases of geographical or altitudinal
clines in the frequencies of variants were found, and
these were correlated with various environmental variables, usually temperature. The most detailed studies
linking the frequencies of variants with their enzymatic
kinetics, physiology, and behavior, while successful in
demonstrating such a relationship, are unable to deal
with the basic issue facing all who study natural selection in natural populations, namely, the question of
which aspects of the organism's biology account for
variance of fitness *in nature*. That is, it may be that,
ceteris paribus, an increase in egg-laying rate of females
would increase the fitness of their genotype, but if females in nature lay so few eggs that differences in physiological potential are irrelevant, then differential physiological fertility is not a significant component of fitness
variance. The challenge of studying adaptive variation
in nature is that one has to know so much about the
biology of the organism. Thus, it would seem that the
second phase of the Dobzhanskian project, to show that
genetic differentiation has occurred by natural selection, seems to evade us. Once again, studies of nucleotide variation have provided a possibility of progress. By
finding short regions of the genome that are markedly
depauperate of nucleotide variation for silent sites and
introns, as compared with other regions in the same
genome, a strong case can be made for a selective gene
fixation in the relatively recent past. A striking example

is the demonstration by BERRY *et al.* (1991) of a selective sweep on the microchromosome of *Drosophila melanogaster*. Of course, we do not know the biological cause of the sweep nor which sites within the region are responsible for it, as opposed to being carried along by hitchhiking. The demonstration of adaptive differentiation can be carried even further to look for evidence of adaptive divergence between species, detected by an excess of amino acid replacements as compared with silent divergences between them (McDONALD and KREITMAN 1991). There is, in principle, no limit to how much of the genome could be investigated in this way, choosing particular genes or gene regions and sequencing them within and between species. We could then estimate, for any collection of populations or related species, how much of their differentiation has been driven by selective sweeps within populations and selective divergences between species. In this way, the second phase of DOBZHANSKY's general scheme could be realized. The only question is whether it is the investigators or the granting agencies that would grow tired first.

The continuation of DOBZHANSKY's program by sequencing studies reveals its original limitation. Although DOBZHANSKY is usually thought of as the founder of experimental population genetics and his 1937 book as the founding document, there is in fact no experiment described there until the last chapter on hybrid sterility, where experimental crosses and backcrosses between *Drosophila pseudoobscura* and *Drosophila persimilis* using marked chromosomes are discussed. The entire body of evidence marshaled on the control of natural variation within populations and the conversion of that variation into genetic differences in time and space is from static data. It depends upon what inferences can be made from the standing patterns of genetic variation in nature. In this case, the testing of hypotheses that we usually associate with experiments is of a special statistical sort, manifest in the 1937 book, in most of DOBZHANSKY's "experimental" (observational) papers, and in the present state of molecular population genetics. By using population genetic theory, either in explicit mathematical form or more heuristically, a prediction is made of what the distribution of genetic variation should look like under some simple model, say no selection and no migration. The observed standing pattern of variation is then compared with this null prediction, and some inference is made from the agreement or disagreement between the observed and the expected. The observations of inversion clines or regional variations in the viability of strains when tested in a standard laboratory condition are, in this respect, of the same evidentiary nature as the comparison of the standing variation within and between species in the ratio of silent to replacement nucleotide substitutions. In 1951 Lamotte attempted to explain the variation in Cepaea by fitting the distribution of colony gene frequencies to a stationary Wrightian distribution. To-

day, molecular population geneticists fit the nucleotide polymorphism and diversity between populations at several loci to the predictions of coalescent theory. Of course, one can attempt to show that a genetic difference observed in nature has some consequence for physiology and selection in a laboratory model, just as DOBZHANSKY showed that inversions would be subject to selection in the laboratory under some conditions. But the success or failure of such experiments does not tell us what forces have operated historically or are now operating in nature. Population genetics, then as now, is an observational and statistical science, not an experimental one. As a consequence, while it can offer statistical evidence supporting the past action of one or another of the evolutionary forces having operated, it cannot cash these inferences out in the form of actual biological mechanisms.

An irony of the intellectual history of *Genetics and the Origin of Species* is that DOBZHANSKY came into evolutionary genetics from the study of morphological diversity in nature and so was able to relate the abstractions of genetic theory to the biology of organisms, yet in the end he and the field he founded became captives of the abstractions. Despite 40 years of study of the chromosomal variation in natural populations of Drosophila, DOBZHANSKY published no observations from nature on the possible biological mediation of the natural selection he had detected. There is, in the entire corpus of 43 papers on the *Genetics of Natural Populations*, no paper on the ecology and life history of *D. pseudoobscura*. The closest he came was to measure the rate of movement of genetically marked, laboratory-raised flies along a trap line of attractive banana bait. Nor did he make any pretense that the demonstration of selection of chromosomal inversions in laboratory population cages was meant to reveal the natural biology of this polymorphism. The purpose of those experiments was to show that the allelic contents of the inversions could, indeed, under some circumstances make a large difference to their fitness and that, in these circumstances, heterozygotes were more fit than homozygotes, as he believed them to be in nature. In fact, although there was selection in the cages at 25°, there was none at 18°.

Thus, we see that *Genetics and the Origin of Species*, like DOBZHANSKY's subsequent research career, although seeming to speak in the language of organisms, had the ultimate effect not of uniting genetics with the natural historical and physiological biology, but of building a science that speaks the language of gene frequencies. One of the consequences of that alienation of population genetics from organismal biology was the failure of the projects of the 1960s to build a unified science of population biology out of the elements of ecology and population genetics.

Another consequence of the way in which DOBZHANSKY constructed the problem of the origin of species has been to remove the problem of the actual speciation process from the concern of most population geneticists. All of the issues of natural selection in relation to adaptation are, for DOBZHANSKY, already dealt with in the problem of adaptive population divergence. The final stage of separation of the species becomes a question of the genetics of reproductive isolation (ORR 1997), a problem in neurobiology and developmental genetics, of why flies don't like each other's looks, or why a particular sperm can't fertilize a particular kind of egg, or why somatic or germline development fails in hybrid embryos. This mechanical view of the problem of ultimate species divergence is already contained in DOBZHANSKY's adherence to a particular view of species. In *Genetics and the Origin of Species* he reaffirms his previous (1935) definition of a species as "that stage of evolutionary process at which the once actually or potentially interbreeding array of forms becomes segregated in two or more separate arrays which are physiologically incapable of interbreeding" (p. 312). By defining it in this way, DOBZHANSKY then created the problematic for the study of speciation, the genetic elucidation of an aspect of developmental and neurobiology. Where are the genes? What are their developmental interactions? What determines when and how they are read? And this is, indeed, the current problematic of speciation studies (COYNE 1992), divorced from the rest of evolutionary genetics until such time as population geneticists finally fold developmental biology into their considerations.

What is now the classical definition of species leads to a problem that DOBZHANSKY acknowledges. What are we to do with all those asexual organisms where this definition of species is irrelevant? He admits that such organisms are not continuously distributed in phenotypic and genotypic space, but that "there are aggregations of more or less distinct biotypes" and that, just like sexually reproducing forms, these biotypes are "clustered around some of the 'adaptive peaks' in the field of gene combinations" and that "the clusters are arranged in a hierarchical order in a way which is again analogous to that encountered in sexual forms." (p. 320). But, he says, they are not species. So what are they, and why do we lavish so much interest on the problem of reproductive isolation? We are never told, because this is the penultimate paragraph in the book. What DOBZHANSKY has done is to finesse one of the most interesting questions in evolutionary biology, which is why organisms occupy the phenotypic state space in the hierarchically clustered pattern that we see, sex or no sex. That is, how do organisms acquire new and quite distinct ways of making a living? This is the antecedent question that makes the problem of reproductive isolation relevant for sexual species. Whatever

the forces are that cluster organisms in state space, that clustering is destroyed by sexual recombination, so an organism that exploits the advantages of sex has a special problem that asexual ones do not have. In order to allow sexual organisms to maintain the clusters against the disruption of sex, they have to develop isolating mechanisms. Those that fail become extinct from too much compromise.

DOBZHANSKY's construction of the problem of speciation as solely the problem of reproductive isolation was a piece of scientific synecdoche, substituting the process of reproductive isolation for the speciation process in its entirety. It is a testimony to the influence that *Genetics and the Origin of Species* has wielded over 60 years that we continue to study the speciation process without reference to the world that organisms construct and occupy.

LITERATURE CITED

BEGUN, D. J., and C. F. AQUADRO, 1992   Levels of naturally occurring DNA polymorphism correlate with recombination rates in *D. melanogaster*. Nature **356**: 519–520.

BERRY, A. J., J. W. AJIOKA and M. KREITMAN, 1991   Lack of polymorphism on the *Drosophila* fourth chromosome resulting from selection. Genetics **129**: 1111–1117.

CAIN, A. J., and P. M. SHEPPARD, 1950   Selection in the polymorphic land snail *Cepaea nemoralis*. Heredity **4**: 275–294.

COYNE, J. A., 1992   Genetics and speciation. Nature **355**: 511–515.

DOBZHANSKY, TH., 1935   A critique of the species concept in biology. Philos. Sci. **2**: 344–355.

DOBZHANSKY, TH., 1937, 1941, 1951   *Genetics and the Origin of Species*. Ed. 1, 2, 3. Columbia University Press, New York.

DOBZHANSKY, TH., and C. EPLING, 1944   *Contributions to the Genetics, Taxonomy, and Ecology of Drosophila pseudoobscura and Its Relatives*. Pub. 554, Carnegie Institute of Washington, Washington, DC.

FISHER, R. A., 1930   *The Genetical Theory of Natural Selection*. Clarendon Press, Oxford.

HALDANE, J. B. S., 1932   *The Causes of Evolution*. Harper and Row, New York.

HUBBY, J. L., and R. C. LEWONTIN, 1966   A molecular approach to the study of genic heterozygosity in natural populations. I. The number of alleles at different loci in *Drosophila pseudoobscura*. Genetics **54**: 577–594.

KREITMAN, M., 1983   Nucleotide polymorphism at the alcohol dehydrogenase locus of *Drosophila melanogaster*. Nature **304**: 412–417.

LAMOTTE, M., 1951   Recherches sur la structure génétique des populations naturelles de *Cepaea nemoralis* (L). Bull. Biol. Fr. Belg., Suppl. **35**: 1–238.

MAYR, E., 1942   *Systematics and the Origin of Species*. Columbia University Press, New York.

MCDONALD, J. H., and M. KREITMAN, 1991   Adaptive protein evolution at the *Adh* locus in Drosophila. Nature **351**: 652–654.

ORR, H. A., 1997   DOBZHANSKY, BATESON and the genetics of speciation. Genetics (in press).

POWELL, J. R., 1987   "In the air"—THEODOSIUS DOBZHANSKY's *Genetics and the Origin of Species*. Genetics **117**: 363–366.

RICHTER, B., M. LONG, R. C. LEWONTIN and E. NITASAKA, 1997   Nucleotide variation and conservation at the *dpp* locus, a gene controlling early development in Drosophila. Genetics **145**: 311–323.

SIMPSON, G. G., 1944   *Tempo and Mode in Evolution*. Columbia University Press, New York.

STEBBINS, G. L., 1950   *Variation and Evolution in Plants*. Columbia University Press, New York.

WRIGHT, S., 1931   Evolution in Mendelian populations. Genetics **16**: 97–159.

The Weaker Sex Is Heterogametic
Seventy-five Years of Haldane's Rule

Cathy C. Laurie

DCMB/Zoology Department, Duke University, Durham, North Carolina 27708

J. B. S. HALDANE (1892–1964) made his greatest contributions to biology in the area of theoretical population genetics, especially the dynamics of natural selection. Along with R. A. FISHER and SEWALL WRIGHT, he is considered one of the founding fathers of population genetics and a major player in the development of the modern synthetic theory of evolution. This work alone identifies HALDANE as one of the great scientists of the twentieth century, but he also made important contributions in an amazing variety of areas including enzyme kinetics (the BRIGGS-HALDANE equation), biochemical genetics, physiology, biostatistics, linkage (the first mapping function), mutation rates in humans, and the origin of life (WHITE 1965; CROW 1992). He also noticed and described an interesting evolutionary pattern that came to be known as HALDANE's rule.

One of HALDANE's earliest papers (1922) is a compilation of data from the literature on sex-specific inviability and sterility in hybrids between animal species. An analysis of 45 Lepidopteran, 10 bird, and six mammalian crosses, as well as a few other types of animal hybrids, led him to formulate a "rule" with only one or two known exceptions: "When in the F_1 offspring of two different animal races one sex is absent, rare, or sterile, that sex is the heterozygous [heterogametic] sex." In birds and Lepidopterans, females (known to be heterogametic) were more often inviable or sterile, while in mammals the heterogametic males were more often affected.

In his 1922 paper, HALDANE stated an earlier suggestion of A. H. STURTEVANT that a deficiency of one sex might be due to inviability or to sexual transformation. He noted that STURTEVANT had demonstrated lethality of male larvae in a Drosophila cross, while GOLDSCHMIDT and HARRISON had shown partial sexual transformation in moth hybrids. He recognized that genetic incompatibilities may result in inviability in hybrids, but did not offer a clear explanation of why the heterogametic sex would be affected more often. With regard to sexual transformation, he suggested that an imbalance of sex-determining factors would be less serious in the homogametic sex, since "the effect of the two Z or X chromosomes will be the average of the parental values."

Although the term "HALDANE's rule" has persisted in the evolutionary genetic literature for the past 75 years, HALDANE himself had very little to say about it after the 1922 paper. In his 1932 book, *The Causes of Evolution,* the rule was mentioned briefly, and a new explanation involving rearrangements of the sex chromosomes (discussed below) was offered. In two articles on the nature of genetic differences between species, sex-specific hybrid effects were not even mentioned (HALDANE 1929, 1938).

After HALDANE's 1922 paper, the development of ideas about the significance and causes of the rule proceeded slowly. There was a great deal of interest and work on the genetic basis of speciation in the 1930s and 1940s, but little attention was focused on the meaning of sex-specific hybrid dysfunction. Although DOBZHANSKY (1937a), in his classic book *Genetics and the Origin of Species,* briefly discussed HALDANE's rule and suggested a cytogenetic explanation based on sex chromosome rearrangements, this idea was not well developed either theoretically or empirically. In MAYR's 1942 book, *Systematics and the Origin of Species,* HALDANE's rule is not dealt with at all. WHITE (1945) suggested that deleterious X-Y interactions could be involved, but noted that this explanation would not apply to *XO* species. The most significant development during this period was MULLER's (1940, 1942) explanation of HALDANE's rule in terms of X-autosome imbalance.

Between the 1940s and the 1980s, HALDANE's rule continued to be a rather neglected topic. For example, in his 1970 book, DOBZHANSKY simply repeated the cytogenetic explanation offered in 1937 without further elaboration or evaluation. M. J. D. WHITE (1973) addressed HALDANE's rule and concluded that it "has so many exceptions that it can no longer be regarded as generally valid," but did not provide data to support this claim.

The stately pace of work on HALDANE's rule abruptly changed in the 1980s, with a remarkable burst of activity that continues to this day. Many of the new ideas have arisen from recent experimental results, while others involve a synthesis and interpretation of data that have accumulated throughout this century. It is the purpose of this article to review current views on the significance and causes of HALDANE's rule, while noting their historical roots wherever possible.

THE GENERALITY OF HALDANE'S RULE

Hybridization data from a vast number of animal species have accumulated steadily since HALDANE's rule was formulated in 1922, but much of this information is scattered and has not been analyzed systematically. However, COYNE (1992) and WU and DAVIS (1993) have provided summaries from four major groups: birds and Lepidopterans (butterflies and moths), which have female heterogamety, and mammals and Drosophila, which have male heterogamety. These summaries show a high degree of compliance with HALDANE's rule. Because this pattern cuts across phylogenetic boundaries (mammals *vs.* insects) and is clearly unrelated to sex per se, it appears to be caused by the difference between heterogametic *vs.* homogametic genotypes.

Recently, READ and NEE (1991) introduced the heretical thought that HALDANE's rule may not be directly related to heterogamety. They pointed out that the data previously summarized involve only four taxa, which require only two independent changes in which sex is heterogametic. Therefore, the association of sex-specific hybrid dysfunction with heterogamety might be due to chance rather than causation. In other words, there could be some property of birds and Lepidopterans other than female heterogamety that predisposes them to evolve female-specific hybrid dysfunction. In response to this suggestion, a few additional cases of HALDANE's rule have been noted in other taxa (COYNE *et al.* 1991; ORR 1997). In amphibians, female heterogamety seems to be ancestral, but Triturus is male heterogametic and follows HALDANE's rule (HILLIS and GREEN 1990; WHITE 1973, p. 558). Among reptiles, where there are cases of both male and female heterogamety, the genus Lacerta follows HALDANE's rule and shows female heterogamety (BULL 1983, p. 20; RYKENA 1991). Finally, the nematode Caenorhabditis has male heterogamety and also follows the rule (BAIRD *et al.* 1992). These cases, along with other hybridization data, are summarized in Table 1.

All of the groups listed in Table 1 show at least one case complying with HALDANE's rule, and those groups with many hybridizations on record show very few exceptions. Because the chromosomal basis of sex determination is variable within many groups (BULL 1983), male heterogamety probably evolved independently in mammals, insects, nematodes, and Triturus, while female heterogamety probably evolved independently in Lepidopterans, birds, and Lacerta. Therefore, it appears very likely that HALDANE's rule is due to heterogamety itself, rather than a chance association. Neverthe-

less, it is important to compile additional hybridization data from diverse groups and to further evaluate the phylogeny of sex chromosome variation. It might be particularly informative to have additional data for taxa like reptiles and amphibians that seem to show multiple changes in the direction of heterogamety. Additional insights might be obtained by comparing groups with different levels of heteromorphism between the two sex chromosomes.

HYPOTHESES ABOUT THE CAUSES OF HALDANE'S RULE

Because HALDANE's rule applies to several diverse animal taxa and is one of the broadest generalizations in evolutionary biology, an attempt has been made to identify a single cause that can account for all, or nearly all, cases. Therefore, in the past, several proposed explanations have been discounted because they do not apply across the board to all taxa or to both viability and sterility. However, in principle, the broad generality of HALDANE's rule could result from a combination of different factors, as repeatedly emphasized by C-I. WU (WU and DAVIS 1993; WU *et al.* 1996). An important consideration here is whether there are more factors that tend to cause heterogametic dysfunction than those causing homogametic dysfunction in any one group, even if some factors operate in one taxon (or on one trait), but not another. This possibility will be kept in mind during the following review of hypotheses.

Before explaining individual hypotheses, it is important to mention the concept of genic incompatibility as a cause of postzygotic isolation, since it forms an integral part of most hypotheses, either implicitly or explicitly. In a classic paper, DOBZHANSKY (1936) suggested that a general cause of hybrid dysfunction is due to "interactions between complementary genetic factors contributed by both parents. If the genetic constitution of one of the parental forms is SStt, and of the other ssTT, the hybrid is SsTt. The assumption is made that the presence of the factor (or the group of factors) S alone, or of the factor T alone, permits unlimited fertility, but that the factors S and T interact in such a manner as to make sterile an organism carrying them simultaneously." He went on to demonstrate such interactions in a very sophisticated genetic analysis of hybrid sterility between *Drosophila pseudoobscura* and *D. persimilis*. Although DOBZHANSKY was not the first to formalize this important concept of a complementary gene pair (ORR 1996), his views and experimental approach were widely recognized and influential.

The following hypotheses are discussed in an order related to the ideas involved rather than by historical precedence. These discussions draw heavily on an excellent series of previous review articles (COYNE and ORR 1989; COYNE 1992; WU and DAVIS 1993; WU and PALOPOLI 1994; WU *et al.* 1996; ORR 1997).

Sexual transformation: As mentioned above, HAL-

TABLE 1

Summary of sex-specific inviability and sterility in F hybrids

Group	Viability[a] $M_I F_V$	Viability[a] $M_V F_I$	Fertility[a] $M_S F_F$	Fertility[a] $M_F F_S$	Sex Determination[b]	Refs[c]
Vertebrates						
Mammalia					XX=F XY=M	1
Complete	0	0	10	0		
Partial	0	1	15	0		
Total	**0**	1	**25**	0		
Aves					ZW=F ZZ=M	1
Complete	2	10	0	14		
Partial	0	11	0	16		
Total	2	**21**	0	**30**		
Amphibia						
Triturus					XX=F XY=M	2
Complete	0	0	1	0		
Reptilia						
Lacerta					ZW=F ZZ=M	3
Complete	0	0	0	1		
Partial	0	0	0	2		
Total	0	0	0	**3**		
Insects						
Diptera						
Drosophila					XX=F XY=M	
Complete	**19**	4	**108**	1		4
Anopheles					XX=F XY=M	5
Complete	0	0	6	0		
Partial	3	1	0	0		
Total	**3**	1	**6**	0		
Glossina					XX=F XY=M	6
Complete	0	0	1	0		
Orthoptera					XX=F XO=M	7
Complete	3	0	1	0		
Partial	0	0	1	0		
Total	**3**	0	**2**	0		
Heteroptera					XX=F XO=M	8
Complete	0	1	6	0		
Partial	0	1	0	0		
Total	**0**	2	**6**	0		
Lepidoptera					ZW=F ZZ=M	9
Complete	1	48	1	12		
Partial	2	20	0	0		
Total	3	**68**	1	**12**		
Nematodes						
Caenorhabditis	**1**	0	0	0	XX=Herm XO=M	10

[a] The F_1 hybrids are between species, semispecies, subspecies or geographically separated populations within a species. Each number represents the outcome of a particular cross. Numbers shown in bold are consistent with HALDANE's rule. Reciprocal crosses are both counted. M, male; F, female; I, inviable; V, viable; S, sterile; F, fertile; Herm, hermaphrodite.

[b] The chromosomal sex determination given is characteristic of the group, but does not necessarily apply to every member. For example, some members of XY groups like Drosophila are XO, while some members of XO groups like the Orthopterans are XY. References: Mammalia, Aves, Lacertidae, Drosophila and Lepidoptera (BULL 1983, p. 17–20); Orthoptera (WHITE et al. 1977); Triturus (HILLIS and GREEN 1990); Anopheles (WHITE 1973, p. 368); Glossina (GOODING 1990); Heteroptera (WHITE 1973; p. 663); Caenorhabditis (BAIRD et al. 1992).

[c] Hybridization data references: 1, Mammalia and Aves (WU and DAVIS 1993); 2, Triturus (WHITE 1973, p. 558); 3, Lacerta (RYKENA 1991); 4, Drosophila references are from BOCK (1984), but original sources were consulted. Among the 19 cases of male inviability, 10 are based on quantitative data (x:0 where x > 5) and nine are based on qualitative statements about the absence of females and presence of males. Among the four cases of female inviability, two are based on quantitative data and two on qualitative data; 5, Anopheles (DAVIDSON 1974; HII 1985; KLEIN et al. 1984; LANZARO et al. 1988; ESTRADA-FRANCO et al. 1993; TAKAI et al. 1987; 6, Glossina (CURTIS 1972); 7, Orthoptera (HARVEY 1979; HEWITT et al. 1987; OHMACHI and MASAKI 1964; BIGELOW 1960; WHITE et al. 1977); 8, Heteroptera (SPENCE 1990; DAVIDSON 1974); 9, The data for Lepidoptera are from a literature survey to be published elsewhere. Among the 48 complete cases of female inviability, 31 are based on quantitative data (0:x where x > 5) and 17 are based on qualitative statements about the absence of females and presence of males. The one case of male inviability is quantitative (27:0). (For the partial cases listed, there is a significant deviation from a 1:1 sex ratio ($P < 0.05$, two-tailed). A similar data set was summarized by WU and DAVIS (1993); 10, Caenorhabditis (BAIRD et al. 1992).

DANE (1922) noted that the absence of one sex in hybrid offspring might be owing to sexual transformation rather than inviability. This idea was inspired by a few observations of intersexes in hybrids between some Lepidopteran species. Later, GOLDSCHMIDT (1934) suggested that half of the all-male progeny from crosses between certain races of *Lymantria dispar* are completely transformed *ZW* (normally female) individuals. However, this suggestion was not supported by CLARKE and FORD (1982), who repeated some of GOLDSCHMIDT's crosses and found that all of the phenotypically male hybrids lack the heterochromatic *W* chromosome found in normal females. So, although many Lepidopteran hybridizations do produce intersexual progeny (ROBINSON 1971, pp. 34, 472), it is not clear whether complete sexual transformation occurs or contributes to HALDANE's rule.

In any case, sexual transformation cannot be a general explanation of HALDANE's rule, since inviability rather than transformation of the heterogametic sex has been demonstrated in many cases. For example, STURTEVANT (1920) showed that, in the cross between *Drosophila melanogaster* females and *D. simulans* males, male hybrids die as larvae and adult female hybrids are all *XX* (based on *X*-linked markers). Furthermore, intersexes are very rare in Drosophila hybrids (PATTERSON and STONE 1952, p. 552). Nevertheless, this factor warrants further investigation, since at least partial transformations occur in some avian and mammalian hybrids, as well as Lepidopterans (WHITE 1945, p. 225; EICHER *et al.* 1982).

Dosage compensation: In Drosophila, dosage compensation occurs by hyperactivation of the *X* chromosome in the heterogametic male, and mutations that interfere with this process cause male-specific lethality (CLINE and MEYER 1996). Sex chromosome-autosome fusions have clearly initiated the evolution of dosage compensation in the neo-*X* chromosomes of some Drosophila species (LUCCHESI 1978), possibly resulting in genic imbalance in interspecific hybrid males (discussed below). It is also possible that the dosage compensation system itself may evolve, even in the absence of sex chromosome rearrangements. Therefore, one potential contribution to HALDANE's rule in Drosophila is a breakdown of dosage compensation in male hybrids (COYNE and ORR 1989).

This hypothesis was evaluated in a very clever experiment by ORR (1989a). In the cross between *D. melanogaster* females and normal *D. simulans* males, male hybrids are inviable while female hybrids are viable but sterile. The normally inviable hybrid males can be rescued by using the Lhr stock of *simulans* (WATANABE 1979). Orr used a mutation of the master control gene *Sxl* to override the initial step in dosage compensation, which is interpretation of the *X:A* ratio. This intervention did not rescue male viability in the cross with normal *simulans* males, nor did it rescue fertility in males from the Lhr *simulans* cross. These results indicate that,

if a breakdown in dosage compensation causes hybrid male inviability, it does not result from steps upstream of *Sxl*. However, it is still possible that a breakdown occurs downstream of *Sxl*. In addition, it is not clear whether male fertility should have been rescued, since whether or how dosage compensation occurs in the germline is unknown (CLINE and MEYER 1996).

Nevertheless, breakdown in dosage compensation is not a good candidate for a general explanation of HALDANE's rule for two reasons. First, as noted by COYNE and ORR (1989), there is some evidence that dosage compensation does not even occur in birds and Lepidopterans (BAVERSTOCK *et al.* 1982; JOHNSON and TURNER 1979). Second, one might expect a breakdown in dosage compensation to affect the homogametic more than the heterogametic sex in some cases. Unlike Drosophila, compensation occurs actively in the homogametic sex in mammals (by inactivation of one *X*; LYON 1961) and in Caenorhabditis (by hypoactivation of the two *X* chromosomes in hermaphrodites; CLINE and MEYER 1996).

Chromosomal rearrangements: HALDANE (1932, p. 75) suggested another possible explanation involving rearrangements of the sex chromosomes. He cited an experimentally induced reciprocal *X-Y* translocation in Drosophila and noted that, in the cross between normal females and males having the translocation, male offspring are sterile because they lack part of the *Y*. At this time, HALDANE thought such rearrangements might be a common cause of the rule. However, this explanation appears unlikely to account for many cases because this type of reciprocal translocation (unlike Robertsonian fusion) would be very difficult to fix within a population (PATTERSON and STONE 1952, pp. 164, 170). Furthermore, some species with *XO* males obey HALDANE's rule (Table 1), which specifically excludes *X-Y* translocation as a mechanism.

DOBZHANSKY (1937a,b) suggested that changes in autosomal *vs.* sex linkage might account for HALDANE's rule. This idea was inspired by crosses between *D. pseudoobscura* and *D. miranda*, which produce inviable males in one direction and morphologically abnormal males in the other, while the female hybrids are viable and morphologically normal. *D. miranda* has a Robertsonian *Y*-autosome fusion, resulting in two *X* chromosomes, one homologous to the single *X* and the other to the third chromosome of *pseudoobscura*. This type of rearrangement does not, in itself, cause duplications or deficiencies in male hybrids. However, in *miranda*, degeneration of the *Y*-linked autosomal material has occurred, along with dosage compensation in most of the neo-*X* (STROBEL *et al.* 1978; STEINEMANN *et al.* 1993). As a result, hybrid males are expected to have either a deficient or an excess level of chromosome *3*-homologous gene expression, relative to the level in homospecific males. DOBZHANSKY did not use the term dosage compensation, but he seems to imply its evolution by stating that the genotype of *D. miranda* has been adjusted by natural selection so that its neo-*X* chromosome is no longer compatible with the autosomes of *pseudoobscura* in hybrid males (and vice versa), while there is no such problem in hybrid females.

Although sex chromosome rearrangement is a potential cause of HALDANE's rule, it appears to be a minimal factor in Drosophila, since many species pairs that do not differ in sex chromosome karyotype show HALDANE's rule. Furthermore, *X*-autosome translocations (other than fusions) are very rare or absent as fixed species differences (PATTERSON and STONE 1952, p. 164). Similarly, *X*-autosome exchanges are rare in mammalian evolution (CHARLESWORTH *et al.* 1987, Appendix).

Y chromosome incompatibilities: A major difference between the heterogametic and homogametic sexes of most species in Table 1 is the occurrence in the former of a largely heterochromatic *Y* (or *W*) chromosome. Therefore, an obvious hypothesis is that *Y-X* or *Y*-autosome incompatibilities contribute to HALDANE's rule (MULLER 1942; WHITE 1945). Several genetic analyses of sterility in hybrids between Drosophila races or species have addressed this issue. In some cases a significant *Y* effect was found, while in others the *Y* appears to play little or no role in hybrid sterility. Significant *Y* effects have been found in hybrids between geographic races of *D. micromelanica* (STURTEVANT and NOVITSKI 1941), between *D. texana* and *D. virilis* (PATTERSON *et al.* 1942; ORR and COYNE 1989; LAMNISSOU *et al.* 1996), between *D. mojavensis* and *D. arizonensis* (VIGNEAULT and ZOUROS 1986; PANTAZIDIS and ZOUROS 1988), and between *D. hydei* and *D. neohydei* (HENNIG 1977; SCHÄFER 1978). In contrast, the *Y* of *D. sechellia* has only subtle effects on male fertility when introgressed into *D. simulans* (JOHNSON *et al.* 1993; ZENG and SINGH 1993). Similarly, there is no detectable effect of the *Y* on sterility in hybrids between *D. virilis* and *D. novomexicana* (ORR and COYNE 1989) or between geographic races of *D. pseudoobscura* (ORR 1989b).

In Drosophila species, the *Y* chromosome is usually required for fertility within a species, as indicated by complete sterility of *XO* males in 17 of 22 species tested (and impaired fertility in others). However, the *Y* generally is not required for viability, since *XO* males are viable in 22 of 23 species tested (VOELKER and KOJIMA 1971). Therefore, one might expect *Y* incompatibilities to contribute to HALDANE's rule for sterility, but not for inviability. So it is not surprising that there are no reports of a *Y* effect on hybrid male viability. There is little evidence concerning the *Y* chromosome in other groups, but if Drosophila species are representative, *Y* incompatibilities frequently (but not always) play an important role in HALDANE's rule for sterility, but do not help explain the rule for inviability.

Meiotic drive: FRANK (1991a) and HURST and POMIANKOWSKI (1991) have suggested that the divergence of meiotic drive systems between species may contribute to the observance of HALDANE's rule. Their argument is briefly as follows: Population genetic theory indicates that the sex chromosomes are particularly susceptible to the rapid evolution of meiotic drive systems, and sex ratio distorters have been found in a number of Dipteran, Lepidopteran, and mammalian species. These distorters frequently have deleterious consequences, leading to rapid evolution of suppressors. When two species, each with a different suppressed system, hybridize, the *X* and *Y* chromosomes in the heterogametic hybrid may drive against each other, leading to sterility. Dysfunctional sex chromosome interactions may even lead to inviability.

This intriguing suggestion has been vigorously attacked (COYNE *et al.* 1991; JOHNSON and WU 1992; CHARLESWORTH *et al.* 1993; COYNE and ORR 1993) and defended (FRANK 1991b; POMIANKOWSKI and HURST 1993). The most persuasive criticism is that there is no evidence that sex ratio distortion occurs in partially fertile hybrids, in spite of several attempts to detect it (JOHNSON and WU 1992; COYNE and ORR 1993). In response, FRANK (1991b) and POMIANKOWSKI and HURST (1993) suggest that drivers unleashed in hybrids are more likely to result in a breakdown of gametogenesis than in drive. Nevertheless, there is still no direct empirical evidence that mutually destructive drive systems contribute to hybrid sterility or inviability.

The dominance theory: Like DOBZHANSKY, MULLER (1940, 1942) viewed hybrid sterility and inviability as a consequence of negative interactions between "complementary genes." MULLER (1942) gave the following example. An ancestral population has the genotype *aabb*, which evolves to *AAbb* in one daughter species and to *aaBB* in the other. When *A* and *B* come together in the *AaBb* hybrid, they may produce a harmful effect, provided that their interaction is not fully recessive. If one of the complementary genes is located in the *X* chromosome, even a completely recessive interaction will produce the harmful effect in the heterogametic sex. For example, the hybrid genotype *AYBb* may be harmful while *AaBb* is not, if the presence of the *a* allele provides protection from the potentially harmful effects of the *A-B* interaction. Therefore, heterogametic hybrids are expected to be affected by more deleterious interactions than the homogametic hybrids. MULLER (1942, p. 89) concluded that "the high frequency of this type of situation is attested to by the widespread applicability of HALDANE's rule . . . ."

MULLER's idea is often called the "*X*-autosome imbalance" hypothesis because he suggested that *X* chromosome genes, when hemizygous in the male, are "especially apt to meet with disharmonies of functioning" in their interactions with autosomal genes (MULLER 1940). Homogametic hybrids have an *X* and autosome from each species (a balanced genotype), while males have an *X* from only one species (unbalanced). This notion of *X*-autosome imbalance was foreshadowed by statements of HALDANE (1922) and DOBZHANSKY (1937a), but MULLER was the first to express it clearly in terms of dominance and recessivity.

MULLER's hypothesis is very important, since it has a generality that is lacking in nearly all of the other hypotheses to explain HALDANE's rule. In principle, it applies equally well to all taxonomic groups, to both male and female heterogamety and to both inviability and sterility. Recently, it was formalized in the development of a simple mathematical model by ORR and TU-RELLI (ORR 1993a; TURELLI and ORR 1995; ORR and TURELLI 1996), referred to as the dominance theory. In the following description of this model, the heterogametic sex will be referred to as male and the homogametic sex as female.

The simplest form of the model directly addresses the difference in sex chromosomal genotypes, while assuming that there is no sex difference in the number of incompatibility factors or in their magnitudes of effect when hemizygous in the male or homozygous in the female. In TURELLI and ORR (1995), each X-autosomal (X-A) incompatibility contributes to an additive scale of hybrid breakdown (S), which maps onto fitness by a nonincreasing function. In males, the contribution to breakdown of the kth X-linked allele from species i (where $i = 1$ or 2) is $b_i(k)$, and the contribution of autosomal-autosomal interactions is ν. The breakdown score of hybrid males (S_m) is given by Equation 1, where n_i is the number of incompatibilities due to X_i.

$$S_m = \sum_{k=1}^{n_i} b_i(k) + \nu \qquad (1)$$

In females, alleles on both X chromosomes contribute to the breakdown, h is the degree of dominance of the X-A interaction in hybrids, and X-X interactions are ignored. The breakdown score of hybrid females (S_f) is given by Equation 2.

$$S_m = \sum_{k=1}^{n_1} b_1(k) h_1(k) + \sum_{k=1}^{n_2} b_2(k) h_2(k) + \nu \qquad (2)$$

HALDANE's rule is favored when $S_m > S_f$. It is clear that a sufficient condition for this inequality is that $h_i(k) < \frac{1}{2}$ for all i and k. In other words, HALDANE's rule will occur if the interactions causing hybrid breakdown are always partially recessive. In addition, TURELLI and ORR (1995) showed that the rule may also hold under less restrictive conditions, depending on n_1, n_2, the distribution of h values, and the covariance of h and b.

A very important result of this analysis was the realization (apparently missed by MULLER) that while hybrid females suffer less than males from each X-A incompatibility (unless it is fully dominant), the presence of two X chromosomes entails twice as many X-A incompatibilities. Thus, additive incompatibilities ($h = \frac{1}{2}$) affect males and females equally, partially recessive ones ($h < \frac{1}{2}$) affect males more than females, while partially dominant ones ($h > \frac{1}{2}$) affect females more than males. Thus, the mere existence of *some* recessive incompatibilities will not necessarily produce HALDANE's rule. They must be recessive on average and/or there must be a tendency for recessive incompatibilities to have greater hemi/homozygous effects (ORR 1993a; TURELLI and ORR 1995). The latter is not unexpected, since within a species, deleterious mutations with large effects tend to be more recessive than those with small effects (SIMMONS and CROW 1977).

Incidentally, HALDANE probably would be very pleased about the fact that this important insight was made while developing a mathematical model of MULLER's verbal argument. Had it been discovered earlier, he might have referred to it in *A Defense of Beanbag Genetics* (HALDANE 1964), a paper in which he defended against an attack by MAYR (1963) on the contributions of population genetic theory. The ORR and TURELLI model is a good example of HALDANE's general point that "not only is algebraic reasoning exact; it imposes an exactness on the verbal postulates made before algebra can start which is usually lacking in the first verbal formulations of scientific principles."

Experimental tests of the dominance theory: Before the development of the mathematical dominance theory, COYNE (1985) performed an important experimental test of the X-autosome imbalance hypothesis, which is summarized in Figure 1a. In the cross of regular *D. simulans* females to either *D. mauritiana* or *D. sechellia* males, male hybrids (genotype 2) are completely sterile, while female hybrids (genotype 1) are fertile. COYNE reasoned that if the sterility of male hybrids is caused by X-autosome imbalance due to hemizygosity of the X chromosome, then unbalanced female hybrids that are homozygous for the same X chromosome should be equally sterile. These unbalanced females were produced through the clever use of an attached-X stock of *D. simulans* (genotype 4) and found to be fertile. COYNE concluded that the X-autosome imbalance hypothesis (which entails recessivity of incompatibilities) could be rejected.

Several years later, this interpretation of the unbalanced female experiment was called into question by ORR (1993b) and by WU and DAVIS (1993), who noted that it fails to consider the fact that male and female fertility are controlled by largely different sets of genes (LINDSLEY and TOKUYASU 1980) that may evolve at different rates. Therefore, the fact that the unbalanced males are sterile, while the unbalanced females are fertile, may reflect a different number of X-autosome incompatibilities affecting male *vs.* female fertility, rather than a lack of recessivity.

ORR (1993b) and WU and DAVIS (1993) noted that the unbalanced female test would be more informative for hybrid inviability than for sterility, since viability genes do not generally have sex-specific effects. Interestingly, the result of one such unbalanced female test for viability has been known for some time (STURTEVANT 1920; BIDDLE 1932; repeated by HUTTER *et al.* 1990; ORR 1993b). When *D. melanogaster* females are crossed with

a. Attached-X experiments

X chromosome genotype of F_1 hybrid		*simulans* ♀ x *mauritiana* or *sechellia* ♂	*melanogaster* ♀ x *simulans* or *mauritiana* ♂	*simulans* ♀ x *teissieri* ♂
(1)	regular female	fertile	viable	viable
(2)	male	sterile	inviable	inviable
(3)	male	sterile	viable	inviable
(4)	$\overset{\wedge}{XX}$ female	fertile	inviable	inviable
	reference	a	b	c

FIGURE 1.—Summary of Drosophila experiments in which male and female hybrids of equivalent genotype are compared. (a) The white chromosomes are from the female parent and the black are from the male parent. Genotypes (1) and (2) represent hybrid progeny from regular females, while (3) and (4) are from attached-*X* females. The *Y* chromosome in Drosophila typically has no effect on female viability or fertility. References are as follows: a, COYNE (1985); b, BIDDLE (1932), HUTTER *et al.* (1990), and ORR (1993b); and c, ORR (1993b). (b) The white chromosomes are from *D. pseudoobscura* and the black are from *D. persimilis*; data from ORR (1987). (c) The white chromosomes are from *D. simulans* and the black segments are from *D. mauritiana*; data from TRUE *et al.* (1996).

b. Backcross hybrids

F_1 (*pseudoobscura* ♀ x *persimilis* ♂) ♀ x *pseudoobscura* ♂

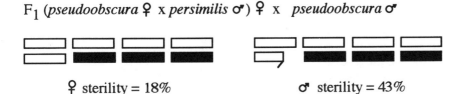

♀ sterility = 18% ♂ sterility = 43%

c. Introgression lines - *mauritiana* into *simulans*

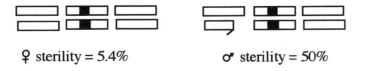

♀ sterility = 5.4% ♂ sterility = 50%

D. simulans males, regular female hybrids of genotype X_mX_s are viable, but X_mY_s males are inviable. In this case, the unbalanced female hybrids ($X_mX_mY_s$) are also inviable (compare genotypes 2 and 4 in Figure 1a). These unbalanced male and female hybrids probably die from the same causes, since they are both rescued by the *Hybrid male rescue* (*Hmr*) mutation (HUTTER *et al.* 1990). A similar result was obtained in an unbalanced female test involving hybrid inviability in the cross between *D. simulans* and *D. teissieri* (ORR 1993b; see Figure 1a).

The unbalanced female results for viability are consistent with the notion that *X*-autosome incompatibilities are recessive or partially recessive on the average. However, we also must consider whether these results are necessarily inconsistent with the hypothesis of additivity or partial dominance. A regular female suffers from *X*-*A* incompatibilities due to alleles fixed in both parental species, while a male suffers from those fixed in a single parental species. Asymmetry between parents in the number (n_i) and magnitude of effects (b_i) is expected and frequently observed in the form of male-specific inviability or sterility in one cross, but not in the reciprocal (WU and BECKENBACH 1983; ORR 1995). This asymmetry can complicate the interpretation of an unbalanced female test.

For the purpose of illustration, assume that there is no variation in the $b_i(k)$ or the $h_i(k)$ in Equations 1 and 2 above. Then if $n_1 > n_2$, recessivity is not required to have the breakdown score of the X_1Y_2 male or the $X_1X_1Y_2$ unbalanced female greater than that of the X_1X_2 regular females [i.e., $(n_1b + \nu) > ((n_1 + n_2)hb + \nu)$]. In fact, this situation will occur whenever $n_1/(n_1 + n_2) > h$. In other words, HALDANE's rule (and a positive unbalanced female test) in one particular cross can occur when $h > \frac{1}{2}$, provided that there is sufficient asymmetry in the contributions of two parental species. However, recessivity is required to get HALDANE's rule in both reciprocal crosses.

Figure 1a shows that asymmetry in the contributions of the two X chromosomes applies to the test involving *D. melanogaster* and *simulans*, in which the unbalanced female is homozygous for the X chromosome from *melanogaster* ($X_mX_mY_s$). The hybrid male X_mY_s is inviable, but the reciprocal male X_sY_m (with the same cytoplasm) is viable, indicating that X_m carries a greater load of incompatibility factors than X_s. [The Y chromosome has no effect on viability in these hybrids (YAMAMOTO 1992).] Therefore, this particular test, while consistent with recessivity, does not rule out additivity or partial dominance. In contrast, both types of hybrid male are inviable in the cross between *D. simulans* and *teissieri*. So, the unbalanced female test in this case can be explained only by recessivity, under the assumption that all incompatibilities causing inviability affect males and females of equivalent genotype equally.

This analysis suggests that hybridizations showing HALDANE's rule for viability in both reciprocal crosses of one species pair provide strong evidence for recessivity (in the absence of sex-specific incompatibilities). Unfortunately, the desired data are scanty, since the viability in hybrids from both crosses is usually unknown because both crosses were not performed, sexual isolation prevented one cross, or inviability of both sexes was not distinguished from prezygotic isolation. In the Drosophila data summarized in Table 1, there are nine species pairs for which hybrid viability is known in both crosses and for which at least one cross shows HALDANE's rule. Among those nine, only one pair shows HALDANE's rule in both crosses. To that can be added the *D. simulans/teissieri* pair described above (not included in the survey of Table 1). Another five of the nine species pairs have male-specific inviability in one cross with inviability of both sexes in the other cross. These cases show a reciprocal difference in hybrid female viability, indicating cytoplasmic- or maternal-zygotic incompatibility (to be discussed below), which is not considered by the dominance theory. Therefore, it may be reasonable to include these five as cases of reciprocal male-specific zygotic inviability, which would bring the total to seven. In the Lepidopteran data there are 18 species pairs with results from both crosses that show HALDANE's rule for at least one cross. Among

those 18, five also show HALDANE's rule in the reciprocal cross.

Therefore, the hypothesis that X-A incompatibilities affecting viability are generally partially recessive is supported by five Lepidopteran species pairs and by at least two (and perhaps seven) Drosophila species pairs. An alternative hypothesis is that X-A incompatibilities are generally partially dominant. This alternative would be supported by the finding of species pairs in which there is homogametic sex-specific inviability in both reciprocal crosses. No such cases were found among the Lepidopterans or Drosophila. However, there is one partial case of this nature in the Heteropteran species pair *Limnoporus notablis* × *L. dissortis*, which has XO males. In one cross the sex ratio was 92 males:zero females and in the other cross 37 males:six females (SPENCE 1990). Thus, at this point, the results of reciprocal crosses favor partial recessivity much more than partial dominance, although such evidence is clearly indirect.

Unfortunately, there is very little direct evidence concerning the dominance of incompatibilities. In some cases, the fact that introgressed chromosomal segments frequently are viable and fertile when heterozygous, but inviable or sterile when homozygous (TRUE *et al.* 1996) has been taken as evidence for recessivity (*e.g.*, BARTON 1996; ORR 1997). However, this result indicates only that the factor(s) contained in those segments are not completely dominant. Quantitative measures of fertility are required to determine whether these factors have a dominance parameter greater or less than one half, which is the critical question in determining whether males having one set of hemizygous X-A incompatibilities are worse off than females having two sets of heterozygous X-A incompatibilities.

One quantitative study of dominance supports the recessivity of incompatibility factors. ORR (1992) measured the fertility of males having a *D. simulans* fourth chromosome either homozygous or heterozygous in an otherwise *D. melanogaster* genetic background. While homozygotes for the *simulans* fourth are completely sterile, heterozygotes have a fertility level comparable to pure *melanogaster* controls.

Rapid evolution of hybrid male sterility: WU and DAVIS (1993) suggested the idea that HALDANE's rule for sterility in Drosophila may be explained by a more rapid rate of evolution of factors that cause hybrid male sterility than those that cause female sterility. Several different experiments support this hypothesis.

As noted earlier, the attached-X experiment of COYNE (1985) involving *D. simulans* and *mauritiana* revealed that $X_sX_sY_m$ hybrid females are fertile, while the genotypically equivalent X_sY_m males are sterile. This experiment clearly shows that the X of *simulans* has an insufficient number of incompatibility factors to cause female sterility even when those factors are made homozygous in a hybrid background. In contrast, the introgression experiments of WU and his collaborators have shown that this X chromosome has many different factors that contribute to hybrid male sterility (WU and PALOPOLI 1994).

A backcross experiment involving *D. pseudoobscura* and *persimilis* also supports a difference between the sexes in the number of incompatibilities affecting fertility (ORR 1987). By making use of mutant markers and inversions that restrict crossing over on the *X*, second, and third chromosomes, genotypes were constructed that closely resemble F₁ hybrids except for homozygosity of the *X* in females (Figure 1b). This comparison of nearly equivalent male and female genotypes shows that males are significantly more sterile than females (43% *vs.* 18%).

Introgression experiments have provided very strong evidence that autosomal factors causing male sterility have accumulated more rapidly than those causing female sterility. In one experiment (TRUE *et al.* 1996), segments of the *D. mauritiana* genome were introgressed into a *simulans* background and made homozygous, producing males and females of equivalent genotype (Figure 1c). In total, 65 autosomal positions were marked with *P*-element insertions, and replicate introgressions were made by repeated backcrossing to *simulans* for 15 generations, providing introgressed segments with an average length of 9.4 cM (about 7% of the genome). An average of 5.4% of replicate lines per insert location were female sterile, compared with 50% for male sterility. One possible caveat in this result is that introgressions were made through heterozygous females, so there could have been some selection against partially dominant female sterility factors during the course of the experiment. However, HOLLOCHER and WU (1996) obtained similar results by backcrossing mainly through heterozygous males rather than females. In this experiment, three large segments of the *mauritiana* or *sechellia* second chromosome were introgressed into *simulans* and made homozygous. In both cases, there were much higher levels of male than female sterility.

The dominance theory has been generalized to accommodate sex differences in the numbers and effects of factors causing incompatibilities, as well as variation in the proportion of incompatibilities attributable to the *X* chromosome (TURELLI and ORR 1995; ORR and TURELLI 1996). In this extension, τ represents the ratio of the cumulative effects of incompatibilities affecting hybrids of the heterogametic sex to those affecting the homogametic sex, p_x represents the fraction of incompatibilities involving *X*-linked loci, and d is a dominance parameter similar to h (assumed to be equal for males and females). (The quantity d equals the expected value of h when the covariance between h and b is zero.) HALDANE's rule is satisfied on the average given the following inequality:

$$d < \frac{\tau p_x}{2[1 - \tau(1 - p_x)]} \tag{3}$$

As noted above, when $\tau = 1$ (*i.e.*, no difference in num-

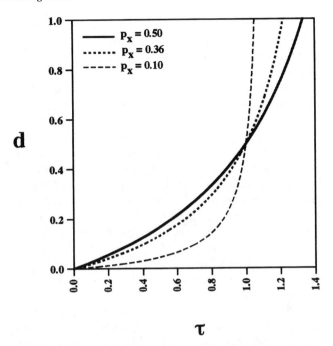

FIGURE 2.—Plot of the relationship in equation line (3) redrawn from ORR and TURELLI (1996). The variable d is a dominance parameter, τ is the ratio of the cumulative effects of incompatibilities affecting hybrids of the heterogametic sex to those affecting the homogametic sex, and p_x is the fraction of incompatibilities involving *X*-linked loci. HALDANE's rule is favored for coordinates below the curve and disfavored above.

ber or effects of male and female factors), a sufficient condition for HALDANE's rule is that the incompatibility factors are recessive or partially recessive ($d < \frac{1}{2}$), regardless of what fraction of the effects are *X*-linked (provided that $p_x > 0$). The effect of variation in τ is illustrated in Figure 2. When $\tau > 1$ (greater effects on the heterogametic than homogametic sex), HALDANE's rule can hold even for complete dominance. As noted by TURELLI and ORR (1995), τ need only be greater than 1.22 to produce HALDANE's rule when $d = 1.0$ and $p_x = 0.36$ (as in *D. simulans* for two locus incompatibilites). Therefore, when factors affecting the heterogametic sex evolve substantially more rapidly than those affecting the homogametic sex, HALDANE's rule is favored regardless of the degree of dominance. However, when $\tau < 1$, hybrid fitnesses that favor HALDANE's rule are obtained only when incompatibility factors are very recessive.

The observation that male sterility factors appear to evolve more rapidly than female factors in Drosophila clearly favors the occurrence of HALDANE's rule in this group, which has heterogametic males. However, if male sterility factors also evolve more rapidly in groups with heterogametic females (such as the Lepidopterans), this process works against the occurrence of HALDANE's rule (but will not prevent it if the incompatibilities are sufficiently recessive). On the other hand, it is possible that factors causing sterility of the heterogametic sex (whether male or female) evolve more rapidly, which could provide an explanation of HALDANE's rule for sterility that applies to both male and female heterogametic species. Three hypotheses have been suggested to account for a sex difference in the rate of evolution of sterility factors.

1. Sexual selection for male reproductive characters: WU and DAVIS (1993) summarized evidence indicating that various male reproductive characters tend to evolve rapidly, perhaps through some form of sexual selection. If the process of spermatogenesis also evolves rapidly, a possible result is the more frequent occurrence of hybrid male than female sterility. This process would favor HALDANE's rule in male heterogametic species like Drosophila, but work against it in female heterogametic species like Lepidopterans. Genetic experiments similar to those done with Drosophila are needed to determine whether Lepidopterans have a higher rate of evolution of male than female sterility factors, as expected under this hypothesis.

2. Special features of gametogenesis: WU and DAVIS (1993) also suggested that hybrid male sterility might evolve rapidly because of special features of spermatogenesis in species with heterogametic males. One important feature is that there appears to be very little or no transcription after meiosis in Drosophila or the mouse (FULLER 1993). The lack of transcriptional regulation during spermiogenesis might cause the system to be very sensitive to an imbalance of gene products in hybrids. Another special feature is the precocious inactivation of the X chromosome relative to the autosomes, which has been observed in many different species with heterogametic males (LIFSCHYTZ and LINDSLEY 1972). Interference with this allocycly is thought to be the reason why a majority of X-autosome translocations in Drosophila and in mice are dominant male steriles, while having no effect on females, even when homozygous. In addition, autosomal rearrangements in mice have much greater deleterious effects on male than female fertility (MATSUDA and CHAPMAN 1994; GROPP *et al.* 1982). This effect may be due to association of asynapsed autosomal segments with the X chromosome, which interferes with X inactivation and/or crossing over between the X and Y, both of which appear to be important for the successful completion of spermatogenesis (MATSUDA and CHAPMAN 1994). Mammalian species frequently differ by autosomal rearrangements that might contribute disproportionately to hybrid male sterility through this type of mechanism (GROPP *et al.* 1982).

Most arguments concerning the special features of gametogenesis apply only to spermatogenesis in species with heterogametic males, which obviously limits the generality as an explanation of HALDANE's rule. However, JABLONKA and LAMB (1991) have suggested that conformational changes in the sex chromosomes in both heterogametic males and in heterogametic females may contribute to HALDANE's rule. They point out that the W chromosome in birds and Lepidopterans, which is heterochromatic in somatic cells, under-

goes decondensation prior to meiosis (JABLONKA and LAMB 1988). They further suggest that problems in this decondensation process could lead to hybrid female sterility. However, they also point out that decondensation of the somatically inactive X occurs in the oogenesis of mammals, even though they are homogametic rather than heterogametic. They suggest that this might lead to mammals obeying HALDANE's rule less frequently than Drosophila, in which the X in females behaves no differently from the autosomes. However, the hybridization data in Table 1 do not support this suggestion.

HALDANE's rule obviously is favored if gametogenesis is more sensitive to genic imbalance or chromosomal rearrangement in the heterogametic than in the homogametic sex. Although there is some evidence that this may be the case in heterogametic males, there is very little, if any, evidence for it in heterogametic females.

3. Rapid evolution of advantageous X-linked recessives: There has been a great deal of discussion in the literature about whether the X chromosome has a greater effect on hybrid incompatibility than the autosomes, how such a difference may have evolved, and how it contributes to HALDANE's rule (*e.g.,* CHARLESWORTH *et al.* 1987; COYNE and ORR 1989; WU and DAVIS 1993). Some digression into the history of these issues is helpful in explaining how a difference in the density of incompatibility factors affecting males and females may evolve owing to selection on advantageous recessive mutations that occur on the X chromosome.

A common experimental design in genetic studies of hybrid male sterility in Drosophila is the standard backcross analysis, which was introduced by DOBZHANSKY (1936). In this design, females with markers on each chromosome are crossed to unmarked males of another species, the heterozygous hybrid females are backcrossed to males of the multiply marked species, and male progeny genotypes are analyzed for differences in sterility level. A general result from studies of this kind is that segregation of the X chromosome appears to have a much larger effect on male sterility than segregation of any of the autosomes (COYNE and ORR 1989). This "large X effect" may be due to a higher density of sterility factors on the X chromosome and/or to a greater expression of recessive X-linked factors owing to their hemizygosity (COYNE and ORR 1989; WU and DAVIS 1993). The relative importance of these two factors in explaining the large X effect in backcross experiments is still unknown. (see TRUE *et al.* 1996; HOLLOCHER and WU 1996; and ORR 1997 for further discussion.)

The possibility that there might be a higher density of X than autosomal incompatibility factors stimulated some theory concerning how such a difference might evolve. In an extension of some early theoretical work of HALDANE (1924), CHARLESWORTH *et al.* (1987) analyzed the conditions under which the rate of substitution of new mutations may differ between the X and autosomes. For favorable mutations that affect the fitness of both sexes, they found that substitution proceeds more rapidly on the *X* when the mutations are recessive or partially recessive on the average. This result indicates that an *X*-autosome difference in density of incompatibility factors can be explained by assuming that most of the fixed differences between species that cause incompatibility originate as recessive advantageous mutations within each of the two parental populations.

(By the way, it is important to distinguish between the dominance of a mutation in the pure species population in which it evolves and the dominance of an incompatibility interaction in an interspecific hybrid. The two dominance parameters may be quite different.)

The mathematical model of TURELLI and ORR (1995) can be used to explore how the relative densities of incompatibility factors on the *X vs.* autosomes may contribute to HALDANE's rule. In this model, p_x is the proportion of incompatibilities involving *X*-linked loci (as opposed to autosomal-autosomal incompatibilities), which is assumed to be the same for both sexes. Figure 2 shows that the effect of p_x depends on the degree of dominance of the incompatibility. For partially recessive factors, increasing p_x favors the occurrence of HALDANE's rule, while for partially dominant factors, it has the opposite effect. When $d = 1/2$, there is no effect. The heterogametic sex suffers less from *X*-linked dominants than the homogametic sex, because the latter has two *X* chromosomes and therefore twice as many incompatibilities. However, the heterogametic sex suffers more from recessives because those effects are sheltered by heterozygosity in the homogametic sex.

This analysis shows that having a greater density of incompatibility factors on the *X vs.* autosomes does not, in itself, have a direct effect on the occurrence of HALDANE's rule. However, the advantageous recessive theory that explains an *X*-autosomal difference can also account for a difference in the density of *X*-linked incompatibility factors that affect males *vs.* females. When some *X*-linked recessives have a sex-specific advantage, those mutations favored in the heterogametic sex will be fixed more rapidly than those favored in the homogametic sex (CHARLESWORTH *et al.* 1987; COYNE and ORR 1989, Appendix). Therefore, this mechanism will favor the occurrence of HALDANE's rule in both male and female heterogametic species. It is most likely to contribute to HALDANE's rule for fertility, since mutations affecting fertility are very likely to have a sex-specific advantage. However, it also may contribute to HALDANE's rule for viability, since not all viability mutations will have the same effect on both sexes.

If this mechanism contributes to HALDANE's rule for fertility in Drosophila, there ought to be an *X*-autosomal difference in the density of male sterility factors. The most direct approach to detecting such a difference is to compare hemizygous *X* introgressions with homozygous autosomal introgressions, so as to avoid complications

due to the possible recessivity of incompatibility factors. Such a comparison has been made for segments of the *D. mauritiana* genome introgressed into a *D. simulans* genetic background. TRUE *et al.* (1996) found that *X* introgressions are more likely to cause male sterility than autosomal introgressions. However, a difference in the size of introgressed segments as a possible explanation of the apparent density difference could not be ruled out. HOLLOCHER and WU (1996) reported that large introgressions on both the *X* and second chromosome cause male sterility, but the large sizes of the segments being compared limit the ability to detect an *X*-autosome difference. Therefore, this issue requires further investigation.

EXCEPTIONS TO HALDANE'S RULE

In principle, there are two situations that would generally favor the occurrence of exceptions to HALDANE's rule in both male and female heterogametic species. As mentioned earlier, when *X*-autosomal incompatibilities are partially dominant, the homogametic sex is affected more severely since they have two *X* chromosomes and therefore twice as many such incompatibilities. A second situation is the occurrence of *X*–*X* incompatibilities. Both of these cases should give an exception to HALDANE's rule in both of the reciprocal crosses between a given pair of species. It has already been noted that no cases of reciprocal exception have been found among the many hybridizations summarized in Table 1, except for the Heteropteran pondskater Limnoporus. Therefore, neither of these situations appears to be a common cause of hybrid inviability or sterility.

In Drosophila and other male heterogametic species, cytoplasmic- or maternal-zygotic incompatibilities involving the *X* chromosome may be a common cause of nonreciprocal exceptions to HALDANE's rule (WU and DAVIS 1993; SAWAMURA 1996). When females of species 1 ($X_1 X_1$) are crossed with males of species 2 ($X_2 Y_2$), the maternal genotype and cytoplasm are always compatible with the X_1 chromosome in the male offspring ($X_1 Y_2$), but may be incompatible with the X_2 in female offspring ($X_1 X_2$). Incompatibilities of this type have been detected by careful genetic analysis in a few Drosophila hybridizations (*e.g.*, PATTERSON and GRIFFEN 1944; SAWAMURA *et al.* 1993a,b).

The maternal/zygotic incompatibility mechanism is not expected to produce exceptions in female heterogametic species and may even favor HALDANE's rule in some cases. A $Z_1 W_1$ female crossed with a $Z_2 Z_2$ male would produce $Z_2 W_1$ female offspring and $Z_2 Z_1$ male offspring. Both hybrid sexes potentially have a maternal/zygotic incompatibility involving the *Z* chromosome. However, female offspring could be affected more if the zygotic component of the incompatibility is recessive.

There is one well-studied exception to HALDANE's rule in Lepidopterans. In the cross of *Heliothis subflexa* females (*ZW*) to *H. virescens* males (*ZZ*), the male hybrids are almost completely sterile, while the females are fertile (PROSHOLD and LACHANCE 1974). When the hybrid females are backcrossed repeatedly to *virescens*, the male progeny are completely sterile, even after more than 170 generations (ROEHRDANZ 1990). These sterile backcross males are expected to have a completely *virescens* genotype. They are produced by mothers with *subflexa* cytoplasm and a *subflexa W* chromosome in an otherwise *virescens* genotype. Evidently there is a cytoplasmic factor (or a maternal effect due to the *W* chromosome) from *subflexa* that is incompatible with a male (*ZZ*) zygotic genotype of *virescens* origin.

In Drosophila, there are well-established cases of cytoplasmic incompatibility causing the death or sterility of males (HURST 1993). For example, in crosses between certain semispecies or races of *D. paulistorum*, hybrid females are fertile, while the males are sterile (EHRMAN and WILLIAMSON 1969). This sterility is clearly due to a microbial endosymbiont, which has been isolated, cultured, and injected into strains that lack it. When newly infected females are crossed to uninfected males from their own strain, the male offspring are sterile while female offspring are fertile (SOMERSON *et al.* 1984). This type of sex-specific cytoplasmic incompatibility specifically affects males (which do not transmit the endosymbiont), but seems to be relatively rare (HURST 1993). Although its operation favors the occurrence of HALDANE's rule in male heterogametic species, it obviously works against HALDANE's rule in female heterogametic species.

CONCLUSIONS

This review has shown that many different factors can cause sex-specific inviability or sterility in interspecific hybrids. As shown in Figure 3, some of these factors favor the occurrence of HALDANE's rule in a general way that applies across taxa, regardless of which sex is heterogametic. Others have a restricted application that sometimes favors and sometimes disfavors HALDANE's rule.

The hypothesis that *X-A* incompatibilities are generally recessive or partially recessive in hybrids provides a very general explanation of HALDANE's rule. It is supported by several cases of reciprocal compliance with HALDANE's rule for viability in both Drosophila and Lepidopterans. In addition, one direct and quantitative estimation of the degree of dominance of a specific incompatibility in Drosophila revealed recessivity (ORR 1992).

Because the dominance theory has such great explanatory power, it is tempting to speculate that recessivity may contribute to all cases of HALDANE's rule, even when additional factors are operating. However, recessivity cannot explain the case of fertile female and sterile male hybrids between *D. simulans* and *D. mauritiana*. The unbalanced female test of COYNE (1985) shows that

I. Factors that favor Haldane's rule regardless of which sex is heterogametic
    A. Affect both fertility and viability
        1. *X-A* incompatibilities are recessive or partially recessive on the average
        2. *X-A* incompatibilities affecting the heterogametic sex evolve more rapidly than those affecting the homogametic sex because new advantageous mutations are sometimes sex-specific and generally recessive
    B. May affect only fertility
        1. *X-Y* translocations
        2. *X-Y* meiotic drive
II. Factors that may favor Haldane's rule when males are heterogametic, but have no effect in female heterogametic species
    A. Rapid evolution of male sterility because spermatogenesis is very sensitive to genic imbalance in *XY* males
III. Factors that may favor Haldane's rule when males are heterogametic, but favor exceptions when females are heterogametic
    A. Rapid evolution of genes causing male sterility due to sexual selection
    B. Cytoplasmic incompatibilities that specifically kill or sterilize males
IV. Factors that may favor Haldane's rule when females are heterogametic, but favor exceptions when males are heterogametic
    A. Maternal/zygotic incompatibilities involving the *X* chromosome
V. Factors that may favor Haldane's rule in some taxa, but favor exceptions in others
    A. Failure of dosage compensation (in some cases related to *X-A* linkage changes)
    B. Rapid evolution of sterility because gametogenesis requires changes in the condensation state of sex chromosomes
    C. Sexual transformation caused by incompatibilities in sex determination
VI. Factors that favor exceptions to Haldane's rule regardless of which sex is heterogametic
    A. Partial dominance of *X-A* incompatibility factors
    B. *X-X* incompatibilities

FIGURE 3.—A classification of factors that cause sex-specific sterility, inviability or transformation in interspecific animal hybrids.

any incompatibility factors that may be present on the *simulans X* chromosome are insufficient to cause female sterility, even when they are made homozygous. On the other hand, introgression experiments clearly show that male sterility factors have accumulated more rapidly than female sterility factors during the divergence of these two species (HOLLOCHER and WU 1996; TRUE *et al.* 1996). It is the absence of female sterility factors, not their recessivity, that is causing HALDANE's rule in this case.

Another generally applicable hypothesis is that *X-A* incompatibilities affecting the heterogametic sex (not just males) evolve more rapidly than those affecting the homogametic sex. This rate difference can occur when new advantageous mutations are sometimes sex-specific and generally recessive within a pure species. While there is strong evidence that male sterility factors evolve more rapidly than female sterility factors in Drosophila, it is not clear whether the advantageous recessive hypothesis accounts for this difference. Unfortunately, this is an *ad hoc* hypothesis formulated to account for an apparently large effect of the *X* chromosome on sterility and inviability in hybrids. There is no independent evidence that new advantageous mutations are generally recessive. Also, further evidence is needed to determine whether incompatibility factors accumulate more rapidly on the *X* than the autosomes, as expected under this hypothesis.

Two additional hypotheses, *X-Y* translocations and *X-Y* meiotic drive, are theoretically applicable to hybrid sterility across taxa, but there is little or no empirical evidence that they occur. Furthermore, it is not clear that either one of these hypotheses can account for HALDANE's rule for inviability.

One process may occur and favor HALDANE's rule when males are heterogametic, but may not occur at all in taxa with heterogametic females. This is the idea that male sterility factors evolve rapidly because spermatogenesis is very sensitive to genic imbalance in *XY* males. The sensitivity may be restricted to *XY* males because there is no transcription after meiosis (perhaps because some meiotic products lack an *X* chromosome) or because of allocycly of the *X* and autosomes. These sensitivity factors may not apply to gametogenesis in female heterogametic species.

Several factors or processes listed in Figure 3 may favor HALDANE's rule under some circumstances, but favor exceptions under other circumstances. Even these factors potentially can contribute to the preponderance of cases that comply with HALDANE's rule, depending on how frequently they operate in male *vs.* female heterogametic taxa and depending on the combination of other factors operating. For example, some types of dosage compensation might be more sensitive to genic imbalance than others, and endosymbionts that cause male-specific cytoplasmic incompatibility might be more prevalent in some taxa than others. Sexual selection on features of spermatogenesis may operate in all groups, but may only contribute to HALDANE's rule in male heterogametic species; its contribution to exceptions in female heterogametic species may be prevented by recessivity. Unfortunately, there is very little evidence concerning whether some of these factors ever operate

(failure of dosage compensation, sexual selection on spermatogenesis) or how frequently others may operate in different groups (male sterilizing cytoplasmic incompatibility, sexual transformation).

In conclusion, it appears very likely that HALDANE's rule is a composite phenomenon with multiple causes. There is good, but largely circumstantial, evidence that recessivity of *X*-autosomal incompatibilities plays an important role. There is also good evidence that sterility factors affecting males evolve more rapidly than those affecting females in Drosophila, but the applicability of this phenomenon to other taxa is unknown. The cause(s) of this rate difference are also unknown. Much more work is needed to determine the relative importance of the many factors that potentially contribute to the widespread occurrence of HALDANE's rule.

During the past 15 years or so, the causes of HALDANE's rule have been hotly debated in the pages of this journal and elsewhere. Strong opinions have been voiced on both sides of many issues in this debate. If HALDANE were alive today, he probably would be delighted with the attention his rule has been getting. He was an outspoken character who loved to argue and was frequently embroiled in controversy (CLARK 1968). However, "in scientific matters, HALDANE was the most undogmatic of men and generally expressed skepticism concerning his own hypotheses" (WHITE 1965). Unlike some of his famous peers, he was not dedicated to the promotion of particular ideas (CROW 1992). So, in spite of all the progress that has been made, I think he would advise us to keep an open mind about the cause(s) of HALDANE's rule.

I thank the members of my laboratory (past and present), especially JOHN TRUE and YUN TAO, for many enlightening discussions about HALDANE's rule. More specifically, YUN TAO provided important insights into the interpretation of unbalanced female tests, and he also compiled the Drosophila data in Table 1. BONNIE LONZE compiled the Lepidopteran data in Table 1. I am also very grateful to BURKE JUDD, BRUCE NICKLAS, ALLEN ORR, MICHAEL TURELLI, and CHUNG-I WU for helpful comments and discussion. This work was supported by U.S. Public Health Service grant GM-47292.

LITERATURE CITED

BAIRD, S. E., M. E. SUTHERLIN and S. W. EMMONS, 1992 Reproductive isolation in Rhabditidae (Nematoda: Secernentea): mechanisms that isolate six species of three genera. Evolution **46**: 585–594.

BARTON, N. H., 1996 Speciation: more than the sum of the parts. Curr. Biol. **6**: 1244–1246.

BAVERSTOCK, P. R., M. ADAMS, R. W. POLKINGHORNE and M. GELDER, 1982 A sex-linked enzyme in birds—Z-chromosome conservation but no dosage compensation. Nature **296**: 763–766.

BIDDLE, R. L., 1932 The bristles of hybrids between *Drosophila melanogaster* and *Drosophila simulans*. Genetics **17**: 153–174.

BIGELOW, R. S., 1960 Interspecific hybrids and speciation in the genus *Acheta* (Orthoptera: Gryllidae). Can. J. Zool. **38**: 509–524.

BOCK, I. R., 1984 Interspecific hybridization in the genus *Drosophila*. Evol. Biol. **18**: 41–70.

BULL, J. J., 1983 *Evolution of Sex Determining Mechanisms*. Benjamin Cummings, Menlo Park, CA.

CHARLESWORTH, B., J. A. COYNE and N. H. BARTON, 1987 The relative rates of evolution of sex chromosomes and autosomes. Am. Nat. **130**: 113–146.

CHARLESWORTH, B., J. A. COYNE and H. A. ORR, 1993 Meiotic drive and unisexual hybrid sterility: a comment. Genetics **133:** 421–424.

CLARK, R. W., 1968 *J. B. S., The Life and Work of J. B. S. Haldane.* Hodder and Stoughton, London.

CLARKE, C., and E. B. FORD, 1982 Intersexuality in *Lymantria dispar* (L.): a further reassessment. Proc. R. Soc. Lond. B **214:** 285–288.

CLINE, T. W., and B. J. MEYER, 1996 Vive la différence: males *vs.* females in flies *vs.* worms. Annu. Rev. Genet. **30:** 637–702.

COYNE, J. A., 1985 The genetic basis of HALDANE's rule. Nature **314:** 736–738.

COYNE, J. A., 1992 Genetics and speciation. Nature **355:** 511–515.

COYNE, J. A., and H. A. ORR, 1989 Two rules of speciation, pp. 180–207 in *Speciation and Its Consequences,* edited by D. OTTE and J. A. ENDLER. Sinauer Associates, Sunderland, MA.

COYNE, J. A., and H. A. ORR, 1993 Further evidence against meiotic-drive models of hybrid sterility. Evolution **47:** 685–687.

COYNE, J. A., B. CHARLESWORTH and H. A. ORR, 1991 Haldane's rule revisited. Evolution **45:** 1710–1714.

CROW, J. F., 1992 Centennial: J. B. S. HALDANE, 1892–1964 Genetics **130:** 1–6.

CURTIS, C. F., 1972 Sterility from crosses between sub-species of the tsetse fly *Glossina morsitans.* Acta Trop. **29:** 250–268.

DAVIDSON, G., 1974 *Genetic Control of Insect Pests.* Academic Press, London.

DOBZHANSKY, T., 1936 Studies on hybrid sterility. II. Localization of sterility factors in *Drosophila pseudoobscura* hybrids. Genetics **21:** 113–115.

DOBZHANSKY, T., 1937a *Genetics and the Origin of Species.* Columbia University Press, New York.

DOBZHANSKY, T., 1937b Further data on *Drosophila miranda* and its hybrids with *Drosophila pseudoobscura.* J. Genet. **34:** 135–151.

DOBZHANSKY, T., 1970 *Genetics of the Evolutionary Process.* Columbia University Press, New York.

EHRMAN, L., and D. L. WILLIAMSON, 1969 On the etiology of the sterility of hybrids between certain strains of *Drosophila paulistorum.* Genetics **62:** 193–199.

EICHER, E. M., L. L. WASHBURN, J. B. W., III and K. E. MORROW, 1982 *Mus poschiavinus* Y chromosome in the C57BL/6J murine genome causes sex reversal. Science **217:** 535–537.

ESTRADA-FRANCO, J. G., M. C. MA, R. W. GWADZ, R. SAKAI, G. C. LANZARO *et al.,* 1993 Evidence through crossmating experiments of a species complex in *Anopheles pseudopunctipennis* sensu lato: a primary malaria vector of the American continent. Am. J. Trop. Med. Hyg. **49:** 746–755.

FRANK, S. A., 1991a Divergence of meiotic drive-suppression systems as an explanation for sex-biased hybrid sterility and inviability. Evolution **45:** 262–267.

FRANK, S. A., 1991b Haldane's rule: a defense of meiotic drive theory. Evolution **45:** 1714–1717.

FULLER, M. T., 1993 Spermatogenesis, pp. 71–148 in *The Development of Drosophila melanogaster,* edited by M. BATE and A. MARTINEZ-ARIAS. Cold Spring Harbor Laboratory Press, Plainview, NY.

GOLDSCHMIDT, R., 1934 *Lymantria.* Bibliogr. Genet. **11:** 1–186.

GOODING, R. H., 1990 Postmating barriers to gene flow among species and subspecies of tsetse flies (Diptera: Glossinidae). Can. J. Zool. **68:** 1727–1734.

GROPP, A., H. WINKING and C. REDI, 1982 Consequences of Robertsonian heterozygosity: segregational impairment of fertility *vs.* male-limited sterility, pp. 115–134 in *Genetic Control of Gamete Production and Function,* edited by P. G. CROSIGNANI, B. L. RUBIN and M. FRACCARO. Academic Press, New York.

HALDANE, J. B. S., 1922 Sex-ratio and unisexual sterility in hybrid animals. J. Genet. **12:** 101–109.

HALDANE, J. B. S., 1924 A mathematical theory of natural and artificial selection. Part I. Trans. Cambridge Phil. Soc. **23:** 19–41.

HALDANE, J. B. S., 1929 The species problem in the light of genetics. Nature **124:** 514–516.

HALDANE, J. B. S., 1932 *The Causes of Evolution.* Longmans, Green and Co., London.

HALDANE, J. B. S., 1938 The nature of interspecific differences, pp. 79–94 in *Essays on Aspects of Evolutionary Biology,* edited by G. R. deBEER. Oxford University Press, Oxford.

HALDANE, J. B. S., 1964 A defense of beanbag genetics. Perspect. Biol. Med. **7:** 343–359.

HARVEY, A. W., 1979 Hybridization studies in the *Schistocerca americana* complex. I. The specific status of the Central American Locust. Biol. J. Linn. Soc. **12:** 349–355.

HENNIG, W., 1977 Gene interactions in germ differentiation of Drosophila. Adv. Enzyme Regul. **XXX:** 363–371.

HEWITT, G. M., R. K. BUTLIN and T. M. EAST, 1987 Testicular dysfunction in hybrids between parapatric subspecies of the grasshopper *Chorthippus parallelus.* Biol. J. Linn. Soc. **31:** 25–34.

HII, J. L. K., 1985 Genetic investigations of laboratory stocks of the complex of *Anopheles balabacensis* Baisas (Diptera: Culicidae). Bull. Entomol. Res. **75:** 185–197.

HILLIS, D. M., and D. M. GREEN, 1990 Evolutionary changes of heterogametic sex in the phylogenetic history of amphibians. J. Evol. Biol. **3:** 49–64.

HOLLOCHER, H., and C.-I. WU, 1996 The genetics of reproductive isolation in the *Drosophila simulans* clade: X *vs.* autosomal effects and male *vs.* female effects. Genetics **143:** 1243–1255.

HURST, L. D., 1993 The incidences, mechanisms and evolution of cytoplasmic sex ratio distorters in animals. Biol. Rev. **68:** 121–193.

HURST, L. D., and A. POMIANKOWSKI, 1991 Causes of sex ratio bias may account for unisexual sterility in hybrids: a new explanation of HALDANE's rule and related phenomena. Genetics **128:** 841–858.

HUTTER, P., J. ROOTE and M. ASHBURNER, 1990 A genetic basis for the inviability of hybrids between sibling species of *Drosophila.* Genetics **124:** 909–920.

JABLONKA, E., and M. J. LAMB, 1988 Meiotic pairing constraints and the activity of sex chromosomes. J. Theor. Biol. **133:** 23–36.

JABLONKA, E., and M. J. LAMB, 1991 Sex chromosomes and speciation. Proc. R. Soc. Lond. B **243:** 203–208.

JOHNSON, M. S., and J. R. G. TURNER, 1979 Absence of dosage compensation for a sex-linked enzyme in butterflies (*Heliconius*). Heredity **43:** 71–77.

JOHNSON, N. A., and C.-I. WU, 1992 An empirical test of the meiotic drive models of hybrid sterility: sex-ratio data from hybrids between *Drosophila simulans* and *Drosophila sechellia.* Genetics **130:** 507–511.

JOHNSON, N. A., H. HOLLOCHER, E. NOONBURG and C.-I. WU, 1993 The effects of interspecific Y chromosome replacements on hybrid sterility within the *Drosophila simulans* clade. Genetics **135:** 443–453.

KLEIN, T. A., B. A. HARRISON, V. BAIMAI and V. PHUNKITCHAR, 1984 Hybridization evidence supporting separate species status for *Anopheles nivipes* and *Anopheles philippinensis.* Mosq. News **44:** 466–470.

LAMNISSOU, K., M. LOUKAS and E. ZOUROS, 1996 Incompatibilities between Y chromosome and autosomes are responsible for male hybrid sterility in crosses between *Drosophila virilis* and *Drosophila texana.* Heredity **76:** 603–609.

LANZARO, G. C., S. K. NARANG, S. E. MITCHELL, P. E. KAISER and J. A. SEAWRIGHT, 1988 Hybrid male sterility in crosses between field and laboratory strains of *Anopheles quadrimaculatus* (Say) (Diptera: Culicidae). J. Med. Entomol. **25:** 248–255.

LIFSCHYTZ, E., and D. L. LINDSLEY, 1972 Sex chromosome activation during spermatogenesis. Genetics **78:** 323–331.

LINDSLEY, D. L., and K. T. TOKUYASU, 1980 Spermatogenesis, pp. 226–294 in *The Genetics and Biology of Drosophila,* edited by M. ASHBURNER and T. R. F. WRIGHT. Academic Press, New York.

LUCCHESI, J. C., 1978 Gene dosage compensation and the evolution of sex chromosomes. Science **202:** 711–716.

LYON, M. F., 1961 Gene action in the X-chromosome of the mouse (*Mus musculus* L.). Nature **190:** 372–373.

MATSUDA, Y., and V. M. CHAPMAN, 1994 X-Y chromosome pairing and hybrid sterility of mice, pp. 257–275 in *Genetics in Wild Mice,* edited by K. MORIWAI, T. SHIROISHI and H. YONEKAWA. Jpn. Sci. Soc. Press, Tokyo.

MAYR, E., 1942 *Systematics and the Origin of Species.* Columbia University Press, New York.

MAYR, E., 1963 *Animal Species and Evolution.* Harvard University Press, Cambridge, MA.

MULLER, H. J., 1940 Bearing of the Drosophila work on systematics, pp. 185–268 in *The New Systematics,* edited by J. HUXLEY. Clarendon Press, Oxford.

MULLER, H. J., 1942 Isolating mechanisms, evolution and temperature. Biol. Symp. **6:** 71–125.

OHMACHI, F., and S. MASAKI, 1964 Interspecific crossing and development of hybrids between the Japanese species of *Teleogryllus* (Orthoptera: Gryllidae). Evolution **18**: 405–416.

ORR, H. A., 1987 Genetics of male and female sterility in hybrids of *Drosophila pseudoobscura* and *D. persimilis*. Genetics **116**: 555–563.

ORR, H. A., 1989a Does postzygotic isolation result from improper dosage compensation? Genetics **122**: 891–894.

ORR, H. A., 1989b Genetics of sterility in hybrids between two subspecies of *Drosophila*. Evolution **43**: 180–189.

ORR, H. A., 1992 Mapping and characterization of a 'speciation gene' in *Drosophila*. Genet. Res. **59**: 73–80.

ORR, H. A., 1993a A mathematical model of HALDANE's rule. Evolution **47**: 1606–1611.

ORR, H. A., 1993b HALDANE's rule has multiple genetic causes. Nature **361**: 532–533.

ORR, H. A., 1995 The population genetics of speciation: the evolution of hybrid incompatibilities. Genetics **139**: 1805–1813.

ORR, H. A., 1996 DOBZHANSKY, BATESON, and the genetics of speciation. Genetics **144**: 1331–1335.

ORR, H. A., 1997 Haldane's rule. Annu. Rev. Ecol. Syst. (in press).

ORR, H. A., and J. A. COYNE, 1989 The genetics of postzygotic isolation in the *Drosophila virilis* group. Genetics **121**: 527–537.

ORR, H. A., and M. TURELLI, 1996 Dominance and HALDANE's rule. Genetics **143**: 613–616.

PANTAZIDIS, A. C., and E. ZOUROS, 1988 Location of an autosomal factor causing sterility in *Drosophila mojavensis* males carrying the *Drosophila arizonensis* Y chromosome. Heredity **60**: 299–304.

PATTERSON, J. T., and A. G. GRIFFEN, 1944 VII. A genetic mechanism underlying species isolation. Univ. Texas Publ. **4445**: 212–223.

PATTERSON, J. T., and W. S. STONE, 1952 *Evolution in the Genus Drosophila*. Macmillan, New York.

PATTERSON, J. T., W. S. STONE and A. B. GRIFFEN, 1942 X. Genetic and cytological analysis of the virilis species group. Univ. Texas Publ. **4228**: 162–200.

POMIANKOWSKI, A., and L. D. HURST, 1993 Genomic conflicts underlying HALDANE's rule. Genetics **133**: 425–432.

PROSHOLD, F. I., and L. E. LACHANCE, 1974 Analysis of sterility in hybrids from interspecific crosses between *Heliothis virescens* and *H. subflexa*. Ann. Entomol. Soc. Am. **67**: 445–449.

READ, A., and S. NEE, 1991 Is Haldane's rule significant? Evolution **45**: 1707–1709.

ROBINSON, R., 1971 *Lepidoptera Genetics*. Permagon Press, Oxford.

ROEHRDANZ, R. L., 1990 Maternal inheritance of a Y chromosome in *Heliothis* could play a role in backcross sterility. J. Hered. **81**: 66–68.

RYKENA, S., 1991 Hybridization experiments as tests for species boundaries in the genus *Lacerta* sensu stricto. Mitt. Zool. Mus. Berl. **67**: 55–68.

SAWAMURA, K., 1996 Maternal effect as a cause of exceptions for HALDANE's rule. Genetics **143**: 609–611.

SAWAMURA, K., T. TAIRA and T. K. WATANABE, 1993a Hybrid lethal systems in the *Drosophila melanogaster* species complex. I. The *maternal hybrid rescue* (*mhr*) gene of *Drosophila simulans*. Genetics **133**: 299–305.

SAWAMURA, K., M.-T. YAMAMOTO and T. K. WATANABE, 1993b Hybrid lethal systems in the *Drosophila melanogaster* species complex. II. The *Zygotic hybrid rescue* (*Zhr*) gene of *D. melanogaster*. Genetics **133**: 307–313.

SCHÄFER, U., 1978 Sterility in *Drosophila hydei* × *D. neohydei* hybrids. Genetica **49**: 205–214.

SIMMONS, M. J., and J. F. CROW, 1977 Mutations affecting fitness in Drosophila populations. Annu. Rev. Genet. **11**: 49–78.

SOMERSON, N. L., L. EHRMAN, J. P. KOCKA and F. J. GOTTLIEB, 1984 Streptococcal L-forms isolated from *Drosophila paulistorum* semis-

pecies cause sterility in male progeny. Proc. Natl. Acad. Sci. USA **81**: 282–285.

SPENCE, J. R., 1990 Introgressive hybridization in Heteroptera: the example of *Limnoporus* Stål (Gerridae) species in western Canada. Can. J. Zool. **68**: 1770–1782.

STEINEMANN, M., S. STEINEMANN and F. LOTTSPEICH, 1993 How Y chromosomes become genetically inert. Proc. Natl. Acad. Sci. USA **90**: 5737–5741.

STROBEL, E., C. PELLING and N. ARNHEIM, 1978 Incomplete dosage compensation in an evolving *Drosophila* sex chromosome. Proc. Natl. Acad. Sci. USA **75**: 931–935.

STURTEVANT, A. H., 1920 Genetic studies on *Drosophila simulans*. I. Introduction. Hybrids with *Drosophila melanogaster*. Genetics **5**: 488–500.

STURTEVANT, A. H., and E. NOVITSKI, 1941 Sterility in crosses of geographical races of *Drosophila micromelanica*. Proc. Natl. Acad. Sci. USA **27**: 392–394.

TAKAI, K., T. KANDA, K.-I. OGAWA and S. SUCHARIT, 1987 Morphological differentiation in *Anopheles maculatus* of Thailand accompanied with genetical divergence assessed by hybridization. J. Am. Mosq. Control Assoc. **3**: 148–153.

TRUE, J. R., B. S. WEIR and C. C. LAURIE, 1996 A genome-wide survey of hybrid incompatibility factors by the introgression of marked segments of *Drosophila mauritiana* chromosomes into *Drosophila simulans*. Genetics **142**: 819–837.

TURELLI, M., and H. A. ORR, 1995 The dominance theory of HALDANE's rule. Genetics **140**: 389–402.

VIGNEAULT, G., and E. ZOUROS, 1986 The genetics of asymmetrical male sterility in *Drosophila mojavensis* and *Drosophila arizonensis* hybrids: interactions between the Y-chromosome and autosomes. Evolution **40**: 1160–1170.

VOELKER, R. A., and K.-I. KOJIMA, 1971 Fertility and fitness of XO males in *Drosophila*. I. Qualitative study. Evolution **25**: 119–128.

WATANABE, T. K., 1979 A gene that rescues the lethal hybrids between *Drosophila melanogaster* and *D. simulans*. Jpn. J. Genet. **54**: 325–331.

WHITE, M. J. D., 1945 *Animal Cytology & Evolution*. Cambridge University Press, London.

WHITE, M. J. D., 1965 J. B. S. HALDANE. Genetics **52**: 1–7.

WHITE, M. J. D., 1973 *Animal Cytology and Evolution*. Cambridge University Press, London.

WHITE, M. J. D., N. CONTRERAS, J. CHENEY and G. C. WEBB, 1977 Cytogenetics of the parthenogenetic grasshopper *Warramaba* (formerly *Moraba*) *virgo* and its bisexual relatives. Chromosoma **61**: 127–148.

WU, C.-I., and A. T. BECKENBACH, 1983 Evidence for extensive genetic differentiation between the sex-ratio and the standard arrangement of *Drosophila pseudoobscura* and *D. persimilis* and identification of hybrid sterility factors. Genetics **105**: 71–86.

WU, C.-I., and A. W. DAVIS, 1993 Evolution of postmating reproductive isolation: the composite nature of Haldane's rule and its genetic bases. Am. Nat. **142**: 187–212.

WU, C.-I., and M. F. PALOPOLI, 1994 Genetics of postmating reproductive isolation in animals. Annu. Rev. Genet. **27**: 283–308.

WU, C.-I., N. A. JOHNSON and M. F. PALOPOLI, 1996 Haldane's rule and its legacy: why are there so many sterile males? Trends Ecol. Evol. **11**: 281–284.

YAMAMOTO, M.-T., 1992 Inviability of hybrids between *D. melanogaster* and *D. simulans* results from the absence of *simulans* X not the presence of *simulans* Y chromosome. Genetica **87**: 151–158.

ZENG, L.-W., and R. S. SINGH, 1993 The genetic basis of HALDANE's rule and the nature of asymmetric hybrid male sterility among *Drosophila simulans*, *Drosophila mauritiana* and *Drosophila sechellia*. Genetics **134**: 251–260.

Seventy Years Ago
Mutation Becomes Experimental

James F. Crow* and Seymour Abrahamson†

* Laboratory of Genetics and †Department of Zoology, University of Wisconsin–Madison, Madison, Wisconsin 53706

IN 1927 H. J. MULLER (1890–1967) published in *Science* a paper entitled "Artificial Transmutation of the Gene." It reported the first experimental production of mutations and opened a new era in genetics. The title is curious. Why *transmutation* rather than *mutation*? The answer emerges from another paper (MULLER 1928a), written in 1926. After reviewing the repeated failure of efforts by many workers to modify the mutation rate, MULLER asked the question: "Do the preceding results mean, then, that mutation is unique among biological processes in being itself outside the reach of modification or control,—that it occupies a position similar to that till recently characteristic of atomic transmutation in physical science, in being purely spontaneous, 'from within,' and not subject to influences commonly dealt with? Must it be beyond the range of our scientific tools?" MULLER thought of his radiation experiments as parallel to those of RUTHERFORD, only a few years earlier, demonstrating experimental transmutation of chemical elements. Like the physicists, who were attracting a great deal of public attention at the time, MULLER had tampered with a fundamental natural process and had succeeded in mastering it. He was an instant celebrity.

The 1927 paper is also curious in another way, for it presented no data–no dosage measurements, no numbers, no statistical analysis. MULLER simply reported qualitative results and rough comparisons, *e.g.*, a mutation-rate increase of "fifteen thousand percent." But a paper without data invited skepticism, and the skeptics included no less than T. H. MORGAN, who was always suspicious of speculations and invariably asked for the data.

MULLER's idea was clearly to establish priority. He noted that many of the mutations were repeats of those found earlier. Most were recessive, but a few were dominant. Many were lethal or sterilizing, and there were dominant lethals, not easy to detect. In addition to gene mutations, MULLER reported a number of chromosome rearrangements, especially translocations. He suggested mutation as a cause of cancer. And in this, his first paper on the subject, he began his lifetime crusade against indiscriminate use of high-energy radiation, a crusade bolstered by the later demonstration that mutation was linearly related to dose, down to doses as low as could be practically studied.

In the summer of 1927 MULLER gave a major paper at the Fifth International Congress of Genetics in Berlin. Typically, he scribbled the paper in transit and was still preparing slides up to the time of its presentation. The talk is said to have been confusing, but the message was clear. This time he gave the full details and the skeptics were silenced. Helpful as he was throughout his life, CURT STERN got the paper typed, and it was published the next year (MULLER 1928b).

Biologists generally accepted mutation as the ultimate basis of evolution. Furthermore, mutation promised a way to get at the nature of the gene. Yet mutations were so rare that there was only anecdotal information. In a few months MULLER found more mutant genes than the total from all Drosophila labs up to that time. His discovery was independently confirmed by L. J. STADLER, who started experiments with barley and other plants at about the same time (ROMAN 1988; STADLER 1997). The slower life cycle in these plants meant that his results appeared somewhat later, but he clearly deserves recognition along with MULLER, although he didn't always receive it. Other geneticists immediately jumped on the bandwagon, and the field of radiation genetics was on its way.

Although he was actively engaged in many aspects of Drosophila genetics and was an active contributor in various ways to the MORGAN group, MULLER's interest centered on mutation. His first experiments started in 1918, so his radiation paper represented the culmination of a decade of work. MULLER's two full reports, one written before the X-ray discovery (1928a) and the other immediately after (1928b), report a remarkable saga. The first paper occupies an entire issue of *Genetics*, 79 pages. In minute detail, he described the various experiments, each successive one being an improvement and coming closer to providing convincing quantitative data. His innovations and their updates are now standard Drosophila methodology.

The problem from the beginning was the rarity of mutations. Early on, MULLER decided that lethals were better material than visible mutations for quantitative study. For one thing, they were far more numerous. For another, the results were unambiguous; with rare exceptions there were no survivors (or only a few pitifully weak ones). The "personal equation" was eliminated; lethals could be identified as well by the average technician as by a sharp-eyed CALVIN BRIDGES. Soon MULLER began devising ways to identify all the lethal mutations on a chromosome, thereby multiplying the per-locus mutation rate by the number of lethal-producing loci on the chromosome.

Early in his work MULLER realized the value of "C factors," crossover suppressors, later proven to be inversions. He exploited these to construct balanced lethal systems in which lethal mutations, in addition to those necessary to keep the system balanced, could be accumulated over many generations. Then, by elaborate mating schemes, he could render the new mutations homozygous and locate their approximate position by linkage with known markers. This permitted further enrichment of the number of mutations by summing the mutations that had accumulated over many generations.

In these accumulation experiments, MULLER foreshadowed the work of MUKAI (1964), who employed this idea to measure the spontaneous rate of mutations with small effects on viability. MULLER had argued that mutations producing small, statistically detected effects on viability and fertility were the most numerous class, and MUKAI showed it.

MULLER's most famous Drosophila stock involved an X chromosome that he called ClB. C stands for a crossover suppressor, l is a recessive lethal, and B is the Bar "gene," later proven to be a duplication. Using the crosses that are now familiar to every student of elementary genetics, MULLER was able to measure the rate of lethal mutation on the X chromosome with almost no ambiguity. MULLER was constantly on the lookout for time-saving methods, and this was one of his best. Since an F_2 culture descended from a new recessive lethal contained no males, it was not necessary to examine the flies in detail, but only enough to ascertain whether males were present. This could be done by examining the flies in the vial with the naked eye or, a bit better, a hand lens sufficed. Figure 1 shows MULLER demonstrating his favorite low-tech instrument. The ClB method provides an easy way to map the location of new lethals, and MULLER quickly exploited this. He showed that lethal mutations are distributed over the entire X chromosome, roughly uniformly, although concentrated at the "left" end.

Another innovation was a "double X experiment," which made use of L. V. MORGAN's strain in which two X chromosomes were attached at the centromere. By crossing treated males to such females, any X-linked visible mutations were immediately apparent in males of the next generation.

From the beginning, MULLER thought that perhaps the best way to get at the question of whether the mutation rate was immutable was to study the effect of temperature. If mutation behaved like ordinary laboratory chemical reactions, the rate should double or triple with each rise of 10°. Therefore, throughout most of the several years of study in the early 1920s, temperature was varied, with increasingly precise results in the later experiments. Controlling temperature was no easy task in those days of poor equipment and poorly supported labs. MULLER did experiments in the MORGAN lab in New York, at Woods Hole in Massachusetts, at Rice Institute in Houston, and at the University of Texas in Austin. It was especially difficult to arrange cool temperatures in the hot Texas summers. He covered the cultures with a wet cloth on which an electric fan blew. Despite the crudity of the experimental conditions, he was able to compare two sets of experiments that, while each varied considerably, differed on the average by about 8°.

By showing that the mutation rate could be influenced, MULLER made mutation a researchable subject. In his words (1928a): "Perhaps the most hopeful feature of the present data is that they show that mutation is indeed capable of being influenced 'artificially'— that it does not stand as an unreachable god playing its pranks upon us from some impregnable citadel in the germ plasm." Later the temperature effect was given a theoretical interpretation (see SCHRÖDINGER 1944).

It is a short intellectual step from realization that the mutation process has a high temperature coefficient to thinking of radiation as a source of activating energy. Although MULLER justly receives great credit for radiation mutagenesis, the greater contribution is his development of techniques whereby mutation could be studied experimentally and measured reproducibly. In three monumental papers—actually only two, since the Science paper gave no details—MULLER provided essentially all the basic techniques used in the burst of radiation experiments done in the next several decades.

In those days, many geneticists thought that best way to get at the nature of the mysterious gene was through mutation. Perhaps the way the gene mutates could tell them what it is. Of course, genetic history has been quite different. The nature of the gene was discovered, not by the kinetics of mutation, but by the identification of DNA as the genetic material, by advances in the chemistry of large molecules, and by some clever model building by WATSON and CRICK. Now the tables are turned; knowledge of the gene is used to understand mutations and mutagens, not the other way around.

It is striking that for two decades after MULLER's discovery, no convincing evidence of chemical mutagenesis was presented. Although many chemicals were tried,

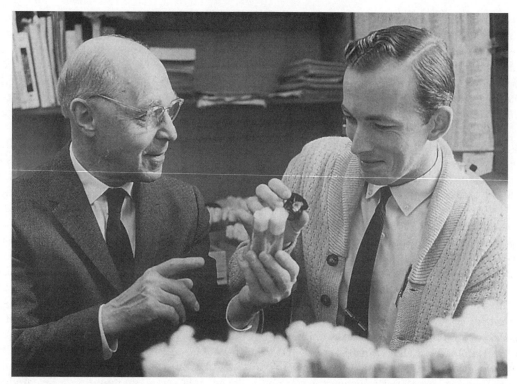

FIGURE 1.—H. J. MULLER and a student, DALE WAGONER, about 1961.

and some experiments would today be regarded as successes, none passed the extreme standards of rigor that the genetics community demanded. If there was an early dogma that mutations could not be induced, there was the new dogma that only radiation could do this. Chemical induction of mutations had to wait for MULLER's protégé, CHARLOTTE AUERBACH, to demonstrate the mutagenicity of mustard gas during World War II (BEALE 1993).

MULLER believed that radiation-induced mutations were essentially the same as spontaneous ones, while STADLER thought, correctly as it turned out, that they were mainly deletions (ROMAN 1988). MULLER hoped that he had discovered a way of inducing mutations important for evolution. Perhaps the hope fathered the belief, for he continued to hold to his original view, despite ever-increasing evidence to the contrary. It is unappealing to consider that we are deleted amoebas.

MULLER's LIFE

HERMAN JOSEPH MULLER, known to his intimates as Joe, was born in 1890 in New York City. His father must have been highly intelligent, for he had graduated number one in the intellectually elite and intensely competitive environment of City College of New York. The senior MULLER had hoped for a scholarly career in the field of international law. But the death of his own father had required that he take over the family business, making metal castings. By all reports he disliked the business, but reveled in his after-hours intel-

lectual pursuits. He took Joe to museums and discussed Darwinism along with his social views. Alas, he died when the boy was nine years old. His busy mother continued to further his interest in nature.

MULLER was able to attend Columbia University, but only by working part time during the school year and in summer jobs. Yet he graduated with honors. His major subject was physiology, but he was attracted by MORGAN and his two brilliant students, A. H. STURTEVANT and C. B. BRIDGES. The excitement in the fly lab was such that it was inevitable for MULLER to gravitate to the group. But although he was associated with the fly group, he never was a real insider. It must have been a busy time for him. On a typical day he rode the subway to Cornell Medical School to teach in a physiology lab, then to Columbia for classes and a visit to the fly lab, then downtown where he taught an evening course in English for foreign students, and then back home by the subway.

The MORGAN lab was a single room, small enough for everyone to participate in the conversation. Everyone knew what everyone else was doing, and it must have been very hard to trace the history of an idea that was so thoroughly batted around. It was a heady environment and must have been intensely exciting for the participants. Drosophila genetics was advancing rapidly, and almost every experiment yielded something new. Yet the environment was not tranquil, for MULLER at least. MORGAN held that the origin of ideas was not important; the important thing was to do the experiment and get the data. Almost certainly MULLER, with his quick mind and creative imagination, contributed more than his share of ideas. And he had a sensitive ego. In any case he began to feel that he was not getting sufficient credit from MORGAN, and the rift persisted.

MULLER completed his thesis, on linkage and crossing over, in 1915 in his usual last-minute frenzy. He accepted a position at Rice Institute with his friend JULIAN HUXLEY. Summers were spent at Woods Hole. He returned to Columbia in 1918 and there began the serious study of mutation. His two-year appointment ended in 1920 and, to his great disappointment, was not extended. So he took a job at the University of Texas.

MULLER was recruited by J. T. PATTERSON, an embryologist, who among other things worked out the embryology of armadillo quadruplets. He provided MULLER with equipment, money, and a student assistant, a contrast to Columbia where he had had to pay for vials and assistance from his own not-too-deep pockets. Later, PATTERSON arranged to get MULLER an X-ray machine. Another Texas faculty member was T. S. PAINTER, a cytologist. Soon both PAINTER and PATTERSON were working with Drosophila.

MULLER worked extraordinarily hard, mainly on his mutation studies, but also on many other things. He discovered a pair of identical human twins that had been reared apart. He discussed the near-absence of polyploidy in animals, the failure of genes to function in spermatozoa, balanced lethals, distribution of crossovers, polyploid segregation, and dosage compensation among other things. He coined the useful words *hypomorph, hypermorph, antimorph*, etc. He formulated his ideas about what the gene had to do, the most remarkable property being to copy errors, that is, to mutate. He was fascinated by bacteriophage and this led to what must be MULLER's most famous statement, a remarkably prophetic one published in 1922:

> If these d'Herelle bodies were really genes, fundamentally like our chromosome genes, they would give us an utterly new angle from which to attack the gene problem. They are filterable, to some extent isolable, handled in test tubes, and their properties, as shown by their effects on the bacteria, can then be studied after treatment. It would be very rash to call these bodies genes, and yet at present we must confess that there is no distinction known between the genes and them. Hence we cannot categorically deny that perhaps we may be able to grind genes in a mortar and cook them in a beaker after all. Must we geneticists become bacteriologists, physiological chemists and physicists, simultaneously with being zoologists and botanists? Let us hope so.

According to MULLER's later recollection, the previous speaker on that occasion thought this was a clever fantasy and congratulated MULLER on his sense of humor. Such farsightedness continued through his life; another often-cited example is his Pilgrim Trust Lecture, delivered in 1945 (LEDERBERG 1991).

Although his research brought him fame, MULLER

was not satisfied at Texas. He felt, correctly, that PATTERSON and PAINTER were exploiting his ideas. Why wasn't he pleased, for he had many more ideas than he could personally test? At the same time he was involved in assorted leftist political activities and sponsored a radical student group. Two Russian geneticists worked in his laboratory. He became increasingly depressed by the racism and inequalities of wealth in the United States.

Germany seemed like a good place to further his socialist ideas, so in 1932 he joined the laboratory of TIMOFÉEFF-RESSOVSKY in Berlin. This was in the Brain Research Institute, headed by OSCAR VOGT. MULLER arrived only a few months before Hitler rose to power. VOGT refused to fire Jews, with the result that there were break-ins at the Institute and at VOGT's home, some of which MULLER witnessed. Staying in Germany became hopeless.

By his leftists activities, MULLER had burned his bridges in Texas, so he accepted a position at the Genetics Institute in Leningrad. The next few years were extremely productive. Salivary chromosomes had been discovered, and MULLER's Russian group became leaders in exploiting this powerful breakthrough. Yet this period of great productivity didn't last long. Genetics came under the diabolical influence of TROFIM LYSENKO, whose extravagant promises of higher crop yields caught Stalin's eye. LYSENKO's Lamarckian views became official and he became the dominant figure in Soviet genetics. The man who brought MULLER to Russia, N. I. VAVILOV, was later imprisoned and died (CROW 1993). So did the two Russians who had worked with MULLER in Texas.

More of MULLER's colleagues disappeared while others remained active "in inverse proportion to their honor." MULLER's plan for getting out of Russia was to take a leave of absence to work in the blood bank of the International Brigade in Spain in the fight against Franco. In this way, he would not seem disloyal to the Soviet regime and this could perhaps protect his surviving Russian friends. It didn't help much. Several perished or were imprisoned and others survived by doing nongenetic work.

After leaving Spain, MULLER had no luck finding a job in the West. Finally in 1937 he got a temporary position in WADDINGTON's Institute at the University of Edinburgh. Compared with the early situation in Russia, conditions were poor. He was without any help and had a hard time in the cold Edinburgh winters; he never was comfortable working with gloves as the others did. A notable event in this period was his supervising CHARLOTTE AUERBACH, who was interested in trying to discover chemical mutagens (BEALE 1993).

MULLER's chronic hard luck continued. Again he was in the wrong place, and when World War II began he tried to return to the United States. Again, no job. He finally obtained a temporary position at Amherst Col-

lege, replacing HAROLD PLOUGH, who was on leave doing War work. Finally, in 1945, FRANK HANSON and WAR-
REN WEAVER of the Rockefeller Foundation suggested
MULLER to FERNANDUS PAYNE, head of the Zoology Department and Dean of the Graduate School at Indiana
University. PAYNE was a Drosophila geneticist who had
worked in the MORGAN lab. He couldn't care less about
MULLER's leftist background, his reputation as a poor
undergraduate teacher, or his "difficult" personality.
He said that he already had several prima donnas on
his staff and one more wouldn't matter. And he knew
that MULLER was good with graduate students, and of
course he was familiar with MULLER's great research.

So, at last in 1945, at age fifty-five, MULLER had a
permanent position with stimulating colleagues, supplies, equipment, assistants, and graduate students. The
Nobel Prize came a year later. Except for three periods
on leave, in Hawaii, at City of Hope in California, and
at the University of Wisconsin, MULLER remained at
Indiana University for the rest of his life. He died in
1967.

MULLER's life was complicated and difficult, one
disappointment after another. He was caught up in
both of the two tragic dictatorships of the century,
each with its way of perverting genetics. His stubborn
idealism and strong personality often led to difficulties. His work was constantly being interrupted. Yet his
work was his life, and usually it meant long days and
seven-day weeks.

Clearly, MULLER was a complicated person. His
great scientific intellect contrasted with his poor social
skills. He could muster overwhelming arguments for
a theory or for a political view, yet he did not realize
that argumentative overkill is not always the way to
win converts. He could be petty in personal relations,
in contrast to his great idealism for mankind in the
large. Even after becoming famous, he was excessively
concerned that he receive credit for all his discoveries,
no matter how minor. Yet, he could be charming,
witty, and above all, a most stimulating conversationalist, be the subject genetics, society, or politics. And all
his personal foibles recede in the glow of his great
scientific achievements.

ELOF CARLSON (1981) has written an excellent full-
length biography of MULLER, on which we have relied
heavily. Some of our material is from CROW (1990).
MULLER, himself, prepared a sampling of his papers
(1962). Although it is impossible to get more than a
small sample of work in a single volume, this is an excellent way to get an idea of the breadth, variety, and depth
of MULLER's contributions. To quote JOSHUA LEDER-
BERG's Foreword, "Thoughtful reader—you will find a
world of rediscovery here."

Several earlier *Perspectives* essays have touched on
MULLER and his work. They include CROW (1988,
1995), GREEN (1996), LEDERBERG (1991), LEWIS (1995),
PAUL (1988), ROMAN (1988), and STADLER (1997).

MULLER AS A PERSON

Each of us was well acquainted with MULLER, both
being his intellectual descendants. One of us (S.A.) was
MULLER's "son," that is, graduate student. The other
(J.F.C.) was a "grandson," having been a student of
one of MULLER's earliest students, W. S. STONE. We here
record a few separate memories.

Some memories of a graduate student (S.A.): When
I entered his laboratory in 1951, MULLER was still a
dynamo of activity—working seven days a week, staying
late into the evenings cloistered in his private office-
laboratory, developing new and ever more complicated
fly stocks to answer still-unresolved mutation questions,
and writing book chapters, papers, and speeches at a
rate that multiplied after the Prize. The lab then had
several research associates, four or five graduate students, and a few laboratory technicians. We students
would often try to corner him for questions in the evening when he was in. His light showed only at the door-
sill level and we would stoop to see if it was on. This
behavior prompted a janitor to ask me why MULLER's
students always bowed before his door, even if he was
a Nobel Prize winner.

Later MULLER used Thursday afternoons for graduate
student appointments to discuss research problems.
There would often be pitched battles in which we defended our results and interpretation as best we could
against his piercing criticisms. However, when either
our experiment or his (if one was a research assistant)
failed, he was mercifully kind and supportive. At the
time I was preparing my thesis draft, he went over it
with me line by line and by the third or fourth draft he
was editing his previous suggestions. When I switched
from cheap yellow to white bond paper, he decided it
was acceptable, probably because he didn't want to
waste expensive paper. For his 65th birthday party his
students prepared songs and poems about him. A few
days later, they came back edited.

When he went on sabbatical to Hawaii in 1953, JIM
TELFER and I were assigned to do his neutron experiments. By frequent mail we received his ever-changing
recommended fly crosses, which we would then expand in order to collect the necessary thousands of
flies. Usually half-way through, he would decide on
an alternate procedure and a mad scramble would
ensue to build up the stocks before we drove from
Bloomington to Oak Ridge for the neutron irradiation. TRACY SONNEBORN likened MULLER to Sturm und
Drang, and this atmosphere was most apparent when
you were the teaching assistant in his genetics laboratory course. Heaven help you if the matings or the
virginal flies were not available on time for the Monday and Friday classes.

Two more memories (J.F.C.): I first met MULLER
in the early 1940s when he was at Amherst College. I
was then teaching naval trainees at Dartmouth Col-

lege, not far away, so we had frequent visits. Of course, I was greatly stimulated by MULLER's deep knowledge and creative mind. Once I happened to visit him during yet another low point in his life, just after he had been notified that his temporary appointment could not be made permanent. I recall being greatly incensed that this great man, in the eyes of many our greatest geneticist, didn't have a job. Some thought he was a communist since he had spent much time in Russia. Others of leftist persuasion called him a fascist, for by this time he was denouncing LYSENKO and Stalin. He laughingly said that at least both could not be correct.

MULLER was very active in the Humanist Society and was once its president. In 1963 he was named "Humanist of the Year" and it was my honor to read a citation. In those days, manned space flights had begun and MULLER was very excited. In fact, in his evolution course he spent much time on the origin of the universe, of the solar system, and of life. Knowing this, I said: "If it were possible to send a man to Mars and bring him back safely and quickly, my candidate would be H. J. MULLER. For one thing, his spirit of adventure is such that he would enjoy the trip. But more important, he would have more interesting, exciting, and scientifically important observations to report than anyone I can think of."

I could see him beaming as I read it.

LITERATURE CITED

BEALE, G., 1993   The discovery of mustard gas mutagenesis by AUERBACH and ROBSON in 1941. Genetics **134**: 393–399.

CARLSON, E. A., 1981   *Genes, Radiation, and Society: The Life and Work of H. J. Muller.* Cornell University Press, Ithaca.

CROW, J. F., 1988   A diamond anniversary: the first chromosome map. Genetics **118**: 1–3.

CROW, J. F., 1990   H. J. Muller, scientist and humanist. Wis. Acad. Rev. **36**: 19–22.

CROW, J. F., 1993   N. I. VAVILOV, martyr to genetic truth. Genetics **134**: 1–4.

CROW, J. F., 1995   Quarreling geneticists and a diplomat. **140**: 421–426.

GREEN, M. M., 1996   The "genesis of the white-eyed mutant" in *Drosophila melanogaster:* a reappraisal. Genetics **142**: 329–331.

LEDERBERG, J., 1991   The gene (H. J. MULLER 1947). Genetics **129**: 313–316.

LEWIS, E. B., 1995   Remembering STURTEVANT. Genetics **141**: 1227–1230.

MUKAI, T., 1964   Spontaneous mutation rate of polygenes controlling viability. Genetics **50**: 1–19.

MULLER, H. J., 1927   Artificial transmutation of the gene. Science **66**: 84–87.

MULLER, H. J., 1928a   The measurement of gene mutation rate in Drosophila, its high variability, and its dependence upon temperature. Genetics **13**: 279–357.

MULLER, H. J., 1928b   The problem of genic modification. Z. Ind. ukt. Abstammungs-Vererbungsl., **Suppl I:** 224–260.

MULLER, H. J., 1962   *Studies in Genetics.* Indiana University Press, Bloomington.

PAUL, D., 1988   H. J. MULLER, communism, and the cold war. Genetics **119**: 223–225.

ROMAN, H., 1988   A diamond in the desert. Genetics **119**: 739–741.

SCHRÖDINGER, E., 1944   *What is Life?* Cambridge University Press, Cambridge.

STADLER, D., 1997   Ultraviolet-induced mutation and the chemical nature of the gene. Genetics **145**: 863–865.

An Oak Ridge Legacy
The Specific Locus Test and Its Role in Mouse Mutagenesis

Allan Peter Davis and Monica J. Justice

Life Sciences Division, Oak Ridge National Laboratory, Oak Ridge, Tennessee 37831–8080

WITHIN the last two decades, mouse genetics has undergone a revolution, an event initiated by breakthroughs in molecular biology and tissue culture techniques. Previous to this explosion, most scientists were content to puzzle over the thousand or so spontaneous mutants, deletion stocks, and specially designed strains of mice that currently existed. This analysis provided a wealth of insight into developmental biology, immunology, and mammalian genetics in general; nonetheless, the nature of the mutation and the gene that was affected often remained unknown. Today, gene targeting is in vogue, with investigators rushing to make "knock-outs" (disrupted alleles) of every cloned gene. This technique allows researchers to focus on specific genes of interest and to work backward to a phenotype, an approach opposite to studying spontaneous mutants. Gene targeting is indisputably a valuable tool for initiating a mutational analysis in the mouse (CAPECCHI 1989). The power of genetic functional analysis, however, lies in collecting an allelic series. A few rare examples do exist where gene targeting is used not to create a knock-out but rather a more subtle lesion, e.g., ZEIHER et al. 1995. For the most part, however, the field today does not often reflect that the early severe phenotype of a disrupted mutation can mask later functions and should only serve as a starting point—as opposed to an end-all—for gene analysis, especially when the allele results in embryonic lethality. Extrapolating from the rampant proliferation of gene targeting papers in the literature, one almost expects the 100,000 or so genes in the mouse to be mutated any day now. Ah, bliss: Every gene knocked-out and a phenotype ascribed to each mouse! In increasing numbers, however, neo-classical geneticists are stepping forward to ask everyone to rethink the analysis.

Backstory: Last November represented the 50th anniversary of the arrival of mouse geneticist WILLIAM (BILL) LAWSON RUSSELL to Oak Ridge, Tennessee. The move was coincident with the great fire in Bar Harbor, Maine, that destroyed most of The Jackson Laboratory, RUSSELL's previous employer (E. S. RUSSELL 1987). At the urging of ALEXANDER HOLLAENDER, BILL—and later his wife LIANE (LEE) BRAUCH RUSSELL, who was finishing her doctorate at the University of Chicago—joined the Biology Division at Oak Ridge National Laboratory to add to HOLLAENDER's vision of determining the effect of radiation on genetic systems (VON BORSTEL and STEINBERG 1995). The research legacy of the RUSSELLS is vast but centers on the creation of a specially designed mouse strain called the T (test) stock that was used as a genetic screen for the mutagenic testing of radiation and chemicals.

The T-stock mouse is a unique genetic tool packed with seven recessive, viable mutations affecting easily recognizable traits. Six influence coat color: a (nonagouti, chromosome 2), b (brown, chromosome 4), c^{ch} (chinchilla at albino, chromosome 7), d (dilute, chromosome 9), p (pink-eyed dilution, chromosome 7), and s (piebald-spotting, chromosome 14); one controls ear morphology: se (short-ear, chromosome 9). RUSSELL created the strain from a stock of NB mice that already harbored six of the recessive alleles. This strain, however, was so highly inbred that its fecundity and viability were dropping fast, and the line risked becoming extinct. To save the stock, RUSSELL had to outcross NB to another mouse. With the recent burning of The Jackson Laboratory, however, mice were next to impossible to locate (E. S. RUSSELL 1987). Any spare animals that existed were being shipped to Bar Harbor to re-establish the mouse colony. Persistent, RUSSELL located a professional photographer in Florida who also dabbled as a "garage" mouse geneticist and breeder. He supplied RUSSELL with animals that carried three of the six recessive alleles and also provided the s mutation.

Corresponding author: Monica J. Justice, Life Sciences Division, Oak Ridge National Laboratory, P.O. Box 2009, Oak Ridge, TN 37831-8080.

Invigorated by this outcrossing, the seven-locus *T*-stock was created in April 1948 (RUSSELL 1989). By packing all of these mutations into a single mouse, RUSSELL built a valuable tool for simultaneously following the genetics of seven traits.

RUSSELL's initial goal at Oak Ridge was not to determine whether radiation caused hereditary changes in mice because GEORGE SNELL and others had shown a decade earlier that chromosomal changes induced by X rays had phenotypic consequences (reviewed in RUSSELL 1954). Rather, he wanted to calculate a rate for heritable gene mutations induced by radiation in germ cells. By using the *T*-stock, he proposed to study a defined set of loci to see how often they mutated. His approach was simple: Wild-type males were divided into two groups, one set irradiated with various doses of X rays and the second set used as controls. All of these males were crossed to his *T*-stock females. Because of the recessive nature of the mutations, the progeny would appear wild type ($a/+$; $b/+$; $p\,c^{ch}/++$; $d\,se/++$; $s/+$). However, a mutation at any one of the specific loci would be immediately recognized in the progeny. This approach, called the specific locus test (SLT), allowed RUSSELL to score the number of specific mutations and to calculate a radiation-induced mutation rate in mammals.

It is important to stress the significance of the *T*-stock mouse. The experiment could have taken several different approaches that did not employ a specially designed tester mouse. In fact, alternative ideas were suggested by H. J. MULLER and RUSSELL's thesis advisor SEWALL WRIGHT during a closed-door meeting in HOL-LAENDER's office (RUSSELL 1989). WRIGHT thought it would be more appropriate to measure the vital statistics, *e.g.*, weight, longevity, and fertility, of the offspring of irradiated males. MULLER feared an SLT in mice would be too difficult to conduct and suggested examining recessive lethals over a larger segment of the genome. RUSSELL argued that was disadvantageous because it would require three generations of breeding. The SLT with the *T*-stock mouse, RUSSELL boasted, would allow an individual to rapidly score in the first generation 2000 loci per hour by focusing on the coat color and ear shape. More importantly, however, the SLT would provide better data on gene mutation rate for comparison with Drosophila. This was critical to him. The human risk-estimates of radiation at that time were almost exclusively based on fly studies, and RUSSELL wanted to make as precise a correlation between Drosophila and mouse as possible. He reasoned that it would be too difficult to compare mutation rates for all dominant visibles in a fly with those in a mouse owing to the "the virtual impossibility of equating morphological and physiological levels of detectability in the two species" (RUSSELL 1951). Instead, the SLT in mice would provide a specific mutation rate for defined loci, a feature especially important because no one had any idea how comparable the two genomes of a mouse and

fly would be. Finally, the SLT allowed the capture and propagation of all of these new mutations in one generation, even those that were lethal when homozygous, allowing many different alleles to be acquired for each locus. By examining each allele individually and in comparison with others, RUSSELL hoped to gain information on the nature of the mutations, initiating a detailed functional genetic analysis in mice.

RUSSELL examined over 85,875 offspring (data rarely matched by today's mouse geneticists) for his first paper on the subject (RUSSELL 1951). In the experiment, he collected 53 new alleles for the seven loci and two spontaneous mutations in the control group, allowing him to calculate a radiation-induced mutation rate per locus for mammals that was 10 times higher than that for Drosophila. In his results, however, RUSSELL discovered a wide range in mutation yield among the seven loci and realized that the data could not be quantitatively extrapolated to the entire genome: Some genes just appeared to be more mutable than others. Because most of the seven loci in RUSSELL's SLT were originally discovered by mouse fanciers and pet owners, they might have an intrinsically higher mutation rate, which would explain why they were easily isolated by amateur breeders (like the photographer in Florida). To test this, a team in Harwell, England, constructed a new *T*-stock, using different loci: *bp* (brachypodism), *fz* (fuzzy), *ln* (leaden), *pa* (pallid), and *pe* (pearl). None of these are known to have been originally collected by mouse fanciers, even though some of them produce coat colors similar to those in RUSSELL's loci. This Harwell-test stock was subjected to the same X-ray treatments that RUSSELL employed. While examining a smaller data set (about 26,000 offspring), the researchers calculated an averaged radiation-induced mutation rate that was four to five times lower than RUSSELL's but still much higher than that of Drosophila (LYON and MORRIS 1966). The value of the SLT approach, however, was not that it could extrapolate to whole-genome mutation rates but that it provided a rapid and defined assay to address the parameters affecting mutagenesis.

The RUSSELLs continued to use the *T*-stock in numerous applications to estimate the genetic hazards of radiation to humans. A seminal paper demonstrated that radiation-induced mutations were dependent on the dose rate, a result in stark contrast to Drosophila studies. In a Herculean task of raising over half a million mice in an SLT, the RUSSELLs found that animals exposed to a chronic dose of radiation produced markedly lower numbers of mutations than mice given the same radiation as an acute dose (RUSSELL *et al.* 1958). To reconcile this effect with Drosophilia, they proposed that in mammals some mutations were "reparable" by an as yet unknown mechanism. Having earlier shown that mouse genes were over 10 times more mutable than those of Drosophila, the RUSSELLs had now demonstrated that "the genetic hazards at least under some radiation conditions may not be as great as those estimated from the mutation rates obtained with acute radiation" (RUSSELL *et al.* 1958).

Several hundred specific locus mutations were scored and collected in a few decades of radiation mutagenesis. Thanks to the foresight of the RUSSELLS, many of these were propagated and maintained for analysis. With dozens of independently induced alleles at each locus, LEE RUSSELL conducted complementation tests that identified sets of overlapping, nested deletions (RUSSELL 1971). This organized the alleles into complementation groups and localized functional units, pioneering a new mapping strategy in the mouse (reviewed in RINCHIK and RUSSELL 1990).

The SLT had other valuable spin-offs. First, radiation-induced translocations between autosomes and the X-chromosome were made visible when coat color markers showed variegated patterning owing to the influence of X-inactivation. Such mutants helped propel the single-active X-chromosome hypothesis (LYON 1961; RUSSELL 1961). Second, specific locus markers allowed LEE to develop the spot test, an assay that quickly scores somatic genetic events such as point mutations, deletions, recombination, and chromosome loss. In the spot test, embryos heterozygous for four of the coat color loci from the SLT were mutagenized and upon birth screened for somatic mutations at these loci by looking for spots of colored fur patches in the pups (RUSSELL and MAJOR 1957). Today, the spot test is still the only general primary *in vivo* screen for mitotic recombination in the mouse and is likely to be revived for today's interest in DNA repair and recombination. Finally, mosaics recovered from the SLT are providing surprising insights into the timing of spontaneous mutations that arise in the germline (RUSSELL and RUSSELL 1996). The analysis of such mice will be invaluable in understanding the basis of human mosaic disease syndromes (reviewed in KENT-FIRST 1997).

Chemical mutagenesis: In addition to study of radiation, the SLT could also be used to assay for harmful effects caused by chemicals. It was already known that certain compounds injected into mice had genetic consequences, *e.g.*, FALCONER *et al.* (1952), and concerns for human safety were raised by J. B. S. HALDANE's "plea" to examine "the mutagenic effect of substances which are frequently added to human food as preservatives" (HALDANE 1956). However, most of the early experiments testing a variety of compounds (from caffeine to diethyl sulfate) provided ineffective at inducing mutations in spermatogonia (reviewed in EHLING 1978). Procarbazine, a drug used in the treatment of Hodgkin's disease, was the most effective chemical found to cause any type of significant spermatogonial mutagenesis in an SLT, yet even this rate was still only one third of the maximum RUSSELL attained with X rays (EHLING and NEUHAUSER 1979). It was almost beginning to appear as if mouse sper-

matogonia were strongly protected against chemical insults or were highly efficient at repairing such lesions. Even diethylnitrosamine (DEN), a compound known to be strongly mutagenic in Drosophila, was completely ineffective in mice (RUSSELL and KELLY 1979). To be mutagenic, however, DEN is enzymatically converted into an alkylating agent, and it was possible either that this activation process was not occurring in mammals or, if it was, that the short-lived metabolite was not capable of reaching the testis in time to be effective. To circumvent this complication, EKKEHART VOGEL suggested that RUSSELL try the experiment again using ethylnitrosourea (ENU), a chemical that forms the same alkylating species as DEN but does not require metabolism. RUSSELL, still disappointed by the DEN results, thought ENU was going to be another long shot, but he set up a small pilot experiment.

A single dose of ENU was injected into a group of male mice, which then underwent temporary sterility owing to massive killing of spermatogonia. Upon recovery about 10 wk later, however, 90 males were crossed to T-stock females and sired 7584 pups. Among this small set of offspring, 35 were mutant for one of the seven loci, yielding an induced mutation rate five times higher than the maximal rate obtained with X rays (RUSSELL *et al.* 1979). Encouraged by these findings, RUSSELL's group showed that if, instead of one large dose, the ENU was fractionated and injected on a weekly schedule to permit a higher total dose to be tolerated, then the mutation frequency jumped to 12 times that of X rays, 36 times higher than procarbazine, and over 200 times the spontaneous rate. When averaged across all seven loci, ENU was now inducing mutations at a frequency of one per locus in every 700 gametes (RUSSELL *et al.* 1982a, 1982b; HITOTSUMACHI *et al.* 1985). Because the spermatogonial stem cells were being affected, the genetic lesions were not restricted to transient stages but could be recovered indefinitely (at least as long as the mutagenized male survived). Additionally, the ENU mutants were slightly different from the ones induced by X rays. First, the phenotypes sometimes appeared intermediate between the wild-type and T-stock alleles. Second, there were never any mutations simultaneously affecting the two closely linked *d* and *se* loci. Third, the number of mutations for the T-stock loci that were lethal when homozygous was very low (RUSSELL 1982). ENU apparently caused subtle intragenic lesions (instead of the X-ray-generated deletions) and was heralded a "supermutagen," deigned the "mutagen of choice for the production of any kind of desired new gene mutations in the mouse" (RUSSELL *et al.* 1979).

ENU as a genetic tool: The earliest application of ENU to create new mouse mutations was in detecting electrophoretic mobility variants of blood proteins, an efficient screen that could easily assay 21 different loci from a single preparation (JOHNSON and LEWIS 1981).

Because the primary structure of many of these proteins had already been biochemically determined, it was of interest to characterize the structure of the ENU-induced variants to identify the molecular basis of mutagenesis. In the first analysis of a hemoglobin variant, a single amino acid substitution was discovered, and it was proposed that ENU had induced an A to T transversion in a histidine codon (Popp *et al.* 1983), supporting the idea that ENU acts as a point mutagen in mice.

Vernon Bode at Kansas State University and William Dove and Alexandra Shedlovsky at the University of Wisconsin used ENU to dissect the properties of the mouse *t-region*, a bizarre genetic locus with many distinctive traits including interaction with *T* (Brachyury) to produce tailless mice, transmission ratio distortion, and male sterility in compound heterozygotes. The analysis of *t* was complicated by the fact that recombination at *t-region* was strongly suppressed, disallowing the locus to be genetically dissected by crossovers. Thus, to study individual functional units, ENU mutagenesis was used to saturate the area and make discrete intragenic lesions (Bode 1984; Justice and Bode 1986, 1988; Shedlovsky *et al.* 1986, 1988).

Realizing the value of the mouse as a model for human diseases, it was now feasible to mutagenize an animal with ENU and screen for phenotypes resembling clinical disorders. Phenylketonuria, one of the first inborn errors of metabolism characterized in humans, was chose by Bode as a disease to reproduce in the mouse with chemical mutagenesis (McDonald *et al.* 1990). Besides creating new mouse models, one of the interesting results from this study was the dramatic frequency at which mutations in the phenylketonuria pathway were collected: an astounding one mutant for every 175 gametes examined (Shedlovsky *et al.* 1993). This value, close to 10 times better than the frequency of other loci, may mean that different genes could have very different induced mutation rates, as Russell's group had noticed in the SLT (Hitotsumachi *et al.* 1985).

The value of ENU alleles and the different types of screens used to capture them are diverse:

1. In the positional cloning of complex genetic lesions, ENU-induced mutations can confirm the functional identity of candidate genes, as was done for the *kreisler*, *quaking*, *eed*, and *Clock* loci (Cordes and Barsh 1994; Ebersole *et al.* 1996; Schumacher *et al.* 1996; King *et al.* 1997b).
2. The easiest screen is a hunt for dominants. These will inherently fall out of any ENU experiment and can yield diverse phenotypes from circling behavior to neoplasia disposition (Moser *et al.* 1990). *Clock*, probably the most famous example, is a dominant, antimorphic, ENU-induced allele captured by carefully assaying mice for abnormal well-running activity, resulting in the first cloned mouse mutation to

disrupt circadian rhythm (Vitaterna *et al.* 1994; Antoch *et al.* 1997; King *et al.* 1997a, 1997b).

3. Alleles of an already known mutation can be recovered by conducting an SLT similar to Russell's, where a mutagenized male is crossed to a female homozygous for the test locus (m/m). ENU mutations specific to the locus (*) will be uncovered and recognized in the F_1 generation (*/m). To fully characterize any one mouse gene, this technique should be applied to any disrupted allele made by gene targeting because a functional analysis can be appreciated only by examining an allelic series. While null mutations are necessary, subsequent alleles generated by point mutations including hypermorphs, hypomorphs, antimorphs, and neomorphs can yield vastly different phenotypes. For example, *eed* is a mouse mutation that causes early embryonic lethality. A hypomorphic allele of *eed* induced by ENU, however, allows the mouse to survive embryogenesis. The hypomorph shows skeletal transformations along the vertebral column and provides insight into *eed* as a regulator of homeotic genes (Schumacher *et al.* 1996). Thus, a knock-out database for the mouse genome should be considered only as a starting point; additional alleles are mandatory to complete the functional analysis.
4. Besides structural mutations, ENU will also induce lesions in regulatory elements, a feature not considered in most gene targeting studies.
5. By exploiting nonallelic noncomplementation, it may be possible to conduct sensitized screens in mice. An induced mutation at another locus that happens to interact with the specific locus of interest might fail to complement (*+; +/m) yet still yield a phenotype reminiscent of the original homozygous mutant (m/m). This approach, reiterated with each new mutation captured, might generate an extensive functional map of genetic interactions.
6. Another application of ENU is in saturation mutagenesis at defined deletions, yielding discrete functional units at any chromosomal site. Eugene Rinchik designed elegant screens exploiting coat color genetics to provide a fine-structure functional analysis for the *c* and *p* loci deletions originally produced in Russell's X-ray treatments in the SLT (Rinchik *et al.* 1990, 1995). Because deletions in the mouse can now be quickly generated in any part of the genome (Ramirez-Solis *et al.* 1995; You *et al.* 1997), the merging of this technology with chemical mutagenesis will undoubtedly be one of the most productive phases of functional genomics starting off the next millennium.

We now stand at an exciting crossroad in mouse genetics. The field has exploded with an infusion of molecular biologists applying their "tricks-of-the-trade" to manipulate the genome. For a while, chemical mutagenesis fell out of favor. It seemed as if knowing the nucleotide lesions in a mutation would be necessary to produce any value to understanding the biology of genetics. Though ENU mutagenesis may produce interesting variants, the nature of its own power, that being a point mutagen, frightened many people who were obsessed by the fear of never being able to clone the affected gene. Instead, pushes were made to sequence genomes, and the concern over function and phenotype would come later. Well, folks, it's later. The tremendous sequencing projects are starting to pay off by now, providing molecular landmarks throughout the mouse genome that can serve as launching points to sequence new mutations. The pendulum has started to swing back to ENU mutagenesis to generate and collect those interesting mice in phenotype-driven screens that will allow an in-depth study of any gene, chromosomal region, or biological system, thanks to the legacy of the RUSSELLS on their 50th Anniversary in Oak Ridge.

LITERATURE CITED

ANTOCH, M. P., E-J. SONG, A.-M. CHANG, M. H. VITATERNA, Y. ZHAO *et al.* 1997 Functional identification of the mouse circadian *Clock* gene by transgenic BAC rescue. Cell **89**: 655–667.

BODE, V. C., 1984 Ethylnitrosourea mutagenesis and the isolation of mutant alleles for specific genes located in the *t* region of mouse chromosome 17. Genetics **108**: 457–470.

CAPECCHI, M. R., 1989 Altering the genome by homologous recombination. Science **244**: 1288–1292.

CORDES, S. P., and G. S. BARSH, 1994 The mouse segmentation gene *kr* encodes a novel basic domain-leucine zipper transcription factor. Cell **79**: 1025–1034.

EBERSOLE, T. A., Q. GHEN, M. J. JUSTICE and K. ARTZT, 1996 The quaking gene product necessary in embryogenesis and myelination combines features of RNA binding and signal transduction proteins. Nat. Genet **12**: 260–265.

EHLING, U. H., 1978 Specific-locus mutations in mice, pp. 233–256 in *Chemical Mutagens*, edited by A. HOLLAENDER and F. J. DESERRES. Plenum Press, New York.

EHLING, U. H., and A. NEUHAUSER, 1979 Procarbazine induced specific-locus mutations in male mice. Mutat. Res. **59**: 245–256.

FALCONER, D. S., B. M. SLIZYNSKI and C. AUERBACH, 1952 Genetical effects of nitrogen mustard in the house mouse. J. Genet. **51**: 81–88.

HALDANE, J. B. S., 1956 The detection of autosomal lethals in mice induced by mutagenic agents. J. Genet. **54**: 327–342.

HITOTSUMACHI, S., D. A. CARPENTER and W. L. RUSSELL, 1985 Dose-repetition increases the mutagenic effectiveness of N-ethyl-N-nitrosourea in mouse spermatogonia. Proc. Natl. Acad. Sci. USA **82**: 6619–6621.

JOHNSON, F. M., and S. E. LEWIS, 1981 Electrophoretically detected germinal mutations induced in the mouse by ethylnitrosourea. Proc. Natl. Acad. Sci. USA **78**: 3138–3141.

JUSTICE, M. J., and V. C. BODE, 1986 Induction of new mutations in a mouse t-haplotype using ethylnitrosourea mutagenesis. Genet. Res. **47**: 187–192.

JUSTICE, M. J., and V. C. BODE, 1988 Three ENU-induced alleles of the murine quaking locus are recessive embryonic lethal mutations. Genet. Res. **51**: 95–102.

KENT-FIRST, M., 1997 A lesson from mosaics: don't leave the genetics out of molecular genetics. J. NIH Res. **9**: 29–33.

KING, D. P., M. H. VITATERNA, A-M. CHANG, W. F. DOVE, L. H. PINTO *et al.*, 1997a The mouse *Clock* mutation behaves as an antimorph and maps within the W^{19H} deletion, distal of *Kit*. Genetics **146**: 1049–1060.

KING, D. P., Y. ZHAO, A. M. SANGORAM, L. D. WILSBACHER, M. TANAKA *et al.*, 1997b Positional cloning of the mouse circadian *Clock* gene. Cell **89**: 641–653.

LYON, M. F., 1961 Gene action in the X chromosome of the mouse (*Mus musculus* L.) Nature **190**: 372–373.

LYON, M. F., and T. MORRIS, 1966 Mutation rates at a new set of specific loci in the mouse. Genet. Res. **7**: 12–17.

MCDONALD, J. D., V. C. BODE, W. F. DOVE and A. SHEDLOVSKY 1990 Pah^{hph-5}: a mouse mutant deficient in phenylalanine hydroxylase. Proc. Natl. Acad. Sci. USA **87**: 1965–1967.

MOSER, A. R., H. C. PITOT and W. F. DOVE 1990 A dominant mutation that predisposes to multiple intestinal neoplasia in the mouse. Science **247**: 322–324.

POPP, R. A., E. G. BAILIFF, L. C. SKOW, F. M. JOHNSON and S. E. LEWIS, 1983 Analysis of a mouse alpha-globin gene mutation induced by ethylnitrosourea. Genetics **105**: 157–167.

RAMIREZ-SOLIS, R., P. LIU, and A. BRADLEY, 1995 Chromosome engineering in mice. Nature **378**: 720–724.

RINCHIK, E. M., and L. B. RUSSELL, 1990 Germ-line deletion mutations in the mouse: tools for intensive functional and physical mapping of regions of the mammalian genome, pp. 121–158 in *Genome Analysis, Volume 1: Genetic and Physical Mapping* edited by K. DAVIES and S. TILGHMAN. Cold Spring Harbor Laboratory Press, Cold Spring Harbor, NY.

RINCHIK, E. M., D. A. CARPENTER and P. B. SELBY, 1990 A strategy for fine-structure functional analysis of a 6- to 11-centimorgan region of mouse chromosome 7 by high-efficiency mutagenesis. Proc. Natl. Acad. Sci. USA **87**: 896–900.

RINCHIK, E. M., D. A. CARPENTER and M. A. HANDEL, 1995 Pleiotropy in microdeletion syndromes: neurologic and spermatogenic abnormalities in mice homozygous for the p^{6H} deletion are likely due to dysfunction of a single gene. Proc. Natl. Acad. Sci. USA **92**: 6394–6398.

RUSSELL, E. S., 1987 A mouse phoenix rose from the ashes. Genetics **117**: 155–156.

RUSSELL, L. B., 1961 Genetics of mammalian sex chromosomes. Science **133**: 1795–1803.

RUSSELL, L. B., 1971 Definition of functional units in a small chromosomal segment of the mouse and its use in interpreting the nature of radiation-induced mutations. Mutat. Res. **11**: 107–123.

RUSSELL, L. B., and M. H. MAJOR, 1957 Radiation-induced presumed somatic mutations in the house mouse. Genetics **42**: 161–175.

RUSSELL, L. B., and W. L. RUSSELL, 1996 Spontaneous mutations recovered as mosaics in the mouse specific-locus test. Proc. Natl. Acad. Sci. USA **93**: 13072–13077.

RUSSELL, W. L., 1951 X-ray-induced mutations in mice. Cold Spring Harbor Symp. Quant. Biol. **16**: 327–335.

RUSSELL, W. L., 1954 Genetic effects of radiation in mammals, pp. 825–859 in *Radiation Biology*, edited by A. HOLLAENDER. McGraw-Hill, New York.

RUSSELL, W. L., 1982 Factors affecting mutagenicity of ethylnitrosourea in the mouse specific-locus test and their bearing on risk estimation, pp. 59–70 in *Environmental Mutagens and Carcinogens*, edited by T. SUGIMURA, S. KONDO and H. TAKEBE. Alan R. Liss, New York.

RUSSELL, W. L., 1989 Reminiscences of a mouse specific-locus test addict. Environ. Mol. Mutagen **14** (Suppl. 16): 16–22.

RUSSELL, W. L., and E. M. KELLY, 1979 Ineffectiveness of diethylnitrosamine in the induction of specific-locus mutations in mice. Genetics **91** (Suppl.): s109–s110.

RUSSELL, W. L., L. B. RUSSELL and E. M. KELLY 1958 Radiation dose rate and mutation frequency. Science **128**: 1546–1550.

RUSSELL, W. L., E. M. KELLY, P. R. HUNSICKER, J. W. BANGHAM, S. C. MADDUX *et al.*, 1979 Specific-locus test shows ethylnitrosourea to be the most potent mutagen in the mouse. Proc. Natl. Acad. Sci. USA **76**: 5818–5819.

RUSSELL, W. L., P. R. HUNSICKER, G. D. RAYMER, M. H. STEELE, K. F. STELZNER *et al.*, 1982a Dose-response curve for ethylnitrosourea-induced specific-locus mutations in mouse spermatogonia. Proc. Natl. Acad. Sci. USA **79**: 3589–3591.

RUSSELL, W. L., P. R. HUNSICKER, D. A. CARPENTER, C. V. CORNETT and G. M. GUINN, 1982b Effect of dose fractionation on the ethylnitrosourea induction of specific-locus mutations in mouse spermatogonia. Proc. Natl. Acad. Sci. USA **79**: 3592–3593.

SCHUMACHER, A., C. FAUST and T. MAGNUSON, 1996 Positional cloning of a global regulator of anterior-posterior patterning in mice. Nature **383**: 250–253.

SHEDLOVSKY, A., J-L. GUÉNET, L. J. JOHNSON and W. F. DOVE

1986 Induction of recessive lethal mutations in the *T/t-H-2* region of the mouse genome by a point mutagen. Genet. Res. **47**: 135–142.

SHEDLOVSKY, A., T. R. KING, and W. F. DOVE, 1988 Saturation germ line mutagenesis of the murine *t* region including a lethal allele at the quaking locus. Proc. Natl. Acad. Sci. USA **85**: 180–184.

SHEDLOVSKY, A., J. D. MCDONALD, D. SYMULA and W. F. DOVE, 1993 Mouse models of human phenylketonuria. Genetics **134**: 1205–1210.

VITATERNA, M. H., D. P. KING, A-M. CHANG, J. M. KORNHAUSER, P. L.

LOWREY *et al.* 1994 Mutagenesis and mapping of a mouse gene, *Clock*, essential for circadian behavior. Science **264**: 719–725.

VON BORSTEL, R. C., and C. M. STEINBERG, 1995 Alexander Hollaender: myth and mensch. Genetics **143**: 1054–1056.

YOU, Y., R. BERGSTROM, M. KLEMM, B. LEDERMAN, H. NELSON *et al.*, 1997 Chromosomal deletion complexes in mice by radiation of embryonic stem cells. Nat. Genet. **15**: 285–288.

ZEIHER, B. G., E. EICHWALD, J. ZABNER, J. J. SMITH, A. P. PUGA *et al.*, 1995 A mouse model for the delta F508 allele of cystic fibrosis. J. Clin. Invest. **96**: 2051–2064.

February 1998

The Engrailed Story

Antonio Garcia-Bellido

Centro de Biologia Molecular, Consejo Superior de Investigaciones Cientificas, Universidad Autonoma de Madrid, Madrid 28049 Spain

IN 1972, a paper on the developmental genetics of the mutation *engrailed* appeared in this journal. PEDRO SANTAMARIA, then a Ph.D. student in my laboratory, and I co-authored it. Being involved, I find it hard to comment on the paper itself, on its impact when it appeared and on its later relevance. I will, therefore, try to navigate along the strait between Scylla and Charybdis, avoiding my own views and considering what others may have thought of the findings.

The story begins at Caltech in 1968. EDWARD B. LEWIS, in charge of the Carnegie Collection of Drosophila mutant stocks, knew their adult phenotypes intimately. One of the many conversations in which we, together with ALFRED H. STURTEVANT, used to indulge was about homeotic genes. Lewis pointed out to me that *engrailed* (*en*) mutants had, in addition to the reported duplicate sex-combs in the male forelegs, a posterior wing margin similar to the normal anterior one. I had made preparations of adult morphogenetic mutant flies from the Caltech collection (mutants were usually observed only under the dissecting microscope) for detailed microscopic examination. Ed was right; under the light microscope there appeared along the posterior margin a secondary pattern of chaetae, typical of the anterior margin. Moreover, the specific corrugation of veins (swellings of the veins, from either a dorsal or ventral aspect) corresponded to a replacement of the posterior venation pattern by the characteristic anterior one. The characteristic chaeta pattern of the legs, including the secondary sex-comb, also showed replacement of the posterior by the anterior half; *engrailed* was clearly a homeotic mutation. And a peculiar one at that; contrary to others, it affected several segments in a homologous way. But many things were happening at that time in the Caltech lab, and I put the *engrailed* problem aside. It was to receive full attention upon my return to Madrid in 1969.

To understand what became interesting in the study of *engrailed*, we have to go back in time for a perspective as to how development and the genes controlling it were conceived. When I arrived at Caltech in 1967, I was invited to give a series of talks in the lab on the state of the art in developmental genetics, in Zurich in particular. I remember talking about determination and transdetermination and prepatterns, morphogenetic fields and blastemata, all terms that appeared metaphysical to Ed, although not to Sturt. In fact, these terms reflected the notions about development at the time, carried out as a continuation of an experimental tradition coming from ROUX and SPEMANN. Blastemata were made of cells, certainly, but the morphogenetic information was in the population of cells. Regeneration experiments repeatedly showed regulative properties that determine, in some mysterious way, what the cells would differentiate into at the last minute before entering into irreversible differentiation. Genes at that time were just alleles with phenotypes that could be modulated by temperature or by many genetic modifiers present in the genome. Mutations led to perturbation of the norm, but there was really nothing else to understand because, after all, evolution was a historically contingent event—the result of changes of alleles to generate fitter morphologies. Researchers described mutants, looking for changes in enzymes or their products that by some complex mechanisms would generate cascades of interactions leading to the abnormality, *i.e.*, "phenogenetic trees of action." Homeotic mutant transformations, for example, supposedly resulted from some abnormalities in the dynamics of growth. Still the central search was for nonautonomous effects of mutations, in transplants or in mosaics, because they could lead to the construction of metabolic pathways.

However, things were changing. "Transdetermination," *i.e.*, a sudden change in prospective differentiation upon regeneration and culture of fragments of imaginal discs, was akin to a homeotic mutant transformation. But it could be experimentally manipulated. It seemed to take place suddenly, in groups of cells, as was experimentally shown later (GEHRING 1967). Thus, transdetermination may result from "assimilative induction" between cells. I had tried in Zurich in 1964–65 to provoke this induction in cell mixtures, after dissociation of imaginal discs. ERNST HADORN had earlier shown that dissociated and reaggregated cells from the same type of disc (from two identical discs labeled with different mutant cuticular markers) did form mixed patterns upon metamorphosis. In 1964, in the HADORN lab ROLF NOTHIGER had shown that cells from different discs sort out, with some exceptional mosaics of isolated cells of one disc trapped in territories of cells of the other disc. Thus, there were no indications of assimilative induction. I showed in a series of experiments that not only do cells of different disc types sort out, but so do cells from different regions within a disc, while if derived from the same region they could partially reconstruct patterns or differentiate unpatterned elements of the region of origin (GARCIA-BELLIDO 1966, 1967). Clearly, the cells of mature imaginal discs of Drosophila already had great personality. They were, singly, determined to form adult pattern elements, and they must have surface labels as to the position in the primordium, which they used for pattern reconstruction in reaggregates. Cells were no longer merely bricks for construction.

Induced mitotic recombination, first used to analyze development in genetic mosaics by CURT STERN and his group, had revealed the cell autonomous response of morphogenetic mutants in genetic mosaics to invariant morphogenetic fields ("prepatterns") (STERN 1954). It could also be used, as HANNAH-ALAVA did, in the foreleg to trace clonal derivations of pattern elements. I used it with JOHN MERRIAM at Caltech to describe the clonal parameters of wing disc development (GARCIA-BELLIDO and MERRIAM 1971). I started with preparations I had made in Madrid of wings heterozygous for multiple wing hairs (mwh) irradiated as larvae and collected every 8 hr at puparium formation. The frequency of X-ray-induced mitotic recombination was reported to be low, and I expected only a few clones. But they would tell me how many cell divisions occur in vivo from mature larvae (the time I had made the cell dissociations) to the point of differentiation. It also had been reported that pupal discs undergo many cell divisions before differentiation, and this was contrary to the observation of a high degree of cell determination found in dissociated cells. To my surprise, adult wings of irradiated mature larvae contained hundreds of clones, each one cell in size. Larvae irradiated 8 hr earlier gave rise to wings with half the number of clones but twice the clone size, and the same trend was true for earlier irradiated larvae, with an average division time of 8 hr. Consequently, development could be described in terms of cells and clones, and in 1967, John and I became engaged in the study of the cell lineages of the wing. One of the first surprises was that clones could transgress neither the wing margin dorso-ventrally, nor the notum/wing boundary since very early in development (GARCIA-BELLIDO 1968b). That meant the existence of determinative decision for cell territories. Chaetal mother cells separated clonally from trichome epidermal cells later, shortly before puparium formation. Thus, cells and cell decisions came to the foreground of developmental descriptions. The obvious next step was to combine cell markers with morphogenetic mutants, or lethals, in mosaics generated by mitotic recombination, at different times of development. I learned the required genetics from John and Ed and started a long project in Madrid of describing development in terms of cells and genes.

Well, not yet in terms of genes. I had come to Caltech to study the behavior of bithorax mutant cells in aggregates. My previous experience with other homeotic mutants, aristapedia and Antennapedia, was confusing (GARCIA-BELLIDO 1968a). True, the homeotic leg cells of the antenna mixed well with leg and not with antenna cells, but the pattern limit of the mixing was more proximal in aggregates than in the mutant fly antenna. More specific limits of transformation were needed to exclude assimilative induction once and for all. This was provided by the two mutations, bithorax (bx) and postbithorax (pbx), with a net separation between wing homeotic tissue and haltere tissue along the middle of both the adult wing and the haltere. When the aggregates were made, the adult transformation boundary was respected; only bx homeotic cells will mix and reconstruct mosaic patterns with anterior wing cells, and the corresponding situation was true for pbx posterior haltere cells. The explanation for Ed was outright and categorical: "haltere posterior cells or haltere anterior cells cannot assimilate to become wing because in the mutant disc either the bx or the pbx cells are wildtype for the complementary region." This apparent tautology was all-revealing. Genes, i.e., their wild-type alleles, were in charge of defining cell states, cell autonomously. For Ed it was clear because he had found gynandromorph mosaics of few Ultrabithorax (Ubx) cells differentiating mesothoracic chaetae in the metanotum (LEWIS 1963). The work on bithorax aggregates was published much later (GARCIA-BELLIDO and LEWIS 1976), delayed by Ed's literary restraint.

Cell mosaics and cell aggregates revealed an undreamed of cell autonomy. These findings allowed the connection between cells, genes, and development, at least in my mind. And this was the title of the final seminar I gave in Caltech in 1968, before coming to Madrid.

One thing is left in the reflections about the background of the engrailed story. Once in Madrid, I gave a seminar in the Centro de Investigaciones Biologicas on my work at Caltech and assembled thereafter three Ph.D. students. One, PEDRO SANTAMARIA, was encouraged to work on the development of tergites (for comparison with the wing), GINES MORATA to work on the clonal analysis of the bithorax mutants; and PEDRO

RIPOLL became engaged in the clonal analysis of lethals and genetic aneuploids in cells. I put myself to work on the dorso-ventral induction in wing vein formation. By so doing, I came to encounter very large wing clones, much larger than the earliest ones initiated in the embryo, but still normal-sized in tergites. How could that be? Early chromosome loss, as in gynandromorphs, but affecting the progeny of wing but not of tergite embryonic cells? I asked GINES to work it out. When he came up with the answer, along with PEDRO RIPOLL who had joined the enterprise, I could not believe it: it was too much cell autonomy, this time for the pace of growth. Clones were large because of a factor that could be mapped in the same chromosome arm of the *mwh* cell marker, and when removed by recombination led the cells to grow faster than their surrounding cells. The mosaic flies developed more slowly and had Minute chaetae, and this reminded me that C. STERN had used Minutes because on this background clones were large and thus could be easily detected under the dissecting microscope. The interesting thing here, however, is that the wing M^+ clones would respect not only the wing margin border, as normal clones do, but would also stop along a mysterious but constant line, running some cell diameters anterior to the fourth longitudinal vein of the wing. This is obviously the anterior-posterior clonal restriction boundary that separates an anterior from a posterior compartment, from the very beginning of development. The wing appeared then to be made of eight compartments consisting of growing cells that do not transgress the corresponding restriction lines after specific moments of development (GARCIA-BELLIDO *et al.* 1973, 1976). Since early gynandromorph mosaics could have male/female boundaries running through the wing, compartments had to be polyclonal in origin.

This was the conceptual background that led to the analysis of *engrailed* (*en*), the real subject of this *Perspectives* essay. The 1972 paper (GARCIA-BELLIDO and SANTAMARIA 1972) contains two different sections. In the first, the clonal analysis of *engrailed* is subdivided into two parts, one describing how the mutant wing grows a "cell lineage", the other what *en* mutant cells do in "morphogenetic mosaics" within *en*⁺ wings. The first part shows that the posterior part of the wing grows like the anterior one, with a very fuzzy clonal separation between anterior and posterior cells. In fact, cell aggregates of posterior regions of *engrailed* wing discs with whole wing disc cells showed mixing in both territories. The second part of the mosaic analysis revealed that mutant cells autonomously differentiate anterior structures in "homologous" posterior positions. In the second section, we showed the phenotype of double mutant combinations of *bx* and *pbx* with *en*, indicating that the duplicated posterior cells do not derive from anterior cells migrating to posterior positions. In the double *pbx en* mutants, the posterior haltere is transformed

into an anterior wing. This observation demonstrated that the specification of the posterior part of the haltere is performed by the combined activity of *pbx*⁺ and *en*⁺ genes.

In the discussion section, in light of the notion of an invariant prepattern for segments and for posterior parts of segments to which mutant cells respond, it is pointed out that prepatterns become entities with no heuristic value in understanding morphogenesis. Thus, if any mutant transformation indicates that the corresponding alternative is its default condition or prepattern, *Contrabithorax* (*Cbx*) alleles, which show a wing to haltere transformation, would reveal the existence of an invariant haltere prepattern, and *Ubx* alleles that of a wing prepattern.

The developmental genetic analysis of *engrailed* and the subsequent one of the *bithorax* complex (MORATA and GARCIA-BELLIDO 1976) were the bases for the notion of selector genes. Systemic transformations, like these homeotic ones, affecting individual cells, meant that the abstract specification of whole cell territories (as to segment or compartment) resided in developmental operations carried out by the individual cells. Moreover, the expression of *engrailed* (and of the *bithorax* genes) is limited to these territories. These two steps required, in turn, other genes in addition. The model was put forward in a Ciba Symposium in 1974 (GARCIA-BELLIDO 1975) that "activator" genes delimit the realm of expression of "selector" genes, which in turn control "realizator" genes, in charge of performing the actual cell behavioral operations that end in final morphologies. Since several selector genes act in combination in the same cell, development results from a combinatorial or parallel processing of specific genetic functions acting in single cells (GARCIA-BELLIDO 1975; GARCIA-BELLIDO *et al.* 1976). Compartments within clonal restrictions were the realm of expression of these genes: *bithorax*, *postbithorax*, and *engrailed*.

The work on *engrailed* has since followed different paths, each paradigmatic. One path extends the notion of selector gene to other segmentation genes, like *bithorax*, *Antennapedia*, *proboscipedia*, and others. Their adult transformations and later the larval phenotypes of lethal null alleles of these genes (first done by Ed for the *bithorax* complex) revealed an underlying logic. Different segments require the function of different selector genes to specify alternatives to an evolutionary primitive segment, made of two parts, both corresponding to the anterior prothorax-mesothorax of the actual flies and by extension of insects (GARCIA-BELLIDO 1977).

The 1972 observation that anterior wing cells and posterior *en* wing cells do not distinguish between each other in aggregates was confirmed by GINES and PETER A. LAWRENCE in clones, as posterior *en* M^+ clones invade the anterior compartments, but not vice versa (MORATA and LAWRENCE 1975). This in turn indicates that *en* is not required in the anterior compartment.

This cell behavior [as well as the phenotype of *Cbx* mutants, corresponding to dominant gain of function alleles of *Ultrabithorax* (*bx* and *pbx*)], strongly suggested that these genes were real morphogenetic genes controlling developmental pathways (a term coined by Ed in contrast to metabolic pathways) in specific territories of the fly, while not active in others. These inferences could only be confirmed later, when it became possible to visualize gene expression patterns, after the advent of molecular techniques applied to the study of these genes.

The molecular analysis of *engrailed* was carried out by THOMAS KORNBERG and his colleagues (POOLE *et al.* 1985) and extended by PATRICK O'FARRELL and his colleagues (KUNER *et al.* 1985). The *en* gene encodes a protein with a homeodomain (similar to that of *Ubx*), a transcription factor that binds to DNA and regulates the expression of other genes. The work of several laboratories analyzed the patterns of embryonic expression of early segmentation genes, corresponding to zygotic lethal mutations discovered by ERIC WIESCHAUS and CHRISTIANE NÜSSLEIN-VOLHARDT in 1978 (NÜSSLEIN-VOLHARD and WIESCHAUS 1980). Three hierarchical classes of genes showed patterns that subdivided the syncytial egg and later the early blastoderm into shorter and shorter regions. Their expression depended on positive and negative controls by the earlier acting genes and, between them, finally specifying cell territories corresponding to embryonic segments. Among these genes were those controlling the limits of expression of *engrailed* and other segmental selector genes. They corresponded to the "activator" genes of the hierarchical model of selector genes. By making use of protein DNA crosslinking and cytological mapping of the *en* protein to salivary chromosomes, the search for the *en* down-stream "realizator" genes started later. It still continues, but among these genes are other selector genes (like *Ubx* and *en* itself) and genes encoding ligands (like *hedgehog*, *hh*) in cell-cell communication. The latter are possibly required to maintain the coherent expression of cell territories specified by *en*. But how these realizator genes control the characteristic behavior of compartment cells, how these systemic signals are converted into compartment-specific morphogenesis, is still unknown.

With the possibilities of manipulating the *en* gene in transgenic flies, it became possible for the first time to express it ectopically; if it is expressed in anterior compartment cells, it causes a transformation of an anterior into a posterior compartment (ZECCA *et al.* 1995).

DNA sequences or antibodies raised against the homeodomain of *engrailed* have found it to be conserved throughout metazoan evolution. The gene *en* or its Drosophila paralog *inv* are expressed in insects and crustacea in the posterior half of embryonic segments, but also in the mesoderm and in certain types of neurons. This expression, related not to territorial domains but to histotypes and cell types, is also conserved. In fact, in the leech, arthropods, and vertebrates, *en/inv* orthologs are expressed in certain cephalic segments in specific neurons, as well as in somites (WEDEEN and WEISBLAST 1991; HOLLAND *et al.* 1997). In vertebrates, midbrain development requires *engrailed*, and how this relates to the insect functions is unclear. The problem of how the evolutionary functions of these selector genes arose and later diversified remains a central issue in metazoan evolution.

Mutations other than those in selector genes cause homeotic transformations in flies or in clones. They correspond to failures in function of genes involved in the activation of selectors or in the maintenance throughout the rest of development of the initial state, active or repressed. Their phenotypes (*e.g.*, *trithorax* or *Polycomb*) correspond to those of alleles of the selector genes. We now know that this maintenance, memory of gene activity, is because of changes in the chromatin organization of the activated selector gene, with positive regulatory feedback loops. These transformations are actual pathway substitutions. But a new type of gene has recently been found whose ectopic expression causes, at least in epidermal structures, the appearance of a complete eye, *i.e.*, a field of ommatidia with perfectly differentiated light receptor cells (HALDER *et al.* 1995). In some mutants of the gene *eyeless* (*ey*) there is complete absence of eyes. This gene is also conserved in metazoans and expressed in primordia of primitive light receptor cells. Those ectopic eye territories result from recruitment of surrounding epidermal cells to differentiate into eyes, another case of assimilative induction. This peculiar behavior of *ey* has led to the coining of a new term, that of "master" genes, to be distinguished from "selectors" because they open developmental pathways, not merely substitute archetypic ones. But there are many cases of genes of the histotypic differentiation class that have similar functions, as *myo-D* for muscle cells (OLSON 1990), the *achaete-scute* complex for neuronal specification (CAMPUZANO and MODOLELL 1992), the *tinman* homologs related to the formation of the heart (LILLY *et al.* 1994), *vestigial* for the wing, and others that could be considered in principle also to be master genes.

engrailed plays a very important morphogenetic role, in addition to acting as a selector gene within compartments. Its function generates the transcription of a signal (*hh*) that releases a cascade of genetic effects on the cells on the other side of the compartment border. Those are mediated by a receptor that activates a nuclear gene, which in turn controls the transcription of another signal, in the wing the ligand *decapentaplegic* (*dpp*) (ZECCA *et al.* 1995). The A/P boundary becomes then a reference for cell proliferation and for cell polarity, with symmetries at both sides of the clonal restriction border. In fact, the embryonic effects of *en* lethal alleles are changes in both the differentiation and the polarity of epidermal segments. For that reason, it is included in the class of segmentation genes called "segment polarity" genes (NÜSSLEIN-VOLHARD and WIESCHAUS 1980). Compartment borders and, in general, clonal restriction borders are associated with both the changes of polarity of cells and the references or signals for cell proliferation. Thus, apterous (*ap*), a recently discovered selector gene for the dorsal compartment of wing and haltere (DIAZ-BENJUMEA and COHEN 1993), also starts a cascade of genetic effects on both sides of the dorso/ventral (D/V) border. Interestingly, *ap* is expressed in the wing primordium before the clonal restriction appears, and only later does its expression become restricted to the dorsal polyclone; mosaics of mutant *ap* cells close to the dorsal border become incorporated into the ventral polyclone (BLAIR et al. 1994). However, when these mosaics appear in central regions of the wing, they cause a D/V duplication growing perpendicular to the wing blade, formed by surrounding wild-type dorsal cells (DIAZ-BENJUMEA and COHEN 1993). Thus, *ap* mutants fail to grow wings, possibly because the D/V border cannot be formed, and hence the signal for cell proliferation emanating from it fails to appear. Similarly, if the gene *engrailed* is ectopically expressed in clones in the anterior compartment of the wing, the associated signals generate a new border and cell proliferation ensues, giving rise to mirror-image duplicated A/P patterns (*e.g.*, veins) made by surrounding normal wing cells (TABATA et al. 1995; ZECCA et al. 1995). Interestingly, the size of these duplications depends on the position of the clone (*en* or *ap*) within the compartment and not on the size of the clone; duplications are larger when the clones arise further away from the corresponding compartment border. These, and results with other types of mutations, indicate that growing compartments are internally heterogeneous, with discontinuities related to presumptive veins (also associated with clonal restrictions) and positional values between them (GARCIA-BELLIDO and deCELIS 1992). This is not the place to go into details, but it is through studies of these discontinuities that we eventually will connect selector function in actual morphogenesis with the species-specificity of sizes and shapes of organs.

We have seen that the *en* embryonic compartment appears in groups of cells. This is so because they result from the subdivision of a continuous blastoderm. Further subdivision of the primordium is also polyclonal for the same reasons. Possibly, the coherence of the territory specified by selector genes results from signals between cells [like *hedgehog* (*hh*)] maintaining the selector activity in all the cells. How these later subdivisions appear, for example, that of *ap* generating the D/V symmetry, is still a mystery. Possibly, it reflects undetected heterogeneities of expression of other genes within the primordium, as happens for *en* and *bx* in the embryo. This may explain why we failed to assimila-

tively induce metathoracic cells to be converted into mesothoracic ones in gynandromorph mosaics of *Ubx* mutant cells in the embryonic metathorax (MIÑANA and GARCIA-BELLIDO 1982). But that cells communicate with each other in genetic specification is evident, for example in the specification of territories with partial transformations owing to homeotic hypomorphic alleles. In these chimeric territories the expression of, *e.g.*, the Ubx protein occurs in contiguous patches not related by clonal origin (BOTAS et al. 1988). We have mentioned that the same applies to transdetermination events, which affect groups of cells. But the cell interactions at work in the transdetermination or in homeotic changes go beyond specifying cell type. The apposition of transdetermined (allotypic) territories to similar (autotypic) territories, owing to cell recognition, is associated with mirror-image copies of their patterns, or their integration into one single pattern, although both cell territories are of different clonal origin (GARCIA-BELLIDO 1972). Thus, the phenomenon of assimilative induction eludes our understanding. Much more knowledge about active genomes defining cell behavior is obviously needed to explain development in terms of genes and cells.

LITERATURE CITED

BLAIR, S. S., D. L. BROWER, J. B. THOMAS and M. ZABORTINK, 1994   The role of apterous in the control of dorsoventral compartmentalization and PS integrin gene expression in the developing wing of Drosophila. Development **120**: 1805–1815.

BOTAS, J., C. V. CABRERA and A. GARCIA-BELLIDO, 1988   The reinforcement extinction process of selector gene activity: a positive feed-back loop and cell-cell interactions in Ultrabithorax patterning. Roux's Arch. Dev. Biol. **197**: 424–434.

CAMPUZANO, S., and J. MODOLELL, 1992   Patterning of the Drosophila nervous system: the achaete-scute gene complex. Trends Genet. **8**: 202–208.

DIAZ-BENJUMEA, F., and S. M. COHEN, 1993   Interactions between dorsal and ventral cells in the imaginal disc directs wing development in Drosophila. Cell **75**: 741–752.

GARCIA-BELLIDO, A., 1966   Pattern reconstruction by dissociated imaginal disc cells of *Drosophila melanogaster.* Dev. Biol. **14**: 278–306.

GARCIA-BELLIDO, A., 1967   Histotypic reaggregation of dissociated imaginal disc cells of *Drosophila melanogaster* cultured in vivo. Wilhelm Roux's Arch. Entwicklungsmech. Org. **158**: 212–217.

GARCIA-BELLIDO, A., 1968a   Cell affinities in antennal homeotic mutants of *Drosophila melanogaster.* Genetics **59**: 487–499.

GARCIA-BELLIDO, A., 1968b   Cell lineage in the wing disc of *Drosophila melanogaster.* Genetics **60**: 181.

GARCIA-BELLIDO, A., 1972   Pattern formation in imaginal disks, pp. 59–91 in *Results and Problems in Cell Differentiation*, Vol. 5, edited by H. URSPRUNG and R. NÖTHIGER. Springer-Verlag, Berlin.

GARCIA-BELLIDO, A., 1975   Genetic control of wing disc development in *Drosophila*, pp. 161–182 in Ciba Found. Symp. 29, *Cell Patterning.*

GARCIA-BELLIDO, A., 1977   Homeotic and atavic mutation in insects. Am. Zool. **17**: 613–629.

GARCIA-BELLIDO, A., and J. F. DeCELIS, 1992   Developmental genetics of the venation pattern of Drosophila. Annu. Rev. Genet. **26**: 277–304.

GARCIA-BELLIDO, A., and E. B. LEWIS, 1976   Autonomous cellular differentiation of homeotic bithorax mutants of *Drosophila melanogaster.* Dev. Biol. **48**: 400–410.

GARCIA-BELLIDO, A., and J. MERRIAM, 1971   Parameters of the wing imaginal disc development of *Drosophila melanogaster*. Dev. Biol. **24**: 61–87.

GARCIA-BELLIDO, A., and P. SANTAMARIA, 1972 Developmental analysis of the wing disc in the mutant engrailed of *Drosophila melanogaster*. Genetics **72**: 87–101.

GARCIA-BELLIDO, A., P. RIPOLL and G. MORATA, 1973 Developmental compartmentalization of the wing disc of Drosophila. Nat. New Biol. **245**: 251–253.

GARCIA-BELLIDO, A., P. RIPOLL and G. MORATA, 1976 Developmental compartmentalization in the dorsal mesothoracic disc of *Drosophila melanogaster*. Dev. Biol. **48**: 132–147.

GEHRING, W., 1967 Clonal analysis of determination dynamics in cultures of imaginal disks in *Drosophila melanogaster*. Dev. Biol. **16**: 438–456.

HALDER, G., P. CALLAERTS and W. J. GEHRING, 1995 Induction of ectopic eyes by targeted expression of the eyeless gene in Drosophila. Science **267**: 1788–1792.

HOLLAND, L. Z., M. KENE, N. A. WILLIAMS and N. D. HOLLAND, 1997 Sequence and embryonic expression of the amphioxus engrailed gene (AmphiEn): the metameric pattern of transcription resembles that of its segment-polarity homolog in Drosophila. Development **124**: 1723–1732.

KUNER, J. M., M. NAKANISHI, A. ZEHRA, B. DREES, E. GUSTAVSON *et al.*, 1985 Molecular cloning of *engrailed*: a gene involved in the development of pattern in Drosophila melanogaster. Cell **42**: 309–316.

LEWIS, E. B., 1963 Genes and developmental pathways. Am. Zool. **3**: 33–56.

LILLY, B., S. GALEWSKY, A. B. FIRULLI, R. A. SCHULZ and E. N. OLSON, 1994 D-MEF2: A MADS box transcription factor expressed in differentiating mesoderm and muscle cell lineages during Drosophila embryogenesis. Proc. Natl. Acad. Sci. USA **91**: 5662–5666.

MIÑANA, F. J., and A. GARCIA-BELLIDO, 1982 Preblastoderm mosaics of mutants of the bithorax-complex. Wilhelm Roux's Arch. Dev. Biol. **191**: 331–334.

MORATA, G., and A. GARCIA-BELLIDO, 1976 Developmental analysis of some mutants of the bithorax system of Drosophila. Wilhelm Roux's Arch. Dev. Biol. **180**: 125–143.

MORATA, G., and P. A. LAWRENCE, 1975 Control of compartment development by the engrailed gene in Drosophila. Nature **255**: 614–617.

NÜSSLEIN-VOLHARD, C., and E. WIESCHAUS, 1980 Mutations affecting segment number and polarity in Drosophila. Nature **287**: 795–801.

OLSON, E. N., 1990 MyoD family: a paradigm for development? Genes Dev. **4**: 1454–1461.

POOLE, S. J., L. M. KAUVAR, B. DREES and T. B. KORNBERG, 1985 The engrailed locus of Drosophila: structural analysis of an embryonic transcripts. Cell **40**: 37–43.

STERN, C., 1954 Two or three bristles. Am. Sci. **42**: 213–247.

TABATA, T., C. SCHWARTZ, E. GUSTAVSON, Z. ALI and T. B. KORNBERG, 1995 Creating a Drosophila wing de novo, the role of engrailed and the compartment hypothesis. Development **121**: 3359–3369.

WEDEEN, C. J., and D. A. WEISBLAST, 1991 Segmental expression of an engrailed-class gene during early development and neurogenesis in an annelid. Development **113**: 805–814.

ZECCA, M., K. BASLER and G. STRUHL, 1995 Sequential organizing activities of engrailed, hedgehog and decapentaplegic in the Drosophila wing. Development **121**: 2265–2278.

Ninety Years Ago
The Beginning of Hybrid Maize

James F. Crow

Laboratory of Genetics, University of Wisconsin–Madison, Madison, Wisconsin 53706

IN early 1908, GEORGE HARRISON SHULL, then at the Cold Spring Harbor Laboratory, published a paper with the unimposing title, "The composition of a field of maize." This marked the beginning of the exploitation of heterosis in plant breeding, surely one of genetics' greatest triumphs. It is appropriate, on this 90th anniversary, to look once again at SHULL's great contribution and its sequelae.

The increased size and vigor of hybrids between plant varieties and species had been known for centuries. A well-known example of hybrid luxuriance was found in crosses between two species of Jimson weed, *Datura stramonium* and *D. tatula*, in which the hybrids were twice as tall as either parent. The most spectacular example that I know of is the radish-cabbage hybrid; a single plant filled a greenhouse and grew out the roof (EAST and JONES 1919, p. 192). It was sterile, however, and only in this century were fertile derivatives obtained by polyploidization. A time-honored showpiece of hybrid vigor is the mule, also sterile, but known for 4000 years for its hardiness and longevity. Even in ancient times it was widely known that inbreeding leads to weakness and small size. The avoidance of incest was practiced by many human societies, and there was speculation about such behavior in animals. ZIRKLE (GOWEN 1952, p. 5) quotes a fanciful mixture of science and myth from none other than Aristotle.

> A story goes that the king of Scythia had a highly-bred mare, and that all her foals were splendid; that wishing to mate the best of the young males with the mother, he had him brought to the stall for the purpose; that the young horse declined; that, after the mother's head had been concealed in a wrapper he, in ignorance, had intercourse; and that, when immediately afterwards the wrapper was removed and the head of the mare was rendered visible, the young horse ran away and hurled himself down a precipice.

The literature of the nineteenth century is full of examples, mostly from plants. As usual, CHARLES DARWIN got in the act. In his words, "Nature thus tells us, in the most emphatic manner, that she abhors perpetual self-fertilization." And, as we have come to expect, his treatment was thorough, careful, and thoughtful. His book, *The Effects of Cross and Self Fertilization in the Vegetable Kingdom,* was published in 1876. Its 490 pages include myriad examples, with the overall conclusion that inbreeding is generally deleterious and cross-fertilization generally beneficial (DARWIN 1876). As pure description, his writings could hardly be improved upon, but an interpretation had to await the rediscovery of MENDEL's laws in 1900.

The development of hybrid maize: In his 1908 paper, SHULL reported that inbred lines of maize showed general deterioration in yield and vigor, but that hybrids between two inbreds immediately and completely recovered (SHULL 1908); in many cases their yield exceeded that of the varieties from which the inbreds were derived. Furthermore, they had a highly desirable uniformity. In a subsequent paper in 1909, he outlined the procedures that later became standard in corn-breeding programs (SHULL 1909).

At the same time, E. M. EAST did similar experiments at Connecticut State College. He also recognized the deleterious effects of inbreeding, but didn't realize the value of crossing inbred lines. Breeding weak parents held no appeal for him until he heard SHULL's report in January 1908. In February, he wrote a letter to SHULL, saying: "Since studying your paper, I agree entirely with your conclusion, and wonder why I have been so stupid as not to see the fact myself." His report (EAST 1908) was characteristically generous to SHULL, and he added considerable corroborating evidence (GOWEN 1952, p. 17).

Nevertheless, EAST was not convinced of the usefulness of the idea, because the puny inbred lines produced such small quantities of seed. The great cost of seed, he thought, negated any increased yield of the hybrids. This led to a strong disagreement with SHULL, but in 1910 they agreed not to let this become an open debate nor to let personalities intrude. They remained true to their word.

The limitation of poor seed production from inbred lines was overcome by an idea from D. F. JONES (1918, 1922), who, while still a graduate student, advocated

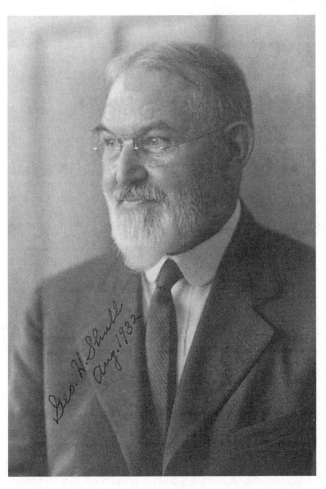

G. H. SHULL in 1932.

using four-way, or double-cross hybrids. This involved crossing two inbred lines and crossing that hybrid with the hybrid of two other inbred lines. The seed-producing strain was thus a heterozygous single-cross, and four-way hybrids yielded about as much as two-way. The abundant seed immediately made the program practical. The four-way crosses were slightly more variable than two-way hybrids, but much less so than randomly mated ("open-pollinated") varieties. EAST and JONES and their role in the history of genetics has been the subject of an earlier Perspectives article (NELSON 1993).

The word "heterosis" was introduced by SHULL (1914) as shorthand for such awkward expressions as "stimulation of heterozygosis." He emphasized that the word was not intended to imply any particular explanation, but was purely descriptive (see also SHULL 1948). The photo above shows SHULL at the time of the 1932 International Genetics Congress.

Hybrid maize invades the Midwest: Meanwhile back in the corn belt, selection for improved yield in open-pollinated varieties was proving to be ineffective. Although qualitative traits could be readily improved by selection, yield was not very responsive. SHULL's idea of crossing inbred lines spread rapidly through the agricul-

tural experiment stations in the 1920s, stimulated especially by JONES' idea of four-way crosses. In 1924, HENRY A. WALLACE, later to be Secretary of Agriculture, Vice President, and in 1948, the Progressive Party's candidate for President, sold a few bushels of seed from his recently developed hybrid crosses, the first commercial sale of hybrid seed (CRABB 1947). Several companies appeared in the next decade. In some regions the inbred lines and crosses were performed by companies who sold the seed each year to farmers. In other areas—Wisconsin was an example—strains were developed at the University Experiment Station and seed was distributed to breeders and farmers.

The transition from open-pollinated to hybrid maize was astonishingly rapid. In Iowa, the proportion of hybrid corn grew from less than 10% in 1935 to well over 90% 4 years later. The transition in other corn-belt states was almost as fast, although somewhat slower in other parts of the United States. But by the 1950s, the great bulk of maize throughout the United States was hybrid. Why was this acceptance so rapid, especially in the corn belt? Substantially better yield is one reason, of course, but how obvious was this to the individual grower? The greater uniformity of hybrids was useful for machine harvesting, and this was undoubtedly a factor. Furthermore, a field of corn in which all the plants are alike, each with a single ear at the same height, is aesthetically pleasing, and this appealed to many corn growers. The hybrids could also incorporate favorable qualitative traits and be adapted to different habitats, especially length of growing season. Another possible reason was the practice of having leading growers demonstrate the robust hybrid plants to their neighbors. Yet another reason for the rapid spread, possibly the most important one, was that 1934–36 was in the dust-bowl period, and the hybrid strains were strikingly more resistant to drought than the open-pollinated varieties then in use (CRABB 1947).

Selection for high-performing hybrids was a vast undertaking involving an enormous number of tests. Inbreds were poor predictors of hybrid performance, and two-way crosses, of four-way yields. Testing of a large number of four-way crosses was a tremendous job, since there were six possible single crosses among the four strains used to produce a double cross. One useful device was due to M. T. JENKINS (CRABB 1947). He suggested predicting four-way yields by the average of the four crosses other than the two used to produce the single crosses. On the average, these mimicked a four-way cross and permitted a considerable saving of testing time and expense. This was only one of many important contributions of this pioneer researcher.

The next major change came with the increasing practicality of single cross hybrids. This was partly indirect: increasingly, breeders used very closely related strains to produce the single crosses, so that the four-way crosses were almost the equivalent of two-way. Eventually, in

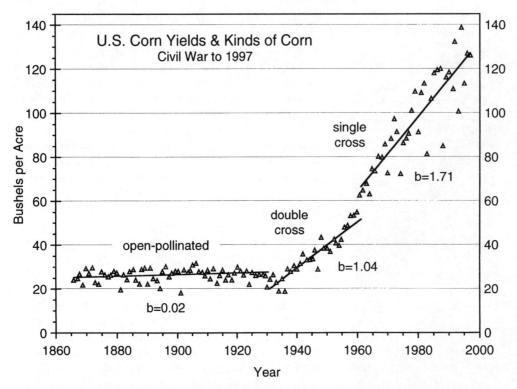

FIGURE 1.—Maize yield in bushels per acre in the United States. The periods dominated by open-pollinated, four-way crosses, and two-way crosses are indicated, along with regression coefficients (bushel/acre). Redrawn with permission from A. FORREST TROYER. Data compiled by the United States Department of Agriculture.

the 1960s, single crosses began replacing double crosses. Selection for higher yield in inbred lines had produced inbreds with yields high enough that they could be used as seed producers. In fact, the inbred lines were as high-yielding as the hybrids of an earlier period. But the single-cross hybrids were better still, and the gap between inbreds and hybrids remained. Not only were the single crosses higher yielding than double crosses, but they were even more uniform.

With the coming of single crosses, not only did the yield show a sudden increase, but the rate of increase improved. Before the introduction of hybrids in the 1930s, there was almost no increase. In the double-cross era, the rate of increase was about 1 bushel per acre per year. After single-crosses predominated, the annual increase was almost 2 bushels per acre. Current yields are some five times what they were in the prehybrid days. Furthermore, there appears to be no reduction in the rate of increase, so there is no reason to expect that the yield will plateau in the foreseeable future (see Figure 1).

But are we giving the hybrid breeding system too much credit? Farm practice did not stand still during this period. Increasing use of fertilizer, greater density of plants, and herbicides all contributed to greater yield. In addition, better machinery made it possible to time the field operations better, thus enhancing efficiency of the operation and reducing waste. Can we separate these effects from those of better genetic strains? RUS-SELL (1974) made a serious attempt to do this. Using hybrid seed preserved from 1930 to 1970 and growing the plants under the same environments, he found a uniform increase in yield from the newer strains. He concluded that 60% or more of the increased performance was genetic. Similar results were reported by DUVICK (1977).

We must not forget that the spread of hybrid maize coincided with the wider use of efficient experimental designs, involving randomization, replication, and better statistical methods, all introduced by R. A. FISHER. FISHER's book, *Statistical Methods for Research Workers*, first appeared in 1925 and went through 14 editions before his death in 1962 (FISHER [1925] 1970). His *The Design of Experiments* first appeared in 1935, and there were 8 editions (FISHER [1935] 1966). In the early 1930s, FISHER spent some time at Iowa State University and exerted a great influence on American agricultural research. Clearly, world agriculture in general and maize in particular owe an enormous debt to FISHER's genius. These better methods increased the rate of improvement of both genetic quality (by more efficient selection) and agronomic practice (by better discrimination among alternative practices). How much of the increase in agricultural productivity should be credited to FISHER, I don't know. But my guess is considerable.

Field techniques have become very sophisticated. Anyone traveling through the corn belt has seen fields in which a few rows of seed-producing plants with pollen-producing tassels removed alternate with one or two rows of pollen-producing plants with tassels intact. De-tasseling of those plants that were intended to produce seed uncontaminated by their own pollen was effective, but inconvenient and expensive. This labor-intensive process was replaced by use of cytoplasmic male sterility, particularly Texas cytoplasm (*cms-T*), along with judiciously used fertility-restoring genes. This saved a great deal of hand labor, and by 1970 more than 85% of U.S. maize carried *cms-T*. But strains with Texas cytoplasm turned out to be susceptible to leaf blight (*Helminthosporium maydis*), which spread through much of the corn belt in a single year (LAUGHNAN and GABBY-LAUGHNAN 1983). The ensuing epidemic was a disaster, especially in humid areas, and the 1970 corn yield dropped from 84 to 72 bushels per acre. By the next year a continuation of the epidemic was avoided, but the maize community had to revert to hand-detasseling. And the message was clear: genetic uniformity has its price.

Why is inbreeding and hybridization so effective? R. A. FISHER (1949, pp. 116–120) stated the issues clearly. The whole process takes place in three stages: (1) foundation individuals chosen to start the process; (2) inbreeding to near homozygosity; (3) crossing chosen lines. If the individuals at each stage are chosen randomly without selection, the hybrids are essentially a random sample of the original population. Actually, of course, selection takes place in all three stages. Selection at the first stage can do little more than has been accomplished in the past by mass selection. Selection during inbreeding is rendered ineffective by the rapid fixation when heterozygosity decreases 50% each generation. So FISHER placed greatest emphasis on the third stage. If there is a great multiplicity of inbred lines, those that combine to produce the best hybrids can be chosen, and in distinction from ordinary breeding methods, those superior genotypes can be reproduced at will. This is the equivalent of choosing the best individual from a large segregating population—best because of a happy combination of genes and their interactions—and doing the equivalent of reproducing it asexually. He emphasized "deliberately planned multiplicity," which is indeed what maize breeders were practicing with their thousands of inbred lines.

The genetic basis of heterosis: Since the early days there have been two alternative, though not mutually exclusive hypotheses of heterosis. The *dominance* hypothesis attributes the greater yield of hybrids to the suppression of deleterious recessives from one parent by dominant alleles from the other. The *overdominance* hypothesis assumes that at key loci the heterozygote is superior to either homozygote. Either hypothesis explains qualitatively the decline of performance with inbreeding and its recovery in hybrids, including the possibility that the better hybrids exceed the average of the original populations before inbreeding.

SHULL believed that there was something about different germ plasms that led to a stimulus; it need not be Mendelian. EAST had similar views, but he increasingly emphasized Mendelian loci in which the heterozygote was superior to either homozygote. Convincing examples of such loci did not exist (instances of interallelic complementation came much later), but nevertheless

EAST (1936) argued for their existence. The alternative dominance hypothesis was also advocated early (KEEBLE and PELLEW 1910; BRUCE 1910). There were two early objections to the dominance hypothesis. One was the failure of selection to produce high-yielding inbreds; if all deleterious recessives could be purged, the inbreds should equal the hybrids. Second, the F_2 distribution was not skewed, as would be expected from the expansion of $(3/4 + 1/4)^n$. But it is clear that with linkage (JONES 1917) and a large number of factors (COLLINS 1921), neither objection holds. On the other hand, overdominance demanded a form of allelic interaction that was rare at best.

The dominance hypothesis held sway until the 1940s. It was clear that it was sufficient to explain the decline with inbreeding and the subsequent recovery when inbred lines were crossed (CROW 1948). It was less clear that this was sufficient to explain the increased performance of hybrids above that of the open-pollinated varieties from which the inbreds were derived. It was argued that purging of deleterious recessives during inbreeding could increase the yield only by an amount equal to the genomic mutation rate (CROW 1948; FISHER 1949, pp. 118–119). Prevailing estimates of mutation rates would place this increase at about 5% or less, not the observed 15–20%. Despite the absence of good examples—sickle-cell hemoglobin was badly overworked—overdominance seemed a possible alternative since a small minority of such loci could suffice.

In the summer of 1950, Iowa State College (as it was then called) held a 5-week conference on heterosis, and the proceedings were published 2 years later (GOWEN 1952). By this time a number of people were interested in overdominance. For many years, FRED HULL had been the leading advocate and presented his views at the meeting. Among other arguments, he emphasized the failure of inbreds ever to equal hybrids and the poor results of mass selection. COMSTOCK and ROBINSON presented a statistical estimate of dominance that was well within the overdominant range. Others (*e.g.*, DICKERSON) suggested breeding schemes that would exploit overdominance (for these and other papers, see GOWEN 1952). Overdominance was in the air, and this conference had a strong influence on both plant and animal breeders.

Within a few years, doubts appeared. More realistic—and higher—estimates of the total mutation rate reduced the force of the mutation rate argument. The COMSTOCK and ROBINSON mating scheme permitted an opportunity for recombination between successive crossing generations, and the dominance estimates dropped from the overdominance to the partial dominance range; seeming overdominance had turned out to be pseudo-overdominance caused by linkage of yield-increasing dominants with deleterious recessives (GARDNER 1963; MOLL *et al.* 1964). Identification of quantitative trait loci (STUBER *et al.* 1992) suggested overdominance, but a more detailed analysis (Cockerham and Zeng 1996) was more consistent with pseudo-overdominance.

G. F. Sprague suggested a particularly simple experiment. Two maize populations were each selected for improved performance of hybrids from crosses with an inbred tester. With overdominance, the two strains should become similar to each other, since each would incorporate alleles that complement those of the inbred tester. A hybrid between them should show decreased yield. In contrast, with additive and dominance effects these hybrids should show increased yield. The experiments were slow, since each generation of selection involved a 3-year cycle, but preliminary results argued against overdominance (Sprague and Russell 1956) and eventually the results were clear (see Sprague 1983). Hybrids between the two selected strains improved over the course of the experiment. In addition, the two selected populations produced increased yields in hybrids with other testers. These offer strong evidence for the sufficiency of additive and dominant effects. Several workers, including me, have changed from preferring overdominance to accepting dominance as sufficient. From the beginning, Sprague has emphasized experimental evidence, and, from the present viewpoint, his early conclusions are correct. In addition, he has made numerous practical and theoretical contributions and is one of the chief architects of modern maize breeding.

The current view, then, is that the dominance hypothesis is the major explanation of inbreeding decline and the high yield of hybrids. There is little statistical evidence for contributions from overdominance and epistasis. But whether the best hybrids are getting an extra boost from overdominance or favorable epistatic contributions remains an open question. The happy side of this story is that, despite ignorance and changing views of this fundamental issue, maize yields have continued to increase, with no sign that the rate of increase is diminishing.

A change of emphasis: In the summer of 1997, a second heterosis conference was held, 47 years after the Iowa State conference. This was sponsored by the International Maize and Wheat Improvement Center (CIMMYT) and took place in Mexico City. The two conferences contrasted in a number of significant ways.

The 1950 conference emphasized mainly maize, along with some discussion of swine and poultry. The 1997 conference included discussions of sorghum, millets, rape seed, sunflowers, wheat, rice, and cotton, along with a number of trees and vegetable crops. There was a major contrast in emphasis. In 1950, the papers were all biological and the emphasis was on getting the highest yields in good environments. The 1997 conference had much more concern for problems in the developing areas. There was more emphasis on ecology: How can we increase food production and at the same time do as little harm to the environment as possible, leaving non-agricultural areas undisturbed? Greater yield per hect-

are leaves more hectares that can be left in pristine condition. A second difference was the current emphasis on varieties that grow well under less favorable conditions, especially drought and poor nutrition. A third difference was greater attention to economic problems—how can there be sufficient capital and appropriate infrastructure for developing better crops for the tropics?

Not always is the maize paradigm the best. For some crops—sunflower appears to be one—crossing inbred lines has produced large increases in yield. For others, this is not true. Even for maize, it may be that open-pollinated varieties are the best in some areas. This may be true, especially in the earlier stages and when locally adapted varieties are already available. Throughout the conference there was an emphasis on empiricism: do what is best for the particular climate, soil, agricultural practice, social structure, and economy.

Back to Shull: G. H. Shull was born April 15, 1874, one of eight children in a sharecropping family. His was a remarkable sibship, for all seven survivors became leading citizens and four were listed in *Who's Who*. The hand-to-mouth farm existence meant that Shull had little chance to go to school and was largely an autodidact. He eventually worked his way through high school and taught in country schools for 2 years. After accumulating the necessary funds, he went to Antioch College, where he served as a janitor while becoming the leading student in his class, graduating at the age of 27. After completing graduate work at the University of Chicago he moved to Cold Spring Harbor in 1904. There he joined C. B. Davenport, a former Chicago faculty member who had been appointed director of the Cold Spring Harbor Laboratory. Since Chicago days, the two had shared an interest in biometrics. In 1915, Shull moved to Princeton University, where he remained. For details of his life and work, see Mangelsdorf (1955).

Shull had wide research interests and worked on a number of plants, especially shepherd's purse and evening primrose. His interest in inbreeding and hybridization started early. At the Iowa State conference, he said that his first personal contact with hybrid vigor was with sunflowers. The hybrids between Western and Russian parents, each 5–6 feet tall, produced hybrids averaging more than twice this height. The tallest plant was more than 14 feet, and he showed a picture of himself in the midst of the hybrids, teetering atop a 6-foot stepladder (Gowen 1952, p. 47). Shull also had an interest in self-incompatibility genes in several plants. Being interested in heterosis, he was attracted to translocations and balanced-lethals in Oenothera as a way of maintaining heterozygosity.

Of special interest to readers of this journal, Shull was the founding editor of Genetics (Mangelsdorf 1955; Crow 1991). He personally arranged for a publisher and assembled an editorial board, and the journal got under way in 1916. He remained editor for 10 years, when he was succeeded by another important figure in maize breeding, D. F. JONES. SHULL did the detailed editing work himself, and the reduction in his output of published papers attests to the amount of time this took. After he ceased to be editor, he retained a strong paternal interest in the journal. Years later, in the 1950s, he apparently was still reading every issue, for the current editors could count on hearing from him if anything did not fit his high editorial standards. He personally contributed the money for the "Galton and Mendel" fund. This was used to defray expenses for extensive tables or illustrations. When this money was used, this fact was to be footnoted with an asterisk and, furthermore, the asterisk was not be used for anything else. A lapse in following this rule brought an immediate letter from SHULL.

I look back with happy nostalgia to hearing him recount the history of his discovery at the 1950 Heterosis Conference (GOWEN 1952, pp. 14–48). True to his 1910 promise, he was generous to his rival, EAST. He had lived to see his idea blossom into a world-wide agricultural revolution. A genial patriarch, he was 76 at the time and clearly enjoyed the well-deserved adulation he received. He died 4 years later, on September 28, 1954.

LITERATURE CITED

BRUCE, A. B., 1910 The Mendelian theory of heredity and the augmentation of vigor. Science **32:** 627–628.

COCKERHAM, C. C., and Z-B. ZENG, 1996 Design III with marker loci. Genetics **143:** 1437–1456.

COLLINS, G. N., 1921 Dominance and vigor of first generation hybrids. Am. Nat. **55:** 116–133.

CRABB, A. R., 1947 *The Hybrid-Corn Makers: Prophets of Plenty.* Rutgers University Press, New Brunswick, NJ.

CROW, J. F., 1948 Alternative hypotheses of hybrid vigor. Genetics **33:** 477–487.

CROW, J. F., 1991 Our diamond birthday anniversary. Genetics **137:** 1–3.

DARWIN, C., 1876 *The Effects of Cross and Self Fertilization in the Vegetable Kingdom.* John Murray, London.

DUVICK, D. N., 1977 Genetic rates of gain in hybrid maize yields during the past 40 years. Maydica **22:** 187–196.

EAST, E. M., 1908 Inbreeding in corn. Rep. Conn. Agric. Exp. Stn. pp. 419–428.

EAST, E. M., 1936 Heterosis. Genetics **21:** 375–397.

EAST, E. M., and D. F. JONES, 1919 *Inbreeding and Outbreeding: Their Genetic and Sociological Significance.* Lippincott, Philadelphia.

FISHER, R. A., [1925] 1970 *Statistical Methods for Research Workers.* Oliver and Boyd, Edinburgh and London.

FISHER, R. A., [1935] 1966 *The Design of Experiments.* Oliver and Boyd, Edinburgh and London.

FISHER, R. A., 1949 *The Theory of Inbreeding.* 2nd ed., 1965. Oliver and Boyd, Edinburgh and London.

GARDNER, C. O., 1963 Estimates of genetic parameters in cross fertilizing plants and their implications to plant breeding, pp. 225–252 in *Statistical Genetics and Plant Breeding,* edited by W. D. HANSON and H. F. ROBINSON. Special Publ. 982, NAS-NRC, Washington.

GOWEN, J. W., editor, 1952 *Heterosis.* Iowa State College Press, Ames.

JONES, D. F., 1917 Dominance of linked factors as a means of accounting for heterosis. Genetics **2:** 466–479.

JONES, D. F., 1918 The effects of inbreeding and crossbreeding upon development. Conn. Agric. Exp. Stn. Bull. 107. 100 pp.

JONES, D. F., 1922 The productiveness of single and double first generation corn hybrids. J. Am. Soc. Agron. **14:** 242–252.

KEEBLE, F., and C. PELLEW, 1910 The mode of inheritance of stature and of time of flowering in peas (*Pisum sativum*). J. Genet. **1:** 47–56.

LAUGHNAN, J. R., and S. GABBY-LAUGHNAN, 1983 Cytoplasmic male sterility in maize. Annu. Rev. Genet. **17:** 27–48.

MANGELSDORF, P. C., 1955 GEORGE HARRISON SHULL. Genetics **40:** 1–4.

MOLL, R. H., M. F. LINDSEY and H. F. ROBINSON, 1964 Estimates of genetic variances and level of dominance in maize. Genetics **49:** 411–423.

NELSON, O. E., 1993 A notable triumvirate of maize geneticists. Genetics **135:** 937–941.

RUSSELL, W. A., 1974 Comparative performance for maize hybrids representing different eras of maize breeding. Proc. 29th Annu. Corn Sorghum Res. Conf., pp. 81–101.

SHULL, G. H., 1908 The composition of a field of maize. Am. Breeders Assoc. Rep. **4:** 296–301.

SHULL, G. H., 1909 A pure line method of corn breeding. Am. Breeders Assoc. Rep. **5:** 51–59.

SHULL, G. H., 1914 Duplicated genes for capsule form in *Bursa bursa-pastoris.* Z. Indukt. Abstammungs u. Vererbungsl. **12:** 97–149.

SHULL, G. H., 1948 What is "heterosis"? Genetics **33:** 439–446.

SPRAGUE, G. F., and W. A. RUSSELL, 1956 Some evidence on type of gene action involved in yield heterosis in maize. Proc. Int. Genet. Symp., Tokyo & Kyoto, pp. 522–526.

SPRAGUE, G. F., 1983 Heterosis in maize: theory and practice. Monogr. Theor. Appl. Genet. **6:** 47–70.

STUBER, C. W., S. E. LINCOLN, D. W. WOLFF, T. HELENTJARIS and E. S. LANDER, 1992 Identification of genetic factors contributing to heterosis in a hybrid from two elite maize inbred lines using molecular markers. Genetics **132:** 823–839.

○ Hershey ○

Franklin W. Stahl

Institute of Molecular Biology, University of Oregon, Eugene, Oregon 97403–1229

ALFRED DAY HERSHEY died at his home, in the Village of Laurel Hollow, New York, on May 22, 1997 at the age of 88. Seven weeks later, a number of Al's friends met at Cold Spring Harbor to commemorate his life. The tributes paid on that occasion have informed this *Perspectives*, and some of them are cited in what follows. Full copies are available from the Cold Spring Harbor Laboratory.

Most students of biology know of HERSHEY—his best known experiment is described in texts of both biology and genetics. This work (HERSHEY and CHASE 1952a) provided cogent support for the hypothesis that DNA is the conveyor of genetic information.

The subject of the "Hershey-Chase experiment" was the bacteriophage T2, composed half of protein and half of DNA, a combination compatible with any of the three competing views of the chemical basis of heredity. T2, like many other phages, is a tadpole-shaped virus that initiates an attack on a bacterium by sticking to it with the tip of its tail. The Hershey-Chase experiment used DNA-specific and protein-specific radioactive labels to show that the DNA of the virus then entered the bacterium while most of the protein could be stripped from the surface of the cell by agitation in a Waring Blender. Such abused cells produced a normal crop of new phage particles. Previous evidence implicating DNA in heredity had shown that a property of the surface coat of the pneumococcus bacterium could be passed from one strain to another via chemically isolated DNA. The observation by HERSHEY and CHASE justified the view that the entire set of hereditary information of a creature was so encoded. This work counted heavily in making HERSHEY a shareholder, with MAX DELBRÜCK (1906–1981) and SALVADORE E. LURIA (1912–1991), of the 1969 Nobel prize for Physiology or Medicine.

In 1934, Al earned his Ph.D. in the Departments of Chemistry and Bacteriology at Michigan State College with a thesis that described separations of bacterial constituents, identified by the quaint definitions of the times. Except for its evident care and industry, the work was unremarkable, merely part of an ongoing study ". . . to arrive ultimately at some correlation between the chemical constitution of [Brucella species], and the various phenomena of specificity by them" (HERSHEY 1934).

Al then assumed an instructorship in Bacteriology and Immunology at Washington University in St. Louis, where he collaborated with Professor J. BRONFENBRENNER. From 1936 to 1939, their papers reported studies on the growth of bacterial cultures. Al certainly had the background for this work; his thesis research had involved not only the preparation of liver infusion growth medium (from scratch, as was routine in those days) but also the testing of 600 better defined media, none of which supported growth of Brucella. From 1940 to 1944, his experiments dealt with the phage-antiphage immunologic reaction and with other factors that influenced phage infectivity. During both those periods, about half of the 28 papers bearing HERSHEY's name were sole-authored. (It was apparently here that Al learned how to handle phage. It may also have been here that Al acquired the idea that authorship belongs to those who do the experiments and should not reflect patronization, rank, title, or even redaction of the manuscript.) Some of these papers may have been important contributions to the understanding of antigen-antibody reactions. To this reviewer they appear original, thoughtful, and quantitative, especially those on the use of phage inactivation to permit the study of the antigen-antibody reaction at "infinite" dilution of antigen (*e.g.*, HERSHEY 1941). But, of course, they interested an audience that did not include many geneticists or others interested in biological replication (except, perhaps, for LINUS PAULING). It took MAX DELBRÜCK to move Al in that direction.

As recounted by JUDSON (1996), DELBRÜCK was attracted by Al's papers. Perhaps he liked their mathematical, nonbiochemical nature. He must have liked their originality, logical precision, and economy of presentation. Max invited Al to Nashville in 1943 and recorded the following impression: "Drinks whiskey but not tea. Simple and to the point . . . Likes independence." Al's first "interesting" phage papers appeared soon thereafter (HERSHEY 1946, 1947).

A *sine qua non* for genetical investigation is the availability of mutants. The ease with which large numbers of phage particles can be handled facilitated the discovery and characterization of mutants that were easily scored. Al recognized that the high infectivity of phage and the proportionality of plaque count to volume of suspension assayed allowed for quantification of mutation far exceeding that possible in most other viral systems. Al measured mutation rates, both forward and back, and demonstrated the mutational independence of *r* (rapid lysis) and *h* (host range). He succeeded also in showing (in parallel with DELBRÜCK) that these mutationally independent factors could recombine when two genotypes were grown together in the same host cells (HERSHEY 1946, 1947). Thus, "Phage Genetics" was born as a field of study, and it became conceivable not only that the basic question of biological replication could be addressed with phage but so could phenomena embraced by the term "Morgan-Mendelism."

Al continued the formal genetic analyses of T2 with investigations of linkage. HERSHEY and ROTMAN (1948) demonstrated that linkage analysis would have to take into account the production of recombinant particles containing markers from three different infecting phage genotypes. The same authors (1949) used "mixed indicators" to enumerate all four genotypes from two-factor crosses involving *h* and *r* mutants. That trick made it feasible to analyze fully the yields from individual mixedly infected bacterial cells. The signal finding was that all four genotypes of phage could be produced by an individual cell but that the numbers of complementary recombinants, which were equal on the average, showed little correlation from cell to cell. This demonstration of apparent nonreciprocality in the exchange process leading to recombination raised the specter that "crossing over" in phages would prove to be fundamentally different from that occurring in meiosis. The desire to unify this and other apparently disparate properties of phage and eukaryotic recombination into a single theoretical framework motivated subsequent studies of recombination by other investigators.

DELBRÜCK tried to make such a unification by algebraic legerdemain and Papal Bull (see below). He formalized phage recombination as a succession of meiosis-like, pairwise exchanges between linear linkage structures (VISCONTI and DELBRÜCK 1953). The resulting algebra embraced some of the major ways in which phage linkage data differed from meiotic data. In particular, it rationalized the "negative interference" between crossovers and the appearance of progeny particles that had inherited markers from three different infecting phage types. VISCONTI and DELBRÜCK assumed that the exchange process involved physical breakage of chromosomes (DNA duplexes) and reciprocal reunion of the resulting fragments. They blamed the failure to see correlated numbers of complementary types in "single bursts" on vagaries of replication and packaging (into proteinaceous "heads") of the complementary recombinant chromosome types subse-

quent to their formation. DELBRÜCK stopped thinking about phage genetics after CHARLEY STEINBERG and I (1958) showed him that his final expressions were independent of both of his two assumptions, reciprocal and break-join. A fully satisfactory conclusion to these issues for T2 came only with MOSIG's and ALBERT's elucidation of the nonreciprocal, replicative mechanism by which recombinants are formed in T-even phages (for review, see MOSIG 1994). More recent advances have established that the various recombinational mechanisms employed by bacteria and their viruses and by eukaryotes are, in fact, pleasingly similar, depending on homologous strategies and enzymes.

By most criteria, individual T2 particles are "haploid"— they contain but one set of genetic material. However, "heterozygous" particles, which contain two different alleles at a single locus, were described by HERSHEY and CHASE (1952b) at the 1951 Cold Spring Harbor Symposium. After the elucidation of DNA as a duplex molecule (WATSON and CRICK 1953), it was possible to propose heteroduplex models for those "heterozygotes." Such models played a central role in all subsequent thinking about recombination, especially that involving relationships between meiotic crossing over and gene conversion.

In 1958, HERSHEY, like LEVINTHAL (1954) before him, expanded on the VISCONTI-DELBRÜCK analysis in an effort to connect observations on heterozygotes, which had molecular implications, with formal concepts proposed to deal with the populational aspects of phage crosses. The effort provided few, if any, answers, but clarified the ambient questions, at least for Al.

In 1950, Al left St. Louis to join the staff of the Carnegie Institution of Washington at Cold Spring Harbor. That move put him at the geographical center of the embryonic field of microbial/molecular genetics, and he soon became the intellectual center of its phage branch. At this time, the fruits of a collaboration conducted at St. Louis were published (HERSHEY *et al.* 1951). This work showed that phage particles were "killed" by the decay of the unstable isotope ^{32}P incorporated within their DNA. After the central importance of DNA to the phage life cycle (and to genetics) had been demonstrated, this "suicide" technique was exploited in other labs in efforts to analyze the phage genetic structure and its mode of replication. Like most early experiments in "radiobiology," these analyses were fun but not much more. From this time on, Al's studies became more down-to-earth (and successful) as he turned from mathematically based genetic analyses to serious studies of phage structure and the biochemistry of phage development. There is no doubt, however, that these studies were informed by Al's acute awareness of the genetical and radiobiological facts that had to be explained. These new studies were jump-started by the "blender" experiment, described above.

Several subsequent papers refined the conclusions of the blender experiment by showing, for i˙ ance, that *some* protein is injected along with the phage DNA (HERSHEY

1955). With Watson-Crickery well established by this time, these studies were interesting but not threatening to the view that the genetic substance was DNA. During this period, Al's lab published works that described DNA and protein production, and relations between them, in infected cells. They provided the biochemical counterpart of the genetically defined notion of a pool of noninfective, "vegetative" phage (Visconti and Delbrück 1953; Doermann 1953). This change of emphasis allowed Hershey (1956) to write:

> I have proposed the ideas that the nucleic acid of T2 is its hereditary substance and that all its nucleic acid is genetically potent. The evidence supporting these ideas is straightforward but inconclusive. Their principal value is pragmatic. They have given rise to the unprecedented circumstance that chemical hypotheses and the results of chemical experiments are dictating the conditions of genetic experiments. This development I regard as more important than the bare facts I have presented, which may yet prove to be of little or no genetic interest.

Biochemical studies on phage development were clouded by the lack of understanding of phage genome structure. It was not even clear how many "chromosomes" (DNA molecules) a phage particle contained. Furthermore, although Watson and Crick had specified what any short stretch of DNA should look like (plectonemically coiled complementary polynucleotide chains), they had been understandably proud of the fact that their model was structurally coherent in the absence of any specification of longitudinal differentiation. For them, it was enough to say that therein lay genetic specificity. For Al, that was not enough, and his lab pursued studies dedicated to the physical description of phage DNA. The results of these studies were succinctly reviewed by Hershey (1970a) in his Nobel Lecture. I'll briefly summarize my view of them, dividing the studies by phage type.

Al developed and applied chromatographic and centrifugal methods to the analysis of T2 chromosome structure (e.g., Mandell and Hershey 1960; Hershey and Burgi 1960). This work systematized our understanding of the breakage of DNA during laboratory manipulation and had its denouement in the demonstration that a T2 particle contains just one piece of DNA (Rubenstein et al. 1961) with the length expected of a linear double helix (Cairns 1962). That conclusion was in apparent contradiction to genetic demonstrations that T4 chromosomes contained more or less randomly located physical discontinuities (Doermann and Boehner 1963). A major insight into the structure of T-even phage chromosomes resulted from attempts to reconcile the apparently contradictory physical and genetic descriptions of T-even chromosomes. The basic idea, elaborated and confirmed in a series of papers orchestrated by George Streisinger, was that the nucleotide sequences in any clone of phage particles were circularly permuted and that the sequence at one end of a given chromosome was duplicated at the other end (the chromosomes were "terminally redundant"). The predicted circular linkage map provided an elegant frame

for displaying the functional organization of the T4 chromosome, as revealed by the pioneering studies of Epstein et al. (1963).

The terminal redundancies of the T-even phage chromosomes provided an additional physical basis for Al's heterozygotes. (See Streisinger 1966 for references and a more detailed recounting.) These insights were exploited and elaborated upon by Gisela Mosig, who spent the years 1962–65 in Al's lab. There she combined her genetic savvy of T4 with studies on the structure of the truncated, circularly permuted DNA molecules that she discovered in certain defective T4 particles. Those studies formed the basis for an elegant demonstration of the quantitative relations between the linkage map of T4 (as constructed from recombination frequencies) and the underlying chromosome (Mosig 1966). Fred Frankel (1963) and Rudy Werner (1968), in Hershey's lab, examined the intracellular state of T-even phage DNA. Their discovery that it was a network undermined analyses of phage recombination as a series of tidy, pairwise, meiosis-like "matings," and well-aimed triparental crosses by Jan Drake (1967) killed the pairwise mating idea once and for all.

Meselson and Weigle (1961) demonstrated that phage λ DNA, like that of Escherichia coli (Meselson and Stahl 1958), is replicated semiconservatively, in agreement with Watson and Crick's proposal that the replication of DNA involves separation of the two complementary strands. However, uncertainties about the structure of the semiconserved entities identified by Meselson prevented those experiments from being taken as proof of the Watson-Crick scheme. Careful measurements of the molecular weight of λ DNA (Hershey et al. 1961) demonstrated that there was just one molecule per particle. That conclusion, combined with Cairns' autoradiographic measurement of the length of λ DNA (1961), established that λ's semiconservatively replicating structure is, indeed, a DNA duplex, putting the issue to rest.

The chromosome of λ also provided a surprise (Hershey et al. 1963; Hershey and Burgi 1965). Though the chromosomes in a λ clone are all identical (i.e., not permuted), each chromosome carries a terminal 12-nucleotide-long segment that is single-stranded and is complementary to a segment of the same length carried on the other end. The complementary nature of the segments gives λ "sticky ends." These ends anneal at the time of infection, circularizing the chromosome, which can then replicate in both theta and sigma modes. The demonstration of a route by which the λ chromosome can circularize provided physical substance to Campbell's (1962) proposal that the attachment of λ prophage to the host chromosome involves crossing over between the host chromosome and a (hypothesized) circular form of λ. And, of course, the understanding of λ's sticky ends, whose annealing creates cos, is exploited by today's gene cloners every time they work with a cosmid.

The nonpermuted character of λ's chromosome made it susceptible to analyses prohibited in T-even phage. For instance, SKALKA *et al.* (1968) demonstrated the mosaic nature of the chromosome; major segments differed conspicuously from each other in their nucleotide composition. (That conclusion foreshadowed our current understanding of the role of "horizontal transmission" in prokaryotic evolution.) HERSHEY's lab demonstrated that these differing segments had distinguishable annealing ("hybridization") behavior. They exploited those differences to identify the approximate location of the origin of replication (MAKOVER 1968) and to identify regions of the chromosome that were transcribed when λ was in the prophage state (BEAR and SKALKA 1969).

Al appreciated that progress in science depends on the development of new methods. Among those to which Al's lab made important contributions were fixed-angle Cs gradients, methylated albumin columns for fractionating DNA, methods of handling DNA that avoid breakage and denaturation, as well as methods that would break phage chromosomes into halves and quarters, and the calibration of methods for measuring molecular weights of DNA. Al confessed that the development of a method was painful; his view of heaven was a "place" where a new method, finally mastered, could be applied over and over. BILL DOVE quoted Al as saying, "There is nothing more satisfying to me than developing a method. Ideas come and go, but a method lasts."

Al occasionally blessed us with his thoughts about the deeper significance of things. His papers "Bacteriophage T2: parasite or organelle" (1957), "Idiosyncrasies of DNA structure" (1970a), and "Genes and hereditary characteristics" (1970b) delighted his contemporaries and can still be read with pleasure and profit.

But how many people really knew Al? From his works, we can say he was interested in this or that, but such a contention might leave the impression that we have adequately summarized his interests. That is hardly likely. Each of Al's contributions was truly original—he never copied even himself! Consequently, each paper was a surprise to us. We can surmise, therefore, that his published works do not begin to saturate the library of ideas available to him. His papers must be but a small sampling of his scientific thoughts.

And the rest of his mind? Who knows? Al exemplified reticence. His economy of speech was greater even than his economy of writing. If we asked him a question in a social gathering, we could usually get an answer such as "yes" or "no." However, at a scientific meeting one might get no answer at all, which was probably Al's way of saying, in the fewest possible words, that he had no thoughts on that subject.

Encounters with Al were rare, considering that he worked at Cold Spring Harbor, which hosted hundreds of visitors every summer. That's because Al spent his summers sailing in Michigan, and, except at occasional Symposia or the annual Phage Meetings, which came early and late in the season, he was not to be seen.

Thus, most of us who valued Al as a colleague and acquaintance didn't really know him. I am one of those, and I suppose that status qualifies me for this assignment; the Al about whom I write is the same Al that most other people did not really know, either.

The Phage Church, as we were sometimes called, was led by the Trinity of DELBRÜCK, LURIA, and HERSHEY. DELBRÜCK's status as Founder and his *ex cathedra* manner made him the Pope, of course, and LURIA was the hard working, socially sensitive priest/confessor. And Al was the saint. Why? How could we canonize Al when we hardly knew him?

Maybe some of the following considerations apply: The logic of Al's analyses was impeccable. He was original, but the relevance of his work to the interests of the rest of us was always apparent; he contributed to and borrowed from the communal storehouse of understanding, casual about labeling his own contributions but scrupulous about attributing the ones he borrowed. He was industrious (compulsively so—each day he worked two shifts). He was a superb editor (*e.g.*, HERSHEY 1971) and critic, devastatingly accurate but never too harsh; he deplored that gratuitous proliferation of words which both reflects and contributes to sloppiness of thought. And his suggestions were always helpful.

Does that qualify him for sainthood? It would do if he was in all other respects perfect. And he may have been. Who could tell? Who among us knew this quiet man well enough to know if there was a dark side? Perhaps canonization was a mark of our deep respect for this quintessential scientist. Maybe, by canonizing Al we could accept the relative insignificance of our own contributions. Maybe we were just having fun.

But, in his papers, Saint Al was *there*. He talked to the reader, explaining things as he saw them, but never letting us forget that he was transmitting provisional understanding. We got no free rides, no revealed truths, no invitation to surrender our own judgment. And we could never skim because *every* word was important. I think this style reflected his verbal reticence, which, in turn, mirrored his modesty. Examples: "Some clarification, at least in the mind of the author, of the concepts 'reversible' and 'irreversible' has been achieved" (HERSHEY 1943). "On this question we have had more opportunity in this paper to discover than to attack difficulties" (HERSHEY 1944). Al's modesty was dramatically documented by JIM EBERT, who recalled that Al, whose research support was guaranteed by the Carnegie Institution, argued with Carnegie directors for the right to apply for National Institutes of Health support so that he might benefit from the critiques of his peers.

In science, Al appeared to be fearless. Fearlessness and modesty might seem an unlikely combination. Not so. Modesty is kin to a lack of pretense. In the absence of pretense, there is nothing to fear.

Tastes of the many flavors of HERSHEY's mind and the accomplishments of his laboratory can be best gained from the Annual Reports of the Director of the Genetics Research Unit, Carnegie Institution of Washington Yearbook. The principal investigators of this unit were HERSHEY and BARBARA McCLINTOCK. In 1963 Al wrote, "Our justification for existence as a Unit, however, resides in the value of our research. We like to think that much of that value is as unstatable and as durable as other human produce that cannot be sold. Some can be put on paper, however. That we offer with the usual human mixture of pride and diffidence." Those who worked with HERSHEY at Cold Spring Harbor included PHYLLIS BEAR, ELIZABETH BURGI, JOHN CAIRNS, CONNIE CHADWICK, MARTHA CHASE, CARLO COCITO, RICK DAVERN, GUS DOERMANN, RUTH EHRING, STANLEY FORMAN, FRED FRANKEL, DOROTHY FRASER, ALAN GAREN, EDDIE GOLDBERG, JUNE DIXON HUDIS, LAURA INGRAHAM, NADA LEDINKO, CY LEVINTHAL, SHRAGA MAKOVER, JOE MANDELL, NORMAN MELECHEN, TEIICHI MINAGAWA, GISELA MOSIG, DAVID PARMA, CATHERINE ROESEL, IRWIN RUBENSTEIN, ANN SKALKA, MERVYN SMITH, GEORGE STREISINGER, NEVILLE SYMONDS, JUN-ICHI TOMIZAWA, NICK VISCONTI, BOB WEISBERG, RUDY WERNER, FRANCES WOMACK, and HIDEO YAMAGISHI.

In his retirement, Al cultivated an interest in computers, and he renewed his youthful interest in music. He is survived by his wife, HARRIET DAVIDSON HERSHEY, and by his son, PETER.

LITERATURE CITED

BEAR, P. D., and A. SKALKA, 1969 The molecular origin of lambda prophage mRNA. Proc. Natl. Acad. Sci. USA **62:** 385–388.

CAIRNS, J., 1961 An estimate of the length of the DNA molecule of T2 bacteriophage by autoradiography. J. Mol. Biol. **3:** 756–761.

CAIRNS, J., 1962 Proof that the replication of DNA involves separation of the strands. Nature **194:** 1274.

CAMPBELL, A., 1962 Episomes. Adv. Genet. **11:** 101–145.

DOERMANN, A. H., 1953 The vegetative state in the life cycle of bacteriophage: evidence for its occurrence and its genetic characterization. Cold Spring Harbor Symp. Quant. Biol. **18:** 3–11.

DOERMANN, A. H., and L. BOEHNER, 1963 An experimental analysis of bacteriophage T4 heterozygotes. I. Mottled plaques from crosses involving six rII loci. Virology **21:** 551–567.

DRAKE, J. W., 1967 The length of the homologous pairing region for genetic recombination in bacteriophage T4. Proc. Natl. Acad. Sci. USA **58:** 962–966.

EPSTEIN, R. H., A. BOLLE, C. M. STEINBERG, E. KELLENBERGER, R. S. EDGAR et al., 1963 Physiological studies of conditional lethal mutants of bacteriophage T4D. Cold Spring Harbor Symp. Quant. Biol. **28:** 375–392.

FRANKEL, F., 1963 An unusual DNA extracted from bacteria infected with phage T2. Proc. Natl. Acad. Sci. USA **49:** 366–372.

HERSHEY, A. D., 1934 The chemical separation of some cellular constituents of the Brucella group of micro-organisms. Ph.D. thesis, Michigan State College. Published in co-authorship with R. C. HUSTON and I. F. HUDDLESON as Technical Bulletin No. 137 of the Michigan Agricultural Experiment Station.

HERSHEY, A. D., 1941 The absolute rate of the phage-antiphage reaction. J. Immunol. **41:** 299–319.

HERSHEY, A. D., 1943 Specific precipitation. V. Irreversible systems. J. Immunol. **46:** 249–261.

HERSHEY, A. D., 1944 Specific precipitation. VI. The restricted system bivalent antigen, bivalent antibody, as an example of reversible bifunctional polymerization. J. Immunol. **48:** 381–401.

HERSHEY, A. D., 1946 Mutation of bacteriophage with respect to type of plaque. Genetics **31:** 620–640.

HERSHEY, A. D., 1947 Spontaneous mutations in bacterial viruses. Cold Spring Harbor Symp. Quant. Biol. **11:** 67–77.

HERSHEY, A. D., 1955 An upper limit to the protein content of the germinal substance of bacteriophage T2. Virology **1:** 108–127.

HERSHEY, A. D., 1956 The organization of genetic material in bacteriophage T2. Brookhaven Symp. Biol. **8:** 6–14.

HERSHEY, A. D., 1957 Bacteriophage T2: parasite or organelle, pp. 229–239 in The Harvey Lectures, Series LI. Academic Press, New York.

HERSHEY, A. D., 1958 The production of recombinants in phage crosses. Cold Spring Harbor Symp. Quant. Biol. **23:** 19–46.

HERSHEY, A. D., 1963 Annual Report of the Director of the Genetics Research Unit, Carnegie Institution of Washington Yearbook **62:** 461–500.

HERSHEY, A. D., 1970a Idiosyncrasies of DNA structure (Nobel Lecture). Science **168:** 1425–1427.

HERSHEY, A. D., 1970b Genes and hereditary characteristics. Nature **226:** 697–700.

HERSHEY, A. D. (Editor), 1971 The Bacteriophage Lambda. Cold Spring Harbor Laboratory Press, Cold Spring Harbor, N.Y.

HERSHEY, A. D., and E. BURGI, 1960 Molecular homogeneity of the deoxyribonucleic acid of phage T2. J. Mol. Biol. **2:** 143–152.

HERSHEY, A. D., and E. BURGI, 1965 Complementary structure of interacting sites at the ends of lambda DNA molecules. Proc. Natl. Acad. Sci. USA **53:** 325–328.

HERSHEY, A. D., and M. CHASE, 1952a Independent functions of viral protein and nucleic acid in growth of bacteriophage. J. Gen. Physiol. **36:** 39–56.

HERSHEY, A. D., and M. CHASE, 1952b Genetic recombination and heterozygosis in bacteriophage. Cold Spring Harbor Symp. Quant. Biol. **16:** 471–479.

HERSHEY, A. D., and R. ROTMAN, 1948 Linkage among genes controlling inhibition of lysis in a bacterial virus. Proc. Natl. Acad. Sci. USA **34:** 89–96.

HERSHEY, A. D., and R. ROTMAN, 1949 Genetic recombination between host-range and plaque-type mutants of bacteriophage in single bacterial cells. Genetics **34:** 44–71.

HERSHEY, A. D., M. D. KAMEN, J. W. KENNEDY and H. GEST, 1951 The mortality of bacteriophage containing assimilated radioactive phosphorus. J. Gen. Physiol. **34:** 305–319.

HERSHEY, A. D., E. BURGI, H. J. CAIRNS, F. FRANKEL and L. INGRAHAM, 1961 Growth and inheritance in bacteriophage. Carnegie Institution of Washington Year Book **60:** 455–461.

HERSHEY, A. D., E. BURGI and L. INGRAHAM, 1963 Cohesion of DNA molecules isolated from phage lambda. Proc. Natl. Acad. Sci. USA **49:** 748–755.

JUDSON, H. F., 1996 The Eighth Day of Creation (Expanded Edition). Cold Spring Harbor Laboratory Press, New York, p. 35.

LEVINTHAL, C., 1954 Recombination in phage T2: its relationship to heterozygosis and growth. Genetics **39:** 169–184.

MAKOVER, S., 1968 A preferred origin for the replication of lambda DNA. Proc. Natl. Acad. Sci. USA **59:** 1345–1348.

MANDELL, J. D., and A. D. HERSHEY, 1960 A fractionating column for analysis of nucleic acids. Anal. Biochem. **1:** 66–77.

MESELSON, M., and F. W. STAHL, 1958 The replication of DNA in Escherichia coli. Proc. Natl. Acad. Sci. USA **44:** 671–682.

MESELSON, M., and J. J. WEIGLE, 1961 Chromosome breakage accompanying genetic recombination in bacteriophage. Proc. Natl. Acad. Sci. USA **47:** 857–868.

MOSIG, G., 1966 Distances separating genetic markers in T4 DNA. Proc. Natl. Acad. Sci. USA **56:** 1177–1183.

MOSIG, G., 1994 Homologous recombination, pp. 54–82 in Bacteriophage T4, edited by J. D. KARAM et al. ASM Press, Washington, DC.

RUBENSTEIN, I., C. A. THOMAS, JR., and A. D. HERSHEY, 1961 The molecular weights of T2 bacteriophage DNA and its first and second breakage products. Proc. Natl. Acad. Sci. USA **47:** 1113–1122.

SKALKA, A., E. BURGI and A. D. HERSHEY, 1968 Segmental distribution of nucleotides in the DNA of bacteriophage lambda. J. Mol. Biol. **34:** 1–16.

STEINBERG, C., and F. STAHL, 1958 The theory of formal phage genetics. Appendix II in Hershey (1958).

STREISINGER, G., 1966 Terminal redundancy, or all's well that ends well, pp. 335–340 in *Phage and the Origins of Molecular Biology*, edited by J. CAIRNS, J., G. S. STENT and J. D. WATSON. Cold Spring Harbor Laboratory, New York.

VISCONTI, N., and M. DELBRÜCK, 1953 The mechanism of genetic recombination in phage. Genetics **38:** 5–33.

WATSON, J. D., and F. H. C. CRICK, 1953 A structure for deoxyribonucleic acid. Nature **171:** 737–738.

WERNER, R., 1968 Initiation and propagation of growing points in the DNA of phage T4. Cold Spring Harbor Symp. Quant. Biol. **33:** 501–507.

See also page 706 in Addenda et Corrigenda.

∘ **Anatomy of a Revolution** ∘

Gerald R. Fink

Whitehead Institute, Massachusetts Institute of Technology, Cambridge, Massachusetts 02142

WITH this volume, GENETICS announces that Arabidopsis has joined the Security Council of Model Genetic Organisms. These favored few form the standard to which all other organisms are compared. Like the Security Council of the United Nations, where there is broad geographical representation, the Security Council of Genetic Organisms seeks broad phylogenetic representation. Therefore, the current membership also includes a virus (lambda), a gram positive bacterium (*Bacillus subtilis*), a gram negative bacterium (*Escherichia coli*), a fungus (*Saccharomyces cerevisiae*), a unicellular alga (*Chlamydomonas reinhardtii*), a worm (*Caenorhabditis elegans*), an arthropod (*Drosophila melanogaster*), a vertebrate (*Mus musculus*), and humans. The idea is that an intense concentration on the genetics of one of the representatives provides a window on the biology of all the other species in that phylum. Arabidopsis has emerged as the flowering plant delegate, presaging dramatic changes in agriculture and the topsy-turvy world of nutritional sciences.

To be elected to the Security Council, a delegate organism must meet objective criteria. It must be amenable to all the classical genetic moves—tests of dominance, complementation, and recombination. Its genome should be sequenced or in the process of being sequenced, and it must be readily transformed with DNA. With all of these techniques in place, geneticists can perform their sacred task: connecting genes with their function. Having said all this, elevation to membership on the Security Council (as with the permanent members of the U.N.) has a strong historical component. Buttressed by 90 years of study, Drosophila is unlikely to be replaced by another Arthropod. And the inclusion of humans smacks of self-interest on the part of the selection committee.

While Arabidopsis fulfills the criteria for membership, its meteoric rise to council rank is still surprising. As few as 10 years ago, most botanists shunned this tiny weed despite the fact that its small size, short generation time, and small genome with little repeated DNA were well advertised (REDEI 1975; PRUITT and MEYEROWITZ

1986). Yet, today there is virtually no major academic institution or agrotech company that does not have an Arabidopsis group; indeed, many formerly disdainful botanists are now among Arabidopsis' most avid proponents. So, what is responsible for this abrupt turnaround? I believe that the rapid rise of Arabidopsis as a premier genetic system is a consequence of the fortuitous confluence of three factors—scientific, social, and economic.

The crucial scientific factors were the concurrent development of Arabidopsis genomics[1] and the technical toolbox of modern molecular genetics. Together, these have made it possible to make mutants, to clone the corresponding gene, and to decipher the function of that gene. Genomic advances include the development of high-resolution physical and genetic maps and the attendant YAC, BAC, and lambda libraries. This genomic infrastructure has accelerated all genetic work and forms the backbone of the global Arabidopsis Sequencing Project. The goal is to have the complete sequence of the roughly 100 Mb in the Arabidopsis genome by the turn of the century.

In addition to these advances in genomics, we also have a panoply of new genetic techniques. There is a convenient transposon tagging system (HEHL 1994; AZPIROZ-LEEHAN and FELDMANN 1997) that permits not only the rapid isolation of mutants, but also the easy acquisition of the corresponding genes. There are also useful enhancer trap and gene trap constructs that facilitate cell and tissue localization for developmental and regulatory analysis (SUNDARESAN *et al.* 1995). But it is the development of a rapid transformation protocol that has propelled Arabidopsis to center stage.

Remarkably, Arabidopsis can be transformed simply by dipping whole plants into a solution of Agrobacterium containing a T-DNA plasmid (BECHTOLD *et al.* 1993; CHANG *et al.* 1994). Plants are inverted and im-

---

[1] Arabidopsis World Wide Web electronic resources: http://genome.www.stanford.edu/Arabidopsis, http://nasc.life.nott.ac.uk/centre.html, Arabidopsis@net.bio.net.

mersed in Agrobacterium, and the combo is placed under vacuum for a brief period. The Agrobacterium infiltrates the tissues and delivers the T-DNA plasmid containing the DNA of interest into cells, where it becomes stably integrated into the genome. As some of the transformed cells develop into gametes, the seeds of these plants give rise to stable transformants in the next generation. Prior to this discovery, transformation in Arabidopsis was a nightmare, requiring a skilled technician to establish cell cultures from plants, transform the cells in culture, and then regenerate them into plants. This painstaking process was slow (4–6 months), cumbersome, and inefficient. More often than not, the few transformants obtained had genetic abnormalities (sterility, somaclonal variation) that made them useless for further analysis.

The *in planta* transformation protocol is easy and avoids all the problems of the cell culture approach. Without much supervision, even a high school student can generate large numbers of fertile transformants. This procedure is now used routinely to identify genes by functional complementation. Once the relevant mutation is localized on the physical map (1 cM = ~200 kb), DNA segments contained within that region can be readily transformed into the plant to identify the one that suppresses the mutant defect. The current protocol makes it practical to scan across a segment of 50 kb (10–15 genes) and to obtain unambiguous gene identification in 2–3 months.

The Arabidopsis transformation system still lacks a reliable method for obtaining homologous integration. This system would permit the simple construction of knockouts and the integration of virtually any DNA segment at a predetermined chromosomal location without rearranging the rest of the genome. This shortcoming has not precluded the election of Arabidopsis to the Security Council, especially since other members, notably Drosophila and the worm, currently suffer from this limitation. However, there are many fascinating plant phenomena that will be understood only when a homologous integration system is developed.

A good example is gene silencing, a phenomenon in which the presence of extra copies of a gene introduced by transformation inactivates both the transgene and the resident homologous gene (FLAVELL 1994; MARTIENSSEN 1996). Silencing is not simply a consequence of transformation because genes that have duplicated spontaneously can also be silenced (BENDER and FINK 1995). This homology-dependent gene inactivation may hold the secret as to how the genome defends itself against rampant gene duplication and the invasion of alien DNAs (viruses and transposons). At least two different types of silencing exist, one operating at the transcriptional and the other at the post-transcriptional level (DEPICKER and VAN MONTAGU 1997). Elucidation of the mechanism of silencing is hampered by the inability to direct a series of diagnostic constructs to the same

chromosomal location. Currently, each construct ends up at a different site, making the results subject to the interpretation that some of the phenotypes may be due to chromosomal position effects. The recent report of a homologous integration event (KEMPIN *et al.* 1997) holds out the hope that this impasse may soon be surmounted.

In addition to these scientific developments, there have also been "extrascientific factors," both social and economic, that were critical to the transcendence of Arabidopsis. A key social factor was the excellent mentoring of students by the scientists who initially populated the field (among them, FRED AUSUBEL, GLORIA CORUZZI, RON DAVIS, ELLIOT MEYEROWITZ, and CHRIS SOMERVILLE). This founding group of molecular biologists transmitted to their students the community spirit that emerged from the lambda, *E. coli*, yeast, worm, and Drosophila traditions. Equally important, these mentors not only allowed but encouraged their students to take their successful projects with them when they embarked upon their own independent careers, creating a web of interacting laboratories. This amicable spirit fostered the rapid dissemination of strains, DNA libraries, techniques, and projects with the consequent rapid acceleration of research.

Another social factor was Cold Spring Harbor's adoption of Arabidopsis as the organism for the plant molecular biology course. The plant's rapid growth and short generation time make it a natural for a brief summer course program. The Cold Spring Harbor imprimatur served simultaneously to advertise the organism and to recruit young scientists to this new and burgeoning field. With the publication of the book, *Arabidopsis* (MEYEROWITZ and SOMERVILLE 1994), Cold Spring Harbor also promoted the codification and dissemination of useful lore and techniques.

Notwithstanding these scientific and social factors, this abrupt turnabout could not have happened without timely financial backing. The church regrettably no longer supports plant science as it did in MENDEL's time. Fortunately, the National Science Foundation (NSF) stepped up to promote Arabidopsis. There are many program directors at NSF who deserve thanks, but it was Dr. DELILL NASSIR who first sensed the zeitgeist and championed Arabidopsis when it was not fashionable to do so. She used discretionary funds, her wise counsel, and influence within the federal funding agencies to get the ball rolling—supporting meetings, identifying the movers and the shakers, and making sure that the best Arabidopsis proposals were supported. We may praise the organism and prize our geniuses, but the role of federal support in the emergence of Arabidopsis cannot be overemphasized.

All of these factors have combined to make Arabidopsis a premier organism with which to study problems of interest to all modern biologists. Many of these topics are covered in this commemorative issue. The central themes of modern biology—development, transcription, cell biology—all can be studied elegantly in Arabidopsis. Some of them, specifically the response to gases, are arguably studied best in Arabidopsis. Moreover, the plant-specific problems of phototropism, gravitropism, photomorphogenesis, and disease resistance, formerly studied by classical genetics or physiological experiments, are now being unraveled at the cellular level by the application of genomics and the molecular genetic techniques discussed earlier. Many of these findings are directly applicable to the improvement of crops, which probably explains why this inedible weed has suddenly become the darling of the agricultural schools.

Advances in the genomics and molecular genetics of Arabidopsis will permit scientists to attack problems that formerly seemed completely beyond their grasp. I would like to address two of these, the first theoretical and the second practical.

Plant movement: One of the key unanswered theoretical questions in biology is: What is the basis for concerted plant cell movements? We know that these dramatic movements are induced by external stimuli (light, gravity, and touch), but we do not have a conceptual framework that permits an understanding of the resulting behaviors. This problem was addressed eloquently by Charles Darwin more than a hundred years ago:

> We believe that there is no structure in plants more wonderful, as far as its functions are concerned, than the tip of the radicle. . . . It is hardly an exaggeration to say that the tip of the radicle thus endowed, and having the power of directing the movements of the adjoining parts, acts like the brain of one of the lower animals; the brain being seated within the anterior end of the body, receiving impressions from the sense organs and directing the several movements.
>
> CHARLES DARWIN, *The Power of Movement in Plants* (1896)

DARWIN's comparison of the tip of the stem to the "brain of the lower animals" focuses squarely on the issue, but his metaphor is inappropriate. Plants have no single organ, like the brain, that can be construed as directing movement. Moreover, movement in animals can be ascribed to the position and connectivity of the underlying anatomical structures—muscles innervated by axons linked to the central nervous system. But plant anatomy has not revealed the equivalent of a neural network that could account for the concerted behavior of some cells but not others.

Although plants do not have the equivalent of neural networks, they have plasmodesmata, channels through the cell walls that provide a continuous cytoplasmic connection between adjacent cells (LUCAS 1995; DING 1997). Plasmodesmata are portals for intercellular communication as shown by their role in the spread of plant viruses; these viruses encode proteins that dilate the channels to enhance their movement throughout the

plant (WAIGMANN and ZAMBRYSKI 1995; HEINLEIN *et al.* 1995). Perhaps cells that respond together for plant movement are united by an underlying network of connectivity via plasmodesmata. This speculation raises many questions. Are there cellular proteins, analogous to the viral movement proteins, that regulate the flow of information through the plasmodesmata in response to external signals? Are there transcellular cytoskeletal structures that extend through plasmodesmata from one cell to another? How do these hypothetical regulatory and cytoskeletal elements coordinate the cell wall expansion that is thought to be necessary for motion?

If plasmodesmata provide the connections for concerted plant movements, then there must be some as yet undiscovered factor(s) that impose the selectivity that permits one group of cells to respond to a stimulus and another to ignore it. Group identity could be conferred by a restricted pattern of intercellular connectivity (only a subset of cells is connected by the same plasmodesmal highway) and specific intercellular molecular signals. This possibility could be revealed by the analysis of mutants defective in response to the stimulus coupled with improved biochemical techniques for the identification of plasmodesmal constituents. Once the relevant molecules have been identified, new imaging techniques applied to wild-type and movement mutants might reveal a structural or chemical network shared by those cells that respond in concert. Thus, the solution to the problem of plant movement raised by DARWIN may not come from a unifying theoretical insight, but rather by stitching together the answers to many diverse puzzles.

The genetics of nutrition: The remarkable developments in Arabidopsis research will form the vanguard of the third revolution in agriculture. As JARED DIAMOND has noted, "Human history's most important event since the last Ice Age was the rise of agriculture in southwest Asia's Fertile Crescent" (DIAMOND 1997). This first tsunami, which occurred in 9000 BC, was followed by another wave that occurred early in this century: the engineering of domesticated plants by the application of Mendelian genetics in the '20s and '30s (see Figure 1). The third wave is building now, with the application of new DNA technologies. Already, introductory botanical texts instruct today's college students that genetic engineering will yield plants that make vitamins and drugs; resist drought, disease, and insects; and "make better tasting food, clean the environment, recycle wastes, prevent tooth decay, and produce antibiotics, biodegradable plastics, and fragrances" (MOORE *et al.* 1998). A few of the more sober predictions already have been realized.

The scientific and social factors are clearly in place for Arabidopsis to lead the third phase of the agricultural revolution, but the economic factor is not. The difficulty is that agricultural research is largely funded by the U.S. Department of Agriculture (USDA), whose policies have

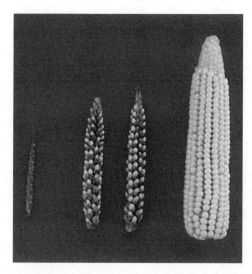

FIGURE 1.—The revolution in agriculture. The photograph illustrates the result of genetic engineering in maize. Teosinte, shown on the left, is the wild grass thought to be the progentor of modern corn. The first revolution involved domestication and selection by natives of the new world. The second depended upon Mendelian genetics to produce the cob on the right. In the center are the F_1 progeny of a cross between teosinte and modern corn. The third revolution may produce plants that look dramatically different from those of the 20th century. The photograph was kindly provided by JOHN DOEBLEY of the University of Minnesota.

remained conservative and unimaginative in the face of the momentous changes that could enable the agency to carry out its mission. Even with well-meaning staff, the USDA has been unable to counteract the political forces that historically have stymied its effectiveness. Its largest competitive grant program, the National Research Initiative Competitive Grants Program, has a woefully inadequate budget of only 97.2 million dollars (FY 1998). Moreover, with an overhead rate of 14% it does not pay the true costs of research, making its grants noncompetitive with those from other federal agencies.

One solution to this problem would be to place the funding of plant engineering within the National Institutes of Health. The creation of a National Institute of Nutrition would house Arabidopsis in the appropriate pantheon of Institutes dedicated to the health of the nation. Such an act would not only provide support to accelerate the revolution, it would bring a breath of fresh air to nutrition, a field fundamental to public health that has so far failed to benefit from the advances in molecular genetics. Despite the enormous interest in diet, there is little critical information about it; the professional journals and the popular press abound with contradictory claims bewildering to both scientists and nonscientists.

The confusion caused by the disarray in nutrition is captured poignantly in WOODY ALLEN's (1973) classic movie *Sleeper*, in which Miles Monroe, the owner of the Happy Carrot Health Food Club, emerges from a 200-year cryogenic immersion in the year 2173. The following is the discussion between two nutritionists observing this modern Rip van Winkle:

Scientist 1: Has he asked for anything special?
Scientist 2: Yes, this morning for breakfast he requested something called wheat germ, organic honey, and tiger's milk.
Scientist 1: Oh yes! Those were the charmed substances that some years ago were thought to contain life-preserving properties.
Scientist 2: You mean there was no deep fat, steak, cream pies, hot fudge?
Scientist 1: Those were thought to be unhealthy. Precisely the opposite of what we now know to be true.
Scientist 2: Incredible!

But it is no joking matter. The problem with research in nutrition is that there is insufficient information about the two components of the system: the plants that are the source of food and the animals that eat them. The ability to alter genetically both parts of the equation would provide a powerful antidote to the current chaos. Although plants are key to our diet, we know little about how they synthesize, metabolize, and deposit the nutrients that are essential to our survival and longevity. Much of this confusion could be remedied by using Arabidopsis as a model for nutritional studies. At the outset, it would be important to unravel the pathways by which fatty acids, vitamins, and other metabolites are produced, how they are regulated, and how their deposition in the various tissues of the plant is controlled.

On the other side of the equation, there is a dearth of knowledge about how we metabolize plant compounds. Superimposed on this shortcoming is the problem that the human population is genetically heterogeneous for the ability to metabolize plant compounds. What's good to eat for one person may be life threatening for another. The inability of people with phenylketonuria to metabolize phenylalanine is emblematic of thousands of other genetically controlled metabolic differences in the human population. This genetic heterogeneity confounds current studies.

It is worth contemplating how the field of nutrition would be changed by genomics and molecular genetics. Think of the power of testing a battery of mouse mutants consuming a diet of well-defined plant mutants. Such experiments would define the critical nutrients that promote good health, longevity, and resistance to infection. But, the benefits go much deeper. For example, one might find that a particular mouse mutant always dies of coronary artery disease when fed a wild-type plant, but survives without complications when fed a mutant plant unable to produce a particular lipid. The ability to perform such experiments would turn nutrition into an exact science.

One objection to this scenario is that Arabidopsis is not an edible plant. But, here the spirit of the Security Council should prevail: *What we learn in Arabidopsis is directly applicable to the engineering of crop plants.* Once we learn to make knockouts and homologous replacements in Arabidopsis these technologies will be quickly adapted to other plants. There seems to be no resistance to applying this idea to rapeseed, a close relative of Arabidopsis that is a source of cooking oil. But, many balk at the idea that Arabidopsis, a dicot, is a good model for the monocots (corn, rice, wheat, and sorghum), which constitute the major source of protein for animals and humans.

However, the new field of genomics has provided data suggesting that perhaps too much has been made of the monocot/dicot distinction (PATERSON *et al.* 1996). Although monocots and dicots are thought to have diverged from each other 130–200 million years ago, there is considerable synteny between the two groups: large tracts of genes in Sorghum are in the same order as they are in Arabidopsis. This colinearity has direct consequences for the engineering of crop plants. Synteny between Arabidopsis and the monocots means that genes in Arabidopsis have functions similar to their orthologues in monocots, and knowing their position in Arabidopsis will aid in their isolation and manipulation in crop plants.

A second objection is that unlike mice, we are not inbred and our genetic diversity will preclude the establishment of a universally applicable diet. True enough. However, with the completion of the human genome project and the attendant technologies for genotyping individuals, it will be possible to identify the alleles associated with many metabolic differences. Once we understand these human differences, it should be possible to design transgenic plants that better meet our needs.

The inclusion of Arabidopsis in the Security Council is noteworthy because it heralds a new era. Although there will be many surprises along the way, one thing is clear: The emergence of a reliable and facile model plant that instructs both basic research and agriculture will alter the course of science and, ultimately, the course of history. And I predict that when *Sleeper*'s Miles Monroe awakens in the future, the nutritionists will want to know his genotype before he dines on the extraordinary plants of the 22nd century.

LITERATURE CITED

ALLEN, W., 1973 *Sleeper*, United Artists.

AZPIROZ-LEEHAN, R., and K. A. FELDMANN, 1997 T-DNA insertion mutagenesis in Arabidopsis: going back and forth. Trends Genet. **13:** 152–156.

BECHTOLD, N., J. ELLIS and G. PELLETIER, 1993 *In planta* Agrobacterium mediated gene transfer by infiltration of adult *Arabidopsis thaliana* plants. C.R. Acad. Sci. Paris **316:** 1194–1199.

BENDER, J., and G. R. FINK, 1995 Epigenetic control of an endogenous gene family is revealed by a novel blue fluorescent mutant of Arabidopsis. Cell **83:** 725–734.

CHANG, S. C., S. K. PAR, B. C. KIM, B. J. KANG, D. U. KIM *et al.*, 1994 Stable genetic transformation of *Arabidopsis thaliana* by Agrobacterium inoculation *in planta.* Plant J. **5:** 551–558.

DARWIN, C., 1896 *The Power of Movement in Plants.* pp. 572–573, Appleton, New York.

DEPICKER, A., and M. VAN MONTAGU, 1997 Post-transcriptional gene silencing in plants. Curr. Opin. Cell Biol. **9:** 373–382.

DIAMOND, J., 1997 Location, location, location: the first farmers. Science **278:** 1243–1244.

DING, B., 1997 Cell to cell transport of macromolecules through plasmodesmata: a novel signaling pathway in plants. Trends Cell Biol. **7:** 5–9.

FLAVELL, R. B., 1994 Inactivation of gene expression in plants as a consequence of specific sequence duplication. Proc. Natl. Acad. Sci. USA **91:** 3490–3496.

HEHL, R., 1994 Transposon tagging in heterologous host plants. Trends Genet. **10:** 385–386.

HEINLEIN, M., B. L. EPEL, H. S. PADGETT and R. N. BEACHY, 1995 Interaction of tobamovirus movement proteins with the plant cytoskeleton. Science **270:** 1983–1985.

KEMPIN, S. S., S. J. LILJEGREN, L. M. BLCOK, S. D. ROUNSLEY, M. F. YANOFSKY *et al.*, 1997 Targeted disruption in Arabidopsis. Nature **389:** 802–803.

LUCAS, W. J., 1995 Plasmodesmata: intracellular channels for macromolecular transport in plants. Curr. Opin. Cell Biol. **7:** 673–680.

MARTIENSSEN, R., 1996 Epigenetic phenomena: paramutation and gene silencing in plants. Curr. Biol. **6:** 810–813.

MEYEROWITZ, E. M., and C. R. SOMERVILLE, 1994 *Arabidopsis.* Cold Spring Harbor Laboratory Press, Cold Spring Harbor, NY.

MOORE, R., W. D. CLARK and D. S. VODOPICH, 1998 *Botany*, p. 16, McGraw-Hill, New York.

PATERSON, A. H., T.-H. LAN, K. P. REISCHMANN, C. CHANG, Y.-R. LIN *et al.*, 1996 Toward a unified genetic map of higher plants, transcending the monocot-dicot divergence. Nature Genet. **14:** 380–382.

PRUITT, R. E., and E. M. MEYEROWITZ, 1986 Characterizaton of the genome of *Arabidopsis thaliana.* J. Mol. Biol. **187:** 169–183.

REDEI, G. P., 1975 *Arabidopsis as a genetic tool.* Annu. Rev. Genet. **9:** 111–127.

SUNDARESAN, V., P. SPRINGER, T. VOLPE, S. HAWARD, J. D. G. JONES *et al.*, 1995 Patterns of gene action in plant development revealed by enhancer trap and gene trap transposable elements. Genes Dev. **9:** 1797–1810.

WAIGMANN, E., and P. ZAMBRYSKI, 1995 Tobacco mosaic virus movement protein mediated protein transport between trichome cells. Plant Cell **7:** 2069–2079.

The Language of Gene Interaction

Patrick C. Phillips

Biology Department, University of Texas, Arlington, Texas 76019-0498

> The study of variation and heredity, in our ignorance of the causation of those phenomena, *must* be built of statistical data, as MENDEL knew long ago; but, as he also perceived, the ground must be prepared by specific experiment. The phenomena of heredity and variation are specific questions. That is where our *exact* science will begin. Otherwise we may one day see those huge foundations of "biometry" in ruins.
>
> W. BATESON (1902)

VERY soon after the rediscovery of MENDEL it was realized that the multilocus nature of inheritance could not be understood solely by examining the action of individual genes and then predicting how these genes would behave in concert simply by combining the separate observations. Frequently genes interact with one another, distorting simple Mendelian ratios and sometimes leading to novel phenotypes. Ninety years ago, WILLIAM BATESON coined the term "epistasis" to describe this sort of interaction (he appears to have first used the term in 1908, although it is most clearly spelled out in BATESON 1909). Epistasis translates directly to "standing upon," and was meant to describe the situation in which the action of one locus masks the allelic effects at another locus, much in the same way that complete dominance (the way in which most genes appeared to work at the time) involves the masking of one allele by another. The locus being masked is said to be "hypostatic" to the other locus.

At the same time that he was investigating all manner of Mendelian segregation ratios, BATESON was involved in a heated battle with the Biometrical school of genetics, exemplified by the views of KARL PEARSON and W. F. R. WELDON (PROVINE 1971). The Biometricians focused on the continuous range of variation among relatives in contrast to the discrete differences studied by the Mendelians. Eighty years ago, in one of the seminal papers in genetics, R. A. FISHER (1918) conclusively ended the debate by showing analytically that Mendelian segregation was compatible with the Biometrician's laws of heredity (something that had been argued qualitatively by a number of others before FISHER). In this same work, he also established several branches of statis-

tics and laid the groundwork for the entire field now known as quantitative genetics. It was quite a paper.

The essential problem with which FISHER had to deal was how to map the discrete segregation of alleles onto the continuous range of measured traits. FISHER noted that in conducting this mapping, it was entirely possible (although, as it was later clear, not likely to his mind), that one would not be able to predict the quantitative phenotype of a particular two-locus genotype by simply adding the effects of two loci together. With undoubted allusion to BATESON's unusual segregation ratios, FISHER called these nonadditive interactions "epistacy." This term rapidly became simply "epistasis," and two related, but distinct meanings of the same word entered the geneticist's vocabulary (WADE 1992a).

It is perhaps telling that this duality in meaning rarely causes much confusion for those using the term. Mendelian and molecular geneticists tend to use epistasis in the strict sense of BATESON, while evolutionary and quantitative geneticists use epistasis to mean just about any form of gene interaction. After briefly tracing the history of the use of "epistasis," I suggest that there is good reason to start thinking about eliminating this potential source of confusion. Some of the difficulty in choosing the right word to describe gene interactions results from the lingering conflict between the Biometrical and Mendelian views of characterizing gene action. The resolution to this difficulty points the way to the possible final synthesis of these two approaches.

EPISTASIS FROM THE MENDELIAN VIEWPOINT

epistasis 1. *Genetics.* An interaction between nonallelic genes, especially an interaction in which one gene suppresses the expression of another.

American Heritage Dictionary of the English Language (1992)

Address for correspondence: Biology Department, Box 19498, University of Texas, Arlington, TX 76019-0498. E-mail: pphillips@uta.edu

Although officially given a name some ninety years ago, the phenomenon of gene interaction was discovered a few years earlier. In their study of the genetics of chicken combs, BATESON and PUNNETT (in BATESON *et al.* 1905) noted that one type of comb, the *single*, was rarely produced in their crosses and that its presence was difficult to reconcile with a simple Mendelian genetic system. Making good use of PUNNETT's recently derived method of creating a matrix, a "Punnett square," to describe all possible combinations of gametes, they concluded that comb inheritance could be described by Mendelian segregation of two factors, with the *single* phenotype appearing only in the rare double-recessive homozygotes. PUNNETT later found similar results in his parallel work on sweet peas (reviewed in PUNNETT 1920). WEINBERG (1910) also noted the possibility of such interactions, calling them *komplizierter polyhybridismus* (complicated polyhybridisms). It is perhaps not surprising that WEINBERG's term did not catch on, and his work unfortunately appears to have been largely ignored.

Despite BATESON's coining of a term to describe this situation and a great deal of coverage of unusual segregation ratios (usually described under the heading "interaction of factors") in early textbooks on genetics, there appears to have been little use of the word "epistasis" in the first few decades of this century [even by PUNNETT (1920) himself; see also CASTLE (1926)]. By the thirties, however, the strength of the Mendelian approach was firmly established and its power illustrated through a description of all manner of segregation ratios, with epistasis being a prime example (*e.g.*, LINDSEY 1932; SINNOTT and DUNN 1932; SNYDER 1935). A menagerie of special cases was collected and given names (Figure 1).

Yet by the fifties, interest in epistasis from a Mendelian point of view appears to have waned substantially. Gene interaction and unusual segregation ratios received diminished attention in textbooks (*e.g.*, COLIN 1956), although newer editions of older texts still maintained wider coverage (SINNOTT *et al.* 1958). Perhaps the decrease in interest in epistasis was because testing the Mendelian paradigm in more complex situations was no longer interesting. It was now self-evident that Mendelian segregation of chromosomes composed primarily of DNA provided an elegant physical mechanism for this segregation. Perhaps it was because variable mortality made Drosophila, still the dominant experimental system, not always the best organism for precise testing of complex segregation ratios. Most likely, geneticists at the time were busy getting on to other things.

Indeed, the next few decades were consumed by the molecular revolution. Since the eighties, however, the analysis of epistasis has made a strong comeback as an important means of ordering genes in developmental pathways (*e.g.*, AVERY and WASSERMAN 1992). This can sometimes include complex bifurcating pathways involving dozens of genes (*e.g.*, THOMAS 1993). The shift back toward epistasis is reflected in an expansion of coverage

Interaction Type	A-B-	A-bb	aaB-	aabb
Classical ratio	9	3	3	1
Dominant epistasis	12		3	1
Recessive epistasis	9	3	4	
Duplicate genes with cumulative effect	9	6		1
Duplicate dominant genes	15			1
Duplicate recessive genes	9	7		
Dominant & recessive interaction	13	3		

FIGURE 1.—Some unusual segregation ratios. Arrows join genotypes with similar phenotypes. After SNYDER (1935) and STANSFIELD (1991).

in recent editions of introductory genetics textbooks (*e.g.*, WEAVER and HEDRICK 1997).

It is clear that the term epistasis in the exact sense in which it was used by BATESON now plays a central role in modern genetics beyond the mere description of segregation ratios and well into the analysis of gene function. In the coming decade, gene interaction, in the very physical sense of the direct interaction between gene products that form molecular machines and signaling pathways, is likely to become more and more central to genetic analysis, and "epistasis" is equally likely to frequent the geneticist's lexicon.

EPISTASIS FROM THE STATISTICAL GENETICS VIEWPOINT

> When we move from Mendelian to biometrical analysis we must retain the concepts which have proved successful and necessary at the old level; but we must be prepared to see them appear, and to use them, in the new way necessitated by the new level of integration at which we are working.
>
> K. MATHER (1949, p. 400)

The impact of FISHER's (1918) paper on the entire field of quantitative genetics has been immense. Almost all of the notation and methods of analysis used today can be traced directly to this point source. It is curious, then, that FISHER's derivative term, epistacy, has not been used to describe quantitative gene interaction. SEWALL WRIGHT, the geneticist most closely identified with championing the importance of gene interactions in evolutionary change, used neither term to describe gene interactions in his most famous papers (WRIGHT 1931, 1932), although a few years later his use of "epistasis" was firmly established (WRIGHT 1935).

The use of epistasis to describe gene interaction in quantitative genetics is ostensibly similar to BATESON's use in describing segregation ratios. The issue here is whether or not the phenotype of a given genotype can be predicted by simply adding (or multiplying, depending on scale) its component single-locus effects. To the extent that this cannot be done, then the leftover bits are called the epistatic deviations. This is much more inclusive than BATESON's original use because many forms of gene interaction can lead to epistatic deviations.

The overall complexity of the situation was sorted out by COCKERHAM (1954, 1956) and KEMPTHORNE (1954). They broke the epistatic deviations into particular components that could be described by a statistical model, leading to terms like additive-by-additive, additive-by-dominance, and dominance-by-dominance epistasis (COCKERHAM 1954). KEMPTHORNE (1954), from the British school, still used "epistacy" in this context, although in his influential book a few years later (KEMPTHORNE 1957) he acknowledged that "epistasis" was the more commonly used descriptor. With this last gasp, the term "epistacy" appears to have winked out of existence.

More recent approaches to dealing with epistasis have focused on FISHER's (1918) most lasting contribution to statistical genetics, the idea that the effect of a gene needs to be estimated within the context of the population from which it is drawn. An alternative approach would be to have a specific model of how genes function and interact and then to construct a building-block description of the phenotype based on the genetic composition of the individual (CROW and KIMURA 1970, pp. 77ff; TACHIDA and COCKERHAM 1989). A similar approach has been suggested by CHEVERUD and ROUTMAN (1995), in what they call physiological epistasis (in contrast to statistical epistasis). The problem with building-block models is that they are still statistical abstractions (as is made clear by TACHIDA and COCKERHAM 1989) and are thus really no closer to the actual physiological mechanism of gene interaction than the effects models. Building-block models are limited by the particular genotypes that happen to be under study (and the particular loci being examined within those genotypes), whereas FISHER was concerned that the total number of possible genotypes could rapidly outpace the total size of any population (see FISHER 1941). The advantage of FISHER's approach is that it yields the parameters that are important for describing evolutionary change while at the same time being relatively insensitive to the particular sample of genotypes under study. The disadvantage of this approach is that the molecular and physiological nature of the gene interactions themselves can be masked by statistical abstraction and vagaries of allele frequencies. Other formulations have been suggested (e.g., SCHNELL 1984; WAGNER et al. 1998), but the best approach is undoubtedly going to be determined by the questions to be answered.

AN EXPANDED LANGUAGE OF GENE INTERACTIONS

epistasis 2. *Medicine.* A film that forms over the surface of a urine specimen. **3.** The suppression of a bodily discharge or secretion.

American Heritage Dictionary of the English Language (1992)

Part of the difficulty in reconciling the Mendelian and statistical formulations of epistasis is that our language for describing gene interactions is currently far too limited. Not all gene interactions are equal from the standpoint of understanding gene action, particularly in their consequences for evolution at those loci (WHITLOCK *et al.* 1995; FENSTER *et al.* 1997). In fact a number of different terms that describe gene interactions do not fit the expectations of classical epistasis and might be overlooked simply because they are not called by the expected name (see Figure 1). For example, compensatory and suppressor mutations clearly involve gene interactions (PHILLIPS 1996; STEPHAN 1996) and may in fact describe the same type of interaction (it is rare for all possible genotypes to be investigated in these cases). Similarly, so-called synthetic phenotypes are sometimes observed when two mutations with apparently separate effects are combined in the same individual. The most extreme case of this is synthetic lethality (DOBZHANSKY 1946), which could potentially be of evolutionary importance (PHILLIPS and JOHNSON 1998), but may be too rare to be significant (TEMIN *et al.* 1969; THOMPSON 1986). Among evolutionary biologists, differentiating reinforcing (or synergistic) from diminishing (or antagonistic) epistasis (CROW and KIMURA 1970, pp. 80–81) is currently a hot topic because of their role in the evolution of sex and recombination (KONDRASHOV 1995). It is important to note that these forms of gene interaction are usually measured as average attributes (OTTO 1997; OTTO and FELDMAN 1997), which may be more illuminating after a careful analysis of the effects themselves (*e.g.*, CLARK and WANG 1997; ELENA and LENSKI 1997). Finally, the genetic incompatibility that drives speciation must be caused by gene interactions, the form of which can be quite complex (WU and PALOPOLI 1994).

When discussing allelic interactions within a locus, it is clear that the consequences of complete dominance, partial dominance, underdominance, and overdominance are quite different, and we have particular terms to describe each situation. To use a single term, epistasis, to describe all gene interactions suggests that we either do not care or do not know how to deal with the complexity that interlocus interactions bring. Different forms of gene interaction have different consequences, and we should move toward elucidating the nature of these consequences and which forms of interaction are most prevalent.

For most of the 80 years since FISHER (1918), these sorts of considerations really did not matter, and the Mendelian and statistical definitions of epistasis could coexist because they rarely crossed paths. This period of separation is appearing to be near an end. Studies of quantitative trait loci (QTL) are beginning to bridge the gap between continuous variation within populations and the genetic mechanisms that generate that variation. In the few studies of this nature that have been conducted, genic interactions have been common (*e.g.*, DOEBLY *et al.* 1995; LONG *et al.* 1995; ROUTMAN and CHEVERUD 1997). With luck in a few particular circumstances, we will no longer be talking about statistical abstractions but instead will be dealing with real loci with particular effects. Especially interesting are studies that actually attempt to physically generate the genotypic decomposition of interactions by targeting particular loci and limiting total genotypic variation to just a few sites (CLARK and WANG 1997; ELENA and LENSKI 1997). While it is possible that epistatic effects discovered using a mutational approach might be expected to be more common and perhaps more extreme as the genetic system is perturbed far from its normal state (CROW 1990), it appears likely that as more and more QTL are investigated, genic interactions will begin to come to the fore in statistical genetics much as they have as a tool for functional analysis in Mendelian genetics. Once freed from being relegated to "epistatic variance" as a nuisance term (with all of the statistical ambiguities that that entails; WADE 1992b), context and interaction may indeed become of the essence (LEWONTIN 1974). However, as FISHER long argued, even if the building blocks display gene interaction, the evolutionary implications of these interactions need not necessarily be profound. The resolution of this conflict awaits more data on the precise nature of the interactions themselves. The debate on the significance of gene interactions has needed the illumination of this sort of data for the last 80 years. It is exciting to note that we appear poised to collect it.

CONCLUSIONS

This definition of 'epistatic' (apparently first used by FISHER in 1918) is a bit more inclusive than what BATESON originally meant. Advancing knowledge of the multiplicity of possible kinds of non-additive interactions of genes has destroyed the distinctness of the original definition. If this broadening of the original definition proves too confusing, perhaps these epistatic deviations will ultimately be called merely 'interactions'.

J. L. LUSH (1940, p. 295)

As statistical and Mendelian genetics begin to slowly converge experimentally (as FISHER allowed them to do conceptually long ago) the question of what to call gene interactions becomes more than mere semantics. It is conceivable that sometime in the near future two articles published in GENETICS will discuss possible epistasis between the same two loci and mean very different things by this, perhaps even coming to different conclusions. It would be a shame to allow semantics to be a barrier to what may well be the final unification of the Mendelian and Biometrical schools.

It is clear that BATESON's more restrictive use of "epistasis" has historical precedence and is still being used in this way by the majority of geneticists. (It is also surprisingly similar in form, if not nuance, to the medi-

cal definitions given above.) The onus is therefore on the statistical geneticists to refine their use of the word. One course of action would be to simply continue using the same word for both meanings, being very careful to allow context to determine which meaning is implied. Alternatively, statistical genetics could return to FISHER's (1918) original descriptor, epistacy. This seems unlikely and is only slightly less confusing. A final solution would be to heed LUSH's advice and simply call the more general case what it is, gene interaction. This might make it clearer that simply detecting an interaction and giving it a general name is insufficient. The actual nature of the interaction is central and is the thing upon which arguments regarding the general significance of gene interactions can be built.

I thank MIKE WHITLOCK for pointing out the dictionary definitions of epistasis. I also thank MIKE WADE and MIKE WHITLOCK for many helpful discussions over the years and NORMAN JOHNSON and MIKE WHITLOCK for comments on the manuscript. Supported in part by National Science Foundation grant number DBI-9722921 and National Institutes of Health grant number GM54185.

LITERATURE CITED

AVERY, L., and S. WASSERMAN, 1992 Ordering gene function: the interpretation of epistasis in regulatory hierarchies. Trends Genet. **8:** 312–316.

BATESON, W., 1902 *Mendel's Principles of Heredity: A Defense.* The University Press, Cambridge.

BATESON, W., 1909 *Mendel's Principles of Heredity.* Cambridge Univ. Press, Cambridge.

BATESON, W., E. R. SAUNDERS, R. C. PUNNETT and C. C. HURST, 1905 *Reports to the Evolution Committee of the Royal Society, Report II.* Harrison and Sons, London.

CASTLE, W. E., 1926 *Genetics and Eugenics,* Ed. 3, Harvard Univ. Press, Cambridge, MA.

CHEVERUD, J. M., and E. J. ROUTMAN, 1995 Epistasis and its contribution to genetic variance components. Genetics **139:** 1455–1461.

CLARK, A. G., and L. WANG, 1997 Epistasis in measured genotypes: Drosophila P-element insertions. Genetics **147:** 157–163.

COCKERHAM, C. C., 1954 An extension of the concept of partitioning hereditary variance for analysis of covariance among relatives when epistasis is present. Genetics **39:** 859–882.

COCKERHAM, C. C., 1956 Effects of linkage on the covariances between relatives. Genetics **41:** 138–141.

COLIN, E. C., 1956 *Elements of Genetics.* McGraw-Hill, New York.

CROW, J. F., 1990 How important is detecting interaction? Behav. Brain Sci. **13:** 126–127.

CROW, J. F., and M. KIMURA, 1970 *An Introduction to Population Genetics Theory.* Burgess, Minneapolis.

DOBZHANSKY, T., 1946 Genetics of natural populations. XIII. Recombination and variability in populations of *Drosophila pseudoobscura.* Genetics **31:** 269–290.

DOEBLY, J., A. STEC and C. GUSTUS, 1995 *teosinte branched1* and the origin of maize: evidence for epistasis and the evolution of dominance. Genetics **141:** 333–346.

ELENA, S. F., and R. E. LENSKI, 1997 Test of synergistic interactions among deleterious mutations in bacteria. Nature **390:** 395–398.

FENSTER, C. B., L. F. GALLOWAY and L. CHAO, 1997 Epistasis and its consequences for the evolution of natural populations. TREE **12:** 282–286.

FISHER, R. A., 1918 The correlations between relatives on the supposition of Mendelian inheritance. Trans. R. Soc. Edinburgh **52:** 399–433.

FISHER, R. A., 1941 Average excess and average effect of a gene substitution. Ann. Eugen. **11:** 53–63.

KEMPTHORNE, O., 1954 The correlation between relatives in a random mating population. Proc. R. Soc. London B **143:** 103–113.

KEMPTHORNE, O., 1957 *An Introduction to Genetical Statistics*. Wiley, New York.

KONDRASHOV, A. S., 1995 Dynamics of unconditionally deleterious mutations: Gaussian approximation and soft selection. Genet. Res., Cambridge **65:** 113–121.

LEWONTIN, R. C., 1974 *The Genetic Basis of Evolutionary Change*. Columbia Univ. Press, New York.

LINDSEY, A. W., 1932 *A Textbook of Genetics*. Macmillan, New York.

LONG, A. D., S. L. MULLANEY, L. A. REID, J. D. FRY, C. H. LANGLEY and T. F. C. MACKAY, 1995 High resolution mapping of genetic factors affecting abdominal bristle number in *Drosophila melanogaster*. Genetics **139:** 1273–1291.

LUSH, J. L., 1940 Intra-sire correlations or regressions of offspring on dam as a method of estimating heritability of characteristics. Am. Soc. Prod. Proc. **33:** 293–301.

MATHER, K., 1949 The genetical theory of continuous variation. Hereditas (**Suppl.**): 376–401.

OTTO, S. P., 1997 Unraveling gene interactions. Nature **390:** 343.

OTTO, S. P., and M. W. FELDMAN, 1997 Deleterious mutations, variable epistatic interactions, and the evolution of recombination. Theoret. Pop. Biol. **51:** 134–147.

PHILLIPS, P. C., 1996 Waiting for a compensatory mutation: phase zero of the shifting-balance process. Genet. Res., Cambridge **67:** 271–283.

PHILLIPS, P. C., and N. A. JOHNSON, 1998 The population genetics of synthetic lethals. Genetics (in press).

PROVINE, W. B., 1971 *The Origins of Theoretical Population Genetics*. The University of Chicago Press, Chicago.

PUNNETT, R. C., 1920 *Mendelism*, Ed. 5, Macmillan, London.

ROUTMAN, E. J., and J. M. CHEVERUD, 1997 Gene effects on a quantitative trait: two-locus epistatic effects measured at microsatellite markers and at estimated QTL. Evolution **51:** 1654–1662.

SCHNELL, F. W., 1984 Modeling basic epistasis for quantitative-genetic studies. Vortr. Pflanzenzuchtg **7:** 1–11.

SINNOTT, E. D., and L. C. DUNN, 1932 *Principles of Genetics*, Ed. 2, McGraw-Hill, New York.

SINNOTT, E. W., L. C. DUNN and T. DOBZHANSKY, 1958 *Principles of Genetics*, Ed. 5, McGraw-Hill, New York.

SNYDER, L. H., 1935 *Principles of Heredity*. D. C. Heath, Boston.

STANSFIELD, W. D., 1991 *Theory and Problems of Genetics*, Ed. 3, McGraw-Hill, New York.

STEPHAN, W., 1996 The rate of compensatory evolution. Genetics **144:** 419–426.

TACHIDA, H., and C. C. COCKERHAM, 1989 A building block model for quantitative genetics. Genetics **121:** 839–844.

TEMIN, R. G., H. U. MEYER, P. S. DAWSON and J. F. CROW, 1969 The influence of epistasis on homozygous viability depression in *Drosophila melanogaster*. Genetics **61:** 497–519.

THOMAS, J. H., 1993 Chemosensory regulation of development in *C. elegans*. BioEssays **15:** 791–797.

THOMPSON, V., 1986 Synthetic lethals: a critical review. Evol. Theory **8:** 1–13.

WADE, M. J., 1992a Epistasis, pp. 87–91 in *Keywords in Evolutionary Biology*, edited by E. F. KELLER and E. A. LLOYD. Harvard Univ. Press, Cambridge.

WADE, M. J., 1992b Sewall Wright: gene interaction and the shifting balance theory, pp. 35–62 in *Oxford Surveys in Evolutionary Biology*, edited by D. FUTUYMA and J. ANTONOVICS. Oxford Press, New York.

WAGNER, G. P., M. D. LAUBICHLER and H. BAGHERI-CHAICHIAN, 1998 Genetic measurement theory of epistatic effects. Genetica (in press).

WEAVER, R. F., and P. W. HEDRICK, 1997 *Genetics*, Ed. 3, Wm. C. Brown, Dubuque, IA.

WEINBERG, W., 1910 Weitere beiträge zur theorie der verebeing. Arch. Rassen. Ges. Biol. **7:** 35–49. (translated by K. MEYER, 1984, pp. 42–79 in *Quantitative Genetics. Part I: Explanation and Analysis of Continuous Variation*, edited by W. G. HILL. Van Nostrand Reinhold, New York).

WHITLOCK, M. C., P. C. PHILLIPS, F. B.-G. MOORE and S. J. TONSOR, 1995 Multiple fitness peaks and epistasis. Annu. Rev. Ecol. Syst. **26:** 601–629.

WRIGHT, S., 1931 Evolution in Mendelian populations. Genetics **16:** 97–159.

WRIGHT, S., 1932 The roles of mutation, inbreeding, crossbreeding and selection in evolution. Proc. 6th Intl. Congr. Genet. **1:** 356–366.

WRIGHT, S., 1935 The analysis of variance and the correlations between relatives with respect to deviations from an optimum. J. Genet. **30:** 243–256.

WU, C.-I., and M. F. PALOPOLI, 1994 Genetics of postmating reproductive isolation in animals. Annu. Rev. Genet. **27:** 283–308.

T. H. Morgan at Caltech
A Reminiscence

Norman H. Horowitz

Division of Biology, California Institute of Technology, Pasadena, California 91125

AT the urging of Professor G. M. McKinley, who taught genetics at the University of Pittsburgh, I applied for graduate school at Caltech, was accepted, and arrived in Pasadena for the opening of the fall term of 1936. It would never have occurred to me to go to a school so far away—3 days by train, in distant California—had it not been for Dr. McKinley, but this was only the first of a series of lucky choices that formed my career.

On arriving at the Caltech campus and locating the Kerckhoff Laboratory of Biology—a building so grand in my eyes that I felt the need to ask a passing student if this was indeed the home of the biology department—I entered and found the office of the Chairman, Thomas Hunt Morgan, on the second floor. I identified myself to Morgan's fearful secretary, Miss Brusstar, and was ushered into Morgan's office. I recognized him immediately from photographs published in 1933, when he won the Nobel Prize. My first encounter with this man who was to have a large influence on my life was brief. I stood in front of his desk, and Morgan looked up at me from a stack of papers in front of him. "Horowitz," he said, "you are going to work with Albert Tyler." He then directed me to Tyler's office. I had never heard of Albert Tyler, but at the moment I was not inclined to ask questions of Morgan, and I went off dutifully to find Albert Tyler's office.

I soon learned that Tyler was an embryologist—what today would be called a developmental biologist. He worked on the early development of sea urchins and other marine invertebrates. He had been Morgan's student at Columbia University and had come to Pasadena with the Morgan group in 1928, when the Biology Division at Caltech was founded. I soon learned that Morgan had long since given up working with Drosophila and had returned to an earlier love, marine animals. Dro-

sophila genetics had become too complex for him. Morgan was a discoverer, not a bookkeeper, and after the basic findings of Drosophila genetics had been made, he left the subject in the competent hands of his students Sturtevant, Bridges, and Muller (and Mrs. Morgan) and moved on to other fields. When I came to know him, he was working on a genetic problem in the primitive marine chordate, Ciona. On most weekends, Morgan and Tyler went to the Kerckhoff Marine Laboratory at Corona del Mar, California, a little over an hour's drive from Pasadena. Being Tyler's graduate student, I would now accompany them.

As an undergraduate, I had done some research on transplantation in salamanders that had resulted in an article in the *Journal of Experimental Zoology*, and this, combined with the fact that I had indicated no preferred field of graduate study in my application, had no doubt determined Morgan's decision to send me to work with Tyler. These events now afforded me the opportunity to become more than casually acquainted with Morgan.

The three of us would leave Pasadena at about nine o'clock on Saturday morning in Tyler's Model-A Ford, with Tyler at the wheel, Morgan in the front passenger seat, and me in the back. We proceeded to the Newport Beach Yacht Club, a few miles up the coast from Corona del Mar. The pilings there were the home of a large population of Morgan's experimental animal, Ciona, an ascidian. We would pull a sufficient number of them off the pilings and take them with us, in a bucket of seawater, to the marine station.

Ciona is hermaphroditic, but self-sterile. The rule is that the sperm of a given individual do not fertilize the eggs of the same individual, but are fertile with the eggs of all other Ciona. Occasional exceptions are found. Morgan perceived here a genetic problem and set himself the task of learning what he could about it. At the marine laboratory, he would set up several experiments, each consisting of a square array of Syracuse dishes containing seawater, 5 to 10 dishes on a side, in which the sperm and eggs from 5 to 10 individuals were crossed in all possible combinations. In some experiments,

This essay commemorates the 70th anniversary of the founding of the Division of Biology at Caltech by Thomas Hunt Morgan in 1928.

acid—which suppressed self-sterility—was added to some of the dishes. Morgan examined each dish under the microscope and noted the result. He did not, as I remember, have a notebook for recording his data, but pulled envelopes and pieces of paper out of his pockets for this purpose. (He must at some point have put his data into more durable form, since he published many papers containing the numerical results of these experiments.) Tyler and I did our own work in the same large laboratory room as Morgan. One of Tyler's roles was to keep an eye on Morgan's experiments. I suspect that he contributed more than a little to saving Morgan's data from chaos.

Morgan worked on Ciona until his death in 1945. He was a tireless experimenter. His last paper appeared in the *Journal of Experimental Zoology* the month he died. He did not solve the problem of self-sterility in Ciona, but he approached a solution. In a paper published in 1944, he summarized his results. From experiments with offspring of selfed animals that he reared in the laboratory, he concluded that at least three—and more likely five—genes, with an indefinitely large number of alleles, were involved.

Morgan's passion for experimentation was symptomatic of his general scepticism and his distaste for speculation. He believed only what could be proven. He was said to be an atheist, and I have always believed that he was. Everything I knew about him—his scepticism, his honesty—was consistent with disbelief in the supernatural.

One of my favorite memories of Morgan is that of a visit he was paid one day by the well-known British author, H. G. Wells. Wells, I had read in the papers, was in Southern California for a reason I have long since forgotten. A few days later, I happened to see him on the sidewalk outside the Kerckhoff Lab, heading for the main entrance. I was immediately struck by his spiffy appearance: the perfect vision of an Englishman abroad, he was wearing a white suit, Panama hat, spats, and a cane. Morgan, who was evidently expecting him, greeted him at the door. In contrast to Wells' elegance, Morgan was his usual unpressed, unstylish self. I got the impression that the two were acquainted and that this was a social call. They moved into the building, and Morgan took Wells on a tour. One could tell where in the course of the tour they were located, because Morgan, who was hard of hearing, assumed that anyone his own age (they were both born in 1866) suffered from the same affliction, and he spoke in a loud voice. Eventually, they went to Morgan's office, and I lost track. It was clear that these two aging gentlemen, so different in appearance, were in fact deeply similar. Both were revolutionaries in their way, and they were united in their passion for biology and in their nonconformist, rationalistic approach to the world.

Morgan was known for his sardonic wit. A famous example were the words he spoke in a speech in 1909 at a meeting of the American Breeders Association (ABA). He had not yet gotten into genetics, and he was critical of it. He said: "In the modern interpretation of Mendelism, facts are being transformed into factors at a rapid rate. If one factor will not explain the facts, then two are invoked; if two prove insufficient, three will sometimes work out. . . ." A year later, he discovered the white-eyed mutation in Drosophila that led, eventually, to the modern chromosomal theory of heredity. I first heard his words to the ABA quoted by the professor (it may have been Ernest Anderson) in a graduate genetics course at Caltech. They served to remind us scientists-to-be that a real scientist changes course when he is forced to do so by evidence. It is instructive to compare the words of Morgan spoken in 1909 to the ABA with those referred to above written in 1944 in summarizing his Ciona results.

Morgan made fun of human gullibility. His attitude was displayed weekly at the General Biology Seminar, held Tuesday evenings at 7:30 in a room in the Kerckhoff Laboratory. The Morgans lived then in a comfortable ranch house on the north side of Kerckhoff, across San Pasqual Street, which traversed the campus. Both the house and the street are gone now. The Morgans would cross the street to Kerckhoff after dinner, carrying with them the *New York Times* that they received daily. The paper came from the East by train, so it was a week old by the time it arrived in Pasadena. Morgan would open the seminar by reading and commenting on stories with a scientific aspect, many of them exhibiting the folly of humankind, and these he treated in his wittiest style. Everyone was amused, except perhaps Calvin Bridges, who was the kindest of men and not easily moved to laugh at the foolishness of others. I recall that among the regular attendees at the seminar were two elderly sisters, both retired school teachers. One had taught biology in high school, and she invariably had one or two uninteresting questions for the speaker of the evening. When she spoke up at the end of the lecture, an almost audible sigh would go up from the audience. Only Bridges, when he was the speaker, could be counted on to reply to her politely and at length. For him, everyone was educable.

Morgan would finally introduce the speaker and then sit down in the front row next to Mrs. Morgan. He was usually asleep by the time the speaker had spoken two sentences. Mrs. Morgan would nudge him and whisper "Tom! Tom!" After a brief nap, he awakened refreshed and frequently had an acute question for the speaker at the end.

I attended these seminars for three years, but I now can remember only the beginning of one of them. That was the lecture Max Delbrück gave shortly after his arrival in 1937 as a Rockefeller Foundation Fellow from Germany. Here was a bright theoretical physicist from the leading European centers of quantum physics, come to Caltech to learn about the wonders and mysteries of

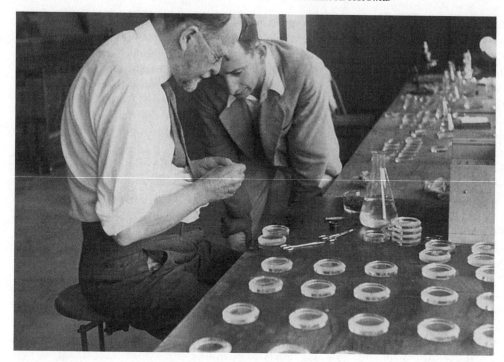

FIGURE 1.—Morgan and Tyler (and Syracuse dishes) at the Kerckhoff Marine Laboratory in 1931 (Courtesy of the Archives, California Institute of Technology).

genetics. He began his talk by drawing a circle on the blackboard and saying, "Let us imagine the cell is a homogeneous sphere." The whole room burst into laughter. Except, perhaps, Bridges.

I am sometimes asked what I know about Morgan's reputed anti-Semitism. I know that there is documentary evidence for anti-Semitic statements by Morgan, but in the years I knew him, I never encountered, or even suspected, any such prejudice on his part. On the contrary, as far as I could see he treated everyone fairly. The fact that he grew up in Kentucky in the 19th century would perhaps incline one to expect some prejudice from him, but if he grew up with prejudices, he had outgrown them by the time I came to know him. I never experienced or even heard of them until after his death. Morgan was a complicated man, and I can easily believe that there were sides of his character that I never saw, but I am certain that during the years I knew him, anti-Semitism was not one of them.

My last memorable encounter with him occurred at the time of my Ph.D. Oral Examination, in 1939. Normally, Albert Tyler would have been chairman of the examining committee, since I had done my thesis with him, but I was informed a day or two before the exam that Morgan would be in charge. I was also told that the Dean of the Graduate School, Richard C. Tolman, would be present. Tolman, a well-known physical chemist, had not yet attended a biology Ph.D. exam and had decided to come to mine, which was scheduled to be the first one held in biology that year. I believe that Morgan's presence as chairman was related to the fact that Tolman would be there. It was his way of welcoming the Dean to the Biology Division. The exam went smoothly. Morgan went through the committee inviting questions, holding Tolman and himself for last. I can now remember only these two last questions. Tolman took the theme of his questions from the title of my thesis, which dealt with the rate of respiration of marine eggs. He asked me to derive the equations for first- and second-order chemical reactions. I had no trouble with the first-order law, but I flubbed the integration step of the second-order equation. (Today, I doubt if I could derive either of them.) Tolman accepted my answer, however, saying that "for a biologist" I had done pretty well.

Finally it was Morgan's turn. Every graduate student knew that Morgan always asked questions about the anatomy and physiology of the experimental animal used by the candidate. To prepare for that I had spent my lunch hour reading Hegner's College Zoology. True to form, Morgan asked me to describe the respiratory system of the sea urchin. I did so perfectly. To my surprise, Morgan said, "No, Horowitz, you have described the starfish." I knew that he was wrong, but the exam was going well, and I didn't want to embarrass him over a triviality, so I kept quiet.

The exam ended, and I was passed. A couple of days later, I ran into Morgan in the hall. He called to me and said he had found that I had been right in the exam. He apologized, and I thanked him. I do not remember ever seeing him again. Not long afterward, newly married, I left with my wife for Stanford University, where I was to work in the laboratory of Morgan's son-in-law, Douglas Whitaker. I had been awarded a National Research Council Fellowship, one of the few postdoctoral fellowships that were available before the war, and one that I have always believed Morgan's influence helped me obtain. Normally, a recipient of that fellowship would have gone to Europe, but war was imminent, and we went to Stanford instead.

The most important thing that happened to me at Stanford was finally to meet George Beadle. Beadle had been on the Caltech faculty when I submitted my application to Caltech in early 1936. Then he left for Paris, where he worked with Boris Ephrussi. After that he moved to Harvard and then Stanford. He told me later that he had voted for my admission as a graduate student because of my undergraduate transplantation paper. He said he had been doing transplantation studies himself, in Drosophila—obviously a bond between us! The meeting with Beadle eventually changed my life, but that is another story.

September 1998

Genes and Chromomeres
A Puzzle in Three Dimensions

Burke H. Judd

411 Clayton Road, Chapel Hill, North Carolina 27514

D ROSOPHILA polytene chromosomes have been used for more than 60 years to explore eukaryotic chromosome organization and the nature of genes. T. S. PAINTER (1934), noting the distinctive and constant chromomeric patterns of the synapsed multistranded chromosomal arms, wrote ". . . it was clear that we had within our grasp the material of which everyone had been dreaming. We found ourselves out of the woods and upon a plainly marked highway with bypaths stretching in every direction. It was clear that the highway led to the lair of the gene." From the banded patterns of these chromosomes, maps of the "highway" were constructed. Mutational and recombinational analyses used in conjunction with these maps have produced a remarkable series of advances in understanding the organization of genes in these chromosomes and have paved the way for molecular cloning and sequencing of individual genes and gene complexes.

Still unresolved, however, is what the chromomeres and interchromomeres represent relative to genes and the structure and organization of chromosomes. It's not that this question has not been addressed. H. J. MULLER in a series of papers throughout his career probed the nature of genes and their arrangement in the chromosome, using X-ray-induced chromosomal rearrangements charted on the polytene maps. He spoke directly to the question as early as 1935 in a paper with A. A. PROKOFYEVA entitled "The individual gene in relation to the chromomere and the chromosome." They selected seven inversion breaks, three of which appeared to be identical, in region 1B of the X chromosome that caused phenotypic changes of the tightly linked genes *yellow*, *achaete*, or *scute*. By obtaining crossovers between rearrangements with different breakpoints, Muller created small deletions and duplications of the genes in the region. The cytological analysis of the breakpoints and the phenotypic effects of left/right combinations

(*i.e.*, deletion or duplication) showed that these genes are arranged in a discontinuous linear order and that the nodes (chromomeres) contain genes. Muller concluded that some chromomeres in the 1B1–7 region appeared to contain clusters of genes, judging from the variety of scute and achaete effects exhibited by some rearrangement combinations. That should have settled the question of the gene-chromomere relationship right there, but it did not. What Muller had opened is an early analysis of what is now known as the *achaete-scute* complex (ASC). More about how this and selected other genes fit within the chromomere-gene concept is discussed below.

Muller and Prokofyeva used the relationships they observed between the numbers of genes and chromomeres in this region of the X chromosome to estimate that the number of genes in the genome of *Drosophila melanogaster* is between 5 and 10 thousand. CALVIN BRIDGES' (1935) inference that faint chromomeres contain 1 gene while the heavy-walled doublets with an interspersed faint band might contain 3 supported this estimate. The detailed polytene chromosome maps (C. B. BRIDGES 1938; P. N. BRIDGES 1942) showed 5072 distinct bands in the four chromosomes. That number has been increased insignificantly through the use of the electron microscope to about 5100 bands (SORSA 1988).

WOLFGANG BEERMANN's (1961, 1962) studies of the puffing patterns in the giant polytene chromosomes of the dipteran Chironomus led him to propose that each puff originates from a single band. His demonstration that a particular secretion granule generated in a lobe of the salivary gland is correlated with the puffing of a specific band supported the concept that the information necessary for production of that protein resides in a single band. It was unresolved, however, whether there was just one or several functions encoded in the DNA of a chromomere.

In search of a eukaryotic operon: I was aware of most of these pioneering studies relating genes and chromomeres, but I did not at first set out to address that

I dedicate this essay to the memory of GEORGE LEFEVRE, who had a strong influence on my scientific career and who was a major figure in advancing the genetics and cytology of Drosophila.

problem. In 1961, I presented a seminar to the genetics group at the University of Texas about the work of MADELINE GANS (1953). It concerned the intriguing manner in which the mutation *zeste* (z^1) repressed the wild-type function of the *white* (*w*) locus in Drosophila females but had no effect on w^+ expression in males. I was studying *white* locus structure at that time, and I wanted to discover more about the interaction between these two tightly linked *X* chromosome genes. The question that interested me then was whether the unique interaction between these two loci is influenced by other elements in the region.

The operon model of gene organization and regulation in bacteria, developed by FRANCOIS JACOB and JACQUES MONOD (1961), was at that time a major advancement in understanding prokaryotic gene organization and expression. The question that intrigued me was whether there is a eukaryotic counterpart to the operon. The far-fetched idea that *zeste* and *white* might be elements of a eukaryotic unit similar to the bacterial operon was a throwaway notion that I raised at the close of the seminar. Later in a discussion of Gans' work with Wilson Stone, the idea that discovering what types of genes occupy the region between *z* and *w* might be worth pursuing developed. That region, according to then-current cytological and recombination maps, consisted of about a dozen bands on the polytene chromosome map and about 0.5 cM linkage units. At that time no genes that definitely mapped to the region were known.

The *zeste-white* region: I had been analyzing the products of recombination events that generated reciprocal duplication and deficiency products in the regions within or flanking the *white* locus (JUDD 1961). These were later demonstrated to be due to recombination involving ectopic pairing and crossingover between interspersed transposable elements (DAVIS *et al.* 1987). One of the deficiencies, designated *Df(1) w^{j1}*, removes the 16-band chromosome segment between 3A1 and 3C2,3 of the polytene chromosome map. The deletion includes the *zeste* locus at 3A3 and the *white* locus at 3C2. I decided to use this deficiency in a genetic screen to saturate the *zeste-white* region with mutations.

The first experiment was designed to generate and recover mutations in all of the indispensable genetic elements located between these tightly linked loci and then to relate their function to *zeste* and *white*. The first series of X-ray experiments was carried out at Harvard University in the summer of 1962. George Lefevre had invited me to spend the summer there working in his lab. That was an exciting time as the first mutants were recovered: 16 lethal mutations composing five complementation groups localized between *z* and *w* (JUDD 1962). That the number of complementation groups was so large surprised me, and George too, as I recall. Early tests failed to show any discernible interactions of the lethals (as heterozygotes of course) with the *zeste-*

white system. The questions then became whether there were indeed an even larger number of loci in that small region of the *X* chromosome and what would be required to identify all of them. Most important, Did any of them relate directly to the interaction of *zeste* and *white*? Answering those questions took on a life of its own as the number of lethals and semilethals identified by the mutation screen grew.

Margaret Shen joined the lab in 1964 and undertook the task of mapping the complementation groups, first into subsets defined by complementation tests against a battery of deletions and duplications. This was followed by the very tedious work of placing each mutation of a subset into an allelic group, which required a very large number of *inter se* complementation tests. The linear order of the genes within and between groups (cistrons) then had to be determined by recombination. This latter operation required the scoring of rare recombinants from many crosses that generated very large numbers of flies. It was Margaret's endless patience and meticulous work that kept this project going.

As the recombination map was worked out, we matched the position of each complementation group to its placement on the polytene chromosome map. This was determined by using overlapping deletions and duplications of the region in complementation tests with each group of lethals. The placement became more precise as the number of available rearrangement breakpoints increased. By the time Thom Kaufman came to the lab in 1967, we had identified and mapped 12 complementation groups flanked by *zeste* at 3A3 and *white* at 3C2. A comparison of the cytological and recombination maps strongly suggested that there was a one-to-one correspondence between the order and position of chromomeres and complementation groups. Judging from the number of allele at each identified complementation group, we calculated that we were approaching saturation of the region. However, since all of the early mutants were X-ray induced, there was concern that we might be failing to mutate some loci with X rays.

Thom began a mutation project to induce mutations with the chemical mutagens nitrosoguanidine and ethyl methanesulfonate. He recovered a large number of mutants but identified no new loci between *z* and *w*. However, his experiments extended the search to include two loci distal to *zeste*, one of which turned out to be the rediscovery of a previously described locus for which the mutants no longer existed. When examining putative lethal cultures, Thom noted one in which some of the third instar larvae that appeared later than normal were very large in size. He thought that possibly the culture had been contaminated with *Drosophila virilis* or *D. hydei*, both rather large flies kept in the Texas collection. Instead of discarding the culture, Thom kept on with his observations and determined that he had induced a semi-lethal mutation in the *giant* locus.

Thom also explored the region proximal to *white* by

an analysis of the mutant phenotypes created by a series of deletions extending into that region. Now with the increased number of mutations, saturation for lethal loci in the z-w region appeared to be very close indeed. I was becoming convinced that we were not going to find any genes that interacted with zeste and white, a feeling that was bolstered by early results from the developmental analysis of the mutation groups by Mary Shannon, a post-doc in the lab, and Thom (SHANNON et al. 1972). The gene-chromomere question now was much more interesting than it had been and soon became a primary focus of the experiments.

Thom made two very interesting discoveries in addition to giant that are indirectly related to the gene-chromomere question and illustrate the value of saturation studies. First, while mapping the X chromosome breakpoints of the inversion In(1)e(bx), he discovered that the distal break created a mutation of zeste that behaved like the null allele, z^a (KAUFMAN et al. 1973). That inversion was induced and described as an enhancer of bithorax years earlier by ED LEWIS (1959). That zeste might play a role in the function of the bithorax complex was surprising and exhilarating. Thom's observation was the beginning chapter of zeste as a major factor in the phenomenon of transvection. But that's another story altogether (for review, see ASHBURNER 1989).

Second, Thom found some semi-lethal alleles of a locus just distal to zeste, the survivors of which exhibited a remarkable behavioral phenotype. When the culture vial was struck sharply on the table, all of the flies convulsed and fell to the bottom of the vial. After a short while they revived and moved about quite normally. We named the locus tko. The tko gene has subsequently been cloned and sequenced by Vince Pirrotta and his collaborators (ROYDEN et al. 1987) and shown to encode a protein similar to a mitochondrial ribosomal protein, S12.

Nonlethal loci: The discovery of the tko phenotype pointed up an important weakness in a part of our search for all of the loci in the z-w region. We were relying on mutations that caused either lethality or observable changes in the morphology of the fly. How many genes might there be that are dispensable to flies raised in the lab or that, when mutated, give no discernible phenotypic change? The work of Seymour Benzer, who had designed a screen for behavioral mutations, was very much on our minds. We had to decide how we could extend our mutation screen to include other categories of changes. Plans for additional experiments were begun as Michael Young came to the lab. He decided to work on a screen to detect mutations that were viable but caused sterility and to detect changes that cause significant reduction in the rate of development, resulting in delayed emergence of the adults.

Rather than delay and wait for Mike's results, we decided that it was time to try to publish the data on the

lethal and semi-lethal loci. Seven years had gone into these studies since that first summer at Harvard (1 year of which I spent pushing papers in the Biology Division of the Atomic Energy Commission). We had already published abstracts of the progress of the work, and the results had attracted quite a bit of attention, particularly among the molecular biologists. We also knew that Ben Hochman was well along with an analysis of the genes in the small chromosome 4 of Drosophila. That analysis would give him an estimate of the number of vital loci in the entire chromosome. His masterful account (HOCHMAN 1971) reported 40 recognized loci in the chromosome distributed among about 50 chromomeres. His positioning of the genes in the chromosome depended entirely on deletion mapping, since there is essentially no recombination in that small chromosome. Nonetheless, his estimate that there were probably 50 or fewer vital loci in chromosome 4 fit well with our data.

We reported (JUDD et al. 1972) finding 16 complementation groups associated with 15 adjacent chromomeres in the 3A1–3C2 segment. The order of the complementation groups, determined by recombination, matched with the position determined by deletion mapping, with the exception of 3 complementation groups in region 3B, where breakpoints separating them were not available. These groups were mapped by recombination, which by our analysis placed 6 complementation groups in region 3B, where we could distinguish only 5 chromomeres. However, HANS BERENDES (1970) had described six bands in 3B from an electron microscope study of the region. If we accepted his map, there was an equal number of genes and chromomeres, and the recombination and deletion maps showed essentially 1 complementation group per chromomere.

As our work progressed, Drosophila workers from other labs sent mutants and rearrangements to be used and tested in the z-w screen. Particularly valuable contributions came from George Lefevre, who sent lethals and a number of deletions and duplications that were crucial to assigning complementation groups to chromomeres. Johng Lim, Mary Louise Alexander, Seymour Abrahamson, Ben Hochman, Bill Welshons, and Raphael Falk also contributed to the pool of lethals.

A concept in flux: Johng Lim played a rather enigmatic role in the rise and fall of the one gene:one chromomere concept. We thought that we had discovered all of the indispensable loci in 3A1-3C2, until LIM and SNYDER (1974) carried out complementation tests on more than 100 lethals they induced in the region with alkylating agents. All but three of their mutations mapped at already known loci. Those three, however, failed to complement with each other but complemented all of the z-w loci we had discovered. Here then was a new lethal locus that mapped in section 3A. Lim and Snyder pointed out that electron microscope chromosome maps by Sorsa and Sorsa (in BEERMANN 1972) showed nine bands in region 3A, one more than we or Bridges had detected. Johng's cytological observations confirmed the existence of the band; furthermore, we discovered by recombination tests that the new locus mapped precisely where the additional band was located.

Was the one gene:one chromomere concept saved? For 3A maybe, but overall, no. During the time that we were working with Johng Lim to position the new locus, we had the results from Mike Young's experiments. The mutations causing delayed adult emergence all proved to be allelic to previously described loci, but Mike also found six mutations that produce female sterility. They formed two tightly linked complementation groups, *fs(1)Y^a* and *fs(1)Y^b*, that mapped to region 3B and were not allelic to any of our known loci. Try as we might to fit them into their own chromomeres, even using Hans Berendes' map, we could not.

In Benzer's lab at Cal Tech, Ron Konopka had discovered a mutant, *per*, that exhibited an abnormal diurnal activity rhythm. KONOPKA and BENZER (1971) had done preliminary mapping showing that *per* was a candidate for inclusion in the *z-w* region. Mike obtained three alleles of *per* from the Benzer lab. With deletion mapping of the mutant activity patterns, he placed the locus between two lethal loci in 3B. We had to conclude that the relationship of loci and bands, although very close to one-to-one, certainly did not hold as a general rule (JUDD and YOUNG 1973; YOUNG and JUDD 1978). However, a much more important question had emerged as we came closer to discovering all of the genes in the *z-w* region: Are genes in Drosophila really as big as these data suggest?

Drosophila genes are large: If our estimate of the total number of genes was accurate, we could calculate the average gene size from measurements of the amount of DNA in this region of the *X* chromosome. GEORGE RUDKIN (1965) had measured the amount of DNA in the polytene *X* chromosome and calculated that in each haploid strand, the average chromomere contains about 3×10^4 nucleotide pairs. If the ratio of genes to chromomeres is about 1:1, a gene of average size in the *z-w* region consists of approximately 20 to 30 kb of DNA. About the same average value is obtained for all Drosophila genes by dividing the amount of DNA in the haploid genome by the total number of chromomeres. There are about 5100 chromomeres, and Charles Laird, then a colleague at the University of Texas, had determined that about 80% of the approximately 1.4×10^8 bp of DNA in the haploid genome are unique copy sequences (LAIRD 1971). On that basis, the size of an average gene comes out to be about 22 kb. Considering that a typical polypeptide chain could be encoded by about 1.2 kb, there is, by that measure, sufficient DNA in the Drosophila genome to encode more than 100,000 different polypeptide chains.

What was then known about the reassociation kinetics

and processing of RNA molecules further complicated the picture. It was evident that very-large-molecular-weight heterogeneous nuclear RNAs (hnRNAs) were transcribed in the nucleus, the sizes of which suggested that most of the DNA of a chromomere might be transcribed. However, most of that hnRNA turned over in the nucleus. The poly(A)-containing messenger RNAs (mRNAs) found associated with polysomes for translation in the cytoplasm were very much smaller and appeared to be derived from the 3' ends of hnRNAs by a series of processing steps. We were not molecular biologists, but clearly those observations caused us to question the possibility that there could be 100,000 different mRNAs generated from *Drosophila melanogaster* DNA sequences.

Considering our cytogenetic data on gene numbers and the molecular studies of the complexity of DNA sequences and the dynamics of RNA metabolism, Mike Young and I (JUDD and YOUNG 1973) proposed the following:

(1) In the most general case, the chromosomal subunit, the chromomere, and the operational unit, the cistron, are coextensive. (2) The majority of the DNA of a chromomere is transcribed. (3) The transcript contains only one or a few structural gene sequences at the 3' end, whereas the remainder contains regulatory information. (4) Adequate processing of the transcription product depends on the integrity of all or most of the regulatory information elements. As a result, mutations derived therein act in a cis-dominant fashion. (5) Some of the 5'-end sequences may be released during processing of the transcript and activate other cistrons of a biosynthetic or developmental pathway. Mutations in these elements may act in pleiotropic fashion.

Speculation, yes, and it caused us to catch a lot of flack. To many molecular biologists of that time, our data suggesting that genes are very large, with only a small fraction of the DNA encoding protein, were hard to accept. Some notable exceptions, however, were Francis Crick and also Roy Britten and Eric Davidson. CRICK (1971), having considered many of the data I have outlined above, including one of our abstracts (SHANNON *et al.* 1970), proposed a general model for chromosomes of higher organisms. He theorized that most of the DNA does not encode protein. His view was that in Drosophila a genetic complementation group usually is contained in a band plus an interband of the polytene chromosomes. He envisioned chromomeres to be globular, unpaired DNA used for gene control. The protein-coding sequences were proposed to be found in the much smaller fraction of fibrous DNA characterizing the interbands. Crick had been stimulated in his considerations by ROY BRITTEN and ERIC DAVIDSON (1969), who earlier in their seminal theory of gene regulation had suggested that large amounts of DNA are devoted to regulatory functions. They proposed five different types of genetic elements, only one class of which, the producer genes, encoded protein. The other classes were envisioned to be sensors, activating RNAs, integrators, or receptors, all of which acted in arrays of varying complexities to regulate the developmental expression of producer genes.

Other genomic regions compared: Despite these theoretical models concordant with our observations, the question concerning whether the density of genes in the z-w region might not be representative of the genome as a whole was raised. LIFSCHYTZ and FALK (1968, 1969) had examined a small region encompassing 5 to 10% of the proximal X chromosome within which they identified 34 functional groups from the analysis of 105 X-ray or EMS-induced lethals. Those studies did not attempt to correlate directly bands with genes, but those data, along with Hochman's, were compatible with our studies. The gene-chromomere relationships and the question of gene size remained open.

In the next few years, however, there were a number of studies of other regions of the Drosophila genome. Several came from George Lefevre, who was a major contributor to the polytene chromosome organization studies. Possibly his most memorable contribution is the outstanding "dream nucleus": a representation of the polytene chromosomes that he compiled as a montage from a number of photographs. That today serves as the standard light microscope photographic map of the *Drosophila melanogaster* genome (LEFEVRE 1976). George approached problems in a variety of interesting and important ways, combining expert cytological analysis with studies of recombination frequency and mutation induction. He and Abraham Schalet published an extensive cytogenetic analysis of the proximal region of the X chromosome (SCHALET and LEFEVRE 1976). This region includes genes located in euchromatic and heterochromatic regions where the cytology is very difficult. Earlier, George studied the frequency of crossing over between two genes relative to the banding pattern of the region to determine whether recombination frequency depends not on the numbers of intervening chromomeres but on their relative sizes, *i.e.*, DNA content (LEFEVRE 1971).

Michael Ashburner also has dealt with polytene chromosomes almost as much as anyone. Examining developmentally programmed puffing patterns, some hormone or heat shock induced, brought him face to face with the issue of chromomeres and the products encoded therein (ASHBURNER 1972). It also made him an early adventurer into chromosome pairing and gene expression, *i.e.*, transvection. Again, that is another story. Michael's major contributions directly to the study of the gene-chromomere relationships come from an exhaustive analysis of the region surrounding the gene for *alcohol dehydrogenase* (*Adh*). Michael and his colleagues published at least seven papers about that region. In the first two, he and Ron Woodruff (WOODRUFF and ASHBURNER 1979a,b) reported finding 21 lethal and 9 visible complementation groups in section 34D-

35C of chromosome 2. Their calculations indicated that a total of about 34 complementation groups are located within that approximately 34-band segment. A complete molecular analysis of *Adh* and surrounding regions, undertaken by Michael and Gerry Rubin and their collaborators, is now almost ready for publication. More about that below.

Janos Gausz and associates, one of whom was Michael Ashburner (GAUSZ *et al.* 1979, 1981), examined the 86F-87C region of chromosome 3 and found that, with the exception of 87C1-3 where no genes mapped and 87C4-5 containing 1, there was apparently 1 complementation group per chromomere. In region 87D-87E,F in 23 to 24 bands, ARTHUR HILLIKER *et al.* (1980) in Art Chovnick's lab found 21 complementation groups. Igor Zhimulev and colleagues (ZHIMULEV *et al.* 1981) analyzed band 10A1-2 and adjoining regions. There also the ratio of genes to bands was near 1:1. Ted Wright and associates (WRIGHT *et al.* 1981) found 12, possible 13, genes in a 7-band segment in 37B10-37C4, clearly not a 1:1 relationship. Further, only 1 gene was found in 37C5-7 and none in 37D1. These cytogenetic analyses showed that the z-w region is quite typical and reinforced the concept that chromomeres and genes, although similar in number, could not be considered strictly coextensive. Most important, the number of genes per unit DNA still indicated that gene size averages about 20 kb.

A large fraction of DNA does not encode protein: What do all these cytogenetic data translate to at the molecular level? That genes contain exons interspersed with noncoding introns, which are spliced out during transcript processing, was not known in the early 1970s. Also, although enhancer and suppressor mutations were known, transcription enhancer and silencer elements that can act at a distance to regulate promoter elements had not yet been described. As molecular techniques for cloning and labeling were developed, the polytene chromosome maps became an important tool in facilitating the analysis of specific genes and chromosome regions. An early attempt to examine the arrangement of genes and their transcripts relative to polytene chromosomes came in 1983 from Pierre Spierer and collaborators (HALL *et al.* 1983). They mapped the transcripts from a 315K-bp segment from 87D5-6 to 87E5-6, which contains about 14 bands. Twenty discrete poly(A) RNA species collected at various stages of development, transcribed from nonrepetitive DNA, were defined. At least 12 complementation groups were recognized in the region. There was good correlation between the position of transcription units, chromomeric units, and complementation groups. Except for two large bands, E1-2 and E5-6, each band contains more than one transcription unit. No detectable transcripts were found from the large E1-2 band. The gene/chromomere number predicted by this analysis does not alter that shown by the cytogenetic studies more than twofold, and it is possible that several transcripts could be related to a single complementation group. Most important, it made clear that much of the DNA does not code for protein. What, then, is the function, if any, of the noncoding DNA?

Lesions with nonmutant effects: Ten years earlier George Lefevre had opened an interesting window to that question when he carried to another level the type of analysis used by Muller. George analyzed cytogenetically both mutant and nonmutant chromosome rearrangement breakpoints to find what proportion of breakpoints cause lethal or detectable morphological changes in the fly. That was a gargantuan undertaking because it required making salivary gland chromosome smears from essentially every individual culture, both mutant and normal, generated from offspring of mutagenized parents. A series of experiments identified almost 150 nonmutant breakpoints, from which George estimated that about 50% of X-ray-induced euchromatic breaks are not associated with lethal or other mutant effects (LEFEVRE 1973).

A similar result, but from a different approach, has now been added by George Miklos and associates (MALESZKA *et al.* 1998). Their molecular analysis of the 6-band 19F region surrounding the *flightless* locus shows 12 genes encoded by just 67 kb of genomic DNA. Seventy-five percent of the 67 kb contributes to 12 transcription units. At least three of the transcripts are alternatively spliced to specify two protein products. Notable, however, is the observation that the simultaneous deletion or disruption of most of the 12 loci results in unobtrusive morphological changes, changes that in all likelihood would not be detected in the usual genetic screens for mutations. They interpret these results to indicate that about 30% of Drosophila loci can mutate to a lethal state, and approximately 20% can produce morphological or behavioral changes. That means that about 50% of loci do not contribute strongly to the morphological phenotype.

Still another approach to the question of gene organization and chromomere structure is to ask whether a gene occupies all or only a part of a band. GEORGE LEFEVRE (1969) analyzed a series of breaks in and around the *vermilion* locus in bands 10A1-2 and showed that breaking a band known to house a specific gene need not always result in a mutation of that gene. This point was also addressed for the *white* locus by SORSA *et al.* (1973), who reached the conclusion that *w* occupied only part of a band. A much more definitive answer comes from the lab of John Sedat (RYKOWSKI *et al.* 1988). These investigators hybridized labeled segments of *Notch* (*N*) locus DNA to stretched preparations of the polytene chromosomes. Using high-resolution, computer-aided optic microscopy, they aligned the molecular map of the gene with the cytological features of band 3C7, the position of *Notch*. This showed that band 3C7 is 34–37 kb in length, within which is found all or most of the 37-kb *Notch* transcription unit. The coding portions and introns are all contained within the band while

the segment positioned 5′ to the transcription start site lies in the open chromatin conformation of the interband between 3C6 and 3C7. Thus, the regulatory sequences are in an interband; Crick's model comes to mind, but with structural and regulatory elements reversed.

Sedat's observations of polytene chromosome structure with computer-assisted analysis of light microscope images give some support to the idea that some of the bands defined by Bridges may consist of smaller subbands separated by very small interbands. This had been suggested previously by several investigators (KEPPY and WELSHONS 1980; LEFEVRE and WATKINS 1986) to account for cytological changes seen at some chromosome breakpoints. This is yet another variable in defining the gene chromomere relationships.

The *cut* locus: *Cut* (*ct*) presents an interesting and possibly extreme view of how a single gene obviously extends across chromomere boundaries. The locus is huge, with mutations mapping over almost 200 kb of genomic DNA in 7B1-2 of the polytene map (JACK 1985). It is a highly mutable locus in which mutations comprise three distinct phenotypic classes. The kinked femur phenotype is characterized by small body size, kinked femurs, and small opaque wings that seldom expand. The cut-wing phenotype consists of incised wing margins of several patterns and some head capsule abnormalities, particularly antennae. The third phenotype consists of three distinct lethal classes. The complementation pattern is complex (LIU *et al.* 1991). All lethal classes fail to complement each other and the cut phenotype mutant class. However, one lethal class complements *kinked femur*, but the other two do not. *Kinked femur* and *cut* mutations all complement each other.

For a locus this big with a complex complementation map, what does the molecular structure look like? In 200 kb of genomic DNA, *kinked femur* lesions map most distally and appear to occupy up to 50 kb. This is difficult to determine because some mutations are deletions that encroach, possibly from outside the locus. The cut phenotype class is caused by changes, many of which are insertions of transposable elements, in about 25 kb just distal to the center of the locus. The lethal classes form three rather clustered groups of lesions positioned over about 70 kb proximal. A cDNA of 8217 bp derived from this 70 kb of genomic DNA has been sequenced. It contains an open reading frame encoding 2175 amino acids in which there is a 60-amino-acid homeodomain. The protein product is required in embryonic and adult organs, regulating sensory organ identities in the wings and various other body parts (JACK *et al.* 1991).

Back in 1979, Terry Johnson and I mapped the various classes of *cut* mutations (JOHNSON and JUDD 1979). On the basis of the complementation patterns, we rather brashly suggested that a very major portion of the locus, where the *kinked femur* and *cut* mutations map, is all regulatory in function and that the structural gene(s) was likely to be found in the proximal region where the lethals map. The molecular work pretty much bears that out. Jo Jack and Yvonne DeLotto (1995) have determined that cis-acting regulatory sequences of cut are spread over the distal and central region more than 85 kb upstream of the transcription start site. Lesions such as retrotransposon insertions in this region block expression of cut in subsets of tissues where normally it would be active. The effect is polar, with lesions farthest from the promoter affecting the fewest tissues.

The achaete-scute complex: I want to return to examining the ASC to relate what has been learned about its structure and expression to what Muller and Prokofyeva discovered about chromomeres and genes more than 60 years ago. Almost all of the ASC complex has now been cloned, restriction mapped, and sequenced. Extensive study has correlated the developmental functions of genes in the complex with transcription units. Antonio Garcia-Bellido (1979) subdivided the ASC complex into four components from the sites of lesions causing mutant phenotypes. A fifth component was added by Dambly-Chaudiere and Ghysen (1987). Nine different transcription units have been identified in the seven-band 1B1-1B7 segment. Some lesions in the region, associated with at least one of the transcripts, affect sex determination and are thus excluded as members of the ASC complex. Four of the transcripts encode helix-loop-helix proteins that can bind as dimers to DNA. These products account for the neurogenic functions attributed to achaete, scute, lethal(1)scute, and asense of the ASC. Three of those transcripts share a 15-nucleotide sequence encoding an acidic amino acid domain on the 3' end. Genetic analysis of the ASC mutations shows that different components specify different but sometimes overlapping subsets of cellular effects. For example, the ac and sc genes have similar patterns of expression in imaginal discs. Juan Modolcll and collaborators (Gomez-Skarmeta et al. 1995) have shown that this coexpression is accomplished by shared, position-specific, enhancer-like elements distributed along most of the approximately 90 kb ASC. Several enhancers located either upstream or downstream of sc drive the expression of the ac and sc promoters. The patterns of ac and sc expression observed when the ac and sc regions are separated, as by the rearrangements selected by Muller and Prokofyeva, show that the enhancer elements with similar specificities are not found in both regions. Also breaks such as the sc⁴ inversion they studied, which has a break inside one of the enhancer elements that disconnect the long downstream region from sc, actually remove expression of both ac and sc from the proneural cell clusters of the imaginal discs.

Muller noted that the rearrangements that appeared to have identical breakpoints in the scute region, but with different proximal breaks in the X chromosome, produced slightly different phenotypic effects. He reasoned this to be due to position effects brought on by placing different neighboring elements adjacent to the sc locus (Raffel and Muller 1940). However, he anticipated the gene complex by noting: "The question is raised of to what extent the breakage in the region of scute in this and other cases where they seem identical in position are really identical, or may be separated by parts of a 'gene-complex' (or 'gene,' according to definition) which, although able to reproduce separately, function to produce bristles only, or mainly, when in proximity to one another, and function normally only when in proper arrangement."

Do the molecular studies significantly change how we view the relationship between genes and chromomeres, or is it confirmation of the cytogenetic data discussed above? Answers to this question may soon be forthcoming. Michael Ashburner and Gerry Rubin and their collaborators, in not-yet-published work, are now analyzing the sequence of about 2.7 mb of DNA surrounding the Adh locus on chromosome arm 2L (34D-36A). The genetic analysis had identified 72 genes, about 50 of which have lethal alleles in these 69 polytene chromosome bands. The computational analysis of the sequence, however, has identified about 109 protein-coding genes. I'm not sure what this means, but it will be very interesting to see how all of this unfolds. It is clear that only about one-third of these genes are detected by even the most thorough genetic tests, and only one-fourth can mutate to lethality. There is clear evidence confirming the cytogenetic data that gene density is far from uniform. Clusters of genes are found in some regions, while long, seemingly empty stretches characterize other parts of the genomic universe.

A summary: The survey I have presented of selected genes, complexes, and extended regions of chromosomes, in my opinion, covers most of the spectrum of gene-chromomere arrangements. What emerges is that the relationship is not a simple one. Clearly, there is no apparent direct correlation between the chromomeric pattern and the numbers and arrangements of genes. In fact, judging from the cytogenetic and molecular maps and evidence from rearrangement breakpoints, genes do not respect chromomeric boundaries. In some regions, clusters of genes are found tightly packed into few bands, and on the other hand there are long stretches of DNA that seem devoid of recognizable genetic elements. Further, even with this nonuniform gene density, it is clear that, overall, a large fraction of the genomic DNA does not encode protein products and that much of the remainder is utilized in the regulation of gene expression. The maps, along with genetic dissection, molecular cloning, and sequencing, have shown us that Drosophila melanogaster genes on average are about an order of magnitude larger than is necessary to encode the polypeptides they specify.

Now, can we estimate how many genes it takes to make a fly? Maybe not with any great accuracy. I say that not just because of the points I have raised about undiscovered genes and bands or how regulatory elements and other apparently noncoding regions fit into the picture, but also because the c-value paradox looms in my mind. The paradox is that there is no direct correlation between the genomic DNA content of an organism and its developmental complexity. That takes the edge off estimating the number of required genes therein. *Drosophila virilis* has about 60% more DNA in its genome than *D. melanogaster*, and the mosquito (Aedes) has six times as much. Maybe here I should also mention, without further comment, that there are many examples of genes that encode proteins that perform two quite different functions. Evolution works, but in mysterious ways.

In the face of uncertainties about the numbers of chromomeres and the probability that many genes remain to be discovered, I am still impressed with just how close the association of genes with chromomeres remains. What has emerged is that the chromomeric map has proven to be one of the most powerful tools available to geneticists, cytologists, and molecular biologists. Genes can be located precisely by these maps, greatly facilitating genetic and evolutionary studies. Chromosome aberrations can be analyzed in great detail and correlated with their effects on genes at or near the breakpoints. Determining the effects of rearrangements in crossover suppression and aberrant chromosome transmission would have been extremely difficult without polytene chromosomes.

The chromomere: I would still like to know what a chromomeric unit is. I surmise that it is an inherent aspect of chromosomal three-dimensional structure, created by winding or folding parallel strands of DNA into tightly packed units, alternating with less dense interchromomeric stretches. The measurements done by John Sedat (RYKOWSKI *et al.* 1988) support the concept that in polytene chromosome chromomeres, the 10-nm nucleosome fiber is wound regularly into a higher-order structure. Band 3C7, where *Notch* is positioned, is not condensed above the level of the 30-nm fiber. As for interbands, their data are consistent with the suggestion by ANANIEV and BARSKY (1985) that interband DNA exists in the 10-nm nucleosome fiber form.

It is clear that breaks in chromosomes can fracture bands and create two condensed segments. From this I conclude that the winding or folding is not unidirectionally determined by sequence information localized at a band margin. With all of the rather extensive sequence data now emerging from analyses of large stretches of Drosophila DNA, there is not yet a clue about band/interband boundary junctions. Somewhere in that one-dimensional nucleotide sequence there certainly resides the necessary three-dimensional information.

I once heard Francis Crick comment after a seminar on transvection that genetic analysis has difficulty dealing with three-dimensional problems. The molecular data do not yet make this any easier.

I am very grateful for the efforts and many stimulating discussions of those who worked in my lab on various aspects of this problem, especially THOM KAUFMAN, MIKE YOUNG, and JO JACK. Also, very special thanks are due to JOHNG LIM for his contributions and discussions and to CATHY LAURIE, who stimulated the genesis of this essay, for her very useful comments. I gratefully acknowledge MICHAEL ASHBURNER's extensive and very helpful comments, and to him and GERRY RUBIN and their collaborators, special thanks for permission to cite the results of work in progress.

LITERATURE CITED

ANANIEV, E. V., and V. E. BARSKY, 1985 Elementary structures in polytene chromosomes of *Drosophila melanogaster*. Chromosoma **93:** 104–112.

ASHBURNER, M., 1972 Puffing patterns in *Drosophila melanogaster* and related species, pp. 101–151 in *Results and Problems in Cell Differentiation, Vol. 4, Developmental Studies on Giant Chromosomes*, edited by W. BEERMANN. Springer Verlag, Berlin/New York.

ASHBURNER, M., 1989 Transvection effects, pp. 915–929 in *Drosophila: A Laboratory Handbook*. Cold Spring Harbor Laboratory Press, Cold Spring Harbor, NY.

BEERMANN, W., 1961 Ein Balbiani-Ring als Locus einer Speicheldrusenmutation. Chromosoma **12:** 1–25.

BEERMANN, W., 1962 *Riesenchromosomen. Protoplasmatologia VI D.* Springer, Wien.

BEERMANN, W. (Editor), 1972 Developmental Studies on Giant Chromosomes. *Results and Problems in Cell Differentiation*, Vol. 4. Springer Verlag, Berlin/New York.

BERENDES, H. D., 1970 Polytene chromosome structure at the submicroscopic level. I. A map of region X, 1-4E of *Drosophila melanogaster*. Chromosoma **29:** 11–13.

BRIDGES, C. B., 1935 Salivary chromosome maps: with a key to the banding of the chromosomes of *Drosophila melanogaster*. J. Hered. **26:** 60–64.

BRIDGES, C. B., 1938 A revised map of the salivary gland X-chromosome of *Drosophila melanogaster*. J. Hered. **29:** 11–13.

BRIDGES, P. N., 1942 A new map of the salivary gland 2L-chromosome of *Drosophila melanogaster*. J. Hered. **33:** 403–408.

BRITTEN, R. J., and E. H. DAVIDSON, 1969 Gene regulation for higher cells: a theory. Science **165:** 349–357.

CRICK, F. H. C., 1971 General model for the chromosomes of higher organisms. Nature **234:** 25–27.

DAMBLY-CHAUDIERE, C., and A. GHYSEN, 1987 Independent subpatterns of sense organs require independent genes of the achaete-scute complex in Drosophila larvae. Genes Dev. **1:** 297–306.

DAVIS, P. S., M. W. SHEN and B. H. JUDD, 1987 Asymmetrical pairings of transposons in and proximal to the *white* locus of Drosophila account for four classes of regularly occurring exchange products. Proc. Natl. Acad. Sci. USA **84:** 174–178.

GANS, M., 1953 Etude genetique et physiologique du mutant z de *Drosophila melanogaster*. Bull. Biol. Fr. Belg. **38** (Suppl.): 1–90.

GARCIA-BELLIDO, A., 1979 Genetic analysis of the achaete-scute system of *Drosophila melanogaster*. Genetics **91:** 491–520.

GAUSZ, J., G. BENCZE, H. GYURKOVICS, M. ASHBURNER, D. ISH-HOROWICZ *et al.*, 1979 Genetic characterization of the 87C region of the third chromosome of *Drosophila melanogaster*. Genetics **93:** 917–934.

GAUSZ, J., H. GYURKOVICS, G. BENCZE, A. A. M. AWAD, J. J. HOLDEN *et al.*, 1981 Genetic characterization of the region between 86F1,2 and 87B15 on chromosome 3 of *Drosophila melanogaster*. Genetics **98:** 775–789.

GOMEZ-SKARMETA, J. L., I. RODRIGUEZ, C. MARTINEZ, J. CULI, D. FERRES-MARCO *et al.*, 1995 *Cis*-regulation of *achaete* and *scute*: shared enhancer-like elements drive their coexpression in proneural clusters of the imaginal discs. Genes Dev. **9:** 1869–1882.

HALL, L. M. C., P. J. MASON and P. SPIERER, 1983 Transcripts, genes and bands in 315,000 base-pairs of Drosophila DNA. J. Mol. Biol. **169:** 83–96.

HILLIKER, A. J., S. H. CLARK, A. CHOVNICK and W. M. GELBART, 1980

Cytogenetic analysis of the chromosomal region immediately adjacent to the rosy locus in *Drosophila melanogaster*. Genetics **95**: 95–110.

Hochman, B., 1971   Analysis of chromosome 4 in *Drosophila melanogaster*. II. Ethyl methanesulfonate induced lethals. Genetics **67**: 235–252.

Jack, J., 1985   Molecular organization of the *cut* locus of *Drosophila melanogaster*. Cell **42**: 869–876.

Jack, J., and Y. DeLotto, 1995   Structure and regulation of a complex locus: the cut gene of Drosophila. Genetics **139**: 1689–1700.

Jack, J., D. Dorsett, Y. DeLotto and S. Liu, 1991   Expression of the *cut* locus in the Drosophila wing margin is required for cell type specification and is regulated by a distant enhancer. Development **113**: 735–747.

Jacob, F., and J. Monod, 1961   On the regulation of gene activity. Cold Spring Harbor Symp. Quant. Biol. **26**: 193–211.

Johnson, T. K., and B. H. Judd, 1979   Analysis of the cut locus of *Drosophila melanogaster*. Genetics **92**: 485–502.

Judd, B. H., 1961   Analysis of products from regularly occurring asymmetrical exchange in *Drosophila melanogaster*. Genetics **46**: 1687–1697.

Judd, B. H., 1962   An analysis of mutations confined to a small region of the X chromosome of *Drosophila melanogaster*. Science **138**: 990–991.

Judd, B. H., and M. W. Young, 1973   An examination of the one cistron: one chromomere concept. Cold Spring Harbor Symp. Quant. Biol. **38**: 573–579.

Judd, B. H., M. W. Shen and T. C. Kaufman, 1972   The anatomy and function of a segment of the X chromosome of *Drosophila melanogaster*. Genetics **71**: 139–156.

Kaufman, T. C., S. E. Tsaka and D. T. Suzuki, 1973   The interaction of two complex loci, zeste and bithorax, in *Drosophila melanogaster*. Genetics **75**: 299–321.

Keppy, D. O., and W. J. Welshons, 1980   The synthesis of compound bands in *Drosophila melanogaster* salivary gland chromosomes. Chromosoma **76**: 191–200.

Konopka, R. J., and S. Benzer, 1971   Clock mutants of *Drosophila melanogaster*. Proc. Natl. Acad. Sci. USA **68**: 2112–2116.

Laird, C. D., 1971   Chromatid structure: relationship between DNA content and nucleotide sequence diversity. Chromosoma **32**: 378–406.

Lefevre, G., Jr., 1969   The eccentricity of vermilion deficiencies in *Drosophila melanogaster*. Genetics **69**: 589–600.

Lefevre, G., Jr., 1971   Salivary chromosome bands and the frequency of crossing over in *Drosophila melanogaster*. Genetics **67**: 497–513.

Lefevre, G., Jr., 1973   The one band-one gene hypothesis: evidence from cytogenetic analysis of mutant and nonmutant rearrangement breakpoints in *Drosophila melanogaster*. Cold Spring Harbor Symp. Quant. Biol. **38**: 591–599.

Lefevre, G., Jr., 1976   A photographic representation and interpretation of the polytene chromosomes of *Drosophila melanogaster* salivary glands, pp. 31–66 in *The Genetics and Biology of Drosophila*, Vol. 1a, edited by M. Ashburner and E. Novitski. Academic Press, London/New York/San Francisco.

Lefevre, G., Jr., and W. S. Watkins, 1986   The question of total gene number in *Drosophila melanogaster*. Genetics **113**: 869–895.

Lewis, E. B., 1959   New mutants report. Dros. Inf. Serv. **33**: 96.

Lifschytz, E., and R. Falk, 1968   Fine structure analysis of a chromosome segment in *Drosophila melanogaster*: analysis of X-ray-induced lethals. Mutat. Res. **6**: 235–244.

Lifschytz, E., and R. Falk, 1969   Analysis of ethyl methanesulfonate-induced lethals. Mutat. Res. **8**: 147–155.

Lim, J. K., and L. A. Snyder, 1974   Cytogenetic and complementation analysis of recessive lethal mutations induced in the X chromosome of Drosophila by three alkylating agents. Genet. Res. **24**: 1–10.

Liu, S., E. McLeod and J. Jack, 1991   Four distinct regulatory regions of the *cut* locus and their effect on cell type specification in Drosophila. Genetics **127**: 151–159.

Maleszka, R., H. G. de Couet and G. L. Gabor Miklos, 1998   Data transferability from model organisms to human beings: insights from the functional genomics of the *flightless* region of *Drosophila*. Proc. Natl. Acad. Sci. USA **95**: 3731–3736.

Muller, H. J., and A. A. Prokofyeva, 1935   The individual gene in relation to the chromomere and the chromosome. Proc. Natl. Acad. Sci. USA **21**: 16–26.

Painter, T. S., 1934   Salivary chromosomes and the attack on the gene. J. Hered. **25**: 465–476.

Raffel, D., and H. J. Muller, 1940   Position effects and gene divisibility considered in connection with three strikingly similar scute mutations. Genetics **25**: 541–583.

Royden, C. S., V. Pirrotta and L. Y. Jan, 1987   The *tko* locus, site of a behavioral mutation in *Drosophila melanogaster*, codes for a protein homologous to prokaryotic ribosomal protein S12. Cell **51**: 165–173.

Rudkin, G. T., 1965   The relative mutabilities of DNA in regions of the X chromosome of *Drosophila melanogaster*. Genetics **52**: 665–681.

Rykowski, M. D., S. J. Parmalee, D. A. Agard and J. W. Sedat, 1988   Precise determination of the molecular limits of a polytene chromosomal band: regulatory sequences for the *Notch* gene are in the interband. Cell **54**: 461–472.

Schalet, A., and G. Lefevre, 1976   The proximal region of the X chromosome, pp. 847–902 in *The Genetics and Biology of Drosophila*, Vol. 1b, edited by M. Ashburner and E. Novitski. Academic Press, London/New York/San Francisco.

Shannon, M. P., T. C. Kaufman and B. H. Judd, 1970   Lethality patterns of mutations in the *zeste-white* region of *Drosophila melanogaster*. Genetics **64**(Suppl.): 58.

Shannon, M. P., T. C. Kaufman, M. W. Shen and B. H. Judd, 1972   Lethality patterns and morphology of selected lethals and semilethal mutations in the zeste-white region of *Drosophila melanogaster*. Genetics **72**: 615–638.

Sorsa, V., 1988   *Chromosome Maps of Drosophila, I and II*. CRC Press, Boca Raton, FL.

Sorsa, V., M. M. Green and W. Beermann, 1973   Cytogenetic fine structure and chromosomal localization of the white gene in *Drosophila melanogaster*. Nat. New Biol. **245**: 34–37.

Woodruff, R. C., and M. Ashburner, 1979a   The genetics of a small autosomal region of *Drosophila melanogaster* containing the structural gene for alcohol dehydrogenase. I. Characterization of deficiencies and mapping of ADH and visible mutations. Genetics **92**: 117–132.

Woodruff, R. C., and M. Ashburner, 1979b   The genetics of a small autosomal region of *Drosophila melanogaster* containing the structural gene for alcohol dehydrogenase. II. Lethal mutations in the region. Genetics **92**: 133–149.

Wright, T. R. F., W. Beermann, J. L. Marsh, C. P. Bishop, R. Steward *et al.*, 1981   The genetics of dopa decarboxylase in *Drosophila melanogaster*. IV. The genetics and cytology of the 37B10-37D1 region. Chromosoma **83**: 45–58.

Young, M. W., and B. H. Judd, 1978   Nonessential sequences, genes, and the polytene chromosome bands of *Drosophila melanogaster*. Genetics **88**: 723–742.

Zhimulev, I. F., G. V. Pokholkova, A. V. Bgatov, V. F. Semeshin and E. S. Belyaeva, 1981   Fine cytogenetic analysis of the band 10A1-2 and adjoining regions. Chromosoma **82**: 25–40.

An Extract from "Memoirs for Family and Friends" [1]

John Tyler Bonner

Department of Ecology and Evolutionary Biology, Princeton University, Princeton, New Jersey 08544

ALL my life I have had this feeling that my ideas are changing, are evolving. I like to think of it as a mental growth, but for all I know it might be just the opposite. Its direct manifestation is a continual desire to see how things fit together and how all parts of biology relate to one another.

There is something about the human brain that makes us want to find some great scheme where all the pieces fit into one great picture. It is an inner need for a satisfactory explanation of everything. Many find God a totally satisfactory answer. If one assumes a supernatural being to be responsible for the existence and placement at any one moment of every pebble and of every living being on earth, everything has a satisfactory explanation. Others, such as myself, seek "natural" laws, where things can be explained without supernatural forces. I know first-hand how common is this desire for all-encompassing syntheses of world order because my writings have elicited a large number of letters, manuscripts, and even a few printed volumes that have been sent to me in the belief that I was a kindred soul and would be able to appreciate their grand schemes. I fear I was not a successful audience; we all like our own schemes best and tend to think of them as the only ones that exist.

If one thinks about it a bit, it is obvious that Darwin's natural selection is just such a world scheme. Darwin's idea explains so much, which is the reason for its success. Its critics complain that it is too simple: For them, world systems that embrace some mystery are far more desirable than rational ones. They say life on earth is much too rich and complex to have a simple explanation.

In my case I did not start with the universe but at the other end, with biological phenomena surrounding my early interest in the development of animals and plants. This was evident in *Morphogenesis* (1952), my first book on development, but then I began to think beyond development as an isolated subject and started to worry about how it fits in with the bigger scheme of things.

I began to see many parallels between the events of development and the components of animal behavior that were being unwrapped at the time by Niko Tinbergen, Konrad Lorenz, and others in the new wave of ethology. In both cases, there was a whole cascading series of actions and reactions, or stimuli and responses, that produced the behavior or the development into adulthood.

I also began to ask myself questions, such as, Why do we have development at all; why go to all that bother of starting as a single cell in the form of a fertilized egg and each generation constructing a large complex adult? It slowly dawned on me that this was something that had arisen, and was maintained, by Darwinian natural selection. To compete successfully, there must be inherited variations, and sexual reproduction is a potent method of handling and disseminating that variation. In a multicellular organism, all the genes of all the cells are the same; each cell has the complete complement of the organism's genes. In every generation there is a mixture of the genes of the two parents, and this can be achieved only by the fusion of one cell from the father (sperm) and one from the mother (egg) to form the new offspring. This led me to the conclusion that development was the inevitable result of sex and size, for if there was selection pressure for an adult larger than the fertilized egg, then there had to be a development.

Just at the time (1955) some of these thoughts were taking shape in my mind, I received an invitation from G. P. Wells to give a course of three lectures at University College in London. "Gyp" Wells, the son of H. G. Wells, was a distinguished professor of invertebrate zoology. I was excited and pleased and immediately began to put some of those grand thoughts together in the form of lectures. I had written up the main ideas, and now I rewrote them completely.

The whole event was a big moment for me. I felt as though I was finally coming into full bloom, but at the same time I was terrified. This was not helped by the fact that as I took the train from Princeton to New York

---

[1] A course of lectures at University College in London, 1956.

to go to the airport, the train came to what seemed like a permanent stop when the drawbridge over a river in New Jersey was stuck and the tracks could not be lined up properly. After an agonizing delay we finally got through and I just caught my flight.

They put me up at the Ciba Foundation on Portland Place, which was supported by the Swiss pharmaceutical company (now Novartis). A number of other scientists from all over were there as guests, and at one memorable breakfast an unidentified Englishman appeared, scowling at everyone. He surveyed all the beautiful Swiss jams and said in a furious tone, "No marmalade—hardly an English breakfast!"

I had splendid reunions with friends who had spent the war with us and were now grown up, and their families, and with Brian Shaffer from Cambridge, a good friend whose work on slime molds I particularly admired. I could hardly believe it when the Ciba Foundation put on a dinner for me the first evening, after which I gave a lecture on my recent work on slime molds that was chaired by the well-known immunologist Peter Medawar, and other distinguished biologists whom I knew only by name were there. Nothing like this had ever happened to me before—I felt like a debutante. And the main show had not yet started.

The day before the first lecture I was so nervous that I decided it might be wise to go to see a play or a film for therapeutic distraction. I found that Agatha Christie's *The Mousetrap* had a matinee—the perfect medicine. It had already been running for years. I was the only man in the audience, and at the intermission tea was served. I was totally distracted.

The first lecture was even more terrifying than I thought possible. I was not allowed to just enter the lecture room, but was marched there by the most magnificent beadle, all dressed in a light blue uniform, rather like the doorman at a very fancy hotel. He carried a huge mace as we proceeded to the lecture hall—I had the impression that I was marching in my own funeral procession. We went to the podium where I sat next to Gyp Wells, who introduced me. The large lecture hall was full, and in the front were people well known to me and others whom I had just met. In the front row I could see a star among neurobiologists, J. Z. Young, and not far from him sat the famous geneticist, J. B. S. Haldane, who positively glowered at me. How I got through the lecture I will never know. Just afterward I rushed to the Gents, and as I was washing my hands, Haldane, behind me, said in his booming voice, "Bonner, we don't make jokes in our lectures in this country." This did nothing to calm me down, but I did manage to say, "Those weren't jokes; I was just nervous."

I had no idea how the first lecture was received. Walking down the street the next day I ran into J. Z. Young, who greeted me with his charming smile as he said, "Well, John, what did you think of your lecture?" I always thought that was a splendid ploy. Later one evening we drank beer in a series of pubs, and while he never said so, he made me feel that my lectures were not a disaster.

The same was true for Haldane, who insisted I come to dinner with him and his wife, Helen Spurway. They both loved to shock and they loved to argue. Helen had just been arrested for a misdemeanor involving someone else's dog. I forget the details, but it was in all the newspapers, and she was reveling in it and the principle she upheld, which I have since forgotten. We ate at a small restaurant in Soho and soon were embroiled in some very spirited arguments. One was about some biological aspect of sex. Mostly they argued with each other, and both of them had very penetrating voices as they became more intense, resulting in all the people at the neighboring tables staring at us. Even though they both appeared to ignore the stir they were causing, I could not help feeling they not only were aware of it, but enjoyed seeing the shock waves travel across the room.

By the time we left the restaurant, we were on to discussing the recent work in animal behavior and its evolutionary implications. It was a subject of concern to all three of us, and indeed it was the central theme of one of my lectures, in which I drew parallels between behavior and development. We all had more to say, so they said they would walk me to Portland Place, but we still had not finished, so I walked them back toward University College. The whole process repeated itself again before we were ready for bed. On one of the laps we passed the BBC building, and on the ground floor a low window was open at the top, and one could hear a radio blaring away. Haldane was talking, and suddenly he veered across the broad sidewalk, stood on his toes, shoved his enormous head into the open window, and yelled with tremendous force, "SHUT UP." He went directly on to his next sentence as he cruised back alongside us without skipping a beat. Apparently he did not like the BBC! And I always wondered what might have been the sensations of the people working in the room.

As a result of that evening and some subsequent meetings during my visit, we began a sporadic correspondence. It was mainly from India, where he and Helen Spurway went to live in 1957. He seemed to enjoy living in India, although he could be as difficult with his new Indian friends as he was with the people he left. I asked him once why he had left Britain, and he said, looking at me as though I did not exist, "Because there are too many damned Americans here, especially damned American soldiers." There probably were, but I don't think that was the reason at all: I think there was quite a bit of the Hindu Brahman in his nature, and he found some peace there for his turbulent mind.

I still have our letters, which span the years from 1959 to 1962. As I reread them I am impressed all over again with how fertile his mind was. He could look at any biological problem with fresh and ingenious insights. He was also not encumbered with a need to flatter. In the early 1960s I had sent him *The Ideas of Biology*, a book that I had written for the layman. Here are some fragments of his replies:

15 November 1960
Dear Bonner,
....You ask about Helen and me coming to Princeton. This is at present impossible for me. I was asked by your government to give a list of all associations to which I have belonged since my 16th birthday (in 1908) with date of joining and leaving, with a threat of jail or fine if I get one wrong. I don't know if I joined the Oxford University Liberal Club in 1912 or 1913. Having a professional regard for truth I am not going to guess. If President Kennedy has the guts to tear down this Iron Curtain I will come when next asked, if I can manage. But I think there are too many officials who have a vested interest in that sort of nonsense.

So you had better come here. There are plenty of molds, especially in the monsoon....

14 February 1962
Dear Bonner,
....Every 15 years or so I write a paranoiac paper. In 1919 I gave the dimensions of a gene, and several other things about genes, not wholly wrong, on very inadequate evidence. In 1928 I gave the general accepted theory of the anaerobic origin of life. I hope Nagy has bust it. In 1944 I produced a cosmological speculation which nobody likes, not even myself. Perhaps it is right....

25 September 1962
Dear Bonner,
Thank you for "The ideas of biology." I have not yet read it, but my first impression is that you have made a number of statements, sometimes for the first time, sufficiently clearly to allow destructive criticism. For example on p. 29...[then he makes five detailed points, all excellent, the last one regarding page 152—the book is only a little over 200 pages!].

Anyway the book is provocative, probably more so than you meant it to be....

I kept wondering what he might have said had he admitted to reading the book!

After giving those 1956 lectures, I received an invitation to spend the weekend with Victor Rothschild, whom I knew slightly, and his family in Cambridge. It was the first time I had seen Cambridge, and I was quite bowled over by its beauty. Both Victor and his wife Tess could not have been kinder, and I had a wonderful time. I had sent the manuscript of my lectures to the Cambridge University Press previously, and they had given me a very discouraging reply. Victor asked about it, and I told him the details. He got up and said wait a bit, then

disappeared into his study. I could hear him distantly on the telephone, and he came back to say that it was all settled: They would publish my book! Victor had not even read it—What could he have possibly said over the telephone, and to whom? Of course I never knew, but they did publish *The Evolution of Development* (1958). Since then, I have always wished that whenever I finish a book, there would be a Lord Rothschild about to speed it on its way.

Even my departure from London after those whirlwind two weeks was an event. On the night I left, the mother of my friends who had stayed with us during the war invited me to a family dinner. She was a celebrated cook and that evening she outdid herself: The food and the wine were a dream. I kept worrying about catching the plane, as I always do, but her son Justin said he would drive me out in plenty of time. We started very late, and by the time we got there almost everyone had boarded. All the regular seats were filled, so they had to put me in First Class. One of the other passengers was the incomparable opera diva Maria Callas, in her splendid elegance. The flight attendant came to me and said that having been upped into First Class, I was to have a steak dinner with champagne. I explained to her that I had just come from a sumptuous dinner and could not do it. She was very upset because I was passing up this chance to have a fantastic meal—and free too! I rode home among the clouds.

BIBLIOGRAPHY

About J. B. S. Haldane:
CLARK, R. W., 1969 *JBS: The Life and Work of J. B. S. Haldane*. Coward-McCann, New York.
CROW, J. F., 1992 Centennial: J. B. S. Haldane, 1892–1964. Genetics **130:** 1–6.
DRONAMRAJU, K. R., 1985 *Haldane: The Life and Work of J. B. S. Haldane with Special Reference to India*. Aberdeen University Press, Aberdeen, Scotland.
NANJUNDIAH, V., 1992 J. B. S. Haldane: his life and science. Curr. Sci. **63:** 582–588.
About or by others:
MEDAWAR, P., 1986 *Memoir of a Thinking Radish: An Autobiography*. Oxford University Press, Oxford.
ROTHSCHILD, V., 1956 *Fertilization*. Methuen, London.
WELLS, H. G., J. S. HUXLEY and G. P. WELLS, 1931 *The Science of Life*. Doubleday-Doran, New York.
YOUNG, J. Z., 1950 *The Life of Vertebrates*. Clarenden Press, Oxford.
References to my own writings:
BONNER, J. T., 1952 *Morphogenesis: An Essay on Development*. Princeton University Press, Princeton, NJ.
BONNER, J. T., 1958 *The Evolution of Development*. Cambridge University, Cambridge.
BONNER, J. T., 1962 *The Ideas of Biology*. Harper & Brothers, New York.

November 1998

Marcus Rhoades and Transposition

Nina Fedoroff

Pennsylvania State University, University Park, Pennsylvania 16802

Barbara McClintock deservedly received the lion's share of recognition for the discovery of transposition, including the 1983 award of an unshared Nobel Prize in Physiology or Medicine (FEDOROFF 1994). But discoveries are punctuation marks in the discourse of science, and many voices impinge on the discoverer's ear. McClintock studied genetics at Cornell. The Cornell genetics group was headed by R. A. Emerson. Marcus Rhoades undertook graduate work at Cornell not long after McClintock's graduation and learned cytogenetics from her (SCHWARTZ 1993). But more than that, Rhoades took important steps on the road to the discovery of transposition before, and quite independently of, McClintock's final sprint. And while hindsight has a certain blinding clarity unavailable to the discoverer, there is always an intellectual framework into which a discovery fits. My purpose is to sketch that framework for the discovery of transposition, here emphasizing Rhoades' work on the *Dotted* (*Dt*) locus of maize. The year 1998 marks the 60th anniversary of the publication of Rhoades' paper in GENETICS reporting seminal work on the properties of a gene with a transposon insertion, carried out a decade before McClintock's identification of the transposable *Dissociation* (*Ds*) locus in maize.

The fact that Rhoades and McClintock were friends and colleagues who corresponded extensively is important to the discovery of transposition. This fertile ground will be tilled in time by historians and, perhaps, biographers. But it is important only because Marcus Rhoades was both an outstanding maize geneticist and because he had himself worked on the genetics of unstable mutations, making observations parallel to those of McClintock. The story doesn't begin with Rhoades either, of course, and a crucial earlier chapter was contributed by Emerson, whose papers were undoubtedly read by both Rhoades and McClintock. Emerson's work, in turn, was rooted in earlier observations on what were initially called "mutable" or "unstable" genes and "ever-sport-

ing" varieties exhibiting variegation for flower and leaf color in plants.

Variegation: Studying pigment variegation in Antirrhinum, de Vries developed the concept of ever-sporting varieties, concluding that the tendency to variegate was heritable (DE VRIES 1905). He noted that the few fully pigmented progeny arising from variegated plants sometimes show heritability of the trait and sometimes give rise instead to progeny that are once again variegated. Correns, working with *Mirabilis jalapa*, and East and Hays, studying variegation in *Zea mays*, reported on the other hand that somatic mutations from a variegated to a fully colored phenotype showed Mendelian inheritance (CORRENS 1910; EAST and HAYES 1911). In any event, the picture was far from clear, and variegation was a phenomenon that was difficult to fit into the newly emerging Mendelian framework. Indeed, EMERSON (1914) opened his first important paper on the genetics of variegation with the striking statement that "Variegation is distinguished from other color patterns by its incorrigible irregularity" (p. 87).

Emerson studied the heritability of pericarp variegation in what was known as "calico" corn (EMERSON 1914). Ears produced on plants grown from variegated kernels generally show one of a variety of patterns of striping, but the red area varies considerably, and both colorless and fully pigmented kernels are produced frequently. Emerson took an approach somewhat different from that of de Vries, asking whether there was a relationship between the amount of red-pigmented tissue in a given kernel and the number of red ears produced upon self-pollination in subsequent generations. The clear answer emerged: the more red there was in the kernels planted, the larger the fraction of red ears in the progeny (EMERSON 1914). Emerson further found that red kernels produced plants that were commonly heterozygous for the red and variegated traits. He concluded: "The development of red in the pericarp is evidently associated with and perhaps due to a modification of some Mendelian factor for pericarp color in the somatic cells" (p. 102).

In this way, Emerson captured variegation within the

Address for correspondence: Biotechnology Institute, Pennsylvania State University, 519 Wartik Lab., University Park, PA 16802-9807. E-mail: nvf1@psu.edu

Mendelian paradigm, adding the important insight that a somatic change could occur in a Mendelian factor, becoming a heritable change that obeyed simple Mendelian principles. But he readily admitted that it was "utterly impossible at the present time to conceive of the cause or even the nature of this change." Nonetheless, he speculated that the genetic factor for variegation might be "a sort of temporary inhibitor, an inhibitor that sooner or later loses its power to inhibit color development, a power that once lost is ordinarily never regained" (EMERSON 1914, pp. 112–113). Emerson's idea was that variegation was due to the association of some kind of a genetic factor with a locus and that its loss was what allowed the gene to be reexpressed. Emerson subsequently reported that occasional variegated kernels appeared on otherwise fully pigmented ears. This suggested that at some low frequency, the inhibitory factor might once again become associated with the gene, then called a "unit factor" (EMERSON 1917). Emerson viewed variegation as a reversible change in an otherwise conventional gene, distinguishing itself from other kinds of mutations by its high frequency. Thus, Emerson had not only made variegation intelligible in a Mendelian context, but had deduced that it was caused by a modification in the structure of the gene.

Emerson later made some puzzling observations that were to remain unexplained until McClintock's studies decades later (EMERSON 1929). First, he made the counterintuitive observation that reversion to wild type was less frequent when the variegating pericarp color gene was homozygous and therefore present in two copies than when it was heterozygous with a stable nonpigmenting allele. Second, he noted that chromosomes carrying a stable, recessive, nonpigmenting allele of the pericarp color locus recovered by segregation from a variegating heterozygote show some ability to suppress variegation when again used to create a variegating heterozygote. As explanations of the latter, he entertained the radical hypothesis that information is transferred between alleles either as "a direct contamination of one allelomorph by another" or by transfer of "distinct gene elements" from one allele to another (EMERSON 1929, p. 506). But he readily admits that he, the writer, "is wholly unable to devise a consistent working hypothesis to account for his results on any such assumption" and suggested the alternative hypothesis of distinct modifiers of variegation, which had already been reported in *Drosophila virilis* (DEMEREC 1928a).

Mutable genes: The view that variegation is attributable to ordinary mutations occurring at a high frequency was challenged over the next decade as mutable genes were studied in both Drosophila and plants (DEMEREC 1928b, 1929, 1931, 1935; STERN 1935; RHOADES 1936; PLOUGH and HOLTHAUSEN 1937; RHOADES 1938, 1941). Goldschmidt proposed that mutations are a consequence of position effects, and both he and Correns believed that mutable genes are sick or diseased genes

and that any conclusions derived from their study were not applicable to other types of mutations (GOLDSCHMIDT 1938). Rhoades and Demerec, on the other hand, shared Emerson's view that there was no clearcut difference between stable and unstable genes.

In 1936, Rhoades reported a seminal observation, one that has withstood the test of controversy and time. He identified and isolated a "dotted" allele of the A_1 locus of *Z. mays* from an ear of Black Mexican sweet corn whose original segregation ratio suggested that the variegating dotted character required both the recessive a_1 allele and a second locus (RHOADES 1936, 1938). He then showed clearly that variegation depends on two different loci, one that he designated the *Dt* locus and the other that appeared to behave like a standard recessive a_1 allele in the absence of the *Dt* locus (RHOADES 1938). Curiously, this apparently new a_1 allele proved indistinguishable from the standard stable recessive a_1 tester allele originally isolated by Emerson and used for two decades without showing evidence of variegation (EMERSON 1918; RHOADES 1938). Rhoades showed that the *Dt* locus was not linked to the *A* locus and that both the standard and newly isolated a_1 alleles exhibited variegation or mutability only in its presence.

Thus, Rhoades had identified a gene that destabilized what appeared to be an ordinary stable mutation. Knowing nothing about the mechanism, he hypothesized that the normally stable a_1 allele mutated to A_1 in the presence of *Dt* (RHOADES 1938). He suggested that each dot of color represented one mutation and, therefore, that the number of dots reflected the mutation frequency and the sizes of the dots reflected their timing in development. Rhoades predicted that mutations that occur in sporogenous tissue that gives rise to gametes should be genetically transmissible. In a plant that was homozygous for a_1 and *Dt* and had the appropriate genetic constitution at other loci affecting pigmentation, Rhoades observed purple anthers and anther sectors. Using pollen from such anthers, he assessed the frequency of transmission of the putative A_1 alleles and observed that half of the fully pigmented anthers he tested were A_1/a_1 heterozygotes. This observation supported his hypothesis. He also noted that, unlike the unstable a_1 allele, the A_1 allele derived by mutation from a_1 was stable and did not revert to the unstable a_1. Rhoades further ascertained that the effect of *Dt* was quite specific to the a_1 allele and had no effect on the mutation frequency of recessive alleles at other loci, including the pericarp color allele Emerson had studied, by then designated P^{vv} (RHOADES 1941).

Rhoades concluded that whether a mutation is stable or unstable can be a function of the genetic background. Having looked for and failed to find chromosomal abnormalities, he dismissed a mechanical explanation, such as chromosome loss or rearrangement, as an explanation for the ability of *Dt* to destabilize the a_1 allele. To explain his observation that the frequency of mutations from a_1 to A_1 increases linearly with the number of a_1 gene copies and exponentially with the number of copies of Dt, he suggested that the Dt gene produced something that accelerated mutation of a_1 to A_1 (RHOADES 1938). Although McClintock's first experience with transposable elements was through the analysis of a chromosome breakage phenomenon rather than an unstable mutation, she knew the behavior of the Dt-a_1 system and recognized the similarities early.

Chromosome breakage: McClintock's discovery of transposition had its origins in her studies on the behavior of broken chromosomes. Her objective was to understand the behavior of a chromosome with a broken end during mitotic divisions and she found that chromosomes lacking telomeres do not separate during replication, thus producing dicentric chromosomes. The dicentric chromosomes break, regenerating chromosomes with broken ends and establishing what McClintock referred to as the "breakage-fusion-bridge" cycle (McCLINTOCK 1938, 1939, 1941a,b, 1942a). From her knowledge of the behavior of broken chromosomes, she developed a method for producing small terminal and subterminal deletions (McCLINTOCK 1942b, 1943).

McClintock undertook a search for new mutations using F$_2$ progeny derived from F$_1$ plants that had received a recently broken chromosome 9 from one parent and the selfed progeny of plants that had received a newly broken chromosome 9 from each parent (McCLINTOCK 1945). She identified a new type of chromosomal behavior in which part of chromosome 9 was lost during development. She also noted the appearance in these cultures of new variegating mutants (McCLINTOCK 1945). It is clear, in retrospect, that these observations were the first emerging indications that transposable elements had been activated in her cultures. McClintock later noted that while reports of the appearance of new mutable genes were relatively rare in maize literature, she had rapidly isolated 14 new cases of such instability and observed more (McCLINTOCK 1946). Continuing to examine the new type of chromosome breakage, McClintock soon understood that breakage occurred repeatedly within a restricted region or at a single site. This was supported by cytological studies that showed a chromosome 9 constitution in which one homologue lacked a large segment of the short arm. McClintock tied the two phenomena together because both variegation in the newly isolated unstable mutants and chromosome breakage showed striking differences in frequency and timing between plants, a resemblance she guessed might be more than coincidental.

By 1947 McClintock was confident enough that the chromosome breakage in the new strain was happening at a single site to name it the *Dissociation* or Ds locus, which she mapped both cytologically and genetically to a position near the centromere on the short arm of chromosome 9 (McCLINTOCK 1947). McClintock also recognized that a second locus was required for chromo-

some dissociation at the Ds locus and she named it *Activator* or Ac, for its ability to activate chromosome breakage at the Ds locus. Turning to the investigation of the mutable loci that had surfaced in her cultures, McClintock soon realized that some were unstable only in the presence of Ac (McCLINTOCK 1947). This began to provide support for her earlier guess that the chromosome breakage and mutability phenomena were related in some way.

Ds transposition: It was at about this time that McClintock recognized the ability of Ds to move (McCLINTOCK 1948). Her first insight came in experiments with a multiply marked short arm of chromosome 9, in which all the markers were distal to Ds and, as a consequence, were lost concomitantly after chromosome breakage. The first clue that something had changed was the observation of two exceptional kernels that did not, as expected and observed for all of the other kernels containing Ac, lose all of the dominant markers distal to Ds simultaneously. Instead, the kernels showed breaks just to the right of the I locus, giving rise to colored sectors (note that I is a dominant inhibitory allele of the C locus, required for anthocyanin pigment biosynthesis). Curiously, there were additional sectors that, in turn, had lost succeeding loci proximal to I sequentially. These observations led McClintock to an intense genetic and cytological analysis from which she concluded that the Ds element had changed its chromosomal location. McClintock also understood that, although the chromosome with the transposed Ds did not lack a telomere, Ds breaks occurring at subsequent cycles of chromosome replication could result in the joining of the two sister chromatids at the Ds insertion site. This generated a dicentric chromosome, which subsequently continued the breakage-fusion-bridge cycle, accounting for the sequential loss of markers observed in the initial odd kernels.

Ds and mutable genes: Although McClintock believed that the response of Ds to Ac and the behavior of the new Ac-controlled mutable alleles were more than coincidentally similar, the relationship was not clear. McClintock's newly isolated mutations shared certain characteristics of the mutable genes studied by both Emerson and Rhoades. Particularly striking was the parallel with Rhoades' Dt-controlled mutable a_1 allele (RHOADES 1938). The solution came when McClintock realized that the Ds element could move. This conclusion emerged from analysis of one new instance of mutability at the C locus emerging in her cultures.

The new mutable allele, designated c-$m1$, arose in a chromosome that carried Ds at its original position and the wild-type C allele. McClintock's crosses revealed that chromosome breakage was now closely linked to the c-$m1$ locus, and she formulated the hypothesis that the c-$m1$ allele originated by transposition of the Ds element into or near the C locus, inactivating it. To test this hypothesis, she selected 16 fully pigmented C kernels arising at a low frequency on *c-m1* ears. Most of the plants grown from such kernels no longer showed evidence of *Ds*-type chromosome breakage. Thus, it appeared that when the *c-m1* allele mutated to the wild-type *C* allele, all evidence of the presence of *Ds* disappeared (MCCLINTOCK 1948, 1949).

Thus, the last piece of the puzzle had fallen into place, explaining the basis of the variegation phenomena that had, by then, been under genetic scrutiny for almost half a century. Unstable mutations of the type analyzed by both EMERSON (1914, 1917) and RHOADES (1938) could be understood as the result of transposable element insertions into a locus, from which it frequently transposed during development, restoring gene function. McClintock was able to make the connection between transposition of a genetic element, the *Ds* locus, and the origin of a mutable gene giving a variegated phenotype, because the particular *Ds* element she first isolated had a second property, chromosome breakage, by which she was able to track the *Ds* element independently. Many of McClintock's original *Ds* insertion mutations were not caused by chromosome-breaking *Ds* elements, which have a special structure (FEDOROFF 1989). Nonetheless, they showed the same relationship to the *Ac* element as Rhoades' *a1* mutation showed to the *Dt* locus: the mutations were unstable *only* in the presence of the second, activating locus. In both cases, the element inserted into the affected gene (*a1*, *c-m1*) was a transposition-defective element. Such mutations are stable because the defective element lacks an intact transposase gene. If supplied with transposase by an intact element at another chromosomal location, such an element can transpose, giving the characteristic variegated phenotype caused by frequent excision of the element from the gene during development.

Soon after, McClintock understood that *Ac* could itself transpose and cause insertion mutations that differed from those caused by a *Ds* element by being inherently unstable (MCCLINTOCK 1949, 1951b). McClintock further found that the dosage of the *Ac* element, as well as more subtle changes in both the *Ds* and *Ac* elements, affected both the timing and frequency of chromosome breaks and transposition (MCCLINTOCK 1949, 1951a,b). The *Ac* dosage effect is a negative one: the more copies, the greater the developmental delay in *Ac*-mediated breakage and transposition. Because *Ac* turned out to be the transposon causing pericarp variegation in Emerson's calico corn, McClintock's findings explained his puzzling observation that there is an inverse relationship between the amount of somatic reversion and the number of copies of the P^{vv} gene (EMERSON 1929).

In contemporary terms, the *Ac* element is a small transposon (4.5 kb) and encodes a single protein, its transposase (FEDOROFF 1989). *Ds* elements are often, although by no means always, internally deleted derivatives of an *Ac* element. There are many additional, structurally different transposons that are mobilized by the *Ac* element. Some share little sequence identity with *Ac*

save the 11-bp terminal inverted repetitions and some subterminal transposase binding sites. By contrast, all *Ac* elements so far isolated are virtually identical in sequence. The chromosome-breaking *Ds* originally identified by McClintock has a unique structure: it consists of two short *Ds* elements that comprise the ends of *Ac*, one inserted in inverted order almost precisely into the middle of the other (FEDOROFF 1989). The ability of this *Ds* element to break chromosomes is related to its replication mechanism and the presence of both ends of the element in both orientations within its structure (ENGLISH *et al.* 1995). Deletion of part of this element can markedly change the timing and frequency of chromosome breakage without abolishing the ability of the element to transpose (FEDOROFF 1989). Most *Ds* and all *Ac* elements are simple in their structure and rarely or never break chromosomes.

As noted above, the element causing instability of the pericarp locus in Emerson's strains and named *Mp* by Brink and his colleagues is the same as *Ac* (BRINK and NILAN 1952; FEDOROFF 1989). Emerson's original observations that a somatic reversion event was almost always stable, except for the occasional reappearance of variegating kernels, probably find their explanation in the observation that *Ac* elements have a propensity to transpose to nearby sites, from which they can, once again, transpose back into the locus of origin (GREENBLATT and BRINK 1962, 1963; GREENBLATT 1984; CHEN *et al.* 1992; MORENO *et al.* 1992). Similarly, chromosome breakage can persist after a chromosome-breaking *Ds* transposes away from a gene if it reinserts nearby on the same chromosome.

Rhoades had identified a different transposon family. The autonomous element of this family, *Dt*, mobilizes a nonautonomous 704-bp element inserted in the A_1 gene to give the *a1* allele (BROWN *et al.* 1989). His suggestion that "the *Dt* gene produces some chemical substance that accelerates the mutation rate of *a1*" appears prophetic in retrospect (RHOADES 1938, p. 395). The "substance" is, of course, transposase, the transposon-encoded protein that is required for transposition and that the intact element *Dt* supplies to the defective element inserted in the *a1* allele. Because of the nature of the mutation that he analyzed, Rhoades was able to go well beyond Emerson's insights and set the stage for McClintock. Rhoades' observation that a second gene was required for instability was very much in McClintock's awareness and important to her growing understanding of transposition as she analyzed chromosome breakage at *Ds* and the mutability of the *c-m1 Ds* insertion mutation, both of which depended on a supply of *Ac*-encoded transposase.

LITERATURE CITED

BRINK, R. A., and R. A. NILAN, 1952 The relation between light variegated and medium variegated pericarp in maize. Genetics **37**: 519–544.

Brown, J. J., M. G. Mattes, C. O'Reilly and N. S. Shepherd, 1989 Molecular characterization of *rDt*, a maize transposon of the "*Dotted*" controlling element system. Mol. Gen. Genet. **215:** 239–244.

Chen, J., I. M. Greenblatt and S. L. Dellaporta, 1992 Molecular analysis of *Ac* transposition and DNA replication. Genetics **130:** 665–676.

Correns, C., 1910 Der Übergang aus dem homozygotischen in einen heterozygotischen Zustand im selben Individuum bei buntblättrigen und gestreifblühenden *Mirabilis*-Sippen. Ber. Dtsch. Bot. Ges. **28:** 418–434.

Demerec, M., 1928a The behavior of mutable genes, pp. 183–193 in *Verhandlungen des V. internationalen Kongresses für Vererbungswissenschaft.*

Demerec, M., 1928b Mutable characters of *Drosophila virilis*. I. Reddish-alpha body character. Genetics **14:** 359–388.

Demerec, M., 1929 Genetic factors stimulating mutability of the miniature-gamma wing character of *Drosophila virilis*. Proc. Natl. Acad. Sci. USA **15:** 834–838.

Demerec, M., 1931 Behavior of two mutable genes of *Delphinium ajacis*. J. Genet. **24:** 179–193.

Demerec, M., 1935 Unstable genes. Bot. Rev. **1:** 233–248.

de Vries, H., 1905 *Species and Varieties: Their Origin by Mutation.* Open Court Publishing, Chicago.

East, E. M., and H. K. Hayes, 1911 *Inheritance in Maize*, Vol. 167. Bul. Conn. Agr. Expt. Sta.

Emerson, R. A., 1914 The inheritance of a recurring somatic variation in variegated ears of maize. Am. Nat. **48:** 87–115.

Emerson, R. A., 1917 Genetical studies of variegated pericarp in maize. Genetics **2:** 1–35.

Emerson, R. A., 1918 A fifth pair of factors A a for aleurone color in maize and its relation to the C c and R r pairs. Cornell Univ. Agric. Exp. Stn. Mem. **16:** 225–289.

Emerson, R. A., 1929 The frequency of somatic mutation in variegated pericarp of maize. Genetics **14:** 488–511.

English, J. J., K. Harrison and J. D. G. Jones, 1995 Aberrant transpositions of maize double *Ds*-like elements usually involve *Ds* ends on sister chromatids. Plant Cell **7:** 1235–1247.

Fedoroff, N., 1989 Maize transposable elements, pp. 375–411 in *Mobile DNA*, edited by M. Howe and D. Berg. American Society for Microbiology, Washington, D.C.

Fedoroff, N., 1994 Barbara McClintock (June 16, 1902–September 1, 1992). Genetics **136:** 1-10.

Goldschmidt, R., 1938 *Physiological Genetics.* McGraw-Hill, New York.

Greenblatt, I. M., 1984 A chromosome replication pattern deduced from pericarp phenotypes resulting from movements of the transposable element, *Modulator*, in maize. Genetics **108:** 471–485.

Greenblatt, I. M., and R. A. Brink, 1962 Twin mutations in medium variegated pericarp maize. Genetics **47:** 489–501.

Greenblatt, I. M., and R. A. Brink, 1963 Transpositions of *Modulator* in maize into divided and undivided chromosome segments. Nature **197:** 412–413.

McClintock, B., 1938 The fusion of broken ends of sister half-chromatids following chromatid breakage at meiotic anaphases. MO Agric. Exp. Stn. Res. Bull. **290:** 1–48.

McClintock, B., 1939 The behavior in successive nuclear divisions of a chromosome broken at meiosis. Proc. Natl. Acad. Sci. USA **25:** 405–416.

McClintock, B., 1941a The association of mutants with homozygous deficiencies in *Zea mays*. Genetics **26:** 542–571.

McClintock, B., 1941b The stability of broken ends of chromosomes in *Zea mays*. Genetics **26:** 234–282.

McClintock, B., 1942a The fusion of broken ends of chromosomes following nuclear fusion. Proc. Natl. Acad. Sci. USA **11:** 458–463.

McClintock, B., 1942b Maize genetics. Carnegie Inst. Wash. Year Book **41:** 181–186.

McClintock, B., 1943 Maize genetics. Carnegie Inst. Wash. Year Book **42:** 148–152.

McClintock, B., 1945 Cytogenetic studies of maize and Neurospora. Carnegie Inst. Wash. Year Book **44:** 108–112.

McClintock, B., 1946 Maize genetics. Carnegie Inst. Wash. Year Book **45:** 176–186.

McClintock, B., 1947 Cytogenetic studies of maize and Neurospora. Carnegie Inst. Wash. Year Book **46:** 146–152.

McClintock, B., 1948 Mutable loci in maize. Carnegie Inst. Wash. Year Book **47:** 155–169.

McClintock, B., 1949 Mutable loci in maize. Carnegie Inst. Wash. Year Book **48:** 142–154.

McClintock, B., 1951a Chromosome organization and genic expression. Cold Spring Harbor Symp. Quant. Biol. **16:** 13–47.

McClintock, B., 1951b Mutable loci in maize. Carnegie Inst. Wash. Year Book **50:** 174–181.

Moreno, M. A., J. Chen, I. Greenblatt and S. L. Dellaporta, 1992 Reconstitutional mutagenesis of the maize *P* gene by short-range *Ac* transpositions. Genetics **131:** 939–956.

Plough, H. H., and C. F. Holthausen, 1937 A case of high mutation frequency without environmental change. Am. Nat. **71:** 185–187.

Rhoades, M. M., 1936 The effect of varying gene dosage on aleurone colour in maize. J. Genet. **33:** 347–354.

Rhoades, M. M., 1938 Effect of the *Dt* gene on the mutability of the *a₁* allele in maize. Genetics **23:** 377–397.

Rhoades, M. M., 1941 The genetic control of mutability in maize. Cold Spring Harbor Symp. Quant. Biol. **9:** 138–144.

Schwartz, D., 1993 Marcus M. Rhoades (1903–1991). Genetics **133:** 1–3.

Stern, C., 1935 The behavior of unstable loci—an hypothesis. Proc. Natl. Acad. Sci. USA **21:** 202–208.

Lionel Sharples Penrose, 1898–1972
A Personal Memoir in Celebration
of the Centenary of His Birth

Renata Laxova

Department of Pediatrics and Medical Genetics, Waisman Center, University of Wisconsin–Madison, Madison, Wisconsin 53706

I T is Friday, mid-morning. You are about to leave the city for a long weekend in the country when you find yourself opening your front door to four bedraggled political refugees. It is difficult for you even to recognize the weary man, woman, and two girls as people whose casual acquaintance you had made on a single previous occasion about 2 months ago, during a brief 3-day work-related visit to their country. You invite them in, show them around and, 15 minutes later, the dazed visitors, now ensconced in your home, are waving good-bye to you as you leave for your weekend in the country.

How many people are there among us who would be willing to entrust their homes, in their absence, to practically complete strangers arriving on their doorstep from a foreign country?

Penrose, the man: That morning in late August 1968, in answer to my telephone call intended merely to inform them that we had escaped from our country, which had been invaded by Soviet forces, Lionel and Margaret Penrose invited my husband, daughters, and me for what we thought would be a polite cup of tea. They met us at the door and, to our amazement, instead of a handshake they handed us their house keys, their only set; characteristically, the spare keys were nowhere to be found. Before they drove off waving breezily, and before we realized what was happening, Margaret managed to show me how to prevent the hot water system from exploding and the contents of the linen closet from toppling over and to give me instructions for Mrs. Lee, the cleaning lady, who was apparently expected to arrive at the house at the beginning of the week. Lionel rather nonchalantly provided my husband with what he called "a few useful telephone numbers"! Subsequently, we found that they enabled us to apply for permission to stay in Britain and to obtain work permits and alien

cards. The children were given books and within 5 minutes were engrossed in some of Lionel's handmade wooden puzzles.

We had met Professor Lionel (Figure 1) and Dr. Margaret Penrose for the first time during a brief working weekend in Brno, Czechoslovakia, the city where Mendel had made his discoveries. The Prof, as we later affectionately learned to call him, gave some talks; we showed him Mendel's monastery and museum, his garden, archives, and documents; and one evening we took them to the opera. That, at the time of our arrival in London, was the extent of our acquaintance with the Penrose family.

In spite of the season (it was August) Lionel and Margaret were both wearing overcoats when they met us at the door. During the three months we lived at 1 Rodborough Road in Golders Green (north London), we found that they frequently wore thick coats in the house to keep warm. It was not until after the Professor's death in 1972 that the large family house was converted into flats and central heating was installed. Thus, it was not unusual to see Lionel spending the afternoon in his study standing at his desk, notebook in hand, peering over his glasses at a problem, coat collar turned up, looking as if he had just arrived or was about to leave. It was in that study where his well-known "reproducible machines" had been constructed (PENROSE and PENROSE 1957) and where he created multiple wooden and other puzzles, among them *Puzzles for Christmas*, published together with son Roger (PENROSE and PENROSE 1958), their purpose "to provide mental stimulation during the academic vacation." The publication included the "impossible staircase," a famous theme in the work of Dutch artist Max Escher; it was the Penroses who, in correspondence with him, had given Escher the idea.

One evening in late autumn, the Prof and I happened to answer the front doorbell simultaneously. A strange young man with a foreign accent thanked us politely and headed confidently past us, into the hall and up

Address for correspondence: Departments of Pediatrics and Medical Genetics, Waisman Center, 1500 Highland Ave., University of Wisconsin, Madison, WI 53706.

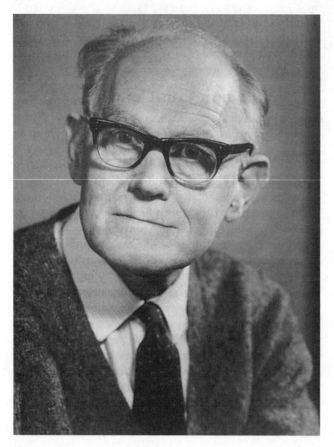

FIGURE 1.—Lionel Sharples Penrose, photograph about 1971. Photo by Godfrey Argent.

the stairs. In answer to the Prof's rather diffident question, he announced that he had lived in the house for over two weeks. He had met Mrs. Penrose in the street late one night and inquired about an address in the neighborhood where a room was available for rent. Rather than give him the complicated directions he sought, she invited him to stay at Rodborough Road. The trivial matter of informing her husband had slipped Margaret's mind.

On another evening during that same fall, the Prof knocked on the door of our room and invited me to his study. Someone wanted to meet me, he said. As I entered, he introduced me simply by my first name. A tall, slender woman came toward me with outstretched arms and, with tears in her eyes, embraced me warmly. I knew I had never seen her before, nor did I recognize either of her two male companions. "So fortunate, my dear," she said, noticing my completely bewildered and uncomprehending facial expression, "that Lionel has such a good memory. You see, I remembered the 'Renata' part and wondered whether it could possibly be you, but it was Lionel who knew your maiden name and so, of course, it *had* to be you!" I learned that the three visitors, like Lionel, his parents, and his family, were longstanding members of the Society of Friends (Quakers). It was they who in 1939 had organized the publica-

tion of a little booklet through which they appealed to their members and other British families to take care of a child seeking refuge from Hitler-occupied Europe. My photograph, at age 7, had been among those in the booklet. Twenty-nine years later Professor Penrose and his visitors recognized my somewhat uncommon name and realized that I had been among the hundreds of children for whom a British home had been found during World War II and whose lives they had helped to save.

Lionel Sharples Penrose was born on June 11, 1898, the second of four brothers. His father was an artist (a portrait painter); one of his brothers was a sailor, and another, Roland, was also an artist and according to family legend introduced Britain to the work of Picasso. For that, Lionel would later quip, Roland was knighted by the Queen. Lionel, the most academically minded of the four, studied the Moral Sciences Tripos (mathematics, philosophy, and psychology) at Cambridge; later, after spending a year in Vienna where he met and explored the work of Freud, Wagner-Jauregg, and others, he became interested in the psychology of mental illness and mental deficiency. However, to learn more thoroughly about brain physiology, Penrose realized that he needed to obtain a degree in medicine. He returned to Cambridge in the late twenties. His subsequent M.D. thesis and his interest in psychiatry resulted in an appointment in 1930 to the position of Research Medical Officer at the Royal Eastern Counties Institution, a residential facility for what was then called the "mentally defective" population. Penrose's charge was to study the causes of mental retardation, with funding provided by the Medical Research Council and the Darwin Trust.

The Colchester Survey, 1931–38: The Royal Eastern Counties Institution was located in Colchester in southeastern England, and Penrose's work there culminated in the incomparable classic, *The Colchester Survey: An Etiological Study of 1280 Cases of Mental Defect*, which became the basis for his lifelong work (PENROSE 1938). His basic concept was that mental retardation (MR) and illness are biologically, not socially, determined. Hence his book *Mental Defect* (PENROSE 1933a) and later three editions of *The Biology of Mental Defect*, the last in 1972 (PENROSE 1972), are unsurpassed in their time for the wealth of original scientific, biological, and genetic information that they contained.

The Colchester Survey included evaluations not only of the residents of the institution but of both parents and siblings whenever available. It took 7 years to complete and contributed an enormous amount to knowledge about multiple aspects of mental retardation, most of which applies to this day. The work was done predominantly by Penrose and one co-worker, Miss D. A. Newlyn; it was prepared for publication by his devoted, loyal, erstwhile secretary, typist of manuscripts, later co-worker, editor, and Cerberus of the office, Miss Helen

Lang-Brown. Every family of the 1280 residents of the institution was visited personally, sometimes more than once; family medical histories were obtained, records reviewed, and IQs tested in every available relative. There were 6629 siblings in addition to parents and other family members. The residents were carefully examined clinically by Penrose himself in an attempt to determine the causes of intellectual impairment in each individual. The end of the survey contains an appendix (still useful) providing detailed information about each of the 1280 propositi and their families. The most important conclusions include the predominance of males among the mentally retarded population, caused in large part, as we now know, by several genes on the X chromosome; the heterogeneous underlying causes of mental defect; the absence of any strict dividing line between mental retardation and "normal" intellectual functioning; the demonstration of the role of environmental as well as genetic factors in the occurrence of certain types of mental retardation (including Down syndrome); and the more frequent recurrence of mental deficiency among children of mildly as opposed to more severely retarded parents. Reproduction among the latter is rare, and causes of severe MR are often *de novo* chromosomal abnormalities or other spontaneous events.

The significance of increased maternal age in families of patients with Down syndrome, which is perhaps among Penrose's best-known discoveries, was mentioned briefly in the Colchester Survey, as were many other topics that subsequently formed the subjects of separate publications in which they were explored in greater detail. For example, the 20 patients at Colchester who had epiloia, or tuberous sclerosis (TS) as it is now better known (an autosomal dominant neurocutaneous disorder characterized by skin changes, seizures, usually benign tumors, and mental retardation), became the basis for the observation by Penrose not only of variable expression in multiple affected members within a single family, but also for one of the first direct estimates of mutation rate in humans. In considering variable expression, Penrose postulated that there had to be "modifier" genes at different loci that altered the expression in different family members. He also observed some individuals who had no other affected relatives within their family, and he suggested that this could be the result of a "fresh" mutation. As the incidence of TS in the mentally retarded population was estimated to be around 1 in 300 and the incidence of MR in the general population about 1%, the incidence of TS in the general population was about 1 in 30,000. In Penrose's study, about one-quarter to one-half of the patients had no affected family members; thus, perhaps the new mutation rate was around 1/240,000 to 1/120,000. This was reported in a joint, now classical paper with Penrose's scientific idol, colleague, and predecessor in the Galton Chair at University College, London, J. B. S. Haldane, who had calculated the mutation rate in hemophilia by the indirect method (HALDANE and PENROSE 1935).

The discovery by Fölling in 1934 of imbecillitas phenylpyruvica, or phenylketonuria (PKU), the designation suggested by Penrose's co-worker, J. H. Quastel, led Penrose to search for patients with the disorder at Colchester. Aware of the characteristic "mousy" odor surrounding such patients, he would visit a room full of residents at any institution for the retarded, look around, sniff for a while, and head straight toward a patient who was usually—though, as Penrose carefully noted, not always—blue eyed and light haired and sitting in a bent-over position, with stereotypic busy "shoe-maker-like" hand movements that distinguished him or her from those around. Since the metabolic block was known to be at the level of phenylalanine, one of the precursors of melanin, patients with PKU were initially thought to be fair skinned and blue eyed because of melanin deficiency. Penrose stressed, however, that since phenylalanine was not the only precursor of melanin and collateral pathways resulted in at least its partial production, the lighter coloring of patients with PKU was due only to a dilution of pigment compared with the rest of their family, not to its complete absence. He was among the first to suggest a diet of fruit, sugar, olive oil, and vitamins to treat it. It led to malnutrition, however, and had to be abandoned. It was at that time that he established, on the basis of several families with similarly affected siblings and one with consanguinity, that PKU was caused by an autosomal recessive gene (PENROSE 1935).

Down syndrome, other aneuploidy, and dermato-glyphics: It was also at Colchester that Penrose's interest in people with Down syndrome was first aroused. They were easily recognizable and formed a more homogeneous group than many others who had mental retardation. The diagnosis was more common than any other and, above all, Penrose enjoyed these patients. He enjoyed their affection for him, and when they could speak, they called him by name. He never ceased to be amused by a story that he told repeatedly about a man with Down syndrome who lived at Harperbury Hospital, where Penrose worked after retirement. The man was walking along the drive and exclaimed to Penrose, with whom he was chatting, "Look, Dr. Penrose, there's another mongol like me, and over there, there are two—they must be bigols!"

There were 63 people in the Colchester Survey who had Down syndrome, and for the rest of his life Penrose studied them and the causes of their condition. Other families with members who had Down syndrome were also included in his investigations. He had initially found that there was a significant correlation between increased maternal and paternal ages and the birth of infants with Down syndrome. However, when he patterned his analysis after that employed by Sewall Wright to assess the causes of polydactyly in guinea pigs (WRIGHT 1926), Penrose determined that there was a highly significant partial correlation between maternal but not paternal age and the occurrence of Down syndrome. To confirm this conclusion further, Penrose used regression analysis to compare paternal and maternal ages, as well as mean maternal and paternal ages at the time of birth of Down syndrome and other offspring within families. After correction for parental age correlations, he found no significant difference between the means of observed and expected paternal ages at the birth of infants with Down syndrome and of other offspring, whereas the difference of the same parameters between those observed and expected for maternal ages was six times the standard error (PENROSE 1933b). He showed that birth order, parity, and length of interval between pregnancies were not significant etiological factors.

Some 30 years later, after the discovery of chromosomal translocations, Penrose returned to his exploration of recurrence risks for Down syndrome within families. He studied "21/D" and "21/G" translocations and subsequently found that the maternal age effect did not apply to either of them. Moreover, he continued to be puzzled by the presence within some families of more than one person with nontranslocational standard Trisomy 21 and apparently normal parental chromosomes. It was Penrose's suggestion that mosaicism could perhaps account for these instances. He studied the dermatoglyphics of such parents, and by comparing them statistically with those in their offspring with Down syndrome, as well as with those in the general population, he concluded that about 10% of mothers of single children with Down syndrome and perhaps 50% of those with more than one were mosaic for Trisomy 21, even in the absence of other phenotypic or intellectual characteristics (BARNICOT et al. 1963).

In 1971, one of Penrose's young co-workers, Peter Ohara (hired as an electron microscopy technician) was the first to observe neurofibrillary tangles in the brains of deceased patients with Down syndrome. Penrose of course immediately noted the connection with similar findings in patients with Alzheimer disease (OHARA 1972). Penrose's lifelong interest in Down syndrome is carefully documented in both editions of the classic, Down's Anomaly (PENROSE and SMITH 1966; SMITH and BERG 1976).

The first instance of human double aneuploidy was described in 1959, shortly after Lejeune's report of Trisomy 21 in a patient who had both Klinefelter and Down syndromes (FORD et al. 1959). Penrose's curiosity about human malformation resulted in the observation of the first instance of human triploidy in an aborted fetus and, astonishingly, in the discovery of a 4-year-old girl with hemihypertrophy and few other physical characteristics who had triploidy in 30% of her blood cells (PENROSE 1963a).

His continuous search for objective quantification whenever possible resulted in a related area of interest, which, like Down syndrome, was also to last for the rest of his life—namely, dermatoglyphics, a science that Penrose considered ideal for the study of normal and pathological variation within and between human and other populations. He contributed more to this area than anyone else in the world, but as the study of dermatoglyphics is rarely used in the current highly technological climate of medicine, I do not discuss it here. Suffice it to say that his most significant contribution was probably the discovery of a negative correlation between the number of X chromosomes and the total dermal ridge count. In other words, he found that, for example, infants with Turner syndrome (a chromosomal complement of $45,X$) had the highest ridge count, whereas those with $49,XXXXX$ had the lowest (PENROSE 1968).

Paternal age effects: The effects of parental age upon the occurrence of abnormalities in offspring never ceased to intrigue Penrose. It was Weinberg who first noted the phenomenon in 1912, and there were others who suggested that it was the father's not the mother's age that played a significant role in the occurrence of infants with, for example, achondroplasia. However, it was Penrose who, again using the partial correlation method employed by Wright, provided the data to prove the hypothesis. His results were a mirror image of those found in families with Down syndrome. In other words, if the maternal age was kept constant, a significantly positive correlation (+0.273) was found between the paternal age and the incidence of achondroplasia, whereas the maternal age effect disappeared completely if the paternal age was regressed out. Furthermore, Penrose noted that the statistical significance of the paternal age effect increased considerably when nonsurviving infants with achondroplasia were excluded from the calculations (PENROSE 1955, 1957). It is possible, although no proof exists from the old data, that the infants with "achondroplasia" who died neonatally or shortly thereafter had different diagnoses of more severe, perhaps lethal, short-limbed dwarfing disorders. The survivors represented true instances of new (paternally derived) mutations of the gene.

Together with Haldane, Penrose also studied the paternal age effect upon mutations of genes located on the X chromosome. Haldane had accurately postulated an increased occurrence of hemophilia in the grandsons of older maternal grandfathers, implying another example of a higher mutation rate in males. Four decades later, it was Crow who finally completed the story by summarizing data showing that, at the molecular level, the rate for base substitutions (the cause of the achondroplasia mutation) is indeed higher in males than in females; he also showed that the phenomenon can be attributed partially to the larger number of cell divisions, estimated to be about 430 at age 30 in the male, as contrasted with the female germ line, in whom there are only about 24 divisions from zygote to egg (CROW 1997a,b). More specifically, the mutation in achondroplasia, in the fibroblast growth factor receptor 3 gene (*FGFR3*) on *4p16.3*, consists of a single substitution of the normal glycine residue by an arginine residue at codon 380. This same Gly380Arg mutation is, surprisingly, present in almost all of the hundreds of patients with achondroplasia who have had mutational analysis to date, and it is of paternal origin in those in which the parental origin could be determined (HORTON 1997). Thus, we owe our understanding of the paternal age factor, its causes as well as underlying mechanisms, to the imaginatively creative minds of three generations of genetics heroes.

Mental illness, 1939–45: As a member of the Society of Friends, Penrose was a conscientious objector and, although he had driven a Red Cross ambulance during World War I and helped to rescue many wounded soldiers from the trenches, it was not a period in his life that he particularly enjoyed discussing. In 1939, after completion and publication of the Colchester Survey and at the beginning of World War II, Lionel, Margaret, and their then three children, Oliver, Roger, and Jonathan, emigrated to London, Ontario, where they stayed for the next 6 years. All three sons, as well as their younger sister, Shirley, born after the war, have made remarkable contributions to science in their respective fields. Oliver, a Fellow of the Royal Society (FRS), is a professor of mathematics and physics; Roger, also a third-generation FRS (after his father and maternal grandfather), now knighted, received the Field prize for mathematics at a very early age; Jonathan, a professor of psychology, was the British chess champion for 10 consecutive years; and Shirley is a distinguished pediatrician and clinical geneticist.

After the arrival of the family in London, Ontario, Penrose was appointed to the position of Director of Psychiatric Research for the Province of Ontario. He gathered data on some 1600 patients, their ages at onset of mental disease, parental ages at birth and onset of disease if applicable, medical histories, and IQs. He used his own nonverbal "pattern perception" test to discriminate between mentally ill and otherwise affected individuals and to compare parent and offspring IQs. These and other data from the Canadian years, published in meticulous tables and appendices, have become the basis for recent studies on evidence for paternal transmission and anticipation in schizophrenia (BASSETT *et al.* 1997).

The Galton Chair, 1945–65: After the war, Penrose was appointed to the Galton Chair of Eugenics and to the directorship of the Galton Laboratory at University College, London. The professional pedigree of the chair was auspicious. Established by Francis Galton in 1911, it was first occupied by Karl Pearson until 1933, when he was succeeded by R. A. Fisher, who held it until 1943. At that time J. B. S. Haldane, who had been head of

the Department of Biometry since 1935, became the head of a united department of Biometry and Eugenics, with Penrose in the Galton Chair from 1945 until his retirement in 1965 at age 67. In 1957, when Haldane moved to India, Penrose became the head of a department called Eugenics, Biometry, and Genetics. He hated the word Eugenics and the philosophies with which it had become synonymous. He said it was "irksome" to be the head of a department of Eugenics and to edit a journal with Eugenics in its title without ever studying or writing a word about eugenics! But it was not until 1954 that he succeeded in officially changing the title of the journal he edited from *Annals of Eugenics* to *Annals of Human Genetics*, and it was only in 1963 that his chair finally became the Galton Professorship of Human Genetics.

The group assembled around Penrose and Haldane in the '50s and '60s, which included several brilliant, enthusiastic, and self-motivated young postdocs, became the future founders of British, European, and some American medical genetics dynasties. A possible reason for this was that Penrose was among the first geneticists of his generation to be medically qualified; hence many of the topics that he selected for study had future medical implications. So, for example, Harry Harris, Penrose's successor to the Galton chair, used paper chromatography as well as gel electrophoresis in the early days to study normal and abnormal polymorphisms in human blood and urine.

Cedric A. B. Smith, the humblest of individuals, was a brilliant mathematician and, according to Penrose, was the firm base upon which the post-war laboratory's reputation was built. For example, Penrose and Smith together simplified the "discriminant function" method of Fisher, conventionally used to discriminate between two populations on the basis of measured characteristics (PENROSE 1945). The older method was cumbersome and required the inversion of the variance-covariance matrix, a calculation that even today is accomplished by computer (then unavailable). Penrose, with Smith (although each gave the other the major credit), devised a method whereby no matrix inversion was required, only a calculation of the difference D between the population means. The loss of efficiency was small (when based on assumptions of normality of distribution). In a later paper, PENROSE (1954) pointed out that the generalized distance between two populations was (approximately) simply the sum of the "size distance" and "shape distance."

Always interested in family as well as population investigations and their formal mathematical analysis, Penrose strongly encouraged linkage exploration despite, as he wrote, "discouraging odds against finding evidence for two genes on the same human autosome" (PENROSE 1967). Three linkages were established in relatively rapid succession, including that by Jan Mohr of Denmark (Lutheran blood groups and secretor status), Sylvia Lawler and Jim Renwick (nail patella syndrome and ABO blood types), and Elizabeth Robson and Harry Harris (transferrin and serum cholinesterase).

Birth weight was another quantifiable, ubiquitous, and variable parameter, applicable to individuals and families, as well as populations, and therefore another obvious target for Penrose's curiosity. Together with M. N. Karn and others, he collected an enormous quantity of data and attempted to correlate birth weight and parity, length of gestation, maternal (and paternal) age, infant survival, etc. They established, among other findings, a genetic tendency toward high (10 lb or more) birth weight in some families (KARN and PENROSE 1961).

Julia Bell, one of Penrose's co-workers at the Galton Laboratory, was a population geneticist interested in the genetics of human disease. She analyzed data from families with dystrophia myotonica (DM) and other diseases (BELL 1947). Although Penrose had great respect for his elder colleague and visited her regularly late into her 90s, he disagreed with her conclusions, which indicated increasing severity and earlier age of onset in successive generations of families with DM. This concept, known as anticipation and defined as a process of progressive worsening of hereditary disease in successive generations, with an earlier onset in offspring than in parents, was initially considered by Penrose to be an artifact of ascertainment rather than a phenomenon of direct biological significance (PENROSE 1948). It took over 40 years to provide one mechanistic explanation of anticipation. It can be explained by unstable DNA, consisting of trinucleotide repeats that increase in number in some families in successive generations and sometimes correlate with the severity and earlier age of onset of disease (SUTHERLAND and RICHARDS 1992).

On the other hand, a myth about Y-linked inheritance really did exist and, before 1958 when Penrose and Curt Stern dispelled it (PENROSE and STERN 1958), it was mentioned in genetics texts as the only example of that form of inheritance in men. It concerned a family of allegedly six consecutive generations of "porcupine" men (the Lambert pedigree) whose bodies were covered with "half-inch scales," sparing face, palms, and soles. Transmission was from father to all sons, with all daughters described as unaffected. Penrose and Stern conclusively showed that the actual family consisted of four, not six, generations with both affected and unaffected males and females and that the disorder, known as ichthyosis hystrix gravior, was inherited through a mutant autosomal dominant, not a Y-linked, gene.

In June 1948, Penrose gave a presentation to a cancer symposium in London on the genetics of breast cancer (PENROSE et al. 1948). He recognized the advantages of studying breast as opposed to other cancers, because it was more easily and accurately diagnosed than other primary tumors. It was common, of public health significance, and accounted for almost 3% of female deaths. Finally, it presented a mathematical and statistical challenge that Penrose addressed with a characteristically simple, yet logical approach.

In spite of the existence of compelling evidence in the form of three- and four-generation pedigrees, previous investigators had been unable to demonstrate a definitive hereditary component in breast cancer. Penrose and co-workers compared deaths from cancer (breast and otherwise) in the relatives of a series of 510 propositae, with the rate by age given in statistics for the general population (available in England and Wales since 1911), thus avoiding the need for a control group. Their second purpose was to attempt to determine the type of inheritance and to rule in or out the possibility of transmission through maternal milk or cytoplasm. Results showed that within the families of the propositae, the same disease occurred with significantly increased frequency in sisters and mothers (and one brother), as compared with the general population. The rate of non-mammary malignant disease was not significantly increased among relatives. The study concludes with an appendix, still useful today, that lists all 510 propositae (by number) with detailed three-generation family histories of breast cancer, including laterality (also found to be genetically determined), pathology, age of onset, and death.

During the Galton Laboratory years, Penrose's overriding interest was the study of patients with mental retardation. He "adopted" one of the large residential institutions for the mentally retarded, Harperbury Hospital, which was located northwest of London in what was then quite seriously called London's "lunatic fringe," now the "green belt." Such institutions were situated in all four directions from the center of London, hence the horrifying term. Harperbury had 1600–1800 residents, two-thirds of whom were male, and it was always Penrose's dream to be located in their midst so that he could study and evaluate them in individual detail.

In 1963, he received an international award from the Joseph P. Kennedy Jr. Foundation for his contributions to the study of mental retardation. He received the award from President Johnson personally in November 1963, shortly after the assassination of John F. Kennedy. A delightful handwritten account exists, entitled "Three trains, three planes, a ship and an etched piece of glass with a silver stand," in which he recorded his impressions of the voyage to America on the Queen Elizabeth II with Margaret and of the ceremony itself.

Issues of social and ethical importance were never far from Penrose's thoughts. Using sound mathematical reasoning, he rarely missed an opportunity for debate with his enthusiastic, eugenically minded peers about their erroneous conceptions of the proliferation of the poor, the mentally ill, and the retarded (e.g., PENROSE 1963b). He also studied crowd behavior and mass hysteria, mostly in connection with the Russian Revolution of 1917 or pre- and "peri"-war Nazi Germany. He sum-

had one vote each. Disregarding votes per capita, which would give no power whatsoever to small countries, Penrose proposed a simple model whereby the power of representative voters was inversely proportional to the square root of the total number of voters in each country. Iceland, Switzerland, and India would then have 1, 3, and 19 votes, respectively, while the United States and (then) Soviet Union would each have 13–14 (PENROSE 1961).

The Kennedy-Galton Centre, 1965–72: When at age 67 he had reached the age of mandatory retirement from University College, Lionel finally saw the realization of his old dream. With the money from the Kennedy award, he established a laboratory and clinic within the grounds of Harperbury Hospital, which he named the Kennedy-Galton Centre for Mental Deficiency Research and Diagnosis.

Penrose's presence at Harperbury was of enormous benefit to the residents and their families, and a more sophisticated replica of the Colchester Survey with clinical, chromosomal, dermatoglyphic, biochemical, and other analyses was completed. It included a study of all females within the institution who had reproduced (1%) and of their offspring, providing a numerical estimate of empiric recurrence risks for "nonspecific" mental retardation, as well as an attempt at a comparable etiologic survey of mental retardation in the school-aged population outside the institution.

The Kennedy-Galton Centre became a mecca for visiting physicians and scientists. All were taken on an educational tour of the residents and acquainted first with them personally and second with their diagnoses. The patients, in turn, enjoyed a great deal of attention, and many of them began to exhibit skills (social, verbal, physical) that had previously not been observed in them.

The most famous of all, however, was Burt, the man with 48 chromosomes who had Klinefelter and Down syndromes. Everyone who came to visit Penrose was first taken to visit Burt to have a discussion about politics. He was the only son of parents who were academics and intellectuals. During our home visit with them, they confessed sadly that in the past they had had dreams for their son who, one day, could become a famous scientist or artist and make a contribution to the world. Instead, he would end his life, forgotten and unknown, in an institution for the retarded. At a memorial symposium for Penrose in the Hague in the fall of 1972, I

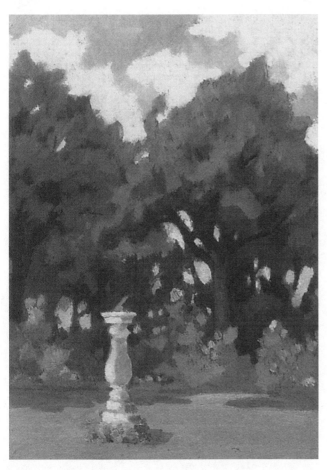

FIGURE 2.—Oil painting on wood of the grounds of the country house in Thorrington, by Penrose.

marized his ideas in a monograph entitled, characteristically, *On the Objective Study of Crowd Behavior* (PENROSE 1952). Later, he published a leaflet, *Hazards of Nuclear Tests,* urging Britain, which he described as a "country aspiring to greatness," to seize the moment and benefit humankind by abandoning its military demonstration of atomic power. In the 1930s he and Margaret had been instrumental in cofounding the Medical Association for the Prevention of War, in which both were active for the rest of their lives.

In 1961, he proposed a more equitable mechanism for representational voting, using the United Nations as a paradigm. It was unfair, he wrote, that member states like Iceland, Switzerland, and India with populations of 150,000, 5 million, and 350 million respectively,

Palindrome in F Major

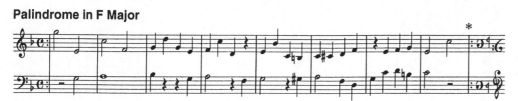

FIGURE 3.—Palindrome in F major, by Penrose.

* Turn upside down and continue.

showed a picture of Burt as an example of one of Penrose's Harperbury friends. The hum of immediate recognition was audible from the audience of some 2000 participants, and I wondered whether the picture of a famous scientist or artist would have evoked a similar reaction from an audience of comparable size. I regretted that Burt's parents were not present to witness his moment of triumph.

The Penrose family owned a lovely old Tudor house in the country in Thorrington, Suffolk, where they spent many weekends, frequently extending their exceptional hospitality to friends and visitors.

Lionel was, among other things, an accomplished artist, and the Thorrington gardens and surrounding countryside were frequent subjects for his oil paintings and his meticulous drawings (see Figure 2). He also played the piano and an antique spinet that stood in his study in Rodborough Road. He considered Bach to be the greatest of all musicians, and as, like many mathematicians, he was intimately acquainted with musical theory, he could analyze Bach's compositions with expertise, insight, and astonishing depth of knowledge. But not even music was safe from his fun-loving, irreverent mind, and his Palindrome in F major combines his ingenuity with his sense of humor (Figure 3).

He died suddenly, unexpectedly, on a Friday evening in May 1972, after having discussed his plans for next week's activities as always with the staff of the Kennedy-Galton Centre.

The 1973 monograph in the series *Biographical Memoirs of Fellows of the Royal Society* (Vol. 19, pp. 521–561) by Harry Harris, entitled *Lionel Sharples Penrose (1898–1972)*, which contains a complete Penrose bibliography, was a helpful resource in the preparation of this manuscript. Deep appreciation goes to Susan Johnson, who patiently typed and retyped with kindness, equanimity, and interest. Finally, I use this opportunity to thank Lionel, Margaret, and their four children for their contributions to the growth of my own family.

LITERATURE CITED

BARNICOT, N. A., J. R. ELLIS and L. S. PENROSE, 1963 Translocations and trisomic mongol sibs. Ann. Hum. Genet. **26:** 279–285.

BASSETT, A. S., L. SCUTT, S. CORREIA, S. KAEGI and J. HUSTED, 1997 Evidence for paternal transmission and anticipation in schizophrenia (Abstr. 1774). Am. J. Hum. Genet. **61**(Suppl.): 4.

BELL, J., 1947 Dystrophia myotonica and allied diseases, pp. 343–410 in *The Treasury of Human Inheritance IV: Nervous Diseases and Muscular Dystrophies*, Chap. 5. Cambridge University Press, London.

CROW, J. F., 1997a The high spontaneous mutation rate: is it a health risk? Proc. Natl. Acad. Sci. USA **94:** 8380–8386.

CROW, J. F., 1997b Molecular evolution—who is in the driver's seat? Nat. Genet. **17:** 129–130.

FORD, C. E., K. W. JONES, J. J. MILLER, U. MITTWOCH, L. S. PENROSE *et al.*, 1959 The chromosomes in a patient showing both mongolism and the Klinefelter syndrome. Lancet **1:** 709–710.

HALDANE, J. B. S., and L. S. PENROSE, 1935 Mutation rates in man. Nature **135:** 907–908.

HORTON, W. A., 1997 Molecular genetics of chondrodysplasias. Growth Genet. Hormones **13:** 4, 49–55.

KARN, M. N., and L. S. PENROSE, 1961 Birth weight and gestation time in relation to maternal age, parity and infant survival. Ann. Eugen. **16:** 147–164.

OHARA, P. T., 1972 Electron microscopical study of the brain in Down's syndrome. Brain **95:** 681–684.

PENROSE, L. S., 1933a *Mental Defect.* Sidgwick and Jackson, London.

PENROSE, L. S., 1933b The relative effect of paternal and maternal age in mongolism. J. Genet. **27:** 219–224.

PENROSE, L. S., 1935 Inheritance of phenylpyruvic amentia (phenylketonuria). Lancet **2:** 192–194.

PENROSE, L. S., 1938 *The Colchester Survey: A Clinical and Genetic Study of 1280 Cases of Mental Defect.* H. M. Stationery Office, Privy Council of Medical Research Council, London.

PENROSE, L. S., 1945 Discrimination between normal and psychotic subjects by revised examination. Bull. Can. Psychol. Assoc. **5:** 37–40.

PENROSE, L. S., 1948 The problem of anticipation in pedigrees of dystrophia myotonica. Ann. Eugen. **14:** 125–132.

PENROSE, L. S., 1952 *On the Objective Study of Crowd Behaviour,* Monograph. H. K. Lewis, London.

PENROSE, L. S., 1954 Distance, size and shape. Ann. Eugen. **18:** 337–343.

PENROSE, L. S., 1955 Parental age and mutation. Lancet **2:** 312–313.

PENROSE, L. S., 1957 Parental age in achondroplasia and mongolism. Am. J. Hum. Genet. **9:** 167–169.

PENROSE, L. S., 1961 Some statistical problems of majority voting. New Sci. **224:** 546–547.

PENROSE, L. S., 1963a A girl with triploid cells. Nature **198:** 411.

PENROSE, L. S., 1963b Limitations of eugenics. Proc. R. Inst. G.B. **39:** 506–519.

PENROSE, L. S., 1967 The influence of the English tradition in human genetics, pp. 13–25 in *Proceedings of the Third International Congress of Human Genetics*, edited by J. F. CROW and J. V. NEEL. Johns Hopkins Press, Baltimore.

PENROSE, L. S., 1968 Dermatoglyphics and mental retardation. Proceedings of the 1st Congress of the International Society for the Scientific Study of Mental Deficiency, Montpellier, France, 1967, pp. 46–55.

PENROSE, L. S., 1972 *Biology of Mental Defect*, Ed. 4. Sidgwick and Jackson, London.

PENROSE, L. S., and R. PENROSE, 1957 A self-reproducing analogue. Nature **179:** 1183.

PENROSE, L. S., and R. PENROSE, 1958 Puzzles for Christmas. New Sci. (Insert).

PENROSE, L. S., and G. F. SMITH, 1966 *Down's Anomaly.* Churchill Livingstone, London.

PENROSE, L. S., and C. STERN, 1958 Reconsideration of the Lambert pedigree (ichthyosis hystrix gravior). Ann. Hum. Genet. **22:** 3, 258–283.

PENROSE, L. S., H. J. MACKENZIE and M. N. KARN, 1948 A genetical study of human mammary cancer. Ann. Eugen. **14:** 234–266.

SMITH, G. F., and J. M. BERG, 1976 *Down's Anomaly*, Ed. 2. Churchill Livingstone, London.

SUTHERLAND, G. R., and R. I. RICHARDS, 1992 Anticipation legitimized: unstable DNA to the rescue. Am. J. Hum. Genet. **51:** 7–9.

WRIGHT, S., 1926 Effect of age of parents upon characteristics of the guinea pig. Am. Nat. **60:** 552–559.

○ **Addenda et Corrigenda** ○

○ **Author Index** ○

○ **Index** ○

Addenda et Corrigenda

Brock, Thomas D. The Value of Basic Research: Discovery of *Thermus aquaticus* and Other Extreme Thermophiles, p. 602

FURTHER REFERENCE

BROCK, T. D., 1998 Early days in Yellowstone microbiology. ASM News **64:** 137–140.

Ely, Bert and Lucy Shapiro. The Molecular Genetics of Differentiation, p. 135

In the decade since the publication of this article, tremendous progress has been made towards understanding cell cycle control and the molecular basis of cell differentiation in Caulobacter. For instance, it has been shown that histidine protein kinases and their cognate response regulators are involved in coordinating cell cycle events. Numerous components of these two-component regulatory systems have been identified and shown to be controlled both temporally and spatially. A central component of this network, the response regulator CtrA, regulates the G1-S transition and is controlled at many levels, including activation by phosphorylation, the transient binding of a CtrA kinase to the cell poles, and cell type-specific proteolysis. Furthermore, the nucleotide sequence of the entire *C. crescentus* genome is near completion, so we anticipate that progress towards understanding the regulatory circuits that control the cell cycle will accelerate dramatically.

Ganetzky, Barry. There's a Whole Lot of Shaking Going On, p. 84

Each of the other leg-shaking mutations discovered by Kaplan has now also been shown to encode a potassium channel polypeptide.

FURTHER REFERENCES

CHOUINARD, S., G. WILSON, A. K. SCHLIMGEN and B. GANETZKY, 1995 A potassium channel β subunit, related to the aldo-keto reductase superfamily, encoded by the Drosophila *Hyperkinetic* locus. Proc. Natl. Acad. Sci. USA **92:** 6763–6767.

DRYSDALE, R. A., J. W. WARMKE, R. KREBER and B. GANETZKY, 1991 Molecular characterization of *eag*, a gene affecting potassium channels in *Drosophila*. Genetics **127:** 497–505.

TRUDEAU, M. C., J. W. WARMKE, B. GANETZKY and G. A. ROBERTSON, 1995 HERG, a human inward rectifier in the voltage-gated potassium channel family. Science **269:** 92–95.

WARMKE, J. W., R. DRYSDALE and B. GANETZKY, 1991 A distinct potassium channel polypeptide encoded by the *Drosophila eag* locus. Science **252:** 1560–1562.

WARMKE, J. W., and B. GANETZKY, 1994 A family of potassium channel genes related to *eag* in Drosophila and mammals. Proc. Natl. Acad. Sci. USA **91:** 3438–3442.

Henikoff, Steven. A Reconsideration of the Mechanism of Position Effect, p. 411

The mechanism of somatic pairing is still unknown. However, structural models have gained in popularity to explain many of the numerous new examples of homology effects (reviewed by WU and MORRIS 1999). Moreover, the notion that pairing underlies heterochromatin formation has received support from reports of homology-dependent transgene silencing in a variety of eukaryotes, suggesting the existence of a surveillance system for detection and silencing of genomic parasites (HENIKOFF and MATZKE 1997).

FURTHER REFERENCES

HENIKOFF, S., and M. A. MATZKE, 1997 Exploring and explaining epigenetic effects. Trends Genet. **13:** 293–295.

WU, C.-T., and J. R. MORRIS, 1999 Transvection and other homology effects. Curr. Opin. Genet. Dev. **9:** 237–246.

Herskowitz, Ira. The Hawthorne Deletion Twenty-five Years Later, p. 76

The decade since publication of this "Perspectives" essay has seen a continuation of beautiful work on mating type interconversion. These studies reveal connections between histones and Sir proteins (HECHT *et al.* 1995), shed new light on the directionality of mating type switching (HABER 1998; SZETO *et al.* 1997), reveal the molecular basis for asymmetric cell division and transcription of the *HO* gene (LONG *et al.* 1997; TAKIZAWA *et al.* 1997), and unravel the mechanism of silencing in fission yeast (GREWAL *et al.* 1998). Hawthorne ploughed fertile ground.

FURTHER REFERENCES

GREWAL, S. I., M. J. BONADUCE and A. J. KLAR, 1998 Histone deacetylase homologs regulate epigenetic inheritance of transcriptional silencing and chromosome segregation in fission yeast. Genetics **150:** 563–576.

HABER, J. E., 1998 A locus control region regulates yeast recombination. Trends Genet. **14:** 317–321.

HECHT, A., T. LAROCHE, S. STRAHL-BOLSINGER, S. M. GASSER and M. GRUNSTEIN, 1995 Histone H3 and H4 N-termini interact with SIR3 and SIR4 proteins: a molecular model for the formation of heterochromatin in yeast. Cell **80:** 583–592.

LONG, R. M., R. H. SINGER, X. MENG, I. GONZALEZ, K. NASMYTH *et al.*, 1997 Mating type switching in yeast controlled by asymmetric localization of ASH1 mRNA. Science **277:** 383–387.

SZETO, L., M. K. FAFALIOS, H. ZHONG, A. K. VERSHON and J. R. BROACH, 1997 Alpha2p controls donor preference during mating type interconversion in yeast by inactivating a recombinational enhancer of chromosome III. Genes Dev. **11:** 1899–1911.

TAKIZAWA, P. A., A. SIL, J. R. SWEDLOW, I. HERSKOWITZ and R. D. VALE, 1997 Actin-dependent localization of an RNA encoding a cell-fate determinant in yeast. Nature **389:** 90–93.

Hodgkin, Jonathan. Early Worms, p. 81

The past 10 years have seen the expected continuing expansion of research on *C. elegans*. In 1998 the worm achieved a special place in scientific history with the publication of an essentially complete DNA sequence for its entire 98 million base pair genome, the first such sequence to be determined for any multicellular organism.

The *C. elegans* research community remains notably integrated and cooperative, as it has been throughout its history. An important early factor in encouraging this communal spirit was the establishment of a *C. elegans* newsletter by R. S. Edgar, who had learned the values and virtues of a strongly interactive research community while working with T4. The first issue of the *Worm Breeder's Gazette* appeared in 1975, and it is still going strong, now in both paper and electronic forms.

Kaiser, Dale. Roland Thaxter's Legacy and the Origins of Multicellular Development, p. 361

Cell-to-cell signaling between bacterial cells has since been widely found; homoserine lactones, peptides, and amino acids are quorum sensors for many bacteria (DUNNY and WINANS 1999). To initiate fruiting body development, myxobacteria use a stringent response, which measures their protein synthetic capacity (HARRIS *et al.* 1998). Maintaining cell-cell interactions is selectively disadvantageous for *M. xanthus* (VELICER *et al.* 1998).

FURTHER REFERENCES

DUNNY, G. M., and S. C. WINANS, eds. 1999 *Cell-Cell Signaling in Bacteria.* American Society for Microbiology, Washington, D.C.

HARRIS, B. Z., D. KAISER and M. SINGER, 1998 The guanosine nucleotide (p)ppGpp initiates development and A-factor production in *Myxococcus xanthus*. Genes Dev. **12**: 1022–1035.

VELICER, G., L. KROOS and R. E. LENSKI, 1998 Loss of social behaviors by *Myxococcus xanthus* during evolution in an unstructured habitat. Proc. Natl. Acad. Sci. USA **95**: 12376–12380.

Kleckner, Nancy. Regulating Tn*10* and IS*10* Transposition, p. 147

A new basic regulatory system for IS*10*/Tn*10* has been elucidated. Architectural protein IHF both stimulates and inhibits intermolecular transposition, and in such a way that intermolecular transposition is favored at low supercoiling levels and disfavored at high supercoiling levels (CHALMERS *et al.* 1998). Known regulatory mechanisms are also now better understood (e.g., MA *et al.* 1994; JAIN and KLECKNER 1993).

Biochemical studies have provided a mechanistic explanation for a group of previously mysterious IS*10*-promoted rearrangements. Two different donor DNA molecules can efficiently synapse and undergo "transposition"; such events could yield adjacent deletions, cointegrates, and "duplicative inversions" (CHALMERS and KLECKNER 1996). Due to dam-mediated regulation (see original "Perspectives"), bimolecular interactions should occur preferentially between sister molecules newly emerged from a replication fork.

Interestingly, in one genetic test system, IS*10*-mediated cointegrate formation requires RecA function and is stimulated by UV irradiation, dependent upon SOS induction (EICHENBAUM and LIVNEH 1998). Perhaps RecA is involved in providing complete products after bimolecular synapsis and strand transfer.

FURTHER REFERENCES

CHALMERS, R. M., and N. KLECKNER, 1996 IS*10*/Tn*10* efficiently accommodates diverse transposon end configurations. EMBO J. **15**: 5112–5122.

CHALMERS, R. M., A. GUHATHAKURTA, H. BENJAMIN and N. KLECKNER, 1998 IHF modulation of Tn*10* transposition: sensory transduction of supercoiling status via a proposed protein/DNA molecular spring. Cell **93**: 897–908.

EICHENBAUM, Z., and Z. LIVNEH, 1998 UV light induces IS*10* transposition in *Escherichia coli*. Genetics **149**: 1173–1181.

JAIN, C., and N. KLECKNER, 1993 Preferential cis action of IS*10* transposase depends upon its mode of synthesis. Mol. Microbiol. **9**: 249–260.

MA, C. K., T. KOLESNIKOW, J. C. RAYNER, E. L. SIMONS, H. YIM *et al.*, 1994 Control of translation by mRNA secondary structure: the

importance of the kinetics of structure formation. Mol. Microbiol. **14**: 1033–1047.

Lederberg, Joshua. Gene Recombination and Linked Segregations in *Escherichia coli*, p. 25

The allusion to Sciara may be mystifying to many current readers, even more than it had been in 1947. It refers to METZ (1938) work on the fly Sciara, where a monocentric meiosis results in substantial ejection of chromatin. For a more accessible and updated review see MILLER (1997).

Page 26, column 2, paragraph 1, 3 lines from bottom: [SCHMIDT] should read [SCHMID]

Page 27, column 2, 4 references from bottom: [SCHMIDT] should read [SCHMID]

FURTHER REFERENCES

METZ, C. W., 1938 Chromosome behavior, inheritance and sex determination in Sciara. Am. Nat. **72**: 485–520.

MILLER, O. J., 1997 Chromosome changes in cell differentiation. Genetics **146**: 1–8.

Lederberg, Joshua. Replica Plating and Indirect Selection of Bacterial Mutants: Isolation of Preadaptive Mutants in Bacteria by Sib Selection, p. 88

Just as this essay was being drafted, "The origin of mutants" (CAIRNS, OVERBAUGH and MILLER 1988) sparked an ongoing controversy about so-called adaptive mutagenesis (CAIRNS 1998; SNIEGOWSKI and LENSKI 1995). It is hard to overestimate the methodological problems entailed in the enumeration of primary mutagenic events. These are typically so rare as to require selective procedures addressed to the change of phenotype, which is distanced by a long and complicated pathway from the original lesion in the DNA. Ten years later, PATRICIA FOSTER (1998), in "Adaptive mutation: has the unicorn landed?" voiced a consensus view that while these mutations "are not 'adaptive' in the original sense . . . a transient mutational state . . . in starving cells could provide a mechanism for adaptive evolution." There remain some holdouts (HALL 1997).

In any case, we can no longer insist on the unqualified randomness of mutation. Site-specific mutagenesis is a matter of daily practice in biotechnology, with DNA-sequence homology to target specific loci (SMITH 1993). Recombinases can effect targeted inversions or deletions of DNA sequences and can be crafted to be responsive to environmental stimuli (CAMILLI, BEATTIE and MEKALANOS 1994). Transposons exhibit a preference for insertion in supercoiled domains of DNA, which in turn may reflect transcriptional activity (GORYSHIN *et al.* 1998). Transcription-coupled DNA repair is a well-established phenomenon (HANAWALT 1995); and it is next to impossible to disentangle biases in primary mutagenesis from the secondary consequences of repair. In sum, DNA sequences can be targeted by any number of site-specific reagents, be they protein enzymes, polynucleotides, or small molecules; and these reagents, as well as the conformation of DNA targets, in turn may be regulated by the physiological state of the cell. The issue is not whether a seemingly adaptive mutagenesis is possible in special cases, but rather whether this is a widely realized capability on which substantial evolutionary capital has been expended.

FURTHER REFERENCES

CAIRNS, J., 1998 Mutation and cancer: the antecedents to our studies of adaptive mutation. Genetics **148**: 1433–1440.

CAMILLI, A., D. T. BEATTIE and J. J. MEKALANOS, 1994 Use of genetic recombination as a reporter of gene-expression. Proc. Natl. Acad. Sci. USA **91**: 2634–2638.

FOSTER, P. L., 1998   Adaptive mutation: has the unicorn landed? Genetics **148:** 1453–1459.

GORYSHIN, I. Y., J. A. MILLER, Y. V. KIL, V. A. LANZOV and W. S. REZNIKOFF, 1998   Tn5/IS50 target recognition. Proc. Natl. Acad. Sci. USA **95:** 10716–10721.

HALL, B. G., 1997   On the specificity of adaptive mutations. Genetics **145:** 39–44.

HANAWALT, P. C., 1995   DNA-repair comes of age. Mutat. Res.-DNA Repair **336:** 101–113.

SMITH, M., 1993   Synthetic DNA and biology. Les Prix Nobel, 123–140.

SNIEGOWSKI, P. D., and R. E. LENSKI, 1995   Mutation and adaptation – the directed mutation controversy in evolutionary perspective. Annu. Rev. Ecol. Syst. **26:** 553–578.

Lederberg, Joshua. The Transformation of Genetics by DNA: An Anniversary Celebration of Avery, MacLeod, and McCarty (1944), p. 384

For a comprehensive archive on O. T. Avery, see: http://profiles.NLM.nih.gov/CC

Page 385, column 2, line 2: [(CLARK and KASTEN 1983)] should read [(KASTEN 1983)].

Page 386, column 2, 5 lines from bottom: [CLARK and KASTEN (1983)] should read [KASTEN (1983)].

Page 387, reference to: [CLARK, G., and F. H. KASTEN, 1983 *History of Staining*. Williams & Wilkins, Baltimore.] should read [KASTEN, F. H., 1983   A history of protein and nucleic acid histochemistry, pp. 186–252 in *History of Staining*, CLARK, G., and F. H. KASTEN. Williams & Wilkins, Baltimore.]

Lederberg, Joshua. Genetic Recombination in *Escherichia coli:* Disputation at Cold Spring Harbor, 1946–1996, p. 545

For additional detail on this encounter and its context, see: http://profiles.NLM.nih.gov/BB

McGinnis, William. A Century of Homeosis, A Decade of Homeoboxes, p. 402

In the past few years, much progress has been made on the unanswered questions posed at the end of this review. Exd/Pbx has been found to be a crucial coactivator protein that binds as a heterodimer with Hox proteins (MANN and CHAN 1996; PINSONNEAULT *et al.* 1997). Solid evidence exists for enhancer sharing between different promoters in Hox clusters, which would maintain the clustered arrangement of Hox genes (GERARD *et al.* 1996; GOULD *et al.* 1997). Finally, human Hox gene mutations have been associated with heritable limb defects (MURAGAKI *et al.*, 1996; MORTLOCK *et al.* 1996).

FURTHER REFERENCES

GERÁRD, M., J.-Y. CHEN, H. GRONEMEYER, P. CHAMBON, D. DUBOULE *et al.*, 1996   In vivo targeted mutagenesis of a regulatory element required for positioning the *Hoxd-11* and *Hoxd-10* expression boundaries. Genes Dev. **10:** 2326–2334.

GOULD, A., A. MORRISON, G. SPROAT, R. A. H. WHITE and R. KRUMLAUF, 1997   Positive cross-regulation and enhancer sharing: two mechanisms for specifying overlapping *Hox* expression patterns. Genes Dev. **11:** 900–913.

MANN, R. S., and CHAN, S.-K., 1996   Extra specificity from *extradenticle:* the partnership between HOX and PBX/EXD homeodomain proteins. Trends Genet. **12:** 258–262.

MORTLOCK, D. P., L. C. POST and J. W. INNIS, 1996   The molecular basis of hypodactyly (*Hd*): a deletion in *Hoxa13* leads to arrest of digital arch formation. Nat. Genet. **13:** 284–289.

MURAGAKI, Y., S. MUNDLOS, J. UPTON and B. R. OLSEN, 1996   Altered growth and branching patterns in synpolydactyly caused by mutations in HOXD13. Science **272:** 548–551.

PINSONNEAULT, J., B. FLORENCE, H. VAESSIN and W. MCGINNIS, 1997   A model for *extradenticle* function as a switch that changes HOX proteins from repressors to activators. EMBO J. **16:** 2032–2042.

Milkman, Roger. Recombination and Population Structure in *Escherichia coli,* p. 596

Given the dramatic mounting documentation of exchange via the "genetic internet," a bacterial species concept may well rest on the difference between intraspecific and extraspecific gene transfer rates, rather than intraspecific versus interspecific (*among close relatives*), as in Ernst Mayr's biological species concept. Important, achievable unfinished business remains: mapping the unmapped MLEE loci.

Additional views and experimental data are now published. Two recombinational replacements, each evidently reflecting a single recent natural intraspecific event, are described in a paper in preparation by R. McBride and R. Milkman.

FURTHER REFERENCES

MILKMAN, R., 1999   Gene transfer in *Escherichia coli*, pp. 291–309 in *Organization of the Prokaryotic Genome*, edited by R. L. Charlebois. American Society for Microbiology, Washington, D.C.

MILKMAN, R., E. A. RALEIGH, M. MCKANE, D. CRYDERMAN, P. BILODEAU *et al.*, 1999   Molecular evolution of the *Escherichia coli* chromosome. V. Recombination patterns among strains of diverse origin. Genetics **153:** 539–554.

Miller, Orlando J. Chromosome Changes in Cell Differentiation, p. 584

Recent papers provide further evidence for the key role of *cis*-acting, nontranslatable RNAs in imprinting and dosage compensation. For example, the four dosage compensation proteins in *Drosophila* bind to the X chromosome, but one of them, MLE, is removed by RNase treatment. The *roX1* and *roX2* genes produce male-specific nontranslatable transcripts that bind to the male X chromosome, probably as essential components of the dosage compensation mechanism (MELLER *et al.* 1997; AMREIN and AXEL 1997).

FURTHER REFERENCES

AMREIN, H., and R. AXEL, 1997   Genes expressed in neurons of adult male Drosophila. Cell **88:** 459–469.

MELLER, V. H., K. H. WU, G. ROMAN, M. I. KURODA and R. L. DAVIS, 1997   roX1 RNA paints the X chromosome of male Drosophila and is regulated by the dosage compensation system. Cell **88:** 445–457.

Morton, Newton E. LODs Past and Present, p. 453

The past 5 years have seen extension of methods for complex inheritance based on relative pairs and variance components, which give weakly parametric LODS in which the genetic parameters for gene frequencies and penetrances are reduced to a single parameter for effect. A similar extension has been made to allelic association, with special interest in a million or so single nucleotide polymorphisms (SNPs). Current effort in optimizing these methods and combining multilocus LODS over samples must soon bring the weakly parametric approach begun by PENROSE (1935) to a successful conclusion that leaves fully parametric LODS most useful for well-characterized genes, both major loci and oligogenes in complex inheritance.

FURTHER REFERENCE

PENROSE, L. S., 1935   The detection of autosomal linkage in data which consist of pairs of brothers and sisters of unspecified parentage. Ann. Eugen. **6:** 133–138.

Oshima, Yasuji. Impact of the Douglas-Hawthorne Model as a Paradigm for Elucidating Cellular Regulatory Mechanisms in Fungi, p. 214

Soon after the publication of this essay, JOHNSTON and CARLSON (1992) described an excellent review on the regulation of galactose and phosphate utilization along with some other regulatory systems in yeast. In 1997 I also summarized the subsequent progress of the phosphatase system (OSHIMA 1997).

FURTHER REFERENCES

JOHNSTON, M., and M. CARLSON, 1992   Regulation of carbon and phosphate utilization, pp. 193–281 in *The Molecular and Cellular Biology of the Yeast Saccharomyces: Gene Expression,* edited by E. W. JONES, J. R. PRINGLE and J. R. BROACH. Cold Spring Harbor Laboratory Press, Plainview, NY.

OSHIMA, Y., 1997   The phosphatase system in *Saccharomyces cerevisiae* (review). Genes Genet. Syst. **72:** 323–334.

Paul, Diane. H. J. Muller, Communism, and the Cold War, p. 51

While there is evidence that Muller's communist past delayed support of his research by the Atomic Energy Commission, the agency ultimately became a major patron, a relationship that lasted until Muller's death in 1966. It is worth noting that Muller was not the only geneticist to fall under political suspicion during the Cold War. The genetic effects of fallout was a national security issue, and geneticists who addressed it, whatever their perspective, attracted attention from the Federal Bureau of Investigation (FBI). Dobzhansky, Wright, Stern, Dunn, and Demerec, among others, also acquired fat FBI files.

Sherman, Fred. Studies of Yeast Cytochrome *c*: How and Why They Started and Why They Continued, p. 157

Additional details on the development and early use of the cytochrome *c* system can be found in SHERMAN (1993). More recently, the cytochrome *c* system has played important roles in determining evolutionary relationships (MELNICK and SHERMAN 1993), mRNA 3′ endforming signals (GUO and SHERMAN 1996), mitochondrial import signal (WANG *et al.* 1996), *N*-terminal processing, etc.

FURTHER REFERENCES

GUO, Z., and F. SHERMAN, 1996   3′ End forming signals of yeast mRNA. Trends Biochem. Sci. **21:** 477–481.

MELNICK, L., and F. SHERMAN, 1993   The gene clusters COR and ARC in the yeast *Saccharomyces cerevisiae* share a common ancestry. J. Mol. Biol. **233:** 371–388.

SHERMAN, F., 1993   My life with cytochrome *c*, pp. 347–357 in *The Early Days of Yeast Genetics,* edited by M. N. HALL and P. LINDER. Cold Spring Harbor Laboratory Press, Plainview, NY.

WANG, X., M. E. DUMONT and F. SHERMAN, 1996   Sequence requirements for mitochondrial import of yeast cytochrome *c*. J. Biol. Chem. **271:** 6594–6604.

Stahl, Franklin W. Hershey, p. 656

The Cold Spring Harbor reference in the first paragraph of this essay is to a volume entitled *We Can Sleep Later,* being published by the Cold Spring Harbor Laboratory Press, Cold Spring Harbor, NY 11724-2211.

Weir, B. S. Quantitative Genetics in 1987, p. 35

In retrospect, the 1987 International Conference on Quantitative Genetics is notable for how nearly it failed to see where the field was moving. Although the term "Quantitative Trait Loci" was coined by GELDERMANN in 1975, only the paper by Soller and Beckmann among the 55 invited papers referred explicitly to QTL mapping. These authors also cited the pioneering 1982 work by TANKSLEY *et al.* on locating genes affecting quantitative traits in the tomato. Readers of this journal will be quite aware of the explosion in QTL mapping activity that has taken place since 1987. The seminal paper will probably be seen to be that of LANDER and BOTSTEIN in 1989, who laid out a statistical approach for locating genes from data on crosses between inbred lines. Their MAPMAKER-QTL software stimulated much theoretical and empirical work. Notable among the theoretical advancements have been those that use the whole genome, rather than single marker intervals, to locate several QTL (e.g., JANSEN 1996; KAO *et al.* 1999). There is parallel activity in human genetics, for data from pedigrees (e.g., ALMASY *et al.* 1999) or from sib-pairs (e.g., ALLISON *et al.* 1999). Quantitative genetics was in good health in 1987, but now it is in excellent health.

FURTHER REFERENCES

ALLISON, D. B., M. HEO, N. KAPLAN and E. R. MARTIN, 1999   Sibling-based tests of linkage and association for quantitative traits. Am. J. Hum. Genet. **64:** 1754–1764.

ALMASY, L., J. E. HIXSON, D. L. RAINWATER, S. COLE, J. T. WILLIAMS *et al.,* 1999   Human pedigree-based quantitative-trait-mapping: localization of two genes influencing HDL-cholesterol metabolism. Am. J. Hum. Genet. **64:** 1686–1693.

GELDERMANN, H., 1975   Investigations on inheritance of quantitative characters in animals by gene markers. 1. Methods. Theor. Appl. Genet. **46:** 319–330.

JANSEN, R. C., 1996   A general Monte Carlo method for mapping multiple quantitative trait loci. Genetics **138:** 871–888.

KAO, C. H., Z. B. ZENG and R. D. TEASDALE, 1999   Multiple interval mapping for quantitative trait loci. Genetics **152:** 1203–1216.

LANDER, E. S., and D. BOTSTEIN, 1989   Mapping Mendelian factors underlying quantitative traits using RFLP linkage maps. Genetics **121:** 185–199. (Correction **136:** 705).

TANKSLEY, S. D., H. MEDINA-FILHO and C. M. RICK, 1982   Use of naturally occurring enzyme variation to detect and map genes controlling quantitative traits in an interspecific backcross of tomato. Heredity **49:** 11–25.

○ **Author Index** ○

Subject Index